D0203141

MEDICAL-SURGICAL NURSING

An Integrated Approach

2nd Edition

MEDICAL-SURGICAL NURSING

An Integrated Approach
2nd Edition

Lois White, RN, PhD

Former Chairperson, Professor
Department of Vocational Nurse Education
Del Mar College
Corpus Christi, Texas

Gena Duncan, RN, MS, MSEd

Assistant Professor and Director of Associate Degree Program
University of Saint Francis
Fort Wayne, Indiana

DELMAR

THOMSON LEARNING

Australia • Canada • Mexico • Singapore • Spain • United Kingdom • United States

Medical-Surgical Nursing: An Integrated Approach, 2nd Edition
by Lois White and Gena Duncan

Business Unit Director:
William Brottmiller

Executive Editor:
Cathy L. Esperti

Acquisitions Editor:
Matthew Filimonov

Senior Developmental Editor:
Elisabeth F. Williams

Editorial Assistant:
Melissa Longo

Executive Marketing Manager:
Dawn F. Gerrain

Channel Manager:
Tara Carter

Project Editor:
Maureen M. E. Grealish

Production Coordinator:
Anne Sherman

Senior Art/Design Coordinator:
Timothy J. Conners

Copyright © 2002 by Delmar, a division of Thomson Learning, Inc. Thomson Learning™ is a registered trademark used herein under license.

Printed in the United States
1 2 3 4 5 6 7 8 9 10 XXX 05 04 03 02 01

For more information, contact Delmar,
3 Columbia Circle, PO Box 15015,
Albany, NY 12212-0515

Or find us on the World Wide Web at http://www.delmar.com

ALL RIGHTS RESERVED. No part of this work covered by the copyright hereon may be reproducd or used in any form or by any means—graphic, electronic, or mechanical, including photocopying, recording, taping, Web distribution or information storage and retrieval systems—without written permission of the publisher.

For permission to use material from this text or product, contact us by
Tel   800-730-2214
Fax   800-730-2215
www.thomsonrights.com

Library of Congress Cataloging-in-Publication Data

White, Lois.
    Medical-surgical nursing, Lois White, Gena Duncan.—2nd ed.
      p. cm.
    Includes bibliographical references and index.
    ISBN 0-7668-2566-3 (alk. paper)
    1. Nursing. 2. Surgical nursing. I. Duncan, Gena. II. Title.
RT41 .M484 2001
610.73—dc21
                                                    2001028702

Notice to the Reader

Publisher does not warrant or guarantee any of the products described herein or perform any independent analysis in connection with any of the product information contained herein. Publisher does not assume, and expressly disclaims, any obligation to obtain and include information other than that provided to it by the manufacturer.

The reader is expressly warned to consider and adopt all safety precautions that might be indicated by the activities herein and to avoid all potential hazards. By following the instructions contained herein, the reader willingly assumes all risks in connection with such instructions.

The Publisher makes no representation or warranties of any kind, including but not limited to, the warranties of fitness for particular purpose or merchantability, nor are any such representations implied with respect to the material set forth herein, and the publisher takes no responsibility with respect to such material. The publisher shall not be liable for any special, consequential, or exemplary damages resulting, in whole or part, from the readers' use of, or reliance upon, this material.

Contents

SECTION 1 FOUNDATIONS OF NURSING

UNIT 1 Factors Affecting Nursing Care 2

UNIT 2 Holistic Nursing Care . . .67

SECTION 2 AREAS OF MEDICAL-SURGICAL NURSING CARE

Reviewers

Diana L. Baker, MSN, RNC
Former Nursing Programs Director
College of Eastern Utah
Price, Utah

Kay Baker, RN, MS
Instructional Faculty (Nursing)
Pima Community College
Tuscon, Arizona

Jan Barrett, PhD, RN
Academic Dean
Deaconess College of Nursing
St. Louis, Missouri

Lou Ann Boose, RN, BSN, MSN
Harrisburg Area Community College
Harrisburg, Pennsylvania

Susan Brooks, RN, BSN, MS, MN
Community College of Southern
  Nevada
Las Vegas, Nevada

Gyl A. Burkhard, RN, BSN, MS
Instructor
OCM BOCES
Syracuse, New York

Brenda Cherry, MSN, FNP
Assistant Professor of Nursing
Georgia Perimeter College
Clarkston, Georgia

David Derrico, MSN, BSN, ASN
Assistant Clinical Professor of
  Nursing
University of Florida
Gainesville, Florida

Sally Flesch, PhD, RN
Department Chair–Allied Health
  Department
Balck Hawk Community College
Moline, Illinois

Kay Rice Francis, RN, BSN, MSN
Woman's Health Nurse Practitioner
Nursing Instructor
Lake Michigan College
Benton Harbor, Michigan

Judith L. Gisondi, RN, BSN, MPS
Career Education Center Hamilton
  Fulton Montgomery BOCES
Johnstown, New York

Esther Gonzales, RN, MSN, MSEd
Associate Professor of Nursing
Del Mar College
Corpus Christi, Texas

Lisa Greenwall
PN Coordinator
Frackville, Pennsylvania

Sheila Guidry, RN, LPNB, BSN, DSN, PhD
Wallace Community College–Selma
Selma, Alabama

Ruth Hall, BA, MA
Augusta Technical Institute
Augusta, Georgia

Marilyn Handley, RN, MSN, PhDc
Instructor
University of Alabama
Capstone College of Nursing
Tuscaloosa, Alabama

Renee Harrison, RN, BSN, MS
Tulsa Community College
Tulsa, Oklahoma

Suellen Klein, RN, BSN, MSN
Nursing Instructor
Lake Michigan College
Benton Harbor, Michigan

Dr. Anne Larson, RN, C PhD
Associate Professor of Nursing
Midland Lutheran College
Fremont, Nebraska

Hope Laughlin, RN, BSN, MS, MSN, EdD
Pensacola Junior College
Pensacola, Florida

Patty Leary, M.ED, RN
Mecosta Osceola Career Center
Big Rapids, Michigan

Mary Lewin, RN, BSN, MSEd
Licensed Practical Nurse Instructor
Orleans Career Technical Education
  Center
Medina, New York

Dr. Bernadette Madara, EdD, APRN
Associate Professor of Nursing
Southern Connecticut State
  University
New Haven, Connecticut

Netta Moncur-Bowen, RN, BSN, MS
ADN Program
Seminole Community College
Sanford, Florida

Carol J. Nelson, RN, BSN, MSN
Spokane Community College
Spokane, Washington

Terrie Ortego, RN, CCM
Louisiana Technical College
T. H. Harris Campus
Opelousas, Louisiana

Dr. Carol Rafferty
Northeast Wisconsin Technical
  College
Green Bay, Wisconsin

Gail J. Smith, RN, BSN, MSN
Miami-Dade Community College
School of Nursing
Miami, Florida

Cynthia Steury-Lattz, MSN, RN, CS
Professor
Kankakee Community College
Kankakee, Illinois

Contributors

Joy E. Ache-Reed, RN, MS
Assistant Professor of Nursing
Indiana Wesleyan University
Marion, Indiana
Chapter 6, Cultural Diversity and Nursing

Carol A. Fetters Andersen, RN, MSN
Director of Mental Health Services
St. Anthony Regional Hospital and Nursing Home
Carroll, Iowa
Chapter 35, Nursing Care of the Older Client

Carma Andrus, RN, MN, CNS
Dauterive Primary Care Clinic
St. Martinville, Louisiana
Chapter 26, Nursing Care of the Client: Sensory System

Diane R. Behrens, RNCS, MA, MSEd
Instructor
University of Saint Francis
Fort Wayne, Indiana
Chapter 22, Nursing Care of the Client: Immune System

Susan L. Bredemeyer, RN, MS
Assistant Professor
Lutheran College of Health Professions
Fort Wayne, Indiana
Chapter 12, Health Assessment

Gyl A. Burkhard, RN, BSN, MS
Instructor
OCM BOCES
Syracuse, New York
Chapter 29, Nursing Care of the Client: Urinary System

Donna J. Burleson, RN, MS
Chair of Health Occupations
Cisco Junior College
Abilene, Texas
Chapter 2, Critical Thinking

Diana L. Case, RN, MA, FNP
Neighborhood Health Clinic
Fort Wayne, Indiana
Chapter 16, Nursing Care of the Surgical Client

Julie Coy, RNC, MS
Pain Consultation Service
The Children's Hospital
Denver, Colorado
Chapter 14, Pain Management

Mary Elias, RNC, BSN, CCE
Instructor
Practical Nursing Program
Ivy Tech State College
Fort Wayne, Indiana
Chapter 30, Nursing Care of the Client: Female Reproductive System

Cheryl Erickson, RN, BSN, MA
Associate Professor
Lutheran College of Health Professions
Fort Wayne, Indiana
Chapter 12, Health Assessment

Mary Ellen Zator Estes, RN, MSN, CCRN
Former Assistant Professor
School of Nursing
Marymount University
Arlington, VA *and*
Former Critical Care Nursing Education Coordinator
The George Washington University Medical Center
Washington, D.C.
Chapter 12, Health Assessment

Michael A. Fiedler, CRNA, MS
Assistant Professor
Applied Health Sciences
University of Alabama at Birmingham
Birmingham, Alabama
Chapter 15, Anesthesia

Mary Frost, RN, BSN
Covington, Louisiana
Chapter 8, Alternative/ Complementary Therapies

Norma Fujise, RN, C, MS
School of Nursing
University of Hawaii
Honolulu, Hawaii
Chapter 21, Nursing Care of the Client: Integumentary System

Cathy Greer, RN, MS
Instructor
Lutheran College of Health Professions
Fort Wayne, Indiana
Chapter 16, Nursing Care of the Surgical Client

Margaret L. Griffin, RN, BSN, MS
Instructor
Lutheran College of Health Professions
Fort Wayne, Indiana
Chapter 21, Nursing Care of the Client: Integumentary System

Susan Halley, RN, MS, FNP
Instructor of Nursing
Ball State University
Muncie, Indiana
Chapter 4, Ethical Responsibilities

Beverly F. Hildebrand, RN, BSN, MS
Former Health Occupations Coordinator
Washington, Saratoga, Warren, Hamilton, & Essex Counties BOCES
Saratoga, New York
Chapter 29, Nursing Care of the Client: Urinary System

Lucille Joel, RN, EdD, FAAN
Professor
College of Nursing
Rutgers, The State University of New Jersey
Newark, New Jersey
Chapter 1, The Health Care Delivery System

Janet Leah Joost, RN, BSN
Instructor
Front Range Community College
Boulder, Colorado
Chapter 18, Nursing Care of the Client: Respiratory System

Denise M. Jordan, RN, BSN, MA
Instructor
Practical Nursing Program
Ivy Tech State College
Fort Wayne, Indiana
Chapter 3, Legal Responsibilities

Janet E. Keith, RN, MSEd
Instructor
Practical Nursing Program
Ivy Tech State College
Fort Wayne, Indiana
**Chapter 24, Nursing Care of the
    Client: Musculoskeletal System**

Mary E. A. Laskin, RN, CS, MN
Clinical Nurse Specialist
Surgical/Orthopedic Services
Kaiser Permanente
San Diego, California
Chapter 14, Pain Management

Celinda Kay Leach, RN, BS, MPH
Program Chair, Practical Nursing
Practical Nursing Program
Ivy Tech State College
Bloomington, Indiana
**Chapter 17, Nursing Care of the
    Oncology Client**

Judy Martin, RN, MS, JD
Nurse Attorney
Louisiana Department of Health
    and Hospitals
Health Standards Section
Baton Rouge, Louisiana
Chapter 3, Legal Responsibilities

Cheryl McGaffic, RN, PhD
Clinical Instructor
College of Nursing
The University of Arizona
Tucson, Arizona
**Chapter 22, Nursing Care of the
    Client: Immune System**

**Robin Theresa McKenzie, RN,
MSN, CCRN**
Assistant Chairman
Navy Medical Center
San Diego, California
**Chapter 26, Nursing Care of the
    Client: Sensory System**

Betty Miller
Staff Development Coordinator
Meadowcrest Hospital
Gretna, Louisiana
Chapter 9, Loss, Grief, and Death

David K. Miller, RNC, BSN, MSEd
ICU/Medical–Surgical Manager
W.S. Major Hospital
Shelbyville, Indiana
**Chapter 22, Nursing Care of the
    Client: Immune System**

Joan Fritsch Needham, RNC, MS
Director of Education
DeKalb County Nursing Home
DeKalb, Illinois
Chapter 9, Loss, Grief, and Death
**Chapter 35, Nursing Care of the
    Older Client**
**Chapter 36, Rehabilitation, Home
    Health, Long-Term Care, and
    Hospice**

Brenda Owens, RN, PhD
Associate Professor
School of Nursing
Louisiana State University Medical
    Center
New Orleans, Louisiana
Chapter 11, IV Therapy

Raymond Phillips, RN, MS, CCRN
Clinical Nurse Specialist
Staff Development Coordinator
U.S. Naval Hospital
Rota, Spain
**Chapter 26, Nursing Care of the
    Client: Sensory System**

Martha Ann Rust, RN, BSN, MSN
Instructor
Lutheran College of Health
    Professions
Fort Wayne, Indiana
**Chapter 25, Nursing Care of the
    Client: Neurological System**

Mary Kay Schultz, RN, MSN, ANP
Instructor
Department of Nursing
Regis University
Denver, Colorado
**Chapter 27, Nursing Care of the
    Client: Endocrine System**

Leslee R. Sinn, RN, BSN
Instructor
Front Range Community College
Boulder, Colorado
**Chapter 28, Nursing Care of the
    Client: Gastrointestinal System**

Russlyn A. St. John, RN, MSN
Associate Professor & Coordinator,
    Practical Nursing
St. Charles Community College
St. Peters, Missouri
**Chapter 27, Nursing Care of the
    Client: Endocrine System**

Susan Stranahan, RN, PhD
Chair, Nursing Department
Indiana Wesleyan University
Marion, Indiana
**Chapter 6, Cultural Diversity and
    Nursing**

John M. White, PhD
Former Chairperson, Professor
Biology Department
Del Mar College
Corpus Christi, Texas
**Chapter 10, Fluid, Electrolyte,
    and Acid–Base Balance**

Lorrie Wong, RN, MS
School of Nursing
University of Hawaii
Honolulu, Hawaii
**Chapter 21, Nursing Care of the
    Client: Integumentary System**

Rothlyn Zahourek, RN, CS, MS
Certified Clinical Nurse Specialist
Amherst, Massachusetts
**Chapter 8, Alternative/
    Complementary Therapies**

Preface

The health care environment is changing. Today's prescriptions of care and prevention are not the same as yesterday's—and tomorrow's needs will be different as well. Practical/Vocational nursing students can confront and adapt to changes in technology, information, and resources by building a solid foundation of accurate, essential information. A firm knowledge base also allows nurses to meet the changing needs of clients. *Medical-Surgical Nursing: An Integrated Approach, 2nd edition* was designed with this goal in mind: helping practical/vocational nurses succeed.

Critical Thinking

Nursing is a challenging subject. There is a large body of information that students must master. The pressures of family and academic life often place a daunting challenge in front of students—even at a time when nurses are needed more than ever! That is why a strong focus on critical thinking continues in this second edition. This important topic helps students think about learning and decision-making. By teaching students "how to think" about nursing and how to solve nursing problems, students will be better prepared to succeed in their studies.

Chapter two, Critical Thinking, outlines the process of critical thinking in easy to understand terms, offering students tips and exercises for comprehension. Chapter 38, Critical Thinking on Multiple Systems, a unique chapter containing several case studies involving multiple body systems, has been expanded. Working through these case studies will help students understand the complexity of human illnesses and that disorders are not textbook-perfect nor are they isolated to one body system. The student's knowledge of all body systems will be challenged.

New to the Second Edition

Health care is changing faster than ever. New technologies, new treatments, new drugs, and new disorders make headlines almost every day. Nursing and nursing textbooks must change to keep pace. To address these new concepts and technologies, seven new chapters were added to the second edition of this market-leading textbook, *Medical-Surgical Nursing: An Integrated Approach*. The new chapters are: (1) The Health Care Delivery System, (8) Alternative/Complementary Therapies, (9) Loss, Grief, and Death, (11) IV Therapy, (13) Diagnostic Tests, (34) Nursing Care of the Client: Substance-Abuse, and (37) Nursing Care of the Client: Responding to Emergencies.

Additional, specific changes to the second edition include:

- Body system chapters are renamed to emphasize the book's holistic approach. Respiratory Disorders, for example, becomes "Nursing Care of the Client: Respiratory Disorders."
- Addition of specific Gerontological Consideration boxes as appropriate to highlight the increasing number of Older Clients nurses are caring for.
- Inclusion of Cultural Consideration boxes to reflect America's changing demographics.
- Nursing Diagnosis, Planning/Goals and Interventions presented in a convenient table format for quick reference.
- The addition of Internet resources.

ORGANIZATION

Medical-Surgical Nursing: An Integrated Approach, 2nd edition consists of 38 chapters grouped into 11 units.

Unit 1, Factors Affecting Nursing Care, provides students with a solid understanding of the basic concepts underlying nursing. This includes chapters on: the health care delivery system, critical thinking, legal responsibilities, and ethical responsibilities.

Unit 2, Holistic Nursing Care, is comprised of chapters that provide the student with concepts of holistic care. Topics presented include: communication, cultural diversity, wellness concepts, alternative/complementary therapies, and loss, grief, and death.

Unit 3, Basic Concepts of Medical-Surgical Nursing, focuses on topics that are essential for students to understand in order to succeed. Specific chapters include: Fluid, Electrolyte, and Acid-Base Balance; IV Therapy; Health Assessment; Diagnostic Tests; Pain Management; Anesthesia; as well as Nursing care of the Surgical and Oncology Client. An in-depth review of the topics in Unit 3 provides students with the basis for understanding many aspects of nursing care.

Unit 4, Oxygenation and Perfusion, through **Unit 8, Reproductive and Sexual Disorders**, follow a systems approach to medical-surgical disorders. Within each chapter there is a thorough review of appropriate anatomy and physiology, a nursing assessment, a discussion of common diagnostic tests and procedures, and relevant therapeutic interventions. Moreover, to aid students, the content of each chapter is presented in a nursing process format, and sample nursing care plans are provided within each of these chapters to help students visualize how textbook content translates into a step-by-step action plan.

Unit 9, Physical and Mental Integrity, addresses the specific and unique issues of mental illness and substance abuse in depth.

Unit 10, Special Areas of Medical-Surgical Nursing, focuses on two vitally important areas of nursing care—care of the older client; and rehabilitation, home health, long-term care, and hospice.

Unit 11, Integration of Body Systems, concludes the text with two chapters on Nursing Care of the Client: Responding to Emergencies; and Critical Thinking on Multiple Systems. This final chapter is a unique presentation of a series of case studies incorporating many of the disorders covered within the text. Each case study leads students through scenarios where the client experiences problems in multiple body systems. Whether used for self-study or as part of classroom discussion, this chapter will help students connect the concepts they have been learning throughout their course of study.

Back matter in the text includes References/Suggested Readings organized by chapter, which allows the student to find the source of the material presented in each chapter and also to find additional information concerning the topics covered. Resources are also listed by chapter and provide names, addresses, and/or telephone numbers of organizations specializing in a specific area of health care. Internet addresses are included as available. The current NANDA diagnosis listing is included in Appendix A. A master listing of all Abbreviations, Acronyms, and Symbols used in the text is provided, as well as an English-Spanish translation chart. A Glossary of the key terms from all of the chapters along with their definitions as used in the text is also provided.

ANCILLARIES

A full supplemental package was created for adopters of *Medical-Surgical Nursing: An Integrated Approach, 2nd edition*.

For the Instructor:

An *Instructor's Manual* (ISBN 0-7668-2570-1) is available for adopters. This manual provides many resources for the LP/VN instructor. It includes lecture approaches and notes, student learning activities, additional resources, web activities, responses to text case studies, and answers to the text Review Questions.

An *Electronic Instructor's CD-ROM* (ISBN 0-7668-3204-X) is also available. This CD-ROM contains many tools useful for the LP/VN instructor. It includes an Image Library of over 600 of the illustrations and photographs used in the textbook. These may be easily printed or edited to create unique classroom handouts. There is also a computerized testbank of over 800 questions on text material.

For the Student:

A *Clinical Companion* (ISBN 0-7668-2567-1) is available for students. This useful, pocket-sized book is a reference for the conditions most frequently encountered in clinical situations. While developed primarily as a supplement to *Medical-Surgical Nursing: An Integrated Approach, 2nd edition*, to which it is cross-referenced, the *Companion* may also be used as a stand-alone reference. It provides nursing students in the clinical area with essential information in an easy-to-follow format.

The *Study Guide* (ISBN 0-7668-2568-X) provides opportunities for additional review on all 38 chapters of the main text. The Study Guide includes Key Term matching review questions, Abbreviation Review, Exercises and Activities, and Self-Assessment Questions.

The *Student Tutorial CD-ROM* (ISBN 0-7668-3823-4) contains flashcard activities to review key concepts on a chapter-by-chapter basis.

Also available is *Delmar's Medical-Surgical Nursing CD-ROM* (ISBN 0-7668-2569-8). This comprehensive resource provides many valuable tools for the student nurse. In addition to 20 cases that build critical thinking skills, the CD-ROM includes an anatomy and physiology review and a module that helps students build their knowledge of auscultation and understanding heart and lung sounds.

Finally, an innovative *Web site* was developed to accompany *Medical-Surgical Nursing: An Integrated Approach, 2nd edition* and *Basic Nursing: Foundations of Skills & Concepts* at no additional charge. Accessed at *www.delmarnursing.com* students may—on a chapter-by-chapter basis—view a multimedia presentation that supports and reinforces the concepts in the book. This is perfect for students whose personal lives may interfere with regular class schedules.

ACKNOWLEDGMENTS

Beth Williams, developmental editor, receives a special thank you from both of us. She has kept us on track and provided guidance with humor and sensitivity. Other members of the team—Matt Filimonov, acquisitions editor; Maureen Grealish, project editor; Tim Conners, art coordinator; Anne Sherman, production coordinator; and Melissa Longo, editorial assistant have all worked diligently for the completion of this textbook. Thank you to all.

A special thank you to consultants Captain Alston Kirk, CHC, USN (retired) and John White, PhD for sharing their expertise in religions and anatomy and physiology respectively. Thank you to the contributors and reviewers for the time and expertise in making this book possible.

About the Authors

Lois Elain Wacker White earned a diploma in nursing from Memorial Hospital School of Nursing, Springfield, Illinois; an Associate degree in Science from Del Mar College, Corpus Christi, Texas; a Bachelor of Science in Nursing from Texas A & I University-Corpus Christi, Corpus Christi, Texas; a Master of Science in Education from Corpus Christi State University, Corpus Christi, Texas; and a Doctor of Philosophy degree in educational administration (community college) from the University of Texas, Austin, Texas.

She has taught at Del Mar College, Corpus Christi, Texas in both the Associate Degree Nursing program and the Vocational Nursing program. For 14 years she was also chairperson of the Department of Vocational Nurse Education. Dr. White has taught fundamentals of nursing, nutrition, mental health/mental illness, medical–surgical nursing, and maternal/newborn nursing. Her professional career has also included 15 years of clinical practice.

Dr. White has served on the Nursing Education Advisory Committee (NEAC) of the Board of Nurse Examiners for the State of Texas and the Board of Vocational Nurse Examiners, which developed competencies expected of graduates from each level of nursing. Serving as an NLN site visitor has given her insight into student and program needs which must be met to provide the best in nursing education. She maintains membership in the Texas Association of Vocational Nurse Educators, Sigma Theta Tau, American Nurses Association, and the National League for Nursing.

Dr. White has been listed in *Who's Who in American Nursing*. She currently serves on the Vocational Nursing Financial Aid Advisory Committee for the Texas Higher Education Coordinating Board.

Gena Duncan has been a maternity nurse, medical-surgical nurse, and assistant head nurse of a medical unit. She taught practical nursing students for 15 years and associate and baccalaureate degree students for 5 years. As a practical nursing instructor, she was a member of the statewide curriculum committee for the Ivy Tech State College. As a faculty member she has served on curriculum committees, a program evaluation committee, and NLN and CCNE accrediting review committees. She is presently an Assistant Professor and Director of the Associate Degree Program in Nursing at the University of Saint Francis in Fort Wayne, Indiana.

She obtained a MSEd and a MS in community health nursing. Her research thesis was entitled *An Investigation of Learning Styles of Practical and Baccalaureate Students*. The results of the study are published in the Journal of Nursing Education. She is a member of Sigma Theta Tau.

Critical thinking and sound nursing judgments are essential in the present health care system. Gena's desire in producing this book is that students will develop into caring, competent nurses.

How to Use this Text

KEY FEATURES

Each chapter includes a variety of learning aids designed to help you, the reader, further your understanding of key concepts.

Each chapter opens with a **Making the Connection** box which guides the reader to other key chapters related to the current chapter. This highlights the integration of the text material.

Learning Objectives are presented at the beginning of each chapter as well. These help students focus their study and use their time efficiently.

A listing of **Key Terms** is provided to identify the terms the student should know or learn for a better understanding of the subject matter.

Each medical-surgical chapter has a **brief review of anatomy & physiology** to review the organs and functions of the system being discussed.

Common Diagnostic Tests are listed in a table for easy reference within each chapter as appropriate. A more comprehensive overview of laboratory and diagnostic tests is provided in chapter 13.

The content of each chapter is presented in a **nursing process format**.

Where appropriate, a **Sample Nursing Care Plan** is provided in the chapter. These serve as models for students to refer to as they create their own care plans based on each chapter's case study.

Nursing Diagnosis, Planning/Goals, and Interventions are presented in a convenient table format for quick reference.

Case Studies are presented at the conclusion of most chapters. These call for students to draw upon the knowledge they have gained and synthesize information to help them develop their own solutions to realistic cases.

Gerontological Considerations provide information related to the care of the older client.

GERONTOLOGICAL CONSIDERATIONS

Asthma and Age

- Asthma attacks usually become more severe and more frequent as the individual ages, and
- Asthma attacks are usually not associated with definite allergens.

CLIENT TEACHING

Thrombophlebitis

- Drink 2 to 3 quarts of water per day.
- Do not to sit with legs crossed.
- Elevate both legs when sitting.
- Avoid sitting or standing for extended periods.
- Wear support hose.
- When standing, shift weight frequently and occasionally stand on tiptoes to stimulate the calf muscle to pump blood.
- Notify the physician immediately if leg pain, tenderness or swelling, difficulty breathing, or chest pain is experienced.

Client Teaching identifies specific items that the client should know related to the various disorders.

Professional Tip offers tips and technical hints for the nurse to ensure quality care.

PROFESSIONAL TIP

Hypertension

Often the hypertensive client may not be experiencing any symptoms and does not see the importance of caring effectively for this condition.

COMMUNITY/HOME HEALTH CARE

Electronic Sphygmomanometers

Electronic sphygmomanometers are used by clients for self-measurements. A stethoscope is not required because the device electronically inflates and deflates the cuff while simultaneously reading and displaying the systolic and diastolic pressures. The electronic device is useful for clients who must monitor their own pressure at home. However, it must be recalibrated routinely to ensure an accurate reading.

Community/Home Health Care describes factors to consider when providing care in the community or in a client's home and adaptations in care that may be necessary.

Web Flash! guides the student to the Internet for the latest information related to the chapter content.

WEB FLASH!

- Search the Internet for HIV and AIDS.
- What new research information is available for clients with HIV and AIDS? What type of drugs are available? Diagnostic tests? Other treatments?
- Search the Web for the resources listed for this chapter at the end of this text. What other information is provided?

CULTURAL CONSIDERATIONS

Impending Surgery

- Special religious rites may be desired by the client before surgery.
- Some clients may not want to receive blood transfusions or other treatments.
- All client beliefs must be respected.

Cultural Considerations share beliefs, manners, ways of providing care, communication, and relationships of various cultural and ethnic groups as a way to provide sensitive and holistic care.

Safety: Iodine Allergy

- Each client must be asked about allergy to iodine.
- If a client is allergic to iodine, document the allergy on the client's record and inform the surgeon and OR personnel so that an iodine-free solution can be used for skin preparation and for other procedures for which iodine is routinely used.

Safety icons emphasize the importance of safety and describe ways to maintain safe care.

Critical Thinking Questions at the end of each chapter allow students to verify and review their understanding of concepts presented in the chapter.

A bulleted **Summary** lists the key concepts and issues presented within the text, allowing students to quickly glance over the content of a chapter.

Multiple choice **Review Questions** at the end of each chapter assist the student in remembering and using the material presented.

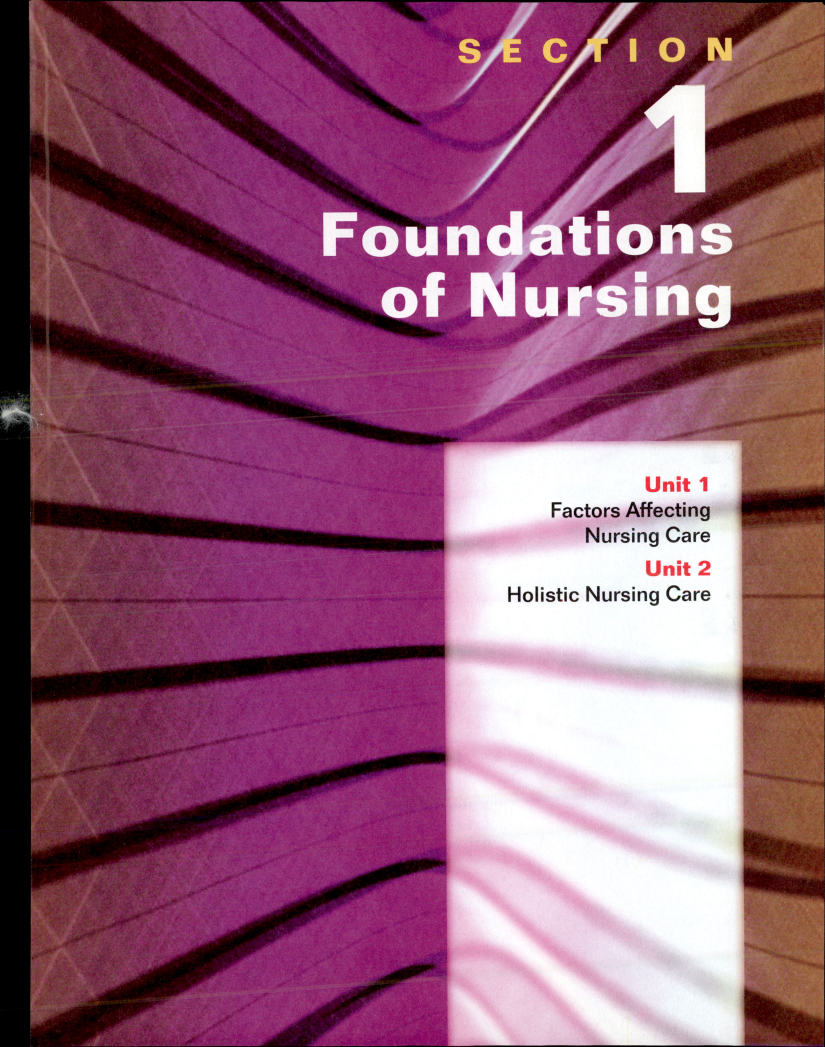

Foundations of Nursing

Unit 1
Factors Affecting
Nursing Care

Unit 2
Holistic Nursing Care

Factors Affecting Nursing Care

THE HEALTH CARE DELIVERY SYSTEM

MAKING THE CONNECTION

Refer to the following chapters to increase your understanding of the health care delivery system:

- **Chapter 3, Legal Responsibilities**
- **Chapter 4, Ethical Responsibilities**
- **Chapter 7, Wellness Concepts**

LEARNING OBJECTIVES

Upon completion of this chapter, you should be able to:
- *Define key terms.*
- *Describe the types of services in the U.S. health care delivery system.*
- *Discuss the various health care settings through which health care services are delivered.*
- *Identify the members of the health care team and their respective roles.*
- *Describe the differences among financial programs for health care services and reimbursement.*
- *Explain the factors that influence health care delivery.*
- *Identify the challenges to providing care.*
- *Discuss nursing's role in meeting the challenges within the health care system.*
- *Describe the emerging trends and issues for the health care delivery system.*

KEY TERMS

capitated rate
comorbidity
exclusive provider
  organization
fee-for-service
health care delivery
  system
health maintenance
  organization
managed care
medical model
preferred provider
  organization
prescriptive authority
primary care
primary care provider
primary health care
prospective payment
secondary care
single-payer system
single point of entry
tertiary care

INTRODUCTION

A **health care delivery system** is a mechanism for providing services that meet the health-related needs of individuals. The U.S. health care delivery system is currently experiencing dramatic change. Health care institutions that once flourished economically are now searching for ways to survive. Health care providers are seeking cost-effective ways to deliver an ever-increasing range of services to consumers. Consumers are demanding greater accessibility to quality health care services that are also affordable. The increase in consumerisms is fueled by the Internet, regulatory changes, the rising popularity of nontraditional therapies, and frustration of clients and their families feeling they have been mistreated by the system (Haugh, 1999).

Nursing is a major component of the U.S. health care delivery system. Consequently, nurses must understand the changes occurring within this system, as well as nursing's role in shaping those changes. This chapter explores the types of health care services available, the various settings where those services are offered, and the members of the health care team. The economics of health care and the challenges within the health care delivery system are also addressed, as is nursing's role in meeting those challenges.

TYPES OF HEALTH CARE SERVICES

Health care services can be classified into three levels: primary, secondary, and tertiary. The complexity of care varies according to the individual's need, the provider's expertise, and the delivery setting. Table 1–1 provides an overview of the types of care. The trend is toward holistic care, that is, care of the entire person

Table 1–1 TYPES OF HEALTH CARE SERVICES

TYPE OF CARE	DESCRIPTION	EXAMPLES
Primary	*Goal:* To decrease the risk to a client (individual or community) for disease or dysfunction *Explanation:* General health promotion Protection against specific illnesses	Teaching Lifestyle modification for health (e.g., smoking cessation, nutrition counseling) Referrals Immunization Promotion of a safe environment (e.g., sanitation, protection from toxic agents)
Secondary	*Goal:* To alleviate disease and prevent further disability *Explanation:* Early detection and intervention	Screenings Acute care Various therapies Surgery
Tertiary	*Goal:* To minimize effects and permanent disability associated with chronic or irreversible conditions *Explanation:* Restorative and rehabilitative activities to attain optimal level of functioning	Education and retraining Provision of direct care Environmental intervention (e.g., advising on necessity of wheelchair accessibility for a person who has experienced a cardiovascular accident [stroke])

including physiological, psychological, social, intellectual, and spiritual aspects.

Primary Care

The major purposes of **primary care** are to promote wellness and prevent illness or disability. Care is coordinated by the office of the primary care provider, usually a family practice physician, pediatrician, internal medicine physician, or family nurse practitioner. Traditionally, the U.S. health care system focused on illness treatment rather than wellness promotion. Within the past two decades, however, focus has shifted to health-promoting behaviors such as regular exercise, reducing fat in the diet, reducing air pollution, and monitoring cholesterol level. Illness prevention activities may be directed toward the individual, the family, or the community.

Under the traditional **medical model**, our health care delivery system was not a *health* care system at all, but, rather, an *illness* care system. Services have traditionally been directed toward caring for an individual after disease or disability has developed rather than emphasizing preventive aspects of care (Pruitt & Campbell, 1994). Today, however, there is more of an emphasis on the holistic promotion of wellness and on the preventive aspects of care.

Secondary Care

Services within the realm of **secondary care**—diagnosis and treatment—occur after the client exhibits symptoms of illness. Acute treatment centers (hospitals) still constitute the predominant site for the delivery of these health care services. However, there is a growing movement to provide diagnostic and therapeutic services in locations that are more easily accessed by the population. These are often satellite care centers of a major hospital, where holistic care is promoted.

Tertiary Care

Restoring an individual to the state of health that existed before the development of an illness is the purpose of **tertiary** (rehabilitative) **care**. In situations where the person is unable to regain previous functional abilities, the goal of rehabilitation is to attain the optimal level of health possible, for example, a client regaining partial use of an arm after experiencing a stroke. Restorative care is holistic in that the physiological, psychological, social, and spiritual aspects of the person are all addressed in the provision of care.

HEALTH CARE DELIVERY SYSTEM

The U.S. health care delivery system is complex, involving myriad providers, consumers, settings, personnel, and services.

Providers/Consumers

Health care services in the United States are delivered by public (including official and voluntary), public/private, and private sectors. Consumers are the individuals who receive the health care services.

Public Sector

Public agencies are financed with tax monies; thus, these agencies are accountable to the public. The public sector includes official (or governmental) agencies and voluntary agencies. Figure 1-1 shows the hierarchy of the official agencies in the public sector of health care delivery.

At the national level, the U.S. Department of Health and Human Services (USDHHS) is administratively responsible for health care services delivered to the public. The U.S. Public Health Service (USPHS) is the major agency that oversees the actual delivery of care services. Table 1–2 lists the USPHS agencies and their purposes. The Veterans Administration (VA) has hospitals and clinics that provide services to veterans of the armed services. These services are also financed with tax monies.

Each state varies in the provision of public health services. Generally, a state department of health coordinates the activities of local health units.

At the local level, services provided include immunizations, maternal–child care, and activities directed toward control of chronic diseases.

Voluntary agencies also constitute an important part of the public sector of the health care delivery system. These not-for-profit agencies (e.g., the National Federation of Licensed Practical Nurses [NFLPN], the American Nurses Association [ANA], the National League for

Table 1–2 AGENCIES OF THE U.S. PUBLIC HEALTH SERVICE

AGENCY	PURPOSE
Health Resources and Services Administration (HRSA)	Provide health-related information Administer programs concerned with health care for the homeless; people with human immunodeficiency virus (HIV) and acquired immunodeficiency syndrome (AIDS); organ transplants; rural health care; and employee occupational health
Food and Drug Administration (FDA)	Protect the public from unsafe drugs, food, and cosmetics
Centers for Disease Control and Prevention (CDC)	Study and prevent the transmission of communicable diseases
National Institutes of Health (NIH)	Conduct research and education related to specific illnesses
Alcohol, Drug Abuse, and Mental Health Administration (ADAMHA)	Serve as clearinghouse for information on substance abuse and mental health issues
Agency for Toxic Substances and Disease Registry (ATSDR)	Maintain registry of certain diseases Provide information on toxic agents Conduct mortality and morbidity studies on defined population groups
Indian Health Service (IHS)	Provide health care services to Native Americans, including health promotion, disease prevention, alcoholism prevention, substance abuse prevention, suicide prevention, nutrition, maternal–child health
Agency for Health Care Policy and Research (AHCPR)	Serve as primary source of federal support for research related to quality of health care delivery

Nursing [NLN], and the American Medical Association [AMA]) can exert significant legislative influence. Other voluntary agencies, such as the American Cancer Society and the American Heart Association, provide educational resources to the general public and to health care providers, such as dietary suggestions along with corresponding recipes. Voluntary agencies are funded in a variety of ways including individual contributions, corporate philanthropy, and membership dues.

Public/Private Sector

A blending of the public and private sectors in many areas of health care has gradually occurred following the inception of Medicare and the diagnosis-related groups (DRGs), discussed in an upcoming section. Federal regulations guide both the care provided to clients in private non-profit and for-profit agencies by private physicians and the reimbursement to both the agencies and the physicians.

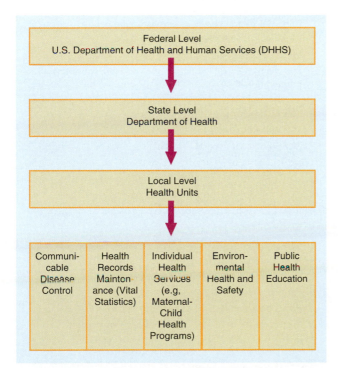

Figure 1-1 The Public Sector of Health Care Delivery (*From Fundamentals of Nursing: Standards & Practice, by S. DeLaune & P. Ladner, 1998, Albany, NY: Delmar. Copyright 1998 by Delmar. Reprinted with permission.*)

Private Sector

The private sector of the health care delivery system is composed primarily of independent health care agencies and providers who are reimbursed on a **fee-for-service** basis (the recipient directly pays the provider for services as they are provided). Fee-for-service clients may have private insurance or use their own financial resources to pay the provider for services rendered.

Settings

The variety of settings where health care is delivered and the roles of nurses in these settings are presented in Table 1–3.

Table 1–3 HEALTH CARE SETTINGS

SETTING	SERVICES PROVIDED	NURSE'S ROLE
Hospital	Diagnosis and treatment of illnesses (acute and chronic) Acute inpatient services Ambulatory care services Critical (intensive) care Rehabilitative care Surgical interventions Diagnostic procedures	Serves as caregiver Educates clients Provides ongoing assessment Coordinates care and collaborates with other health care providers Maintains client safety Initiates discharge planning Can specialize in a variety of areas: • Cardiology · Obstetrics • Critical care · Oncology • Dialysis · Orthopedics • Emergency · Pediatrics • Geriatrics · Psychiatry • Infection control · Rehabilitation • Neurology · Surgery • Nursery
Extended-care (long-term care) facilities (e.g., nursing homes, skilled nursing facilities)	Intermediate and long-term care for people who have chronic illnesses and are unable to care for themselves Restorative care until client is ready for discharge home	Provides care directed toward meeting basic needs (e.g., nutrition, hydration, comfort, elimination) Provides teaching and counseling Plans and coordinates care Administers medications, treatments, and other therapeutic modalities
Home health care agencies	Wide range of services, including curative and rehabilitive	Provides skilled nursing care Coordinates health-promotion activities (e.g., education)
Hospices	Care of individuals who have terminal illnesses Improving the quality of life until death	Promotes comfort measures Provides pain control Supports grieving families Educates family/client
Out-patient settings (clinics, physician's offices, ambulatory treatment centers)	Treatment of illness (acute and chronic) Diagnostic testing Simple surgical procedures	*Traditional role:* Checks vital signs Assists with diagnostic tests Prepares client for examination *Expanded role:* Provides teaching and counseling Performs physical (or mental status) examination In some settings, advanced practice registered nurses (APRNs) act as primary care providers
Schools (school-based clinics [SBCs])	Federally funded to provide physical and mental health services in middle and high schools	Coordinates health-promotion and disease prevention activities Treats minor illnesses Provides health education

continues

Table 1–3 HEALTH CARE SETTINGS *continued*

SETTING	SERVICES PROVIDED	NURSE'S ROLE
Industrial clinics	Maintain health and safety of workers	Coordinates health-promotion activities Provides education for safety Provides urgent care as needed Maintains health records Conducts ongoing screenings Provides preventive services (e.g., tuberculosis testing)
Managed care organizations	Reimbursement for health care services	Serves as case manager Uses triage to determine the most appropriate intervention for various clients
Community nursing centers	Direct access to professional services	Treats client's responses to health problems Promotes health and wellness
Rural primary care hospitals (RPCHs)	Stabilize clients until they are physiologically able to be transferred to more-skilled facilities	Performs assessments and provides emergency care

Personnel and Services

Many personnel and services exist within the various health care settings. Large hospitals provide the greatest number of services. Other health care settings may provide some but not all of these same services. The service departments most commonly found in the various settings include nursing units, specialized client care units, diagnostic departments, therapy departments, and support services.

Nursing Units

Nursing units are composed of client rooms, where most nursing care is provided. Units often serve one particular type of client such as cardiac, orthopedic, diabetic, surgical, pediatric, or obstetric. The nurse responsible for the unit may be called by several different titles, such as unit coordinator, nurse manager, or head nurse. Registered nurses (RNs), licensed practical/vocational nurses (LP/VNs), and nursing assistants provide the nursing care.

Specialized Client Care Units

Specialized units provide nursing care for specific needs of the clients. The LP/VN may work in these areas depending on experience, further education, the size and location of the hospital, and the number of RNs available. Examples of specialized units include the following:

- Emergency department (ED): provides care to clients involved in all types of accidents and those confronted with medical emergencies such as heart attack or stroke
- Intensive care unit (ICU): provides care to critically ill clients until they are stabilized and can be managed with routine nursing interventions on a regular nursing unit
- Coronary care unit (CCU): provides care to clients who have had a heart attack or who have had heart surgery such as coronary artery bypass or valve replacement
- Mental health unit: provides care to clients who are having difficulty with relationships, coping with everyday demands, or dealing with a crisis
- Psychiatric unit: provides care to clients diagnosed as having mental illness
- Rehabilitation unit: provides care to clients who must learn to regain the highest level of self-care possible following injury, accident, or illness such as heart attack or stroke
- Dialysis unit: provides care to clients who need dialysis because of renal failure
- Hospice unit: provides both care to clients who are dying and support to their families; may be a unit in a hospital or a free standing unit
- Outpatient unit: provides care to clients when admission to the hospital is unnecessary
- Home care: provides care to clients in their homes when professional supervision and/or minimal care is required; has been added to many hospitals to provide continuity of care
- Client education unit: provides teaching to clients, either individually or in groups, about specific client conditions or other health-related issues

Surgical Units

Care of the client just before, during, and after surgery is performed by the operating room (OR) and recovery room (RR) personnel. In addition to the main surgical unit, many hospitals also have a day surgery/ambulatory surgery unit. Clients come in a couple of hours before their scheduled surgeries and leave when recovered from the anesthesia. Total length of stay is shorter than 24 hours.

Diagnostic Departments

Diagnostic departments provide specialized tests that assist the physician in making a diagnosis for the client.

Clinical Laboratory Clinical laboratory personnel examine specimens of tissues, feces, and body fluids such as blood, sputum, urine, amniotic fluid, and spinal fluid. Testing assesses values of normal components as well as abnormal components of these specimens.

Radiology Department X-ray studies are performed in the radiology department, sometimes called nuclear medicine. This department also performs computed tomography (CT) scans, mammography, ultrasound, arteriograms, venograms, echocardiograms, and magnetic resonance imaging (MRI).

Other Diagnostic Services Other diagnostic services may include the following:

- Sleep center: provides observation, testing, and monitoring of clients as they sleep, to identify sleep-related problems
- Electroencephalography (EEG): records brain waves and ascertains electrical activity in the brain
- Electrocardiogram (ECG): records electrical activity in the heart
- Electromyogram (EMG): records electrical activity in body muscles

Therapy Departments

The function of the various therapy departments is to provide specialized treatments and/or rehabilitation services to clients to improve functional level in a specific area. Most hospitals have respiratory therapy and physical therapy departments. Some large teaching hospitals also have occupational therapy and speech therapy departments.

Support Services

Support services meet various other needs in providing care to clients.

Pharmacists mix and dispense medications to the various client care units. Nurses then administer the medications to the clients.

Dietitians supervise food preparation for all clients. They specifically choose the foods and calculate the amounts for special diets and provide client teaching for those clients on special diets.

Social workers help clients deal with psychosocial problems, providing assistance in areas such as housing, finances, and referrals to support groups.

Chaplains provide individual counseling to clients and support to families and assist clients in meeting spiritual needs.

The admission department handles the admission process by preparing necessary paperwork and ensuring that the ordered preadmission laboratory testing and x-rays are performed.

The business office oversees insurance and financial affairs upon client discharge from the health care agency.

Medical records, also called health information systems, maintains and stores all medical records for every client ever cared for by the health care agency.

Housekeeping and maintenance keep the physical facilities and equipment clean, in good repair, and in proper working order.

HEALTH CARE TEAM

Health care services are delivered by a multidisciplinary team (Figure 1-2). Table 1–4 lists the various health care team members, their educational requirements, and their roles. Because nurses work with the other team members on an ongoing basis, it is necessary to understand the role of each team member.

The nurse fulfills a variety of roles in assisting clients to meet their needs. Table 1–5 defines the most common roles of nurses. Nurses function in independent, interdependent, and dependent roles. In the independent role, the nurse requires no direction or order from another health care professional, for example, in deciding that a client's edematous arm should be elevated. In the interdependent role, the nurse works in collaboration with other health care professionals,

Figure 1-2 Members of the health care team work together for the benefit of the client.

Table 1–4 HEALTH CARE TEAM MEMBERS

TEAM MEMBER	EDUCATION	FUNCTION/ROLE
Nurse (LP/VN, RN, and APRN)	LP/VN: 1 year RN: 2 to 4 years APRN (Advanced Practice Registered Nurse): 1 to 3 years post-RN	Emphasizes health (wellness) promotion With a holistic approach, assists clients in coping with illness or disability by providing nursing care, health and health care education, and discharge planning Formulates nursing diagnoses to guide plan of care Addresses the needs of the client (individual, family, or community) Assists physician Functions may vary by state and specialization
Physician (medical doctor [MD])	8+ years	Formulates medical diagnoses and prescribes therapeutic modalities Performs medical procedures (e.g., surgery) May specialize in a variety of areas (e.g., gynecology/obstetrics, oncology, surgery)
Physician assistant (PA)	2 years (plus a master's degree for PA licensure, required in many states)	Provides medical services under the supervision of a physician
Registered pharmacist (RPh)	5 to 6 years	Prepares and dispenses drugs for therapeutic use May be involved in client education
Dentist (both doctor of dental surgery [DDS] and doctor of dental medicine [DMD])	8+ years	Diagnoses and treats conditions affecting the mouth, teeth, and gums Performs preventive measures to promote dental health
Registered dietitian (RD)	4+ years	Plans diets to meet special needs of clients Promotes health and prevents disease through education and counseling May supervise preparation of meals
Social worker (SW)	4 years	Assists clients with psychosocial problems (e.g., financial, housing, marital) May assist with discharge planning Makes referrals to support groups
Respiratory therapist (RT)	2 years	Administers pulmonary function tests Performs therapeutic measures to assist with respiration (e.g., oxygen administration, ventilation) Provides various treatments for respiratory illnesses and conditions
Physical therapist (PT)	4 years	Works with clients experiencing musculoskeletal problems Assesses client's strength and mobility Performs therapeutic measures (e.g., range of motion, massage, application of heat and cold) Teaches new skills (e.g., crutch walking)
Occupational therapist (OT)	4 years	Works with clients who have functional impairment to teach skills for activities of daily living
Speech therapist	4 years	Assists clients who have speech impairments to speak understandably or to learn another method of communication
Chaplain	8 years	Assists clients in meeting spiritual needs Provides individual counseling Provides support to families Conducts religious services

Table 1–5 NURSING ROLES

ROLE	DESCRIPTION
Caregiver: **LP/VN and RN**	Traditional and most essential role Functions as nurturer Provides direct care Is supportive Demonstrates clinical proficiency Promotes comfort of client
Teacher: **LP/VN and RN**	Provides information Serves as counselor Seeks to empower clients in self-care Encourages compliance with prescribed therapy Promotes healthy lifestyles Interprets information
Advocate: **LP/VN and RN**	Protects the client Provides explanations in client's language Acts as change agent Supports client's decisions
Manager: **LP/VN and RN**	Makes decisions Coordinates activities of others Allocates resources Evaluates care and personnel Serves as a leader Takes initiative
Expert: **RN**	Advanced practice clinician Conducts research Teaches in schools of nursing Develops theory Contributes to professional literature Provides testimony at governmental hearings and in court
Case manager: **RN**	Tracks client's progress through the health care system Coordinates care to ensure continuity
Team member: **LP/VN and RN**	Collaborates with others Possesses excellent communication skills

for example, in a client care conference where several members of the health care team together plan ways to meet the client's needs. In the dependent role, the nurse requires direction from a physician or dentist, for example, medications must be ordered by a physician or dentist before a nurse may administer them to the client. The degree of autonomy nurses experience is related to client needs, nurse expertise, and practice setting.

ECONOMICS OF HEALTH CARE

The reform movement in health care has been motivated primarily by costs. Control of costs has shifted from the health care providers to the insurers, with the result being increasing constraints on reimbursement. For years, the predominant method of covering health care costs was fee for service, and there was little, if any, incentive for cost-effective delivery of care (Chamberlain, Chen, Osuna, & Yamamoto, 1995). All that is changing.

The U.S. health care system has a diverse financial base, composed of both private and public funding. As a result, administrative costs for health care reimbursement are higher in this country than in countries with a **single-payer system** (a model wherein the government is the only entity to reimburse health care costs, such as in Canada). The level of U.S. health care expenditures is higher than that of any other nation, and previous cost-containment measures have been ineffective in slowing the growth in expenditures (Schieber, Poullier, & Greenwald, 1997). Despite the enormous expenditure of public funds, the United States has not found a way to provide health care coverage for all citizens. Figure 1-3 shows the sources of the nation's health dollars in 1998.

Private Insurance

The system for financing health care services in the United States is based on the private insurance model. Private insurance companies constitute one of the largest sectors of the health care system. Currently, more than 1,000 private insurance companies exist

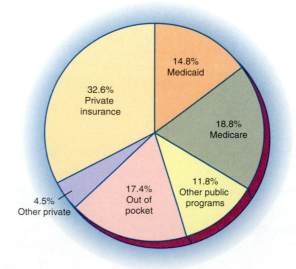

Figure 1-3 Source of the Nation's Health Dollar in 1998. (*Health Care Financing Administration, 2000*)

(Feldstein, 1999). Payment rates to health care providers vary among insurance companies.

In the United States, insured individuals pay substantial monthly premiums for insurance coverage having high deductibles for health care services. For many, these costs may prove barriers to procuring necessary insurance coverage and health services. In addition, insurers will no longer pay for services that *they* deem unnecessary, effectively taking client care decisions out of the hands of physicians. The quality of care provided is now being monitored not only by providers (physicians), but by third-party payers (insurance companies) and, ever increasingly, by consumers.

Managed Care

Managed care is a system of providing and monitoring care wherein access, cost, and quality are controlled before or during delivery of services. The goal of managed care is the delivery of services in the most cost-efficient manner possible. Managed care organizations combine the financing and delivery of health care services. Managed care seeks to control costs by monitoring delivery of services and restricting access to expensive procedures and providers.

Managed care was designed to provide coordinated services with an emphasis on prevention and primary care (ANA, 1995). The rationale behind managed care is to give consumers preventive services delivered by a **primary care provider** (a health care provider whom a client sees first for health care; typically, a family practitioner, internist, or pediatrician). The primary care provider is responsible for managing or coordinating all care of a client when illness makes referrals necessary. This is supposed to result in less expensive interventions.

Managed care has been in existence for years; however, it is only within the past 20 years that it has enjoyed national prominence (Society for Ambulatory Care Professionals, 1994). The Health Maintenance Organization Act (passed in 1973) implemented two mandates. First, federal grants and loans were made available to **health maintenance organizations** (HMOs) (prepaid health plans that provide primary health care services for a preset fee and that focus on cost-effective treatment measures) that complied with strict federal regulations as opposed to the less-restrictive state requirements. Second, large employers were required to provide to employees an HMO as an option for health care coverage (Society for Ambulatory Care Professionals, 1994). From their inception, HMOs have constituted a viable alternative to the traditional fee-for-service system.

Managed care is not a place but, rather, an organizational structure with several variations. One such variation is the HMO, which is both provider and insurer. Other variations are **preferred provider organiza-**

Table 1–6 COMPARISON OF INDEPENDENT PRACTICE AND MANAGED CARE	
TYPE	**DESCRIPTION**
Independent Practice	Fee for service or salary
	Functions within socially prescribed boundaries (professional ethics)
	Free choice of provider
	Disease-oriented philosophy
Managed Care	
Health maintenance organizations (HMOs)	Provide services to a group of enrolled persons
	Preset and prepaid fees
	Limited to certain providers
Preferred provider organizations (PPOs)	Networks of providers that give discounts to sponsoring organization
	Members' choice of physician not mandated, but lesser reimbursement if physician is outside of the network
Exclusive provider organizations (EPOs)	No benefit if member is treated outside of the network
	Usually regulated by state insurance laws

tions (PPOs), wherein members must use providers within the system in order to obtain full reimbursement but may use other providers for lesser reimbursement, and **exclusive provider organizations** (EPOs) wherein care must be delivered by the providers in the plan in order for clients to receive any reimbursement. In the past decade, there has been a great shift on the part of the population from private insurance to HMOs and PPOs (Feldstein, 1999). Table 1–6 compares independent practice and managed care organizational structures.

Health Maintenance Organizations

Health Maintenance Organizations often maintain primary health care sites (although not necessarily) and commonly employ provider professionals. They use **capitated rates** (preset flat fees based on membership in, not services provided by, the HMO), assume the risk of clients who are heavy users, and exert control over the use of services. Health maintenance organizations have been noted for using advanced practice registered nurses (APRNs) as primary care providers and using precertification programs to limit unnecessary hospitalization. Further, HMOs emphasize client education, health promotion and self-care.

Another common feature of HMOs is **single point of entry** (entry into the health system through a point designated by the plan which primary care is delivered. **Primary health care** is the client's point of entry into the health care system and includes assessment, diagnosis, treatment, coordination of care, education, preventive services, and surveillance. It comprises the spectrum of services provided by a family practitioner (nurse or physician) in an ambulatory setting. Primary care providers (PCPs) serve as "gatekeepers" to the health care system, in that they determine which, if any, referrals to specialists are needed by the client. To reduce costs, HMOs purposely limit direct access to specialists. Managed care plans assume a significant portion of the risk of providing health care and, consequently, encourage prudent use by both consumers and providers. In 1976, there were 175 HMOs in the United States; by 1995 there were 591 (Feldstein, 1999).

Preferred Provider Organizations

The most common managed care systems are PPOs. A PPO represents a contractual relationship between hospitals, providers, insurers, employers, and third-party payers to form a network wherein providers negotiate with group purchasers to provide health services for a defined population at a predetermined price (Feldstein, 1999). Care received within the network is associated with the highest reimbursement; care received outside the network is associated with lower reimbursement, with the client paying the difference. Preferred provider organizations have been very popular in the United States. In fact, the number of PPOs has increased from fewer than 10 in 1981 to over 700 in 1994 (Feldstein, 1999).

Exclusive Provider Organizations

Exclusive provider organizations create a network of providers (such as physicians and hospitals) and offer the incentive of consumer services for little or no copayment if the network providers are used exclusively. If a member receives treatment outside of the network, no benefit is paid. For instance, a member who becomes ill and receives treatment while visiting relatives in another state would receive no benefits for the treatment.

Federal Government Insurance Plans

The federal government became a third-party payer for health care services with the advent of Medicare and Medicaid in 1965. The Health Care Financing Administration (HCFA) is a federal agency that regulates Medicare, Medicaid, and Children's Health Insurance Program (CHIP) expenditures. There are many public programs for the financing of health care, with Medicare and Medicaid being the predominant ones. Medicare is the federally funded program that provides health care coverage for elderly persons and disabled persons. Medicaid pro-

vides health care coverage for the poor. Children's Health Insurance Program is a partnership between the federal and state governments to cover previously uninsured children.

With the ultimate goal of curtailing spending for hospitalized Medicare recipients, the federal government created diagnosis-related groups (DRGs) to categorize the average cost of care for each diagnosis. A prospective payment system was then created based on the DRGs. **Prospective payment** is a predetermined rate paid for each episode of hospitalization based on the client's age and principal diagnosis and on the presence or absence of surgery and **comorbidity** (simultaneous existence of more than one disease process in an individual). Hospitals are reimbursed the predetermined amount regardless of the actual cost of providing services to the client. The prospective payment system, originally designed for Medicare, has been adopted by other agencies and insurance companies.

Medicare

When Medicare was established in 1965, it was intended to protect individuals over the age of 65 years from exorbitant health care costs. In 1972, Medicare was modified to also cover permanently disabled individuals and those with end-stage renal disease. Because many individuals over the age of 65 do not have employee-paid insurance, public funds cover the majority of health care services for elderly persons (USDHHS, 1993).

Medicaid

Medicaid is the largest third-party payer of nursing home health care expenditures (Feldstein, 1999). Medicaid is a shared venture between the federal and state governments. Each state has latitude in determining who is "medically indigent" and, thus, qualifies for pub-

PROFESSIONAL TIP

Impact of Prospective Payment System and DRGs

- Decreased length of client stay in hospitals
- More emphasis on preventive care
- Increased concern about consumer's (client's) response to care
- An increased number of critically ill clients in hospitals
- Clients sicker upon discharge from hospital
- An increase in outpatient care
- Client and family more responsible for care
- Greater need for home health care
- Mergers or closures of hospitals because of inordinate competition

lic monies. Minimal services covered by Medicaid are defined by the federal government and include inpatient and outpatient hospital services, physician services, laboratory services (including x-ray), and rural health clinic services. States may elect to cover other services, such as dental, vision, and prescription drug.

Children's Health Insurance Program

Children's Health Insurance Program was created in 1997 as part of the Balanced Budget Act. The program is designed to provide health care to uninsured children, many of whom are members of working families that earn too little to afford private insurance on their own but earn too much to be eligible for Medicaid.

FACTORS INFLUENCING HEALTH CARE

Despite cost-containment efforts (such as DRGs, established by the federal government, and managed care, established by the insurers), the U.S. health care system still has problems with issues of cost, access, and quality. These issues are important for nurses to understand and are integral to any effort toward health reform.

Cost

Cost has been a driving force for change in the health care system as evidenced by the strength and numbers of managed care plans, increased use of outpatient treatment, and shortened hospital stays. These market forces (to maximize profits by minimizing costs) are dominating the current changes in the health care system.

The cost of providing health care has risen dramatically during the past 15 years. The U.S. government spends more on health care per person than does any other country (O'Neil, 1993). The increasing consumption of federal funds for health care means that resources are being moved from other areas of need, such as education, housing, and social services (Grace, 1997). Figure 1-4 illustrates health care expenditures.

The most cost-efficient programs in terms of administration are Medicare and Medicaid (HCFA, 1998). It should be noted that the administration of these programs is subcontracted to private agencies and organizations. In contrast, some private plans, particularly small business plans, use over 40 cents of each dollar for administration. The cost of employee health care benefits is thus an expensive commitment for small businesses.

Three major factors increase the cost of health care: (1) an oversupply of specialized providers (fees are raised to maintain provider income in light of fewer clients); (2) a surplus of hospital beds (empty beds are a cost liability); and (3) the passive role assumed by

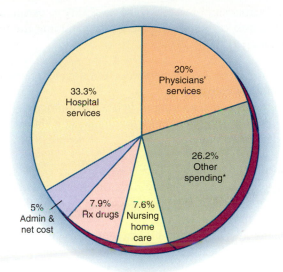

Figure 1-4 Health Care Expenditures in 1998. *Note:* Other spending included dental services, other professional services, home health, durable medical products, OTC medicines and sundries, public health, research, and construction. (*Health Care Financing Administration, 2000*)

most consumers (when someone else pays the bill, consumers typically are less concerned about cost) (Feldstein, 1999). Other factors that contribute to the high cost of health care are the aging of the population, the increased number of people with chronic illnesses, the increase in health-related lawsuits and the associated unnecessary use of services (e.g., additional diagnostic testing), and advanced technology that has allowed more people to survive formerly fatal illnesses even though those people require extensive and lifelong care.

Access

Related to the issue of cost is that of access to health care services, which carries serious implications for the functioning of the health care system. As a result of high costs, health care for many people is crisis oriented and fragmented. Numerous people in the United States are unable to gain access to health care services because of inadequate or no insurance; thus, illness among these people may progress to an acute stage before intervention is sought. Services used by individuals during acute illnesses are typically provided by emergency departments. Emergency room and acute care services are expensive when compared to early intervention and preventive measures.

Only a small portion of the medically indigent are covered by Medicare. In addition, many individuals are underinsured. These people are neither poor nor old but, rather, are middle-class unemployed Americans or those who have jobs lacking adequate health care benefits. In addition to poverty and unemployment, other factors can hinder a person's ability to obtain insurance and/or health care services, including the following:

- Lack of insurance provision by employer because of prohibitive costs
- High costs of obtaining individual insurance
- Certain preexisting conditions making it difficult to obtain insurance
- Cultural barriers
- Shortages of health care providers in some geographic areas (especially rural or inner city areas)
- Limited access to ancillary services (e.g., child care and transportation)
- Status as single-parent or two-income family, making it difficult for parents to take time from work to transport children to health care providers

Quality

It is estimated that 30% to 40% of diagnostic and medical procedures performed in this country are unnecessary (Lee, Soffel, & Luft, 1997). This inappropriate use of resources can be traced to several factors, including:

- The litigious environment and resultant tendency toward defensive practice (e.g., ordering all possible tests instead of only those that the provider deems truly necessary).
- The widely held American belief that more is better.
- Lack of access to and continuity of services and the subsequent misuse of acute care services.

The greatest number of health care dollars are expended in the last days of life, with 40% of in-hospital days and 35% of prescription medications being used

CULTURAL CONSIDERATIONS

Barriers to Health Care Services

Certain cultural beliefs and values may prevent individuals from seeking health care. These may include the following:

- Belief in Divine healing
- Refusal of care on holy days
- Belief that the individual taking the ill person to a health care facility is responsible for the ill person for the rest of that person's life after recovery
- Belief that illness is a result of sins committed in previous life
- View of prayer as a tool for deliverance from illness
- Belief that illness is God's punishment

by elderly persons. Twelve percent of the U.S. population is aged 65 years or older and uses 33% of health care expenditures (Rowe, 1996).

In an attempt to provide universal access to services in a cost-effective manner, quality may be sacrificed. For example, hospitals that are reducing the numbers of nurses ("downsizing") risk endangering quality. Safety and quality are frequently compromised by the inappropriate substitution of unqualified personnel for LP/VNs and RNs in direct care of clients. Cross-training of staff, increased use of unlicensed personnel, and reductions in full-time positions for nurses are affecting the type of care delivered in hospitals. Any movement toward reform must focus on providing quality nursing care to all consumers.

CHALLENGES WITHIN THE HEALTH CARE SYSTEM

The major challenges facing the U.S. health care delivery system—which also happen to impact the control of costs—include the public's disillusionment with providers; providers' and consumers' loss of control over health care decisions; decreased use of hospitals and the accompanying negative impact on quality of care; changing practice settings; ethical issues; and vulnerable populations.

Disillusionment with Providers

Greed and waste have been identified as major problems of the U.S. health care system (Maraldo, 1997). Whether these problems are caused by defensive practice, consumer demand, or professional economics is irrelevant to the public. Success in reform depends on starting where the public expects reform should begin: eliminating the greed of providers and the waste in the health care system. Further, people in the United States have become suspicious of health care providers. The high level of esteem in which medicine has traditionally been held has eroded over the past few years. Consumers, increasingly tired of paying the high cost of care, are questioning medical practices and fees (Zerwekh & Claborn, 1997). However, the public is not disillusioned with nurses (Kellogg Foundation, 1994). As reported in the *American Journal of Nursing* (AJN) (2000) a November 1999 Gallup poll reported that almost three-quarters of those surveyed rated the honesty and ethics of nurses as "high" or "very high." Nursing received higher ratings than any other profession including other health care professionals. Nurse Week and Sigma Theta Tau International commissioned another survey. It revealed that 92% of the public trust health information provided by registered nurses. This positive perception of nurses will be important as patterns of reform are established.

Positive Perception of Nurses

Several studies (ANA, 1993a; Kellogg Foundation, 1994) verify the public's trust in nurses. The public sees nurses as part of the solution, not the problem, and believes that if nurses were allowed to use their skills, they would significantly enhance quality and reduce costs. One survey (ANA, 1993a) inquired about consumer receptivity to nurses' taking on expanded responsibilities. Respondents supported **prescriptive authority** (legal recognition of the ability to prescribe medications) for RNs and endorsed the role of nurses in performing physical examinations and managing minor acute illnesses. Nurses should expand their focus on holistic care and spend as much time as possible on prevention of illness and wellness issues.

Loss of Control

Providers feel they have lost control over the care they provide to their clients. Increasingly, the insurance companies or the managed care organizations decide which care can and which care cannot be provided to the client.

Consumers express feeling terrorized by the health care delivery system. They feel they have lost personal control over their health care. Many stay in their current jobs because of their health care benefits or give up employment mobility out of fear of being denied a new policy because of preexisting conditions.

Decreased Hospital Use

In the early 20th century, hospitals focused on providing care to those who had no caregivers in the family or community. The focus of these early institutions was care as opposed to cure (Grace, 1997). The focus of hospitals changed in the mid-1940s as a result of technological changes and the passage by Congress in 1946 of the Hill–Burton Act, which provided funding for the renovation and construction of hospitals. One unanticipated outcome of this act was a substantial oversupply of hospital beds. Health care costs escalated because of the need to keep the hospital beds occupied: Everyone was put in the hospital, for everything from a complete physical examination, to specific diagnostic testing, to acute care or surgery.

From 1945 to 1982, the demand for hospital beds steadily increased. After 1982, however, a steady decline in the number of hospital admissions and the average length of stay occurred (Grace, 1997). In 1995, there were 23.7% fewer inpatient days than in 1985 (Feldstein, 1999). Many small hospitals have had to close their doors because they could no longer compete with the large hospitals.

Currently, hospitals continue to be the nucleus of the health care delivery system in the United States. Hospitals account for the largest proportion of expenditures and employ the majority of health care workers. Hospitals have fewer clients today because of the trend toward rapid discharge and a greater number of procedures being performed in outpatient settings. The clients who are hospitalized require more nursing care because of greater complexity of needs and severity of illness. Additional factors that have contributed to the decreased hospital population include:

- Shorter length of stays,
- Greater availability of outpatient facilities,
- Technological advances,
- An increased number of services available in outpatient settings, and
- Expectations/demands of third-party payers.

As a result of the changes in reimbursement practices, hospitals are restructuring (also referred to as redesigning and reengineering). Examples of restructuring activities include mergers with larger institutions; development of integrated systems that provide a full range of services focusing on continuity of care, such as preadmission, outpatient, acute inpatient, long-term inpatient, and home care; and the substitution of multiskilled workers for nurses.

Changing Practice Settings

Most nurses currently practice in hospitals and will continue to do so in the future (Aiken, 1995). The increasing presence of severely ill clients requires that nurses who work in hospitals possess technical expertise, critical thinking skills, and interpersonal competence. Outside the hospital setting, there is an ever-increasing need for nurses in different areas of practice. Home health services, in particular, will need to continue expanding in order to meet the growing needs of the steadily increasing elderly population (Hull, 1997). Social and political changes are affecting nurses by creating the need for expanded services and settings. Because of these changes, demand for nursing care fluctuates: For example, nursing employment outside the hospital continues to increase. More nurses will be needed in the future because:

- The growing elderly population will require more health care services.
- The number of people admitted to nursing homes is steadily growing.
- The number of homeless individuals, who are most often denied access to health care, is increasing rapidly.

As initial reform occurs, some nurses may be displaced from their current jobs. But overall, many more jobs will be created by the demand for greater access to health care services. Some examples of areas where larger numbers of nurses will be required are primary care, public health, extended care, and home care.

COMMUNITY/HOME HEALTH CARE

Cost of Home Health Care

- Since the advent of Medicare and Medicaid, home health care has grown rapidly. Because it is much less costly to provide home care, clients are sent home to recuperate.
- Expenditures for health care in the home are greatly increasing.

Ethical Issues

The United States is struggling with a major ethical conflict of cost containment versus compassionate care. According to Hicks and Boles (1997), no country, regardless of wealth, can provide all citizens with every health care service they desire or need. Today, the U.S. health care delivery system is faced with the dilemma of citizens' needs being greater than available resources. Thus, some difficult choices must be made to determine which needs will be met and which will remain unmet.

The national mentality reflected in the expectation that everything must be done to save a dying person has created an enormous drain on the health care resources of the United States and represents one example of ethical issues related to health care. As decisions are made regarding how scarce resources are to be allocated, there will be much debate about the ethics involved. The appropriateness of futile life-sustaining measures—those that only keep the client in a vegetative state—must be addressed (Rowe, 1996). Nurses must strongly advocate for just and ethical distribution of resources as health care reform progresses.

Vulnerable Populations

Meeting the health care needs of underserved populations is especially challenging. Groups that may be unable to gain access to health care services include children, rural residents, people with AIDS, and the homeless and others living in poverty. An increase in poverty further strains hospitals because Medicaid is no longer adequate to meet the needs of the medically indigent.

Our current health care system neglects the overall needs of children. Children are more likely than adults to be uninsured or underinsured. Children who are covered by health insurance have a greater degree of well-being.

Many parents have their children immunized only when the children are ready to start school, because immunization is a requirement for entry into the public school system. Preventive health care should be encouraged and made available to children of all ages,

with an emphasis on early immunization. The ANA and a coalition of allied nursing associations are working together in an attempt to immunize all children in the United States.

Traditionally, rural areas have had fewer health care providers and facilities that are easily accessible than have their urban counterparts. Approximately 45% of those over the age of 65 years live in rural areas (Vrabec, 1995). Because people in rural areas tend to work for small businesses or be self-employed, many of them have no health insurance.

As of December 1997, 641,086 people in the United States have been diagnosed with AIDS, and estimates suggest that 650,000 to 900,000 persons in the United States are now living with HIV (CDC, 1998). It is estimated that at least 40,000 new infections occur each year (CDC, 1998). The most rapid spread of the disease is occurring among women, children, and intravenous drug users and their sexual partners. Women who have AIDS have a higher mortality rate than do men, and decreased access to health care may be one contributing factor (Tlusty, 1994). Although the cost of this epidemic is unmeasurable in terms of human suffering, approximately $10.5 billion was spent on care of people with AIDS in 1994 alone (Hull, 1997). Not only will additional funding be necessary, but outpatient care settings (such as hospices, home care, and clinics) must be expanded to care for those affected by this epidemic.

The homeless and others living in poverty are often mobile, having no permanent address. They may not know which services are available to them or how to access the system except through inner city hospitals. This creates a significant financial burden on these health care agencies. Illegal aliens, because of fears of being arrested and deported, may enter emergency departments under false identities and in acute distress, receive treatment, and then disappear.

NURSING'S RESPONSE TO HEALTH CARE CHALLENGES

As the United States continues to look for ways to address the issue of health care reform, the implications for nursing will continue to increase. Some nurses feel threatened by impending changes, whereas others are excited about the possibility of transforming the health care system into something better. The nursing profession has responded to the myriad challenges in health care delivery by proposing a plan for reform.

Nursing's Agenda for Health Care Reform

In 1991, in response to the problems of high cost, limited access, and eroding quality that were affecting the U.S. health care system, the nursing community

GERONTOLOGICAL CONSIDERATIONS

Rural Elders

Health care barriers experienced by elderly persons living in rural areas include the following:

- Inadequate financing of rural health care facilities. Medicare's lower reimbursement rates for rural hospitals than for urban hospitals has been a contributing factor to the closure of some hospitals in rural communities.
- Decreased availability of health care providers.
- Greater geographic distances that must be traveled in order to obtain services.

Table 1–7 NURSING'S AGENDA FOR HEALTH CARE REFORM

Nursing's agenda for health care reform includes several basic tenets, including the following:

- All citizens and residents of the United States must have equitable access to essential health care services.
- Primary health care services must play a very basic and prominent role in service delivery.
- Consumers must be the central focus of the health care system. Assessment of health care needs must be the determining factor in the ultimate structuring and delivery of programs and services.
- Consumers must be guaranteed direct access to a full range of qualified health care providers who offer their services in a variety of delivery arrangements at sites that are accessible, convenient, and familiar to the consumer.
- Consumers must assume more responsibility for their own care and become better informed about the range of providers and potential options for services.
- Health care services must be restructured to create a better balance between the prevailing orientation toward illness and cure and a new commitment to wellness and care.
- The health care system must ensure that appropriate, effective care is delivered through efficient use of resources.
- A standardized package of essential health care services must be provided and financed through an integration of public and private sources.
- Mechanisms must be implemented to protect against catastrophic costs and impoverishment.

From Nursing's Agenda for Health Care Reform, *by American Nurses Association, 1991, Kansas City, MO: Author.*

created a public policy agenda that is currently endorsed by more than 70 organizations. *Nursing's Agenda for Health Care Reform* (ANA, 1991) provides a valid framework for change in health care policies and establishes nursing's legislative program, through which these changes can be implemented. Table 1–7 lists the major tenets of this agenda. A cornerstone of nursing's proposal is the delivery of health care services in environments that are easily accessible, familiar, and consumer friendly. Another essential part of nursing's agenda is the empowerment of consumers in the area of self-care. This goal has enormous implications for nurses as health educators and for the use of incentives for increasing personal accountability for one's own health status.

Standards of Care

Another approach to the challenges of the health care delivery system has been the move toward standardization of care. In December 1990, the Agency for Health Care Policy and Research (AHCPR) was established with the specific charge of achieving consensus within the medical/health care community regarding the usual treatment of high-volume and expensive disease conditions that differ in therapeutic management despite substantial research. More simply put, there is significant variation in the diagnosis and treatment of certain illnesses and diseases. The medical justification for such variance has been that every client is an individual and that the choice of treatment is a private decision involving client and physician. Prostatic hypertrophy (enlarged prostate gland) and breast cancer are examples of high-volume diagnoses that have been studied by the AHCPR but for which appropriate diagnostic tests and treatments of choice have not yet been conclusively determined. The AHCPR aims to identify the standards of treatment to which the health care community can be held. Currently, 18 AHCPR-

published guidelines are available to the public and should be integral to nursing practice.

Advanced Practice

The advanced practice of nursing has evolved as nursing has become more complex and specialized. Since the late 1960s, nurse practitioners (NPs), clinical nurse specialists (CNSs), certified nurse midwives (CNMs), and other advanced practice registered nurses (APRNs) have provided primary health care services to individuals, many of whom would have otherwise had inadequate or no access to services (Brown & Grimes, 1993). The APRN possesses advanced skills and in-depth knowledge in specific areas of practice (Stafford & Appleyard, 1997). Although there are differences among various advanced practice roles, all APRNs are experts who work with clients to prevent disease and promote health.

There are more than 100,000 APRNs in the United States (ANA, 1995). Nurses in advanced practice are also moving toward independent practice. Data suggest that APRNs can independently diagnose and resolve over 80% of the primary health care problems of the American public (ANA, 1993a). The NP facilitates access to and continuity of care and provides high-quality care (Brown & Grimes, 1993). Advanced practice registered nurses prescribe less-expensive diagnostic tests, the length of their visits is comparable to that of physicians', and they charge less for services because of the comparatively lower cost of professional liability insurance (ANA, 1993b). Despite repeated proof of the cost efficiency and therapeutic effectiveness of APRNs, obstacles to this role for nurses persist. In a recent Division of Nursing report on APRNs, the single most formidable obstacle to practice is that most people are unaware of what APRNs offer (Washington Consulting Group, 1994).

Recent progress has been made on the access issues that constrain APRNs. Reimbursement is now available to some segments of the advanced practice community in every federal entitlement program (HCFA, 1998).

Currently, all states except Minnesota, Tennessee, and Wisconsin award APRNs some type of prescriptive authority (National Council of State Boards of Nursing [NCSBN], personal communication, 2000). In 15 states, this authority is complete and unrestricted, is unassociated with physician oversight, and includes all classes of drugs (Pearson, 1996). The ANA (through the JCAHO and the HCFA) began the groundwork for professional staff privileges for APRNs in its revision of the official definitions of professional staff that include a broad range of providers.

Public vs. Private Programs

The combination of public sector and private sector health care resources seems to be beneficial for U.S. residents. The competition between the two sectors has encouraged quality and progress. Each setting offers benefits as well as drawbacks to health care recipients.

The nursing profession supports an integration of public and private sector programs and resources. Public dollars are required to help the poor and those who do not receive health care benefits through the workplace. Actual services should be available through a variety of public and private sources. To safeguard the health care system from becoming a two-tiered process based on personal resources, both the poor and nonpoor and the privileged and nonprivileged must be enrolled in the same programs.

Finally, the basic required package of services must be defined in the same way in each state and required as the minimum for both public and private sector programs. Minimal national standards should be set, but local planning and implementation should be promoted.

The states' rights philosophy prevalent in the United States creates an obstacle to national standards, which are necessary for several areas of assurance. Some coast-to-coast consistency in the cost of services, with room for local adjustments, is needed.

Public Health

During the past several years, public health has perceptibly eroded. Public health includes services such as immunizations, prenatal care, environmental concerns (conditions that may affect health), and analysis of the prevailing disease patterns in a community. Current public health problems include:

- Appearance of new fatal diseases (e.g., AIDS and the Ebola virus),
- Emergence of drug-resistant strains of tuberculosis, and
- Presence of toxic environmental conditions.

Community Health

Parris and Hines (1995) recommend a commitment to a community-based approach to reforming the system of health care delivery. Community-based care focuses on prevention and primary care. Successful movement toward a healthy and empowered consumer requires access to community-based primary health care. Nursing has a rich heritage of providing such community services, as evidenced by the work of pioneers such as Lillian Wald and Mary Breckenridge.

TRENDS AND ISSUES

As current trends continue, the delivery of health care services will continue to change. Table 1–8 lists factors that will continue to shape reform of the health care delivery system.

Table 1–8 TRENDS AFFECTING DELIVERY OF HEALTH CARE SERVICES

- The aging of the U.S. population
- Increasing diversity in the U.S. population
- Increased number of single-parent families and of children living in poverty
- Continued growth in outpatient settings and a greater demand for primary care providers
- Advances in technology with resultant ability to perform more services in outpatient settings (including the home)
- More states using managed care models to deliver services to the medically indigent
- Incentives for individuals who participate in preventive activities
- Federal funding of health care provider education focusing on service to underserved populations and areas
- The system as a union of both public and private sector resources and services
- Managed care dominating as the context for service delivery
- Continued focus on quality improvement

GERONTOLOGICAL CONSIDERATIONS

Meeting the Needs of Elderly Clients

In 1992, the HCFA funded community nursing organizations (CNOs) to help meet the needs of elderly persons in four communities. These four projects yielded the following results:

- A high degree of client satisfaction
- Decreased Medicare expenditures associated with home care
- Use of less-expensive equipment
- Decrease emergency department costs (ANA, 1995)

As health care reform occurs, some professions will experience opportunities for growth whereas others will experience layoffs (O'Neil, 1993). The challenge is to improve the nation's delivery of health care services by positioning nursing to preserve its integrity and to guarantee its preferred future. Nurses must be at the forefront of change.

SUMMARY

- The three levels of health care services can be categorized as primary, secondary, and tertiary.
- Health care services are delivered and financed by the public (official, voluntary, and nonprofit agencies), public/private, and private (hospitals, extended-care facilities, home health care agencies, hospices, outpatient settings, schools, industrial clinics, managed care organizations, community nursing centers, and rural hospitals) sectors.
- The health care team is composed of nurses, nurse practitioners, physicians, physician's assistants, pharmacists, dentists, dietitians, social workers, therapists, and chaplains.
- Managed care organizations seek to control health care costs by monitoring the delivery of services and restricting access to costly procedures and providers.
- Managed care plans include health maintenance organizations, preferred provider organizations, and exclusive provider organizations.
- The primary federal government insurance plans are Medicare, the program that provides health care coverage for elderly persons and disabled persons, and Medicaid, the jointly administered program that provides health care services for the poor.
- To achieve equity for all Americans, health care reform must address the three critical issues of cost, access, and quality of health care services.

- The challenges that the health care delivery system must overcome are the public's disillusionment with providers; the public's loss of control over health care decisions; the decreased use of hospitals and the related impact on quality of care; the change in practice settings; ethical issues, and the health care needs of vulnerable populations.
- *Nursing's Agenda for Health Care Reform* outlines nursing's proposals for easing the current problems in health care delivery.
- The Agency of Health Care Policy and Research aims to identify therapeutic standards to which the health care community can be held.
- A primary goal of the nursing profession within the areas of public health, community health, and long-term care is to provide health care services that emphasize prevention and primary health care for clients in these settings and thus help reduce costs and increase quality of health care.

Review Questions

1. When the goal of a health care service is to decrease the risk to clients for a disease or dysfunction, the type of care is called:
   a. primary.
   b. tertiary.
   c. exclusive.
   d. secondary.

2. Identified members of the health care team include:
   a. nurses, pharmacists, chaplains.
   b. nurses, physicians, ward clerks.
   c. therapists, housekeeping personnel, dietitians.
   d. dentists, social workers, maintenance personnel.

3. The primary federal government insurance plan(s) is (are):
   a. Medicaid and welfare.
   b. Medicaid and Social Security.
   c. Medicaid and diagnosis-related groups.
   d. Medicare and Children's Health Insurance Program.

4. Cost, access, and quality of health care services are the three critical issues that must be addressed by:
   a. schools.
   b. hospitals.
   c. health care reform.
   d. managed care plans.

5. The nursing role that protects the client and supports the client's decisions is:

   a. teacher.
   b. advocate.
   c. caregiver.
   d. team member.

6. The major health care problem for children is:

   a. living in poverty.
   b. having no transportation.
   c. receiving substandard health care.
   d. not receiving immunizations as infants.

Critical Thinking Questions

1. The U.S. health care system is first in technological advances, biomedical research, and state-of-the-art clinical equipment and facilities. Yet, even given these advantages, many consider the system to be in crisis. From your perspective, is the health care system in a state of strength or weakness? Why or why not?

2. What factors do you think have contributed to a positive perception of nurses? A negative perception? What can you do specifically to promote positive images of nurses among the public?

3. Think about the ethical ramifications of determining medically necessary therapeutics. Is rationing of scarce resources the answer to our health care dilemma?

 WEB FLASH!

- Search the Internet for information regarding Oregon's plan for allocating resources. What are the main points of the plan?
- Research health care reform on the Web. What is its status? What are the future plans for health care reform?

CRITICAL THINKING

MAKING THE CONNECTION

Refer to the following chapter to increase your understanding of critical thinking:

- **Chapter 5, Communication**

LEARNING OBJECTIVES

Upon completion of this chapter, you should be able to:
- *Define key terms.*
- *State five characteristics of the person who uses critical thinking.*
- *Identify behaviors that illustrate the traits of a nurse who is a critical thinker.*
- *Assess personal strengths and weaknesses in relation to critical thinking skills.*
- *Develop a personal plan for the enhancement of personal critical thinking and reasoning skills.*

KEY TERMS

concept	logic
critical thinking	opinion
discipline	reasoning
disciplined	reflective
judgment	standard
justify	

INTRODUCTION

Thinking as a nurse involves much more than gathering an assortment of facts and skills. Critical thinking in nursing education is not a separate component of the curriculum. It is "an approach to inquiry where both students and faculty examine clinical and professional issues and search for more effective answers" (Miller & Malcolm, 1990).

Nursing is part of a rapidly changing and increasingly complex society. Anyone who expects to have a successful career in nursing, at any level, must be able to compete effectively. This means that practical/vocational nurses must have good problem-solving skills and make quality decisions related to the client care they deliver. Over the past 15 years, increasing attention has been paid to the need for graduates of educational programs at every level and in every **discipline** (branch of learning, field of study, or occupation requiring specialized knowledge) to develop better thinking skills. Nurse educators have been among the leaders in the current movement to find ways to improve the thinking ability of their students. Nurses in clinical practice have also been challenged to improve their ability to reason clearly and logically. Because of these movements, you, as a beginning nursing student, will need to develop your critical thinking skills.

CRITICAL THINKING

The first step in improving the ability to think well is to develop an understanding of **critical thinking**. This involves much more than memorizing a simple definition of this process. The ability to think critically requires a great deal of effort and time. Many questions must be asked as you begin the process of learning to assess your own thinking and the quality of the thinking of others (Figure 2-1). In fact, memorizing an exact definition of critical thinking would be detrimental to the full development of an understanding of this **disciplined** (trained by instruction and exercise) type of thinking. The **concept** of critical thinking includes the basic idea that one becomes a better thinker by developing specific attitudes, traits, and skills. A concept is a mental picture of abstract phenomena that serves to organize observations related to that phenomena. Each person must learn to be **reflective**, or introspec-

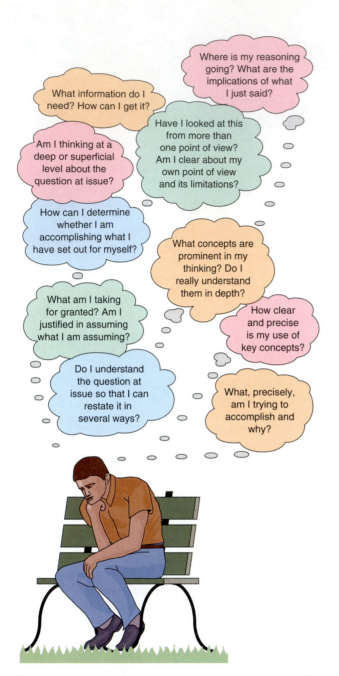

Figure 2-1 Assessing Our Own Thinking (*Courtesy of The Foundation for Critical Thinking, Santa Rosa, CA*)

tive, about his or her own thinking. Critical thinking was briefly described in this way in a workshop presented by Richard Paul (Paul & Willsen, 1993): "Critical thinking is that mode of thinking—about any subject, content, or problem—in which the thinker improves the quality of his or her thinking by skillfully taking charge of the structures inherent in thinking and imposing intellectual **standards** (or a level or degree of quality) upon them." To ensure integrity and consistency of the presentation in this chapter, the criteria, standards, and materials developed by the Center for

Critical Thinking have been used as the organizing framework.

Penny Heaslip (1994), in a newsletter designed for nurse educators interested in the use of critical thinking within the nursing curriculum, presents a definition of critical thinking. This definition serves as a basis for your development of strategies and tactics as you begin the exciting experience of learning to think more clearly, and in a disciplined manner, about nursing. A comprehensive definition of critical thinking is the disciplined, intellectual process of applying skillful clinical **reasoning** (use of the elements of thought to solve a problem or settle a question) and self-reflective thinking as a guide to belief or action in nursing practice (Heaslip, 1994; Norris & Ennis, 1989; Paul, 1990).

Table 2–1 presents some definitions of critical thinking. Review them and compare the elements that are common to all of them and the elements that are different.

Most of the authors who have written about critical thinking have addressed instructors. This chapter is written for you, the student. It is designed to guide your process of reflecting on and evaluating your own thinking. While your instructors want to help you with the process, you are ultimately responsible for your own thinking.

Many students enter nursing programs unprepared to think critically. Many educators believe this inability may be the result of a lack of instruction in thinking. The result is similar to what would happen to you if you tried to play soccer without knowing the rules or having had a chance to learn the basic skills of the game. Quality thinking is like any skill; it takes practice and discipline to learn. This is a good time to do a self-evaluation related to your current ability to perform the four basic critical thinking processes: reading for meaning, listening critically, writing clearly, and speaking in a logical, coherent manner. These four skills are discussed in the next section. If your basic education program did not emphasize all of these skills, decide now to develop these abilities.

Table 2–1 DEFINITIONS OF CRITICAL THINKING

- "Reflective and reasonable thinking that is focused on deciding what to believe or do" (Ennis, 1985).

- "An investigation whose purpose is to explore a situation, phenomenon, question, or problem to arrive at a hypothesis or conclusion about it that integrates all available information and that can therefore be convincingly justified" (Kurfiss, 1988).

- "The attentive commitment to a self-reflective process of examining one's thoughts, ensuring that the thinking occurring meets intellectual standards" (Heaslip, 1993).

New Information

The quantity of new information that you must be prepared to master may be a barrier to the development of critical thinking skills. Many students (and instructors) focus so intently on the content of a course that they allow little time to think about the material. The ability to think critically about the knowledge base of nursing is essential for learning the content of your nursing courses. The discipline of nursing has an organizing **logic**, or formal principles of a branch of knowledge, that serves to define the appropriate facts and methods required to produce effective nursing practice. This logic serves as a framework within which the student can construct a unique, meaningful system for the practice of nursing. Your nursing program probably has a philosophy and a statement of the main concepts that the nursing faculty uses to present the course material in a logical framework.

Activity

If you have not yet reviewed your program's philosophy and main concepts for the purpose of helping you understand your program of study, this would be a good time to do so. Most programs of nursing include a philosophy statement, organizing concepts, and program outcomes in the student handbook or other document provided to students. To use these resources to help you use your own logic to discover the logic of nursing as presented in your program, try the following activities:

1. Identify the major concepts (such as nursing, learning, caring) that provide structure for your program's philosophy and organization.
2. Discuss the components, or parts, of each major theme with your classmates and instructors.
3. Use your own words to see how your mental pictures of these ideas may be the same or different from those in your program materials.
4. Review the material you have already covered in your nursing program to identify how the major parts of each course relate to these concepts.
5. Look at the objectives for this course and the topics in this textbook to see how they will relate to the main ideas you have discovered in this activity.

Student Responsibility

Finally, many students find the process of becoming responsible for their own thinking painful. For many students the education processes that were part of their basic school preparation were based on a very structured approach to acquiring selected facts and skills; the students' recall was then tested by "objective" tests. If this was your experience, you may view learning as being the result of the teacher's presenting what must be learned and devising "fair" tests. You may thus believe your own input to the learning process to be of less importance than that of the teacher. You, along with many other students, may find that you are uncomfortable when asked to decide what is important or to be able to defend your **opinions** (subjective beliefs) and **judgments** (conclusions based on sound reasoning and supported by evidence). You may prefer to be told, with no ambiguity, what you need to know.

Nursing, however, does not take place in predictable, highly structured situations. Practical/vocational nurses are required to make decisions at many levels. Knowing how to make good decisions begins with developing the essential skills, traits, and attitudes associated with critical thinking.

SKILLS OF CRITICAL THINKING

Four basic skills are necessary for the development of higher-level thinking skills. These skills are part of the process of developing and using thinking for problem-solving and reasoning. Your abilities in these four areas can be measured by the extent to which you are achieving the universal intellectual standards (UIS). These standards are discussed in the following section and are illustrated in Table 2–2. The four basic skills are critical reading, critical listening, critical writing, and critical speaking.

Critical Reading

Reading for meaning is basic to the acquisition of knowledge from textbooks and journals. The student who can read critically will also do better on tests. Study time will be reduced and retention of material

---

Table 2–2 THE SPECTRUM OF UNIVERSAL INTELLECTUAL STANDARDS

Clear	Unclear
Precise	Imprecise
Specific	Vague
Accurate	Inaccurate
Relevant	Irrelevant
Consistent	Inconsistent
Logical	Illogical
Deep	Superficial
Complete	Incomplete
Significant	Insignificant
Adequate	Inadequate
Fair	Unfair

Adapted from The Foundation for Critical Thinking, Santa Rosa, CA.

will be enhanced. An exercise that can help build reading skills is to use a highlighter pen to mark the main idea of a sentence. Students who have not learned to read critically will find that they have marked most of the text. Joining a study group may help you identify main ideas by comparing with others the various main ideas each of you have derived from the same material. During test reviews, you can make sure to note when misreading or misinterpretation caused you to make an error on the test. By making a conscious effort to identify your individual weaknesses, you will improve your critical reading skills.

Another tactic you can try is to practice restating the main idea to yourself or to another student. As you read the text, have a dialogue with yourself, which could go something like this: "What is the reason for studying this material? How does this relate to what I already know? This does not seem to fit. Did I misunderstand? Can I say this in my own words?" Worrell (1990) has developed a useful tool for guiding your dialogue. It is illustrated in Table 2–3.

Critical Listening

Communication skills, especially listening skills, receive a great deal of emphasis in the nursing curriculum. Even so, many persons do not have effective listening skills. One reason is that many persons have developed the habit of tuning in only occasionally to orally presented material. The result is that the meaning of the oral communication is lost. A way to improve your listening skills is to try to restate the points made in a discussion with another student and have that student give feedback about how accurately you have restated her position. Critical listening also requires that you carry on a mental dialogue with the speaker. For instance, as you listen, focus on what the speaker is saying, listen for key points, notice anything that seems confusing to you as well as those points you already understand (Figure 2-2).

Figure 2-2 Effective listening skills are essential to all client interactions.

Table 2–3 STRATEGIC READING LIST

The following questions serve as a guide for self-talk when reading texts or journal articles. An effective reader is an active, strategic reader! Soon you will find yourself automatically using these and other questions that you have developed, no longer needing the checklist.

PREREADING QUESTIONS

____ 1. Have I previewed (skimmed) the title, headings, subheadings, objectives, and overview?

____ 2. Do the headings/subheadings identify main ideas?

____ 3. What is the chapter about?

____ 4. How is the content related to what I already know?

____ 5. How has the author organized the material? How will this organization help me?

____ 6. Will I need other resources as I read?

____ 7. Based on previewing, what questions should I formulate to guide my reading?

QUESTIONS DURING READING

____ 1. Does this make sense to me?

____ 2. Do I need to look up any unfamiliar words?

____ 3. Do I need to reread difficult material? Or will this be explained further if I read on?

____ 4. Is the author using signal words (*first, next, therefore, as a result,* etc.)?

____ 5. How is this information related to what I know?

____ 6. How is this section linked to the previous section?

____ 7. Can I summarize this section before going any further?

____ 8. Can I answer my prereading questions? Can I formulate new questions?

QUESTIONS AFTER READING

____ 1. Do I understand the main points?

____ 2. Can I outline the content?

____ 3. How is this related to previous learning?

____ 4. How would I use or apply this information?

____ 5. Are there points that I need to clarify? How will I do this?

____ 6. What questions would likely be on an exam from this material?

____ 7. Can I answer my questions, paraphrase the content, and link main points without looking at my notes or text?

From Metacognition: Implications for instruction in nursing education, by P. J. Worrell, 1990, Journal of Nursing Education, *29(4). Reprinted with permission of* Journal of Nursing Education, SLACK Incorporated, Thorofare, NJ.

Critical listening requires that you make a conscious commitment to focus on the topic of discussion. This means that you should actively attend to the words and meanings of the speaker. Your ability to recognize things that distract your attention is valuable in increasing your listening skills. Some typical distractions for students include attempting to take word-for-word notes, focusing on the mannerisms or appearance of the speaker, and daydreaming. As in all areas, a good thinker is not afraid to identify weaknesses and strengths in order to improve.

Critical Writing

The ability to state one's thoughts coherently, clearly, and concisely is basic to good thinking skills. Many students arrive at college unable to write well. The quality of thinking is improved by the discipline required to state facts and judgments well. Many students are afraid to write down their thoughts, because they feel that writing is too revealing. Writing is important for the improvement of thinking because it can be reviewed using the UIS to evaluate the quality of the thinking reflected in the writing (Figure 2-3). These standards are discussed in greater detail later in the chapter. You may also refer back to Table 2–2.

One technique for improving the quality of your thinking through writing is to summarize, in your own words, the main idea in a reading assignment. Next, use that main idea in relation to a client care problem from the material you are studying. Then, put the writing away until the next day and reread it. Can you understand it? Submit it to a friend for critique. Can your friend understand what you meant to say? How could you improve what you have written? Improving your writing skills may not seem like fun, but it is an effective and vital process for improving the quality of your own thinking.

Critical Speaking

Perhaps the most neglected skill is disciplined speaking. We do not hear many examples of clear, logical, accurate spoken communication. Oral communication is different from written communication. It is usually more spontaneous and must be carefully presented because, unless recorded, it is present only for the moment. Ambiguous statements are misleading. Personal biases influence what the other person hears. Practicing in a small group and soliciting feedback from the listeners can help a student assess and improve this skill.

STANDARDS FOR CRITICAL THINKING

The simple definition of critical thinking used in the preceding section includes the provision that the assessment of your own thinking relies on the use of universal standards for quality thinking. As you begin to develop and apply critical thinking to nursing, the first requirement is to become familiar with these standards. The Spectrum of Universal Intellectual Standards developed by The Center for Critical Thinking is used in this discussion because it provides a valid and

Figure 2-3 Effective writing skills are integral to critical thinking.

reliable measure for the quality of thinking. Whether you are reading the assigned material from a textbook, listening to an oral presentation, writing a paper, answering test questions, or presenting ideas in oral form, the following standards should be applied.

Clarity vs. Lack of Clarity

Fundamental to quality thinking is the ability to think clearly. Thinking clearly means that you can place the facts and ideas of course content into a logical and coherent framework. The measure for the degree to which this is true is the degree to which you can state these relationships orally or in writing so that others can understand your position. One tactic for increasing your clarity of thought is to pay particular attention to the exact meaning of the words encountered. The year that you spend in the practical/vocational nursing program is filled with many new terms and concepts. Time spent in practicing the proper use of these terms and in applying concepts appropriately will result in improved clarity of thought and increased retention of content. You can use small study groups to challenge one another to write and speak clearly as you review content together.

A review of the words used in the preceding paragraph may illustrate how the meaning of words can be misunderstood. For example, think about the word *clarity*. When you look up this word in a dictionary, you find that there are several shades of meaning. Look up the word for yourself and decide which of the definitions applies to the use of clarity in describing a standard for critical thinking.

Think about some expressions you use every day. Would someone who is from another part of the country understand them? An example is the use of the term *this evening*, which is common in some parts of the country. If someone told you that she would visit you "this evening," when would you expect her? In some places, the person might arrive in the early afternoon; in other places, at night. When speaking to clients, families, and other health team members, the nurse must be sure that the words used clearly express the intended message. When reading or listening, do not assume that you understand a term. Take the time to verify the meaning.

Precision vs. Imprecision

Sometimes, we have a "ballpark" mentality. That is, we learn enough about a subject to be "in the ballpark," but not enough to hit a home run. The result is a general idea of the meaning of a fact or idea, but not enough understanding to apply it or to use the information for problem-solving or promoting communication of an idea to someone else. You may be making this mistake if you find yourself saying something like this: "I knew that, but on the test, it was stated differently." Precision of thought means that the meaning of a concept is clearly understood in terms of its relationship to other concepts and to its practical implications, so that the thought is exact, accurate, and definite (Paul & Willsen, 1993).

Specificity vs. Vagueness

Specificity means that the student can be concrete or exact in stating or applying a fact. An example of vagueness, which can be commonly ascribed to nursing students, occurs during the use of the planning phase of the nursing process when students do not write concrete nursing interventions. For example, a student may state that the nursing action will "provide support to the client and his family." It is difficult to explain exactly what this statement means, either in general or in relation to this client and this nurse. Appropriate planning involves deciding on definite, well-stated nursing diagnoses, goals, and nursing actions. The use of the nursing process requires that the student learn the degree of specificity required for each nursing situation. State or itemize the nursing actions to be performed.

Accuracy vs. Inaccuracy

Accuracy means being correct and within the proper parameters. Nursing students can readily understand the need for accurate calculation of a drug dose or accurate measurement of blood pressure. In the same way, the collection and interpretation of data must be accurate. Accuracy usually implies the use of some measuring instrument. In the case of blood pressure, this is easy to see. In the case of accuracy in thinking, it may be harder to conceptualize. An example would be when the nurse uses the term *hypertension* to mean someone who is anxious and hyperactive instead of the actual meaning, an elevation of blood pressure above the accepted normal maximum. When dealing with more abstract concepts, accuracy of interpretation and understanding are equally important. Students can

improve the accuracy of their thinking by trying to write new information in their own words and having another student interpret the meaning. Inaccurate information will become evident.

Accurate recording of findings during client care is essential to quality care. Accurate understanding of the concepts underlying each part of your nursing courses, plus understanding of the ways whereby each part of your nursing course relates to any given client, will enable you to be more accurate in your thinking.

There are degrees of accuracy. For example, you might measure a client's temperature using a thermometer that can measure to the 0.01 degree, but this degree of accuracy may be unnecessary. On the other hand, when figuring a pediatric dosage, a difference of 0.01 can be important. One of your challenges is to increase your awareness of the degree of accuracy required in given nursing situations.

Relevance vs. Irrelevance

Relevance refers to needed information as opposed to information that is not needed at the moment. Students must be able to separate the two; otherwise, they may spend time arguing for a position that does not matter. For instance, students may get sidetracked from the purpose of an exercise by failing to limit their responses to the central issue or heart of the question or problem to be solved. It is also important to be able to recognize when sufficient relevant information is not available. An example of failing to recognize relevant information might be ignoring a client's comment that his rash began the day after starting a new medication. On the other hand, the nurse may assume that a client is depressed about being in the hospital and so may fail to ask him why he seems sad.

During the study process, you can ask yourself how a particular concept is relevant to the application of the nursing process to client care. **Justify** (prove or show to be valid) your ideas to yourself and to another student.

Consistency vs. Inconsistency

Consistency means using principles and concepts appropriately for related applications. For instance, if you are using a particular nursing diagnosis based on accepted indicators, it should be applied when those indicators are present and should not be used when the indicators are not present. Failure to follow this standard results in inconsistent use of the nursing diagnosis.

Consistency can also refer to recognizing and using basic concepts appropriately whenever they apply. For example, knowing the basic actions of epinephrine will enable you to predict client responses to the administration of the drug. It will also help you understand that the client has the same response when an increased secretion of epinephrine is released by the client's kidneys.

Logical vs. Illogical

To be logical means to build one idea upon another so that the conclusion is based on a sequence of steps. Each step should be reasonable and related to the step before it and the step after it. Many symptoms that clients exhibit can be understood logically based on your knowledge of normal physiology and the changes produced by the client's given disease or malady. The successful student will make more efficient use of study time by identifying the logical basis of the material being presented.

The author of a nursing textbook uses nursing logic to organize the content of the book. You must use your own logic to grasp the meaning of the material. Do this by discovering the logic of the author. In this way you will begin to think within the logic of nursing.

Depth vs. Superficiality

Busy students may be tempted to rely on the specific learning objectives and the teacher's pre-test review as indicators of the amount of material they must master. This, however, may result in only a superficial understanding of basic processes and principles. Students can improve their ability to recognize the depth to which they must explore concepts and ideas. There is no easy way to do this, but knowing that different material requires different depth of study can assist the student. With time, these decisions will be easier to make. Your instructor and the learning aids within your textbook are useful guides. The more you use them, the better you will become at identifying relevant information and the appropriate depth of knowledge required to make good clinical decisions.

Completeness vs. Incompleteness

During the assessment phase of client care it is important that the nurse know when the client database is sufficient. Proper nursing care is based on identification of priority needs. The nurse will provide care only for those problems that have been identified. Although the physician orders treatments related to the medical diagnosis, these orders are not meant to direct all required care. Nursing care is essential to client well-being. Incomplete information or analysis of client needs will result in inappropriate or inadequate nursing care. Of course, your ability to identify and prioritize client care problems depends on the completeness of your knowledge base. This standard is related to accuracy. An incomplete database leads to inaccurate conclusions.

Significance vs. Triviality

When making decisions or sorting out information it is important for the nurse to identify information that is necessary for good decision making. Being able to recognize irrelevant facts or data that are not helpful for the problem at hand is an important skill. It is easy for a student to view all the material in a textbook as equally significant. Learning to identify significant (important) concepts will minimize the chances of your being distracted by trivial materials.

Adequacy vs. Inadequacy

In solving problems or exploring a subject, adequacy refers to the degree to which the available information is sufficient for the purpose and the amount of time and effort spent on the matter. When making clinical decisions, the nurse must be able to recognize when there is sufficient information upon which to base a decision. Premature closure of the process or the inability to decide because of fear that there is not enough information are equally detrimental to quality thinking.

As you study each chapter you will be given information that will help you identify the basic information required to care for each client. Knowing that good client care decisions are based on good preparation by the nurse can help you fit information into the logic of nursing.

Fairness vs. Bias

You, along with other students, come to the educational setting with a set of beliefs, opinions, and points of view. People are predisposed to believe that what they think is true must be true. The improvement of the quality of your thinking depends on your ability to identify the biases present in your thinking and the biases present in the thinking of others. Commitment to fairness will lead a person to challenge conclusions in the light of the presence or absence of personal bias. A nursing example would be the assessment of a person in pain. Each individual has learned a way to respond to pain: Some become quiet, some complain loudly, some are stoic, and some are emotional. When a nurse who has a stoic response to pain assesses a person who has an emotional response to pain, it is possible that the nurse will allow personal values to influence the assessment. This can lead to stereotyping a client as a "cry baby," with the result being that the nurse provides inadequate pain control for the client.

REASONING AND PROBLEM-SOLVING

Reasoning has been defined as the process of figuring things out by using critical thinking skills. Although reasoning involves thinking, all thinking is not reasoning. A human being is thinking when daydreaming, jumping to conclusions, stereotyping, or deciding to listen to music. None of these activities can be called reasoning. In order to use reasoning, to figure things out, or to problem-solve, the student must become

Table 2–4 THE ELEMENTS OF THOUGHT IN REASONING

1. All reasoning has a PURPOSE.
   - Take time to state your purpose clearly
   - Distinguish your purpose from related purposes
   - Check periodically to be sure you are still on target
   - Choose significant and realistic purposes
2. All reasoning is an attempt TO FIGURE SOMETHING OUT, TO SETTLE SOME QUESTION, TO SOLVE SOME PROBLEM.
   - Take time to clearly and simply state the question at issue
   - Express the question in several ways to clarify its meaning and scope
   - Break the question into subquestions
   - Identify whether it is a factual question, a preference question, or a question that requires reasoning
3. All reasoning is based on ASSUMPTIONS.
   - Clearly identify your assumptions and check for their probable validity
   - Check the consistency of your assumptions
   - Reexamine the question at issue when assumptions prove insupportable
4. All reasoning is done from some POINT OF VIEW.
   - Identify your own point of view and its limitations
   - Seek other points of view and identify their strengths as well as their weaknesses
   - Strive to be fairminded in evaluating all points of view
5. All reasoning is based on DATA AND INFORMATION.
   - Restrict your claims to those supported by sufficient data
   - Lay out the evidence clearly
   - Search for information against your position and explain its relevance
6. All reasoning is expressed through, and shaped by, CONCEPTS.
   - Identify each concept that is needed to explore the problem, and precisely define it
   - Explain the choice of important concepts and the implications of each
   - Define when concepts are used vaguely or inappropriately
7. All reasoning contains INFERENCES by which we draw CONCLUSIONS and give meaning to data.
   - Tie inferences tightly and directly from evidence to conclusions
   - Seek inferences that are deep, consistent, and logical
   - Identify the relative strength of each of your inferences
8. All reasoning leads somewhere and has IMPLICATIONS AND CONSEQUENCES.
   - Trace out a variety of implications and consequences that stem from your reasoning
   - Search for negative as well as positive consequences
   - Anticipate unusual or unexpected consequences from various points of view

Courtesy of The Foundation for Critical Thinking, Santa Rosa, CA.

familiar with the components of reasoning. These elements are purpose, the question at issue, assumptions, point of view, data and information, concepts, inferences and conclusions, and implications and consequences (Paul & Willsen, 1993). Table 2–4 illustrates the elements of thought in reasoning.

Purpose

All reasoning is directed toward some specific purpose. This is one way whereby reasoning is different from daydreaming. In the case of the nursing student, the purpose of reasoning is to effectively solve client care problems. During your formal education process, you will use reasoning to discover the logic of the practice of nursing.

The Question at Issue

The reasoning process has as its purpose the solution to some problem. This problem must be clearly defined. At the beginning of each study period, you must be able to state clearly the particular problems presented by this particular material. In the clinical setting, good clinical judgment begins with the clear statement of the problems presented by each client. One purpose of the nursing process is to identify client problems in a sufficiently clear and simple manner to enable appropriate responses by the nurse.

Assumptions

Assumptions are those ideas or things that are taken for granted. In the process of reasoning, you must be aware of the assumptions that are made in contrast to the facts that are known. Assumptions are accepted as being true without examination. Assuming certain things may be helpful in problem-solving, but an attempt should be made to recognize the assumptions. An example of an assumption is that nursing makes a difference in the outcome of a client's illness. It is evident that this is a necessary assumption for the nurse to make in order to engage in problem-solving related to client care needs; but it is also important for the nurse to examine this assumption from time to time. One of the issues in nursing today is the question of what nurses do and what preparation is necessary.

It is important to remember that assumptions that have proven reliable can help in decision making. It is just as true that faulty assumptions may cause you to draw faulty conclusions and may lead to poor problem-solving. Learn to recognize your own assumptions and those of others. Never be afraid to challenge your own assumptions or to ask others to clarify the assumptions they are using.

Point of View

Each person reasons using his own logic. Logic consists of previous experience, the quality of thinking already acquired, available information, and many other factors. These factors work together to give each person a unique way of thinking and a unique perspective. This unique perspective determines the individual's point of view. This can be conceptualized by thinking about what a person can see from a small window as compared to a view of the same landscape from an airplane. Each person will see things differently. They may both see a house but each person's view of the house may differ. In the same way, the individual's point of view determines what facts and information will be noticed, the relative importance assigned to each bit of information, and even the acceptable solutions to the problem. You must take the time to recognize your own point of view and to affirm the right of others to have their own points of view (Figure 2-4).

Data and Information

Data and information are the basic materials of reasoning. These are needed in order to define the problem under consideration and to find the solution. During the nursing education program, you may often feel overwhelmed by the quantity of data and information that is presented to you. The result may be that you attempt to practice rote memorization. If data and information are seen as the evidence for reasoning and for problem-solving, however, the process will be more than an exercise in memory. There is a logical relationship between the ideas and facts that compose the content of the nursing course. This logic can be discovered by reasoning. Once the logic is found, the

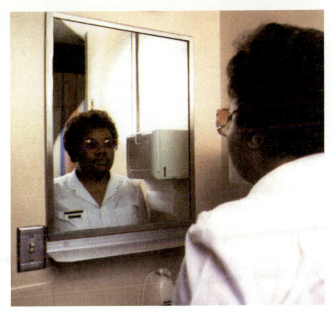

Figure 2-4 To be effective problem-solvers and critical thinkers, nurses must first take a good look at their own ideas and beliefs.

information can be used for problem-solving. Be sure to also look for evidence against your position.

Concepts

The evidence given in support of a conclusion consists of one or more statements relating the conclusion to the problem and to the supporting facts. Reasons must be logically related to the information; in other words, the conclusion cannot be based on something apart from the reasoning process. The concepts (such as pain, adaptation, and so on) that support the nursing process must be part of the evidence supporting a nursing judgment.

Inferences and Conclusions

Reasoning requires interpretation of facts and information. The interpretation must be justifiable in light of the relevant facts. It must be supported by logical connections to the problem and to appropriate data and information. Such interpretation can be called a judgment or inference. Too many times, students state opinions as judgments or inferences. This occurs when interpretations are based on personal preferences rather than on the information that is pertinent to the solution of the problem and on accepted authoritative information.

Properly drawing judgments or inferences is basic to thinking well. An inference results from the following kind of thinking: "Because that is true, then this must be true." For example, you have learned that when the body's temperature goes above normal, the body's metabolic rate increases. You also know that increased metabolism requires more oxygen for the tissues. One way more oxygen can be delivered to the tissues is to increase the heart rate. From these facts, you can infer that an elevated body temperature may result in an increased heart rate.

The product of reasoning is a conclusion in regard to the problem. The conclusion is the answer to the question that began the process. The conclusion must be logical and must answer the question. It must be based on the proper information and be logically related to the question.

Implications and Consequences

As an outcome of the reasoning process, more than one solution will usually be apparent. At this point, it will be necessary to examine the implications of each solution. This may require thinking about the ease with which a solution can be applied, the ability of a person to carry out the required actions, or the risks involved.

The outcomes of a particular approach to a problem under consideration are important. Consequences can result from action or inaction. Responsible problem-solving requires that all known consequences be acknowledged. Of course, it is not possible to predict all consequences; but the possible outcomes should be examined as completely as possible.

TRAITS OF A DISCIPLINED THINKER

The presentation in this chapter of some of the requirements of critical thinking will not make anyone think critically. By incorporating the idea that thinking about the quality of your own thinking in relation to UIS is a desirable goal, you can improve your own thinking. Improved thinking is not something that can

PROFESSIONAL TIP

Critical Thinking

Critical thinking is far more than an academic exercise. As a nurse, you are responsible for helping clients achieve and maintain their optimal level of health. To help sharpen your critical thinking skills, get in the habit of asking yourself several times throughout the day while caring for clients questions such as "Why is this procedure being done?", "What are its benefits?", and "Do I see alternatives that might result in better client outcomes?" Training yourself to think critically about all client care and interactions will help you to become a more skilled and compassionate professional.

be acquired in a day or two. It is like any high-level skill; it takes time, effort, and disciplined practice. The result is well worth it, however. Consistent efforts to improve your thinking can result in the acquisition of the traits of an educated person (Paul & Willsen, 1993). These traits or habitual characteristic ways of thinking can be recognized by others and can enable a person to compete successfully in the high-tech world.

Reason

The educated person will be reasonable. This simply means that the person values reasoning in himself and in others. This person will not be interested in placing blame or dodging responsibility. There will be a commitment to problem-solving and to cooperative efforts aimed at logically solving the problems encountered in the workplace.

Humility

Another quality that results from consistent efforts to practice disciplined thinking is intellectual humility. To be intellectually humble means that an individual is aware of how much he does not know. There will be a willingness to examine conclusions and beliefs based on new evidence. There will be respect for the thoughts and ideas of others and a sense of continually learning and improving one's own thinking.

Courage

The thinking person will be intellectually courageous. One of the characteristics of this trait is a willingness to take unpopular positions based on reasoning. Conclusions and beliefs that direct activities will thus be the result of disciplined thinking, rather than the opinions of the group.

Integrity

Integrity refers to the constancy of one's actions, meaning that based on reasoning, the same standards are applied consistently and are not changed to suit circumstances or personal prejudices. The result is a person whose behavior is in harmony with his thinking.

Perseverance

The thinking person will be capable of intellectual perseverance; meaning a willingness to undertake the challenge of completing hard intellectual tasks. Not giving up, pursuing a solution until its conclusion, and maintaining the quality of thinking are the qualities related to this trait.

Fairmindedness

The fairminded person considers all viewpoints without referring to feelings or vested interests, adheres to intellectual standards, and is impartial.

CASE STUDY

At this point in subsequent chapters, you will be given a client scenario or case study. This activity is designed to give you an opportunity to apply the knowledge and skills you have gained. This means that you will be expected to use critical thinking skills as you explore selected nursing situations. For this chapter, the scenario is to be written by you and about you.

1. Review the four basic skills of critical thinking: reading, writing, listening, and speaking.

2. Identify specifically the precise skills you want to improve. Write in your own words what you want to accomplish in terms of positive skills you will possess when you have implemented your plan and accomplished your goal. This means that you will identify both specific performance measures for your reading, writing, speaking, and listening skills, and time frames for points at which you will evaluate your performance. For example, if you set a goal of being able to identify the main points of an assigned reading, how would you measure that? In comparison with others in your study group? By your test performance? Write down your evaluation criteria and the time frames for evaluation.

3. When you have clearly stated in writing which basic skills you will work on, review the material in this chapter or from other resources to identify possible ways to work on those skills. Choose the most appropriate methods for you. Write down your plan. Be precise and specific.

4. Your next step is to actually put your plan into action by doing what you have planned to do.

5. Evaluate your actions to see whether they have resulted in the desired outcome. In order to perform a valid evaluation, you must evaluate your performance based on the evaluation criteria and goals you outlined in number 2.

6. Realize that you must know yourself well. If the processes of critical thinking and reasoning are new to you, select only one or two things on which to work. If you feel more adventurous, use the suggested process to explore your thinking in relation to the universal standards of thought and to the traits of a thoughtful person. Assess your problem-solving style in relation to the elements of thought in reasoning.

CRITICAL THINKING AND THE NURSING PROCESS

The purpose of the nursing education program is to help you develop the logic of nursing. Another way to state this is to say that you will learn to think like a nurse. The method that nurses have adopted to implement the practice of nursing is called the nursing process. The nursing process is an application of the problem-solving process to the practice of nursing. A form of the problem-solving process is part of every scientific or human service discipline. The use of the nursing process requires critical thinking. If you can find the relationship between the content of the textbooks and the logic of nursing you will find the study of nursing to be an exciting and challenging process. Use of the nursing process will thus become the means by which the quality of your thinking is improved. The use of reasoning will enhance your use of the nursing process.

SUMMARY

- Critical thinking is a disciplined way of thinking that the nursing student can begin to develop. The effective use of the nursing process depends on the ability to think well.

- There are many ways to define critical thinking. Essential components of any definition should emphasize self-assessment of the quality of one's own thinking according to standards of excellence and careful use of the elements of reasoning.

- Four basic intellectual skills are essential to quality thinking: critical reading, critical listening, critical writing, and critical speaking.

- The spectrum of Universal Intellectual Standards (UIS) can be the measure of competence in each of the basic skills.

- Reasoning is the process of applying critical thinking to some problem so as to find an answer or to figure something out. Therefore, reasoning has a purpose. The process of reasoning requires that attention be paid to the elements of thought in reasoning and to the UIS.

- When students begin to be aware of their own thinking and begin to assume responsibility for it, they will begin to use their own logic to discover the logic of nursing. The result will be better learning and the ability to make high-quality decisions related to client care.

- Consistent attention to improving the quality of thinking will produce the traits of an educated nurse. The student will become intellectually reasonable, humble, and courageous and will possess intellectual integrity and perseverance.

Review Questions

1. A branch of learning or field of study is called a:
   a. career.
   b. movement.
   c. principle.
   d. discipline.

2. Fundamental to quality thinking is the ability to think:
   a. clearly.
   b. effectively.
   c. quantitatively.
   d. with ambiguity.

3. The person who is concrete or exact when stating or applying a fact is practicing the standard for critical thinking called:
   a. accuracy.
   b. precision.
   c. consistency.
   d. specificity.

4. The person who has the ability to separate needed information from information not needed at the present time is practicing the standard for critical thinking called:
   a. logic.
   b. relevance.
   c. adequacy.
   d. significance.

5. Ideas or things that are taken for granted are called:
   a. evidences.
   b. inferences.
   c. assumptions.
   d. implications.

6. The person who is willing to take an unpopular position based on reasoning is said to have:
   a. courage.
   b. humility.
   c. integrity.
   d. perseverance.

Critical Thinking Questions

1. Of the four basic skills of critical thinking, which one are you able to do best? Why? How do you know?

2. How do you take responsibility for your own thinking?

WEB FLASH!

- Search the Web for sites dealing with critical thinking. What date is the oldest entry? What date is the newest entry?
- Search the web using the names of the major nursing organizations such as National Federation of Licensed Practical Nurses (NFLPN), National Association of Practical Nurse Education and Service, Inc. (NAPNES), and the National League for Nursing (NLN). Do they have web sites that include pages that might offer information on critical thinking?

LEGAL RESPONSIBILITIES

MAKING THE CONNECTION

Refer to the following chapters to increase your understanding of legal responsibilities:

- **Chapter 4, Ethical Responsibilities**
- **Chapter 9, Loss, Grief, and Death**
- **Chapter 34, Nursing Care of the Client: Substance Abuse**

LEARNING OBJECTIVES

Upon completion of this chapter, you should be able to:
- *Define key terms.*
- *Describe the difference between public law and civil law.*
- *State the purpose and identify various sources of standards of practice.*
- *Discuss the difference between intentional and unintentional torts.*
- *Discuss the importance of accurate documentation.*
- *Discuss ways that informed consent relates to nursing practice.*
- *Discuss the concept of advance directives.*
- *State the purpose and correct utilization of an incident report.*
- *Discuss ways the nurse can reduce personal liability.*
- *State the benefits of having one's own malpractice insurance policy.*
- *List steps to be taken when suspecting a colleague of being impaired by drugs or alcohol.*

KEY TERMS

administrative law	incident report
advance directive	informed consent
assault	law
battery	liability
civil law	libel
confidential	living will
constitutional law	malpractice
contract law	misdemeanor
criminal law	negligence
defamation	nursing practice act
durable power of attorney for health care	peer assistance program
expressed contract	privacy
false imprisonment	public law
felony	restraint
formal contract	slander
fraud	standard of practice
Good Samaritan law	statutory law
impaired nurse	tort
implied contract	tort law

INTRODUCTION

Nursing, which embodies a concern for the client in every aspect of life, encompasses a great responsibility—one that requires knowledge, skill, care, and commitment. As society advances and technology changes, the issues that affect nursing practice also change. We continue to recognize the importance of informed consent, the right to decide what is best for one's self, and belief in the client's bill of rights. However, difficult issues, such as living wills, advance directives, do-not-resuscitate (DNR) orders, and impaired nurses, now confront the profession of nursing. Nurses in the past did not have to contend with these controversial topics. Today's nurse must be informed on these and other issues. This chapter provides a general overview of many legal concepts that affect nursing.

BASIC LEGAL CONCEPTS

Because it is useful to have working definitions of some basic legal concepts before applying them to a health care setting, a discussion of pertinent legal concepts follows.

Definition of Law

Laws are rules of conduct that guide interactions among people. Laws are binding, enforceable, and necessary so that people can live and work together. If laws are broken, a penalty is incurred.

The word **law** is derived from an Anglo-Saxon term meaning "that which is laid down or fixed." The two types of law are **public law**, which deals with the individual's relationship to the state, and **civil law**, which deals with relationships among individuals.

Sources of Law

The four sources of public law at the federal and state levels are constitutional, statutory, administrative, and criminal. The three sources of civil law at the federal and state levels are contracts, torts, and protective/reporting laws.

Public Law

Constitutional law, set forth in the U.S. and state constitutions, defines and limits the powers of government. **Statutory law** is enacted by legislative bodies. State boards and professional practice acts, such as nursing practice acts, are created and governed under statutory laws.

Administrative law (regulatory law) is developed by those persons appointed to governmental administrative agencies. These persons are entrusted with enforcing the statutory laws passed by the legislature. Administrative law gives state boards of nursing the power to make rules and regulations governing nursing as set forth in the nursing practice acts. In these administrative rules, nursing boards identify the specific processes for educational programs; licensure; grounds for disciplinary proceedings; and the establishment of fees for services and for penalties rendered by the board.

Criminal law, the most common example of public law, addresses acts or offenses against the safety or welfare of the public. Under criminal law, there are two types of crime: **felony** (crime of a serious nature that is usually punishable by imprisonment at a state penitentiary or by death or crime in violation of federal statute and involving punishment of more than 1 year incarceration) and **misdemeanor** (offense that is less serious than a felony and may be punishable by a fine or a sentence to a local prison for less than 1 year). Table 3–1 outlines the types of public law.

Civil Law

Civil law addresses crimes against a person or persons in such legal matters as contracts, torts, and protective/reporting law (Table 3–2). Most cases of malpractice fall under the civil law of torts (Flight, 1998).

Contract law is the enforcement of agreements among private individuals. There are three essential elements in a legal contract.

- Promise(s) between two or more legally competent individuals that state what each individual must do or not do
- Mutual understanding of the terms and obligations the contract imposes on each individual
- Compensation for lawful actions performed

The terms of a contract may be agreed on orally or in writing. However, a **formal** (written) **contract**

Table 3–1 TYPES OF PUBLIC LAW		
TYPE	**FEDERAL**	**STATE**
Constitutional law	U.S. Constitution Civil Rights Act	State Constitutions Law
Statutory law	None	State boards and professional practice acts such as nursing practice acts
Administrative law	Food, Drug, and Cosmetic Act Social Security Act National Labor Relations Act	Rules and regulations governing nursing as set by state boards of nursing
Criminal law	Controlled Substance Act Kidnapping	Criminal codes (defining murder, manslaughter, criminal negligence, rape, fraud, illegal possession of drugs, theft, assault, and battery)

Adapted from Fundamentals of Nursing: Standards & Practice, *by S. DeLaune and P. Ladner, 1998, Albany, NY: Delmar. Copyright 1998 by Delmar. Adapted with permission.*

Table 3-2 TYPES OF CIVIL LAW

TYPE	FEDERAL	STATE
Contract law	None	Employment contracts Business contracts with clients Contracts with allied groups Uniform Commercial Code
Torts	Federal Torts Claims Act	State Torts Claims Act (allows claims against the state) Negligence (common law claim) Malpractice statutes (professional liability) Assault Battery False Imprisonment Invasion of privacy Defamation (libel and slander) Fraud
Protective/ reporting laws	Child Abuse Prevention and Treatment Act Privacy Act of 1974	Age of consent statutes (medical treatment, drugs, sexually transmitted disease) Privileged Communication Statute Abortion statute Good Samaritan Act Abuse statutes (child, elderly, domestic violence) Involuntary Hospitalization Act Living will legislation

Adapted from Fundamentals of Nursing: Standards & Practice, *by S. DeLaune and P. Ladner, 1998, Albany, NY: Delmar. Copyright 1998 by Delmar. Adapted with permission.*

cannot be changed legally by an oral agreement. An **expressed contract** gives, in writing, the conditions and terms of the contract. An **implied contract** recognizes a relationship between parties for services.

In accord with U.S. Contract Law, the nurse is legally required to:

- Adhere to the employer's policies and standards unless they conflict with federal or state law,
- Fulfill the terms of contracted service with the employer, and
- Respect the rights and responsibilities of other health care providers, especially in areas that promote continuity of client care.

Along with these legal responsibilities, the nurse has a right to expect:

- Adequate and qualified assistance in providing care,
- Reasonable and prudent conduct from the client,
- Compensation from the employer for services rendered,
- A safe work environment with the necessary resources to render services, and
- Prudent, reasonable conduct from other health care providers.

A **tort** is a civil wrong committed by a person against another person or property (Zerwekh & Claborn, 1997). **Tort law** is the enforcement of duties and rights among individuals independent of contractual agreements.

The protective/reporting law may be considered criminal law, depending on the state classification. Two examples of protective law are The Americans with Disabilities Act (ADA) and the Good Samaritan Act.

The ADA was passed by the U.S. Congress in 1990. It prohibits discrimination in employment, public services, and public accommodations on the basis of disability. The ADA defines a disability as a physical or mental impairment that substantially limits one or more of the major life activities. Disabilities that may be covered by the ADA include the following:

- Mental impairments
    Learning disabilities
    Psychiatric disorders
    Organic brain syndrome
    Retardation
- Physical impairments
    Addiction
    Cancer

Cerebral palsy
Diabetes
Epilepsy
Heart disease
Human immunodeficiency virus (HIV, sympto-
  matic or asymptomatic)
Multiple sclerosis
Muscular dystrophy
Orthopedic, visual, speech, and hearing impair-
  ments
Tuberculosis

All fifty states and the District of Columbia have enacted **Good Samaritan** laws which protect health care
providers by ensuring immunity from civil **liability**
(obligation one has incurred or might incur through
any act or failure to act) when care is provided at the
scene of an emergency and the caregiver does not intentionally or recklessly cause the client injury (Brown,
1999).

The Good Samaritan law applies only in emergency
situations, usually those outside the hospital setting. It
stipulates that the health care worker must not be acting for an employer or receive compensation for care
given. There is also a federal Good Samaritan law that
protects health care providers who voluntarily give
care to a person in distress during an airplane flight
(Brown, 1999).

In most states, health care professionals are not required to stop at the scene of accidents. If they do
stop, however, they are held to higher standards than
is a lay person. Health care professionals are expected
to use their specialized body of knowledge when providing care. They are expected to act as would most
other professionals with the same background and education.

PROFESSIONAL TIP

Good Samaritan Laws

Good Samaritan laws vary in coverage from state
to state and may be amended periodically by legislation. It is the responsibility of caregivers to know
the law for their respective jurisdictions (Brown,
1999).

NURSING PRACTICE
AND THE LAW

Nursing practice falls under both public law and
civil law. In most states, nurses are bound by rules and
regulations stipulated by the **nursing practice act** as
determined by the legislature. For licensed practical/
vocational nurses (LP/VNs) four states, Texas, Cali-

PROFESSIONAL TIP

Nursing Practice Act/Title Act
- Nursing practice acts state those things that the
  nurse can and cannot do.
- Title acts state who can be called an LP/VN.

fornia, Tennessee, and South Dakota, have title acts as
opposed to practice acts.

Public laws are designed to protect the public. If
these laws are broken, the nurse can be punished by
paying a fine, losing her license, or being incarcerated.
An example would be a nurse guilty of diverting drugs,
which is considered a crime against the state. The offending nurse could lose her license to practice and
could be sent to jail.

Civil laws deal with problems that occur between a
nurse and the client. For example, if a nurse catheter-
izes a client and perforates the bladder, the client may
bring a civil suit against the nurse. No law affecting the
population as a whole has been broken, but the client
has sustained injury. This is a problem between individuals—the nurse and the client or the nurse, the
client, and the nurse's employer. The client may receive
compensation for injuries, but no jail time is incurred
by the nurse.

Multistate nursing practice has become common with
the increasing presence of telehealth, transporting of
clients across state lines, and being employed by
staffing companies that operate in several states (Ventura, 1999b). Many states are considering a licensure
system facilitating interstate nursing practice.

Standards of Practice

The state boards of nursing have been assigned the
responsibility of determining and regulating nursing
practice. The boards indicate what nursing is and is
not, defines registered nursing and practical nursing,
and sets educational guidelines for each program.

The state boards of nursing also stipulate who may
practice nursing in their respective states (licensure).
The related criteria usually involve graduating from a
state-approved or -accredited program, passing the
National Council Licensure Exam (NCLEX), and meeting certain moral and legal standards. The boards have
the authority to bring disciplinary action against a
nurse for violation of its rules and regulations. Disciplinary action can include suspension or revocation of a
nurse's license and/or a fine.

Under the auspices of the nursing practice acts,
guidelines have been developed to direct nursing care.
These guidelines are called **standards of practice** or
standards of care.

Standards of practice are derived from a variety of sources. As stated, they are usually defined by the board of nursing and described in the nursing practice act. However, professional organizations like the American Nurses Association (ANA) for the registered nurse (RN) and the National Federation of Licensed Practical Nurses (NFLPN) for the LP/VN also develop standards of practice. Books on nursing care planning, especially for specialized areas, are additional resources for the development of practice standards.

Policy and procedure manuals also represent standards of practice. Each facility, based on a rigorous review process, has identified specific ways of performing procedures such as passing medications, inserting catheters, and collecting specimens. The nurse employed by the facility is expected to follow the guidelines as laid out by the policy and procedure manuals. For situations not covered in the policy and procedure manuals, the nurse is expected to exercise good judgment in the planning and providing of client care. In other words, the nurse is expected to act in a reasonable and prudent manner.

Liability

What is meant by reasonable and prudent? In the case of nursing, it means that the nurse is expected to act as would other nurses at the same professional level and with the same amount of education or experience. If most nurses would respond to a particular situation in a certain way, and the nurse in question does so also, the nurse would be acting in a reasonable and prudent manner. However, if most nurses would respond differently than the nurse in question, the nurse would not be behaving in a reasonable and prudent manner and can be held liable or responsible for damages. Liability is determined by whether the nurse adhered to the standards of practice.

Legal Issues in Practice

Many aspects relating to nursing practice and areas of nursing are subject to liability, including physician's orders, floating, inadequate staffing, critical care, and pediatric care.

Physician's Orders

The physician is in charge of directing the client's care, and nurses are to carry out the physician's orders for care, unless the nurse believes that the orders are in error or would be harmful to the client. In this case, the physician must be contacted to confirm and/or clarify the orders. If the nurse still believes the orders to be inappropriate, she should immediately contact the nursing supervisor and put in writing why the orders are not being carried out. A nurse who carries out an erroneous or inappropriate order may be held liable for harm experienced by the client. *Nurses are responsible for their actions regardless of who told them to perform those actions.*

Floating

Nurses sometimes are asked to "float" to an unfamiliar nursing unit. The supervisor should be informed about a float nurse's lack of experience in caring for the type of clients on the new nursing unit. The nurse should be given an orientation to the new unit and will be held to the same standards of care as are the nurses who regularly work on that unit.

Inadequate Staffing

The Joint Commission on Accreditation of Healthcare Organizations (JCAHO) has established guidelines for determining the number of staff needed for any given situation (staffing ratios) (JCAHO, 1995). When there are not enough nurses to meet the staffing ratio and provide competent care, substandard care may result, placing clients at physical risk and the nurse and institution at legal risk. The nurse in this situation should provide nursing administration with a written account of the situation. *A nurse who leaves an inadequately staffed unit could be charged with client abandonment.*

Critical Care

Because the monitors used in critical care units are not infallible, constant observation and assessment of the clients are required. This makes a one-to-one or a one-to-two nurse–client ratio imperative. Furthermore, equipment must be checked regularly, and on a schedule, by the biomedical department.

Pediatric Care

Legislation in each state requires that suspected child abuse or neglect be reported. Legal immunity is provided to the person who makes a report in good faith. When suspected child abuse or neglect is not reported by health care providers, legal action, civil or criminal, may be filed against them.

NURSE–CLIENT RELATIONSHIP

A variety of situations can develop between a nurse and a client that may require legal intervention. The following is a discussion of the types of torts that may arise.

Torts

When a case is brought against a nurse, it is usually a civil action that falls under tort law. Torts can be intentional or unintentional (Table 3–3). The person who commits an intentional tort violates the civil rights of another individual knowingly and willfully. Examples of intentional torts are assault and battery, defamation (libel and slander), fraud, false imprisonment, and

Table 3–3 SELECTED TORTS: DEFINITIONS AND EXAMPLES

TYPE OF TORT	DEFINITION	EXAMPLE
Intentional		
Assault and battery	Threaten or attempt to touch another person. Unconsented touching.	Nurse who unjustifiably forces a treatment against the client's will and in the absence of consent
False imprisonment	Unwarranted restriction of the freedom of an individual.	Nurse who uses the restraints on a client who is of sound mind and is not in danger of inflicting injury on self or another
Quasi-intentional		
Invasion of privacy	All individuals have the right to privacy and may bring charges against any person who violates this right.	Nurse who either discloses information about a client that is considered private or photographs a client without consent
Defamation (libel and slander)	Verbal (slander) or written (libel) remarks that may cause the loss of an individual's reputation.	Nurse who makes a statement that could either ruin the client's reputation or cause the client to lose his or her job
Unintentional		
Negligence	Failure to use such care as a reasonably prudent person would use under similar circumstances, which leads to harm.	Nurse who loses client's property Nurse who makes a medication error Nurse who burns a client via the improper use of equipment Nurse who fails to observe and/or report a change in the client's condition. Nurse who inaccurately counts sponges in the operating room
Malpractice	Failure of a professional to use such care as a reasonably prudent member of the profession would use under similar circumstances, which leads to harm.	Nurse who makes an inaccurate nursing diagnosis and implements the wrong treatment Nurse who does not follow physician orders Nurse who does not question physician's clearly erroneous order

Adapted from Nursing Perspectives and Issues *(5th ed.), by P. R. Mitchell and G. M. Grippando, 1993, Albany, NY: Delmar. Copyright 1993 by Delmar. Adapted with permission.*

invasion of privacy. Unintentional torts are those actions that cause harm to the client and that result from a carelessness or negligence on the part of the nurse. If found liable, the nurse generally must pay monetary damages. Prison terms are rare.

Intentional Torts

Assault and battery, defamation, fraud, false imprisonment, and invasion of privacy are types of intentional torts.

Assault and Battery Assault and battery, though frequently used together, are actually two separate terms. **Assault** is the threat to do something that may cause harm or be unpleasant to another person. **Battery** is the unauthorized or unwanted touching of one person by another.

Fear and intimidation are the key elements in assault. The person assaulted must believe that the threat made can and will be carried out, for example, a client who is confined to a wheelchair and told, "If you do not finish your meal, you are going to sit there all night." The client complies because he believes the health care worker will leave him to sit for an uncom-

 CULTURAL CONSIDERATIONS

Assault and Battery Charges

To prevent assault and battery charges:

- Respect the client's cultural values, beliefs, and practices with regard to "touching."
- African Americans sometimes view touching another person's hair as offensive.
- Asian Americans usually do not touch others during conversations. Touching someone on the head is considered disrespectful because the head is considered sacred.
- European Americans employ handshakes for formal greetings.
- Hispanic Americans are very tactile and may embrace and shake hands when greeting one another.
- Native Americans prohibit touching a dead body. This may leave the offender open to charges of assault.

fortable period of time. The worker is in a position to carry out this threat, and the client knows it.

The key factor regarding battery is consent. People have the right to be free of unwanted handling of their person. Striking a client is battery. Performing a procedure without the client's consent is battery. Forcing a person to take medication they do not want is battery. Any unwanted touching, regardless of outcome, can be construed as battery.

Defamation **Defamation** is the use of words to harm or injure the personal or professional reputation of another person. If the words are written down, they constitute **libel**. If the information is communicated verbally to a third party, it constitutes **slander**.

Nurses must be discreet as to the ways that they characterize clients, peers, and other health care professionals. Negative or derogatory comments that are untrue leave the nurse no defense against charges of defamation. If comments are true, the relevance of the information is important. The most common examples of this tort are giving out inaccurate or inappropriate information from the medical record; discussing clients, families, or visitors in public areas; or speaking negatively about coworkers (Zerwekh & Claborn, 1997).

Fraud **Fraud** is a wrong that results from a deliberate deception intended to produce unlawful gain. Common forms of fraud in health care include illegal billing and deceit in obtaining or attempting to obtain a nursing license (Flight, 1998).

False Imprisonment **False imprisonment** refers to making the client wrongfully believe that she cannot leave a place. The most common example of this tort is telling a client not to leave the hospital until the bill is paid (Zerwekh & Claborn, 1997). Any mechanism used to confine a client or to restrict movement can be considered a restraint and a form of false imprisonment. This includes threats, locked doors, physical restraints such as wrist or vest restraints, side rails, geriatric chairs, and psychotropic drugs.

Nurses may find themselves in a quandary in situations where a client chooses to leave the health care facility, and no discharge order has been written. It is possible that the health care problem has not been resolved, and the nurse feels that it is not in the best interest of the client to leave. If the client is of sound mind, however, he has the right to make this decision, regardless of what others think is best. Detaining the individual could result in charges of false imprisonment.

Documentation is very important in these situations. The nurse should document the client's reasons for leaving the facility and include any teaching or interventions related to the situation. Facility policy usually requires that the client sign a form indicating that he is leaving against medical advice (AMA), which releases the facility of any liability. If the client is angry and refuses to sign the AMA form, the client's refusal should be documented, and the nursing supervisor and the client's physician should be notified.

As indicated, any device used to restrict movement is called a **restraint**. To safeguard against possible charges of false imprisonment, the nurse should carefully assess the situation and include the client or significant other in the care planning process. If it is determined that a restraint is needed, the purpose and use of the restraint should be explained, including the way the restraint fits into the plan of care, the length of time the restraint may be necessary, and the expected outcome. The planning session should be documented in the client's medical record.

The client in restraints must be assessed frequently. Documentation must show that:

- Restraints were checked hourly and released every 2 hours,
- The client was toileted,
- The client received food and water, and
- The client had position changes.

In acute care settings, restraints can usually be applied temporarily as a nursing measure for client safety; however, in most states, a physician's order must be immediately obtained. In long-term care settings, a physician's order is required prior to utilizing any restraints.

Invasion of Privacy **Privacy** includes the right to be left alone, to choose care based on personal beliefs, to govern body integrity, and to choose when and how sensitive information is shared (Badzek & Gross, 1999). People are entitled to **confidential** (nondisclosure of information) treatment regarding health care. All information gleaned from working with a client or his medical records must be kept confidential. Therefore, a client's health status may not be discussed with a third party, unless either the client is present and has given verbal permission or permission has been obtained in writing. This does not apply to nurses' discussing a client's health status with other health care workers involved in the care of the client.

Invasion of privacy occurs when a person's private affairs become public knowledge without the person's permission. Photographing a client without his consent is an invasion of privacy. Failing to pull curtains to shield the client when performing personal or intimate care also constitutes an invasion of privacy.

A common mistake made by health care personnel is discussing clients in public areas. It is difficult to gauge who may overhear when comments are made while sitting in the cafeteria or waiting for the elevator (Figure 3-1). The results can be detrimental if the client is embarrassed by this loss of privacy: The client's job or family situation may be compromised, depending on the nature of the information. For example, news of an abortion, positive HIV status, or venereal disease may be socially damaging to some clients. Clients or their health care status should never be discussed in public areas or with those persons not directly involved in the care of the client.

Figure 3-1 The nurse should not discuss clients, families, or coworkers in public areas.

All clients have the right to be free of unwanted public exposure. Permission should be obtained before going through a client's belongings. Doors should be kept closed and curtains pulled when providing personal care. People not involved in the performance of a procedure should not be invited to watch unless the client has given permission. Clients cannot be photographed or videotaped without their permission and a release form must be signed. Confidentiality should not be breached by using a client's full name on care plans, case studies, or other assignments that a student may have during clinical experience; only initials should be used. This helps protect the client's privacy should the papers be lost. The client's chart and other materials should not be left lying around, making a client's private information public knowledge.

Unintentional Torts

Negligence and malpractice are considered to be unintentional torts.

Negligence **Negligence** is a general term referring to negligent or careless acts on the part of an individual who is not exercising reasonable or prudent judgment. All nurses, including student nurses, are expected to use good judgment when providing client care. This means, for instance, that side rails should not be left down on confused clients' beds, and sedated clients should not be allowed to smoke unattended. To prevent falls, puddles and spills are cleaned up immediately, rather than waiting for housekeeping to take care of the matter. Any person, with or without the specialized knowledge required for nursing, could make these determinations. Should a nurse fail to protect a client in such a situation or in one requiring similar judgments, the nurse could be found negligent.

Malpractice Negligent acts on the part of a professional can be termed **malpractice**, or professional negligence. More specifically, malpractice relates to the

conduct of a person while acting in a professional capacity.

Negligent or careless acts on the part of a nurse frequently come from not meeting the standards of care, in other words, from not doing what a reasonable and prudent nurse would do under similar circumstances. A nurse can be charged with malpractice for acts committed or acts omitted. Failure to properly assess a client or to act on assessment information are examples of omission. Giving a client the wrong medication because of improper identification procedures (not checking the armband) or improper setup (not using the medication administration record) are acts of commission.

Malpractice can include attempting a procedure with which the nurse is unfamiliar or improperly performing a procedure that results in client injury. Malpractice differs from negligence in that anyone can be accused of negligence; only professionals can be accused of malpractice.

Several factors must hold true for a nurse to be found guilty of malpractice:

- The nurse owed a special duty to the client; in other words, a nurse–client relationship existed.
- The nurse failed to meet the standards of care. Policy, procedure, or standards of care were not followed.
- Injury occurred as a result of the nurse's action or inaction, a direct cause and effect.

The prudent nurse is protected by adhering to facility policy and procedure and attempting to meet the standards of care at all times. The case study discussed in Figure 3-2 illustrates some of the difficulties in distinguishing between malpractice and negligence.

Documentation

The source of information regarding the client's clinical history is the medical record, or the chart. The chart should accurately reflect diagnosis, treatment, testing, clinical course, nursing assessment, and intervention. According to the law, "If it was not charted, it was not done." If a chart ever winds up in court, this is the standard the jury applies when trying to determine what happened and who is at fault.

The nurse should not chart medications before they are given or treatments before they are completed. Either constitutes a direct violation of the standards of practice for documentation and medication administration. The standard of practice is that medications are documented *after* they are administered. All client care, including treatments, is documented after being provided.

Documentation must be accurate and objective. The nurse should describe what is seen and done. Nurses' notes should reflect facts, not inferences or opinions, about the client. Furthermore, it is not enough to chart

Case Study: Standard of Care—Malpractice or Ordinary Negligence?

Facts: A 75-year-old client fell and fractured a hip while in the hospital. The client had been medicated with castor oil and a sleeping pill, and the nurse failed to raise the side rails on the bed. During the night, the client got out of bed to go to the bathroom and fell, fracturing the hip. The client sued, alleging that the nurse had been negligent in failing to raise the side rails and in failing to tell the client that a bedpan would be brought to the client when needed.

Holding: The nurse's conduct constituted negligence. Unlike a malpractice action, no expert testimony was necessary to establish the applicable standard of care. The duty to raise side rails on a bed and to instruct the client to use the call button beside the bed if assistance were needed did not involve the failure to render professional nursing or medical services requiring special skills. The jury, therefore, could evaluate the nurse's conduct under the standard of "the reasonably prudent person," rather than "the reasonably prudent nurse."

Norris v. Rowan Memorial Hospital, North Carolina Court of Appeals 1974

Comment: This case points out the difficulties even courts have in drawing the line between ordinary negligence and malpractice. Cases involving a nurse's failure to raise bed rails are decided under the standard of ordinary negligence as often as they are decided under the standard of professional malpractice.

Figure 3-2 Case Study: Standard of Care—Malpractice or Ordinary Negligence?

Incomplete Documentation: Mrs. Drew

Mrs. Drew, 85 years old, was a resident on a transitional care unit. She lost 15 pounds over a 3 month period. When her chart was reviewed, the auditor targeted the weight loss as a problem. She examined the chart to discover what the nurses did to try to correct this situation.

The nurses had carefully documented the percentages Mrs. Drew had eaten at each meal, her lack of appetite, and the pattern of weight loss. They thought they had covered all bases. They were wrong.

The auditor referred to the standards of practice on weight loss in long-term care facilities. She questioned, "Did the nurses follow the guidelines?" No interventions were charted, so it was presumed that nothing was done.

In fact, the nurses had called the dietitian to see this client several times to discuss her food preferences and a calorie count was initiated. Student nurses assigned to Mrs. Drew sat with her at mealtimes to encourage her to eat. The nurses had spoken with the doctor and Mrs. Drew's family about their concern over her lack of appetite and loss of weight. However, none of this was charted. There was no proof, other than the dietitian's entries, that any attempt had been made to intervene in this client's nutritional deficit.

Figure 3-3 Incomplete Documentation: Mrs. Drew

nursing assessment or identified problems. The nurse must complete the task by documenting any actions taken, including nursing interventions and physician's orders implemented.

Entries must be neat, legible, spelled correctly, written clearly, and signed or initialed. It is illegal to go back and change a chart. If an error in charting is made, a line should be drawn through the incorrect entry and the nurse should initial it. Blacking out entries or using correction fluid is not acceptable, as this renders the original entry illegible. Sloppy, misspelled charting might discredit excellent nursing care.

Figures 3-3 and 3-4 reflect situations where nurses identified client problems. In Figure 3-3, documenta-

tion was incomplete. In the situation presented in Figure 3-4, the nurses clearly identified the problem, the client's response, and the actions taken.

INFORMED CONSENT

Informed consent refers to a competent client's ability to make health care decisions based on full disclosure of the benefits, risks, potential consequences of a recommended treatment plan, and alternate treatments, including no treatment and the client's agreement to the treatment as indicated by the client's signing a consent form. This detailed explanation, provided by the physician, allows the client to make intel-

Complete Documentation: Roberta Wilson

Roberta Wilson is a 44-year-old woman with a history of diabetes mellitus controlled by diet. She was admitted 2 days ago for abdominal pain. Ms. Wilson has been designated nothing by mouth (NPO) since midnight for an ultrasound scheduled at 9:30 A.M. The doctor instructed that she was to remain NPO until seen by a consultant. Her 11 A.M. accucheck revealed a blood sugar of 44. She was experiencing no symptoms of hypoglycemia.

What needed to be done and what needed to be documented to protect everyone involved? Hospital protocol stipulated giving 4 ounces of Coke for blood sugars less than 60, then repeating the accucheck in approximately 30 minutes. The nurses contacted the physician to cancel the NPO order, then administered the Coke. Roberta's blood sugar at 11:40 A.M. was 93. She was served an 1,800 calorie ADA (American Dietetic Association) diet for lunch.

What was charted?

2/08/00	11:10 A.M.	Accucheck 44. Client's skin is warm and dry, denies nausea, tremors, or confusion. States she feels "fine." Physician notified of low blood sugar and client condition. Orders received to discontinue NPO status and resume previous orders.
2/08/00	11:15 A.M.	4 ounces of Coke given.
2/08/00	11:40 A.M.	Blood sugar 93. Served 1,800 calorie ADA diet for lunch. Blood sugar to be repeated at 4 P.M.

Figure 3-4 Complete Documentation: Roberta Wilson

ligent decisions about treatment options. The issue of informed consent deals with the right of the client to determine what happens to his or her person. Consent to treatment also helps protect the health care worker from unwarranted charges of battery.

Individuals who are declared incompetent have a guardian or someone who has power of attorney to make heath care decisions and give consent for treatment.

Nurses must obtain consent for nursing procedures. Each client, on admission, signs a general care consent form. The nurse is obligated to explain what is to be done to the client and to receive at least implied consent, as indicated by lack of objection on the part of the client. It is the physician's responsibility to obtain consent for medical or surgical treatment. The disclosure about the risks and benefits of treatment generally takes place at a time when the nurse is not present, often in the physician's office. It is usually on the basis of this discussion that the client decides whether to accept the treatment recommendation and sign the consent form. Confusion arises, however, because nurses are often delegated the duty of collecting the signature

for invasive procedures such as surgery, cardiac catheterization, and other diagnostic procedures. Student nurses should neither ask the client to sign a consent form, nor witness a consent form.

When a nurse has a client sign a consent form, the nurse is verifying the following three things:

- The client's signature is authentic.
- The client has the mental capacity to understand the things discussed with the physician.
- The client was not coerced into signing the form.

If the nurse is unsure about the client's understanding or if the client still has questions, the client should not sign the form. The nurse should document the client's lack of understanding and contact the physician. Further clarification is needed, and it must come from the physician.

Clients over the age of 18 years may give consent for their own health care. Parents or guardians give consent for minor children. In most states, however,

CLIENT TEACHING

Informed Consent

Consent may be withdrawn, either verbally or in writing, at any time.

PROFESSIONAL TIP

Consent in Emergencies
- Consent is implied when immediate action is necessary to save a life or prevent permanent physical harm. Written consent is waived.
- After the emergency is over, consent must be obtained for further care.

CLIENT TEACHING

Advance Directives

- Advance directives should be discussed with the family and physician so that everyone understands the client's wishes, and conflicts are less likely to occur at a later time.
- An advance directive may be changed by the client as long as the client is competent.

minors who are married, live on their own, become pregnant, or require treatment for sexually transmitted diseases, mental illness, or substance abuse may give consent for themselves.

Complex situations occur when minors refuse treatments to which parents have consented, or parents refuse consent or treatment that has been deemed medically necessary for their minor children. The court has had to intervene in such cases. In situations such as these, the child may be made a ward of the court and the decision-making capacity temporarily taken away from the parents. An example would be the child of Jehovah's Witnesses who needs a blood transfusion but whose parents refuse treatment on the basis of religious beliefs.

Invasive procedures or those that may have serious consequences, such as surgery, cardiac catheterization, or HIV testing, require written consent. Figure 3-5 illustrates a typical consent form used to obtain client permission for the performance of invasive medical, surgical, or diagnostic procedures. Consent for procedures that are not invasive can be either given verbally or implied. The client implies consent when he cooperates with the procedure offered. For example, if the orderly says, "Mr. Jones, I am here to take you for your chest x-ray," and Mr. Jones gets into the wheelchair, consent is implied by Mr. Jones' cooperation.

PROFESSIONAL TIP

Consent in Special Situations

- If a client is unable to consent and the family is too far away, consent may be received over the telephone, according to agency policy (usually, two persons must hear the consent being given).
- A client who has already received preoperative or preprocedure medication is not competent to sign a consent. When this situation arises, the surgery or procedure may have to be postponed.
- For blood transfusions, some facilities require that a denial form be signed if the client indicates *No* on the consent form.

ADVANCE DIRECTIVES

An **advance directive** is a written instruction for health care that is recognized under state law and is related to the provision of such care when the individual is incapacitated. Advance directives emphasize the right of the client to self-determination. They are instructions about health care preferences regarding life-sustaining measures. These instructions may indicate who may make health care decisions for the client should he become unable to do so for himself. In essence, they express the client's wishes about the kinds of medical treatment wanted and not wanted.

A client of sound mind retains the right to make all health care decisions and even reverse previous decisions. Should a situation arise when the person becomes incapable of making decisions, however, advance directives serve as a guide to family members concerning those kinds of treatment that should or should not be allowed. Advance directives permit those involved in the decision-making process to know what the client prefers. Although these instructions are best put in writing, this is not always done. Sometimes, health care preferences are shared verbally with family members or friends. Such verbal instructions can be interpreted differently by different people, creating difficulty for all involved—the physician, the health care facility, and the family. Thus, it is best to get this information in writing. When an advance directive indicates that the client does not wish to have cardiopulmonary resuscitation (CPR) performed in the event of cardiac arrest, the physician must write a DNR order, also referred to as a "No Code."

All health care facilities that receive Medicare or Medicaid monies are required to offer to all competent clients on admission the opportunity to execute advance directives. The client should also be told about the purpose and availability of a living will and durable power of attorney for health care (discussed following). If desired, assistance in completing these documents should be offered to the client. In addition, the medical record must show that the client was offered the opportunity to complete these documents. The documentation must indicate decisions made or not made at that time. Clients cannot be coerced into signing advance directives, nor can they be discriminated against should they choose not to sign an advance directive.

Facility policies vary as to who provides the information on advance directives. Many health care facilities assign this responsibility to the admissions office or social services; others have the nurses do it. Regardless of which department is assigned this task, the nurse is frequently called on to assist the client in understanding this information.

Before discussing advance directives with a client, the nurse must be familiar with the Patient Self-Determination Act of 1990. In the role of client advocate, the nurse

TO THE PATIENT: You have the right as a patient to be informed about your condition and the recommended surgical, medical, or diagnostic procedure to be used so that you may make the decision whether or not to undergo the procedure after knowing the risks and hazards involved. This disclosure is not meant to scare or alarm you, but is simply an effort to make you better informed so you may give or withhold your consent to the procedure. Any questions or concerns you may have with respect to the proposed procedure, its risks, complications, or benefits should be directed to your treating physician.

I (we) voluntarily request Dr. _____ as my physician, and such associates, technical assistants and other health care providers as they may deem necessary to treat my condition, which has been explained to me as: _____

I (we) understand that the following surgical, medical, and/or diagnostic procedures are planned for me, and I (we) voluntarily consent and authorize these procedures: _____

I (we) understand that my physician may discover other or different conditions which require additional or different procedures than those planned. I (we) authorize my physician, and such associates, technical assistants, and other health care providers, to perform such procedures which are advisable in their professional judgment.

I (we) [DO] [DO NOT] consent to the use of blood and blood products as deemed necessary.

I (we) understand that no warrant or guarantee has been made to me as a result or cure.

Just as there may be risks and hazards in continuing my present condition without treatment, there are also risks and hazards related to the performance of the surgical, medical, and/or diagnostic procedures planned for me. I (we) realize that common to surgical, medical, and/or diagnostic procedures is the potential for infection, blood clots in veins and lungs, hemorrhage, allergic reactions, and even death. I (we) realize that the following risks and hazards may occur in connection with this particular procedure:

(Additional Consent Information On Back.)

INITIAL: _____

CHRISTUS SPOHN HEALTH SYSTEM

DISCLOSURE AND CONSENT
MEDICAL AND SURGICAL PROCEDURES
PATIENT CARE SERVICES

2704980   NEW: 05/82
              REVISED: 10/99

3025

I (we) understand that anesthesia involves additional risks and hazards, but I (we) request the use of anesthetics for the relief and protection from pain during the planned and additional procedures. I (we) realize the anesthesia may have to be changed, possibly without explanation to me (us).

I (we) understand that certain complications may result from the use of any anesthetic, including respiratory problems, drug reaction, paralysis, brain damage, or even death. Other risks and hazards which may result from the use of general anesthetics range from minor discomfort to injury to vocal cords, teeth, or eyes. I (we) understand that other risks and hazards resulting from spinal or epidural anesthetics include headache, chronic pain, remote possibility of nerve injury, hematoma, infection, septic and aseptic meningitis, nausea, vomiting, itching, and urinary retention.

I (we) consent to the photographing of the operations or procedures to be performed, including appropriate portions of the body, for medical, scientific, or educational purposes, provided my identity is not revealed by descriptive texts accompanying the picture.

I (we) consent to the disposition by hospital authorities of any tissues or parts which may be removed.

I (we) have been given the opportunity to ask questions about my conditions, alternative forms of anesthesia and treatment, risks of non-treatment, the procedures to be used, and the risks and hazards involved, and I (we) believe that I (we) have sufficient information to give this informed consent.

My physician has discussed the alternatives, risks and benefits, of the proposed procedures. I (we) certify that this form has been fully explained to me; that I (we) have read it or have had it read to me; that the blank spaces have been filled in, and that I (we) understand its contents.

_____
PHYSICIAN'S SIGNATURE

DATE: _____ TIME: _____ A.M./P.M.

_____
Witness (Signature of witness/print name of witness)

_____
Patient/Other Legally Responsible Person
(Minor patient and parent/guardian signature)

Figure 3-5 Disclosure and Consent—Medical and Surgical Procedures (*Courtesy Christus Spohn Health System, Corpus Christi, TX*) explains the different types of advance directives to the client and family members. Terms such as *palliative care, supportive care, comfort measures,* or *nutrition and hydration* may not be understood by the client. The nurse can define those concepts more clearly and emphasize that the client has the right to choose what he believes is best for himself.

The nurse may suggest that the client discuss personal preferences with the physician and family members. When the client does so, problems may be prevented later. If the wishes of the family are different from those of the client, the health care team is caught in the middle, the concern being that the family may bring a lawsuit against the facility and the physician. The advance directive serves as a guide from the client. The facility's ethics committee may also be involved. The nurse should emphasize that these advanced directives only go into effect should the individual become incompetent or have a terminal illness, or death is imminent.

Durable Power of Attorney

A **durable power of attorney for health care** (DPAHC) is a legal document designating who may make health care decisions for a client when that client is no longer capable of decision making. This health care representative is appointed by the client and is expected to act in the best interests of the client. This appointment can be revoked any time the competent client chooses.

For example, if a client lapses into a coma and the prognosis is poor, the health care representative or the person appointed DPAHC can either give consent for certain types of treatment or withhold consent for treatment, even if the lack of treatment results in the client's death. It is expected that the health care representative has discussed treatment preferences with the client and thus knows the client's wishes. The DPAHC is activated only when the client is no longer competent to make health care decisions.

The person who has power of attorney or the authority to make decisions for a client in some areas does not necessarily have the same authority regarding health care issues. The granting of the right to make health care decisions has to be specified in the power of attorney agreement, or a DPAHC must be signed (Figure 3-6). Because of a possible conflict of interest, the health care representative may be different from the individual assigned the power of attorney.

A person who stands to benefit from the client's estate cannot be appointed health care representative. If a decision to terminate life support would benefit the designee financially, for instance, a conflict of interest would exist. This person could have the right to make decisions about the client in matters not pertaining to health care, however.

Living Will

A **living will** is a legal document that allows a person to state preferences about the use of life-sustaining measures should she be unable to make her wishes known. These preferences can be expressed either with a living will or a Life-Prolonging Procedure Declaration. These documents allow the client to specify, in advance, those life-sustaining measures that are to be done or not done.

The living will states that certain life-prolonging treatments are not to be used and that the individual prefers to die naturally. Food, fluids, and comfort measures are continued, and the person is not abandoned. However, artificial means of sustaining life, such as ventilators or feeding tubes, are not to be used.

Although not all states currently recognize living wills, the client's requests should be given due weight when making health care decisions. The nurse must be knowledgeable about living will legislation in her state. A sample living will is shown in Figure 3-7.

The Life-Prolonging Procedure Declaration indicates that the person wants all possible procedures done to delay the dying process (Figure 3-8). This can include the use of ventilators and any other methods to keep the person alive by artificial means.

Where a form for a living will, durable power of attorney, and/or health care representative is provided by statute, it should be utilized, because health care providers are familiar with it. However, variations of the forms, if all the required elements are included, may also be legal.

INCIDENT REPORTS

An **incident report** is a risk management tool used to describe and report any unusual event that occurs to a client, visitor, or staff member. It is used to help the facility identify or track problem areas and alert the legal department to possible lawsuits. An incident report is not meant to be a punitive device, although it is often perceived in that manner.

Incident reports are completed to document such events as falls, medication errors, forgotten treatment, injuries—anything that happens out of the ordinary. Another name for an incident report is a variance report or an occurrence report. The following three examples illustrate the types of occurrences that should be documented in an incident report.

- Mrs. Duncan had blood drawn for various laboratory tests. It was later discovered that the laboratory work had been ordered on Mrs. Falson, not Mrs. Duncan. The requisition had been stamped with the wrong name.
- Mrs. Barnes was given Lasix 20 mg PO at 9 A.M. When reviewing the physician's orders, the evening

Part I. Durable Power of Attorney for Health Care

• If you do NOT wish to name an agent to make health care decisions for you, write your initials in the box [Initials]

This form has been prepared to comply with the "Durable Power of Attorney for Health Care Act" of Missouri.

1. Selection of agent. I appoint:
Name:_____
Address:_____

> It is suggested that only one Agent be named. However, if more than one Agent is named, anyone may act individually unless you specify otherwise.

Telephone:_____
as my Agent.

2. Alternate Agents. Only an Agent named by me may act under this Durable Power of Attorney. If my Agent resigns or is not able or available to make health care decisions for me, or if an Agent named by me is divorced from me or is my spouse and legally separated from me, I appoint the person(s) named below (in the order named if more than one):

First Alternate Agent	Second Alternate Agent
Name:_____	Name:_____
Address:_____	Address:_____
_____	_____
Telephone:_____	Telephone:_____

> This is a Durable Power of Attorney, and the authority of my Agent shall not terminate if I become disabled or incapacitated.

Part I. Durable Power of Attorney for Health Care (Continued)

3. Effective date and durability. This Durable Power of Attorney is effective when two physicians decide and certify that I am incapacitated and unable to make and communicate a health care decision.

• If you want ONE physician, instead of TWO, to decide whether you are incapacitated, write your initials in the box to the right. [Initials]

4. Agent's powers. I grant to my Agent full authority to:

A. Give consent to, prohibit, or withdraw any type of health care, medical care, treatment, or procedure, even if my death may result;

• If you wish to AUTHORIZE your Agent to direct a health care provider to withhold or withdraw artificially supplied nutrition and hydration (including tube feeding of food and water), write your initials in the box to the right. [Initials]

• If you DO NOT WISH TO AUTHORIZE your Agent to direct a health care provider to withhold or withdraw artificially supplied nutrition and hydration (including tube feeding of food and water), write your initials in the box to the right. [Initials]

B. Make all necessary arrangements for health care services on my behalf, and to hire and fire medical personnel responsible for my care;

C. Move me into or out of any health care facility (even if against medical advice) to obtain compliance with the decisions of my Agent; and

D. Take any other action necessary to do what I authorize here, including (but not limited to) granting any waiver or release from liability required by any health care provider, and taking any legal action at the expense of my estate to enforce this Durable Power of Attorney.

5. Agent's Financial Liability and Compensation. My Agent acting under this Durable Power of Attorney will incur no personal financial liability. My Agent shall not be entitled to compensation for services performed under this Durable Power of Attorney, but my Agent shall be entitled to reimbursement for all reasonable expenses incurred as a result of carrying out any provision hereof.

Part II. Health Care Directive

• If you DO NOT WISH to make a health care directive, write your initials in the box to the right, and go to Part III. [Initials]

I make this HEALTH CARE DIRECTIVE ("Directive") to exercise my right to determine the course of my health care and to provide clear and convincing proof of my wishes and instructions about my treatment.

If I am persistently unconscious or there is no reasonable expectation of my recovery from a seriously incapacitating or terminal illness or condition, I direct that all of the life-prolonging procedures which I have initialed below be withheld or withdrawn.

I want the following life-prolonging procedures to be withheld or withdrawn:

• artificially supplied nutrition and hydration (including tube feeding of food and water)	[Initials]

• surgery or other invasive procedures. . . . . [Initials]

• heart-lung resuscitation (CPR) . . . . [Initials]

• antibiotic. . . . . [Initials]

• dialysis. . . . . [Initials]

• mechanical ventilator (respirator). . . . . [Initials]

• chemotherapy. . . . . [Initials]

• radiation therapy. . . . . [Initials]

• all other "life-prolonging" medical or surgical procedures that are merely intended to keep me alive without reasonable hope of improving my condition or curing my illness or injury. . . . . [Initials]

However, if my physician believes that any life-prolonging procedure may lead to significant recovery, I direct my physician to try the treatment for a reasonable period of time. If it does not improve my condition, I direct the treatment be withdrawn even if it shortens my life. I also direct that I be given medical treatment to relieve pain or to provide comfort, even if such treatment might shorten my life, suppress my appetite or my breathing, or be habit forming.

IF I HAVE NOT DESIGNATED AN AGENT IN THE DURABLE POWER OF ATTORNEY, THIS DOCUMENT IS MEANT TO BE IN FULL FORCE AND EFFECT AS MY HEALTH CARE DIRECTIVE.

Part III. General Provisions Included in the Directive and Durable Power of Attorney

YOU MUST SIGN THIS DOCUMENT IN THE PRESENCE OF TWO WITNESSES. IN WITNESS WHEREOF, I have executed this document this_____day of _____, year____.

_____
Signature

Print name _____
Address _____

The person who signed this document is of sound mind and voluntarily signed this document in our presence. Each of the undersigned witnesses is at least eighteen years of age.

Signature_____	Signature_____
Print name _____	Print name _____
Address _____	Address _____

> ONLY REQUIRED FOR PART I — DURABLE POWER OF ATTORNEY

STATE OF MISSOURI   )
) as
_____OF _____   )

On this _____day of _____, year_____, before me personally appeared to me known to be the person described in and who executed the foregoing instrument and acknowledged that he/she executed the same as his/her free act and deed.

IN WITNESS WHEREOF, I have hereunto set my hand and affixed my official seal in the County of _____, State of Missouri, the day and year first above written.

_____
Notary Public

My Commision Expires:_____

Figure 3-6 Durable Power of Attorney for Health Care and Health Care Directive (*Reprinted with permission of The Missouri Bar*)

Sample Living Will

Declaration made this _____ day of _____, year_____.

I, _____, willfully and voluntarily make known my desire that my dying not be artificially prolonged under the circumstances set forth below, and I do hereby declare:

If at any time I have a terminal condition and if my attending or treating physician and another consulting physician have determined that there is no medical probability of my recovery from such condition, I direct that life-prolonging procedures be withheld or withdrawn when the application of such procedures would serve only to prolong artificially the process of dying, and that I be permitted to die naturally with only the administration of medication or the performance of any medical procedure deemed necessary to provide me with comfort care or to alleviate pain.

It is my intention that this declaration be honored by my family and physician as the final expression of my legal right to refuse medical or surgical treatment and to accept the consequences for such refusal.

In the event that I have been determined to be unable to provide express and informed consent regarding the withholding, withdrawal, or continuation of life-prolonging procedures, I wish to designate, as my surrogate to carry out the provisions of this declaration:

Name: _____
Address: _____
_____ Zip Code:_____
Phone: _____

I wish to designate the following person as my alternate surrogate, to carry out the provisions of this declaration should my surrogate be unwilling or unable to act on my behalf:

Name: _____
Address: _____
_____ Zip Code:_____
Phone: _____

Additional instructions (optional):

I understand the full importance of this declaration, and I am emotionally and mentally competant to make this declaration.
Signed: _____

Witness 1:
    Signed: _____
    Address: _____

Witness 2:
    Signed: _____
    Address: _____

Figure 3-7 Sample Living Will (*Reprinted by permission of Choice in Dying, 200 Varick Street, New York, NY 10014*)

CAYLOR-NICKEL MEDICAL CENTER   Date of Birth   Clinic #

LIFE PROLONGING PROCEDURES
DECLARATION

Patient
Name:

Declaration made this _____ day of _____ (month, year).

I, _____, being at least eighteen (18) years old and of sound mind, willfully and voluntarily make known my desires that if at any time I have an incurable injury, disease, or illness determined to be a terminal condition, I request the use of life-prolonging procedures that would extend my life. This includes appropriate nutrition and hydration and the administration of medication and the performance of all other medical procedures necessary to extend my life, to provide me with comfort care, or to alleviate pain.

Other instructions:

In the absence of my ability to give directions regarding the use of life-prolonging procedures, it is my intention that this declaration be honored by my family and physician as the final expression of my legal right to request medical or surgical treatment and as acceptance of the consequences of the request.

I understand the full impact of this declaration.

Signed _____

City, County, and State of Residence

The declarant has been personally known to me, and I believe (him/her) to be of sound mind. I did not sign the declarant's signature above for or at the direction of the declarant. I am not a parent, spouse, or child of the declarant. I am not entitled to any part of the declarant's estate and/or financially responsible for the declarant's medical care. I am competent and at least eighteen (18) years old.

Witness _____ Date_____
Witness _____ Date_____

Forward to social service department

Figure 3-8 Life-Prolonging Procedures Declaration (*Courtesy Caylor-Nickel Medical Center*)

nurse discovered that Losec 20 mg had been ordered. Mrs. Barnes received the wrong medication.

- Mrs. Gomez was visiting her daughter, who had just given birth to the family's first grandchild. While walking down the hall, Mrs. Gomez slipped and fell, injuring her right hip.

All of the previous examples are incidents or variances that may typically occur in health care settings. For each situation, an incident report must be completed and channeled to the risk management department. Under the auspices of risk management, a subgroup comprising representatives from various departments, such as nursing administration, dietary services, environmental safety, and others, reviews the incident report. This group tries to identify those factors, if any, that contributed to the incident. Examples of questions asked include "Can the causal factors be eliminated or reduced?" "Does the possibility of a lawsuit exist as a result of the incident?" and "What can be done to prevent this incident from occurring again?"

Incident reports are filed by the person who was responsible for, who witnessed, or who discovered the incident. The report should state what was observed, as opposed to what is supposed. It should be factual and concise. In the third example given previously, if the nurse did not witness the actual fall, the correctly worded report would read: "Mrs. Gomez found lying on floor outside room 222. Several puddles of liquid found under and around her; paper cup lying nearby." An incorrect, presumptuous, and potentially damaging report might read: "Mrs. Gomez tripped and fell outside room 222. She slipped in a puddle of water." Mrs. Gomez may have spilled the cup of water she was carrying during the fall. However, this second note implies that Mrs. Gomez slipped in water that was already on the floor, thus implicating the facility.

Incident reports should include a description of the care given to the client or individual, and the name of the physician who was notified. The incident should be charted in the client's medical record, but the incident report should not be referred to in any way. Although the incident report is not a part of the medical record, the details described in the medical record and in the incident report should be the same.

When completing an incident report, the nurse should be sure to include the date and time of the incident; assessments; and interventions. The time that family members and physicians were notified should also be included. The nurse should refer to nursing administration policy and procedure regarding follow-up documentation.

PROFESSIONAL LIABILITY

Many nurses believe they do not need their own malpractice or liability insurance. They assume the coverage provided by their employer is adequate. This may be a misconception.

Nurses claim to be competent and knowledgeable health care providers. The health care consumer has heard this message and thus holds the nurse accountable for her actions. As a result, nurses are named as defendants in malpractice suits. Under the doctrine of *Respondeat Superior,* employers are responsible for the actions of their employees. However, this responsibility stops when the employee leaves work. Also, if the nurse violates policy and the employer is forced to pay damages, the employer has the right to sue the nurse to recover losses.

Having a professional liability policy provides the nurse with an attorney, someone who will represent that nurse in court. An attorney representing the facility or a group of employees will be most concerned about the employer; the needs of an individual nurse will be secondary. The decision to settle a case or pursue a particular course of action may be based on the needs of the employer. The individual nurse is better represented in court by private counsel.

Frequently, family members and friends ask a nurse for advice or assistance in health care matters. This advice is sought because of the nurse's knowledge, experience, and role. Should the family members or friends later take issue with the results of the advice or treatment given by a nurse, they might bring a suit against the nurse.

Despite the fact that no money was exchanged for information or services, the nurse is still accountable for the advice given. If the situation ends up in court, the nurse needs legal representation. Legal representation is costly as can be judgments against the nurse. A professional liability insurance policy protects the nurse by providing legal representation and paying the judgments.

There are two basic types of liability protection: the claims made policy and the occurrence policy. The claims made policy protects the nurse against claims made during the time the policy is in effect. If a claim is made after the policy has been terminated, the nurse is not covered. Occurrence policies protect the nurse against events that took place during the period of time the policy was active, even if a claim is filed after the policy is terminated. Occurrence policies seem to offer better protection for the nurse.

Opinions differ as to whether nurses should carry individual liability insurance. Some attorneys and health care professionals believe this practice encourages lawsuits. Nurses must compare the cost and the benefits of having professional liability insurance against the cost of potential legal fees and loss of personal assets. When securing liability insurance, the nurse should validate the company's reputation. Most nursing organizations offer group professional liability insurance.

IMPAIRED NURSE

One of the more sensitive issues in the nursing profession today is the subject of the impaired nurse. By definition, an **impaired nurse** is a nurse who is habitually intemperate or is addicted to the use of alcohol or habit-forming drugs. Although job performance may not be immediately compromised, substance abuse does eventually interfere with clinical judgment and performance. Because of the high level of job-related stress and the accessibility of drugs, the chemical dependency rate among nurses is greater than that among the general public.

In cases of impaired health care workers, the primary concern is client care. In the role of client advocate, a nurse cannot let loyalties to co-workers interfere with duty to the client. It is difficult reporting a coworker. No one wants to be a "squealer." In many states, however, the board of nursing requires nurses to report impaired coworkers. Nurses suspected of being under the influence of drugs or alcohol must be reported to the proper authority at the place of employment. The second consideration is getting help for the impaired nurse and taking action to correct the problem.

A nurse who suspects a coworker of diverting drugs or abusing alcohol should:

1. Document the dates, times, and observed behavior. Specific and descriptive accounts of what was observed are critical. For example:

   > January 3, l999. P.P. working 3–11 shift. Client A and Client B verbalized unrelieved postoperative pain. Documentation by P.P. stated both clients were comfortable after administration of Demerol 75 mg IM. Narcotic count at shift change satisfactory.

   > January 4, l999. Client C and Client D verbalized unrelieved pain. Documentation by P.P. indicated both clients stated pain was relieved after administration of Demerol 100 mg IM. Narcotic count at shift change okay.

   > January 5, l999. Narcotic count showed 1 Demerol 100-mg syringe listed as broken and 1 Demerol 75-mg syringe listed as wasted, "client changed her mind." P.P. signed the narcotic sheet.

   or

   > March 1–2, l999. S.L. working the night shift. Strong odor of alcohol on his breath.

   > March 3, l999. S.L. observed walking with unsteady gait, speech is slurred, strong odor of alcohol on breath.

2. Go to the supervisor and report concerns. Providing a copy of the documentation about the suspicious incidents is helpful. The supervisor will take responsibility for confronting the suspected employee. Intoxication requires immediate removal from the clinical area. In other situations, the supervisor will devise a plan before confronting the nurse.

3. Refrain from approaching or confronting the coworker. The impaired coworker may become defensive and deny the problem or make threats. Also, once aware that someone is suspicious, the nurse may become more secretive, making detection less likely. Frequently, the nurse will quit one facility and go to another, repeating the same pattern.

Some employers offer an employee assistance program to rehabilitate the impaired nurse. In addition, most states have **peer assistance programs** (rehabilitation programs designed to provide an impaired nurse with referrals, professional and peer counseling support groups, and assistance and monitoring for reentry into nursing). These peer assistance programs operate under the auspices of the state nurses association and in conjunction with the board of nursing. The goals of assistance programs are to protect the public from impaired nurses, provide the needed assistance to the impaired nurse, assist the nurse to reenter nursing, and monitor the nurse's compliance. With the

help of the peer counselor, the impaired nurse develops a contract for treatment. Compliance is monitored, and confidentiality is ensured. Successful completion of the program allows the nurse to return to the practice setting.

Participation in employer and peer assistance programs is optional. If the nurse chooses not to cooperate, however, employment may be terminated, and sanctions by the board of nursing may follow, including revocation of the license to practice.

SUMMARY

- Laws are rules that guide personal interaction. They are derived from several sources and can be classified as public or civil.
- Within most states, the nursing practice act indicates the scope of practice for nurses. Standards have been developed to guide nursing practice.
- The nurse should be familiar with client rights. Care should be taken not to falsely imprison a client or violate the client's right to privacy.
- The client's chart is a legal document and should accurately reflect client status and care. Entries should be neat and timely.
- Informed consent is more than just signing a form. It requires an understanding of the risks, benefits, and alternatives to treatment.
- Whether to purchase malpractice insurance is a personal decision. However, having one's own policy provides both coverage off the job and individual legal counsel.
- Impaired nurses are everyone's concern. Dates and times of inappropriate behaviors should be documented and reported to the immediate supervisor.
- Incident reports are a risk management tool. They are not meant to be used for punitive purposes.
- Advance directives are instructions about health care preferences. They both protect the rights of the client and guide the family through difficult decisions.

Review Questions

1. Standards of practice are:
   a. different for each school of nursing.
   b. guidelines to direct nursing care.
   c. not legally binding.
   d. specific criteria on how to perform procedures.

2. Immunity for nurses giving care in emergency situations is provided under the:
   a. Care and Good Faith Act of 1937.
   b. Good Samaritan Act.
   c. state nursing practice act.
   d. Patient Self-Determination act.

CASE STUDY

Mr. Jones is admitted for congestive heart failure. He is 66 years old, newly diagnosed, and acutely ill at this time. A student LP/VN is assisting the RN with the admission. The student notes that Mr. Jones has a living will. Later, she asks the RN, "Will you have to contact the doctor regarding a No Code status for Mr. Jones? He's got a living will, so he doesn't want anything done."

1. List factors that the nurse should explain to assist the student in understanding the concept of a living will.

2. Describe how a cardiac arrest might affect this situation.

Mr. Jones' wife speaks privately with the RN, stating, "I want everything possible done to save my husband. I don't care what it takes."

3. Describe how Mrs. Jones' statements may or may not affect the living will requests that Mr. Jones has made.

4. Delineate how the nurse might respond in this situation.

When Mr. Jones refuses a recommended treatment option, Mrs. Jones disagrees and tells the doctor to go ahead with the recommended treatment plan.

5. How does the Patient Self-Determination Act affect Mr. Jones' refusal of treatment?

6. List the parameters that allow Mrs. Jones to consent or refuse treatment for her husband.

Jamal Wilkins came to the hospital for outpatient diagnostic testing. Passing an open door, he saw his high school principal, Mr. Jones, lying in a bed. A respiratory therapist was giving Mr. Jones a treatment, and there seemed to be tubes and bags hanging everywhere. Alarmed, Jamal went to the nurse's station seeking information. He pointed to Mr. Jones' name and room number, which were listed on the board, and began asking questions.

7. Discuss ways to calm Jamal's fears without violating Mr. Jones' right to privacy.

8. Identify those ways that this client's privacy has already been violated.

---

3. Select the situation that violates client privacy.
   a. copying information from the chart for a case study
   b. discussing client status with clinical instructor
   c. shutting the door and closing the curtain during a procedure
   d. talking in the cafeteria about an interesting client

4. To make the best use of time in the clinical area, the nurse should:
   a. chart events as they happen.
   b. chart in a block at the end of the shift.
   c. have a coworker who is not busy chart for her.
   d. sign off all meds at the beginning of the shift.

5. The responsibility for informed consent rests with the:
   a. nurse.
   b. client.
   c. physician.
   d. unit clerk.

6. Informed consent occurs when the:
   a. nurse discusses the surgical procedure with the client.
   b. client gives consent verbally.
   c. client understands the risks, benefits, and alternatives to treatment.
   d. client signs the consent form.

7. If a coworker is suspected of diverting drugs, the nurse should:

   a. approach the coworker and tell him what she thinks.
   b. document dates, times, and observed behavior and report same to the supervisor.
   c. say nothing; it is none of her business.
   d. tell coworkers what she thinks so that they can help watch for suspicious behavior.

8. Advance directives:

   a. are binding only if written.
   b. cannot be changed once they are notarized.
   c. guide family members through difficult decisions.
   d. prevent clients from determining the course of their health care.

9. The health care representative or durable power of attorney for health care:

   a. is appointed by hospital administrators to make medical decisions for the client.
   b. can give or withhold consent for treatment.
   c. is contacted to override the decisions the client makes for himself.
   d. is the client's physician or health care provider.

10. Which of the following situations reflects inappropriate use of an incident report?

    a. Mrs. Khamel falls in the hall while visiting her daughter.
    b. A student nurse gives Losec instead of Lasix.
    c. The safety committee reviews incident reports regarding falls on the 3–11 shift on A-wing.
    d. An instructor, frustrated with a disorganized student nurse, fills out an incident report because the student gave a 9 A.M. medication at 9:25.

Critical Thinking Questions

1. How would you explain advance directives to your family?

2. How would you know whether a client gave informed consent?

WEB FLASH!

- What organizations or professional journals could you search to obtain information on nursing and legal issues?
- Search the Web sites of certain law schools, such as Harvard or the University of Texas, for information pertaining to nurses or health care.
- What resources are available on the Web for nurses needing legal advice?
- Search for information about the Good Samaritan law, malpractice, and professional liability insurance.

ETHICAL RESPONSIBILITIES

MAKING THE CONNECTION

Refer to the following chapters to increase your understanding of ethical responsibilities:

- **Chapter 2, Critical Thinking**
- **Chapter 3, Legal Responsibilities**

- **Chapter 6, Cultural Diversity and Nursing**

LEARNING OBJECTIVES

Upon completion of this chapter, you should be able to:
- *Define key terms.*
- *Explain the relationship among the concepts of ethics, morality, and law.*
- *Discuss the ethical theories of teleology and deontology.*
- *Describe the major ethical principles that have an impact on health care.*
- *Explain the link between ethics and values and the process involved in reconciling the potential conflicts between them.*
- *Relate the ethical codes developed by the National Federation of Licensed Practical Nurses and the International Council of Nurses to daily nursing practice.*

- *Identify the rights of the client as established by the American Hospital Association.*
- *Apply the steps identified in the framework for ethical decision making to issues such as euthanasia, refusal of treatment, and scarcity of resources.*
- *Discuss the roles of the nurse as client advocate and whistleblower in the delivery of ethical nursing care.*

INTRODUCTION

Every day, nurses encounter situations wherein they must make decisions based on the determination of right and wrong. How do they make such decisions? Whose values determine the rightness of an action?

The delivery of ethical health care is becoming an increasingly difficult and confusing issue in contemporary society. Nurses are committed to respecting their clients' rights in terms of providing health care and treatment. This desire to maintain clients' rights, however, often conflicts with professional duties and institutional policies. Nurses must thus learn to balance these potentially conflicting perspectives so as to achieve the primary objective—the care of the client.

In considering the situations presented throughout this chapter, one must realize that there are no absolute right answers. Dealing with the gray areas (ambiguities) causes much discomfort for many nurses. Because clients and nurses are humans, no two situations, no matter how similar, can ever be exactly alike. This chapter explores the concept of ethics, including ethical principles and theories; ethics and values; ethical codes; the client's rights; ethical dilemmas; ethical decision making; and the application of ethical guidelines to nursing practice.

KEY TERMS

active euthanasia	fidelity
assisted suicide	justice
autonomy	material principle of
beneficence	justice
bioethics	nonmaleficence
categorical imperative	passive euthanasia
client advocate	teleology
deontology	utility
ethical dilemma	value system
ethical principle	values
ethical reasoning	values clarification
ethics	veracity
euthanasia	whistleblowing

CONCEPT OF ETHICS

Ethics is the branch of philosophy concerned with determining right from wrong on the basis of a body of knowledge rather than on just the basis of opinions. Ethics deals with one's responsibilities (duties and obligations) as defined by logical argument. Ethics is *not* a religious dogma. Ethics looks at human behavior—which things people do under which types of circumstances. But ethics is not merely philosophical in nature; ethical persons put their beliefs into action.

Ethics in Health Care

The application of general ethical principles to health care is referred to as **bioethics**. Ethics affects every area of health care, including direct care of clients, allocation of finances, and utilization of staff. As Aroskar (1994) states:

Ethics encompasses the whole of life: our conduct and behavior toward ourselves, toward others, and toward the environment. Ethics in nursing and health care is not just about terrible dilemmas at the beginning or end of life. Most human activity involves an ethical dimension even if it is not recognized or articulated.

Ethics does not provide easy answers, but it can help provide structure by raising questions that ultimately lead to answers.

Ethical practice is gaining ever-increasing importance in health care today. Several factors contribute to the increased need to provide health care in an ethical manner. Some of these factors are:

- An increasingly technological society. The nature of advanced technology creates situations involving complicated issues that never had to be considered before. As a result of technological advances:

  Many newborns are surviving at earlier gestational ages, and many of them have serious health problems.
  People are living much longer than ever before.
  Organ transplants and the use of bionic body parts are becoming more common.
- The changing fabric of our society. Family structure is moving from extended families to nuclear families, single-parent families, and nonrelated groups living together as families.
- Clients are becoming more knowledgeable about both their health and health-related interventions. As consumer demand for information increases, health care providers must adapt quickly. The result is a focus on the consumer-driven system.

Every day, nurses face situations wherein they must make decisions that transcend technical and professional concerns. These situations may or may not be life threatening. Such situations raise complex problems that cannot be answered completely with technical knowledge and professional expertise. The way that nurses relate to clients, families, and other health care providers is the true demonstration of ethical behavior.

ETHICAL PRINCIPLES

Ethical principles are codes that direct or govern actions. They are widely accepted and generally based on the humane aspects of society. Ethical decisions are principled, that is, they reflect what is best for the client and society. Table 4–1 summarizes the major ethical principles. Each principle is discussed in detail in the following paragraphs.

By applying ethical principles, the nurse can become more systematic in solving ethical conflicts. Ethical principles can be used as guidelines in analyzing dilemmas; they can also serve as justification (rationale) for the resolution of ethical problems. It should be emphasized that these principles are not absolute; there can be exceptions to each principle in any given situation.

Autonomy

The principle of **autonomy** refers to the individual's right to choose and the individual's ability to act on that choice. The individuality of each person is respected. This respect for personal liberty is a dominant value in U.S. society.

Nurses must respect the client's right to decide and must protect those clients who are unable to decide for themselves. Although the legal definition of competency varies among states, the ethical principle of autonomy reflects the belief that every competent person has the right to determine his own course of action. The right to free choice thus rests on the client's competency to decide.

Table 4–1 OVERVIEW OF ETHICAL PRINCIPLES	
PRINCIPLE	**EXPLANATION**
Autonomy	Respect for an individual's right to self-determination; respect for individual liberty
Nonmaleficence	The obligation to do or cause no harm to another
Beneficence	The duty to do good to others and to maintain a balance between benefits and harms
Justice	The equitable distribution of potential benefits and risks
Veracity	The obligation to tell the truth
Fidelity	The duty to do what one has promised

PROFESSIONAL TIP

Autonomy

- Competent clients have a right to self-determination, even if their decisions may result in self-harm.
- Probably one of the most difficult things for nurses to accept is that clients are ultimately responsible for themselves; they will do what they want to do.

Informed consent is based on the client's right to decide for herself. Upholding autonomy means that the nurse accepts the client's choices, even those choices that are not in the client's best interests or those choices that conflict with the nurse's values. Following are examples of autonomous behavior on the part of the client that can impair recovery or treatment:

- Smoking after a diagnosis of emphysema or lung cancer
- Refusing to take medication
- Continuing to drink alcohol after being diagnosed with cirrhosis of the liver
- Refusing to receive a blood transfusion because of religious beliefs

Nonmaleficence

Nonmaleficence is the obligation to cause no harm to others. Harm can take many forms: physiological, psychological, social, financial, and/or spiritual. Nonmaleficence refers to both intentional harm and the risk of harm. The principle of nonmaleficence helps guide decisions about treatment approaches; the relevant question is "Will this treatment modality cause more harm or more good to the client?" Determining whether technology is harmful to the client is not always a clear-cut process. Factors to consider when choosing a treatment include:

- A reasonable prospect of benefit, and
- Lack of excessive expense, pain, or other inconvenience.

Nonmaleficence requires that the nurse act thoughtfully and carefully, weighing the potential risks and benefits of research or treatment. It is sometimes easier to weigh the risk than to measure the benefit. Further, it is possible to violate this principle without acting maliciously and without ever being aware of the harm, making the principle of nonmaleficence closely related to the concept of negligence. When upholding the principle of nonmaleficence, the nurse practices according to professional and legal standards of care.

Table 4–2 VOCATIONAL NURSE'S PLEDGE

God being my Witness and Judge and the Light whereby my life is patterned, do solemnly pledge myself to keep the following vows:

I shall endeavor in all ways so to live and to conduct myself, at home and abroad, that my vocation shall be uplifted in the eyes of all people.

I shall help to elevate the standards of my vocation by doing my work, where ever I may be, at least a little better on each tomorrow than I was able to do it on each today.

I shall put the welfare of my patients above all else.

I shall not engage in idle talk about other vocational nurses, professional nurses, or doctors, for we are united in our care of the patient and gossip destroys unity.

So let me live that I may be of service to Him Who "so loved the world that He gave His only begotten Son that whosoever believeth in Him should not perish but have everlasting life."

Author unknown: Used over 30 years by the Department of Vocational Nurse Education, Del Mar College, Corpus Christi, TX.

Nonmaleficence is considered a fundamental duty of health care providers. The Vocational Nurses's Pledge (Table 4–2), The Practical Nurse's Pledge (Table 4–3), and the Nightingale Pledge (Table 4–4) all profess the same basic philosophy of nursing care. Some clinical examples of nonmaleficence are:

- Preventing medication errors (including drug interactions),
- Being aware of potential risks of treatment modalities, and
- Removing hazards (e.g., obstructions that might cause a fall).

Table 4–3 PRACTICAL NURSE'S PLEDGE

Before God and those assembled here, I solemnly pledge:

To adhere to the code of ethics of the nursing profession.

To cooperate faithfully with the other members of the nursing team and to carry out faithfully and to the best of my ability the instructions of the physician or the nurse who may be assigned to supervise my work.

I will not do anything evil or malicious and I will not knowingly give any harmful drug or assist in malpractice.

I will not reveal any confidential information that may come to my knowledge in the course of my work.

And I pledge myself to do all in my power to raise the standards and the prestige of practical nursing.

May my life be devoted to service, and to the high ideals of the nursing profession.

Reprinted with permission of the National Association for Practical Nurse Education and Services Inc., Silver Spring, MD.

Table 4–4 NIGHTINGALE PLEDGE

I solemnly pledge myself before God and in the presence of this assembly: To pass my life in purity and to practice my profession faithfully.

I will abstain from whatever is deleterious and mischievous, and will not take or knowingly administer any harmful drug.

I will do all in my power to maintain and elevate the standards of my profession, and will hold in confidence all personal matters committed to my keeping, and all family affairs coming to my knowledge in the practice of my profession.

With loyalty will I endeavor to aid the physician in his work, and devote myself to the welfare of those committed to my care.

Beneficence

Beneficence is the duty to promote good and to prevent harm. Beneficence is often viewed as the core of nursing practice. The nurse serves as a client advocate and promotes the rights of the client. The nurse nurtures the client and incorporates the desires of the client into the plan of care. Sometimes, it is difficult to determine what is "good," especially when doing good causes the client discomfort. For example, a client who has been in a serious car accident may resist performing painful range of motion exercises and become angry at the nurse for insisting. The nurse understands the long-term value of performing the exercises, yet understands the client's physical and psychological pain.

Justice

The principle of **justice** is based on the concept of fairness extended to each individual. The major health-related issues of justice involve the way people are treated and the way resources are distributed. Justice considers action from the point of view of the least fortunate in society. As a result of equal and similar treatment of people, benefits and burdens are equally distributed. The distribution of scarce resources is commonly decided according to individual need (Davis & Aroskar, 1997).

The ethical principle of justice requires that all people be treated equally unless there is a justification for unequal treatment. The **material principle of justice** is the rationale for determining those times when there can be unequal allocation of scarce resources. This concept specifies that resources be allocated:

- Equally,
- According to need,
- According to individual effort,
- According to the individual's merit (ability), and
- According to the individual's contribution to society (DeLaune & Ladner, 1998)

An example of the application of the material principle of justice (according to the individual's contribution to society) is the Veterans Affairs (VA) Medical Centers. Only individuals who gave to their country by serving in the military are eligible to receive health care through the VA in ambulatory, acute care, and psychiatric facilities.

In health care institutions, the principle of justice is being strenuously tested on the issue of allocating one important resource: nursing personnel. Many institutions and agencies are downsizing their professional staff as a cost-containment measure. As a result, some health care facilities are so poorly staffed or have such a high ratio of underqualified personnel providing care, that quality of care is being severely compromised (Schildmeier, 1997).

Veracity

Veracity means truthfulness (neither lying nor deceiving others). Deception can take many forms: intentional lying, nondisclosure of information, or partial disclosure of information. Veracity often is difficult to achieve. It may not be hard to tell the truth, but it can be very hard to decide how much truth to tell. Exceptions to truth-telling are sometimes upheld by the principle of nonmaleficence, when the truth does greater harm than good. The act of giving placebo medications is an example of when telling the truth does greater harm than good.

Fidelity

The concept of **fidelity** (which is the ethical foundation of nurse–client relationships) means faithfulness and keeping promises.

Clients have an ethical right to expect nurses to act in their best interests. As nurses function in the role of **client advocate** (a person who speaks up for or acts on behalf of the client), they are upholding the principle of fidelity. Fidelity is demonstrated when nurses:

- Represent the client's viewpoint to other members of the health care team,
- Avoid letting their own personal values influence their advocacy for clients, and
- Support the client's decision, even when it conflicts with their own preferences or choices.

Within the nurse–client relationship, nurses should be loyal to their responsibilities, keep promises, maintain privacy, and meet resonable expectations of clients. Nurses also have a duty to be faithful to themselves. Conflict between commitments can complicate matters for the nurse, who may question who is owed fidelity. Although maintaining client centeredness may help clarify this question, it may not resolve the conflict. For example, if the mother of a frightened teenage girl tried to pressure the nurse into revealing the results of the daughter's pregnancy test after the daughter had already requested that her mother not be told, although the nurse may believe that the mother has the girl's best interests at heart, the nurse must protect the client's right to privacy.

ETHICAL THEORIES

Ethical theories were debated by ancient philosophers such as Plato and Aristotle, and the debate continues today. Whereas ethical theories can be used as a way to analyze ethical problems, no theory in and of itself can provide the "correct" answer to any single ethical conflict. Common ethical theories include teleology, deontology, situational theory, and caring-based theory.

Teleology

Teleology is an ethical theory that states that the value of a situation is determined by its consequences. Thus, the outcome of an action—not the action itself—is the criterion for determining the goodness of that action. An example would be immunizations—receiving an injection is not "good," but preventing the illnesses is.

This theory (also called the consequentialist theory) was advocated by the philosopher John Stuart Mill. The principle of **utility** is a basic concept of teleology; utility states that an act must result in the greatest degree of good for the greatest number of people involved in a given situation. "Good" refers to positive benefit. Thus, any act can be ethical if it delivers positive results. Concepts considered inherently good for all members of a society include health, strength, truth, freedom, security, and peace (Edge & Groves, 1999). Every alternative is assessed for its potential outcomes, both positive and negative. The selected action is the one that results in the most benefits and the least amount of harm for all those involved. A major disadvantage is that minority and individual rights may be ignored for the benefit of the masses.

Safety: Immunizations

- The outcome of immunizations is the prevention of given illnesses in the individual and, thus, the prevention of the spread of those illnesses to the community.
- The greatest good for the greatest number of persons is achieved with immunizations.

Deontology

Deontology is an ethical theory that considers the intrinsic significance of an act itself as the criterion for determination of good. That is, in determining the ethics of a situation, a person must consider not the consequences of the act, but the motives of the individual performing the act. This theory (also called formalism) was postulated by the philosopher Immanuel

CULTURAL CONSIDERATIONS

Smoke-Free Facilities
- Declaring health care facilities "smoke free" results in the most benefit and least harm for everyone.
- The minority group of smokers and the individual's right to smoke are ignored.

Kant. Kant established the concept of the **categorical imperative**, which states that a person should act only if the action is based on a principle that is universal (that is, everyone would act in the same way in a similar situation). The categorical imperative also mandates that a person should never be treated as a means to an end. Adherence to this concept may pose an ethical problem for health care researchers, who sometimes might be willing to risk the well-being of a person participating in an experimental procedure for the sake of finding, for example, a drug that will save many victims from suffering.

Situational Theory

The situational theory holds that there are no set rules, norms, or majority-focused results. Each situation must be considered individually, with an emphasis on the uniqueness of the situation and a respect for the person involved. Decisions made in one situation cannot be generalized to another situation (Pappas, 1997).

Caring-Based Theory

Caring-based theory is founded on the premise that people do not make ethical decisions based on principles. Decisions are made with respect to relationships, caring, communication, a desire not to hurt others, and responsiveness. Caring-based theory focuses on emotions, feelings, and attitudes (Figure 4-1). This theory is sometimes referred to as the "voice of care" and is contrasted with the "voice of justice." Justice and caring are not considered mutually exclusive and can, in fact, be complementary (Beare & Myers, 1998).

ETHICS AND VALUES

The close relationship between ethics and values both illuminates and complicates the nurse's approach toward balancing the ethical principles of the health care profession with those of the client. Nurses must examine their own value systems to ascertain the best approach in managing the care of clients whose values may be different from their own. In order to practice ethically, nurses must understand their own values.

Figure 4-1 Caring-based theory is expressed by this nurse, who is supporting the client through caring.

Values are different from principles, in that they influence the development of beliefs and attitudes rather than behaviors, although they might, and usually do, indirectly influence behaviors. A **value system** is an individual's collection of inner beliefs that guides the way the person acts and helps determine the choices the person makes in life. Although nearly nothing in life is value free, the impact of values on decisions and resultant behaviors is often not considered. Values are similar to the act of breathing; one does not think about them until a problem arises.

Nurses often care for clients whose value systems conflict with their own. "Rarely do diagnostic and treatment decisions occur without reference to values" (Gordon, Murphy, Candee, & Hiltunen, 1994). For example, a client with a value system of "grin and bear it" may be insulted by a nurse's attempts to offer pain medications. In order to ascertain those things that are meaningful to the client, the nurse must have an understanding of the client's value system (Figure 4-2). Furthermore, nurses must be aware of their own values, especially when they conflict with the values of clients.

Values Clarification

Values clarification is the process of analyzing one's own values to better understand those things that are truly important. Through values clarification, nurses can increase self-awareness and become better

PROFESSIONAL TIP

Values Clarification

It is the nurse's responsibility to make known to the supervisor any personal values that may influence or interfere with client care. For instance, a nurse who believes abortions should not be performed would find a conflict in working on a unit where abortions are performed. The nurse with this belief should make her values known to the employer before employment so that an assignment to that unit would not be made.

able to care for clients whose values differ from their own. In their classic work *Values and Teaching*, Raths, Harmin, and Simon (1978) formulated a theory of values clarification and proposed a three-step process of valuing, as follows:

- Choosing: Beliefs are chosen freely (that is, without coercion) from among alternatives. The choosing step involves analysis of the consequences of the various alternatives.
- Prizing: The beliefs that are selected are cherished (that is, prized).
- Acting: The selected beliefs are demonstrated consistently through behavior.

Nurses must understand that values are individual rather than universal and that, therefore, the nurse should not try to impose personal values on clients. The provision of ethical nursing care is directly related to one's values. For example, the nurse who strongly

Figure 4-2 Clients' values determine those things that are meaningful to them.

values the sanctity of life may experience an ethical conflict when caring for a terminally ill client who refuses treatment that may extend life for a short time.

ETHICAL CODES

One hallmark of a profession is the determination of ethical behavior for its members. Several nursing organizations have developed codes as guidelines for ethical conduct. The Code for Licensed Practical/Vocational Nurses, developed by the National Federation of Licensed Practical Nurses (NFLPN), is presented in Table 4–5. This code, adopted by NFLPN in 1961 and revised in 1979 and in 1991, provides a motivation for establishing, maintaining, and elevating professional standards. Each LP/VN, upon entering the profession, inherits the responsibility to adhere to the standards of ethical practice and conduct as set forth in this code.

The Code for Nurses (Table 4–6) was developed by the International Council of Nurses (ICN). The American Nurses Association (ANA) has also established a code for ethical conduct of registered nurses. Although a code of ethics, which provides broad principles for determining and evaluating nursing care, is not legally binding, most state boards of nursing have authority to reprimand nurses for unprofessional conduct that results from violation of the ethical code.

Figure 4-3 Clients have the right to information that will enable them to make decisions regarding their care.

THE CLIENT'S RIGHTS

The concept of rights is often misused, overused, and abused. Our society tends to take rights for granted. Rights and obligations are culturally defined. The dominant culture in the United States, however, holds the ethnocentric perspective that our rights and values are shared globally.

Clients have certain rights that apply regardless of the setting for delivery of care. These rights include, but are not limited to, the right to:

- Make decisions regarding their care (Figure 4-3),
- Be actively involved in the treatment process, and
- Be treated with dignity and respect (Figure 4-4).

When clients are admitted to short-term acute care agencies or extended care facilities, they are also entitled to certain rights. In 1972, the American Hospital Association (AHA) established *A Patient's Bill of Rights*, which outlines the rights and responsibilities of clients receiving care in hospitals (Table 4–7). This document, revised in 1992, increases health care providers' awareness of the need to treat clients in an ethical manner and encourages all health care providers to protect the rights of clients.

Table 4–5 THE CODE FOR LICENSED PRACTICAL/VOCATIONAL NURSES

1. Know the scope of maximum utilization of the LP/VN as specified by the nursing practice act and function within this scope.
2. Safeguard the confidential information acquired from any source about the patient.
3. Provide health care to all patients regardless of race, creed, cultural background, disease, or lifestyle.
4. Refuse to give endorsement to the sale and promotion of commercial products or services.
5. Uphold the highest standards in personal appearance, language, dress, and demeanor.
6. Stay informed about issues affecting the practice of nursing and delivery of health care and, where appropriate, participate in government and policy decisions.
7. Accept the responsibility for safe nursing by keeping oneself mentally and physically fit and educationally prepared to practice.
8. Accept responsibility for membership in NFLPN and participate in its efforts to maintain the established standards of nursing practice and employment policies which lead to quality patient care.

From Nursing Practice Standards for the Licensed Practical/Vocational Nurse, *by National Federation of Licensed Practical Nurses, Inc. (NFLPN), 1996, Garner, NC: Author. Copyright 1996 by Author. Reprinted with permission.*

 COMMUNITY/HOME HEALTH CARE

The Client's Rights

The client's rights as outlined in Table 4–7 must be respected regardless of the setting for delivery of care. For care delivered in the home environment, for instance, the home health care nurse should discuss the client's rights with the client during the initial assessment (Figure 4-5).

Table 4–6 INTERNATIONAL COUNCIL OF NURSES' CODE FOR NURSES

The fundamental responsibility of the nurse is fourfold: to promote health, to prevent illness, to restore health, and to alleviate suffering.

The need for nursing is universal. Inherent in nursing is respect for life, dignity, and rights of man. It is unrestricted by considerations of nationality, race, creed, color, age, sex, politics, or social status.

Nurses render health services to the individual, the family, and the community and coordinate their services with those of related groups.

Nurses and People

The nurse's primary responsibility is to those people who require nursing care.

The nurse, in providing care, promotes an environment in which the values, customs, and spiritual beliefs of the individual are respected.

The nurse holds in confidence personal information and uses judgment in sharing this information.

Nurses and Practice

The nurse carries personal responsibility for nursing practice and for maintaining competence by continual learning. The nurse maintains the highest standards of nursing care possible within the reality of a specific situation.

The nurse uses judgment in relation to individual competence when accepting and delegating responsibilities.

The nurse, when acting in a professional capacity, should at all times maintain standards of personal conduct that reflect credit upon the profession.

Nurses and Society

The nurse shares with other citizens the responsibility for initiating and supporting action to meet the health and social needs of the public.

Nurses and Coworkers

The nurse sustains cooperative relationships with coworkers in nursing and other fields. The nurse takes appropriate action to safeguard the individual when his care is endangered by a coworker or any other person.

Nurses and the Profession

The nurse plays the major role in determining and implementing desirable standards of nursing practice and nursing education.

The nurse is active in developing a core of professional knowledge.

The nurse, acting through the professional organization, participates in establishing and maintaining equitable social and economic working conditions in nursing.

From ICN Code for Nurses: Ethical Concepts Applied to Nursing, *by International Council of Nurses (ICN), 1973, Geneva, Switzerland: Imprimeries Populaires. Copyright 1973 by ICN. Reprinted with permission.*

Figure 4-4 Clients have the right to dignity and respect and may keep personal articles in their rooms.

Figure 4-5 A home health nurse explains a client's rights.

Table 4–7 A PATIENT'S BILL OF RIGHTS

Introduction

Effective health care requires collaboration between patients and physicians and other health care professionals. Open and honest communication, respect for personal and professional values, and sensitivity to differences are integral to optimal patient care. As the setting for the provision of health services, hospitals must provide a foundation for understanding and respecting the rights and responsibilities of patients, their families, physicians, and other caregivers. Hospitals must ensure a health care ethic that respects the role of patients in decision making about treatment choices and other aspects of their care. Hospitals must be sensitive to cultural, racial, linguistic, religious, age, gender, and other differences as well as the needs of persons with disabilities.

The American Hospital Association presents *A Patient's Bill of Rights* with the expectation that it will contribute to more effective patient care and be supported by the hospital on behalf of the institution, its medical staff, employees, and patients. The American Hospital Association encourages health care institutions to tailor this bill of rights to their patient community by translating and/or simplifying the language of this bill of rights as may be necessary to ensure that patients and their families understand their rights and responsibilities.

Bill of Rights*

1. The patient has the right to considerate and respectful care.

2. The patient has the right to and is encouraged to obtain from physicians and other direct caregivers relevant, current, and understandable information concerning diagnosis, treatment, and prognosis. Except in emergencies when the patient lacks decision-making capacity and the need for treatment is urgent, the patient is entitled to the opportunity to discuss and request information related to the specific procedures and/or treatments, the risks involved, the possible length of recuperation, and the medically reasonable alternatives and their accompanying risks and benefits. Patients have the right to know the identity of physicians, nurses, and others involved in their care, as well as when those involved are students, residents, or other trainees. The patient also has the right to know the immediate and long-term financial implications of treatment choices, insofar as they are known.

3. The patient has the right to make decisions about the plan of care prior to and during the course of treatment and to refuse a recommended treatment or plan of care to the extent permitted by law and hospital policy and to be informed of the medical consequences of this action. In case of such refusal, the patient is entitled to other appropriate care and services that the hospital provides or transfer to another hospital. The hospital should notify patients of any policy that might affect patient choice within the institution.

4. The patient has the right to have an advance directive (such as a living will, health care proxy, or durable power of attorney for health care) concerning treatment or designating a surrogate decision maker with the expectation that the hospital will honor the intent of that directive to the extent permitted by law and hospital policy. Health care institutions must advise patients of their rights under state law and hospital policy to make informed medical choices, ask if the patient has an advance directive, and include that information in patient records. The patient has the right to timely information about hospital policy that may limit its ability to implement fully a legally valid advance directive.

5. The patient has the right to every consideration of privacy. Case discussion, consultation, examination, and treatment should be conducted so as to protect each patient's privacy.

6. The patient has the right to expect that all communications and records pertaining to his/her care will be treated as confidential by the hospital, except in cases such as suspected abuse and public health hazards when reporting is permitted or required by law. The patient has the right to expect that the hospital will emphasize the confidentiality of this information when it releases it to any other parties entitled to review information in these records.

7. The patient has the right to review the records pertaining to his/her medical care and to have the information explained or interpreted as necessary, except when restricted by law.

8. The patient has the right to expect that, within its capacity and policies, a hospital will make reasonable response to the request of a patient for appropriate and medically indicated care and services. The hospital must provide evaluation, service, and/or referral as indicated by the urgency of the case. When medically appropriate and legally permissible, or when a patient has so requested, a patient may be transferred to another facility. The institution to which the patient is to be transferred must first have accepted the patient for transfer. The patient must also have the benefit of complete information and explanation concerning the need for, risks, benefits, and alternatives to such a transfer.

9. The patient has the right to ask and be informed of the existence of business relationships among the hospital, educational institutions, other health care providers, or payers that may influence the patient's treatment and care. The patient has the right to obtain information as to the existence of any professional relationships among individuals, by name, who are treating him.

10. The patient has the right to consent to or decline to participate in proposed research studies or human experimentation affecting care and treatment or requiring direct patient involvement, and to have those studies fully explained prior to consent. A patient who declines to participate in research or experimentation is entitled to the most effective care that the hospital can otherwise provide.

11. The patient has the right to expect reasonable continuity of care when appropriate and to be informed by physicians and other caregivers of available and realistic patient care options when hospital care is no longer appropriate

12. The patient has the right to be informed of hospital policies and practices that relate to patient care, treatment, and responsibilities. The patient has the right to be informed of available resources for resolving disputes, grievances, and conflicts, such as ethics committees, patient representatives, or other mechanisms available in the institution. The patient has the right to be informed of the hospital's charges for services and available payment methods.

The collaborative nature of health care requires that patients, or their families/surrogates, participate in their care. The effectiveness of care and patient satisfaction with the course of treatment depend, in part, on the patient's fulfilling certain responsibilities. Patients are responsible for providing information about past illnesses, hospitalizations, medications, and other matters related to health status. To participate effectively in decision making, patients must be encouraged to take responsibility for requesting additional information or clarification about their health status or treatment when they do not fully understand information and instructions. Patients are also responsible for ensuring that the health care institution has a copy of their written advance directive if they have one. Patients are responsible for informing their physicians and other caregivers if they anticipate problems in following prescribed treatment. *continues*

Table 4–7 A PATIENT'S BILL OF RIGHTS *continued*

Patients should also be aware of the hospital's obligation to be reasonably efficient and equitable in providing care to other patients and the community. The hospital's rules and regulations are designed to help the hospital meet this obligation. Patients and their families are responsible for making reasonable accommodations to the needs of the hospital, other patients, medical staff, and hospital employees. Patients are responsible for providing necessary information for insurance claims and for working with the hospital to make payment arrangements, when necessary.

A person's health depends on much more than health care services. Patients are responsible for recognizing the impact of their lifestyle on their personal health.

Conclusion

Hospitals have many functions to perform, including the enhancement of health status, health promotion, and the prevention and treatment of injury and disease; the immediate and ongoing care and rehabilitation of patients; the education of health professionals, patients, and the community; and research. All these activities must be conducted with an overriding concern for the values and dignity of patients.

*These rights can be exercised on the patient's behalf by a designated surrogate or proxy decision maker if the patient lacks decision-making capacity, is legally incompetent, or is a minor.

A Patient's Bill of Rights *was first adopted by the American Hospital Association (AHA) in 1973. This revision was approved by the AHA Board of Trustees on October 21, 1992. Copyright 1992 by the American Hospital Association, 840 North Lake Shore Drive, Chicago, Illinois 60611. Printed in the U.S.A. All rights reserved. Reprinted with permission of the American Hospital Association. Copyright 1992.*

ETHICAL DILEMMAS

An **ethical dilemma** occurs when there is a conflict between two or more ethical principles—when there is no "correct" decision. Ethical dilemmas are situations of conflicting requirements; something ought to be done and ought not to be done at the same time. When an ethical dilemma occurs, the nurse must make a choice between two alternatives that are equally unsatisfactory. Ethical analysis is not an exact science. In some cases, even after a dilemma seems to have been resolved, questions remain. This ambiguity makes it emotionally painful for the persons involved. Three areas where ethical dilemmas are possible are euthanasia, refusal of treatment, and scarcity of resources.

Euthanasia

Most people hope to experience a peaceful, gentle death when their "time comes." The word *euthanasia* comes from the Greek word *euthanatos*, which literally means "good, or gentle, death." In current times, **euthanasia** refers to intentional action or lack of action that causes the merciful death of someone suffering from a terminal illness or incurable condition.

Active euthanasia refers to taking deliberate action that will hasten the client's death, such as removing from a respirator a client who is in a vegetative state. In contrast, **passive euthanasia** means cooperating with the client's dying process. Passive euthanasia is "a decision made not to prolong life. . . . It is the omission of an action that would prolong the dying process" (Sumodi, 1995). An example is not putting in a feeding tube to provide nourishment when the client cannot or will no longer eat.

Assisted suicide is a form of active euthanasia whereby another person provides a client with the means to end his own life. Recently, physician-assisted suicide has been the topic of much controversy. Nurses have differing opinions regarding assisted suicide. Some look on it as a violation of the ethical principles on which the practice of nursing is based: autonomy, nonmaleficence, beneficence, justice, veracity, and fidelity. Regardless of a nurse's personal viewpoint, assisted suicide is still illegal. Other nurses may see assisted suicide as an ethical dilemma; they agree that it violates some ethical principles but question whether it violates others. For example, in answer to the question "Does assisted suicide violate the principle of autonomy?" one might argue that it is *refusal* to assist a suicide that violates a client's autonomy.

Refusal of Treatment

The client's right to refuse treatment is based on the principle of autonomy. In fairness, the client can refuse treatment only after the treatment methods and their consequences have been explained. A client's rights to refuse treatment and to die challenge the values of most health care providers.

> Honoring the refusal of treatments that a patient does not desire, that are disproportionately burdensome to the patient, or that will not benefit the patient is ethically and legally permissible (Curtin, 1995).

One possible ethical dilemma in this area relates to the use of ventilators for clients who would otherwise die. Medical technology makes it possible for these clients to continue breathing as long as they are connected to the machine. But one might ask "What are the emotional, physical, psychological, and fiscal costs?" and "What is the quality of a life prolonged by technology?"

Scarcity of Resources

With the current emphasis on containing health care costs, the use of expensive services is being closely examined. The use of specialists, organ transplants, and distribution of services are being influenced by social and political forces. For example, the length of stay in a hospital and the number of office visits allowable for individual clients are already predetermined by many third-party payers. In addition to economics, the availability of goods (such as organs) is contributing to a scarcity of resources.

In many situations, clients wait extended periods before receiving donated organs. The allocation of scarce resources is emerging as a major ethical dilemma: Who should receive the benefit of such a scarce and precious resource as a living organ? How should the determination be made? Currently, the selection of organ recipients is based on objective criteria such as organ availability, donor/recipient match, the degree of the recipient's need, and the recipient's willingness to commit to a lifetime of drug therapy and follow-up care. But should only objective criteria be used in determining who receives a donated organ, or should moral judgments also be made?

ETHICAL DECISION MAKING

Nurses must understand the basis on which they make their decisions. **Ethical reasoning** is the process of thinking through what one ought to do in an orderly, systematic manner based on principles. Ethical decisions cannot be made in a scattered, unorganized manner based entirely on intuition or emotions. Ethical decision making is a rational way of making decisions in nursing practice. It is used in situations where either the right decision is not clear or conflicts of rights and duties exist. A framework for resolving ethical dilemmas follows.

Framework for Ethical Decision Making

"After a moral conflict has been formulated, the nurse must differentiate the relevant parts of the conflict and resolve it" (Gordon et al., 1994). When making an ethical decision, the nurse must consider the following relevant questions:

- Which theories are involved?
- Which principles are involved?
- Who will be affected?
- What will be the consequences of the alternatives (ethical options)?

To resolve ethical dilemmas, the nurse must be able to make decisions in a systematic fashion. Figure 4-6 illustrates a method for making ethical judgments.

The first step of ethical analysis is to gather relevant

Determination of claims and parties

Identification of problem: Statement of the ethical dilemma

Consideration of priorities of claims;
Generation of alternatives for resolving the dilemma;
Consideration of the consequences of alternatives

Carrying out selected moral actions

EVALUATION

Evaluation of the outcome of moral actions;
"Were the actions ethical?"
"What were the consequences?"

Figure 4-6 Ethical Decision-making Model *(Adapted from Fundamentals of Nursing: Standards & Practice, by S. DeLaune and P. Ladner, 1998, Albany, NY: Delmar. Copyright 1998 by Delmar. Adapted with permission.)*

data in order to identify the ethical problem and to determine which type of ethical problem exists: Do principles conflict with principles? Do actions conflict with actions? Do actions conflict with principles? What are the claims?

Next, all the people involved (the parties) must be considered. What are their rights, responsibilities, duties, and decision-making abilities? Who is the most appropriate person to make the decision? Whose problem is it? It is important to identify several possible alternatives and predict the outcome of each. Then, and only then, can a course of action be selected—one that, it is hoped, ends in resolution of the problem. The final step of ethical decision making is evaluation of the resolution process.

ETHICS AND NURSING

As professionals, nurses are accountable for protecting the rights and interests of the client. Consequently, sound nursing practice involves making ethical decisions. Ethics affects nurses in every health care setting, and each practice setting presents the nurse with its own set of ethical concerns. Whatever the setting, nurses must balance their ethical responsibilities to each client as an individual with their professional obligations. Often, there is an inherent conflict.

Ethics Committees

The provision of ethical health care requires both self-examination on the part of the care provider and dialogue among health care providers. Many health care agencies now recognize the need for a systematic manner whereby to discuss ethical concerns (Figure 4-7). Multidisciplinary committees (also referred to as institutional ethics committees) constitute one arena for dialogue regarding ethical dilemmas. In addition to serving as a forum where ethical issues are discussed, ethics committees can lead to the establishment of policies and procedures for prevention and resolution of dilemmas.

Figure 4-7 Ethics Committee Meeting *(Photo courtesy of Photodisc)*

COMMUNITY/HOME HEALTH CARE

Client Autonomy

With the increased acuity level of clients cared for in the home setting, home health nurses face ever-increasing ethical challenges.

Clients who are being cared for at home have more control over their decisions and actions than those who are institutionalized. . . . Client autonomy becomes a much stronger influence in the outcome of care than it does in institutional settings, because the provider has less control over what the client does on a day-to-day basis at home. . . . [Home health care] represents a power reversal in which the client's autonomy takes on greater significance. (Kristoff, Sellin, & Miller, 1994)

PROFESSIONAL TIP

Providing Ethical Care

- Initiate dialogue concerning the client's wishes. Do more listening than talking. (For example, the following is a question you might ask to help determine the client's wishes: "If your heart stopped, would you want us to try to start it again?")
- Assess the client's understanding of the illness and the available treatment options.
- Allow time for the client to explore values and to communicate.
- Facilitate communication of the client's desires to family and other health care providers.

Nurse as Client Advocate

When acting as a client advocate, the nurse's first step is to develop a meaningful relationship with the client. The nurse is then able to make decisions with the client based on the strength of the relationship. The nurse's primary ethical responsibility is to protect clients' rights to make their own decisions.

Nurses have an ethical obligation to do everything possible to prevent anyone from taking advantage of vulnerable patients—or clouding objectivity so that the patients' best interests fade from sight. (Haddad, 1995)

Nurse as Whistleblower

The term **whistleblowing** refers to calling public attention to unethical, illegal, or incompetent actions of others. Whistleblowing is based on the ethical principles of veracity and nonmaleficence. As professionals, nurses are expected to monitor coworkers' abilities to perform their duties safely. Although nurses are expected to "blow the whistle" on incompetent health care providers, many are reluctant to do so because there are inherent risks in whistleblowing. Haddad (1999b) identifies some of the questions a person should consider before reporting unethical or incompetent behavior:

- Has the behavior in question created or is it likely to create serious harm?
- Have I gathered all appropriate information, and am I competent to judge this behavior?
- Do others confirm my information and judgment?
- Have all internal resources been exhausted to resolve the problem?
- Is it likely that past wrongdoing will be corrected or future damage prevented after the problem is reported?

CASE STUDY

Janice is a 45-year-old woman who is pregnant with her fourth child. The pregnancy was unplanned and distressed Janice and her husband at first, but now they have accepted it and look forward to the delivery of their child. Janice has been receiving prenatal care from her family practice physician since her second month of pregnancy. She is now in her seventh month.

During her sixth month of pregnancy, the physician ordered laboratory tests, and the results indicated a fetal abnormality. The physician requested to perform further diagnostic testing on the fetus during the seventh month. Janice and her husband refused further fetal testing. Although the physician explained the importance of the testing, the couple continued to refuse it.

After the couple left the office, the physician turned to the nurse and stated, "Since they will not follow my suggestions, write them a letter and tell them I am terminating our relationship. Tell her to see a specialist." No arrangements for a referral were made for Janice by the doctor, who feared that the high-risk delivery predisposed him to a lawsuit.

The following questions are related to the case study.

1. Based on the information presented, what are the primary ethical issues?
2. What are your personal values in relation to the situation?
3. What course of action would you recommend for the nurse and why? What ethical principles would guide you?
4. To what extent, in your opinion, is Janice noncompliant?
5. Was the medical intervention adequate? Is the nurse to judge medical care?
6. What is the nurse's responsibility to ensure follow-up care?

- Is the harm created by whistleblowing likely to be less than the harm done by the behavior in question?

The False Claims Act (FCA) encourages whistleblowers to report evidence of fraud against the federal government (Polston, 1999).

Federal law and state laws (to varying degrees) provide protection, such as privacy, to whistleblowers. Unfortunately, however, the inclination to protect one's coworkers and the fear of reprisal may deter a nurse from fulfilling the ethical obligation to report substandard behaviors.

SUMMARY

- Ethics is the branch of philosophy concerned with the distinction of right from wrong on the basis of a body of knowledge rather than on just opinions. It is the study of the rightness of conduct.
- Ethics examines human behavior—those things that people do under a given set of circumstances.
- There is a connection between acts that are legal and acts that are ethical. Professional nursing actions are both legal and ethical.
- Teleology is an ethical theory that states that the value of a situation is determined by its consequences.

- Deontology is an ethical theory that considers the intrinsic significance of an act itself as the criterion for determination of good.
- Ethical decisions are based on principles such as autonomy, nonmaleficence, beneficence, justice, veracity, and fidelity.
- Because ethics and values are so closely associated, nurses must explore their own values in order to acknowledge the value systems of their clients.
- Ethical codes that have been developed by nursing organizations such as the NFLPN, the ICN, and the ANA establish guidelines for the ethical conduct of nurses with clients, coworkers, society, and the nursing profession.
- The Patient's Bill of Rights is designed to guarantee ethical care of clients in terms of their decision making about treatment choices and other aspects of their care.
- Nurses must apply the process of ethical reasoning to resolve ethical dilemmas wherein conflict exists between principles and duties.
- The roles of client advocate and whistleblower enable nurses to protect their clients' rights and ensure the ethical and competent actions of their peers within the nursing profession.

Review Questions

1. Nurses would use the Code for Licensed Practical/ Vocational Nurses to:

   a. solve an ethical dilemma.

   b. develop a nursing care plan.

   c. seek an answer to a client care problem.

   d. understand the professional expectations required of them.

2. Values influence the nurse–client relationship because:

   a. the client's values take precedence over the nurse's values.

   b. every individual has a personal value system that helps determine actions.

   c. the nurse must help the client clarify his values in order to ensure effective nursing care.

   d. the nurse cannot effectively care for a client who has values that differ from those of the nurse.

3. Values clarification is a useful exercise for the nurse to perform because it helps the nurse:

   a. make ethically sound decisions.

   b. stay informed of new developments.

   c. avoid conflicts with clients and coworkers.

   d. establish policies about proper and improper client care.

4. An ethical dilemma is a:

   a. choice to be made between right and wrong.

   b. problem with two equally unsatisfactory solutions.

   c. series of problems that the nurse encounters in each client care situation.

   d. problem the nurse cannot solve without the intervention of a physician.

5. Active euthanasia means a person:

   a. helps a client to die.

   b. has an advance directive.

   c. limits the amount of care.

   d. chooses to stop pain therapy.

Critical Thinking Questions

1. A client delivers a baby with multiple congenital defects. The prognosis is poor, with the infant not being expected to live longer than 12 months at most. The mother says, "We can't afford to pay for the baby's care." Who should determine the degree of intervention? Should the cost of care be the foremost basis for the decision?

2. An 80-year-old woman is in a persistent vegetative state as a result of a cardiovascular accident. She has always talked about "someday" signing a living will requesting that heroic measures not be taken, but her family wants "everything to be done that can be done." Whose wishes should prevail? What ethical principles would come into play in this decision process?

WEB FLASH!

- What organizations or professional journals can you locate for information on nursing and ethical issues?
- What resources and references can you find when you search under healthcare ethics as related to organ donation, euthanasia, scarcity of resources, or refusal of treatment?

UNIT
2
Holistic Nursing Care

COMMUNICATION

MAKING THE CONNECTION

Refer to the following chapters to increase your understanding of communication:

- **Chapter 2, Critical Thinking**
- **Chapter 3, Legal Responsibilities**
- **Chapter 6, Cultural Diversity and Nursing**
- **Chapter 9, Loss, Grief, and Death**
- **Chapter 12, Health Assessment**

LEARNING OBJECTIVES

Upon completion of this chapter, you should be able to:
- *Define key terms.*
- *Describe the process of communication and factors that influence it.*
- *Differentiate between verbal and nonverbal communication.*
- *Utilize therapeutic communication.*
- *Understand the psychosocial aspects of communication.*
- *Demonstrate proper telephone communication.*
- *Communicate effectively with clients and families.*
- *Demonstrate communicating with special clients who are visually impaired, hearing impaired, speech impaired, unconscious, and non-English speaking.*
- *Communicate effectively with terminally ill clients and their families.*
- *Communicate effectively with other members of the health care team.*

KEY TERMS

active listening	hearing
aphasia	listening
communication	nonverbal communication
congruent	proxemics
dysarthria	rapport
dysphasia	telemedicine
empathy	therapeutic communication
feedback	verbal communication

INTRODUCTION

Why study communication? Students in a nursing program have generally had a minimum of 17 years of communicating. Have you ever told another person a story and then heard the story repeated by someone else? Or have you ever played the game of "telephone," where a message is whispered from one person to another and the last one states the message out loud? In both situations, when you hear the story or message again, it typically has changed from the original. When communicating with a client, family, or another member of the health care team, it is important that the message be sent and received accurately.

This chapter addresses the process of communication; methods of communicating, including verbal and nonverbal communication and factors that influence communication, such as age, culture, education, language, attention, emotions, and surroundings. Techniques that promote effective (therapeutic) communication are also described, as are barriers to communication, and examples of both are presented. Also explored are psychosocial aspects of communication, such as style, gestures, meaning of time, meaning of space, cultural values, and political correctness, and their importance to the health care system. Finally, communication with the client, family, and health care team as well as self-communication is discussed.

PROCESS OF COMMUNICATION

The simplest definition of **communication** is the sending and receiving of a message. The six aspects of communication are: sender, message, channel, receiver, feedback, and influences.

Sender

The sender of a message is the person who has a thought, idea, or emotion to convey to another person. Messages stem from a person's need to relate to others, to create meanings, and to understand various situations.

Message

The message is the thought, idea, or emotion one person sends to another person. It is a stimulus produced by the sender and responded to by the receiver.

Channel

The person sending the message must decide how to send the message. The channel, or medium, through which a message is transmitted may be auditory, visual, or kinesthetic.

The auditory channel involves the verbal (speaking) method for the sender and the **hearing** (act or power of perceiving sounds) and/or **listening** (interpreting sounds heard and attaching meaning to them) modes of transmission for the receiver.

The visual channel involves the verbal (writing) and/or nonverbal methods for the sender and the sight, reading, observation, and perception modes of transmission for the receiver.

The kinesthetic channel involves touch for the sender and experience of sensation for the receiver (Table 5–1).

Receiver

The physiological component involves the processes of hearing, seeing, and the reception of the touch stimulus. The psychological processes may enhance or impede the receiving of messages. For example, anxiety may cause an individual to experience alterations in hearing, sight, or feeling.

The cognitive aspect is the "thinking" part of receiving. It involves interpreting stimuli and converting them into meaning.

Feedback

Feedback is a response from the receiver that enables the sender to verify that the message sent was the message received. If this is not the case, additional messages are sent and received until an understanding of the primary message is reached between the sender and receiver.

Influences

Both the sender and receiver are influenced by their education, culture, emotions, and perceptions and by the situation within which they find themselves. These elements are collectively referred to as a person's frame of reference. Sometimes these influences help communication, and sometimes they hinder communication. Figure 5-1 shows the process of communication and the influences on the sender and receiver.

Table 5–1 COMMUNICATION CHANNELS

CHANNEL	MODE OF TRANSMISSION	OUTCOME	EXAMPLE
Auditory (verbal)	• Hearing	Receiving an auditory stimulus	Hearing the client say, "I feel fine"
	• Listening	Interpreting sounds heard and attaching meaning to them	Hearing loud moaning in a client's room, the nurse enters the room to check whether the client is in pain
Visual (nonverbal or verbal)	• Sight	Receiving a visual stimulus	Watching the rise and fall of a client's chest while counting respirations
	• Reading		Reading the client's record
	• Observation	Interpreting a visual stimulus by making note of accompanying sounds	Making note of sounds of labored breathing while counting respirations and concluding that breathing is abnormal
	• Perception	Assigning meaning to a visual event	Diagnosing an alteration in oxygenation related to respiratory distress
Kinesthetic (tactile or nonverbal)	• Procedural touch	Performing nursing procedures and techniques	Giving the client a bed bath
	• Caring touch	Conveying emotional support	Holding the client's hand

Adapted from Fundamentals of Nursing: Standards & Practice, *by S. DeLaune and P. Ladner, 1998, Albany, NY: Delmar. Copyright 1998 by Delmar. Adapted with permission.*

Figure 5-1 Process of Communication

METHODS OF COMMUNICATING

There are two methods of communicating: verbally and nonverbally. Which is better? The answer is neither, or more accurately, it depends on what the sender is trying to communicate. Seldom is a spoken message sent without some accompanying nonverbal aspects. Some experts believe that nonverbal communication is more honest than is verbal communication because it usually is conveyed unconsciously by the sender.

Verbal Communication

Verbal communication is the use of words, either spoken or written, to send a message. Methods of verbal communication include speaking, listening, writing, and reading.

Speaking/Listening

Most commonly, speaking is thought of as verbal communication. The receiver of a spoken message must listen. Speaking and listening must both occur in order for there to be communication. Have you ever sent a spoken message to someone in the same room with you and received nonmeaningful, senseless feedback from that person, or no feedback at all? More than likely, the other person was only hearing the message but not listening.

Communication experts say that people speak at a rate of 125 to 150 words per minute (WPM) but hear at a rate of 400 to 800 WPM. This extra time allows for distractions. Listeners are generally distracted because they are not concentrating on what is being said. Listening is one of the most difficult skills to learn and execute well.

Writing/Reading

The other mode of verbal communication is writing. The receiver of the written message must read the words. The reader must understand the words and attach meaning to them. With a written message, immediate feedback is generally not available. Therefore, great care should be taken to ensure clarity when composing a written message. Charting is a good example. The physician may read the chart after the caregivers who did the charting go off duty, allowing little chance for immediate feedback. In such an instance, if a chart read that a client was "uncooperative," for example, the physician would have little idea exactly what the caregiver meant. An entry of "refused to eat lunch, refused to get out of bed and sit in chair," however, is far more exact, illustrating the clarity in writing that is essential to good communication.

Nonverbal Communication

Nonverbal communication, sometimes called body language, is the sending of a message without using words. There are many ways we communicate without words, including gestures, facial expressions, posture and gait, tone of voice, touch, eye contact, body position, and physical appearance.

Nonverbal communication is generally unconscious—part learned behavior and part instinct. Because there is little conscious control involved in nonverbal communication, feelings are generally most honestly expressed nonverbally.

Clients seem to believe and are particularly sensitive to nonverbal messages. Nurses must thus make an effort to be aware of the nonverbal messages they may be sending to clients. For example, consider those aspects of nursing care that are not pleasant but must be done. Think how the client would feel if a nurse were to register an expression of disgust or revulsion on her face when changing a surgical dressing.

Nurses must also be sensitive to the client's nonverbal messages. Many clients do not want to bother "busy" nurses. Such clients may say they are fine or do not need anything when this is in fact not the case. An astute nurse, however, will observe nonverbal signs such as stiff posture, clenched fists, or a frowning facial expression and know that something is not right. Further assessment would then be undertaken to determine why the client is sending such nonverbal clues.

Gestures

Gestures are often referred to as "talking with hands." Gestures may be used to help clarify a verbal message, to emphasize an idea, to hold other's attention, or to relieve stress. Fingertapping, fidgeting, or ring twisting generally indicates tension, nervousness, or impatience. Shaking a fist indicates anger, whereas pointing may be used to clarify directions.

Facial Expressions

Although some people have very expressive faces, others do not. A big smile is easily interpreted as indicating happiness. Eyebrows can be very expressive, showing surprise, worry, thoughtfulness, or displeasure. The manner in which the forehead is wrinkled also sends a message.

Nurses must be very aware of their own facial expressions, especially when caring for a client under "unpleasant" conditions, such as when a client is vomiting or suffering from bowel incontinence. An expression of displeasure manifested as a "curled up" nose or disgust is easily identified by the client. The client, often already embarrassed at requiring such care, is likely to feel even worse should the nurse's facial expressions indicate anything but caring, concern, and empathy.

Posture and Gait

Good posture, with the head held up, and a purposeful gait are usually interpreted as meaning self-confidence, competence, and a positive self-image. Stooped shoulders, a downward-held head, and a shuffling gait generally convey low self-esteem, depression, and lack of confidence.

Tone of Voice

Tone of voice has been estimated to convey 23% of the context of a message. When the same words are said in different tones of voice, they can have very different meanings. Tone of voice might be pleasant, sincere, sorrowful, sarcastic, joyful, or angry.

Touch

Touch is a simple yet powerful form of nonverbal communication that even a newborn infant can understand. Touch can communicate caring, understanding, encouragement, warmth, reassurance, or affection. Of course, touch can also communicate anger, displeasure, or a lack or caring and understanding. Sometimes touch can hurt or be harmful to the person being touched.

While some people are natural "touchers," others are not. The use of touch can be learned, however. Many nursing tasks involve touching the client. If the nurse is uncomfortable touching a client, the touch along with other nonverbal communication such as facial expression, posture, eye contact, and tone of voice will all convey the nurse's discomfort. Most clients accept touch as an integral part of nursing care when it is done appropriately and professionally.

Eye Contact

Eyes, it is said, mirror the soul. Have you ever seen joy, sadness, pain, or laughter in someone's eyes? It is very difficult to control these messages of the eyes.

Eye contact is generally interpreted as indicating interest and attention, whereas lack of eye contact is thought to indicate avoidance, disinterest, or discomfort.

CULTURAL CONSIDERATIONS

Eye Contact

In some cultures it is considered rude or disrespectful to make direct eye contact.

Body Position

Body position is often a good indicator of a person's attitude. For example, crossed arms generally indicate withdrawal, although the person could just be cold. Open body positions, with the arms held freely at the sides, are usually taken to mean a receptive attitude.

Physical Appearance

A person's physical appearance says a great deal about that person. A clean, neat, appropriately dressed individual conveys a positive self-image, knowledge, and competence. A dirty, sloppy, or inappropriately dressed person conveys the message of "I don't care how I look," with the potential further implication of "maybe I am not too knowledgeable or competent," or "I am sloppy in what I do."

It is very important for every nurse to be clean, neat, and professionally dressed. Clients and families understand the nonverbal message that appearance conveys. Appearance does influence communication.

INFLUENCES ON COMMUNICATION

Communication involves more than just the sending and receiving of verbal and nonverbal messages. How a person sends or receives a message is influenced by such factors as age, education, emotions, culture, and language. Attention to the message and the surroundings are other influences. These factors must be taken into account for accurate communication to take place.

Age

Factors related to age affect communication. For instance, communicating with a child is different from communicating with an adult and is dependent on the age of the child. Nonverbal communication, particularly touch, and facial expression can be understood by infants. Before learning to understand words, a child can interpret tone of voice and gestures. Preschool children respond well to communication involving toys or play situations. They should be allowed some choices, but no more than two alternatives should be offered. As the child's vocabulary increases, more verbal communication can take place.

Elderly persons may have some degree of hearing loss or a slowed response time. The nurse should face the elderly client when speaking and allow time for a response. The client should be addressed as "Mr." or "Ms." unless he or she asks to be called by his or her first name. Elderly clients should be treated with respect and not talked to as if they were children; they are individuals with special needs (Figure 5-2).

Education

Education is another strong influence on communication. The more educated a person, the greater the vocabulary of that person. Highly educated persons are generally able to discuss and understand concepts and abstract ideas, whereas persons of lesser education generally communicate in a more literal and less abstract way.

Emotions

A person's emotional state greatly influences how messages are sent or received. Someone who is very anxious or upset, for example, may not hear what is said or may interpret the message differently than the sender intended. This same person typically speaks in an abrupt manner, loudly, and in harsh tones. The depressed person, on the other hand, typically says very little, speaking only one or two words or in very short sentences.

Culture

Each culture has its own standards of communication, especially with regard to nonverbal behavior. In the United States, for example, eye contact is considered a sign of openness and honesty. Those of Spanish heritage, however, believe eye contact to be disrespectful. Similarly, in many parts of Europe, a kiss on the cheek between two men is accepted. People from other parts of the world, however, may look suspiciously on this behavior.

Language

Language certainly influences communication. Speaking the same language assists people in understanding each other, although regional accents or dialects of a language can inhibit communication and understanding. When verbal communication comes to a standstill, nonverbal communication is often employed to assist. Any nurse who works in an area where there is a predominate second language should learn a few words or phrases in that language to help put clients at ease and to facilitate their understanding.

Attention

The amount of attention each individual focuses on a given communication greatly affects the outcome. In selective listening, the receiver hears only what he

Figure 5-2 When addressing elderly clients, face them directly and allow adequate response time. A warm touch on the hand or arm will communicate caring and respect.

wants or expects to hear. Pain or discomfort, physical or mental, may result in preoccupation, limiting the attention given to the communication.

Surroundings

Most people do not want to talk about the intimate details of their health care concerns in public (Figure 5-3). Thus, privacy should be provided. If the client occupies a room alone, the nurse should close the room door; if the client shares a room, the nurse should take the client to a conference room or other private place, if possible, to discuss personal information.

The nurse should respect the client's current "home" (e.g., the hospital room) as she would any person's home, knocking on the door before entering the room, not sitting on the bed without permission, and asking before moving any personal articles that are in the way. These simple courtesies show respect for the client as a person. When the client feels respected, communication is enhanced.

CONGRUENCY OF MESSAGES

It is important that verbal and nonverbal communications be **congruent**, or in agreement. Saying, "I really appreciate what you just did," in a happy tone of voice while smiling is congruent and clear; saying the

Figure 5-3 Provide privacy when discussing personal or intimate health concerns with clients.

same words in a disgusted tone of voice while frowning is incongruent and, thus, potentially unclear. The receiver may not know whether the sender is genuinely pleased with what was done or is displeased and being sarcastic. Messages such as these can confuse the receiver, who then may require feedback in order to correctly interpret the message.

It is important for the nurse to watch for congruency between verbal and nonverbal messages and to ask for clarification when incongruity exists.

LISTENING/OBSERVING

Listening and observing are two of the most valuable skills a nurse can have. These two skills are used to gather the subjective and objective data for the nursing assessment. Because the nursing diagnoses and nursing interventions are based on the assessment, it is imperative that the assessment be accurate.

The term **active listening** has been used to describe this behavior of listening and observing; it reflects the process of hearing spoken words and noting nonverbal behavior. It takes energy and concentration. The nurse who is at eye level with the client, who leans slightly forward toward the client, and who makes eye contact is showing undivided attention to the client and will be able to listen and observe more accurately. Responses from the nurse such as "go on," "tell me more," "yes," "what else?" or "mmhm" both encourage the client to continue and communicate that the nurse is really listening.

THERAPEUTIC COMMUNICATION

Therapeutic communication, sometimes called effective communication, is purposeful and goal di-

rected, creating a beneficial outcome for the client. One person is the helper (nurse) and the other is being helped (client). The focus of the conversation is the client, the client's needs, or the client's problems, not the needs or problems of the nurse.

Goals of Therapeutic Communication

There are several goals or purposes of therapeutic communication. One or more of these goals guide every therapeutic communication in the nurse–client relationship. The goals are: obtain or provide information, develop trust, show caring, and explore feelings.

Obtain or Provide Information

The nurse obtains information from the client about general health and specific health problems. It is with this information that the nurse can make an accurate assessment and plan of care.

The nurse provides information to the client from admission to discharge, beginning with the orientation of a new client to the hospital policies and routines. Information provision continues throughout the hospital stay as the nurse explains procedures, treatments, and tests; teaches the client self-care; clarifies instruction from other health care workers; and answers client questions. The discharge instructions constitute the final stage of information provision.

Develop Trust

Client and nurse are generally strangers at the time of their first meeting. The nurse must work to establish trust with each client. Answering questions honestly, responding to call lights promptly, and following through are examples of ways to build trust. Trust develops faster when caring is shown. Mutual trust established between client and nurse is termed **rapport**.

Show Caring

Fluffing a pillow or offering a drink of water without being asked are two ways to show caring. Taking time to always greet the client by name and knocking on the room door before entering are other ways.

Explore Feelings

Once rapport is established, the nurse can encourage the client to explore feelings. Generally, most clients are anxious about illness. Some fear the results of diagnostic tests, and some are anxious about the hospital environment. Many clients do not want to admit they are anxious or fearful. By using therapeutic communication techniques, the nurse is often able to help the client talk about feelings and reduce anxiety. Sometimes, a clarifying statement is all that is needed to alleviate fear or anxiety. Other times, allowing the client to talk about the fear or anxiety reduces that fear or anxiety.

Behaviors/Attitudes to Enhance Communication

Some behaviors and attitudes enhance therapeutic communication. Included are: self-disclosure, caring, genuineness, warmth, active listening, empathy, and acceptance and respect.

Self-Disclosure

Self-disclosure means sharing something about yourself such as thoughts, expectations, feelings, or ideas. It does not mean sharing your personal problems. When the nurse shares something, such as future goals in nursing, it shows that the client is trusted with that knowledge. The more the client feels trusted, the more the client will trust the nurse and therapeutic communication is enhanced.

Caring

Caring is not only a goal of therapeutic communication but also an attitude that enhances communication. Caring is the foundation of a nurse–client relationship. A caring attitude is easily identified by the client. Make the client feel important. Table 5–2 gives some examples of ways to show caring.

Keller and Baker (2000) identify four steps to help communicate a caring attitude to clients.

Table 5–2 WAYS TO SHOW CARING

ACTIVITY	STATEMENTS TO USE WITH ACTIVITY
Cover the client with a blanket.	"It feels chilly in here. Perhaps this blanket will help."
Assist the client to dress.	"I noticed you're having a little trouble getting your robe on. Perhaps I can help."
Serve a tray to the client.	"It's time to eat. I hope you're hungry because it really looks good."
Offer assistance.	"Here, let me help you. Perhaps together we can arrange these flowers."
When leaving the room.	"Is there anything more I can do for you before I go?" or "I'm leaving now, but I'll be back in 20 minutes."
Move the client up in bed.	"You look so uncomfortable. Let me move you up in bed."
Make the client's bed.	"Now you have a nice fresh bed."
Regulate environmental temperature.	"It seems very warm in here. Perhaps if I turn the air conditioner up, it will help."
Turn the client in bed.	"Changing position really makes a difference, doesn't it?"
Straighten a pillow.	"Let me straighten your pillow for you."

Adapted from Mental Health Concepts (4th ed.), by C. Waughfield, 1998, Albany, NY: Delmar. Copyright 1998 by Delmar. Adapted with permission.

- **Connect with the client.** Make eye contact; be at eye level when speaking to client; address client by last name.
- **Appreciate the client's situation.** Listen carefully; focus on what client is saying; acknowledge client's point of view; express concern.
- **Respond to client needs.** Clarify what is being asked; respond in ordinary language; let client know what to expect.
- **Empower the client.** Find out what client knows about condition and acknowledge opinions; work as partner to develop plan of care; allow choices as appropriate; encourage questions.

Genuineness

Effective communication must be genuine. The nurse must be himself. It means being honest about one's feelings. Sometimes it is "ok" to cry with a client.

It means being truthful and never attempting to answer a question when the answer is not known. The nurse should admit not knowing but offer to find the answer and then do so.

Being genuine builds trust. However, the nurse must use good judgment when expressing negative thoughts or confronting a client, family member, or another health care worker.

Warmth

Warmth makes the client feel welcomed, relaxed, and unjudged. It is expressed predominantly by nonverbal communication. A smile helps the client feel relaxed.

Touch is an important method to show warmth, but it must be used appropriately. Society dictates the type of touching that is appropriate in different situations. Holding a client's hand or putting a hand on the shoulder can greatly enhance communication by providing a connection between the nurse and the client. Touch may not always be welcomed by the client.

Active Listening

As the words imply, listening is an active process requiring energy and concentration. It involves listening to the words spoken as well as being aware of nonverbal messages. The nurse listens to both the words spoken and the nonverbal messages.

Active listening requires responses from the listener. This indicates that the nurse is really listening to the client. It is important for the nurse to concentrate on the interaction at hand and not let other thoughts become a distraction (Figure 5-4).

Empathy

Empathy is the capacity to understand another person's feelings or perception of a situation. It is an objective awareness of, or a sensitivity to, another person's feelings and thoughts. Although the nurse does

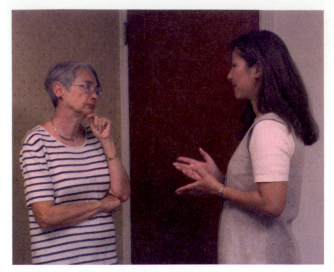

Figure 5-4 Active listening, concentrating on the interaction with the client, enhances communication.

not share the thoughts and feelings of the client, with empathy the nurse is able to understand and accept the thoughts and feelings of the client. Sympathy and empathy are not the same. In sympathy, the nurse becomes involved in the feelings and thoughts of the client, which are generally related to a loss.

Acceptance and Respect

Accepting clients as individuals with beliefs and values of their own is an attitude that enhances communication. The nurse must be nonjudgmental, that is, accepting of the client at face value. It is acceptable to privately disagree with the client's values and beliefs, but the nurse must accept that the client has different values and beliefs.

The nurse shows acceptance by not expressing differing values or beliefs and by simply accepting the statements or complaints of clients. Clients may then feel free to communicate and cooperate in their care.

Respect follows acceptance. Accepting clients in a nonjudgmental way leads to understanding them as unique individuals. Acceptance and respect on the part of the nurse let clients know that they can be themselves; they can then feel that they will still receive the best quality care, even though they have different values and beliefs than the nurse. The nurse also shows respect by introducing himself and addressing the client by name (preceded by "Mr.," "Mrs.," or "Ms.").

Techniques of Therapeutic Communication

Certain techniques promote therapeutic communication. These techniques should be learned and incorporated into the nurse's manner of communicating.

Clarifying/validating

Clarifying or validating are used when the nurse is not sure of the meaning of a message. Clarifying is the technique used to understand verbal messages. For example:

"Do you mean . . . ?"

Validating is used to establish truth or accuracy. It is used for nonverbal as well as verbal messages. Examples are as follows:

"Are you saying that you did not get your medication today?"

"You are holding your side. Are you having pain there?"

Open Questions

Open questions encourage clients to express their own thoughts and feelings. *How, when, where,* and *what* are words with which to begin an open question. Open questions cannot typically be answered with "yes" or "no" or with just one or two words. For example:

"How has this medication affected your vision?"

"What did the doctor tell you about going home?"

Indirect Statements

An indirect statement calls for a response from the client. Because it is a statement and not a question, the client does not feel quizzed. Indirect statements allow the client to determine the direction of the conversation, thus helping the client maintain a feeling of independence. Examples of indirect statements are as follows:

"Tell me about your physical therapy today."

"You were telling me about. . . ."

Reflecting

Reflecting is repeating all or part of a message back to the sender. Often, reflecting focuses on feelings and helps the sender "hear" the message from the receiver. This allows the sender a chance to clarify the message and shows that the listener is trying to understand the message. Reflecting can be a very useful technique if not overused. Examples include the following:

Client: "I'm really nervous about my surgery tomorrow. My friend got an infection after her surgery. I'm very frightened."

Nurse: "You are anxious about your surgery and afraid of getting an infection?"

Paraphrasing

Paraphrasing is restating the message in the receiver's own words. This lets the sender know how the receiver interpreted the message. Clarification can then be done if necessary. The sender is aware that the receiver is listening and trying to understand the message. For example:

Nurse: "You are afraid that you might have complications from your surgery?"

Summarizing

Summarizing in a sentence or two the major points of a conversation lets the sender know what was heard. The sender can then add more information or clarify what was originally heard. An example might be as follows:

"Let me see, we have discussed. . . ."

Focusing

Keeping communication focused on the topic being discussed can sometimes be difficult. Clients may wander off to other topics, or the topic may shift to the nurse. It is important to keep the focus on the client and not the nurse. For example the nurse could say:

"We can discuss that in a minute, right now I'd like to discuss. . . ."

"A minute ago you mentioned that you'd had an upset stomach after taking your medication. Tell me more about that."

Silence

Silence is one of the most difficult techniques to use. In the dominant U.S. culture, most people are uncomfortable with silence and feel the urge to fill the gap by saying something. Silence can be a valuable therapeutic technique, however, allowing the client time to gather thoughts or check emotions. Silence also gives the nurse a chance to decide how best to continue the interaction. If the nurse employs behaviors to enhance communication during the silence, the client will often verbalize thoughts or feelings.

Barriers to Communication

Employing behaviors and attitudes to enhance communication will be of little use if the nurse also employs barriers to communication. Although the communication process is sensitive, it should not be threatening. The purpose in learning about those things that block communication is to enable the nurse to identify them and avoid using them. Many mistakes can be corrected when identified. A simple "I'm sorry, I shouldn't have said that" will often take care of the situation. Practice helps sharpen communication skills. The most common barriers are discussed following.

Closed Questions

Questions that can be answered with "yes" or "no" or with only one or two words are considered closed.

PROFESSIONAL TIP

Therapeutic Communication

Practice the techniques of therapeutic communication with family, classmates, friends, and instructors. This may seem artificial and uncomfortable at first; but it will become easier with practice. If you begin using the techniques of therapeutic communication now, you will have incorporated them into your manner of communication by the time you begin clinical experience.

After the one- or two-word answer, communication is usually ended; there is no other avenue for the communication to follow. This type of question is appropriate in certain circumstances, however, such as when taking a health history or in an emergency. Examples of closed questions are as follows:

"Is the pain gone?"

"Did you sleep well?"

Clichés

Clichés are overused, trite phrases that are almost meaningless. They are impersonal and often used when individuals are at a loss for anything better to say. They are used without thinking of the impact on the other person, and often seem disrespectful of the client's individual circumstances. Examples include the following:

"Hang in there, tomorrow is another day."

"It could be worse."

False Reassurance

False reassurance is often used in an effort to cheer up the client regardless of the facts, giving false hope about the outcome of a situation. False reassurance can be especially traumatic to a terminally ill client who may be desperate to believe assurances even if they are not founded in reality. An example of false reassurance is as follows:

"Don't worry, I'm sure everything will be fine."

Judgmental Responses

Judgmental responses are based on the nurse's personal value system and imply right or wrong. Such responses allow no room for further discussion. For example:

"You shouldn't feel that way."

Agreeing/Disagreeing or Approving/Disapproving

Whether the nurse is agreeing/approving or disagreeing/disapproving, offering an opinion implies that one belief is right and the other wrong. Clients are thus prevented from sharing their feelings and may feel pressured to express the same values and opinions as the nurse. One example is as follows:

"I wouldn't do it that way."

Giving Advice

Giving advice involves offering personal rather than professional opinion. When the nurse does this, the client's responsibility for making decisions is diminished. Furthermore, some clients may end up feeling unable to make their own choices and may therefore become more dependent on the nurse. One example might be:

"I think you should. . . ."

Stereotyping

Stereotyping occurs when individual differences are ignored and a person is automatically put into a specific category. The stereotype may have either a positive or negative connotation. For example:

"Someone your age shouldn't worry about that."

"Boys aren't supposed to cry."

Belittling

Belittling conveys to a person that his thoughts or feelings really have no value, that it is silly to think or feel a certain way, or that he is no different from other individuals in similar circumstances. Examples include the following:

"Many people have it much worse."

"Yes, everyone feels like that."

Defending

Defending is a response to a feeling of being directly or indirectly threatened. The nurse may make statements in defense of self, another nurse, a doctor, or the health care facility. Defending implies that the client is not permitted to criticize or express feelings. This may be one of the most difficult communication barriers to overcome. No one likes to be criticized or to hear coworkers criticized. A natural first response is to defend why something was said, done, or not done. An example of defending is as follows:

"No one on this unit would say that."

Requesting an Explanation

It can be very intimidating for a client when a nurse asks for an explanation of behaviors, feelings, or thoughts. Often, the client does not know the "why." The usual results are increased anxiety and an end to communication. Examples are as follows:

"Why did you do that?"

"Why do you feel that way?"

Changing the Subject

An abrupt change of subject by the nurse generally indicates to the client that the nurse is uncomfortable or anxious about the topic under discussion. It often is used to avoid listening to a client's fear, distress, or problems and is interpreted by the client as a lack of interest.

Client: "I don't think I'll ever get well."

Nurse: "Isn't it a beautiful day?"

PSYCHOSOCIAL ASPECTS OF COMMUNICATION

The psychosocial aspects of communication include: style, gestures, meaning of time, meaning of space, cultural values, and political correctness. These aspects are based on individuality and culture and will influence the nurse–client relationship. It is important to understand these aspects and how they vary in different persons and cultures.

PROFESSIONAL TIP

Understanding Communication Barriers
Take measures to become aware of communication barriers. For instance, join a classmate in pointing out the barriers that each of you use, then discuss how you each feel when confronted with these communication barriers.

PROFESSIONAL TIP

When Clients Block Communication
In instances when clients block communication, keep the following things in mind:

- The client may not wish to discuss the topic introduced by the nurse or may not wish to talk at all. Everyone needs time alone to think.
- Accept and respect the client's desires to not communicate at a particular time.
- Let the client know that you are ready to listen whenever she is ready to talk.

Style

Each person has a style of communication that reflects the personality and self-concept of that person. According to Jack (1997), style can be divided into three common types: passive, aggressive, and assertive. It is important to remember that a person's style of communication is learned and reinforced over the years. The fact that communication style is learned indicates it can change.

When a person becomes a client in the health care system, fear and anxiety may change the person's style of communication, causing the client's communication style to become passive or aggressive.

Passive

The person who uses the passive style of communication does not stand up for himself, is not able to share feelings or needs with others, has difficulty asking for help, and feels hurt and angry at others for taking advantage of him. This person uses apologetic words; has a weak, soft voice; makes little eye contact; and is often fidgety. The person with a passive style of communication will often go along with others without expressing a personal desire for an alternate plan of action. The client who has a passive style of communication is generally very compliant, asks for nothing, and gets little attention.

Aggressive

The person who uses the aggressive style of communication puts his own feelings, rights, and needs first and communicates them in a haughty or angry way. The voice is often demanding, and the eyes expressionless. Such a person also has an attitude of superiority, works to control or manipulate others, and shows no concern for anyone else's feelings.

Assertive

The person who uses the assertive style of communication stands up for himself without violating the basic rights of others. He expresses true feelings in an honest, direct manner and does not allow others to take advantage of him. His voice is firm and confident, and he makes appropriate eye contact. Such a person also respects the rights, needs, and feelings of others;

CULTURAL CONSIDERATIONS

Gestures

The meaning of gestures is not universal. For instances, in many places, a small circle made with the thumb and forefinger means "okay." This is not true in Japan and France, however, where this gesture means "money" and "zero," respectively. And in Brazil and Turkey, this gesture is a symbol for female genitalia and is considered an insult.

takes responsibility for the consequences of his actions; and behaves in a manner that enhances self-respect.

A person using the assertive style of communication effectively lets others know his thoughts, feelings, and needs. He also listens to and acknowledges the other person's thoughts, feelings, and needs. If the thoughts, feelings, or needs of the persons communicating are in conflict, a compromise acceptable to both can usually be worked out.

Gestures

Gestures are movements of the hands and arms. Some gestures are known globally, such as applause to indicate approval. Some gestures, however, have entirely different meanings in various countries. The nurse must be sensitive to cultural variances and exercise good judgment when caring for clients of different backgrounds and heritages.

Meaning of Time

In the United States, great emphasis is placed on time and schedules. Being on time is very important. Time is precious. The clock tells us what we are to do and where we are to be every hour of the day and night. A person is considered dependable when scheduled appointments are kept.

People of some cultures know a day has passed only because the sun has risen, set, and is rising again. In fact, some cultures do not even have an instrument for telling time. They have different ways of perceiving and dividing time. Scheduling in such cultures may mean "when they get around to doing it."

PROFESSIONAL TIP

Being Assertive

"I" messages—I think . . . , I expect . . . , I feel . . . , I need . . .—are excellent ways to begin practicing assertive communication. Such messages indicate ownership of the thought, feeling, or need—a fact with which no one can argue.

PROFESSIONAL TIP

Time Orientation

Be sensitive to the fact that clients of different cultural backgrounds may value time differently than you do. Do not jump to conclusions that the client who is always late is lazy or inconsiderate of schedules.

Meaning of Space

Edward T. Hall (1959) has for many years studied **proxemics**, the study of space between people and its effect on interpersonal behavior. Hall says that humans, like other animals, are territorial. Some examples of human territoriality include the following: On a beach, people mark territory with a towel or blanket; in waiting rooms, people mark space with a jacket, hat, luggage, or newspaper; in a classroom, students generally sit in the same place and expect others to respect that space.

How close do you like to be to another person? Generally, this distance varies with the person and the situation. Age, gender of those interacting, and cultural values all influence the distance at which one person is comfortable with another person. Hall (1959) categorizes these comfort zones as intimate, personal, social, and public space.

- Intimate—touch to 18 inches; usually limited to family and close friends; necessary when performing most nursing procedures.
- Personal—18 inches to 4 feet; used with friends and coworkers; effective for many nurse–client interactions involving interviewing or data gathering.
- Social—4 to 12 feet; preferred distance with casual acquaintances.
- Public—12 feet or more; generally used with strangers in public places.

The distances associated with the comfort zones vary from person to person. Some people are comfortable being quite close in space to the person with whom they are interacting. Others prefer a greater distance. Nurses must always be aware of the client's comfort level with regard to space (Figure 5-5).

Much of nursing care involves touching the client, yet on admission, the nurse and client generally do not know each other. Thus, in a very short span of time, the nurse moves from the client's public space to the client's intimate space when giving care. Care given competently and professionally will help the client feel comfortable when the nurse occupies the client's intimate space.

Cultural Values

It is important that the nurse be familiar with the cultural values of the people in the nurse's region of employment, especially when those values differ from the values of the dominant culture. For example, optimal health for all is the focus of the dominant U.S. culture. In some cultures, however, health is not a major concern, and little financial or political effort is dedicated to health. Likewise, individualism is stressed in our culture. In many other cultures, however, the social group, not the individual, is the primary focus.

As another example, consider that a number of cultural groups have learned to enjoy what they have and do not feel the need to keep working for some goal or material object. This contrasts with the dominant U.S. culture, where persons must work hard, achieve, and keep busy in order to be considered successful. Finally, in the dominant U.S. culture, cleanliness is closely related to optimal health and is a dominant value. Few cultural groups emphasize cleanliness in the way the U.S. culture does, however. In fact, many have no problem with being dirty, and some even see it as a positive value.

Political Correctness

To be politically correct in communication means to use language that shows sensitivity to those who are different from oneself. It is intended to help eliminate prejudice by avoiding the use of language that offends. Politically correct language is designed to replace terms that suggest inferior status for members of minority groups and terms that exclude women, older people, and those with handicaps. Racist and bigoted language perpetuates prejudice and false ideas and often leads to violence.

Importance to Health Care System

It is important for nurses to understand the psychosocial aspects of communication and be aware of them with regard to individual clients. Communication is more effective when these aspects are taken into consideration.

Effective communication has a positive influence on a client's well-being. Furthermore, clients often judge nurses' competence by their communication skills. Good communication skills also result in increased client satisfaction, and increased client satisfaction leads to increased compliance with the therapeutic regimen.

Communication, then, is a key factor in the client's perception and evaluation of the health care services provided.

Figure 5-5 A distance of up to 4 feet is appropriate for interviewing and data gathering.

NURSE–CLIENT COMMUNICATION

One of the most important aspects of nursing care is communication. Whether the nurse is gathering admission information, taking a health history, teaching, or implementing care, good communication skills are essential.

Nurses have both an ethical and moral responsibility to use any information gathered from the client in the client's best interest. Information that affects the health status or care of the client should be shared with other members of the health care team. All information concerning a client is confidential and should never be discussed in elevators, the cafeteria, the hallways, or other public places outside the health care facility.

Formal/Informal Communication

Formal communication is purposeful and is employed in a structured situation such as information gathering on admission or scheduled teaching sessions (Figure 5-6). Specific items are covered in a planned sequence. In this way, more information can be given or received in the shortest amount of time.

Informal communication does not follow a structured approach, though it often reveals information that is pertinent to the client's care. For instance, a client may comment that the tape holding her bandage in place is irritating to her skin. This would lead the nurse to assess the wound area and take action to correct the problem. This interaction, although not planned or structured, was nonetheless helpful in ensuring quality nursing care.

Social Communication

Social communication is the everyday conversations held with family, friends, and acquaintances. Topics are generally those of interest to both parties and reflect the social relationship of those involved. Both parties share information, thoughts, and feelings. When getting acquainted with clients, social communication provides a way to learn about each other and to begin a nurse–client relationship.

Although social communication is not considered therapeutic communication, it is part of nurse–client communication. Because it is nonthreatening, social communication puts the client at ease; it also allows the nurse to get to know the client and what is important to the client. Clients often interpret social communication as expressions of caring on the part of the nurse—that is, the nurse cares enough about the client to spend some time communicating on a person-to-person level rather than on a nurse-to-client level.

Interactions

Nurse–client interactions and relationships progress through three phases. The amount of time spent on each phase depends on the purpose of the interaction.

Introduction Phase

The beginning of any interaction is usually fairly short. The client is greeted by name, and the nurse introduces himself and defines his role. Expectations of the interaction are clarified, and mutual goals are set. A good format might be:

"Good morning, Mrs. Jamal. My name is Paul Farrell. I am a student practical (vocational) nurse and I will be caring for you today and tomorrow. I would like to teach you some breathing and coughing exercises that you will be asked to do after your surgery tomorrow."

Working Phase

The working phase generally constitutes the major portion of any interaction. It is used to accomplish the goal or objective defined in the introduction. The nurse should always ask for feedback to ensure understanding on the part of the client. In the previously presented scenario, the client's demonstrating the breathing and coughing exercises and verbalizing why the exercises are necessary would indicate understanding.

Termination Phase

The final phase of any interaction is the termination phase. Seldom do nurses have unlimited time to spend with one client, and there are several ways for the nurse to indicate the end of an interaction. The nurse may ask whether the client has any questions about the topic discussed. Summarizing the topic is another good way for the nurse to indicate closure.

Factors Affecting Nurse–Client Communication

As mentioned previously, factors such as age, education, emotions, culture, language, attention, and surroundings, affect both parties in a communication. In

Figure 5-6 Formal Interaction, Admission Interview

nurse–client communications, additional factors relating to both the nurse and client also come into play. The nurse must be sensitive to these factors and to personal biases in order to provide appropriate nursing care.

Nurse

Many personal factors pertaining to the nurse can influence nurse–client communication. Past experiences as a nurse, state of health, home situation, workload, and staff relations can all impact the thinking, concentration, attitude, and emotions of the nurse. These in turn influence how the nurse sends and receives messages. Self-awareness is very important for the nurse when communicating.

Client

Factors related to the client that must be considered include: social factors, religion, family situation, visual ability, hearing ability, speech ability, level of consciousness, language proficiency, and state of illness.

Social Factors Some health concerns are easy to discuss because they are socially acceptable, such as having the gallbladder or appendix removed or having the flu. It may be more difficult, however, to communicate with a woman who is having a breast removed. The symbolic meaning of the breast may make its removal hard for the client to accept and may influence how she relates to others. A person with a sexually transmitted disease or one who is HIV positive may be very reluctant to discuss any aspect of the illness.

Religion Members of some religions seek healing through faith and not through conventional medical services. Others will not receive blood transfusions when an accident or disaster places these individuals in the health care system. When religious beliefs conflict with those of the health care team, communication can be difficult.

A client may have a priest, minister, or rabbi visit. Privacy for such visits should be provided if at all possible.

Family Situation Illness often unites family members around the client. If the family has not been close to or supportive of the client before the illness, communication between the family and client may be strained. Such stress may be noticed in the course of nurse–client interactions. If so, the nurse must be careful not to discuss aspects of the client's condition or treatment in front of family members. In fact, it is best to ask family members to step out of the room when any nursing care is being given. This applies whether assessing the client, providing physical care, or gathering information. The client's right to privacy and confidentiality is thus maintained.

Sometimes the client expresses a desire for a specific person to remain in the room. Unless contraindicated, this is usually allowed.

Visual Ability Communicating with clients who are visually impaired may not seem to be a challenge at first. However, because the nonverbal part of any message, such as facial expressions, gestures, and other body language, is missed, an important part of every message is lost to the client.

Persons who are visually impaired generally speak only when spoken to. Their speech may be loud if they are not sure where the other person is. Silence makes them uncomfortable if they are not sure of another person's presence in the room.

The nurse must include an explanation of "hospital sounds" when orienting a new client who cannot see. The room must be described in detail and the client guided around the room if possible. It is important for nurses to always speak and identify themselves when entering the room. As with any client, all procedures should be explained. Each step of the procedure as well as any touching should be described before it is initiated. As with any client, the nurse should always inform the client who is visually impaired before touching so as not to startle him.

PROFESSIONAL TIP

Caring for the Client Who Is Visually Impaired

- Look directly at the client when speaking.
- Use a normal tone and volume of voice.
- Advise the client when you are entering or leaving the room.
- Orient the person to the immediate environment; use clock hours to indicate positions of items in relation to the client.
- Ask for permission before touching the client.

Adapted from Health Assessment & Physical Examination *(2nd ed.), by M. E. Z. Estes, 2002, Albany, NY: Delmar. Copyright 2002 by Delmar. Adapted with permission.*

GERONTOLOGICAL CONSIDERATIONS

Nurse–Client Communication
- Assess for sensory disturbances.
- Face the client when speaking.
- Have patience, response may be slow.
- Show respect and be considerate of the older client's personal dignity.

PROFESSIONAL TIP

Caring for the Client Who Is Hearing Impaired

- Check to see whether the client wears a hearing aid. Be sure it is in working order and turned on.
- Make every effort to move the client to a setting with minimal background noise.
- Always face the client.
- Speak in a normal tone and at a normal pace.
- Determine whether the client uses sign language. If signing is used, enlist the assistance of an interpreter.
- Pay particular attention to nonverbal cues of the client and to your own nonverbal behavior.
- Provide a pen and paper to facilitate communication, if necessary.

Adapted from Health Assessment & Physical Examination *(2nd ed.), by M. E. Z. Estes, 2002, Albany, NY: Delmar. Copyright 2002 by Delmar. Adapted with permission.*

Hearing Ability Many persons who are hearing impaired can communicate by sign language, but few hearing persons can understand or use sign language. If the person who is hearing impaired is able to read, writing may be the easiest method of communication. Many persons who are hearing impaired have learned, at least to some degree, to speechread, formerly known as lipread. Communicating with a client who is hearing impaired requires time and patience.

The nurse should face the client and speak slowly and deliberately using slightly exaggerated word formation. Gesturing can also be very effective. Check to see whether the client has a hearing aid and, if so, encourage its use during the communication.

The frustration of trying to communicate can make the client who is hearing impaired stubborn or even hostile. Such frustration generally stems more from trying to understand others rather than from trying to be understood. Touching the client's arm when entering the room lets the client know that someone is there and helps prevent feelings of paranoia.

Speech Ability **Dysphasia**, the impairment of speech, and **aphasia**, the absence of speech, both can result from a brain lesion, although they are most commonly seen as the result of a stroke. Other neurological diseases such as Parkinson's disease may also cause dysphasia. A dysfunction of the muscles used for speech is termed **dysarthria**, which makes a person's speech difficult, slow, and hard to understand. Dysphasia, aphasia, and dysarthria create communication problems.

The person with dysphasia has difficulty both putting thoughts and feelings into words and sending messages. It should be noted, however, that seldom does the person with dysphasia have difficulty receiving and interpreting messages; thus, explanations should be given before doing anything. If the client can write, a magic slate or paper and pencil can be used for communication. A picture board, word board, or letter board may also be employed, as can a computer, assuming that one is available and that the client is able to use a computer. A person with any of these speech impairments may feel frustrated and helpless. Establishing some method of communication for the client provides hope and maintains self-esteem while at the same time minimizing or preventing feelings of depression, anger, and hostility.

Level of Consciousness True communication cannot be accomplished with unconscious or comatose clients. It should be remembered, however, that unconscious or comatose clients can hear even though they cannot respond. Caregivers should speak to these clients just as they would to alert clients. Always greet the client by name, identify yourself, and explain why you are in the room (i.e., what you are going to do). Then let the client know when you are leaving and, if possible, when you will return. Although one-sided, this interaction is important to the client.

Language Proficiency The client's ability to communicate effectively through the spoken language also influences the nurse–client interaction. Clients who do not speak English are generally from another culture. It is important to learn about the other culture, especially about the values and beliefs. Doing so will help prevent the nurse from violating those values and beliefs.

If a family member speaks English, that person could be used as an interpreter, as shown in Figure 5-7. Sometimes another health care worker on the nursing unit may speak the same language as does the client. As long as it does not interfere with his or her work, this person could also be used as an interpreter.

Pictures or a two-language dictionary are often helpful. If the other language is prevalent in the community, the nurse should learn some phrases in the language that are useful in client assessment and in care. Remember, gestures and other nonverbal communication send messages without the use of language.

Stage of Illness The stage of a client's illness may influence the client's desire to communicate with the nurse. Clients in the early stages of illness may be eager to learn all they can about the illness or may express anger and resentment at their current state of health.

Terminally ill clients may pose special challenges for the nurse. Most terminally ill clients know they are dying and are concerned about those whom they love. It is thus important for the nurse to have the client

Figure 5-7 A family member interprets communications with non-English speaking client.

identify those persons the client considers to be "family." Family and nurses often struggle with the proper way to speak with those who are dying; no one can escape death, but many people do not want to discuss it. Death is often considered a defeat by health care workers and therefore is not a prime subject for discussion. It is important to remember that listening and silence are both part of communication.

Anytime a client initiates a conversation regarding death the nurse must be willing to participate. Too often nurses hesitate to communicate with the terminally ill for fear of saying the wrong thing. When the client wants to talk, a good listener is needed. Let the client guide the conversation. Try not to give advice, just listen and accept what the client says. This may be very difficult to do.

CULTURAL CONSIDERATIONS

Family Interaction Patterns
- In some families the male members make all the decisions.
- In some families, decisions are made jointly, with all members (or all adults) participating.
- In some families, unrelated persons such as godparents or special friends are involved in decision making.

PROFESSIONAL TIP

Objectivity

The nurse must remain objective and nonjudgmental when the client's idea of family is different from the nurse's idea of family.

The nurse and the family must work together to understand the ways that the terminally ill client communicates. It can take persistence and insight to identify and decipher some messages. "Listening" to the client's gestures and facial expressions helps facilitate understanding of messages.

COMMUNICATING WITH THE HEALTH CARE TEAM

Providing care to clients is a team effort. For the team to work efficiently and effectively and to provide continuous quality care to clients, effective communication is necessary. This communication may be oral or written, individual or group, or even on computer.

Oral Communication

Oral communication among the health care team is necessary for the appropriate planned care of the client and for the efficient and effective functioning of the nursing unit. In order to provide continuity of care, all persons who provide direct care to clients must communicate orally with each other concerning that care.

Nurse–Nurse

Nurse–nurse communications can be either peer–peer or superior–subordinate communication. Peer–peer communication takes place many times every day. If each nurse uses effective communication with peers as well as clients, the unit will run more efficiently, and client care will be more effective. Superior–subordinate communication often directs the client care to be performed by the subordinate. The way whereby this communication is handled affects both the attitude of the subordinate and the client care given.

Nurse–Nursing Assistant

The nurse is responsible for informing the nursing assistants of their duties. Taking time to answer questions and providing reasons for specific activities requested helps establish a relationship of trust and mutual respect.

An experienced nursing assistant can be of considerable assistance to the new graduate (whether an RN or LP/VN). Nursing assistants are often much more comfortable and confident in providing bedside care. Given that they also often have creative solutions to problems, they should be included in planning care.

Nurse–Student Nurse

Student nurses must communicate not only with the clinical instructor but also with the staff nurses. How well the staff nurses interact with student nurses depends on how the staff nurses were treated as students and on the experiences the staff nurses have had with other student nurses. Student nurses are involved in the clinical facility for specific learning experiences selected by the instructor and related to classroom topics. They must have time to review client records, observe others performing procedures, and communicate with and care for their clients. Students are limited in their nursing activities depending on how far they have progressed through the nursing curriculum. Because staff nurses retain responsibility for the care of clients even when clients are assigned to students, communication between student nurses and staff nurses is essential. Generally, a complementary relationship develops between nursing students and staff nurses.

Nurse–Physician

Nursing education and expertise have evolved over the years to a professional level. Nurses are responsible for their own actions even when under the direction of a physician.

When the term *nursing diagnosis* was introduced, many physicians had difficulty understanding how nurses could make a diagnosis. Whereas medical diagnoses focus on disease conditions, nursing diagnoses focus on human needs. Nurses must communicate openly and honestly with physicians, demonstrating their competence in assessments, nursing skills, and provision of quality care.

Nurse–Other Health Professionals

Communication with professionals in other departments should always be on a peer basis. Clarification of goals for each client and of ways to meet those goals should be the focus of communication. Listening to those in other departments and establishing mutual respect for each other's area of expertise provides the client with top quality care.

Group Communication

Client care conferences may be scheduled regularly or whenever the need arises. Some conferences may be solely for the staff of a particular nursing unit; others may include members of other departments. In either case, only those persons directly involved with the care of the client should be invited (Figure 5-8).

The conference leader should establish the objectives of the conference and make all necessary arrangements. A conference room or other private place should be used as a meeting site. One person should be designated to record the discussion. If the conference is about a specific client, only facts should be documented on the client's chart. If the topic is general and not related to a specific client, only a record of the discussion is needed.

Telephone

When a student nurse is the only person available to answer a telephone call, the call should be answered with the name of the department or floor and the student's full name and position (i.e., student nurse). The

Figure 5-8 Nurses work together to plan client care.

caller should then be informed that an appropriate person will be found to take the call. If a message must be taken, the student nurse should write it down and read it back to the caller and ask for the caller's name and for the caller to spell out his or her name. The nurse must never give out any information about clients.

Written Communication

Most written communication relates to the client's chart. All aspects of a client's care are recorded on that client's chart.

Requisitions to x-ray or to physical or respiratory therapy and requests for laboratory services for a client are all forms of written communication. The reports resulting from these requests become a part of the client's chart.

One type of written communication not pertaining to a specific client is the interdepartmental memo requesting equipment, supplies, maintenance, or housekeeping. Such documents are necessary to keep the nursing unit functioning efficiently and effectively.

Electronic Communication

Computers are being used extensively in the business offices of health care agencies and have been so for years. The introduction of computers into the departments of direct client care has been slower, however. Nonetheless, in many places, computers are used by client care departments to send requisitions to other departments and to receive test results. Some hospital pharmacies use computer programs that show safe dosages and drug interactions. There are also programs to aid physicians in diagnosing and treating some conditions. With the expanding use of computers in health care and the corresponding potential for increased use, it is important for all health care workers to have some knowledge about computers.

COMMUNITY/HOME HEALTH CARE

Use of Telemedicine

- From the office, a home health nurse can watch a client at home change a dressing or self-administer insulin.
- During a video consult, a home health nurse might assist by manipulating the peripherals or actually performing a physical assessment.

PROFESSIONAL TIP

Telemedicine Confidentiality

- Avoid sending or receiving client data by e-mail unless the computer has encryption capabilities.
- During a two-way video consultation, inform the client of any other people who are present in the room, but off camera. Try to ensure that only those persons who must know about the client's condition are present (Granade, 1997).

Although the computerized patient record (CPR) as envisioned by the Institute of Medicine (IOM) is not yet available in the United States, parts of the CPR have been implemented. The IOM defines the CPR as an "electronic record that resides in a system specifically designed to support users through availability of complete and accurate data, practitioner reminders and alerts, clinical decision support systems, links to bodies of medical knowledge and other aids." This moves the client record from simply tracking client care to serving as a resource for health care delivery (Zolot, 1999).

Before there is widespread use of the CPR, many questions must be be answered, including: How can changes to the data entered be prevented? How will charting errors be corrected? What happens when the computers are down? How will security be maintained? What are the legal implications of electronic or digital signatures? According to Zolot (1999), all client records must be confidential, accurate, secure, and protected from unauthorized access and disclosure, regardless of the form.

Telemedicine

The Telemedicine Research Center (1997) defines **telemedicine**, also called telehealth, as the use of communications technology to transmit health information from one location to another. Included is the transmission of radiographic (teleradiology) and pathologic (telepathology) images, telemetry, and telephone triage.

The use of two-way video allows the client and health care provider to see, hear, and talk to each other. A stethoscope or otoscope (called peripherals) can be included in the hookup so that the sounds and visual images can be transmitted (Granade, 1997). This allows physician specialists in large medical centers to examine a client many miles away.

California and Arizona have both passed legislation requiring providers to obtain written and verbal informed consent before providing any nonemergency care via telemedicine. Oklahoma is also considering such legislation (Granade, 1997).

Nurses should document all activities, assessment findings, information provided by the client, and any

instructions given to the client. All data transmissions (e.g., telemetry printouts or videotapes) should be stored in the client's record. Most telemedicine laws require that existing confidentiality rules be maintained.

COMMUNICATING WITH YOURSELF

Whether they admit it or not, people talk to themselves every day. Oftentimes, such communication takes the form of thoughts rather than spoken words. What people say to themselves influences their personalities and, therefore, how they interact with others. Sherman (1994) describes self-talk as positive or negative.

Positive Self-Talk

Practicing positive self-talk is the key to positive self-esteem. Send positive thoughts to yourself about yourself. Better yet, say the thoughts out loud. Thinking, saying, and hearing positive statements about oneself reinforces positive self-esteem. Remind yourself of your good attributes and accomplishments. When you have had a difficult day, whether in the classroom or clinical area, pat yourself on the back for what you did accomplish. Each day verbally tell yourself what you learned or what good care you gave to your client(s).

Positive self-talk reinforces the desire to succeed. Memories of successes can serve as positive influences, especially when things are not going well and frustration sets in.

Positive affirmation is a positive thought or idea on which a person consciously focuses to produce a desired result. Positive affirmation can be used to change negative inner messages to positive messages. Instead of saying, "I don't know if I can pass this test," for instance, say, "I know I can pass this test." Of course, positive affirmation is not a substitute for studying and preparing for the test. Positive affirmation merely serves to modify your attitude about the test—or about any other situation.

CASE STUDY

Martha, a 25-year-old Mexican American female, is admitted for severe abdominal pain. Martha clings to her mother's arm when the nurse asks the mother to leave the room during the admission procedure. The mother asks to stay in the room. The nurse looks at Martha, who smiles but says nothing.

Consider the following:

1. What do you think may be causing Martha to cling to her mother?
2. What can the nurse do to communicate with Martha?
3. What subjective and objective data should the nurse gather?

Negative Self-Talk

Whenever you say to yourself, "I can't do . . . ," you are decreasing your self-esteem with the negative self-talk. Negative self-talk may originate within you, or you may be replaying things that others have said about you. Negative self-talk is self-destructive. Your self-image is lowered by your own criticism, and you begin to see yourself as a failure.

SUMMARY

- Communication is influenced by age, education, emotions, culture, language, attention, and surroundings.
- Nonverbal messages are generally more accurate in communicating a person's feelings.
- Verbal and nonverbal messages must be congruent for clear communication to take place.
- Techniques of therapeutic communication should be practiced and incorporated into the nurse's communication.
- Barriers to communication should be identified and avoided when communicating.
- People have four comfort zones of closeness: intimate, personal, social, and public.
- Therapeutic communication is purposeful and goal directed.
- Psychosocial aspects of communication may aid or hinder communication.
- Almost every nurse–client interaction should involve therapeutic communication.
- Nurse–client communication is influenced by both the nurse and the client.
- The nurse is often a role model for the family in terms of communicating with the terminally ill client.
- Accurate communication among the health care team is necessary for continuity of care.

Review Questions

1. Mr. George is looking out the window, with his back to the door. A nurse opens the door and says, "You will not be able to eat or drink after supper because of tests tomorrow." Then the nurse leaves. Did communication take place?

   a. No; there was no feedback.
   b. No; there was no eye contact.
   c. Yes; Mr. George had to hear the message.
   d. Yes; there was a sender, receiver, and message.

2. What is the best way to communicate?

   a. verbally
   b. nonverbally
   c. it depends on what the message is
   d. verbally and nonverbally together

3. Initial client assessment related to communication would include:

   a. vital signs.
   b. visual ability.
   c. ambulatory ability.
   d. complete health history.

4. When performing a nursing procedure on a client, the nurse should:

   a. only listen to what the client says.
   b. be aware of her own nonverbal messages.
   c. always have someone witness the procedure.
   d. tell the client how fortunate he is to be the nurse's client.

5. The nurse is aware that most nursing procedures are performed in which spatial comfort zone?

   a. public
   b. social
   c. personal
   d. intimate

6. Which of the following are all examples of verbal communication?

    a. singing, dancing, smiling
    b. reading, writing, listening
    c. shaking hands, reading, grimacing
    d. whispering, making eye contact, answering

7. When a client says, "I'm not sure how I'll handle all this;" which response of the nurse represents clarification?

    a. "Handle all this?"
    b. "Well, you can ask your sister to help."
    c. "Oh, you'll be able to handle things. You're an intelligent person."
    d. "I'm not sure I understand what it is you're concerned about being able to handle."

8. The statement "I'm sure you'll feel much, much better after your surgery" is an example of:

    a. advice.
    b. false reassurance.
    c. a judgment.
    d. excessive emotionalism.

9. That phase of an interview during which goals and objectives are identified is called the:

    a. working phase.
    b. interview phase.
    c. termination phase.
    d. introduction phase.

10. The most effective technique the nurse can use to facilitate communication is:

    a. giving.
    b. focusing.
    c. listening.
    d. questioning.

11. Which of the following represents the best way for a nurse to show caring?

    a. constantly staying with the client
    b. doing everything for the client
    c. assisting the client in learning self-care
    d. relaying to the physician everything the client says

12. A terminally ill client denies there is anything wrong and talks constantly about going back to work. The nurse should:

    a. listen but not comment.
    b. acknowledge the client's hopes and wishes.

    c. advise the client that it will be impossible to return to work.
    d. assist the client in planning when to return to work.

13. The nurse uses therapeutic communication with the client to:

    a. cure the client of fear.
    b. discuss personal problems.
    c. obtain or provide information.
    d. relieve the client of all concerns.

14. The nurse is aware that communication among members of the health care team is necessary because it:

    a. provides for continuity of care.
    b. identifies who provides better care.
    c. allows team members to become friends.
    d. promotes competition between departments.

15. Mrs. Banc tells the nurse that she would rather die than have radiation. To whom should the nurse report this communication?

    a. the physician only
    b. everyone on the nursing unit
    c. the physician and charge nurse
    d. no one; the communication is confidential

Critical Thinking Questions

1. How can you communicate with an unconscious adult?

2. Which barriers to communication do you use? How can you change?

WEB FLASH!

- Search for information on the Web about the Telemedicine Research Center. What are the latest reports?
- How much information about telemedicine is available on the Internet?
- To what sites can a client go to find out about telemedicine?

CULTURAL DIVERSITY AND NURSING

MAKING THE CONNECTION

Refer to the following chapters to increase your understanding of cultural diversity and nursing:

- **Chapter 4, Ethical Responsibilities**
- **Chapter 5, Communication**
- **Chapter 7, Wellness Concepts**

- **Chapter 8, Alternative/Complementary Therapies**
- **Chapter 14, Pain Management**

LEARNING OBJECTIVES

Upon completion of this chapter, you should be able to:
- *Define key terms.*
- *Describe the components and characteristics of culture.*
- *Describe the impact of cultural beliefs on health and illness.*
- *Compare and contrast diverse health beliefs of major cultural groups in the United States.*
- *Describe specific differences of cultural groups in relation to time and space.*
- *Identify nutritional preferences held by various cultural groups.*
- *Identify the general beliefs that account for the differences among religions.*

- *Describe the way that the nurse's religious beliefs or lack thereof can influence nursing care.*
- *Discuss the nurse's role in meeting the spiritual needs of the client and family.*
- *Analyze personal cultural beliefs and values.*
- *Perform a cultural assessment.*

INTRODUCTION

Every aspect of one's life—including attitudes, beliefs, and values—is influenced by one's culture. Behavior, including behavior affecting health, is culturally determined. As the population of the United States continues to diversify, recognition of cultural differences and their impact on health care becomes more critical. Nurses provide health care to culturally diverse client populations in a variety of settings. Knowledge of culturally relevant information is thus essential for delivery of competent nursing care. This chapter discusses the various concepts related to culture, the influence of culture on health, the relationships between culture and health beliefs, cultural aspects and the nursing process, and illnesses associated with ethnic groups.

CULTURE

Each individual is culturally unique. Behavior, self-perception, and judgment of others all depend on one's cultural perspective. To provide holistic care, the nurse needs a thorough understanding of concepts relating to culture.

KEY TERMS

acculturation	minority group
agnostic	oppression
atheist	race
cultural assimilation	religious support system
cultural diversity	spiritual care
culture	spiritual need
dominant culture	stereotyping
ethnicity	yin and yang
ethnocentrism	

In society, **culture** refers to dynamic and integrated structures of knowledge, beliefs, behaviors, ideas, attitudes, values, habits, customs, languages, symbols, rituals, ceremonies, and practices that are unique to a particular group of people. This structure provides the group of people with a general design for living.

Individuals often acquire cultural beliefs unconsciously throughout the process of growth and maturation (Giger & Davidhizar, 1999). People are exposed to culture at an early age through the observance of traditions (established customary patterns of thought and behavior). Cultural beliefs, values, customs, and behaviors are transmitted from one generation to another through interaction, daily activities, and celebrations. For instance, the birth of a child is celebrated according to the family's cultural norms and customs, which may include prayers, blessings, special naming ceremonies, religious rites, and so forth. Grandparents, other elders, and parents all teach children cultural expectations and norms through role modeling, demonstration, and discussion (Figure 6-1).

CULTURAL CONSIDERATIONS

Sharing Culture

Cultural messages are transmitted in a variety of settings such as homes, schools, religious organizations, and communities. The various media, such as radio and television, are also powerful transmitters and shapers of culture.

Culture is not static nor is it uniform among all members within a given cultural group. Culture represents adaptive dynamic processes learned through life experiences. Diversity among and within cultural groups results from individual perspectives and practices. Consider, for example, the way that a family deals with a crisis. A crisis may cause a family that is part of a culture with a strong sense of responsibility to family and blood relatives to become closer; conversely, the same situation may cause a family that is from a culture that values independence and individuality to withdraw and create distance among its members. These reactions are rooted in the family's cultural background and heritage.

Ethnicity and Race

Ethnicity is a cultural group's perception of itself, or a group identity. Ethnicity is a sense of belongingness and a common social heritage that is passed from one generation to the next. Members of an ethnic group demonstrate their shared sense of identity through common customs and traits. Ethnic identity can be expressed in many ways, including dress; for instance, many African Americans display ethnic pride by choosing clothing that highlights their ethnic origin and shared heritage.

Race refers to a grouping of people based on biological similarities. Members of a racial group have similar physical characteristics such as blood group, facial features, and color of skin, hair, and eyes. There is often overlap between racial and ethnic groups because the cultural and biological commonalities support one another (Giger & Davidhizar, 1999). The similarities of people in racial and ethnic groups reinforce a sense of commonality and cohesiveness.

Cultural Diversity

Cultural diversity refers to the differences among people that result from racial, ethnic, and cultural variables. Within the United States exist a variety of rich cultural heritages. The vast potential of human resources with divergent viewpoints and behaviors enriches the sociopolitical climate. New and varied ideas, viewpoints, and problem-solving approaches and increased tolerance are all outcomes of a diverse population.

Figure 6-1 This child is celebrating his Native American heritage by participating in a traditional ceremony that has been passed down through the generations. *(Photo courtesy of Smithsonian Institution)*

Figure 6-2 Areas of Cultural Diversity (*From* Fundamentals of Nursing: Standards & Practice, *by S. DeLaune and P. Ladner, 1998, Albany, NY: Delmar. Copyright 1998 by Delmar. Reprinted with permission.)*

There are also some disadvantages associated with living and working in such a culturally diverse society. Problems arise when differences across and within cultural groups are misunderstood. Misperception, confusion, and ignorance often accompany people's expectations of others. Figure 6-2 illustrates the many areas in which individuals may differ.

Members of some cultural groups have historically and globally experienced bias or prejudice in the forms of racism (discrimination based on race and biological differences), sexism (discrimination based on gender), and classism (prejudice based on perceived social class). These biases are perpetuated (consciously and unconsciously) by society. The basic underlying premise of these biases is that one way is better or "right," and every other way is inferior. **Ethnocentrism**, an assumption of cultural superiority and an inability to accept other cultures' ways of organizing reality, results in oppression. **Oppression** occurs when the rules, modes, and ideals of one group are imposed on another group. Oppression is based on cultural biases, which stem from values, beliefs, traditions, and cultural expectations.

Stereotyping is the belief that all people within the same racial, ethnic, or cultural group will act alike and share the same beliefs and attitudes. Stereotyping results in labeling people according to cultural preconceptions, thereby ignoring individual identity.

A **dominant culture** is the group whose values prevail within a given society. The dominant culture of the United States is that composed of white, middle-

class Protestants of European ancestry. The European value orientation has greatly influenced U. S. culture, as illustrated by the following beliefs held by the dominant culture:

- Achievement and success
- Individualism, independence, and self-reliance
- Activity, work, and ownership
- Efficiency, practicality, and reliance on technology
- Material comfort
- Competition and achievement
- Youth and beauty

Frequently, these dominant values conflict with the values of minority groups. A **minority group** is a group of people that constitutes less than a numerical majority of the population. Because of their cultural, racial, ethnic, religious, or other characteristics, such groups are often labeled and treated differently from others in the society. Minority groups are usually considered to be less powerful than the dominant group (Giger & Davidhizar, 1999).

People assume the characteristics of the dominant culture through **acculturation**, which is the process of learning norms, beliefs, and behavioral expectations of a group. **Cultural assimilation** occurs when individuals from a minority group are absorbed by the dominant culture and take on the characteristics of the dominant culture.

Components of Culture

Stewart has identified five components of culture that organize the way people think about life (as cited in Lock, 1992).

- Activity: identifies how people organize and value work
- Social relations: explains the importance and structure of friendships, gender roles, and class
- Motivation: describes the value and methods of achievement
- Perception of the world: refers to the interpretation of life events and religious beliefs
- Perception of self and the individual: refers to personal identity, value, and respect for individuals

 CULTURAL CONSIDERATIONS

Individuality

Remember that each person is first and foremost an individual, and secondly a member of a cultural group. While similarities may exist within an ethnic or culture group, individual differences must also be respected.

This model is particularly helpful to the nurse who is planning care for a client from another ethnic group. Work, social relationships, success, religion, and self-identity influence both the definition cultural groups attribute to health and illness and the cultural group's response to health events. For example, if a culture values relationships more than work, the culture may sanction an extended period of illness and a lengthy time away from the employment site. However, if a culture measures achievement by output at work, illness may be interpreted in a negative manner. Members of the latter culture may deny illness and delay seeking appropriate health care.

Characteristics of Culture

Spradley and Allender (1996) have identified five characteristics shared by all cultures.

- Culture is learned. Patterns of behavior are acquired as children imitate adults and develop actions and attitudes acceptable by others in society.
- Culture is not inherited or innate, but, rather, culture is integrated throughout all the interrelated components. Activities, relationships, motivations, world views, and individuality are permeated with consistent patterns of behavior to form a cohesive whole.
- Culture is shared by everyone who belongs to the cultural group. Behavioral patterns are not individually defined, but, rather, are accepted and practiced by all.
- Culture is tacit (unspoken), in that acceptable behavior is understood by everyone in the cultural group, regardless of whether beliefs are written down or spoken. Cultural beliefs are commonly known and adopted.
- Culture is dynamic; it is constantly changing. Each generation experiences new ideas that may generate different standards for behavior.

CULTURAL INFLUENCES ON HEALTH CARE BELIEFS AND PRACTICES

It is common for cultural groups to have a body of knowledge and beliefs about health and disease. Cultural practices can positively and negatively affect health and disease distribution. In cultures where raw foods are not consumed, for instance, the incidence of shigellosis may be lower than cultures where consumption of raw meat and fish is common. On the other hand, cultural taboos against eating protein during pregnancy have a harmful or destructive effect on fetal development. Human responses to illness are defined by cultural values. Whether an individual seeks professional care when ill and complies with prescribed treatment depends on cultural values.

PROFESSIONAL TIP

Cultural Sensitivity

Nurses must be able to provide culturally appropriate care to a diverse population of clients. Cultural diversity presents special challenges for nurses who must provide care that is incongruent with personal beliefs and values. Nurses caring for clients who differ from themselves must remember to ascertain the client's perception of the event (illness), including the significance (meaning) that the client assigns the event. The nurse must honor individual differences and understand that culture influences the way clients are viewed and treated within health care settings.

Beliefs and patterns of behavior affect attitudes about various aspects of health. Beliefs about the definition of health; etiology (cause and origin of disease); health promotion and protection practices; and health practitioners and remedies are all influenced by cultural background. Clients tend to define wellness and illness in the context of their own culture (Estin, 1999).

Definition of Health

The most widely accepted definition of health, developed by the World Health Organization (WHO), purports that health is not only the absence of disease, but also complete physical, mental, and social wellness. While this definition of health is broad enough to be global, that which is understood to be physical, mental, and social wellness is culturally defined. Any deviation from that which is culturally understood to be normal health is considered illness. For example, a biological disease of immediate etiology might not be interpreted as an illness by some cultures; intestinal parasites are so common in some areas in Africa that the presence of ascaris in stools is considered normal. When the cultural group does not recognize certain behaviors or symptoms as illness, individuals are not likely to seek medical intervention when these symptoms appear. In such cases, disease conditions may persist untreated to an irreversible state.

Etiology

Peter Morley, a noted medical anthropologist, presents four views of the origin of disease: supernatural, nonsupernatural, immediate, and ultimate (Morley & Wallis, 1978). The supernatural view of disease traces disease to metaphysical forces such as witchcraft, sorcery, and voodoo. In this view, an individual might ascribe illness to evil spirits or to a curse by a powerful spiritual person. The nonsupernatural view holds that diseases have an accepted cause-and-effect relationship, even though that relationship may lack scientific rationale. For example, people of many cultures believe that colic in an infant is caused by breast milk rendered impure when a nursing mother has sexual relations. In such cultures, sexual relations are prohibited for nursing mothers. The immediate view of disease traces diseases to known pathogenic agents, such as chickenpox is caused by *Herpes varicella;* and the ultimate view describes determinates for diseases, such as smoking resulting in lung cancer. Most cultural groups support a multietiologic origin, borrowing from three or all four explanations for how and why diseases occur.

Health Promotion and Protection

Strategies for achieving and maintaining good health vary by cultural group. For example, the dominant U.S. culture has come to endorse a low-fat, high-fiber diet; regular exercise; and appropriate immunizations as means to promote and protect health. Other cultures may place greater value on meditation, prayer, and restored relationships, particularly those cultures wherein health protection and disease prevention are closely linked to beliefs about disease etiology. For example, preventing disease may require paying homage to ancestral spirits in order to avoid offending them and provoking their revenge through illness.

Practitioners and Remedies

Variety in health/illness care providers is a natural extension of culturally diverse concepts of etiology and definitions of health and illness. Alternative remedies and practitioners are characteristic of culturally diverse groups. When a scientific rationale for the etiology of disease is not accepted by a cultural group, standard medicine may not be accepted as treatment. In order to enhance client compliance with treatment regimens health care providers must make efforts to base therapy and prescribe treatments that respect culturally traditional remedies. Clients who trace disease etiology to a supernatural cause are more likely to seek interventions from spiritual leaders or traditional healers.

The folk medicine system categorizes illnesses as either natural or unnatural (Giger & Davidhizar, 1999). The classification of an illness determines the type of treatment and healer used. Because the folk medicine system (also referred to as alternative medicine) can present challenges to nurses caring for clients from diverse cultures, knowledge of basic beliefs about illness, factors contributing to illness, and home remedies is necessary.

Folk healers are knowledgeable about cultural norms and customs (Edelman & Mandle, 1998). Table 6–1 lists both the various healers within the five dominant cultural groups in the United States (European American, African American, Hispanic American, Asian American, and Native American) and the common folk

healing practices within these cultures. Nurses must be able to relate care and treatment to the client's cultural context and incorporate informal caregivers, healers, and other members of the client's support system as allies in treatment.

Beliefs of Select Cultural Groups

While the population of the United States encompasses innumerable ethnic groups—European Americans, African Americans, Hispanic Americans, Asian Americans, and Native Americans together represent a majority. These groups form the basis for the following brief discussion of specific health beliefs affected by culture.

European American

In 1990, Americans of European descent represented 75% of the U.S. population; this figure is expected to be only 53% by the year 2020, however (U.S. Department of Commerce, Bureau of the Census, 1999). The prevailing value system for many European Americans is based on what is referred to as the white, Anglo-Saxon, Protestant (WASP) ethic (Sue & Sue, 1999). This ethnic group traces its origins to the Caucasian Protestants who came to this country from Northern Europe over 200 years ago. Values that still dominate the Caucasian American middle-class ethic include independence, individuality, wealth, comfort, cleanliness, achievement, punctuality, hard work, aggression, assertiveness, rationality, orientation toward the future, and mastery of one's own fate (Andrews & Boyle, 1998; Edmission, 1997).

Traditionally, most Caucasian Americans have wanted to be recognized as individuals rather than as members of groups. Thus, Caucasian Americans, unlike members of many other cultures, tend to be competitive rather than cooperative with each other. Mainstream American culture also values the nuclear family and its traditions (Luckmann, 1999).

African American

The African American population currently represents the largest minority group in the United States (U.S. Department of Commerce, Bureau of the Census,

CULTURAL CONSIDERATIONS

Subculture

Many Caucasian Americans do not belong to the mainstream culture, but, instead, belong to ethnic subcultures that hold strong values of their own (e.g., Irish, Jewish, German, Italian, Norwegian, Appalachian, and Amish subcultures).

Table 6–1 FOLK MEDICINE: HEALERS AND PRACTICES

CULTURAL GROUP	TRADITIONAL HEALERS	HEALING PRACTICES
European American	• Nurse • Physician	• Exercise • Medications • Modified diets • Amulets • Religious healing rituals
African American	• Elderly women healers • "Community Mother" or "Granny" • "Root doctor" • Voodoo healer ("Mambo" or "oungan") • Spiritualist	• Herbs, roots, oils • Poultices • Religious healing through rituals (e.g., laying on of hands) • Talismans worn around the wrist or neck or carried in a pouch to ward off disease
Hispanic American	• Curandero • Espiritualista • Yerbero (herbalist) • Brujo (healer who uses witchcraft) • Sobadora • Santiguadora	• Hot and cold foods to treat some conditions • Herbal teas, such as manzanilla, to treat gastrointestinal problems, insomnia, and menstrual cramps • Prayers and religious medals • Massage • Azabache, a black stone, worn as a necklace or bracelet to ward off the "evil eye" • Among some Haitian mothers, the "three baths" ritual (bathing for the first 3 postpartum days in water boiled with special leaves)
Asian American	• Herbalist • Physician	• Hot and cold foods • Herbs, soups • Cupping, pinching, and rubbing • Meditation • Acupuncture • Acupressure • Application of tiger balm (a salve) to relieve muscular pains • Energy to restore balance between yin and yang
Native American	• Shaman • Medicine man/woman	• Plants and herbs • Medicine bundle or bag filled with herbs that have been blessed by a medicine man/woman during a healing ceremony • Sweet grass (herbs) burned to purify the ill person • Estafiate (dried leaves) boiled to produce a tea for treating stomach disorders • The Blessingway ceremony (a healing ritual conducted by the medicine man/woman) • In some Navajo tribes, sand paintings made by the medicine man/woman for diagnostic purposes

Data compiled from Cultural diversity and community health nursing practice, by C. Degazon, in Community Health Nursing: Promoting Health of Aggregates, Families, and Individuals *(4th ed.), by M. Stanhope and J. Lancaster (Eds.), 1996, St. Louis: Mosby;* Transcultural Nursing: Assessment and Interventions *(3rd ed.), by J. Giger and R. Davidhizar, 1999, St. Louis, MO: Mosby; and "Cultural dimensions in home health nursing," by D. Grossman, 1996, AJN, 96(7).*

1999). African American ancestors came to North America from various African countries and the Caribbean as either slaves or free immigrants. The different countries of origin as well as disparate educational levels, income, occupations, and religious beliefs explain the heterogeneous (different) cultural practices among African Americans today.

Some African American beliefs about health and illness are linked to either a supernatural or a nonsupernatural view of disease. In traditional African societies, disease may be viewed as caused by disharmony in relationships. Discord may occur between a client and ancestral spirits, evil spirits, or living relatives. For example, if, following a wedding, a man were to refuse to finish making bride-price payments to his in-laws and the man were subsequently to become ill, his illness may be attributed to the break in relations with his wife's family caused by his outstanding debt. Healing comes with restoration of harmony and may be achieved through prayer, meditation, or activities considered to be therapeutic, such as offering a gift, wearing a charm, or confessing a wrong.

Disease may also be viewed as sent by God or another higher power as a punishment for a serious infraction against Him or another person. Evil forces may be thought to account for illness in other cases. Treatments may be found in herbs and home remedies, consultation with a local healer, and prayer.

Hispanic American

Hispanic Americans constitute the second largest minority ethnic group in the United States. The majority of this group has origins in Mexico, Puerto Rico, and Cuba. Although the Spanish language is common to most Hispanics, cultural patterns vary due to the different countries of origin. In general, the Hispanic American belongs to a large extended-family system within which females are seen as subservient to males but as having a major role in family cohesiveness (Giger & Davidhizar, 1999).

The influence of religion on culture is particularly evident in Hispanic populations. Most Hispanic Americans have roots in Catholicism blended with traditional Indian beliefs. Illness may be viewed as having a natural cause, as "an act of God" as punishment for sin, or as the result of witchcraft or a curse by an enemy. Diseases may be traced to an imbalance between "wet" and "dry" or "hot" and "cold" forces. Treatment depends on the cause. Western medicine is appropriate for some diseases, whereas the native healer (curandera) may have to intervene for illnesses having supernatural causes. Treatment may consist of herbal potions, diets based on hot and cold foods, or religious ceremonies.

Asian American

Asian Americans have origins in the Pacific-rim countries: Korea, Vietnam, Laos, the Philippines, Cambodia, China, and Japan. Generalization of a specific Asian culture is not possible among peoples from such a diversity of countries; however, certain similarities exist. Asian cultures are typically patrilineal, that is, family relations are traced through males. Males are the heads of household, and decision-makers, and elders are respected. Only physical complaints are acceptable, and maintaining eye contact is considered disrespectful (Estin, 1999).

Asians hold to a yin (cold) and yang (hot) etiology of disease. **Yin and yang** are opposing forces that when in balance yield health (Figure 6-3). Illness occurs as a consequence of an imbalance in these forces.

Figure 6-3 Yin and Yang

Foods are identified as either hot or cold and are used in treatment. For example, if yang is overpowering yin, hot foods are avoided until balance is restored. Illness may also be viewed as being caused by supernatural powers such as God, evil spirits, or ancestral spirits. In this situation, healing might be attained through prayer or treatment by a traditional healer. Many Asian Americans rely on herbal remedies, acupuncture, and cupping and burning, a treatment that draws blood to the skin's surface when a warmed cup is placed on the skin. In cupping, the inside and rim of a cup are heated with a candle flame. The rim of the cup is then applied directly to the client's skin, and, as the cup cools, blood is drawn to the surface of the skin, causing a bruised appearance. Cupping is used to draw out evil or illness in order to restore yin and yang. The nurse must be aware of these cultural practices so they are not viewed as abuse but, rather, as important cultural customs.

Native American

The fourth major minority ethnic group in the United States is Native Americans (U.S. Department of Commerce, Bureau of the Census, 1999). These peoples form a very diverse group, stemming from over 200 different tribes across the United States. Although many Native Americans have assumed Euro-American practices with regard to health, some still use traditional practices. Health is believed to result from a harmonious relationship with nature and the universe. Illness is frequently traced to a supernatural origin and discord with the forces of nature. Use of witchcraft can cause illness, and treatment may require exorcism of evil spirits. Prevention may be attained through prayer, charms, and fetishes (objects having power to protect or aid the owner). Remedies often include herbal drinks. "Medicine men" are persons thought to have supernatural powers of healing. Through prayers, rituals, ceremonies, and herbal drinks, health may be restored.

CULTURAL AND RACIAL INFLUENCES ON CLIENT CARE

Clients' cultural backgrounds and preferences influence the manner whereby they interact with other people and with the world around them. In an unfamiliar situation, such as admission to a health care setting, cultural differences may seem even greater, because in times of stress, most people hold tightly to that which is familiar in order to protect themselves from the unknown. The nurse can show caring in such a situation by acknowledging the expression of these differences and encouraging the client to retain what is familiar.

The influences of culture and race can be viewed through the phenomena of communication, space and time orientation, social organization, and biological variations.

Communication

Although language is common to all human beings, not everyone shares the same language. This cultural difference can lead to misunderstanding and frustration. The nurse must realize that a client who speaks a different language or with an accent, simply has a different means of expressing needs. When communication is restricted because of language differences, alternative methods of communication such as gestures and flash cards can be used.

The client's family may be able to assist when there is a block in communication. Family members can interpret procedures and instructions for the client and communicate the client's thoughts and questions to the nurse (Figure 6-4). If no family members are avail-

Figure 6-4 Family members often serve as interpreters to help clients who do not speak English understand procedures and instructions and to communicate the client's thoughts and questions to the nurse.

PROFESSIONAL TIP

Non-native Speakers
When interacting with someone who does not understand English well, many people will try to compensate for the lack of understanding by speaking more loudly. Speaking slowly, distinctly, and in a normal volume are more effective measures to ensure communication.

able, the hospital social worker may be able to find an interpreter.

Orientation to Space and Time

Orientation with regard to space and to time represents two other culturally influenced variables that may affect a client's attitude toward care. Territoriality, or interpretation of personal space, is a pattern of behavior resulting from an individual's belief that certain spaces and objects belong to that person. The distance that a person prefers to maintain from another is determined by one's culture. In general, people of Arabic, Southern European, and African origin frequently sit or stand relatively close to each other (0 to 18 inches), whereas people from Asian, Northern European, and North American origin are more comfortable with a larger personal space (more than 18 inches).

Affection and caring behavior are not communicated by touch in some cultures. For instance, among Asians, adults seldom touch one another, and the head is believed to be sacred. The nurse should thus not touch an Asian client's head without permission to do so. When working with clients from cultures where personal touch is viewed negatively, the nurse should use the universal sign of caring: the smile.

People in U.S. society tend to be future oriented: They plan for the future, establish long-term goals, and, increasingly, are concerned with prevention of future illnesses. In daily life, they are oriented to time of day, constantly referring to clock time for everything from meal time to time of appointments with health care professionals as well as other obligations. The nurse must also be very attentive to time. Medications are given at scheduled times, and work begins and ends at specified times. Other groups that tend to be future oriented are Japanese, Jews, and Arabs. These groups tend to view time as a commodity for achieving future goals.

Not all cultural groups are future oriented, however. People of some cultures (e.g., Asians) may be oriented to the past. For Asians, this orientation is reflected in the roles that ancestor worship and Confucianism play in the present. Members of other cultural groups, such as Native Americans, tend to be present oriented. Many Native Americans do not own clocks, and they live one day at a time, showing little concern for the future (Giger & Davidhizer, 1999). Mexican Americans and African Americans often value relationships with people in the present more than in the future. African Americans tend to be present oriented in health care behaviors as well. They often express the fatalistic belief that "it's going to happen anyway, so why bother" and fail to seek medical attention until a disabling condition occurs. The African American culture often teaches flexible attention to schedules; whatever is happening currently is most important. Explanations about the necessity of time scheduling, for instance, the need for strict schedules for medication requiring therapeutic blood level maintenance, must be given to the client.

How does time orientation affect health care? An individual's orientation to time may affect promptness or attendance at health care appointments, compliance with self-medication schedules, and reporting the onset of illness or other health concerns. Clients might not see the necessity for preventive health care measures if they experience no difference in their health today when they follow a special diet or exercise programs. The nurse must both teach clients when timing is critical in health care situations and practice patience when working with people whose background differs from that of the dominant culture.

Social Organization

Social organization refers to the ways whereby cultural groups determine rules of acceptable behavior and roles of individual members. Examples of social organization include family structure, gender roles, and religion.

Family Structure

The definition of family has changed dramatically through the years (Doherty, 1992). Until 1920 the norm was the "institutional family," which was organized around economic production and the kinship network. Marriage was a functional, not a romantic, relationship. Family tradition and loyalty were more important than individual goals or romantic interests. The chief value was responsibility.

CULTURAL CONSIDERATIONS

Environmental Control

Environmental control refers to the relationships between people and nature and to a person's perceived ability to control activities of nature, such as factors causing illness. One's cultural background and heritage influence one's perception of environmental control.

PROFESSIONAL TIP

Families

Each individual defines family differently. These definitions are shaped by personal experience and observation of other families. You must remain objective and nonjudgmental when the client's family is different from your idea of family. Have the client identify family members, so you know exactly who the client considers to be family.

From 1920 to 1960, the norm was the "psychological family." Family affairs were more private and less tied to the extended kinship network. Family was based on personal satisfaction and fulfillment of the individual members in a nuclear, two-parent arrangement. The chief value was satisfaction.

The social changes of the 1960s, including gender equality and personal freedom, caused changes in the family. The increased divorce rate may have resulted from the sexual revolution and the attitude that the individual deserves more and owes less to the family.

Today, no single family arrangement has a monopoly. Many types of families have emerged and are accepted. The chief value is flexibility. Family no longer necessarily implies biological relation, but rather has come to mean members of a shared household who have similar values and participate in shared goals. Fawcett (1993) cites the following characteristics of family:

- Love and affection
- Caring and compassion
- A sense of belonging and connectedness
- A history and linkage to posterity
- Rituals of rejoicing
- A sense of place
- Acceptance of members, including shortcomings
- Honor of elders
- A system of earning and spending money
- A competent manner of parenting or caretaking
- Division of chores and labor

According to systems theory, families are considered to be interdependent, interacting individuals related by birth, marriage, or mutual consent (Sherman, 1994). Examples of families with varying lifestyles today are two-parent nuclear, single-parent, blended (through remarriage), extended (including grandparents), cohabitating (couple having never married), gay or lesbian, divorced, adoptive, multi-adult, and mixed or interracial families (Figure 6-5).

Gender Roles

Gender roles vary according to cultural context (Figure 6-6). For example, in families organized around

Figure 6-5 Families come in all shapes, sizes, and configurations.

a patriarchal structure (with the man being the head of the household and chief authority figure), the husband/father is the dominant member. Such expectations are typically the cultural norm in Latino, Hispanic, and traditional Muslim families. The husband/father is the one who makes decisions regarding health care for all family members. Also, in such cultures, the wife is responsible for child care and household maintenance, whereas the father's role is to protect and support the family members (Grossman, 1996).

Religion

Anthropologists have identified the strength of the influence of religion on culture. In many cases, culture

COMMUNITY/HOME HEALTH CARE

Culturally Sensitive Care

To provide culturally sensitive care in the home:

- Remember that the setting for care is controlled by the client and family, not by the health care provider.
- Be sensitive to the fact that the nurse is often viewed as a guest by the client and family. Social chatter may be necessary to facilitate rapport.
- Be nonjudgmental about the condition of the home (e.g., presence of clutter and disarray).
- Show respect and consideration for the client. For example:
  - Wipe your feet before entering the home.
  - Ask permission to use the sink or bathroom to wash your hands.
  - Ask permission before moving the client's belongings and replace items after you have finished the task.
- Take advantage of the home environment to assess cultural values and norms. Clues to cultural values may include:
  - Decor and possessions on display in the home.
  - Assignment of family roles and tasks.
  - Types of interactions among family members.
  - Value placed on privacy.
  - Value placed on possessions.

Figure 6-6 One example of changing gender roles is fathers assuming more responsibility in caring for children.

and tradition have been maintained and preserved through religious beliefs. Religion often includes the formal organizational structures for social behavior.

Spiritual and religious beliefs are important in many individuals' lives. These beliefs can influence lifestyle, attitudes, and feelings about life, pain, and death. Some organized religions specify practices about diet, birth control, and appropriate medical care. Spiritual beliefs often assume a greater significance at the time of illness than at any other time in a person's life. These beliefs help some people accept their own illnesses and help explain illness for others. Spiritual beliefs often help people plan for the future. Religion can both help people live fuller lives as well as strengthen or console people during suffering and in preparation for inevitable death. By providing meaning to life and death, religion can supply the client, the family, and the nurse with a sense of strength, security, and faith during a time of need.

Spiritual needs are identified as an individual's desire to find meaning and purpose in life, pain, and death. The spiritual realm is often considered a very private area. In order to provide holistic care, however, the nurse must pay attention to the spiritual dimension of each client, recognizing spiritual needs and assisting the client in meeting them (Figure 6-7).

Although spiritual needs are recognized by many nurses, **spiritual care** (recognition of spiritual needs and the assistance given toward meeting those needs) is often neglected. Spirituality is characterized as an individual's search to find meaning and purpose in life. The goal of spiritual nursing care is to enable clients to identify and utilize their spiritual beliefs as coping mechanisms when faced with a health crisis. Among the reasons that nurses fail to provide spiritual care are the following:

- They feel that spirituality is a private matter.
- They are uninformed about the religious beliefs of others.
- They have not identified their own spiritual beliefs.
- They view meeting the spiritual needs of the client as a family or clergy responsibility, not a nursing responsibility.

Spiritual nursing care is appropriate when the nurse cares about the client's emotional, physical, and psychosocial health. The nursing diagnosis, *Spiritual Distress,* can be apparent in a client who is unable to practice religious or spiritual rituals due to illness or confinement in a health care institution.

The **religious support system** is a group of ministers, priests, rabbis, nuns, mullahs, shamans, or laypersons who are able to meet clients' spiritual needs in the health care setting. The nurse has the responsibility of working with these individuals, including them in the client care team.

Nurses must be aware of the general philosophies of their clients' spiritual beliefs, and also be aware that some individuals do not believe in a higher being or practice a specific religion. **Agnostics** believe that the existence of God cannot be proved or disproved, whereas **atheists** do not believe in God or any other deity.

It is important to identify particular beliefs from various religions that can influence client care activities. Some of these beliefs concern holy day practices, dietary restrictions, birth, death, and organ donation.

Protestant Many separate denominations (over 1,200) constitute the group known as Protestant. Protestant groups include such denominations as Baptist, Episcopal, Lutheran, Methodist, Presbyterian, and Seventh Day Adventist. The majority worship on Sunday, and their primary written reference is the Holy Bible.

Baptist Baptists do not practice infant baptism. For them, baptism is a rite to be performed only after a believer reaches an age of understanding and confesses his acceptance of the saving work of Jesus Christ. Communion is a spiritual act and symbolizes the suffering, death, and resurrection of the Lord.

Episcopal Episcopalians have a number of sacraments including confession, anointing of the sick (Holy Unction), communion, and baptism. Holy Unction is most often given as a healing sacrament. Episcopalians believe that a dying infant should be baptized, and the nurse may perform the rite. The usual administration of these sacraments is by an Episcopal priest.

Lutheran Traditionally, Lutherans practice baptism of infants and adults by sprinkling. Emergency baptisms may be performed by any baptized Christian. The Lutheran churches recognize two sacraments, baptism and Holy Communion. Holy Communion is understood

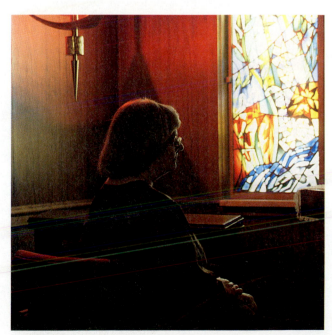

Figure 6-7 Spiritual needs often increase when individuals are sick.

as the body and the blood of the Lord and is often administered to those who are ill or awaiting surgery. Central to the Lutheran belief is the doctrine of "justification by faith." People are redeemed by God solely on the basis of God's grace, which they receive through faith or acceptance of what God has done for them.

Methodist Methodists practice both infant and adult baptism. They believe that religion is a matter of personal belief, and they use the conscience as a guide for living.

Presbyterian Presbyterians also practice communion, remembering the death of Jesus Christ for them and baptism. Salvation is believed to be a gift from God.

Seventh Day Adventist Seventh Day Adventists do not believe in infant baptism, but baptize individuals when they reach an age of accountability. They follow some dietary restrictions. Their Sabbath worship is observed from sunset on Friday to sunset on Saturday. They do not pursue their jobs or worldly pleasures during this time.

Roman Catholic Various rites known as Sacraments (sacred) are performed by the priest at appropriate times in the life of the Catholic. Sacraments that might be encountered in the health care setting are: baptism, the Eucharist (Communion), confession, and sacrament of the sick. Baptism, administered only once in the life of a Catholic, is believed to be absolutely necessary for salvation. A client preparing to take communion is normally asked to abstain from food or drink for an hour before the rite, although water and medications are allowed at any time. Confession is a rite for the forgiveness of sins. It is a very private matter and should be respected. The Sacrament of the Sick, in which the client is anointed with holy oil, was formerly known as the "last rites" given to someone near death.

Orthodox The Orthodox churches express their love of God through worship liturgies. It is important to the church that they remain faithful to the teachings of the ancient church. Holy Unction is practiced using oil to anoint the body for healing of bodily and spiritual infirmities. Baptism is also important; in life-threatening situations involving an unbaptized child an emergency baptism is performed.

Jehovah's Witness Jehovah's Witnesses are prohibited from receiving any blood or blood products, including plasma. They also will not eat anything containing blood. Blood volume expanders are permissible if they are not derivatives of blood. In some cases, children have been made wards of the court so that they could receive blood when a medical condition requiring blood transfusion was life-threatening. They have a special observance of the Lord's Supper.

Mormon (Church of Jesus Christ of the Latter Day Saints) Mormons do not believe in baptizing infants, but will baptize at the age of eight years. If necessary, baptism of the dead will be performed for adults. Mormons wear a special undergarment that has special significance symbolizing dedication to God. This garment may be worn under the hospital gown.

Christian Science Christian Scientists generally believe that illness can be eliminated through prayer and spiritual understanding. Healing is considered an awakening to this belief. When a critically ill Christian Scientist client is admitted to a health care facility they may wish to have a Christian Science practitioner contacted to give treatment through prayer. Christian Scientists ordinarily do not use medicine, agree to surgical procedures, or accept blood transfusions.

American Indian Religions All life is sacred and all things are interconnected is the central belief of the various religions. Community importance is emphasized. The individual who is able to communicate with the spirits or the Great Spirit is the spiritual leader. There are no written religious books. Religious traditions are passed on orally and through participation in ceremonies and festivals. Illness may be the result of a sin or a spirit or god who is unhappy.

Judaism Judaism is both a religious faith and an ethnic identity. The religion is based on the five books of Moses called the Torah. Culture and religion are deeply interwoven in the Jewish faith. As a result, ritual, tradition, ceremony, religious and social laws, and the observance of holy days are major influences in the Jewish daily life.

There are three groups in Judaism: Orthodox, Conservative, and Reformed. All share the fundamental teachings of Judaism but vary in how strictly they follow the traditions. Orthodox Jews strictly observe all traditional practices. The Conservative group observes many of the traditional practices, and the Reformed group interprets traditions loosely.

The rabbi is the spiritual leader of the Jewish congregation and is the representative to be informed when a client of the Jewish faith requests it.

The Jewish Sabbath, the day of worship, begins at sunset on Friday and ends at sunset on Saturday.

Circumcision is a religious custom in Judaism that is performed on the male infant eight days after birth. It may be done by the pediatrician or by the Mohel who may be a rabbi.

Islam The religion of Muslims is Islam. They believe that Allah is the supreme deity and that Mohammed, the founder of Islam, is the chief prophet. The Muslim's holy day of worship extends from sunset on Thursday to sunset on Friday. Some Muslims may desire to pray to their god Allah five times a day (after dawn, at noon, at mid-afternoon, after sunset, and at night). If the client requests that he face Mecca, the holy city of Islam, a bed or chair may be positioned facing the southeast direction (if in the continental United States). The Muslim client may be wearing an article of writing from the Koran on a piece of string around his neck, arm, or waist. This should not be allowed to get wet or to be removed. Rules of cleanliness include eating with the right hand and cleansing self with the left hand after urinating or defecating. Medications or other materials should be handed to the Muslim client with the right hand so as not to offend them, as they consider the left hand dirty.

Some Islamic females prefer to be clothed from head to ankle. During the physical examination, they may prefer to undress one body part at a time. They may refuse to be cared for by male nurses or physicians.

Buddhism Buddhism is a general term that indicates a belief in Buddha, "the enlightened one." Nirvana, a state of greater inner freedom and spontaneity, is the goal of existence. When one achieves Nirvana, the mind has supreme peace, purity, and strength. Buddhism does not dictate any specific practices or sacraments. There are no religious restrictions for therapy or special holy days. Buddhists do not believe in healing through faith. The religious support system for the sick is the priest. The Buddhist believes in reincarnation. Figure 6-8 shows the inside of a Buddhist temple.

Hindu Hinduism has no common creeds or doctrines that bind Hindus together. The major distinguishing characteristic is the social caste system. The religion of Hinduism is founded on the Scripture called the Vedas. Brahma is the principal source of the universe and the center from which all things proceed and to which all things return. Reincarnation is a central belief in Hindu thought. The goal of existence is freedom from the cycle of rebirth and death and entrance into what the Hindus, like the Buddhists, call Nirvana. Hindu temples are dwelling places for deities to which people bring offerings. Some Hindus believe in faith healing; others believe that illness is God's way of punishing a person for sins.

Biological Variation

Biological variations distinguish one cultural or racial group from another. Common obvious biological variations include hair texture, skin color, thickness of lips, eye shape, and body structure (Degazon, 1996). Biological variations that are less obvious include enzymatic differences and susceptibility to disease (Andrews & Boyle, 1998; Giger & Davidhizar, 1999). Enzymatic differences account for diverse responses of some groups to dietary therapy and drugs (Table 6–2).

Table 6–2 EFFECTS OF BIOLOGICAL VARIATIONS ON SELECT DRUGS	
CULTURAL GROUP	**EFFECT OF BIOLOGICAL VARIATION ON DRUG ACTION**
European American	• Due to liver enzyme difference, caffeine is metabolized and excreted faster than by people of other cultural groups.
African American	• Isoniazid (drug used to treat tuberculosis) is rapidly metabolized, thus becoming inactive quickly: occurs in approximately 60% of population. • An enzyme deficiency interferes with metabolism of primaquine (used to treat malaria); occurs in approximately 35% of population. • Antihypertensive drugs (e.g., propranolol) must be administered in higher doses to produce same effects as in European Americans.
Hispanic American	None noted
Asian American	• Isoniazid is rapidly metabolized, thus becoming inactive quickly; occurs in approximately 85% to 90% of population. • Rapid metabolism of alcohol results in excessive facial flushing and other vasomotor symptoms. • Chinese men need only approximately half as much propranolol (antihypertensive drug) to produce same effects as in European American men.
Native American	• Isoniazid is rapidly metabolized, thus becoming inactive quickly; occurs in approximately 60% to 90% of population. • Rapid metabolism of alcohol results in excessive facial flushing and other vasomotor symptoms.

Data from Transcultural Nursing: Assessment and Intervention (3rd ed.), *by J. Giger and R. Davidhizar, 1999, St. Louis: Mosby.*

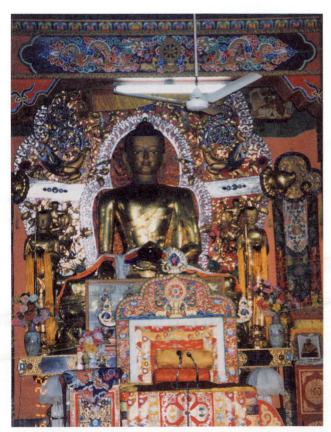

Figure 6-8 Inside of a Buddhist Temple. (*Photo courtesy of John White.*)

CULTURAL ASPECTS AND THE NURSING PROCESS

Each individual comes from a cultural background that, in some way, influences behavior and attitudes about health and illness. Personal attitudes and behaviors determine not only the ways that clients interpret health events and utilize health care, but also the ways that nurses interpret health events and provide health care. The central role that culture plays in determining perception compels health care providers to evaluate their personal views about health and illness before examining those of clients from other cultural groups. Nurses must be able to recognize the way that culture affects the health care needs of clients and respond appropriately.

Assessment

Culturally sensitive nursing care begins with an examination of one's own culture and beliefs. It is followed by an assessment of the client's cultural beliefs and background.

PROFESSIONAL TIP

Culturally Diverse Coworkers

Many nursing units represent a mix of nationalities and cultures. While such a mix has the potential of improving nursing care, in practice it often leads to conflict and poor teamwork. The same cultural differences discussed in relation to clients may also be found among coworkers. Grensing-Pophal (1997) suggests five ways to successfully manage diversity in the workplace:

- Be aware of your own biases, and strive to avoid stereotyping others.
- Be aware of the way the things you do and say affect others.
- Help others to be more sensitive and help correct misconceptions.
- Learn to welcome different opinions and viewpoints.
- Be open to feedback.

Learn more about your coworkers and remember that respect for individual differences reflects acknowledgment of each person's uniqueness. Have a unit conference focusing on a cultural assessment of each other. Grossman and Taylor (1995) suggest having a potluck lunch, with everyone bringing a typical ethnic dish. Such strategies might also work well in a nursing program where various cultures are represented.

Personal Cultural Assessment

Spradley and Allender (1996) identify five areas to be examined in assessing one's own culture and the influence it may have on personal beliefs about health care.

- Influences from own ethnic/racial background
- Typical verbal and nonverbal communication patterns
- Cultural values and norms
- Religious beliefs and practices
- Health beliefs and practices

They suggest that the nurse should gather as much information as possible on each issue and then validate this information with one or two other persons from the same cultural group.

Client Cultural Assessment

Having examined one's own culture and the influences it may have had in developing personal beliefs about sickness and health, the next step to providing culturally appropriate care is to assess the client's cultural background (Figure 6-9). Data about various cultures may be collected from members of the culture to be studied, from others familiar with the culture, or from the local library.

Spradley and Allender (1996) identify six categories of information necessary for a comprehensive cultural assessment of the client. These categories may also be useful in organizing interviews with representatives from the culture.

- *Ethnic or racial background.* Where did the client group originate, and how does that influence the status and identity of group members?
- *Language and communication patterns.* What is the preferred language spoken, and what are the culturally based communication patterns?
- *Cultural values and norms.* What are the values, beliefs, and standards regarding such things as roles, education, family functions, child-rearing, work and leisure, aging, death and dying, and rites of passage?
- *Biocultural factors.* Are there physical or genetic traits unique to the ethnic or racial group that predispose group members to certain conditions or illnesses?
- *Religious beliefs and practices.* What are the group's religious beliefs, and how do they influence life events, roles, health, and illness?
- *Health beliefs and practices.* What are the group's beliefs and practices regarding prevention, causes, and treatment of illnesses?

Nursing Diagnosis

Any nursing diagnosis may be appropriate for a client of any cultural group. When cultural variables

Cultural Assessment Interview Guide

Name: _____

Nickname or other names or special meaning attributed to your name: _____

Primary language:

    When speaking _____

    When writing _____

Date of birth: _____

Place of birth: _____

Educational level or specialized training: _____

To which ethnic group do you belong? _____

To what extent do you identify with your cultural group? _____

Who is the spokesperson for your family? _____

Describe some of the customs or beliefs that you have about the following:

    Health _____

    Life _____

    Illness _____

    Death _____

How do you best learn information?

☐ Reading

☐ Having someone explain verbally

☐ Having someone demonstrate

Describe some of your family's dietary habits and your personal food preferences: _____

Are there any foods forbidden from your diet for religious or cultural reasons? _____

Describe your religious affiliation: _____

What role do your religious beliefs and practices play in your life during times of good health and bad health? _____

On whom do you rely on for health care services or healing, and to what type of cultural health practices have you been exposed? _____

Are there any sanctions or restrictions in your culture about which the person taking care to you should know? _____

Describe your current living arrangements: _____

How do members of your family communicate with each other? _____

Describe your strengths: _____

Who /what is your primary source of information about your health? _____

Is there anything else that is important about your cultural beliefs that you want to tell me? _____

Figure 6-9 Cultural Assessment Interview Guide (*From* Fundamentals of Nursing: Standards & Practice, *by S. DeLaune and P. Ladner, 1998, Albany, NY: Delmar. Copyright 1998 by Delmar. Reprinted with permission.*)

are identified during assessment, the nurse should be as specific as possible when asking questions and determining appropriate nursing diagnoses, so that interventions can be individualized with respect to the client's cultural beliefs. For instance, *Cardiac Output, Decreased* may be viewed by the nurse or physician as having a medical or physical cause, whereas the client may attribute the origin to an imbalance of yin and yang. Table 6–3 lists select nursing diagnoses that are most likely to have cultural implications.

Planning/Outcome Identification

Cultural variables must be taken into consideration when establishing goals and planning interventions. Care will be most effective when the client and family are active participants in planning care, and when cul-

Table 6–3 NURSING DIAGNOSES WITH CULTURAL IMPLICATIONS

Anxiety
Body Image Disturbance
Breastfeeding, Ineffective
Communication, Verbal, Impaired
Coping, Family, Ineffective, Compromised
Coping, Individual, Ineffective
Decisional Conflict
Fear
Grieving, Anticipatory
Health Maintenance, Altered
Health-Seeking Behaviors
Noncompliance
Nutrition, Altered, More Than Body Requirements
Pain
Role Performance, Altered
Sleep Pattern Disturbance
Social Interaction, Impaired
Spiritual Distress

tural preferences are respected. Potter and Perry (1999) suggest the following goals to consider when cultural factors are involved:

- Client will express health care needs to family and caregiver.
- Client will maintain cultural health practices as appropriate.
- Client and family will understand the effect that health care beliefs have on health status.

Implementation

Cultural aspects are always a factor in a nursing care plan, and effective communication and client education are important nursing responsibilities that can enhance cultural understanding and appreciation. Interventions should be carried out in a manner that will respect, to the degree possible, the preferences and desires of the client. When a client does not speak or understand the native language well, the nurse should arrange to have an interpreter present to explain procedures and tests.

Evaluation

Evaluation should include feedback from the client and family to determine their reaction to the interventions. Revisions to the plan of care should be made with client and family input, and alternative sources and resources brought in when needed to enhance communication and exchange of information. Nurses should also perform self-evaluations to identify their attitudes toward caring for clients from diverse cultures.

CLIENT TEACHING

Culturally Sensitive Teaching Guidelines

When caring for clients from diverse cultures, consider the following guidelines for client teaching:

- Determine the client's cultural background.
- Evaluate the client's current knowledge base by asking the client to state what he knows about the specific topic.
- To identify the client's perception of need, ask the client and family what they need and want to learn.
- Observe the interaction between the client and family to determine family roles and authority figures. Ask the client whether the dominant family member should be included in teaching and care sessions.
- Use language easily understood by the client, avoiding jargon and complex medical terms.
- Clarify your verbal and nonverbal messages with the client.
- Have the client repeat the information. If feasible, have the client do a return demonstration of the material taught.

PROFESSIONAL TIP

Culturally Appropriate Care
- Respect clients for their different beliefs.
- Be sensitive to behaviors and practices different from your own and respond accordingly.
- Accommodate differences if they are not detrimental to health. For example, a client might believe that eating onions will resolve his respiratory infection. While eating onions may not be therapeutic, it is also not likely to negatively impact health.
- Listen for cues in the client's conversation that relay a unique ethnic belief about etiology, transmission, prevention, or some other aspect of disease. For example, a client might say, "I knew I would be sick today. I heard an owl last night."
- Use the occasion to teach positive health habits if the client's practices are deleterious to good health. For example, when asked about her diet, a pregnant woman might reply that she never eats meat or eggs while pregnant because she believes that gaining too much weight will increase her risk of a difficult delivery. Such a situation offers the nurse an opportunity to provide nutritional instruction.

SAMPLE NURSING CARE PLAN

THE FAMILY WITH INEFFECTIVE COPING

Mrs. Chang, a 74-year-old Asian American housewife, was admitted to the hospital with complaints of nausea and difficulty keeping food down related to treatment for recurrent breast cancer with bone metastasis. For the past few weeks, her appetite has been decreasing. She is able to drink some fluids.

Mrs. Chang's husband of 53 years remains at her bedside, as do their two grown daughters. Mrs. Chang insists that they remain at her bedside so that she does not have to bother the nurses for her basic care and insists that the oldest daughter bathe her and walk her to the bathroom. Mr. Chang leaves her bedside only to go home and shower; when he does so, both daughters remain with Mrs. Chang.

The nurses notice that Mr. Chang is looking exhausted and appears to have lost weight. The daughters have tried to relieve their father at night to allow him to go home and rest, but he insists on remaining at the hospital.

Although Mrs. Chang never voices discomfort, she has her husband and daughters constantly massaging her back and legs. She changes position slowly and grimaces with each movement. She does not verbalize to the nursing staff, but lets her family do the talking for her. She denies pain when questioned by the nurse, but she complains of pain to her family. She does not sleep well.

Mrs. Chang's treatment plan is supportive. The hospital staff has mentioned the idea of hospice care to the family. Mrs. Chang has stated that she wants to go home.

Nursing Diagnosis *Compromised Family Coping related to prolonged disease or disability progression that exhausts the supportive capacity of significant people as evidenced by Mr. Chang's looking exhausted.*

PLANNING/GOALS	NURSING INTERVENTIONS	RATIONALE	EVALUATION
Family will plan a specific rotation schedule to meet each other's needs for rest and support while caring for Mrs. Chang.	Provide empathy and support for the husband and daughters. Provide them with unlimited visitation, adequate space for members who stay overnight, and privacy. Assess family members for signs of fatigue or overexertion. Explore with husband and daughters other possible extended family members who would be willing and be accepted by Mrs. Chang to keep her company and give her support.	The family is one of the most important factors in the life of the Asian American. A sense of obligation to intervene and assist is highly valued. Casual help from strangers is avoided. Asian Americans value self-control and self-sufficiency. To ask for help would mean loss of face and dignity. This family will not be able to keep up this vigil for an unknown period of time. Family obligations take precedence over individual desires.	Family is sharing bedside care responsibilities. Husband and eldest daughter remain at bedside during daytime hours. Youngest daughter rests at home during the day and exchanges places with the father and eldest sister at night. Mrs. Chang is agreeable.

continues

PLANNING/GOALS	NURSING INTERVENTIONS	RATIONALE	EVALUATION
Client and family will maintain open communication.	Develop trusting and respectful relationships with Mrs. Chang and family members.	Asian Americans tend to be reserved with those whom they view as being in authority. The nurse should remember that this family needs to establish a caring, trusting relationship before they participate in self-disclosure.	Mr. Chang meets with both daughters to discuss their mother's plan of care. He includes the primary care nurse in the discussion.
	Encourage Mr. Chang to have family meetings as necessary to discuss realistic plans and expectations of other family members, using health care providers as needed.	Asians traditionally value authoritarian styles of leadership, where the father makes unilateral family decisions. Authority and communication come from the top down. Discouragement of verbal communication, avoidance of discussion of personal problems, and limited expression of emotion have been noted as common patterns in the traditional Asian family.	
	Encourage and assist family to explore outside resources to assist them in dealing with the crisis.	This family structure cannot maintain bedside attendance without help. The outside resource might take the form of extended family, sisters, brothers, nieces, or nephews of Mrs. Chang who live in the neighborhood.	
Family members will perform client care without compromising their own physical and emotional health.	Assess whether basic physical and emotional needs of Mrs. Chang and family members are being met.	The ideal pattern of communication in Asian society is silent communication. Stoic reactions to pain and other uncertain situations is common. Direct expression of negative feelings is unusual. The nurse will need to assess for nonverbal clues indicating the status of needs.	Mr. Chang and his daughters continue to provide the physical care for Mrs. Chang. Mr. Chang appears more rested and has gained back some weight. The daughters express gratefulness that their father is stronger and has taken on the leadership role.
	Monitor ability of family members to carry out treatment plan and provide safe care.	When care is provided by family members who are exhausted, safety is always an issue. The	*continues*

PLANNING/GOALS	NURSING INTERVENTIONS	RATIONALE	EVALUATION
		nurse is ultimately responsible for the well-being of the client.	
	Teach coping strategies for managing tension and strain in the event of previous techniques losing their effectiveness.	Coping strategies to maintain healthy emotional and psychological health may be necessary. This is especially true for individuals from a culture that discourages placing individual needs or emotions ahead of those of the family.	

CASE STUDY

Maria Garcia brings her Catholic, 18-year-old sister, Rosa, to the hospital emergency room. Rosa has a high temperature and chills, is vomiting, and complains of right-lower-quadrant pain. Maria also brings her three children, ages 3, 2, and 1 year old, with her. Maria understands and speaks broken English, but Rosa is fluent in Spanish only. The nurse directs Maria to the waiting room with her children, then takes Rosa to the examination room. Rosa is examined by a male nurse, who promptly complains at the nurses' station about how uncooperative Rosa was during the physical examination. Rosa is admitted for inpatient care and is diagnosed with appendicitis requiring emergency surgery. Maria is left in the waiting room, unaware of the difficulty that the nursing staff has had in communicating with Rosa. Rosa is taken upstairs to her room to await her surgical preparation. Maria is notified that she can go upstairs for a few minutes but must then leave because her children do not meet the age requirement for visitor privileges. Maria finds Rosa weeping, nearly hysterical. The physician walks in and asks Maria why she waited so long to bring Rosa in for treatment. He informs her that Rosa's appendix was close to rupturing and that treatment should have been started 3 days ago, when her symptoms first began. Maria informs him that she had taken Rosa to the curandero, who had given her some herbal tea to drink. When that did not help, she had brought Rosa to the hospital.

The following questions will guide your development of a nursing care plan for the case study.

1. Why was communication among Maria, Rosa, and the health care professionals problematic?
2. What Mexican American cultural diversities were not addressed by the health care professionals?
3. What needs of Maria and Rosa are being ignored by the health care professionals?
4. What questions do you feel must be asked by the health care professionals to give them a better understanding of this situation?
5. Identify two individualized culturally sensitive nursing diagnoses and goals for Rosa.
6. Formulate pertinent nursing interventions for the diagnoses and goals identified in question 5.
7. List resources that the nurses could use to assist Rosa in her recovery.
8. List at least two successful client outcomes for Rosa.

SUMMARY

- Culture is composed of beliefs about activity, relations, motivation, perception of the world, and perception about self.
- Culture is learned, integrated, shared, unspoken, and dynamic.
- Beliefs about concepts of health, disease etiology, health promotion and protection, and practitioners and remedies are influenced by culture.
- Unlike opinions, preferences, and attitudes, which can change, cultural characteristics are deeply rooted and are thus difficult to change. Clients reflect their cultural and ethnic heritage every time they interact with the world around them.
- Culture is influenced by religion, which in turn affects beliefs and practices about health and illness.
- Spiritual and religious beliefs are important in many people's lives. They can influence lifestyle, attitudes, and feelings about illness and death.
- The nurse should not make assumptions about clients based on the client's religious and cultural affiliations. Individuality exists among all peoples.
- The focus of nursing care is to help the client maintain his own beliefs in the midst of a health care crisis and to use those personal beliefs to strengthen coping patterns.
- Understanding and encouraging client differences are important aspects of nursing.
- Response to health and illness varies depending on cultural origin.
- Culturally appropriate care begins with an understanding of one's own cultural beliefs.
- Client cultural assessment is a prerequisite to providing appropriate nursing care.

Review Questions

1. A mother is observed breastfeeding her 4-year-old son, who is a client in the pediatrics wing of the hospital. A nurse is overheard talking in the nursing station about the "weird" way the mother has continued to breastfeed a 4-year-old. She comments that the American way is the best. The nurse is guilty of:

   a. ethnocentrism.
   b. stereotyping.
   c. unusual break behavior.
   d. not insisting that the mother stop breastfeeding.

2. Which religious group teaches that physical healing comes exclusively through prayers and readings?

   a. Roman Catholic
   b. Jewish
   c. Christian Science
   d. Seventh Day Adventist

3. Which religious group observes the Sabbath from sunset Friday until sunset Saturday?

   a. Mormons
   b. Jews
   c. Presbyterian
   d. Muslims

4. A client of this religion would most likely refuse a blood transfusion, even if his life were in jeopardy.

   a. Hindu
   b. Jehovah's Witness
   c. Jew
   d. Mormon

5. The nursing diagnosis that might be used for a client who is hospitalized and has religious practices that conflict with hospital practice is:

   a. *Emotional Depression.*
   b. *Guilt and Misery.*
   c. *Spiritual Distress.*
   d. *Spiritual Manipulation.*

6. It is important for the nurse to know the client's religion in order to:

   a. chart it on his record.
   b. give holistic care.
   c. meet his physical needs.
   d. know how to pray for him.

7. Which of the following is a characteristic of culture?

   a. Culture is learned.
   b. Culture stays the same.
   c. Culture is biologically inherited.
   d. Culture is individually determined.

8. Which of the following is descriptive of Hispanic Americans?

   a. They are culturally homogeneous.
   b. Their culture is not based on religion.
   c. Illness may be viewed as a punishment from God.
   d. They always seek Western medical intervention.

9. When a client says to the nurse, "I need to pray with my pastor in order to get well," the most appropriate response from the nurse is:

   a. "The medicine you take will make you well."
   b. "When you are released from the hospital, you can go to church and pray."
   c. "May I call your pastor for you and ask him to visit you?"
   d. "Why do you think prayer will make you well?"

10. It is important to be aware of cultural aspects of health and disease because:

    a. some cultural groups are represented in greater numbers than others.
    b. cultural groups respond differently to illness.
    c. differences in care should not be based on culture.
    d. reimbursement is related to ethnicity.

Critical Thinking Questions

1. How does your culture influence your beliefs about health practices?

2. Suppose one of your clients practiced the custom of placing an amulet (religious icon and necklace) around a newborn's neck. You are concerned about the risk of strangulation this presents. How would you approach this client to discuss your concerns?

WEB FLASH!

- Search "cultural diversity" on the Web. What related topics do you find?
- Can you locate health-related Web sites specific to European Americans, African Americans, Hispanic Americans, Asian Americans, and Native Americans?

WELLNESS CONCEPTS

MAKING THE CONNECTION

Refer to the following chapters to increase your understanding of wellness concepts:

- **Chapter 6, Cultural Diversity and Nursing**
- **Chapter 9, Loss, Grief, and Death**
- **Chapter 30, Nursing Care of the Client: Female Reproductive System**
- **Chapter 31, Nursing Care of the Client: Male Reproductive System**
- **Chapter 34, Nursing Care of the Client: Substance Abuse**
- **Chapter 35, Nursing Care of the Older Client**

LEARNING OBJECTIVES

Upon completion of this chapter, you should be able to:
- *Define key terms.*
- *Discuss guidelines for healthy living.*
- *Describe the scope of prevention.*
- *Explain the importance of Healthy People 2010.*
- *Make a teaching plan for ways to promote and maintain wellness.*

KEY TERMS

health
prevention
primary prevention
secondary prevention
tertiary prevention
wellness

INTRODUCTION

The responsibility for maintaining health rests squarely on the shoulders of each individual adult. Parents are responsible for maintaining their children's health and teaching them a healthy lifestyle. Health maintenance involves the whole person and the person's whole life. It includes the prevention of disease and the early detection and treatment of disease. Main-tenance of health requires constant effort and a focus on all aspects of a person's life.

Simon (1992) quotes Dr. Wood Hutchinson, who wrote in the *Journal of the American Medical Association* that "our system's philosophy might be condensed in the motto 'millions for health care and not a penny for prevention'." This was written in 1896. Over 100 years have passed and we still spend less than 3 cents of each health dollar on prevention and education.

The United States is the world leader in medical science and education yet is only 16th among nations in life expectancy. We spend more for health care than any other country, yet we rank 24th in infant mortality. In 1991, there were 82,902 positions for residents in specialty areas and only 202 in preventive medicine. Many doctors have not incorporated preventive medicine into their practices (Simon, 1992).

There is no profit in prevention. Insurance premiums buy illness insurance, not health insurance, given that insurance companies often will not pay for preventive testing and treatment. Compensation for clinical care makes illness the priority, not wellness. Diagnosis and treatment of illnesses are what insurance pays for, not health maintenance.

HEALTH

A widely accepted definition of **health** comes from the World Health Organization (WHO), which defines health as a state of complete physical, mental, and social well-being, not merely the absence of disease or infirmity.

Other concepts of health focus on motivation. A eudaemonistic approach to health (from the Greek word *eudaimonia,* meaning "fortunate or happy") views the individual as being motivated by joy and self-fulfillment: Health is the full realization of potential, and illness is an impediment to that realization.

Those who hold the adaptive view of health are motivated by altering the risks in self or the environment through such means as dietary and exercise programs or reducing exposure to environmental hazards. Illness results when the individual is unable to cope with the risks and stresses of daily life.

Some individuals are motivated by being able to meet responsibilities at home, at work, at play, and in the community: Their health focus is role performance. Health is considered achieved when the individual fulfills the obligations and responsibilities to family, job, and community.

Other individuals are motivated by the absence of disease: Theirs is a clinical health focus. As long as no disease is present, the individual considers himself healthy. Personal definition of health influences life choices and personal health decisions.

WELLNESS

Wellness is defined as a state of optimal health wherein an individual moves toward integration of human functioning, maximizes human potential, takes responsibility for health, and has greater self-awareness and self-satisfaction. Floyd, Mimms, and Yelding-Howard (1995), Hafen and Hoeger (1997), and Seiger, Vanderpool, and Barnes (1995) describe the behaviors exhibited by individuals in a state of wellness. These researchers outline seven areas of wellness: emotional, mental, intellectual, vocational, social, spiritual, and physical wellness. Various areas of wellness overlap and none is mutually exclusive.

CLIENT TEACHING

Suppressed Anger in Women

Research has shown that middle-aged women who suppress anger and have hostile attitudes may be at greater risk for developing cardiovascular disease (Matthews, 1998). Nurses can help such women minimize this risk by encouraging them to learn to express negative feelings in a constructive manner, to talk calmly about their feelings, to find other women who may share some of the same concerns and stressors, and to engage in regular exercise routines to relieve stress and tension.

Emotional Wellness

Emotions bridge the gap between mind and body. The person who is emotionally well understands his own feelings and knows when to express them appropriately. This individual accepts his limitations, has the ability to adjust to change, copes with stress in healthy ways, enjoys life, is optimistic and happy, and shows respect and affection to others.

Mental Wellness

The individual who is mentally well is alert, creative, logical, curious, open-minded, clear thinking, and accepting of others. This person also exhibits common sense, a good memory, and a desire for continual learning.

Intellectual Wellness

Intellectual wellness manifests as the ability to think, to process information, and to solve problems. The intellectually well person questions and evaluates information and situations, learns from life experiences, and is flexible, creative, and open to new ideas.

Vocational Wellness

The individual who is satisfied in school and/or job and who works in harmony with others enjoys vocational wellness (Figure 7-1).

Figure 7-1 Vocational wellness means being content and satisfied with your occupation.

CULTURAL CONSIDERATIONS

Spiritual Well-Being

Oman and Reed (1998) studied nearly 2,000 persons age 55 years and older for 5 years. They found that those persons who attended religious services were 24% less likely to have died in those 5 years than were those who did not attend services. This underscores the importance of religion and spiritual wellness to an individual's overall state of health.

Social Wellness

Social wellness is evident when a person shows concern, fairness, affection, and respect for others; communicates effectively; has satisfying relationships; and interacts well with others. This person has a network of family and friends, is a member of various organizations, and works with a spirit of teamwork. Other behaviors exhibited are honesty, loyalty, confidence, and tolerance.

Spiritual Wellness

Spiritual wellness gives meaning, direction, and purpose to life by way of values, ethics, and morals. The spiritually healthy person has faith, optimism, and high self-esteem.

Physical Wellness

Physical wellness is noted in the person who avoids risky sexual behavior; tries to limit exposure to environmental contaminants; and restricts the intake of alcohol, tobacco, caffeine, and drugs. Regular exercise, a well-balanced diet, and regular physical examinations also enhance physical wellness (Figure 7-2).

HEALTH PROMOTION

Health promotion means more than preventing illness: It means assisting individuals to enhance their health, well-being, and functioning and to maximize their potential. Health promotion focuses on adopting healthy behaviors rather than on avoiding illness. The goal is for individuals to control and improve their health. Health promotion is appropriate for the individual and the population as a whole.

The concept of self-responsibility is important to health promotion, and it must be accepted and acted on in order for wellness to become a reality for an individual. No one else can make a person live a healthy life; self-responsibility is the only way to make changes. An individual can be given information relating to health and wellness, but only that person can change unhealthy or destructive habits. With the exception of small children, each individual must take responsibility

Figure 7-2 Individuals must learn to achieve physical wellness in a manner that accommodates their lifestyle and physical abilities.

for behaviors leading to health and wellness (Figure 7-3). Objectives for healthy living are outlined in the Healthy People 2000 and Healthy People 2010 documents issued by the federal government.

Healthy People 2000

In 1980 and again in 1990, the United States Department of Health and Human Services (USDHHS) released a list of objectives for disease prevention and health promotion in 22 priority areas (USDHHS, 1990). In 1990, more than 10,000 individuals representing 300

PROFESSIONAL TIP

Predictors of Healthy Aging

The most consistent predictors of healthy aging are low serum glucose, normal blood pressure, avoidance of smoking, and maintenance of target weight for height (Reed, 1998). To prevent disease in later years, young adults and even adolescents must keep these four factors in check. Remind clients that it is never too late to modify these four factors to improve health.

Figure 7-3 Families can engage in activities together to achieve wellness.

national organizations were involved in developing the health objectives for the year 2000. More than 300 health objectives for the nation to achieve by the year 2000 evolved. These objectives were published in a document titled *Healthy People 2000: National Health Promotion and Disease Prevention Objectives,* which addresses three important issues:

- Personal responsibility: Each individual must be health-conscious and must practice responsible, informed health behaviors.
- Health benefits for all people: Everyone must have health benefits in order for the nation to be healthy.
- Health promotion and disease prevention: Health care must change from a treatment focus to a prevention focus to cut costs and to increase the quality of life.

The overall goals include:

- Increasing the span of healthy life for Americans,
- Reducing health disparities among Americans, and
- Achieving access to preventive services for all Americans.

A sample of the objectives is found in Table 7–1. The entire document may be ordered from the United States Department of Health and Human Services, Washington, DC, DHHS Publication No. (PHS) 91–50212.

The USDHHS (2000b) reported on the progress made in meeting the 319 objectives of Healthy People 2000. In 1997, 15% of the goals had been reached or surpassed, and progress had been made in another 44%. Eighteen percent had fallen short of target, 6% showed mixed results, and 2% showed no change. Eleven percent now have baseline data but no data to evaluate progress, and baselines have not yet been established for 3% of these goals (USDHHS, Healthy People 2000).

Healthy People 2010

The Healthy People 2000 Consortium met in November of 1996 to discuss necessary improvements and modifications to be made for Healthy People 2010 objectives. Over the past 4 years, the consortium worked with a wide range of representatives of national membership organizations, state governments, managed care organizations, and private businesses through focus groups, public meetings, and the Healthy People 2010 website. Several themes that emerged from the meetings and focus groups were earmarked to be addressed in the revised objectives. These include the:

- need to address morbidity and mortality in setting objectives,
- value of packaging the 2010 document into different formats for multiple audiences,
- necessity of linking objectives to community-based health improvement initiatives, and
- importance of using language that is understandable to the general public.

Two goals for the 2010 objectives emerged as a result of these sessions: (1) "Increase Years of Healthy Life," which was retained from the Healthy People 2000 goal, and (2) "Eliminate Health Disparities," a stronger version of the Healthy People 2000 goal "Reduce Health Disparities." These two goals will be supported by four enabling goals concerned with promoting healthy behaviors, protecting health, achieving access to quality health care, and strengthening community prevention. A comparison of select 2000 objectives is presented in Table 7–1, along with baselines, targets, and 2010 objectives.

The 467 objectives for 2010 are grouped into 28 focus areas. New focus areas include disability; people with low income; race and ethnicity; chronic diseases; and public health infrastructure (USDHHS, 2000a).

To expand the ability to track the objectives, new strategies are being developed to improve data collection, especially at the community level, and to improve the ability to measure access and quality of health services.

Healthy People 2010 was released in January 2000.

ILLNESS PREVENTION

Prevention (hindering, obstructing, or thwarting a disease or illness) incorporates both old and new ideas. The taboos, dietary laws, and traditions of various

Table 7–1 SELECTED OBJECTIVES FROM HEALTHY PEOPLE 2000 AND 2010

OBJECTIVE	BASELINE	YEAR 2000 TARGET	REPORT	YEAR 2010 TARGET
Physical Activity and Fitness				
• Increase the proportion of people who engage regularly in light to moderate physical activity for at least 30 minutes per day	22% (1985)	30%	23% (1995) (+)	30%
• Increase the proportion of young people in grades 9 to 12 who participate in daily school physical activity	42% (1991)	50%	27% (1997) (−)	50%
Nutrition				
• Increase the proportion of people aged 2 years and older who meet the Dietary Guidelines average daily goal of no more than 30% of calories from fat	34% (1989–91)	30%	33% (1994–96) (−)	75%
• Reduce the prevalence of BMI at or above 30.0 among people ages 20 years and older	24% males 27% females (1976–80)	20% both groups	34% males 37% females (1988–94) (−)	15%
Tobacco				
• Increase the proportion of cigarette smokers ages 18 years and older who stopped smoking cigarettes for a day	34% (1986)	50%	45.8% (1995) (+)	75%
• Increase the proportion of worksites with a formal smoking policy that prohibits smoking or limits it to separately ventilated areas at the workplace	NA	NA	59% of worksites with 50 or more employees (1992)	100%
Substance Abuse				
• Decrease alcohol-related motor vehicle crash deaths	9.8/100,000 (1987)	5.5/100,000	6.5/100,000 (1997)	3.5/100,000
• Reduce drug-related deaths	3.8/100,000 (1987)	3/100,000	4.7/100,000 (−) (1998)	1.3/100,000
Family Planning				
• Reduce the proportion of individuals ages 15 to 17 who have ever had sexual intercourse	33% of males 27% of females (1988)	15%	27% of males 22% of females (1999)	15%
• Increase the proportion of all females ages 15 to 44 at risk of unintended pregnancy who use contraception	88.2% (1982)	95%	92.5% (1999)	95% (modified to "use effective contraception")
Mental Health and Mental Disorders				
• Reduce suicide rates	11.7/100,000 (1987)	10.5/100,000	11.3/100,000 (1996)	9.6/100,000
Injury/Violence Prevention				
• Reduce firearm-related deaths	14.6/100,000 (1990)	11.6/100,000	13.5/100,000 (1996)	Fewer than 11.6/100,000
• Increase use of bicycle helmets of 9th- to 12th-grade students who ride bicycles		50%	8% (1995)	50%
Maternal, Infant, Child Health				
• Increase the proportion of all pregnant women who begin prenatal care in the first trimester of pregnancy	78.9% (1993)	90%	82.5% (1999)	90%
• Reduce the cesarean delivery rate	24.4/100 (1987)	15/100	21.8/100 (1999)	15/100
Cancer				
• Reduce cancer deaths		130/100,000	130/100,000 (1998) (=)	103/100,000

continues

Table 7–1 SELECTED OBJECTIVES FROM HEALTHY PEOPLE 2000 AND 2010 *continued*

OBJECTIVES	BASELINE	YEAR 2000 TARGET	REPORT	YEAR 2010 TARGET
AIDS/HIV Infection				
• Confine annual incidence of diagnosed AIDS cases among adolescents and adults	29.8/100,000 (1994)		28/100,000 (1998) (+)	12/100,000
• Increase the proportion of those with positive HIV tests who return for counseling	72.5% (1989)	80%	83% (1995) (+)	none
Sexually Transmitted Diseases				
• Reduce prevalence of *Chlamydia trachomatis* infections among 14–24 year olds	12.5% (1996)	5%	10.9% (1998)	3%
• Eliminate sustained domestic transmission of primary and secondary syphillis	84% higher than 1997 (1990)	4/100,000	3.2/100,000 (1998) (+)	0.25/100,000
Immunizatons and Infectious Diseases				
• Reduce indigenous cases of vaccine preventable diseases				
– Diphtheria		0	4 (1997)	0
– Polio		0	0 (1997)	0
– Measles	3,058 (1988)	0	135 (1997)	0
– Rubella	225 (1988)	0	161 (1997)	0
– Mumps	4,866 (1988)	500	612 (1997)	0
– Pertussis	3,450 (1988)	1,000	6,568 (1997) (−)	2,000
• Increase proportion of contacts completing course of preventive therapy for tuberculosis	66.3% (1987)	85%	65.4% (1995) (−)	85%
Environmental Health				
• Reduce exposure of children age 6 and younger who are regularly exposed to tobacco smoke	39% (1986)	20%	27% (1997)	15%

(+) Exceeding target
(−) Receding from target
(=) Met target

Data from U.S. Department of Health & Human Services (USDHHS), Public Health Service (PHS). (2000b). 1998–1999 Progress Review (On-line) Available: http://odphp.osophs.dhhs.gov/pubs/hp2000.

cultural, ethnic, and religious groups were initiated for a reason. If scientific research has not proved these incorrect or harmful, there is no reason not to practice the old ways. New methods of illness prevention emerge as technology expands and health awareness increases.

All stages of life should embody the tenets of preventive health. It must begin before conception with healthy parents and prenatal care and continue through the life span. Scientific advice based on firmly established medical data and reasonable probability should be heeded. Interventions for disease prevention range from lifestyle changes that cost little or nothing to high-tech procedures that are very expensive.

Before the full impact of illness prevention can be discovered, major changes are needed in health care delivery, funding, and insurance coverage. The health care system must insist on more research relating to prevention and must then apply the results of the research to insurance practices. Prevention practices must be supported and funded by the health care system in order for a change from illness treatment to illness prevention to occur. The rewards of such a shift will be enhanced health, longer life expectancy, and a population that feels better, looks better, and functions better.

Illness prevention must be viewed according to the type of prevention and the health care team responsible for its implementation.

Types of Prevention

Prevention extends to all stages of health. There are three types of prevention: primary, secondary, and tertiary. Primary prevention has not historically been supported by our health care system, whereas secondary and tertiary prevention have been, and still are, the main focus. They are also the most expensive.

Primary Prevention

Primary prevention includes all practices designed to keep health problems from developing. Following recommended childhood immunization schedules, not smoking to prevent lung cancer, and eating calcium-rich foods to prevent osteoporosis are all examples of primary prevention. Primary prevention should be the focus for every individual and health care provider. It is usually the least expensive intervention and provides the greatest benefits.

Secondary Prevention

Secondary prevention refers to early detection, diagnosis, screening, and intervention to reduce the consequences of a health problem. That is, disease or illness is identified before the individual has any symptoms or functional impairment. Screening for tuberculosis and performing monthly breast self-examinations are both examples of secondary prevention. When no known methods of primary prevention exist for a specific disease or illness (such as breast cancer), the focus should be on performing self-examinations, and having a regular physical exam, and testing.

Tertiary Prevention

Tertiary prevention refers to caring for a person who already has a health problem; the illness or disease is treated after symptoms have appeared so as to prevent further progression. For example, taking antibiotics for an ear infection should eliminate the infection. Furthermore, potential complications and the disability of hearing impairment are prevented. Rehabilitation is an important aspect of tertiary prevention; this refers to preventing deterioration of a person's condition and minimizing the loss of function. One example is providing range of motion exercises to a client who has had a stroke, to encourage circulation and maintain function in the extremities.

Prevention Health Care Team

The prevention health care team consists of the individual assisted by nurses and the primary physician.

Individual

The individual is the center of the prevention health care team. It is the individual who must incorporate the knowledge related to preventive health care and make the behavioral changes necessary to live a more healthy life.

Individuals should decide those things that they want and expect from health care. Honesty with self, the nurses, and physician is necessary. Clients must be assertive and ask questions of the physicians and nurses and be active, informed health care consumers. The ultimate responsibility for health care belongs with the individual.

Nurses

Nurses, especially nurse practitioners, often do the initial health screening in clinics and physicians' offices. This provides a great opportunity to inquire about lifestyle and the preventive health habits of the client. Nurses can use their excellent listening skills to give clients time to discuss health care habits and ask questions. Nurses are also great teachers of preventive health habits and health promotion activities.

Primary Physicians

Primary physicians generally are family practitioners, pediatricians, or internists: These are the family doctors, the physicians seen on a regular basis. They have the opportunity and obligation to discuss and inquire about preventive health habits. When necessary, they refer clients to specialists for specific problems. After the problem has been resolved, the client returns to the primary physician for further care.

FACTORS AFFECTING HEALTH

A great many factors affect health. They can be categorized into four broad topics:

- Genetics and human biology
- Personal behavior
- Environmental influences
- Health care

Genetics and Human Biology

Inherited traits and the way the human body functions have an impact on an individual's state of health and wellness. An individual's genetic make up may include inherited disorders, such as sickle-cell anemia, or chromosomal anomalies, such as Down syndrome. Both of these may ultimately affect the individual's quality of life and level of health.

Human biology affects health because normal body functioning prevents some illnesses and makes us more susceptible to others. Production of the female and male hormones, estrogen and testosterone, respectively, are responsible for many of these effects (Hoffman, 1996) (Table 7–2).

Personal Behavior

Personal behavior is the area having the most factors affecting health and wellness, and they are controlled entirely by the individual. It is the individual's decision to use or not to use these factors to promote health and wellness. Factors typically deemed to be under the individual's control include diet, exercise, personal care, sexual relationships, level of stress, tobacco and drug use, alcohol use, and safety.

Table 7–2 EFFECTS OF ESTROGEN AND TESTOSTERONE ON SPECIFIC TISSUES

| | HORMONE | |
Tissue	Estrogen (Female)	Testosterone (Male)
Cardiovascular	• Increases arterial dilation • Causes vascular spasms • Improves cardiac function	• Increases size of heart
Liver	• Inhibits production of triglycerides, low-density lipoprotein (LDL) (bad) cholesterol, and free glucose • Decreases drug metabolism, prolonging action	• Produces triglycerides, LDL (bad) cholesterol, and free glucose • Increases drug metabolism, shortening action
Fat	• Encourates fat deposits in breasts, hips, and thighs and suppresses the movement of fat from these areas	• Encourages fat deposits in the abdomen
Gastrointestinal	• Slows motility and favors formation of gallstones	
Respiratory	• Increases respiratory rate and basal body temperature	
Musculoskeletal	• Enhances bone density	• Ensures bone density and strength
Immune	• Enhances antibody production and suppresses T cell-mediated processes (prevents rejection of sperm and fetus)	
Blood	• Suppresses red blood cell (RBC) development • Lowers hemoglobin (Hgb) level • Increases coagulation	• Increases RBC development • Increases Hgb level
Integumentary	• Enhances skin vitality • Increases collagen and water content	• Promotes body hair

Adapted from Our Health, Our Lives, *by E. Hoffman, 1996, New York: Pocket Books. Copyright 1996 by Pocket Books.*

Diet

Healthy eating habits and a proper diet greatly enhance an individual's overall state of health and well-being. Eating both fulfills the basic biological needs of sustenance, nutrition, and hydration and allows individuals to meet social and interpersonal needs (Figure 7-4). All of these factors contribute to overall wellness.

Exercise

Integrating physical activity into daily life is one of the best ways of promoting health. Exercise improves circulation, muscle strength, and emotional well-being; lowers blood pressure; increases endurance; and reduces the chances of heart attack, stroke, and osteoporosis. The individual who exercises regularly looks healthier and feels better.

Many people have joined health clubs in an effort to meet their need for exercise. Health clubs can be a wonderful source of regular exercise, but, also, a source

Figure 7-4 Sharing meals together is a wonderful means of meeting both physical and interpersonal needs.

CULTURAL CONSIDERATIONS

Parents' Beliefs about Feeding Children

Many parents:

- Begin feeding cereal and other solid foods earlier than recommended, believing that milk alone will not satisfy their babies' hunger,
- Use food to soothe or console children,
- Believe a heavier child is a healthier child, and
- View having a heavy infant or toddler as evidence of parental competence (Baughcum, 1998).

Nurses can work with these clients by respecting their cultural beliefs while enforcing the notion that a healthy child is a child who is satisfied following a meal and who shows a healthy, normal physical and emotional growth pattern. These factors, not plumpness, are indicators of wellness.

of disease, as reported in *Health-Club Hygiene* (Nov. 6, 1995). For example, perspiration on exercise machines is a prime source of impetigo. Clients should be made aware of such dangers so that they can practice safety precautions, such as wearing thigh-length shorts and always keeping a towel between the body and the exercise equipment.

CLIENT TEACHING

Dietary Guidelines for Americans

Aim for fitness
- Aim for a healthy weight.
- Be physically active each day.

Build a healthy base
- Let the Pyramid guide your food choices.
- Choose a variety of grains daily, especially whole grains.
- Choose a variety of fruits and vegetables daily.
- Keep food safe to eat.

Choose sensibly
- Choose a diet that is low in saturated fat and cholesterol and moderate in total fat.
- Choose beverages and foods to moderate your intake of sugars.
- Choose and prepare foods with less salt.
- If you drink alcoholic beverages, do so in moderation.

From Home and Garden Bulletin No. 232 *(5th ed.), by U.S. Department of Agriculture and U.S. Department of Health and Human Services, 2000.*

CLIENT TEACHING

Preventing Food-Borne Diseases

Share the following tips with clients to educate them in ways to prevent food-borne diseases:

- Allow cooked foods to sit at room temperature for no more than 2 hours
- Date leftovers, refrigerate, and eat within 5 days
- Wash dirty dishes in hot (120°F) water, as dirty dishes are an ideal place for bacteria to multiply
- Keep dishcloths and sponges clean and allow to dry between uses
- Use a bleach solution to clean cutting boards and countertops
- Wash all fruits and vegetables in a diluted bleach solution (a bleach to water ratio of 1:100)

Personal Care

The skin protects the body from outside elements. It works with the immune system to defend the body against harmful bacteria, fungi, viruses, and allergens. Regular skin, hair, and nail care will enhance wellness and foster self-esteem. Personal care also includes such wellness habits as proper posture, proper body mechanics, adequate sleep, and dental hygiene.

Sexual Relationships

Establishing intimacy and a sexual relationship with another person is a natural step in growth and development. To maintain health and wellness, the individual will use values, ethics, and morals to guide the development of the relationship. A healthy sexual relationship is based on mutual satisfaction of the parties, a consensual approach to pleasurable activities, and mutual respect for preferences and personal choices.

Level of Stress

Not all stress is harmful. Limited stress makes one more alert and raises one's energy level. The way one responds to or copes with stressors dictates whether the situation is healthy or harmful. For instance, whereas one individual may enjoy the challenge of balancing work and family, another may feel torn by these seemingly conflicting demands and will therefore experience undue stress. Stress results not from an individual's life situation, but from that individual's reaction to and perception of the life situation.

Tobacco and Drug Use

Refraining from tobacco use is a strong step towards health promotion and maintenance. Even when a long-time smoker gives up the habit, the health risks begin to decrease at once; although it will take 10 to 15 years to eliminate all the effects of smoking from the lungs. The person who smokes exhales secondhand smoke, which presents a health risk to those who do not smoke.

PROFESSIONAL TIP

Moderate Exercise Reduces Stroke Risk

- Individuals who burn 1,000 to 1,999 calories per week by exercising moderately have a 24% lower risk of suffering a stroke than do those who burn less.
- Individuals who burn 2,000 to 2,999 calories per week by exercising moderately have a 46% lower risk.
- Burning over 2,999 calories a week through moderate exercise lowered the risk of having a stroke by only 20%.
- Moderate exercise includes activities such as brisk walking, dancing, and cycling (Lee & Paffenbarger, 1998).

Abuse of both illegal and prescription drugs is a serious medical and social problem in our society. Drugs prescribed by a physician are abused if they are not taken as directed, or if they are taken by anyone other than the client for whom they were prescribed. Many prescribed drugs can be addictive if not taken as directed. Health can be maintained when clients understand the effects, indications, side effects, and interactions of the prescription medications they are taking.

Alcohol Use

The decision to consume alcohol is a personal choice that can influence an individual's state of health. The amount of alcohol consumed will affect sobriety, decision-making ability, and, in many instances, safety. The use of alcohol can play a significant role in drownings, adult fire deaths, traffic fatalities, falling fatalities, and suicides.

Safety

Personal choices concerning safety affect many areas of an individual's life and can be viewed collectively more as a lifestyle choice than individually as separate acts to promote safety. For example, individuals who embrace safety as a fundamental element of health and well-being will ensure safety in their homes by having smoke detectors, fire extinguishers, carbon monoxide detectors, practiced escape plans, locked medicine cabinets, and gates blocking dangerous stairways. These individuals will also most likely buckle their car seat belts, secure their children in child car seats, and obey speed limits when driving. All these elements of safety add up to a healthy lifestyle.

Environmental Influences

Environmental factors that may influence health are numerous, can be natural or man-made, and vary de-

pending on geographic location and living conditions. Exposure to or ingestion of certain natural biological irritants can cause disease, such as results from exposure to poison ivy, and even death, such as results from ingestion of poison mushrooms. Exposure to chemicals such as asbestos in older buildings, lead in paint in older houses, and mercury in polluted water sources, can also pose health hazards. Radiation from the sun and certain types of machinery can be harmful in large doses; extreme, prolonged exposure to solar radiation can even result in death. Natural disasters such as hurricanes, floods, volcanic eruptions, droughts, heat waves, blizzards, and other extreme weather conditions pose health risks, as do man-made environmental crises including wars, bombings, pollution, and overpopulation.

Health Care

Most people use the health care system when they are ill, for the treatment of their disease or condition. A more effective use of the health care system, however, is health promotion and disease prevention. Routine physical examinations with minimal testing are invaluable for maintaining health and preventing disease (Figure 7-5). Healthy adults should consider health care services based on factors related to family health history, personal health history, personal habits, or the presence of symptoms that may alter the time frame for suggested health care services.

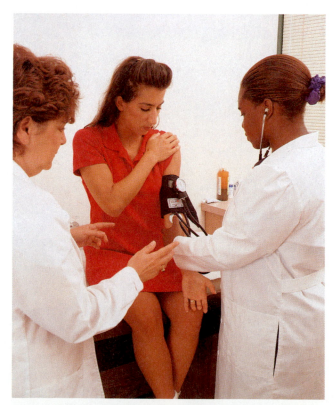

Figure 7-5 Routine physical examinations are essential to maintaining health and preventing disease.

Physical Exam

The physical examination should begin with a review of family health history, personal health history, personal habits (tobacco, alcohol, and drug use, sexual practices), and concerns or questions the client may have. Before visiting the physician, the client should write down questions and concerns so that none will be forgotten. Individuals between the ages of 20 and 39 years should have a complete physical exam every 1 to 3 years; those 40 to 49 years of age, every 1 to 2 years; and those over 50 years of age, every year. Women should have a breast exam with every physical exam obtained before age 40 and yearly thereafter. Men should have a testicular exam with every physical exam and should have a rectal exam to check the prostate at every physical exam obtained after age 40.

Immunizations

Adults who have not had the recommended immunizations as children should discuss this with their primary physicians. Depending on the client's risk factors, the physician may recommend having the immunizations as an adult.

Each adult should have a tetanus booster immunization every 10 years for life. Those at high risk of exposure, such as health care workers and college students; those who have chronic pulmonary, heart, or kidney disease; those who have diabetes; and those 65 years of age and older should have an influenza immunization every year and a pneumococcal pneumonia immunization every 6 years.

Tests

The following tests should be done with every physical exam: complete blood count, blood sugar, cholesterol, urinalysis, stool for blood, and, for women, a Papanicolau (Pap) smear. An electrocardiogram (EKG

PROFESSIONAL TIP

Mammograms

The Centers for Disease Control and Prevention (CDC) (1998) reports that 70.9% of insured women over 40 years of age had a mammogram in 1996–1997, but only 46.2% of uninsured women over age 40 had a mammogram in the same years.

or ECG) should be done at ages 20 years and 40 years and every 5 years thereafter (and yearly if the client is at high risk). Women should have a baseline mammogram (Figure 7-6) at age 40 and yearly thereafter. Men should have a testicular exam and rectal exam of the prostate at each physical exam. Each woman should perform a breast self-exam after every menstrual period. Each male should perform a testicular self-exam on a monthly basis.

Dental Exam

A dental exam, prophylaxis, and needed treatment should be performed every 6 to 12 months throughout life.

Eye Exam

An eye exam, including tonometry for glaucoma, should be performed every 2 to 3 years from ages 40 to 49 years and every 1 to 2 years after the age of 50.

PROFESSIONAL TIP

Hepatitis B Vaccine

Health care personnel who may be exposed to blood and body fluids are at risk for contracting the hepatitis B virus. Health care employers are required by law to offer the hepatitis B vaccination without cost to employees who are in direct care positions. Employees have the option of having or refusing this immunization. The vaccine is not contraindicated during pregnancy, and there are no apparent adverse effects to developing fetuses; however, the vaccine may cause shock in individuals who are allergic to baker's yeast.

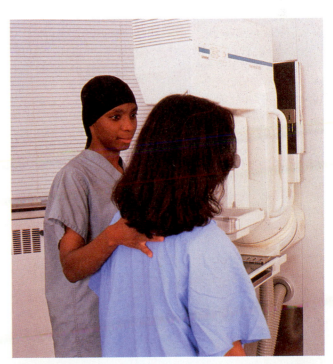

Figure 7-6 Mammograms are a key element to wellness promotion for all women over the age of 40 years.

CLIENT TEACHING

Crucial Health Practices

Simon (1992) states that all the medical progress in the United States from 1900–1990 increased the life span of an average adult by 4 years; but that simple lifestyle changes increased the life span of an average adult by 11 years. He describes 10 crucial health practices:

- Do not use tobacco and drugs.
- Do not consume more than 2 ounces of alcohol per day.
- Eat a diet low in fat, cholesterol, and salt but high in fiber, fruits, vegetables, and fish.
- Exercise regularly—1 hour each week is helpful, 3 is ideal.
- Stay lean.
- Drive cars with air bags and wear seatbelts; drive prudently, and never drink before driving.
- Avoid excessive stress.
- Minimize exposure to radiation, ultraviolet rays, chemical pollutants, and other environmental hazards.
- Protect self from sexually transmitted diseases.
- Obtain regular medical care including immunizations and screening tests.

GUIDELINES FOR HEALTHY LIVING

Because of their education and training, nurses are in a unique position to practice healthy living habits themselves and to promote such habits in their clients. Table 7–3 outlines select causes of death and the controllable lifestyle factors that most contribute to these types of deaths. While it is important to remember that certain health variables such as gender and race cannot be controlled or changed, others such as diet and tobacco use result from individual choice. These lifestyle choices are based on individual preference, and nurses can help clients make the best choices to promote wellness and optimal functioning. Following is a list of select guidelines, for nurses and their clients, to promote healthy living and wellness in daily life.

Heart Disease:
- Eat a diet low in fat and cholesterol and high in fiber
- Exercise regularly, 30 minutes three to five times a week (walking, swimming, cycling)
- Quit smoking or do not start to smoke
- Handle stress appropriately; use relaxation or meditation
- Do not use caffeine or alcohol excessively
- Maintain appropriate weight for height

Table 7–3 CONTROLLABLE FACTORS FOR TOP 10 CAUSES OF DEATH

CAUSE OF DEATH	CONTROLLABLE FACTORS
Heart disease	Tobacco use, high blood pressure, high cholesterol, lack of exercise, excessive stress, diabetes, obesity
Cancer	Tobacco use, radiation, alcohol abuse, improper diet, environmental exposure
Stroke	Tobacco use, high blood pressure, high cholesterol, lack of exercise
Chronic lung disease	Tobacco use, environmental exposures
Accidents	Alcohol abuse, drug abuse, tobacco use, failure to use seat belts, fatigue, stress, recklessness
Pneumonia and influenza	Chronic lung disease, environmental exposures, tobacco use, alcohol abuse, lack of immunization
Diabetes	Obesity, improper diet, lack of exercise, excessive stress
AIDS	Unsafe sex, neglecting condom use
Suicide	Excessive stress, alcohol abuse, drug abuse
Liver disease	Alcohol abuse, exposure to toxins (ingested and environmental), lack of immunizations

Top 10 data from National Center for Health Statistics (1997) monthly vital statistics report. 45 (1152) 23, 40–43. [On-line] Available: www.youfirst.com/risks.htm

- Maintain normal blood pressure
- Have a regular physical exam

Osteoporosis:
- Throughout life, eat calcium-rich foods (milk and milk products) and a balanced diet
- Get plenty of exercise
- Discuss with the primary care physician the need for a calcium supplement and estrogen replacement therapy (females)
- Do not smoke

Cancer:
- Do not smoke
- Avoid exposure to unnecessary radiation
- Protect skin from ultraviolet rays; use sunscreen
- Avoid exposure to harmful chemicals
- Minimize exposure to pesticides, herbicides, and poisons

- Limit alcohol intake
- Eat a well-balanced diet with adequate fiber
- Exercise
- Practice safe sex
- Have cancer screening tests—mammogram, Pap smear, fecal occult blood test, and rectal exam—with each physical exam

Low-Back Pain:
- Exercise regularly
- Practice good posture
- Use proper body mechanics

Colds and Flu:
- Wash hands frequently
- Use paper tissues and dispose of properly
- Have flu shots yearly
- Follow the Dietary Guidelines for Americans for a balanced diet
- Drink plenty of fluids

Breast Cancer:
- Eat a diet low in fat
- Exercise regularly
- Limit alcohol and caffeine intake
- Perform monthly breast self-examinations
- Have mammograms as recommended by the American Cancer Society

Sexually Transmitted Diseases:
- Practice monogamous sex between noninfected individuals
- Use latex condoms

Tuberculosis (especially for health care workers):
- Mantoux test
- Isoniazid preventive therapy—any newly exposed and infected individual taking a full course of therapy (Reichman & Mangura, 1996)

Urinary Tract Infections:
- Drink plenty of water
- Empty bladder frequently, especially before and after sexual intercourse
- Wear underwear with a cotton crotch
- Wipe from front to back
- Drink cranberry juice
- Avoid bubble bath, douches, and scented or colored toilet paper

Sickle-Cell Anemia and Thalassemia:
- Request genetic screening and counseling if a high-risk group

Cataracts:
- Wear sunglasses and a hat with a brim
- Eat a well-balanced diet
- Do not smoke

Glaucoma:
- Have tonometry performed
- Have an optic nerve exam

Sunburn:
- Always wear suncreen (with a minimum SPF of 15) when out in the sun

Dental Caries and Periodontal Disease:
- Brush after each meal; floss daily
- Use fluoride toothpaste
- Have a professional cleaning twice a year
- Have a dental exam yearly

Home Safety:
- Lock cupboards containing medicines and cleaning materials
- Maintain working smoke alarms and fire extinguishers
- Use a carbon monoxide alarm in the presence of gas appliances and heaters
- Plan escape routes in case of fire and have fire drills
- Safety proof home against falls
- Know water safety rules

Work Safety:
- Follow workplace safety regulations
- Report unsafe equipment or practices

Travel Safety:
- Wear a seat belt
- Do not drink and drive
- Drive safely and defensively
- Use infant and child seats and restraints
- Wear a helmet when riding a bicycle or motorcycle
- Never swim alone

Weight:
- Follow the Dietary Guidelines for Americans for a balanced diet
- Exercise 30 minutes daily
- If overweight, eat the least number of servings recommended
- If needed, use raw fruits or vegetables as snacks between meals
- If underweight, eat the largest number of servings recommended
- Eat a nutritious snack between meals

Stress:
- Identify sources of stress
- Establish realistic goals and expectations
- Be flexible
- Express thoughts and feelings
- Do not depend on alcohol or drugs for relaxation
- Exercise
- Practice deep breathing and muscle relaxation
- Get enough sleep
- Have a sense of humor—laugh
- Obtain professional help when needed

SUMMARY

- Wellness includes prevention, early detection, and treatment of health problems.
- The best way to maintain health is to follow the Dietary Guidelines for Americans, exercise regularly, reduce stress, prevent accidents, and receive routine health exams.
- The leading causes of death can be significantly reduced by lifestyle changes.
- Physical, mental, emotional, social, and spiritual aspects play a key role in the ability to resist disease and maintain health and wellness.

Review Questions

1. The person responsible for health maintenance and disease prevention is the:

    a. nurse.
    b. physician.
    c. individual.
    d. nurse practitioner.

2. The Healthy People 2000 objectives:

    a. are related only to physical fitness.
    b. are related only to disease conditions.
    c. address the treatment of disease conditions.
    d. address the issue of personal responsibility for health behaviors.

3. Primary prevention:

    a. begins with the physician.
    b. is curing a disease in a week.
    c. takes place before disease begins.
    d. includes all diseases or conditions.

4. The prevention health care team is composed of the:

    a. dietitian, nurses, and pharmacist.
    b. individual, physician, and nurses.
    c. physician, pharmacist, and laboratory.
    d. radiology, laboratory, and individual.

5. Health is improved by:

    a. not smoking.
    b. drinking alcohol.
    c. eating more sweet foods.
    d. sleeping 3 to 4 hours each night.

6. How often should an individual have a physical exam?

    a. Every year.
    b. Every two years.
    c. Every three years.
    d. It depends on the person's age.

7. A genogram is used for:

    a. building a family tree.
    b. identifying potential health problems.
    c. preventing most diseases and illnesses.
    d. identifying the genes a person inherits.

8. Colds and flu can best be prevented by:

    a. smoking.
    b. staying warm and dry.
    c. washing hands frequently.
    d. having a flu shot every three years.

Critical Thinking Questions

1. How can you assist a client in identifying potential health problems?

2. What kind of preventive health care should be received by a person 20 years old, 42 years old, and 65 years old?

3. How does the nurse's state of health affect client care?

 WEB FLASH!

- What information does the Internet provide about Healthy People 2010?
- What information/resources can be found about wellness?

ALTERNATIVE/ COMPLEMENTARY THERAPIES

MAKING THE CONNECTION

Refer to the following chapters to increase your understanding of alternative/complementary therapy:

- **Chapter 6, Cultural Diversity and Nursing**
- **Chapter 7, Wellness Concepts**

LEARNING OBJECTIVES

Upon completion of this chapter, you should be able to:

- *Define key terms.*
- *Describe the historical influences on current alternative/complementary modalities.*
- *Discuss the connection between mind and body and the effect of this relationship on a person's health.*
- *Explain the concept of the nurse as an instrument of healing in holistic nursing practice.*
- *Identify the various mind-body, body-movement, energetic-touch healing, spiritual, nutritional, and other modalities that can be used as complementary therapies in client care.*
- *Discuss the use of alternative/complementary modalities.*

KEY TERMS

acupressure	healing touch
acupuncture	hypnosis
alternative therapy	imagery
antioxidant	instrument of healing
aromatherapy	meditation
biofeedback	neuropeptide
bodymind	neurotransmitter
centering	phytochemical
complementary therapy	psychoneuro-immunology
curing	shaman
energetic-touch therapy	shamanism
free radical	therapeutic massage
healing	therapeutic touch
	touch

INTRODUCTION

Western society tends to think of health and healing in terms of medical, surgical, and other technological interventions. However, in many other cultures—both past and present—healing has been promoted by faith, magic, ritual, and other nonmedical approaches.

The use of **alternative therapies** (therapies used *instead of* conventional or mainstream medical modalities) and **complementary therapies** (therapies used *in conjunction with* conventional medical therapies) is becoming more prevalent among the general public (Keegan, 1998).

This chapter addresses alternative/complementary treatment methods that are currently being used in ho-

listic nursing practice. Nurses are encouraged to think critically before recommending or implementing any of these approaches. Whether they simply discuss alternative/complementary therapies with clients or perform these therapies, nurses should understand the ramifications.

Because more and more states are regulating alternative/complementary therapies, nurses must know the laws that govern these therapies in the states in which they work. Some states have outlawed certain therapies or consider them experimental procedures, whereas other states require licensure or certain educational standards before allowing practitioners to perform alternative/complementary therapies. Nurses who perform alternative/complementary therapies not in accordance with the laws of their respective states could have legal charges filed against them (Brooke, 1998).

Employer policy and the nurse's job description must also be checked to confirm that performing alternative/complementary therapies is within the nurse's scope of practice at that agency. Employer malpractice insurance policies typically do not cover situations where a client is injured as a result of an alternative/complementary therapy. The financial risk of any nurse who engages in alternative/complementary therapies will be lowered by having insurance that specifically covers those therapies.

HISTORICAL INFLUENCES ON CONTEMPORARY PRACTICES

For as long as history has been recorded, people have tried to cure ills and relieve pain. Early cave drawings depict healers practicing their art. Primitive healers attributed the cause of mysterious diseases to magic and superstition; as a result, religious beliefs and health practices became intertwined. Remedies and practices that are based in ancient traditions are being rediscovered and used by contemporary holistic healers. A brief look at ancient Greek, Far Eastern, Chinese, Indian, and Shamanistic practices will highlight their influences on modern alternative/complementary modalities.

Ancient Greece

In the ancient Greek culture, health was perceived as the maintenance of balance in all dimensions of life. In Greek mythology, Asclepius was the god of healing. Temples (called Ascleipions) were beautiful places for people (regardless of ability to pay) to rest, restore themselves, and worship. The elaborate healing system consisted of myths, symbols, and rites administered by rigorously trained priest-healers. Illnesses were treated by restoring balance to a person's life through music, art, baths, massage, laughter, herbs, and simple surgery (Keegan, 1994). Many of our current therapies such as massage, art therapy, and herbal therapy have origins in ancient Greek traditions.

The Far East

Healing systems from the Far East have traditionally integrated mind, body, and spirit into a system of balanced energy between the individual and the universe. The concept of a life force or life energy "has been recognized in many cultural traditions. . . . What is universally agreed on is that the more [life energy] you have, the more vital your mental and bodily processes" (Chopra, 1998). The origins of some energetic-touch therapies can be traced to the Far East.

China

The traditional Chinese healing system is based on the belief in the oneness of all things in nature. Life energy (chi) flows through both the universe and the person, thus creating a wholeness among all things and people. Chi provides warmth, protection from illness, and vitality. Chi flows along an invisible system of meridians (pathways) that link the organs together and connect them to the external environment and, therefore, to the universe. Illness and injury can alter the flow of this energy. The energy flow can be influenced by stimulating points along the meridians.

Herbalism is an essential component of traditional Chinese healing practice. In seeking to promote balance, healers use herbs for dual purposes. For example, the herb dan qui relaxes the uterus when it is contracted (as in preterm labor) and tightens it if it is too relaxed (when normal labor needs to be enhanced). A complete discussion of the use of herbs in contemporary health practices appears later in this chapter.

Many contemporary Western health care providers are studying and now using traditional Chinese healing techniques. **Acupuncture**, one technique used in traditional Chinese medicine, is the application of heat and needles to various points on the body to alter the energy flow (Figure 8-1). Acupuncture is helpful in relieving headache and low back pain (Eisenberg, 1993) and is used to treat a variety of chronic and acute conditions.

India

Practiced for more than 4,000 years by the people of India, Ayurvedic medicine emphasizes prevention and a holistic approach to life (Keegan, 1994). The term *ayurveda* (meaning "the science of life") refers to India's traditional medicine and has an underlying spiritual basis. The life energy (prana) is transported through the body by a "wind" or vata. Vata regulates every type of movement.

Figure 8-1 Acupuncturist, Nurse, and Client

Vata, Kapha, and Pitta are the three metabolic principles (doshas) that provide life to all living things (Chopra, 1998). Kapha is the energy responsible for body structure, and pitta is the transformative process between vata and kapha. Each person is born with a unique balance of the three doshas. One predominates, and that dosha determines body type, temperament, and susceptibility to certain illnesses.

In the Ayurvedic system, chakras are areas of energy concentration in the body. Like the Chinese pathways (or meridians), these areas can become stagnant and blocked, thus causing illness. Ayurvedic healers seek to activate chakra energy for self-healing.

Prevention of illness and restoration of health through inner search and spiritual growth are the primary goals in the Ayurvedic system. Union of the Divine and the Truth occurs through the physical and meditative practice of yoga. In contemporary practice, Ayurvedic intervention may consist of yoga, herbs, diet, and exercise; methods to cleanse the body, such as steam baths, cathartics, and detoxifying massage; and nasal purging.

Shamanistic Tradition

A need to understand and explain life processes (i.e., birth, health, illness, and death) is part of being human. In many cultures, both modern and ancient, ritualized practices have been used to keep peace with the great spirits, to harness their power, to promote power, and to prevent death.

Shamanism refers to the practice of entering altered states of consciousness with the intent of helping others. The **shaman** is a folk healer-priest who uses natural and supernatural forces to help others and who has an extensive knowledge of herbs, is skilled in many forms of healing, and serves as guardian of the spirits. Illness is considered to be the result of spirit loss; shamans have the power to heal by working with the spirits to encourage their full return to the individual. The shaman functions as both healer and priest and one who has access to the supernatural.

Seeking wisdom about the universe, establishing a relationship with the creator, and avoiding death are all feats accomplished through ritualized processes performed by the shaman. The shaman's practice incorporates special objects such as power animals, totems, and fetishes as well as ritual songs, dances, food, and clothing. Sleep deprivation, ritual chants, isolation, imagery, drumming, and hallucinogenic drugs may be used to create a trance-like state that is the vehicle through which the shaman contacts the spirit world. The contemporary practices of hypnosis and guided imagery have roots in Shamanistic traditions.

MODERN TRENDS

The public perception of alternative/complementary treatment methods has been changing over the past few decades. In the late 1960s and early 1970s, the "natural," "new age," and "self-help" movements began to attract followers, first among consumers and later among health care practitioners. During that time period, there was a growing trend toward rejection of traditional medicine because of its perceived invasiveness, painfulness, cost, and ineffectiveness. A rekindled interest in Eastern religions, lifestyle, and medicine has fueled the development of contemporary holistic, alternative/complementary modalities. Clients are seeking out alternative/complementary therapies because most such therapies are noninvasive, holistic, and, in many instances, less expensive than going to a physician (Keegan, 1998).

Astin (1998) reports that 40% of the U.S. population now uses some type of complementary/alternative therapy in addition to standard medical treatment, spending about $13 billion each year on these therapies. In 1992, the U.S. government established the Office of Alternative Medicine (OAM) at the National Institutes of Health and allocated $2 million to disseminate information about complementary and alternative medicine to practitioners and the public. Congress increased the OAM's budget to $20 million for fiscal year 1998 (National Institutes of Health, 1998).

Then in late 1998, Congress established the National Center for Complementary and Alternative Medicine (NCCAM), which replaced the Office of Alternative Medicine. Their budget for the fiscal year 2000 is $68.7 million (National Institutes of Health, 2000). The NCCAM has the added responsibility of investigating the application of treatments shown to be effective.

Mind/Body Medicine and Research

The traditional medical model is founded on the belief that the mind, body, and spirit are separate entities. A relatively new field of science, however, called **psychoneuroimmunology** (PNI), is studying the complex relationship among the cognitive, affective, and physical aspects of humans. Psychoneuroimmunologists are investigating the way the brain transmits signals along the nerves to enhance the body's normal immune functioning. This research supports the idea that the human mind can alter physiology.

All body cells have receptor sites for **neuropeptides**, amino acids that are produced in the brain and other sites in the body and that act as chemical communicators. Neuropeptides are released when **neurotransmitters** (chemical substances produced by the body that facilitate nerve-impulse transmission) signal emotions in the brain. Pert, of the National Institutes of Health, wrote in 1986 that "the more we know about neuropeptides, the harder it is to think in the traditional terms of a mind and a body. It makes more sense to speak of a single integrated entity, a 'body-mind'" (Pert, 1986).

Thus, it is possible for cells to be directly affected by emotions. In other words, people can affect their health by what they think and feel. There are many examples of terminally ill persons hanging on to life until the occurrence of a specific event such as a child coming to visit or a grandchild's graduation or marriage.

The intermeshed, complex system of psyche and body chemistry is now referred to as the **bodymind**, the inseparable connection and operation of thoughts, feelings, and physiological functions. According to psychologist Earnest Rossi (1993), because all body systems are interconnected, mental images can be converted into neurotransmitters in the autonomic nervous system, hormones in the endocrine system, and white blood cells in the immune system. These three systems (nervous, endocrine, and immune) are interactive, thus modulating the activity of each other (Rossi, 1993). This helps explain how some alternative/complementary therapies allow the calming influences of the parasympathetic system to take over during stress-inducing situations such as illness (Dossey, 1995b).

Holism and Nursing Practice

The expansion of the holistic health movement has been based on the growing acceptance of the concept that body, mind, and spirit are interconnected. Nursing in its broadest sense (theory, concept, and practice) is truly holistic in nature. Holism encompasses consideration of the physiological, psychological, sociocultural, intellectual, and spiritual aspects of each individual. Holistic nursing can be described as the art and science of caring for the whole person, knowing that each person is unique in all expressions of self. This means that the nursing assessment must include eliciting information regarding client use of complementary/alternative therapies (Hodge and Ullrich, 1999).

As holistic caregivers, nurses may employ alternative/complementary techniques to promote clients' well-being. The focus of care in these practices is healing, as opposed to curing. The word **healing** is derived from the Anglo-Saxon word *hael*, meaning "to make whole, to move toward, or to become whole." It is important to establish that healing is not the same as **curing** (ridding one of disease), but is instead a process that activates the individual's forces from within. As a healing facilitator, the nurse enters into a relationship with the client and can assist the client by offering to be a guide, change agent, or **instrument of healing** (a means by which healing can be achieved, performed, or enhanced).

When the nurse serves as an instrument of healing, the objective is to help the client call forth inner re-

sources for healing. In order to accomplish this goal, nurses must develop the following attributes:

- Knowledge base: initially established in nursing school and then continuously expanded through lifelong learning
- Intentionality: having a conscious direction of goals, essential in helping the healer to focus
- Respect for differences: demonstrated by honoring clients' culturally based health beliefs
- Ability to model wellness: tending to one's own needs and attempting to stay as healthy and balanced as possible

ALTERNATIVE/ COMPLEMENTARY INTERVENTIONS

Many alternative/complementary interventions are used in holistic nursing practice. These interventions are categorized as mind/body, body-movement, energetic-touch, spiritual, nutritional/medicinal, and other methodologies (Table 8–1). Although different in technique, many of the alternative/complementary therapies have common ideological threads, as follows:

- The *whole system* must be considered if the *parts* of the individual are to be helped to function.
- The person is integrated and related to the surroundings.
- There exists some life force or energy that can be used in the healing process.
- Ritual, prescribed practice and skilled practitioners are integral parts of holistic healing interventions.

PROFESSIONAL TIP

Use of Alternative/Complementary Therapy

Practical ways for nurses to use alternative/complementary therapies include:

- Having a nonjudgmental attitude about these therapies;
- Asking clients whether they use any nontraditional therapies and, if so, asking which therapies, why, and how the therapies have worked;
- Getting adequate instruction in these therapies before trying to administer them;
- Trying one or two basic therapies such as massage or guided imagery; and
- Discussing a therapy with the client *before* using it (Keegan, 1998).

Table 8–1 CATEGORIES OF ALTERNATIVE/COMPLEMENTARY INTERVENTIONS

MIND/BODY	BODY MOVEMENT	ENERGETIC TOUCH	SPIRITUAL	NUTRITIONAL/ MEDICINAL	OTHER
Meditation	Movement and exercise	Touch	Faith Healing	Phytochemicals and antioxidants	Aromatherapy
Relaxation	Yoga	Therapeutic massage	Healing Prayer	Macrobiotic diet	Humor
Imagery	Tai chi	Therapeutic touch	Shamanism:	Herbal therapy	Pet Therapy
Biofeedback	Chiropractic therapy	Healing touch	• Sand painting		Music therapy
Hypnosis		Acupressure	• Sweat lodges		
		Reflexology	• Drumming		

Adapted from Fundamentals of Nursing: Standards & Practice, *by S. DeLaune and P. Ladner, 1998, Albany, NY: Delmar. Copyright 1998 by Delmar. Adapted with permission.*

Mind/Body (Self-Regulatory) Techniques

Self-regulatory techniques are methods by which an individual can, independently or with assistance, consciously control some functions of the sympathetic nervous system (for example, heart rate, respiratory rate, and blood pressure). When the client is learning the way to perform these techniques, an assistant is involved; later, however, the client can perform them independently. Self-regulatory techniques include meditation, relaxation, imagery, biofeedback, and hypnosis.

Meditation

The practice of **meditation**, quieting the mind by focusing the attention, can bring about remarkable physiological changes. People who meditate strive for a sense of oneness within themselves and a sense of relatedness to a greater power and the universe.

A person can be guided into a meditative or relaxed state with breath coaching (assisting the client to become aware of or focus on breathing and thus slow it). Meditation has proved particularly beneficial for clients in labor. Nurses can teach this modality to clients by using verbal cues, counting the client's inhalations and exhalations, and showing the client the way to take slow, deep breaths. According to Borysenko and Borysenko (1994), some therapeutic benefits of meditation are:

- Stress relief,
- Relaxation,
- Reduced level of lactic acid,
- Decreased oxygen consumption,
- Slowed heart rate,
- Decreased blood pressure, and
- Improved functioning of the immune system.

Relaxation

In 1975, cardiologist Herbert Benson studied the effects of meditation on individuals. He then incorporated

CLIENT TEACHING

Progressive Muscle Relaxation

After explaining the purpose and process of progressive muscle relaxation, instruct the client to:

- Assume a comfortable position in a quiet environment.
- Close eyes and keep them closed until the exercise is completed.
- Breathe in deeply to a count of 4.
- Hold breath for a count of 4.
- Breathe out to a count of 4.
- Continue to breathe slowly and deeply.
- Tense both feet until muscle tension is felt.
- Hold a gentle state of tension in both feet for a count of 3.

Caution the client to tighten the muscles only until the muscles are tensed, not to the point of pain.

- Slowly release the tension from the feet.
- Fully experience the difference between tension and relaxation.
- Repeat the previous three steps.
- Gently tense the muscles of both lower legs.
- Continue this procedure with all the muscle groups in a toe-to-head direction.
- After tensing and releasing all muscle groups, take in a few more deep relaxing breaths and scan your body for any areas that remain tense. Concentrate on tensing and relaxing the muscles in those areas.
- Breathe in deeply to a count of 4.
- Hold breath for a count of 4.
- Breathe out to a count of 4.
- Resume your usual breathing pattern.
- Slowly stretch and open your eyes.

To be effective, this procedure requires approximately 20 to 30 minutes. Like all other relaxation exercises, progressive muscle relaxation is most effective with repetition.

the basic elements of meditation into the therapeutic process he called the *relaxation response* (Benson, 1975). Benson employed the relaxation response with individuals experiencing high blood pressure and heart disease. Benson discovered that the techniques were more effective if individuals focused on an inspirational prayer or phrase. The basic elements of the relaxation response are:

- A quiet environment,
- A comfortable position,
- Focused attention,
- A passive attitude, and
- Practice.

One method for achieving relaxation is progressive muscle relaxation (PMR), which is the alternate tensing and relaxing of muscles. Clients are instructed to concentrate on a certain body area (the jaw, for instance), tense the muscles for a count of five, then relax the muscles for a count of five. This process is repeated for muscle groups over the entire body until the client has achieved a state of overall relaxation.

Nurses can use relaxation techniques in their work with clients to reduce pain and stress. Relaxation techniques are also an essential aspect of cognitive behavioral therapy when treating people with phobias, fear, and depression.

Imagery

Imagery is a technique of using the imagination to visualize a pleasant, soothing image. The practitioner encourages the client to use as many of the senses as possible in order to enhance the formation of vivid images. Table 8–2 presents examples of incorporating all five senses into imagery.

Nurses can create guided imagery for many clients who are capable of hearing and understanding the nurse's suggestions of meaningful and physiologically correct images. For example, a nurse can show a chart of the stages of bone healing to a client who has suffered a fracture and ask the client to imagine this sequential activity in his body.

Table 8–2 INCORPORATING ALL FIVE SENSES INTO IMAGERY

SENSE	IMAGERY
Visual	See the dark blue sky
Auditory	Hear the babbling brook
Kinesthetic	Feel yourself floating on a cloud
Gustatory	Taste the tartness of a freshly cut lemon
Olfactory	Smell the salt air at the ocean

CLIENT TEACHING

Guided Imagery

After explaining the purpose and process of guided imagery, instruct the client to:

- Assume a comfortable position in a quiet environment.
- Close your eyes and keep them closed until the exercise is completed.
- Breathe in deeply to a count of 4.
- Hold breath for a count of 4.
- Breathe out to a count of 4.
- Continue to breathe slowly and deeply.
- Think of your favorite place and prepare to take an imaginary journey there. Select a place in which you are relaxed and at peace.
- Picture in your mind's eye your favorite place. Look around you and see all the colors, the light and shadows, and all the pleasant sights.
- Listen to all the sounds. Pay attention to what you hear.
- Feel all the physical sensations . . . the temperature . . . the textures . . . the movement of the air.
- As you take in a deep breath, smell the aromas of your favorite place.
- Taste the foods and drinks you usually consume in your favorite place. Savor each taste fully.
- Focus all your attention totally on your favorite place.
- Breathe in deeply to a count of 4.
- Hold breath for a count of 4.
- Breathe out to a count of 4.
- Resume your usual breathing pattern.
- Slowly open your eyes and stretch, if desired.

This procedure works best when all five senses are used. Like all other relaxation exercises, guided imagery becomes more effective with repetition.

"The nurse using guided imagery can promote a sense of well-being in clients and help them change their perceptions about their disease, treatment, and healing ability" (Dossey, 1995a). Studies have found that a combination of medication and guided imagery decreases physical tension, anxiety, and the adverse effects of chemotherapy (Keegan, 1998). In addition to being a tool for distraction when a person is confronting pain, discomfort, and fear, imagery is also a powerful mechanism for making decisions and for altering behaviors, as it allows the client to try out decisions and behaviors before actually implementing them. The power of the human imagination is limitless, and helping clients to use that power can be a rewarding role for the nurse.

Biofeedback

Biofeedback is a measurement of physiological responses that yields information about the relationship between the mind and the body and helps clients learn ways to manipulate those responses through mental activity. Biofeedback allows a person to see the effect of the mind on the body. While attached to sensitive devices that measure bodily responses such as skin temperature, blood pressure, galvanic skin resistance, and electrical activity in the muscles, the individual imagines stressful experiences. The individual's physiological responses are then measured and recorded, as are the individual's physiological responses to relaxation. The individual receives an interpretation of these responses and is taught methods for practicing relaxation to control reactions to stressful experiences.

Biofeedback is used as a restorative method in rehabilitation settings to help clients who have lost sensation and function as the result of illness or injury. Machines that can detect a person's internal bodily functions translate them into a form that the client can detect, such as a light or beep. After training with the machine, clients are able to alter their responses without the machine. Biofeedback also enhances relaxation in tense muscles, relieves tension headaches and backache, and reduces bruxism (grinding of the teeth) and the pain associated with temporomandibular joint syndrome (Association of Psychophysiology and Biofeedback, 1998). Temperature biofeedback is useful in training clients to purposefully warm their hands to treat Raynaud's disease (a circulatory disorder), to lower blood pressure, and to prevent or relieve migraine headaches.

Hypnosis

The practice of hypnosis was once overshadowed by mystery and misconception. Today, with our expanding knowledge of the human mind, hypnosis is becoming a more common nursing intervention (Zahourek & Larkin, 1995). Therapeutic **hypnosis** induces an altered state of consciousness or awareness resembling sleep and during which the person is more receptive to suggestion. Hypnosis also enhances the client's ability to form images.

Nurses wishing to use hypnosis in their practices must be aware of the guidelines concerning this modality with regard to the scope of practice as defined by their respective state boards of nursing. They also should receive advanced training in the art of hypnosis (Kolkmeier, 1995).

Body-Movement (Manipulation) Strategies

As the name implies, body-movement therapies employ techniques of moving or manipulating various body parts to achieve therapeutic outcomes. Modalities such as movement and exercise, yoga, tai chi, and chiropractic treatment are discussed in the following sections.

Movement and Exercise

Movement, as a therapeutic intervention and health-promoting activity, is associated with athletic exercise, dance, celebration, and healing rituals. Although the primary goal of exercise is fitness (muscle strength, flexibility, endurance, and cardiovascular and respiratory health), there are many other positive outcomes of exercise, such as feeling more energetic and sleeping better.

Nurses can help clients use movement as therapy in a variety of ways such as range of motion exercises, water exercises, physical therapy, and stretching exercises. Movement is an effective method through which people of all ages can improve their level of functioning. Exercise has also been documented to improve functional ability in people with arthritis (Budesheim, Neuberger, Kasal, Vogel-Smith, Hassanein, & DeViney, 1994).

Yoga

Many cultures believe that particular forms of movement keep the body's life forces in correct balance and flow. Yoga and tai chi are examples of ancient ritual movements that enhance overall health including spiritual enlightenment and well-being. Both of these approaches require concentration and the use of symbolic movements.

A form of meditative exercise, yoga rejuvenates, promotes longevity and self-realization, and speeds the natural evolution of the person toward self-enlightenment. Traditional yoga has always been primarily concerned with healthy individuals and promoting health by maintaining the balance and flow of life forces.

Yoga therapy is an effort to integrate traditional yogic concepts and techniques with Western medical and psychological knowledge (Feuerstein, 1998). The focus of yoga therapy is to holistically treat various psychological or somatic dysfunctions ranging from back problems to emotional distress.

Both yoga and yoga therapy are based on the understanding that the human being is an integrated body/mind system that best functions in a state of dynamic

GERONTOLOGICAL CONSIDERATIONS

Exercise and the Very Old

Those of very advanced ages (95 years and older) are achieving positive results from regular exercise and weight lifting, including increased physical strength and flexibility and improved mental status in areas such as memory and depression (Mills, 1994).

balance (Feuerstein, 1998). Studies regarding benefits of yoga practice have found that mentally challenged individuals become more aware of their bodies and enjoy improved coordination, while clients with osteo-arthritis of the hands experience less pain (Keegan, 1998). Claims made by yoga authorities range from a beneficial effect on physical flexibility, muscle tone, and stamina to a reduction in obesity, back pain, hypertension, various respiratory diseases, anxiety, and memory loss (Feuerstein, 1998).

Tai Chi

Tai chi is based on the philosophy of the quest for harmony with nature and the universe through the laws of complementary (yin and yang) balance. When perfect harmony exists, everything functions effortlessly, spontaneously, perfectly, and in accordance with the laws of nature. If one moves to the right, then one must also move to the left. Tai chi consists of a series of sequential, dance-like movements connected in a smooth-flowing process. The movements, accompanied by deep breathing, improve flexibility, range of motion, muscle strength, and balance (Cerrato, 1999d).

People who regularly perform tai chi believe that it enhances stamina, agility, and balance and that it boosts energy and confers a sense of well-being. Tai chi has been shown to reduce blood pressure and the risk of falling in the elderly, and significantly reduced discomfort of clients with low back pain (Cerrato, 1999).

Chiropractic Therapy

The major principle underlying chiropractic therapy is that the brain sends vital energy to every organ in the body via the nerves originating in the spinal column. Dis-ease, body disharmony, or malfunction results from vertebral subluxation complex (spinal nerve stress). The body is rebalanced and realigned using chiropractic "spinal adjustment" techniques.

The goal of chiropractic care is to awaken the client's own natural healing ability by correcting any areas of vertebral subluxation complex. Vitality, strength, and health are thus promoted. Chiropractic Arts Center (1998) reports case histories of clients recovering from heart trouble, hyperactivity, fatigue, digestive problems, and many other conditions.

Stedman (1999) explains that chiropractic practitioners fall into one of two groups, the "straights" and the "mixers." The straights believe in the chiropractic therapy just described, despite the fact that no scientific evidence exists to support the claims. The mixers use spinal adjustments mainly to relieve back pain, neck stiffness, and headaches, conditions that have sometimes been shown to be alleviated by chiropractic therapy. Most mixers are willing to work closely with a client's medical doctor.

PROFESSIONAL TIP

Preparing for Chiropractic Therapy
As with any alternative/complementary intervention, nurses should encourage clients who are considering the use of chiropractic services to first undergo comprehensive health assessment to rule out any contraindications.

Chiropractic services have gained increasing acceptance in the United States. Chiropractors are licensed in all 50 states, and 41 states require insurance reimbursement for chiropractic services (Japsen, 1995).

Energetic-Touch Therapies

One category of alternative/complementary therapies that has been incorporated into nursing practice in the past 20 years is the **energetic-touch therapies**, techniques of using the hands to direct or redirect the flow of the body's energy fields and thus enhance balance within those fields. These modalities are effective interventions for many problems and can be used to restore harmony in all aspects of a person's health. Energetic-touch therapies can be used with persons of all ages and all stages of wellness and illness.

Energetic-touch therapies have their roots in traditional Chinese, ancient Eastern, and Native American philosophies. The fundamental concept is that individuals are composed of a life force, a source of energy that is not confined to physical skin boundaries. Figure 8-2 illustrates the energy field that extends beyond a person's physical body.

An individual's energy field consists of energy layers in constant flux. These energy layers can be diminished or otherwise adversely affected by any type of illness, trauma, or distress. The energy system can also be positively affected by the intentionally directed use of a practitioner's hands. The primary focus of the nurse using an energetic-touch therapy is "to restore the optimal flow of life energy through the field" (Cowens, 1996).

Many energetic-touch therapies are being used by nurses today. Touch, therapeutic massage, therapeutic touch, and healing touch are some examples. Other modalities include acupressure and reflexology, techniques that involve deep-tissue body work and require advanced training on the part of practitioners.

Touch

One of the most universal alternative/complementary modalities is touch. **Touch**, simply defined, is the means of perceiving or experiencing through tactile

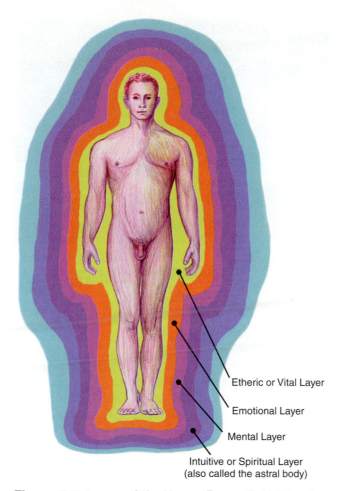

Etheric or Vital Layer

Emotional Layer

Mental Layer

Intuitive or Spiritual Layer
(also called the astral body)

Figure 8-2 Layers of the Human Energy Field Extending Beyond the Physical Boundaries

sensation. Although it was used in all ancient cultures and shamanistic traditions for healing, the advent of scientific medicine and Puritanism led many healers away from the purposeful use of touch. It should be noted that touch carries with it taboos and prescriptions that are culturally dictated. Some cultures are very comfortable with physical touch; others specify that touch may be used only in certain situations and within specified parameters.

Because touch involves personal contact, the nurse must be sure to convey positive intentions. When in doubt, the nurse should withhold touch until effective communication with the client has been established.

CULTURAL CONSIDERATIONS

Touch

- Ask permission before touching a client.
- Tell the client what is going to happen.
- The meaning of touch and the body areas acceptable to touch vary from culture to culture.

PROFESSIONAL TIP

Contraindications for Touch

It is important to know when *not* to touch.

- It may be difficult for persons who have been neglected, abused, or injured to accept touch therapy.
- Touching those who are distrustful or angry may escalate negative behaviors.
- Persons with burns or overly sensitive skin may not benefit from touch.

Touch has several important uses in nursing practice, in that it:

- Is an integral part of assessment;
- Promotes bonding between nurse and client (Figure 8-3);
- Is an important means of communication, especially when other senses are impaired;
- Assists in soothing, calming, and comforting; and
- Helps keep the client oriented.

Therapeutic Massage

Therapeutic massage is the application of pressure and motion by the hands with the intent of improving the recipient's well-being. It involves kneading, rubbing, and using friction.

Massage therapy is now recognized as a highly beneficial modality and is prescribed by a number of physicians. In addition, many states now have licensing requirements for massage practitioners.

Traditionally, back rubs have been administered by nurses to provide comfort to hospitalized clients. Massage techniques can be used with all age groups and are especially beneficial to those who are immobilized. A back rub or massage can achieve many results, including relaxation, increased circulation of the blood and lymph, and relief from musculoskeletal stiffness, pain, and spasm.

 Safety: Precautions for Massage

- Massage should be used with caution on people with heart disease, diabetes, hypertension, or kidney disease, because increased circulation may be harmful in the presence of these conditions.
- Massage should never be attempted in areas of circulatory abnormality, such as aneurysm, varicose veins, necrosis, phlebitis, or thrombus, or in areas of soft-tissue injury, open wounds, inflammation, joint or bone injury, dermatitis, recent surgery, or sciatica.

Figure 8-3 Touch promotes bonding between nurse and client.

Figure 8-4 A Nurse Administering Therapeutic Touch to a Client

Therapeutic Touch

Therapeutic touch, which is based on ancient healing practices such as the laying on of hands, consists of assessing alterations in a person's energy field and using the hands to direct energy to achieve a balanced state. Therapeutic touch is based on four assumptions:

- A human being is an open energy system.
- Anatomically, a human being is bilaterally symmetrical.
- Illness is an imbalance in an individual's energy field.
- Human beings have natural abilities to transform and transcend their conditions of living (Krieger, 1993).

The therapeutic touch process is readily learned in workshops, can be done with hands either on or off the body, complements medical treatments, and has demonstrated reasonably consistent and reliable results (Figure 8-4). Table 8–3 outlines the five-phase process of therapeutic touch.

The relaxation response may be apparent in the client as quickly as 2 to 5 minutes after a therapeutic touch treatment has begun, and some clients may fall asleep or require less pain medication after a treatment. When done correctly, the practice of therapeutic touch can be mutually beneficial, energizing and increasing feelings of wellness in the practitioner as well as in the client (Mackey, 1995).

Research has documented the effectiveness of therapeutic touch in numerous areas. Therapeutic touch has been shown to accelerate wound healing of infections after cesarean section delivery (Wetzel, 1993); promote relaxation, increase energy, enhance a sense of well-being, and improve immunological functioning (Quinn, 1993); decrease anxiety in hospitalized psychiatric clients (Gagne & Toye, 1994); reduce postoperative pain, thereby decreasing the need for medication (Meehan, 1993); enhance the relaxation response, pain management, and immune function (Wilson, 1995); and alleviate generalized anxiety (Olsen & Sneed, 1995).

Healing Touch

Healing touch is an energy-based therapeutic modality that alters the energy field through the use of touch, thereby affecting physical, mental, emotional, and spiritual health (Keegan, 1995b). Healing touch was developed in the 1980s by Janet Mentgen, a nurse. In 1990, healing touch was established as a certification program of the American Holistic Nurses' Association (AHNA). The curriculum includes varied techniques in general balancing of the body's energy field, relaxation, and specific problems such as headaches, spinal problems, and pain.

Healing touch can be administered in a few minutes or, ideally, in a session lasting one full hour (Mentgen, 1995). Implicit in this therapy is the need for follow-up or sequential treatments as well as discharge planning and referral to assist the client in adequately meeting goals.

In both therapeutic touch and healing touch, the practitioner uses **centering** (a process of bringing oneself to an inward focus of serenity) before initiating treatment. Centering is a valuable tool to use before performing any treatment or before any situation that may be stressful or difficult (such as a major school examination).

Shiatsu and Acupressure

Shiatsu, from the word meaning "finger pressure," is a Japanese form of acupressure. Both shiatsu and acupressure are based on the Chinese meridian theory, which states that the body is divided into meridian channels through which energy (*Qi*, pronounced "chi") flows. Cold, damp, fire, bacteria, or viruses may block the flow of Qi, causing disease in the body. **Acupressure** is a technique of releasing blocked energy within an individual when specific points (Tsubas)

Table 8–3 PHASES OF THERAPEUTIC TOUCH

PHASE	DEFINITION	TECHNIQUES
Centering	• Bringing body, mind, and emotions to a quiet, focused state of consciousness • Being still • Being nonjudgmental	Become centered: • Controlled breathing, • Imagery, and • Meditation.
Assessment ("scanning")	• Using the hands to determine the nature of the client's energy field • Being attuned to sensory cues (e.g., warmth, coolness, static, pressure, tingling) to detect changes in the client's energy	• Hold the hands 2 to 6 inches from the client's energy field while moving the hands from the head to the feet in a rhythmic, symmetrical manner.
Unruffling ("clearing")	• Facilitating the symmetrical and rhythmic flow of energy through the field	• Use slightly more vigorous hand movements from midline while continuing to move in a rhythmic and symmetrical manner from the head to the feet.
Treatment ("balancing," "rebalancing," or "intervention")	• Projecting, directing, and modulating energy on the basis of the nature of the living energy field • Assisting to reestablish order in the system.	• Because each practitioner experiences the living energy field uniquely, the law of opposites serves as a guideline for intervening (e.g., if a pulling or drawing sensation is detected, energy is directed to the depleted area until it feels replenished). • Continue to assess, clear, and balance the field while remaining centered.
Evaluation	• Using professional, informed, and intuitive judgment to determine when to end the session	• Reassess the field. • Elicit feedback from the client. • Give the client an opportunity to rest and integrate the process.

The phases, although learned sequentially by beginners, are dynamic and often performed concurrently and repetitively by experienced practitioners.

Adapted from Therapeutic Touch: Teaching Guidelines: Beginner's Level Krieger/Kunz Method, *by Nurse Healers-Professional Associates, Inc., 1992, New York: Author.*

along the meridians are pressed or massaged by the practitioner's fingers, thumbs, and heel of the hands. When the blocked energy is freed, the disease subsides. The most commonly treated conditions include muscular pains, joint pains, depression, digestive disturbances, and respiratory disorders (Lanfranco, 1997).

Shiatsu primarily focuses on health maintenance rather than on treatment of illness (Keegan, 1995b); that is, it is used to make sure the Qi is able to flow freely so that the individual does not become ill. When practicing shiatsu, nurses must be self-aware and grounded (focused on their inner energy). This focus enables the practitioner to concentrate completely on promoting the client's comfort.

Reflexology

Reflexology is rooted in ancient healing arts. The fundamental concept of reflexology is that the body is divided into 10 equal, longitudinal zones that run the length of the body, from the top of the head to the tip of the toes. These 10 zones are correlated with the 10 fingers and toes. The foot is thus viewed as a microcosm of the entire body. Reflexology theory posits that illness manifests itself in calcium deposits and acids in the corresponding part of the person's foot. The pressing of specific points on the foot stimulates energy movement and produces relaxation, reduces stress, and promotes health by relieving pressures and accumulation of toxins in the corresponding body part (Figure 8-5).

Reflexology can be used as a complementary method for managing chronic conditions such as asthma, sinus infections, migraines, irritable bowel syndrome, kidney stones, and constipation. After the pressure points are learned, the nurse can massage the areas of the client's foot to relieve pain and produce relaxation.

Spiritual Therapies

A state of wholeness or health is dependent on one's relationship not only to the physical and interpersonal environments, but also to the spiritual aspects of self. The idea that there is a relationship between spirituality and health is not new. "From the earliest time of the shaman we have witnessed the mysterious spiritual element of healing . . . the connection of the healer with the divine" (Keegan, 1994).

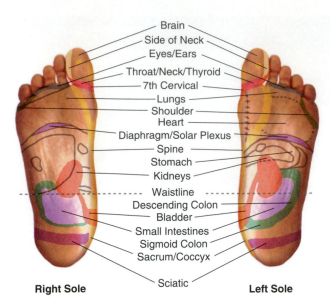

Brain
Side of Neck
Eyes/Ears
Throat/Neck/Thyroid
7th Cervical
Lungs
Shoulder
Heart
Diaphragm/Solar Plexus
Spine
Stomach
Kidneys
Waistline
Descending Colon
Bladder
Small Intestines
Sigmoid Colon
Sacrum/Coccyx
Sciatic

Right Sole   **Left Sole**

Figure 8-5 Foot Reflexology Charts *(Reproduced with permission from* Better Health With Foot Reflexology. *Copyright 1983 by Dwight C. Byers, Ingham Publishing, Inc., POB 12642, St. Petersburg, FL 33733-2642.)*

The role of the spirit in healing is witnessed in all cultures. The inseparable link between the state of one's soul (life energy or spirit) and the state of one's health is accepted by many cultures. Scientists (especially psychoneuroimmunologists) are beginning to validate that individuals have inner mechanisms of healing. Many of the major religions have ideologies relating to health, illness, and healing.

Faith Healing

At the heart of spiritual or faith healing is the belief that practitioners must purify themselves and reach a state of unity with God or a Higher Power before faith healing can occur. This process, based on religious belief, is usually accomplished through prayer. During preparation for healing, the practitioner adapts a passive and receptive mood in order to be a channel for divine power. The ill person's belief enhances, but is not crucial to, the success of healing.

Healing Prayer

When individuals pray, they believe they are communicating directly with God or a Higher Power. Prayer is an integral part of a person's spiritual life and, as such, can affect well-being. Florence Nightingale recognized that prayer helps connect individuals to nature and the environment (Nightingale, 1969). Medical research is currently investigating the effects of prayer on physical health.

A study conducted by Byrd and Sherrill (1995) investigated the effects of prayer on clients in critical care units. The results showed that clients who received standard medical treatment with the addition of intercessory prayers had fewer complications, required less medication, and improved faster than did clients in the control group, who received standard medical care and no prayers. Findings reported by Marwick (1995) showed that religious involvement may lead to improved physical health status.

Shamanism

Shamanism was discussed earlier in this chapter.

Nutritional/Medicinal Therapies

In the past 20 to 30 years, nutritional interventions for prevention and treatment of disease have generated increasing interest among consumers and health care providers. This section addresses the alternative/complementary nutritional and medicinal approaches.

Phytochemicals

Currently, certain foods are being studied for their medicinal value. **Phytochemicals** are nonnutritive, physiologically active compounds present in plants in very small amounts (Simons, 1997). *Phyto* is the Greek word for "plant." Therefore, phytochemicals are plant chemicals. These chemicals have several functions including storage of nutrients and provision of structure, aroma, flavor, and color. Phytochemicals protect against cancer and prevent heart disease, stroke, and cataracts. Phytochemicals are found in fruits and vegetables.

No single fruit or vegetable contains all phytochemicals. The consumption of a wide variety of fruits and vegetables provides the best supply. The major sources of phytochemicals are onions, garlic, leeks, chives, carrots, sweet potatoes, squash, pumpkin, cantaloupe, mango, papaya, tomatoes, citrus fruits, grapes, strawberries, raspberries, cherries, legumes, soybeans, tofu, and the cruiciferous vegetables (broccoli, cauliflower, brussels sprouts, and cabbage). Nurses can use this information to encourage clients to eat more fruits and vegetables.

Antioxidants and Free Radicals

Antioxidants are substances that prevent or inhibit oxidation, a chemical process whereby a substance is joined to oxygen. In the body, antioxidants prevent tissue damage related to **free radicals**, which are unstable molecules that alter genetic codes and trigger the development of cancer growth in cells. Vitamins C and E, beta-carotene (which is converted to vitamin A in the body), and selenium are antioxidants. Antioxidants may prevent heart disease, some forms of cancer, and cataracts. Free radicals contribute to cardiovascular disease by oxidizing low-density lipoproteins (LDLs) and allowing cholesterol to adhere to vessel walls. Antioxidants help repair eye tissue damaged from sunlight and thus prevent cataract formation (Simons, 1997).

Other vitamins, minerals, trace elements, and enzymes are being investigated for their possible therapeutic value. Phytosterols (plant sterols) are the active ingredients in the new lipid-lowering margarines. These inhibit absorption of dietary cholesterol and slow down the reabsorption of cholesterol secreted in bile (Cerrato, 1999a).

Macrobiotic Diet

In the 1960s, macrobiotic (from the Greek words *makro,* meaning "long," and *bios,* meaning "life") diets became popular because of a heightened interest in "natural" and more spiritual approaches to managing health and illness. The basis of macrobiotics is the Taoist concept of balance between opposites as achieved through food intake. Food has the qualities of *yin* (associated with death, cold, and darkness) and *yang* (associated with immortality, heat, and light). For example, tropical sweet foods are yin, and meat and eggs are yang. Overindulgence in either type causes difficulties; for example, too much yin food yields worry and resentment, whereas too much yang food leads to hostility and aggression. People need balance and, therefore, should consume foods that balance yin and yang.

Because brown rice and whole grains are categorized as balanced foods, they are major staples of a macrobiotic diet. The diet should be flexible and related to the season and should consist of foods indigenous to the area where the individual lives. Foods to be avoided include processed and treated foods, red meat, sugar, dairy products, eggs, and caffeine. The macrobiotic diet generally conforms to the recommendations of the American Dietary Association in terms of the guidelines for low-fat, low-cholesterol, high-fiber diets (Guinness, 1993).

Herbal Therapy

Herbal medicine has been a powerful tool in folk healing for centuries. Medicinal herbs have been catalogued for thousands of years and have probably been used in every culture. Many drugs commonly used today were, in an earlier time, tribal remedies derived from plants. Herbal medicine, also known as botanical medicine or phytotherapy, uses plant extracts for therapeutic outcomes.

Learning about herbal treatment is similar to learning pharmacology. Many holistic practitioners incorporate the use of herbs into their practices. Herbs work because of their chemical composition. Different herbs contain different compounds that can strengthen the immune system, alter the blood chemistry, or protect specific organs against disease. Table 8–4 lists medicinal values of commonly used herbs.

Others

S-adenosylmethionine (SAMe) is a modified amino acid produced naturally by the body; however, the level decreases with age. Controlled research has shown that SAMe may work at least as well as certain antidepressants and may benefit clients with osteoarthritis by assisting in cartilage repair (Cerrato & Rowell, 1999).

Omega-3 fatty acids, found in salmon, trout, sardines, walnuts, canola oil, and flax seeds help reduce the threat of cardiac arrhythmias. Research has also shown that the omega-3 fatty acids suppress inflammation of rheumatoid arthritis and may improve glucose control in Type 2 diabetes (Cerrato, 1999b).

Other Methodologies

The mind/body, body-movement, energetic-touch, spiritual, and nutritional/medicinal treatment modalities are not the only available alternative/complementary therapies. Others such as aromatherapy, humor, pet therapy, music therapy, and play therapy are also used by holistic practitioners.

Aromatherapy

Aromatherapy is defined as the therapeutic use of concentrated essences or essential oils that have been extracted from plants and flowers. When diluted in a carrier oil for massage or in warm water for inhalation, essences may be stimulating, uplifting, relaxing, or soothing. The following are some popular essential oils (Keville & Green, 1995):

- *Lavender* is said to have anti-inflammatory, antidepressant, and antibacterial effects.
- *Eucalyptus* is claimed to act as a decongestant, antimicrobial, and stimulant.
- *Chamomile* is believed to benefit the gastrointestinal tract, relieve allergies, and act as a sedative.
- *Marjoram* is purported to work as an antiseptic and anti-inflammatory agent and to relieve muscle spasms.
- *Peppermint* is believed to improve digestion and act as an antiseptic and decongestant.
- *Rosemary* is said to stimulate the circulation.
- *Geranium* is thought to balance the mind and body.

Aromatherapists use concentrated oils derived from the roots, bark, or flowers of herbs and other plants to treat specific ailments. The aromas cause physiological,

PROFESSIONAL TIP

Use of Medicinal Plants

Nurses are cautioned against the casual use of plants to treat self or others. "Natural" substances can be harmful. In fact, if not processed properly, many plants (including some herbs) can be poisonous.

Table 8–4 MEDICINAL VALUE OF HERBS

HERB	MEDICINAL VALUE	HERB	MEDICINAL VALUE
Aloe vera	• Promotes wound healing • Soothes minor cuts, abrasions, and burns	Ginkgo	• Enhances cerebral blood flow • Helps lessen mild depression • Eases dementia • Combats impotence • Decreases peripheral vascular insufficiency • Relieves premenstrual syndrome symptoms • Decreases vascular fragility
Calendula	• Promotes healing of cuts, abrasions, minor burns, sunburn, acne, and athlete's foot • Soothes oral thrush (as a mouthwash) and vaginal thrush (as a douche)		
Celery	• Lowers cholesterol • Decreases dizziness • Relieves headache	Peppermint	• Relieves headache • Eases sinus congestion • Reduces muscle spasms
Chamomile	• Produces a calming effect • Relieves nausea • Eases tension headache	Sage	• Acts as an antibacterial
		Saint John's Wort	• Relieves mild to moderate depression • Lessens severity of viral infections
Eucalpytus	• Acts as an antibacterial • Acts as a decongestant	Thyme	• Acts as an antimicrobial • Helps relieve symptoms of common cold • Acts as an antispasmodic on bronchioles • Relieves cystitis • Acts as an antifungal (especially when applied as a lotion for athlete's foot) • Used as a mouthwash for oral thrush
Garlic	• Acts as an antimicrobial remedy for intestinal worms • Helps protect against and treat respiratory infections • Used as expectorant in cases of bronchitis or a cold		
Ginger	• Eases nausea (especially effective for motion sickness and morning sickness associated with pregnancy) • Stimulates circulation in feet and hands • Acts as expectorant • Helps relieve indigestion and flatulence • Relieves diarrhea		

Note: This information is not intended to serve as a guide for self-medication or the treatment of others. Consult a health care practitioner trained in the use of herbs before consuming or giving any herb for medicinal purposes.

From Herbs for health, by S. Foster, 1995, The Herb Companion, 8(1), Down to Earth: An ancient herb for a modern garden, by J. Long, 1995. The Herb Companion, 8(1), 22; Eight healing herbs, 1995–1996, by M. Polunin and C. Robbins, 1995, Holistic Health Directory, The Backyard Medicine Chest: An Herbal Primer, by D. Schar, 1995, Washington, DC: Elliot & Clark; Spontaneous Healing: How to Discover and Enhance Your Body's Natural Ability To Maintain and Heal Itself, by A. Weil, 1996, New York: Alfred A. Knopf; and Herbal Medicines, by C. O'Neil, J. Avila, & C. W. Fetrow, (1999), Nursing99, 29(4).

psychological, and pharmacological reactions (Trevelyan, 1993). Some essential oils have antibacterial properties and are found in a wide variety of pharmaceutical preparations. Essential oils should be used intelligently and with caution.

A clinical study reported by Wilkinson (1995) concluded that massage oil that incorporated the essential oil Roman chamomile reduced anxiety and improved the quality of life of cancer clients to a greater extent than did unscented oil. Another study found that postcardiac surgery clients receiving foot massages with neroli oil (from orange flowers) experienced greater and more lasting psychological benefits than did those receiving massages without neroli oil (Stevenson, 1994). Weiss and James (1997), however, report clients with allergic contact dermatitis to essential oils.

Some contraindications for aromatherapy are listed in Table 8–5.

 GERONTOLOGICAL CONSIDERATIONS

Essential Oils

Essential oils should be used with caution in elderly persons. These clients are usually more sensitive to essential oils than are adults and teenagers and thus require smaller amounts and less-concentrated forms of the essence.

Table 8-5 AROMATHERAPY CONTRAINDICATIONS

ESSENTIAL OIL	CONTRAINDICATION
Sweet fennel	Epilepsy
Rosemary, sage, thyme	Hypertension
Peppermint, rose, rosemary	First trimester of pregnancy
	Use only in well-diluted form in later stages of pregnancy
Arnica, basil, celery, sage, cypress, jasmine, juniper, marjoram, myrrh, sage, thyme	Pregnancy
Camomile, lavender	Use with care in pregnancies carrying the risk of bleeding or miscarriage

From Aromatherapy, by J. Trevelyan, 1993, Nursing Times, 89(25), 39.

Safety: Aromatherapy

- Essential oils are very potent and should never be used in an undiluted form, be used near the eyes, or be ingested orally.
- Because some people are allergic to certain oils, a small skin-patch test should be done before generalized application.

Humor

Of all the complementary interventions addressed in this chapter, humor is the one that can be used most often by nurses to benefit clients. "Humor is probably one of the least understood, easiest to do, and most beneficial of the nonpharmacologic interventions" (Mornhinweg & Voignier, 1995).

To avoid giving offense, it is important to determine the client's perception of what is humorous. Whether a given situation is considered humorous or offensive will vary greatly from culture to culture and person to person. Good taste and common sense should serve as guides.

Nurses can use humor with clients in a variety of ways. A humor cart (portable cart or carrier filled with cartoon and joke books, magic tricks, and silly noses) is easy to use and allows clients to select their own humor tools for health. A "humor room" may be made

PROFESSIONAL TIP

Use of Humor

Never do or say anything that gives clients the idea that you are laughing *at* them as opposed to *with* them (McGhee, 1998).

available, where clients can watch comedy videos or play fun games with visitors or other clients.

Humor has many therapeutic outcomes. Norman Cousins, former chairman of the Task Force in Psychoneuroimmunology at the School of Medicine at UCLA, relates how he enhanced his recovery from an incurable connective tissue disorder, ankylosing spondylitis, by the daily watching of films and movies that made him laugh (Cousins, 1979). Humor can be used effectively to relieve anxiety and promote relaxation, improve respiratory function, enhance immunological function, and decrease pain by stimulating the production of endorphins.

Pet Therapy

The use of pets to enhance health status has a long history. In Britain in the 18th and 19th centuries, pets were used in institutions to give a sense of meaning and purpose to people institutionalized because of developmental delays (i.e., mental retardation). Pet therapy was also used during the Crimean War and World War II (Mornhinweg & Voignier, 1995). Pet therapy is currently used as adjunctive treatment for people in both acute and long-term care settings (Figure 8-6).

Pet therapy has many applications including overcoming physical limitations, improving mood, lowering blood pressure, and improving socialization skills and self-esteem.

Figure 8-6 Pet therapy provides health benefits. *(Photo courtesy of John White)*

CULTURAL CONSIDERATIONS

Music and Culture

- Each culture and each generation within each culture has its own preferred type of music.
- Music that is soothing to one client may be irritating to another.
- Either ask which type of music the client would prefer or allow the client to bring music.

Music Therapy

Music enters the bodymind through the auditory sense. Therapeutic use of music consists of playing music to elicit positive changes in behavior, emotions, or physiological response. Music complements other treatment modalities and encourages clients to become active participants in their health care and recovery.

Music is a good adjunct to use with imagery, as it can enhance the relaxation response and, therefore, heighten images. Different types of music elicit different responses, but all music stimulates the neurotransmitters that evoke chemical changes in the bodymind (Achterberg, Dossey, & Kolkmeier, 1994). Music-thanatology is a holistic and palliative method of using music with dying clients (Schroeder-Shecker, 1994). It is used to help dissipate obstacles to the client's peaceful transition to death.

Music on audiocassette and heard via a tape player and headphones can be a very useful tool for clients who are immobilized, who must wait for diagnostic tests, or who are undergoing the perioperative experience (Figure 8-7). Some facilities allow clients to choose the type of music played while they undergo procedures such as cardiac catheterization. Clients may request that their music and tape player accompany them during surgery. Pleasurable sound and music can reduce stress, perception of pain, anxiety, and feelings

Figure 8-7 Music therapy helps client relax.

of isolation. Music can also be especially useful in helping adolescent clients relax.

Play Therapy

Play therapy is especially useful with children. Toys are used to allow children to learn about what will be happening to them and to express their emotions and their current situations. Drawing and art work also provide a way for children to share their experiences. When language ability is reduced or not yet well developed, play therapy and drawings constitute a method for children to communicate their needs and feelings to care providers.

NURSING AND ALTERNATIVE/COMPLEMENTARY APPROACHES

Some methods labeled by Western society as "alternative" (e.g., acupuncture) have already been validated by having been used successfully for centuries. Other alternative/complementary methods such as biofeedback have been proven through research. Still other alternative/complementary modalities such as therapeutic touch need further investigation and validation. Nurses play an important role in educating consumers about nontraditional interventions appropriate throughout the life cycle (Table 8–6) by providing information about the safety and efficacy of such methods. The following are terms frequently used to describe various treatment modalities:

- *Proven:* have been scientifically tested in clinical trials
- *Experimental:* are undergoing Food and Drug Administration (FDA) investigations to ascertain safety and efficacy
- *Untested:* have not been investigated by the FDA with regard to safety and efficacy
- *Folklore:* have been passed from one generation to another as remedies, many of which have therapeutic value
- *Quackery:* have not proven effective, may result in harm to consumers, and are usually marketed with numerous unfounded promises (e.g., as "cure-all" products or therapies) (Brown, Cassileth, Lewis, & Renner, 1994)

According to Keegan (1998), research has documented the effectiveness of specific alternative/complementary therapies:

- Meditation combined with guided imagery decreases physical tension, anxiety, and the adverse effects of chemotherapy.
- Nutrition, exercise, and meditation—without the use of medication or surgery—can reverse coronary heart disease.

Table 8–6 CORRELATION OF SELECTED STAGES OF LIFE CYCLE WITH RECOMMENDED COMPLEMENTARY THERAPIES

STAGE OF LIFE CYCLE	RECOMMENDED COMPLEMENTARY THERAPIES
Adolescents	All modalities discussed in this chapter, as appropriate to the condition
Adults	All modalities discussed in this chapter, as appropriate to the condition
Elders	• Massage (lighter pressure and other modifications for body's status) • Aromatherapy (with precautions) • Any other modalities discussed in this chapter, as appropriate to the condition and with precautions
Terminally ill	• Massage • Reflexology • Energetic-touch therapies • Music-thanatology • Prayer • Any other modalities discussed in this chapter, as appropriate to the condition and with precautions

Adapted from Fundamentals of Nursing: Standards & Practice, *by S. DeLaune and P. Ladner, 1998, Albany, NY: Delmar. Copyright 1998 by Delmar. Adapted with permission.*

- Yoga can help mentally challenged individuals become more aware of their bodies and improve coordination.
- Yoga can help reduce pain in clients with osteoarthritis of the hands.

Numerous alternative/complementary interventions can be incorporated into nursing practice. As Frisch (1997) states:

> While holistic nurses use many alternative and complementary approaches to care, it is not the alternative modality that makes us holistic; it is our presence, our caring, and our willingness to put the client first.

Putting the client first means individualizing every intervention on the basis of the client's unique needs. From the time before birth until the moment of death, people of all ages experience trauma, stress, and life challenges and have needs in all dimensions. Nurses are challenged to discover and meet those needs.

The power of the nurse's presence with any client should never be underestimated. Many of the alternative/complementary modalities require further study and advanced training. However, nursing students already have the ability to listen, to touch, and to care. Clients can benefit from intent, compassion, and something as simple as having another person present with them.

CASE STUDY

Mr. Vincent, who is receiving chemotherapy for colon cancer, tells the nurse that he is seeing both an aromatherapist to relieve his pain and nausea and a practitioner of healing touch to cure his cancer. He also says that he does not know whether he will come back for his next chemotherapy session because it makes him feel bad. The other therapies make him feel better.

Consider the following:

1. What should the nurse do with this information?
2. How should the nurse respond?
3. What assessments should the nurse make?
4. Identify a nursing diagnosis and goal for Mr. Vincent.
5. List three nursing interventions for this nursing diagnosis.
6. Identify sources for information about the therapies.

SUMMARY

- Ever-increasing numbers of health care consumers are using nontraditional treatment modalities.
- Psychoneuroimmunology is the study of the way that the body and mind are connected and the way that beliefs, thoughts, and emotions affect health.
- Holistic nursing practice encompasses consideration of each client as a unique and whole being with many aspects: physiological, psychological, sociocultural, intellectual, and spiritual.
- Healing is not curing but, rather, is regaining balance and finding harmony and wholeness as changes take place from within the individual.
- No one can heal another, but a nurse can act as a guide, support system, or instrument of healing for the client.
- Some of the mind/body modalities that nurses use are meditation, relaxation, imagery, biofeedback, and hypnosis.
- Body-movement modalities include movement and exercise and chiropractic therapy.
- Energetic-touch therapies can be used with persons of all ages and in various stages of illness and wellness.
- Energetic-touch therapies include therapeutic massage, therapeutic touch, healing touch, shiatsu, acupressure, and reflexology.
- Spiritual therapies such as faith healing, healing prayer, and laying on of the hands are helpful modalities to use in caring for clients.
- Nutritional/medicinal therapies include the use of antioxidants, macrobiotic diets, and herbal therapy.
- Other modalities such as aromatherapy, humor, pet therapy, music therapy, and play therapy are valuable adjuncts to conventional treatment.

Review Questions

1. Therapies that are used instead of mainstream medical practice are called:

    a. alternative therapies.
    b. contemporary therapies.
    c. complementary therapies.
    d. nontraditional therapies.

2. Therapies that are used in conjunction with conventional medical therapies are called:

    a. alternative therapies.
    b. contemporary therapies.
    c. complementary therapies.
    d. nontraditional therapies.

3. The Office of Alternative Medicine:

    a. investigates nontraditional treatment methods.
    b. refers persons to practitioners of nontraditional therapies.
    c. monitors the number of people using nontraditional therapies.
    d. grants a license to those who practice nontraditional therapies.

4. Healing is:

    a. curing a disease.
    b. treating a disease.
    c. making a client well.
    d. a process that activates internal forces.

5. Imagery is a:

    a. balancing of life forces.
    b. relaxation technique using the five senses.
    c. measurement of physiological responses when dreaming.
    d. blocking of the body's energy fields with unhappy thoughts.

6. One of the most universal alternative/complementary modalities is:

    a. touch.
    b. massage.
    c. nutrition.
    d. faith healing.

7. Learning about herbal treatments can be compared to learning about:

    a. hypnosis.
    b. nutrition.
    c. reflexology.
    d. pharmacology.

8. Clients using pet therapy:

    a. play with a cat.
    b. have no other companions.
    c. experience a decrease in blood pressure.
    d. show an increase in physical limitations.

9. The complementary therapy recommended for all ages in the life cycle is:

    a. massage.
    b. hypnosis.
    c. reflexology.
    d. aromatherapy.

Critical Thinking Questions

1. Your close friend has AIDS and is experiencing a great deal of pain and discouragement. She wants to find alternative methods to ease the pain. She confides in you that she believes there may be a cure available at the holistic health center. How do you best help your friend in this situation? What do you advise?

2. A client asks the nurse to rub his foot in a particular spot because that is where his reflexologist rubs to relieve his abdominal pain. How should the nurse handle this situation?

WEB FLASH!

- Are there specific sites listed under alternative therapies or complementary therapies?
- Search the Web for the organizations listed as resources for this chapter at the end of the book. What information do they provide?
- What resources (books, videos, discussion forums) are available through the Internet for clients interested in a specific alternative/complementary therapy?

LOSS, GRIEF, AND DEATH

MAKING THE CONNECTION

Refer to the following chapters to increase your understanding of loss, grief, and death:

- **Chapter 3, Legal Responsibilities**
- **Chapter 4, Ethical Responsibilities**
- **Chapter 6, Cultural Diversity and Nursing**

- **Chapter 8, Alternative/Complementary Therapies**
- **Chapter 36, Rehabilitation, Home Health, Long-Term Care, and Hospice**

LEARNING OBJECTIVES

Upon completion of this chapter, you should be able to:
- *Define key terms.*
- *Describe various losses that affect individuals at different stages of the life cycle.*
- *Describe the characteristics of an individual experiencing grief.*
- *Differentiate adaptive grief and pathological grief.*
- *Discuss theoretical perspectives of loss, grief, and death.*
- *Discuss use of the nursing process with a grieving individual.*
- *Discuss the holistic needs of the dying person and his family.*
- *Define the purpose of hospice care.*
- *Develop a plan of care for a dying client.*
- *Discuss nursing responsibilities when a client dies.*
- *Describe ways that nurses can cope with their own grief.*

KEY TERMS

algor mortis	hospice
anticipatory grief	life review
autopsy	liver mortis
bereavement	loss
breakthrough pain	maturational loss
Cheyne-Stokes respirations	mortuary
	mourning
complicated grief	palliative care
death rattle	post-mortem care
disenfranchised grief	resuscitation
dysfunctional grief	rigor mortis
grief	shroud
grief work	situational loss
Health Care Surrogate Law	uncomplicated grief

INTRODUCTION

In contemporary society, individuals constantly experience loss. Frequent episodes of terrorism, natural disaster, and personal crises result in the universal experience of loss. It can be overwhelming to think about real and potential losses. Nurses must be aware of the potential for loss in today's world, as well as the processes whereby individuals react and adapt to losses.

Throughout the life cycle, people are faced with loss, without which growth would not continue. Many people consider loss only in terms of death and dying; however, loss of every type occurs daily.

Every day, nurses encounter clients who are responding to grief associated with losses. Nurses must have an understanding of the major concepts related to loss and grieving. Grief is a response to losses of all types. However, this chapter focuses on grief as a response to death. Nurses also care for dying clients. Thus, this chapter also provides information on meeting the special needs of terminally ill clients and their families.

LOSS

Loss is any situation, either actual, potential, or perceived, wherein a valued object or person is changed or is no longer accessible to the individual. Because change is a major constant in life, everyone experiences losses. Loss can be actual (e.g., a spouse is lost through divorce) or anticipated (a person is diagnosed with a terminal illness and has only a short time to live). A loss can be tangible or intangible. For example, when a person is fired from a job, the tangible loss is income, whereas the loss of self-esteem is intangible.

Losses also occur as a result of moving from one developmental stage to another. An example of such a **maturational loss** is the adolescent who loses the younger child's freedom from responsibility. Other examples of losses associated with growth and development are discussed later in this chapter. A **situational loss** occurs in response to external events usually beyond the individual's control (such as the death of a significant other).

Types of Loss

Not everyone responds to loss in the same way because the significance of the lost object or person is determined by individual perceptions. There are many types of loss, including:

- *Actual loss:* loss of someone or something, such as the death of a loved one or the theft of one's property.
- *Perceived loss:* sense of loss felt by an individual but not tangible to others, such as the perceived loss of self-esteem of a student who was not accepted into a nursing program.
- *Physical loss:* loss of a part or aspect of the body, such as the loss of an extremity in an accident, scarring from burns, or permanent injury.
- *Psychological loss:* emotional loss, such as a woman feeling inadequate after menopause and resultant infertility.

There are four major categories of loss: loss of external objects, loss of familiar environment, loss of aspects of self, and loss of significant other.

Loss of an External Object

When an object that a person highly values is damaged or changed or disappears, loss occurs. The significance of the lost object to the individual determines the type and amount of grieving that occurs. For instance, an individual who loses a family heirloom in a fire may react not only to the lost financial value of the piece, but also to the lost sense of history and heritage that the piece represented.

Loss of Familiar Environment

The loss of a familiar environment occurs when a person moves away from familiar surroundings, for instance to another home or a different community, to a new school, or to a new job. A client who is hospitalized or institutionalized may also experience loss when faced with new surroundings. This type of loss evokes anxiety related to fear of the unknown.

Loss of Aspect of Self

Loss of an aspect of self can be psychological or physiological. Examples of psychological aspects of self that may be lost include ambition, a sense of humor, or enjoyment of life. These feelings of loss may result from life events such as losing a job or failing at a task that the individual deems important. Physiological loss includes loss of physical function or loss resulting from disfigurement or disappearance of a body part, as is the case with amputation or mastectomy. Loss of a physiological aspect of self can result from illness, trauma, or treatment methodologies such as surgery.

Loss of Significant Other

The loss of a loved one is a significant loss. Such a loss can result from separation, divorce, running away, moving to a different area, or death. This chapter focuses on the loss of a significant other as a result of death.

GRIEF

Grief, a series of intense physical and psychological responses that occur following a loss, is a normal, natural, necessary, and adaptive response to a loss. Loss leads to the adaptive process of **mourning,** the period of time during which grief is expressed and resolution and integration of the loss occur. **Bereavement** is the period of grief following the death of a loved one (Figure 9-1).

Figure 9-1 Older adults may grieve intensely over the loss of a person or situation that has been a part of their life for many years.

Theories of the Grieving Process

Several theoretical models describe grieving. The theories of Erich Lindemann, George L. Engle, John Bowlby, and J. William Worden are discussed in the following sections.

Lindemann

Following the Coconut Grove fire in Boston in 1944, Lindemann studied survivors and their families. Lindemann coined the phrase **grief work**, which is still used today to describe the process experienced by the bereaved. During grief work, the person experiences freedom from attachment to the deceased, becomes reoriented to the environment where the deceased is no longer present, and establishes new relationships (Lindemann, 1944). Lindemann's classic work is the basis of current crisis and grief resolution theories. Lindemann (1944) and Roach and Nieto (1997) describe Lindemann's theory of a person's reactions to normal grief as:

- *Somatic distress:* The bereaved experience episodic waves of discomfort in durations of 10 to 60 minutes; multiple somatic complaints; fatigue; and extreme physical or emotional pain.
- *Preoccupation with the image of the deceased:* The bereaved experience a sense of unreality, emotional detachment from others, and an overwhelming preoccupation with visualizing the deceased.
- *Guilt:* The bereaved consider the death to be a result of their own negligence or lack of attentiveness; they look for evidence of how they could have contributed to the death.
- *Hostile reactions:* The bereaved's relationships with others become impaired owing to the bereaved's desire to be left alone and the bereaved's feelings of irritability and anger.
- *Loss of patterns of conduct:* The bereaved exhibit generalized restlessness and an inability to sit still; they continually search for something to do.

Engle

Grief is a typical reaction to loss of a valued object. According to Engle, there are three stages of mourning, and progression through each stage is necessary for healing. The grieving process, which may take several years to complete, cannot be accelerated. The goal of the grieving process is for the mourner to accept the loss and let go of the deceased. Engle (1961, 1964) and Roach and Nieto (1997) outline Engle's theory of grief as follows:

- *Stage I: Shock and Disbelief* (can last from minutes to days)
    Disorientation
    Feeling of helplessness

Denial, which provides protection until the person is able to face reality

- *Stage II: Developing Awareness* (may last from 6 to 12 months)
    Guilt
    Sadness
    Isolation
    Loneliness
    Feelings of helplessness
    Possible anger and hostility toward others
    Increasing emotional pain in response to increasing reality of loss
    Recognition that one is powerless to change the situation

- *Stage III: Restitution and Resolution* (marks the beginning of the healing process; may take up to several years)
    Emergence of bodily symptoms
    Possible idealization of the deceased
    Beginnings of coming to terms with the loss
    Establishment of new social patterns and relationships

Bowlby

According to Bowlby, grief results when an individual experiences a disruption in attachment to a love object. His theory proposes that grief occurs when attachment bonds are severed. The four phases of grieving as cited by Bowlby are:

- Numbness,
- Yearning and searching,
- Disorganization and despair, and
- Reorganization (Bowlby, 1982)

Worden

Worden has identified four tasks that an individual must perform in order to successfully deal with a loss:

- Accept the fact that the loss is real
- Experience the emotional pain of grief
- Adjust to an environment without the deceased
- Reinvest the emotional energy once directed at the deceased into another relationship (Worden, 1991)

Types of Grief

Grief is a universal, normal response to loss. Grief drains people, both emotionally and physically. Because grief requires so much emotional energy, relationships may suffer (Wong, 1996). There are different types of grief, including uncomplicated ("normal"), dysfunctional, anticipatory, and disenfranchised grief.

Nurses play an important role in assisting mourners to develop and understand the normal grieving process and the complex feelings exhibited when grief becomes more complicated. Nurses with a sound knowledge base of both normal grief and dysfunctional grief are better prepared to assist survivors than are nurses who mistakenly believe that all grief is the same.

Uncomplicated Grief

Uncomplicated grief is what many individuals would refer to as *normal grief*. Engle (1961) states that the grief reaction is similar to other physical conditions and draws a parallel between a disease process and the grief process. Both include:

- A common etiologic factor (e.g., loss precipitates grief),
- A predictable symptomatology and course,
- Functional impairment for a period of time, and
- Distress and inability to function normally.

Engle (1961) proposed use of the term **uncomplicated grief** to describe a grief reaction that normally follows a significant loss. Uncomplicated grief runs a fairly predictable course that ends with the relinquishing of the lost object and the resumption of the duties of life. Some of the common reactions experienced by grieving individuals are cited in Table 9–1.

Many grieving people experience feelings of anger or blame; these feelings may be directed toward those perceived to have caused or contributed to the death. Often, the anger associated with grief is directed at one's self, that is, expressed as guilt or depression. Even though the bereaved have done nothing to cause the death, "they often believe that somehow they should have been able to prevent it" (MacGregor, 1994). Some survivors have a strong need to assign blame. If someone else can be blamed, the survivors can rid themselves of any responsibility (Figure 9-2).

Figure 9-2 Anger is often a response to grief. This nurse is trying to help this client work through the anger she feels following a loss.

Dysfunctional Grief

Dysfunctional grief is a demonstration of a persistent pattern of intense grief that does not result in reconciliation of feelings. Persons experiencing dysfunctional (or pathological) grief do not progress through the stages of overwhelming emotions associated with grief and may fail to demonstrate any behaviors commonly associated with grief. The person experiencing pathological grief continues to have strong emotional reactions, does not return to a normal sleep pattern or work routine, usually remains isolated, and displays altered eating habits. The bereaved may have the need to endlessly tell and retell the story of loss but without subsequent healing. The pathologically

---

Table 9–1 REACTIONS COMMONLY EXPERIENCED DURING GRIEF (ENGLE)

PHYSICAL REACTIONS	PSYCHOSOCIAL REACTIONS	COGNITIVE REACTIONS	BEHAVIORAL REACTIONS
• Loss of appetite • Insomnia • Fatigue • Decreased libido • Decreased immune functioning (increased susceptibility to illness) • Multiple somatic complaints (e.g., headache, backache) • Restlessness	• Profound sadness • Helplessness • Hopelessness • Denial • Anger • Hostility • Guilt • Nightmares • Ennui (overwhelming sense of emptiness) • Preoccupation with lost object • Loneliness	• Inability to concentrate • Forgetfulness • Impaired judgment • Decreased problem-solving ability	• Impulsivity • Indecisiveness • Social withdrawal • Distancing

PROFESSIONAL TIP

Identifying Dysfunctional Grief

The difference between normal and dysfunctional grief is that the person experiencing dysfunctional grief is unable to adapt to life without the deceased person.

Dysfunctional grief can take several forms, specifically absent grief, distorted grief, or converted grief.

Absent grief is the inability of the person to incorporate the reality of the death into his life. This blocking of reality leads to an incapacity to feel.

Distorted grief blocks the progress of adaptive grieving. The person becomes "stuck" in feelings of guilt and anger, two emotions that are most likely to become distorted. This type of dysfunctional grief usually occurs when the relationship with the deceased was ambivalent or dependent and issues were left unresolved.

Converted grief occurs when the anxiety is expressed as distressing symptoms without the bereaved's being aware of the relationship between the symptom and the loss. The manifestations have no organic basis and can consist of:

- Somatic symptoms: fatigue, headache, tension, sleep changes, weight fluctuations, loss of libido;
- Psychological symptoms: anger, mood instability, diminished coping ability, depression, loss of sense of humor, inability to relax;
- Attitudinal changes: rigid thinking, cynicism, criticism, lack of concern, apathy; and
- Relational differences: irritability, decreased frustration tolerance, distancing.

grieving person is unable to reestablish a routine. Visits to the gravesite or mausoleum may be made often or not at all. A person experiencing dysfunctional grief continues to focus on the deceased, may overvalue objects that belonged to the deceased, and may engage in depressive brooding.

The professional caregiver must be aware of these behaviors and refer the pathologically grieving person to professional counseling.

Anticipatory Grief

Anticipatory grief is the occurrence of grief work before an expected loss actually occurs. Anticipatory grief may be experienced by the terminally ill person as well as the person's family. This phenomenon promotes adaptive grieving and, therefore, frees up the mourner's emotional energy necessary for problem solving. Although anticipatory grieving may be helpful in adjusting to the loss, it also has some potential disadvantages. For example, in the case of the dying client, anticipatory grieving may lead to family members' distancing themselves and not being available to provide support. Also, if the family members have separated themselves emotionally from the dying client, they may seem cold and distant, and, thus, not meet society's expectations of mourning behavior. This response can, in turn, prevent the mourners from receiving their own much needed support from others (Prichett & Lucas, 1997b).

Disenfranchised Grief

Doka, Rushton, and Thorstenson (1994) describe **disenfranchised grief** as "grief that is not openly acknowledged, socially sanctioned, or publicly shared." Grief can become disenfranchised when an individual either is reluctant to recognize the sense of loss and develops guilt feelings or feels pressured by society to "get on with life." An example of disenfranchised grief is extreme sadness over the loss of a pet when this mourning might be viewed by others as excessive or inappropriate. A mother's sadness over a miscarriage might also be considered disenfranchised grief, as a lengthy period of mourning may not be publicly expected despite the mother's intense feelings of loss and despair.

Factors Affecting Loss and Grief

Studies (Corless, Germino, & Pittman, 1995) conducted to determine factors that influence grieving identify the following variables as possibly affecting the intensity and duration of grieving:

- Developmental stage
- Religious and cultural beliefs
- Relationship with the lost object
- Cause of death

Developmental Stage

Depending on the client's place on the age/development continuum, the grief response to a loss will be experienced differently. Nurses practice in many settings where children, adolescents, and adults, as a result of growth and development, experience changes that result in loss. For example, a pregnant woman will, to some degree, experience loss after delivery of a first child (loss of freedom, independence, and self-focused life), even when the child is normal and healthy. Certain kinds of loss at key developmental points may have a profound effect on a person's ability to both work through the resulting grief and achieve the tasks of the given developmental stage. For example, an adolescent who has lost a parent may have difficulty forming an intimate relationship with members of the opposite sex.

Early Adulthood In the young adult, grief is usually precipitated by loss of role or status. For example, unemployment or the breakup of a relationship may cause significant grief for the young adult. The concept of death in this age group is primarily a reflection of cultural values and spiritual beliefs.

Middle Adulthood During middle adulthood, the potential for experiencing loss increases. The death of parents often occurs during this developmental phase. As an individual ages, it can be especially threatening when peers die, because these deaths force acknowledgment of one's own mortality.

Late Adulthood During late adulthood, most individuals recognize the inevitability of death. It is challenging for elders to experience the death of age-old friends or to find themselves the last one of their peer group left living. Older adults often turn to their children and grandchildren as sources of comfort and companionship. Cultivating friendships in all age groups helps prevent loneliness and depression.

Religious and Cultural Beliefs

Religious and cultural beliefs can have a significant effect on an individual's grief experience. Every culture has certain religious beliefs about the significance of death, as well as rituals for care of the dying. Beliefs about an afterlife, a supreme being, redemption of the soul, and reincarnation are important aspects that can assist one in grief work.

Relationship with the Lost Person or Object

In general, the more intimate the relationship with the deceased, the more intense the grief experienced by the bereaved. The death of a child poses a particular risk for dysfunctional grieving:

> One of life's saddest and deepest losses is the death of a child. . . . Without denying the seriousness of the loss in any death, there is an increased understanding that, at least in our culture, loss of a child represents a more severe and longer-lasting kind of injury and, because of this, is more difficult for the parents to process and resolve. (MacGregor, 1994)

The death of a child is generally thought to be exceptionally painful because it upsets the natural order of things; parents do not expect their children to die before them.

Individuals experiencing parental grief usually have intense reactions and responses (Figure 9-3). The uniqueness of parental grief for a deceased child may lie in the loss of the perceived potential of that child. It is the loss of the hopes of the parents for the child, for "the things that could have been." Table 9-2 suggests some characteristics of parents of infants who have died.

CULTURAL CONSIDERATIONS

Rituals following Death

- Judaism practices burial of the dead within 24 hours. A 7-day period of mourning, called *Shiva*, begins the day of the funeral.
- In the Muslim faith, men wash the body of a man and women wash the body of a woman after death.
- Buddhists believe that after death, the body should not be disturbed by movement, talking, or crying.
- Hindus pour holy water into the mouth of the dying person. The eldest son arranges for the funeral and cremation within 24 hours of death. Embalming is forbidden.
- Jehovah's Witnesses believe that the soul dies with the body, but 144,000 will be resurrected at the end-time and will be born again as spiritual sons of God.
- Native Americans believe that the spirit lives on after death. Ancestor worship is practiced.

(*From* Health Assessment & Physical Examination, *by M. E. Z. Estes, 1998, Albany, NY: Delmar. Copyright 1998 by Delmar.*)

The death of a parent or a sibling can pose a major challenge for children. The child's feelings may often go unrecognized by adults who fail to understand the child's need to mourn.

Cause of Death

The intensity of the grief response also varies according to the cause of death, be it unexpected, traumatic, or a suicide.

Unexpected Death The loss occurring as a result of an unexpected death poses particular difficulty for the bereaved in achieving closure. As Roach and Nieto

Figure 9-3 This couple discusses grief over the loss of a child.

Table 9–2 CHARACTERISTICS OF PARENTS WHOSE CHILDREN DIE

TYPE OF DEATH	PARENTAL CHARACTERISTICS
Miscarriage and stillbirth	• Parents, especially the mother, may have feelings of intense sadness, anger, or guilt. The death is often inadequately recognized by others, especially if the loss occurs in early weeks of pregnancy. • The death may be considered a personal failure. • Parents may dwell on details, designating blame to themselves or others. • Grief from previous miscarriages may be relived. • Anticipatory grief may occur if the condition of the infant is known early in the pregnancy. • Ambivalence about being pregnant, experienced early in the pregnancy, may increase grief. • Hopes for the future must be modified or changed. • Despair may peak when the parents must leave the hospital or birthplace without the baby.
Neonatal death	• Feelings are similar to those associated with stillbirth. • Parents have had the time to form a bond with the infant, intensifying the grief. • Grief may be intense for both parents.
Sudden infant death syndrome (SIDS)	• Parents are in a state of shock. • Pain is increased by lack of knowledge and misinformation. • Because SIDS usually occurs during the first 6 months of life, parental bonding is complete. • Guilt may be present. • Police may investigate, adding to the guilt. • Grief is acute, because the death is sudden and the parents are not prepared for the loss. • Parents, especially the mother, may be preoccupied with the details of the death.
Abortion	• Shame, secrecy, and guilt may accompany grief. • Highly ambivalent feelings may be present. • Little support or comfort is offered by others. • Feelings of relief are expected, but despair and depression may surface. • No guilt may be felt, especially if the woman did not want a child.

From Healing and the Grief Process, by S. S. Roach and B. C. Nieto, 1997, Albany, NY: Delmar. Copyright 1997, by Delmar.

(1997) state, any death, even an anticipated death, is a traumatic experience to the surviving loved ones. Unanticipated death, such as a death from a heart attack, aneurysm, or stroke, leaves survivors shocked and bereaved. Most often, the bereaved are capable of working through the grieving process without complications.

Traumatic Death Complicated grief is associated with traumatic death such as death by homicide, violence, or accident. Although traumatic death does not necessarily predispose the survivor to complications in mourning, survivors often suffer emotions of greater intensity than those associated with normal grief.

When loved ones die violently, the bereaved may suffer from traumatic imagery, that is, reliving the terror of the incident or imagining the feelings of horror felt by the victim. Traumatic imagery is a common occurrence in cases of traumatic death. Such thoughts, coupled with intense grief, can lead to post-traumatic stress disorder (PTSD) in the survivors. Nurses must be aware of the possibility of PTSD and be alert for the presence of symptoms, which may include:

• Sleep disturbances, such as recurrent, terror-filled nightmares;
• Psychological distress; and
• Chronic anxiety.

Unless this problem is recognized and the survivors are encouraged to express their intense feelings, they will not be able to progress through the normal, adaptive grieving process.

Suicide The loss of a loved one to suicide is frequently compounded by feelings of guilt among the survivors. They feel guilty for failing to recognize clues that may have enabled the victim to receive help. These feelings of guilt and self-blame can transform into anger at the victim for inflicting such pain, at themselves, and at caregivers. Feelings of shame for having a suicide in the family may also be present. The negative stigma of suicide may prohibit survivors from successfully resolving their grief.

Nursing Care of the Grieving Client

Resolution of a loss is a painful process and must be done by clients in their own way. Nurses can assist by providing support as the client moves through the process of mourning. Rodebaugh, Schwindt, and Valentine (1999) suggest that grief be thought of as a journey through four broad categories titled reeling, feeling, dealing, and healing. Clients are reeling when experiencing shock or disbelief. Feelings may be expressed in various emotions and behaviors. Dealing occurs when they begin to adapt to the loss. Things do not necessarily get better; they just get different. Healing is when the loss becomes part of them, and the acute anguish lessens; it does not mean forgetting. Grief changes people by affecting self-esteem, triggering the development of new ways of coping, and precipitating a new lifestyle without the deceased.

Nurses can play an active role in assisting people to grieve by encouraging clients to do their grief work, that is, to experience their feelings to the fullest in order to work through them. Providing support and explaining to the bereaved that it will take time to grieve the loss and to gain some closure to the relationship are both important nursing responsibilities (Figure 9-4).

Assessment

A thorough assessment of the grieving client and family begins with a determination of the personal meaning of the loss. Another key assessment area is deciding the person's progress in terms of the grieving process. The nurse understands that the stages of grieving are not necessarily mastered sequentially, but, instead, that individuals may vacillate in progression through the stages of grief.

Nursing Diagnosis

The North American Nursing Diagnosis Association (NANDA) defines *Dysfunctional Grieving* as "extended, unsuccessful use of intellectual and emotional responses by which individuals, families, communities attempt to work through the process of modifying self-concept based upon the perception of loss" (NANDA, 2001). Another diagnosis that may be applicable is *Anticipatory Grieving,* defined as "intellectual and emotional responses and behaviors by which individuals, families, communities work through the process of modifying self-concept based on the perception of potential loss" (NANDA, 2001).

Planning/Outcome Identification

It is important to clarify the expected outcomes when planning care for the grieving client. Listed below are some expected goals for the person experiencing grief:

- Verbalize feelings of grief
- Share grief with significant others
- Accept the loss
- Renew activities and relationships

Some of these expected outcomes will take a long period of time to achieve, and some must be achieved before others are mastered. For example, to accept the loss, the person must begin to share grief with others by verbalizing those feelings. Two of the expected outcomes are discussed below.

Acceptance of the Loss Only by going through grief work are individuals able to reach some acceptance and, ultimately, resolution of feelings about the loss. Often, people try to find some meaning in their

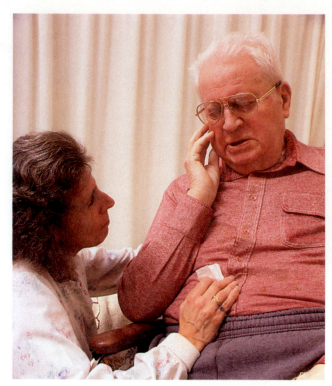

Figure 9-4 The nurse provides support to this client to help him through the grief process.

situations. This search involves introspection, for which spiritual support may be therapeutic.

Renewal of Activities and Relationships The very core of grief work revolves around acceptance of the fact that the needs met by key people in our lives can be met in other ways and by other people. The deceased cannot be replaced; however, enough healing must occur so that new relationships can be initiated.

Implementation

Therapeutic nursing care is based on an understanding of the significance of the loss to the client. To understand the client's perspective, the nurse must

PROFESSIONAL TIP

Adaptive Grieving

How long does the process of adaptive grieving take? The length of time necessary for grief resolution is as individual as the person experiencing it and depends on the intensity of the grief. Grief is considered to be a "long-term process" (Corless, Germino, & Pittman, 1995). Grief work takes time. There are no definite time frames within which grief should occur. Each person grieves in his own way and at his own pace.

spend time listening. As the client expresses feelings, the nurse must demonstrate acceptance, even if the client is not responding according to the nurse's expectations or belief system. The nurse's nonjudgmental, accepting attitude is essential during the bereaved's expression of all feelings, including anger and despair. The nurse communicates an understanding of the client's anger and avoids personalizing and using defensive behaviors. "Caregivers must demonstrate, verbally and through nonjudgmental attitudes and behaviors, that the expression of grief is not only appropriate but essential for therapeutic resolution of the loss" (MacGregor, 1994).

Grieving people need reassurance, counseling, and support. One mechanism of support on a long-term basis is support groups. The nurse must be informed about the availability of such groups within the community in order to make appropriate referrals. When bereaved people join support groups, they will be with others who have experienced similar losses. This sharing decreases the feelings of loneliness and social isolation so common in the grief experience.

Evaluation

People follow their own time schedule for grief work. In general, it takes months or years for grief resolution. Therefore, nurses usually do not have an opportunity to be with the bereaved family when grief work is completed. However, the nurse has a unique opportunity to lay the foundation for adaptive grieving by encouraging the bereaved to share their feelings and to continue to verbalize their experience with significant others. The goals mutually established with client and family are the foundation for evaluation. It is important for nurses to teach grieving individuals that resolution of the loss is generally a process of life-long adjustment.

DEATH

Historically, death has been considered as natural as birth, as simply the last stage of life. The last three decades have brought about significant changes in the cultural perception of death, however. In some cases, dying and death are no longer simple matters but are issues involving ethical concerns and, in some cases, legal intervention by the court system.

Just as each person lives a unique life, each person dies a unique death. Death may be sudden and unexpected, caused by heart attack or accident, for example, or death may be prolonged, coming after a distressing long-term illness. Death may come quietly for the older person who dies during sleep. And some deaths are planned by those who choose to die on their own terms by way of suicide.

Health care workers must understand the legal and ethical issues surrounding dying and death. Under-

standing the stages of death and dying and the signs of impending death will help prepare the nurse to render sensitive, effective care, both to the client and family and to the client's body after death. Nurses must also come to terms with their own mortality and feelings about death if they are to provide comfort to dying clients and their families. Health care workers can learn a great deal about life from the dying client.

Legal Considerations

The *Patient Self-Determination Act* (PSDA) was incorporated into the Omnibus Budget Reconciliation Act (OBRA) of 1990. The act was intended to provide a legal means for individuals to determine the circumstances under which life-sustaining treatment should or should not be provided to them. The individual's choices are validated by advance directives. An advance directive is any written instruction, including a living will or durable power of attorney for health care, that is recognized under state law (Taylor, 1995). The act applies to hospitals, long-term care facilities, home health agencies, hospice programs, and certain health maintenance organizations (HMOs). According to the PSDA, all clients entering the health care system through any of these organizations must be given

CULTURAL CONSIDERATIONS

Cultural Influences and Advance Directive Decisions

African American Clients
- Are more likely to select aggressive interventions.
- Are less likely than European American or Hispanic American clients to have documented their end-of-life health care wishes

European American Clients
- Are much more likely to have written advance directives than are members of other cultures.
- Select "no code" more than do Hispanic American or African American clients but less than do Asian American clients

Asian American Clients
- Select "no code" more than do all other groups
- Are less likely to have advance directives

Hispanic American Clients
- Are less likely than are European American or Asian American clients to have written directives
- Are least likely of all groups to select "no code"

(*Data from "Meeting the Challenge of Advance Directives," by P. Haynor, 1998,* AJN, 98(3), 27–32.)

information and the opportunity to complete advance directives if they have not already done so. Clients need to know that in many states, just signing these documents may not be adequate for carrying out their wishes. They may also need to indicate their wishes in regard to artificial feeding, intubation, chemotherapy, surgery, blood transfusions, and transfer to the hospital (for residents in skilled care facilities).

Although the living will and durable power of attorney for health care are legal documents, they do not preclude the need for **resuscitation** (support measures to restore consciousness and life). The medical record must have a written do-not-resuscitate (DNR) order from a physician if this is in agreement with the client's wishes and with the advance directives. In the absence of such an order, resuscitation will be initiated.

Many states also have a **Health Care Surrogate Law** which is implemented in the absence of advance directives. This law varies from state to state. Basically, it provides a legal means for specific individuals to make decisions for the client when the client can no longer do so. The law has developed a hierarchy of individuals who would act in the interests of the client. The spouse is the first person in the hierarchy, followed by children in the event that there is no spouse.

Ethical Considerations

Death is often fraught with ethical dilemmas that occur almost daily in health care settings. Many health care agencies have ethics committees to develop and implement policies to deal with end-of-life issues. Ethics committees are interdisciplinary and may have attorneys and clergy in addition to health care providers as members. Ethical decision making is a complex issue. One of the most difficult dilemmas is determining the difference between killing and allowing someone to die by withholding life-sustaining treatment methods.

The American Nurses Association (ANA) distinguishes relieving pain and mercy killing (euthanasia or assisted suicide). Pain relief is a central value in nursing, whereas euthanasia is viewed as unethical. The ANA's position is that increasing doses of medication to control pain in terminally ill clients is ethically justified, even at the expense of maintaining life (ANA, 1992).

Stages of Dying and Death

In her classic works, Elizabeth Kübler-Ross (1969, 1974) identified five possible stages of dying that are experienced by clients and their families (Table 9–3). Not every client moves sequentially through each stage. These stages are experienced in varying degrees and for varying lengths of time. The client may express anger, and then, a few minutes later, express acceptance of the inevitable, and then express anger again. The value in Kübler-Ross' work is that it helps increase sensitivity to the needs of the dying client.

PROFESSIONAL TIP

Care of the Dying Client

Dying was once considered to be a normal part of the life cycle. Today, it is often considered to be a medical problem that should be handled by health care providers. Technological advances in medicine have lead to depersonalized and mechanical care of those who are dying. Technological advances, the institutionalization of medical practice, legislative regulations, and societal changes have "in many ways depersonalized the process of dying, while engendering growing new fears of death" (Thompson, 1994).

Our highly technological world calls for application of high-touch interventions with the dying. In other words, appropriate care of the dying is administered by compassionate nurses who are both technically competent and able to demonstrate caring.

Table 9–3 KÜBLER-ROSS' STAGES OF DYING AND DEATH	
STAGE	**EXAMPLE**
First Stage: **Denial**	*Verbal:* "This can't be happening to me!" *Behavioral:* Client is diagnosed with terminal lung cancer; client continues to smoke two packs of cigarettes daily.
Second Stage: **Anger**	*Verbal:* "Why me?" *Behavioral:* Client strikes out at caregivers.
Third Stage: **Bargaining**	*Verbal:* Client prays, "Please, God, just let me live long enough to see my grandchild graduate." *Behavioral:* Client tries to "make deals" with caregivers or god.
Fourth Stage: **Depression**	*Verbal:* "Go away. I just want to lie here in bed. What's the use?" *Behavioral:* Client withdraws and isolates self.
Fifth Stage: **Acceptance**	*Verbal:* "I feel ready. At least, I'm more at peace now." *Behavioral:* Client gets financial or legal affairs in order. Client says goodbye to significant others.

Data from On Death and Dying, *by E. Kübler-Ross, 1969, New York: Macmillan. Copyright 1969 by Macmillan.*

Denial

In the first stage of dying, the initial shock can be overwhelming. Denial is a useful tool in coping. It is an essential and protective mechanism that may last for only a few minutes or may manifest for months.

In some clients, denial manifests as "doctor shopping" (not to imply that second opinions are not sometimes necessary) or insisting that there must have been a mix-up or mistake in the diagnostic tests. In other clients, denial manifests as simply avoiding the issue. They go about their daily routines as though nothing in their lives has changed. Most people, given the time, will eventually move past the stage of denial.

Clients may choose to be selective in the use of denial. For example, clients may use denial with certain family members or friends because they are trying to protect those people from the truth. Clients may also use denial from time to time to set aside thoughts of illness and death in order to focus on living.

Anger

The initial stage of denial is often followed by anger. The client's security is being threatened by the unknown. All the normal daily routines have become disrupted. This stage is typically very difficult for family and caregivers because they may feel powerless or useless in terms of helping their loved one through the situation. The client has no control over the situation and, thus, becomes angry in response to this powerlessness. The anger may be directed at self, God, others, the environment, and the health care system. In the client's eyes, whatever is done is not the right thing. Family members may be greeted with silence or with outbursts of anger. Their response, in turn, may be anger, guilt, or despair.

Bargaining

The anticipation of the loss through death may bring about bargaining, through which the client attempts to postpone or reverse the inevitable. The client's bargaining represents an attempt to postpone death and usually has self-imposed limitations. For example, the client will ask to live just long enough to see her first grandchild born in exchange for a promise to perform some service for the church. Most clients bargain in silence or in confidence with their spiritual leader. Caregivers who have cared for terminally ill clients will agree that it is not uncommon for a client to live long enough for some special event (a wedding or birth), only to die shortly afterwards.

Depression

When the realization comes that the loss can no longer be delayed, the client moves to the stage of depression. This depression is different from dysfunctional depression in that it helps the client detach from life and, thus, be able to accept death. Depression in

PROFESSIONAL TIP

Reactions to Impending Death

- Persons of all ages generally experience the same feelings and emotions as they progress through a terminal illness.
- Persons of any age who have endured a long illness may view death as a release from their suffering.
- Persons of any age may find it difficult to reach acceptance if they have unfinished business.
- Many people receive satisfaction from **life review** (a form of reminiscence wherein a client attempts to come to terms with conflict or to gain meaning from life and die peacefully).

this sense is a therapeutic experience for the dying person. Clients sometimes feel abandoned, as persons who were once friends begin to visit less and less, sometimes severing ties with the client even before death; this may compound the client's feelings of depression and hopelessness.

Acceptance

The final stage, acceptance, may not be reached by every dying client. With acceptance comes growing peace and contentment. The feeling that all that could be done has been done is often expressed during this stage. Reinforcement of the client's feelings and sense of personal worth are important during this stage. Many clients will make an effort to get all of their personal and financial affairs in order.

The client may sleep more, not to avoid reality, but because sleep is needed to fill a physical and emotional need. The client may limit visitors to a few people with whom he feels safe and comfortable. The most significant form of communication at this time is moments of silence.

Nursing Care of the Dying Client

Nursing care of clients who are terminally ill or who are facing and preparing for their own death can be both challenging and rewarding. The death process is typically a very emotional time for clients and their

GERONTOLOGICAL CONSIDERATIONS

Death

- Elderly clients may welcome death, especially if they have outlived everyone who was near and dear to them.

families; compassionate and sensitive nursing care that respects clients' wishes as well as meets their physical needs can help bring peace and dignity to this natural process.

Assessment

Nursing interventions are based on a thorough assessment of the client's holistic needs. Assessment of the dying client includes an ongoing collection of data regarding the strengths and limitations of the dying person and the family.

Nursing Diagnoses

The nurse's assessment of the dying client may lead to any number of diagnoses. One NANDA-approved nursing diagnosis that is applicable for many dying clients is *Powerlessness,* that is, "the perception that one's own action will not significantly affect an outcome; a perceived lack of control over a current situation or immediate happening" (NANDA, 2001). Another response that is often experienced by the dying is described by the diagnosis *Hopelessness,* "a subjective state in which an individual sees limited or no alternatives or personal choices available and is unable to mobilize energy on own behalf" (NANDA, 2001). The client may also exhibit *Death Anxiety,* "apprehension, worry, or fear related to death or dying" (NANDA, 2001).

Planning/Outcome Identification

The major goals of nursing care are the physical, emotional, and mental comfort of the client. The goals of nursing care for the dying client are the same as those goals developed for all clients who are unable to meet their own needs. The dying client must be treated as a unique individual worthy of respect, rather than as a diagnosis to be cured. Many dying clients do

PROFESSIONAL TIP

Information Needed in Assessment of the Dying Client

- Client and family goals and expectations
- Client's awareness of the terminal nature of illness
- Availability of support systems
- Current stage of dying
- History of previous positive coping skills
- Client perception of unfinished business to be completed

(Adapted from Death and Dying, by K. Pritchett and P. Lucas, 1997. In Psychiatric–Mental Health Nursing: Adaptation and Growth (4th ed., pp. 206–207), by B. S. Johnson (Ed.), 1997, Philadelphia: Lippincott.)

PROFESSIONAL TIP

Planning Care for the Dying Client

- Schedule time to be available to the client
- Identify areas that are of special concern to the client and make referrals if appropriate (e.g., social worker consult for information on financial assistance)
- Promote and protect individual self-esteem and self-worth
- Balance the client's needs for independence and assistance
- Meet the physiological needs of the client and family
- Respect the client's confidentiality
- Answer all questions and provide factual information to the client and family
- Offer to contact clergy or other spiritual leader

(Adapted from Death and Dying, by K. Pritchett and P. Lucas. In Psychiatric–Mental Health Nursing: Adaptation and Growth (4th ed., p. 208), by B. S. Johnson (Ed.) (1997) Philadelphia: Lippincott.)

not fear death but are anxious about a painful death or dying alone.

Promoting optimal quality of life means treating the client and family in a respectful manner and providing a safe environment for the expression of feelings. Planning focuses on meeting the holistic needs of the client and family. These needs are specified in the Dying Person's Bill of Rights (Figure 9-5), which is as relevant today as when it was written in 1975. In planning care, the nurse should make every effort to be sensitive to the dying client's rights.

Implementation

The nurse's first priority is to communicate a caring attitude to the client. A recent study (Czerwiec, 1996) quoted family members of recently deceased hospitalized clients as stating that "the factor that most strongly affects family satisfaction [is] perceiving the staff to have a caring attitude toward the patient and to be acting on his behalf."

When a client is in denial, it is important for the nurse to approach the client with understanding and the knowledge that moving between the stages of dying is enhanced by a trusting nurse–client relationship. Establishment of rapport facilitates the client's verbalization of feelings (Figure 9-6). The nurse establishes a safe environment wherein the client does not feel embarrassed or chastised for experiencing those feelings. Nurses must understand that clients are not angry with them, but, rather, with the situation they are experiencing.

The Dying Person's Bill of Rights

- I have the right to be treated as a living human being until I die.
- I have the right to maintain a sense of hopefulness, however changing its focus may be.
- I have the right to be cared for by those who can maintain a sense of hopefulness, however challenging this might be.
- I have the right to express my feelings and emotions about my approaching death in my own way.
- I have the right to participate in decisions concerning my care.
- I have the right to expect continuing medical and nursing attention even though "cure" goals must be changed to "comfort" goals.
- I have the right not to die alone.
- I have the right to be free from pain.
- I have the right to have my questions answered honestly.
- I have the right not to be deceived.
- I have the right to have help from and for my family in accepting death.
- I have the right to die in peace and dignity.
- I have the right to retain my individuality and not be judged for my decisions, which may be contrary to beliefs of others.
- I have the right to expect that the sanctity of the human body will be respected after death.
- I have the right to be cared for by caring, sensitive, knowledgeable people who will attempt to understand my needs and will be able to gain some satisfaction in helping me face my death.

Figure 9-5 The Dying Person's Bill of Rights *(From "The dying person's bill of rights," by A. J. Barbus, 1975,* AJN, *75(1).)*

Terminally ill clients are often given **palliative care**, or care that relieves symptoms, such as pain, but does not alter the course of disease. A primary aim of palliative care is to help the client feel safe and secure. The nurse can do much to increase the client's feelings of safety by being available when needed. Holding the client's hand and listening are therapeutic measures. Ufema (1995a) suggests asking the client three questions: What do you want? From whom do you want it? and When do you want it? The client needs to know that he has the nurse's support as an advocate for his care and well-being.

Physiological Needs According to Maslow's hierarchy of needs, physiological needs must be met be-

Figure 9-6 Establishing a caring and trusting relationship helps the client come to terms with a terminal illness.

fore others, because they are essential for existence. Areas that are often problematic for the terminally ill client are respirations; fluids and nutrition; mouth, eyes, and nose; mobility; skin care; and elimination.

Respirations Oxygen is frequently ordered for the client experiencing labored breathing. Suctioning may be needed to remove secretions that the client is unable to swallow.

Fluids and Nutrition The refusal of food and fluids is almost universal in dying clients. It is believed that the client is not feeling thirst and hunger. Although the issue of permitting dehydration in terminally ill clients is often met with great resistance, the literature supports the concept that forced nutrition has questionable value and may even exacerbate the client's condition (Taylor, 1995). Artificial nutrition often increases the client's agitation, leads to increased use of limb restraints, and increases the risk of aspiration pneumonia (Rhymes, 1993). Hospice nurses have indicated that withholding artificial nutrition is not painful. Regardless, in every situation, the client's own wishes must always take precedence. If the comatose client has not previously made his wishes known, family members must be given accurate and truthful information. For the person in irreversible coma, withholding of artificial nutrition does not cause death; rather, it allows life to take its natural course (Taylor, 1995). Several professional groups have issued statements regarding artificial nutrition and hydration. The American Medical Association, the American Dietetic Association, and the ANA agree that it is legally, ethically, and professionally acceptable to discontinue nutritional support if the terminally ill client so requests (Taylor, 1995).

Mouth, Eyes, and Nose Oral discomfort is the only documented side effect of dehydration in the terminally ill client (Taylor, 1995). Both the administration of oxygen and mouth breathing increase the need for meticulous oral care. Caregivers can use saliva substitutes and moisturizers to alleviate discomfort. The regular use of toothpaste and a toothbrush may be adequate. The tongue must be given the same attention as is the rest of the mouth, with gentle brushing. Ice chips and sips of favorite beverages should be offered frequently, and petroleum jelly applied to the lips. Oral care must be given every 2 to 3 hours to maintain the client's comfort.

The eyes may become irritated due to dryness. Artificial tears can alleviate this discomfort. A cotton ball should be used to gently wipe the eye from inner to outer canthus (one wipe per cotton ball) to remove any discharge.

The nares may become dry and crusted. Oxygen given by cannula can further irritate the nares. A thin layer of water soluble jelly applied to the nares will help alleviate discomfort. The elastic strap of the oxygen cannula should not be applied too tightly, lest it cause discomfort.

Mobility As the client's condition deteriorates, mobility decreases. The client becomes less able to move about in bed or to get out of bed and requires more assistance. Physical dependence increases the risk of complications related to immobility, such as atrophy and pressure ulcers. Attentive nursing care can prevent the onset of these complications, which increase both client discomfort and the cost of care.

The client should be repositioned at least every 2 hours. It is important to keep in mind that the client may have other disorders that contribute to discomfort related to mobility, such as arthritis or lung disease. The nurse can help the client maintain body alignment with the use of pillows and other supportive equipment and can use positioning techniques to facilitate ease of breathing. Passive range of motion exercises should be performed at least twice a day to prevent stiffness and aching of the joints. The client may prefer to be assisted into a reclining type of chair at intervals throughout the day. Using a wheelchair can also increase the client's environmental space, giving the client more mobility, control, and independence.

Skin Care The prevention of pressure ulcers is a priority. Pressure ulcers are painful, can cause secondary complications such as sepsis, and are costly to treat. Regular repositioning and passive range of motion exercises are two preventive measures. In addition, keeping the skin clean and moisturized will promote healthy tissue. The skin should be inspected once or twice daily, with special attention paid to pressure points and areas where skin surfaces rub together. Gentle massages with soothing lotion are comforting. Bed baths are adequate if the client cannot get into the tub or sit in a shower chair.

Elimination Constipation may occur due to side effects of pain medications and to lack of physical activity. Fluids and foods with high-fiber content can be effective preventive measures for clients with adequate oral intake. Constipation can also be alleviated by maintaining a scheduled time for bowel elimination and administering suppositories, if necessary. A commode with padded arms can be more comfortable than a toilet.

The client may become incontinent of bladder and bowel, so the nurse must check the client frequently, clean the skin with peri-washes, and apply a moisture barrier after each incontinent episode. Incontinent undergarments may increase the client's comfort, especially when the client is out of bed.

Indwelling catheters are never a first choice for bladder management. However, for some clients, the need for frequent cleaning, the discomfort of using a bedpan, or getting out of bed to use the toilet or commode may cause agonizing pain. In these circumstances, the benefits of a catheter greatly outweigh the risks.

Comfort The primary activities directed at promoting physical comfort include pain relief, keeping the client clean and dry, and providing a safe, nonthreatening environment. The nurse who demonstrates a respectful, caring attitude promotes the client's psychological comfort by establishing rapport. The fear of a painful death is almost universal. Pain is a subjective, personal experience, and the client is the best judge of the severity of the pain. Many, though certainly not all, dying clients experience pain. In its position statement on pain relief for the terminally ill, the ANA states that promotion of comfort is the major goal of nursing care (ANA, 1992). Comfort should be maximized by management of pain and other discomforting factors.

The client needs to know that caregivers accept and believe complaints of pain and that they will intervene to prevent and alleviate the pain. The nurse should ask the client to rate the pain on a scale from 0 to 10, with 0 being no pain, and 10 being severe pain. Medication must be given around the clock and not "as needed." A nonnarcotic analgesic may be effective in early stages for mild, intermittent pain. As the pain increases, the client may need to be started on morphine, titrated at increments until adequate pain relief is achieved without severe side effects. Titrating the analgesic dose and interval means finding the lowest dose and the longest interval that will relieve pain. The dosage that should be used is the one that controls the pain to the satisfaction of the client and that causes minimal side effects. For some clients, this may be 10 mg of oral morphine sulfate (MS) every 4 hours. For other clients, it may be 480 mg MS intravenously per hour. The question for the nurse is, what dose can be safely given? No maximum number of milligrams applies to every individual.

The nurse must monitor the client's responses with regard to pain rating and respiratory rate. For example, 10 mg MS given IM may afford pain relief, but if the respiratory rate drops from 12 to 6 per minute, the next

PROFESSIONAL TIP

Adjuvant Therapy

Adjuvant therapy may be effective. Nonsteroidal anti-inflammatory agents are beneficial for bone metastases; tricyclic antidepressants and anti-seizure medications for neurogenic pain, and steroids for headaches related to cerebral edema (Rhymes, 1993). Nonpharmacological techniques can be used along with medication. Relaxation techniques, guided imagery, massages, and repositioning may enhance the action of the medications.

dose should be reduced. If the same dose given to another client provides minimal relief, and the client is alert and displays no change in respirations, the next dose should be increased (McCaffery & Pasero, 1999).

The client must be monitored for **breakthrough pain**, or sudden, acute, temporary pain that is usually precipitated by a treatment or procedure or by unusual activity of the client. A supplemental dose of medication is required. If the precipitating factor is known (dressing changes, for example), a dose should be given 30 to 60 minutes before the procedure.

Physical Environment A soothing physical environment can significantly increase the client's comfort. Soft lighting enhances vision without causing the discomfort associated with harsh, glaring light. Complying with the client's request for a night light is also helpful in creating a pleasant and non-threatening environment. If possible, the client should be offered the opportunity to have the bed or a chair near a window to increase the range of the environment. As the client's circulation becomes more sluggish, body temperature will fall. Lightweight comforters will increase warmth without adding uncomfortable weight. The nurse can help eliminate environmental odors by ensuring adequate ventilation, daily cleaning of the room, removal of leftover food, and frequent linen changes. Noise can be distracting and anxiety provoking, so the nurse and visitors should comply with the client's wishes with regard to the use of radio and television. The telephone can be removed from the room, if the client finds the ringing disturbing.

Psychosocial Needs Death presents a threat to not only one's physical existence, but to one's psychological integrity. As deBlois (1994) states:

We are all too familiar with the scene of the dying person tethered to tubes and electronic gadgetry in an intensive care unit. Held captive in a tangle of technology, the person is kept at a distance from the supportive presence and touch of family and friends by well-meaning but technologically oriented healthcare professionals.

Technology does not replace touch, concern, compassion, and human companionship. Nurses, through their presence, can humanize the dying person's environment. Families should be encouraged and invited to participate in the client's care, if they desire to do so and the client is willing.

For many clients, maintaining a well-groomed appearance is important. When the client can no longer make requests or give directions for care, caregivers should presume that the client would prefer to maintain the same grooming habits as were previously preferred. Shaving the male client's beard or cleaning and trimming the client's fingernails and toenails, for instance, will help the client maintain a well-groomed appearance and will also promote client dignity. Combing and brushing the hair not only improves appearance, but is also a comforting and relaxing activity for many clients.

Dressing and undressing may become a cumbersome, frustrating, and fatiguing activity. The client who spends time up and about may choose attractive pajamas, housecoats, dusters, or exercise suits. Nurses should advise individuals who may be purchasing clothing for the client to select items that are loose fitting, have few fasteners, and are washable.

Spiritual Needs Nurses play a major role in promoting the dying client's spiritual comfort. "Dying persons are among the most vulnerable members of the human family. The moral health and integrity of the broader community can be measured in part by the

COMMUNITY/HOME HEALTH CARE

Equipment To Increase Client Comfort

The following equipment can be rented and may qualify for payment by Medicare or private insurance.

- An electric hospital bed with overhead trapeze, to give the client more control of the environment
- A commode, to extend the client's independence in elimination
- A lifting device, to facilitate getting the dependent client out of bed
- Remote control, for the client who enjoys television
- Portable telephone
- Shower chair and hand-held shower for the bathtub
- Comfort devices such as special mattresses for the bed and cushions for chairs
- Overbed table, for eating or hand activities
- Comfortable chairs close to the bed, to facilitate visits of family and friends

way we respond to their needs" (deBlois, 1994). Dying persons may experience confusion, anger at their god, crises of faith, or other types of spiritual distress.

Dying is a personal and, frequently, lonely process. "People living impoverished spiritual, social, intellectual lives lack the resources for a meaningful experience with dying" (Thompson, 1994). Table 9–4 provides information on the views of various religions with regard to withdrawal of life support; death; and

organ donation. The nurse can serve as a sounding board for the client who expresses values and beliefs related to death. The following are therapeutic nursing interventions that address the spiritual needs of the dying client:

- Communicate empathy
- Play music
- Use touch

Table 9–4 RELIGIONS AND DYING AND DEATH ISSUES

RELIGION	LIFE SUPPORT WITHDRAWAL	DEATH	ORGAN DONATION
Judaism	Allowed under the right circumstances (when life support is serving only to impede a natural death).	• Suicide is forbidden. • Burial should occur within 24 hours. • Cremation is forbidden.	• Permitted because the procedure saves life. • Rejected by Orthodox Jews. • Autopsy is permitted if it will save future lives.
Islam	Permitted if only serving to prolong death or if client's condition is medically hopeless.	• Suicide is forbidden. • Relatives and friends are present. • Autopsy is permitted to solve a crime or provide further medical knowledge.	• Permitted.
Catholicism/ Orthodoxy	Controversial; permitted if client's condition is hopeless.	• Prayers are offered at time of death. • Burial and cremation are permitted. • Autopsy is permitted.	• Permitted.
Protestantism	Permitted if client's condition is hopeless.	• Prayers are offered at time of death. • Burial and cremation are permitted. • Autopsy is permitted.	• Permitted, although may be rejected by some Baptists or Pentecostals.
Jehovah's Witnesses	Permitted if serving only to prolong death or if quality of life is nonexistent.	• Suicide is not approved. • Autopsy is permitted if legally necessary.	• Individual choice.
Buddhism	Acceptable for those on threshold of death.	• Suicide is criticized. • Cremation is common.	• Controversial.
Hinduism	Supported to allow a natural death.	• Prefer to die at home. • Embalming is forbidden. • Autopsy is discouraged. • Suicide is forbidden.	• Forbidden.
Mormons	A client or family decision.	• Cremation is discouraged. • Autopsy is a family decision.	• A family decision.
Native Americans	Life support is viewed as unnatural and, therefore, unnecessary.	• Complex beliefs about death and treatment of the body.	• Discouraged.

Data from Health Assessment & Physical Examination *(2nd. ed.), by M. E. Z. Estes, 2002, Albany, NY: Delmar. Copyright 2002 by Delmar.*

- Pray with the client
- Contact clergy, if requested by the client
- Read religious literature aloud, at the client's request.

Support for the Family Family members need to be involved in the care of their dying loved one. Guilt may be increased by feelings of powerlessness. Involving family members in the treatment is a helpful intervention (MacGregor, 1994). Families facing the impending death of a loved one require much support from nurses and other caregivers. The nurse's presence, just being there with the family, is extremely important. A recent study showed that "family members indicated that when a loved one is dying, they'd like to know that a nurse will make a special effort to be . . . available" (Czerwiec, 1996).

Each family group has its unwritten rules, its leaders and followers, and its methods for coping with crises. The family's equilibrium is threatened by the impending death. If family members have limited coping skills and inadequate support systems, they need assistance and guidance from the caregivers. Nurses must remember that the rules and coping mechanisms used by the family may not always coincide with the values and beliefs of the staff and that the client's and family's wishes must be respected to the extent possible.

Each family member will grieve the approaching death in her own way. The nurse must be supportive and nonjudgmental. The family needs to know that the staff cares about them as well as the client.

The relationship with the family does not always end with the client's death. Staff members may attend visitations, funerals, or memorial services. If a hospice was involved, the family may participate in a bereavement support program. If the client was a resident in a long-term care facility, family members may return to visit other residents with whom they became acquainted.

Learning Needs Bereaved families need much support and information. The nurse's role is to teach family members what they need to know. For instance, families must be assisted with acquiring the tools that will help them help their loved one. An example might be the need for the family to understand that the dying person needs to conserve energy. Some simple actions on the part of the family could be to schedule activities after a rest period or early in the morning, when the client is strongest. The nurse may need to point out to the family this type of common sense approach, as simple interventions such as these can be overlooked during this highly charged emotional time.

Client and family knowledge deficits can relate to:

- Insufficient information about physical condition,
- Information about the treatment regimen,

CLIENT TEACHING

Guidelines for Teaching a Family Caregiver
- Discuss the nature and extent of the disease process
- Use adult-education principles
- Reinforce material frequently
- Clearly explain the purpose of palliative care while maintaining a sense of realistic hope
- Inform client and family of available community resources; reassure them that they are not alone
- Teach steps for caregiver to follow if an emergency arises at home
- Provide written instructions for caregiver to follow, including important telephone numbers and persons to be contacted
- Inform about the purpose of hospice

- Inability to anticipate medical crises,
- Inexperience with personal threat of death, and
- Unfamiliarity with protocol to follow in case of the need for emergency care outside of the hospital

Hospice Care **Hospice**, a type of care for the terminally ill, is founded on the concept of allowing individuals to die with dignity and surrounded by those who love them. Clients enter hospice care when aggressive medical treatment is no longer an option or when the client refuses further medical intervention.

Home Care A dying person is often not given the opportunity to be surrounded by family and friends. "More than 80% of all reported deaths in the United States occur in healthcare institutions where people die in unfamiliar, and sometimes intimidating, surroundings" (deBlois, 1994).

Impending Death

No one can predict how long a client will be in the terminal stages of illness. A client may exhibit signs of impending death and then rally to live for several more days. It is not uncommon for clients to endure until a member of the family arrives for a last good-bye. The client who has had a long and troublesome illness may be ready to die but needs "permission" to die from a loved one, who says, "It's okay, you can go now." A client may not wish to die when others are present and will wait to take the last breath until everyone has left the room.

Even when death is expected, it is never easy for the family. The family should be thoroughly informed, in simple terms, about what will happen before and after the client's death, including:

An Alternative for the Dying Client

- Family members should be physically and emotionally able to provide care.
- Health care providers should share the responsibility of home care with the family. This sharing could include respite time and frequent visits.

- Physical changes that will occur just before and following death
- Pronouncement of death
- Post-mortem care
- Removal of the body

Impending death is signaled by a series of irrevocable events (Durham & Weiss, 1997):

- The lungs become unable to provide adequate gas diffusion.
- The heart and blood vessels become unable to maintain adequate tissue perfusion.
- The brain ceases to regulate vital centers.

Cheyne-Stokes respirations (breathing characterized by periods of apnea alternating with periods of dyspnea) most often herald pulmonary system failure. Secretions accumulate in the larynx and trachea, causing noisy respirations, often called the "**death rattle**."

The heart fails in its pumping function, resulting in poor perfusion, ischemia, and cell death. The skin becomes cool and, possibly, very pale, cyanotic, jaundiced, or mottled. The pulse becomes rapid, irregular, weak, and thready. Death is several hours away if a peripheral pulse is strong and easily palpated. Cold, cyanotic extremities and irregular respirations indicate that death may be expected within an hour or two (Durham & Weiss, 1997).

Inadequate cerebral perfusion hinders the brain's ability to integrate vital functions. The client may be confused and lethargic and may respond only to direct visual, auditory, or tactile stimulation. Pupils no longer react to light and become fixed. The client may "talk" to dead loved ones. A frown or tight facial muscles may indicate pain or discomfort. A client in a coma will move only in response to deep pain. Analgesics should not be withdrawn from a client in a coma.

The care of the client does not cease during this final stage of life. The nursing actions previously described should be continued. The nurse should tell the client in brief, simple terms what is happening as care is rendered. The family should be allowed and encouraged to continue their participation, if that is their wish. The nurse should caution family members that the dying client can hear even in the absence of verbal

When the Client Dies at Home (Expected Death)

The family must:

- Have a list of telephone numbers readily available,
- Have the name and telephone number of the funeral director,
- Know whom to call (physician or hospice nurse or funeral director),
- Know whom not to call (ambulance and emergency services),
- Record the time of death,
- Record the last medications given,
- Record the condition of the client during the last few hours, and
- Record the last time the client was seen by the nurse.

response, so all comments and conversation should continue to be respectful.

There may be other indications that death is near. The client may report seeing angels (Ufema, 1995b) or hearing beautiful music. These experiences should be accepted as a natural step in the process of dying. When the final breath is taken, the heart stops beating. Within a few minutes, cerebral death (the point at which brain cells die) occurs, and brain activity ceases.

Care after Death

Caring for the deceased body and meeting the needs of the grieving family are nursing responsibilities. The body of the deceased must be treated in a way that respects the sanctity of the human body (Barbus, 1975). Nursing care includes maintaining privacy and preventing damage to the body. **Post-mortem care** is given immediately after death but before the body is moved to the mortuary.

Several physiological changes occur after death. Body temperature decreases, resulting in a lack of skin elasticity (**algor mortis**). In order to avoid skin breakdown, the nurse must therefore use caution when removing tape from the body. Another physiological change, **liver mortis**, is a bluish-purple discoloration of the skin, usually at pressure points, that is a byproduct of red-blood-cell destruction. This discoloration occurs in dependent areas of the body; the nurse should therefore elevate the head to prevent discoloration associated with pooling of blood. Approximately 2 to 4 hours after death, **rigor mortis** occurs: The body stiffens due to contraction of skeletal and smooth muscles. To prevent disfiguring effects of rigor

PROFESSIONAL TIP

Post-Mortem Care

- Treat the body with respect and dignity
- Bathe and put a clean gown on the body—and place an incontinent pad under the client's hips
- Remove dressings and tubes, unless these must remain in place for an autopsy
- Place the client in body alignment with the extremities straight
- Place dentures in the mouth, if the client normally wore them
- Comb the client's hair

mortis, as soon as possible after death, the nurse should close the client's eyelids, insert dentures (if applicable), close the mouth, and position the body in a natural position.

In preparing the body for family viewing, the nurse strives to make the body look comfortable and natural. This means removing all tubes (if allowed) and preparing and positioning the body as previously described. After the family has viewed the body, identification tags are placed on the body's toe and wrist. The body is then placed in a plastic or fabric **shroud** (a covering for the body after death), and the shroud is tagged. Next, the body is transported to the morgue according to the agency's policy, where it is kept until it can be transported to a **mortuary** (funeral home). In some institutions, the body is kept in the room until the funeral director arrives. The nurse is also responsible for returning the deceased's possessions, such as jewelry, eyeglasses, clothing, and all other personal items, to the family.

Legal Aspects

In most states, the physician is legally responsible for determining the cause of death and signing the death certificate. The nurse may, in certain situations, be the person responsible for certifying the death. It is important for nurses to know their legal responsibilities, which are defined by their respective state boards of nursing.

Autopsy

An **autopsy** (examination of the body after death, by a pathologist to ascertain the cause of death) is mandated in situations where an unusual death has occurred. For example, an unexpected death and a violent death are circumstances that would necessitate an autopsy. Families must give consent for an autopsy to be performed in other situations. The funeral director must know whether an autopsy is to be performed.

Organ Donation

The donation of organs for transplantation is a matter that requires compassion and sensitivity from the caregivers. Health care institutions are required to have policies related to the referral of potential donors to organ procurement agencies. It is important that families of the deceased know the need for and process of organ donation. There is an inadequate supply of organs and tissues to meet the demand for transplants. The following organs and tissues are used for transplantation:

- Kidneys
- Heart
- Lungs
- Liver
- Pancreas
- Skin
- Corneas
- Bones (long bones and middle ear bones)

At the time that the family gives consent for donation, the nurse notifies the donor team that an organ is available for transplant. Time is of the essence, because the organ or tissue must be harvested and transplanted quickly to maintain viability.

Care of the Family

At the time of death, the nurse provides invaluable support to the family of the deceased. Informing the family of the circumstances surrounding the death is extremely important. The nurse provides information about viewing the body, asks the family about donating organs, and offers to contact support people (e.g., other relatives, clergy). Sometimes, the nurse must help the family with decision making regarding a funeral home, transportation, and removal of the deceased's belongings. Sensitive and compassionate interpersonal skills are essential in providing information and support to families.

Nurse's Self-Care

Working with dying clients can evoke both a personal and a professional threat in the nurse. Because many nurses are confronted with death and loss daily, grief is a common experience for nurses. Smith-Stoner and Frost (1998) describe a part of the psyche called the shadow self, where stresses are stored. Unresolved sadness is called shadow grief. Everyone has a shadow self and may have some shadow grief. Nurses often have a great deal of shadow grief, which, if not released, may cause illness and burnout. Frequent exposure to death can interfere with the nurse's effectiveness because of subsequent anxiety and denial.

Whether working in a hospice, a hospital, a long-term care facility, or the home, nurses are at particular risk for experiencing negative effects from caring for the dying. Often, nurses do not want to confront their grief and will use some of the common defenses against grieving: keeping busy, taking care of others, being strong, and suffering in silence. Nurses must avoid pretending that they do not experience grief and subsequent suffering and must instead talk about the intense emotions associated with caregiving. According to Smith-Stoner and Frost (1998), shadow grief may be starting to overwhelm a person if that person experiences the following:

- A loss of energy, spark, joy, and meaning in life
- Detachment from surroundings
- A feeling of being powerless to make a difference
- Increased smoking or drinking
- Unusual forgetfulness
- Constant criticism directed toward others
- Consistent inability to get work done
- Uncontrolled outbursts of anger
- Perception of clients and their families as objects
- Surrender of hobbies or interests

To cope with their own grief, nurses need support, education, and assistance in coping with the death of clients. Staff education should focus on decreasing staff anxiety about working with grieving clients and families; ways to seek support; and ways to provide support to coworkers. Smith-Stoner and Frost (1998) suggest the following ways to cope.

- Take time to cry with and for clients.
- Get physical: run, walk, bicycle, play tennis.
- Ask colleagues to help with tasks; do not try to be "Supernurse."

- Connect to place of worship; pray.
- Look for joy in work. Laughter is a great healer.
- Create a caring circle of friends.
- Listen to music.

Often, the nurse's fears and doubts about death and its meaning surface, causing anxiety related to feelings about mortality. Even though such feelings are normal, caring for the dying client and the client's family can be emotionally draining. Nurses must therefore remember to care for themselves.

PROFESSIONAL TIP

Care for Yourself during Grief

- Do what you do so well: care. By helping the family, you will counter your feelings of helplessness.
- Set aside some time for your own grieving.
- Allow for crying to help ease the pain.
- Know when to ask your coworkers for help.
- Call on someone you can trust, and express your feelings of grief to that person.
- Use support from within your agency—counselors, clergy, support groups.
- Find a way to say goodbye to the deceased client. Rituals bring closure, which is a necessary part of grieving.

(*Adapted from "Please Cry with Me: Six Ways to Grieve," by C. D. Reese, 1996, Nursing96, 26[8], 56.*)

SAMPLE NURSING CARE PLAN

THE CLIENT WITH A TERMINAL ILLNESS/CANCER OF THE LUNG

Mrs. O'Riley, a 78-year-old widow, was diagnosed with cancer of the lung 6 months ago. After a right lower lobectomy, she was discharged to a local skilled-care facility with plans to go home after completing her treatment. Mrs. O'Riley was transported to a cancer center for radiation therapy. After completing the treatments, she resisted the idea of going home, and discharge plans were discontinued. Mrs. O'Riley's condition is deteriorating. She now requires pain medication, is frequently short of breath, has dyspnea, and needs moderate assistance with activities of daily living because of fatigue. She frequently grimaces and says, "Oh, it hurts." Her nutritional intake is marginal because of difficulty swallowing. Mrs. O'Riley is in bed most of the day, getting up only to use the commode. She has two adult children and three grandchildren who live nearby and visit often. They are willing to help their mother get her affairs in order but she resists their efforts. The family very much wants to make their mother's remaining time as comfortable and serene as possible. However, Mrs. O'Riley sometimes defies their attempts to do so.

continues

Nursing Diagnosis 1 *Chronic Pain related to disease progression as evidenced by verbal statements, body language, and the need for pain medication*

PLANNING/GOALS	NURSING INTERVENTIONS	RATIONALE	EVALUATION
Mrs. O'Riley will verbalize relief from pain.	Give analgesics as ordered.	Administering regular doses of medication is more effective than waiting until the pain begins.	Mrs. O'Riley's body language and verbal statements indicate freedom from pain.
	Ask client to rate pain on a scale of 0 to 10, with 0 being no pain and 10 being severe pain, to assess the need for beginning morphine. Give morphine as ordered, titrated at increments until adequate pain relief is achieved.	Morphine is the drug of choice for severe pain associated with cancer. The client should begin morphine as soon as it is necessary.	
	Monitor for signs of sudden, acute, temporary pain (breakthrough pain). If the precipitating factor is known, give medication 30 to 60 minutes before the event. For unpredictable breakthrough pain, give the medication as soon as possible.	Breakthrough pain is often precipitated by activity or stress and requires supplemental medication.	
	Assure Mrs. O'Riley that the nurses will help her manage the pain and keep it under control. Give back massages and reposition as necessary for comfort. Assist with progressive relaxation techniques if client agrees.	Clients need reassurance that everything possible will be done to manage the pain.	
	Monitor bowel elimination.	Pain medication may cause constipation.	

continues

Nursing Diagnosis 2 *Ineffective Breathing Pattern related to diminished lung function as evidenced by dyspnea and shortness of breath*

PLANNING/GOALS	NURSING INTERVENTIONS	RATIONALE	EVALUATION
Mrs. O'Riley will be free from moderate or severe dyspnea.	Teach breathing exercises and effective coughing techniques.	Breathing exercises and coughing techniques enhance gas exchange in the alveoli.	Mrs. O'Riley breathes with ease. Dyspnea does not interfere with activities.
	Allow adequate time for physical activities. Postpone activity if dyspnea is present. Provide as much assistance as needed.	Physical exertion increases dyspnea.	
	Administer low-flow oxygen if blood gases indicate need.	Oxygen will ease the effort to breathe but will not be effective unless blood gases indicate the need.	
	Encourage client to drink 8 to 10 glasses of fluid each day.	Adequate fluid intake liquifies respiratory secretions and promotes hydration.	
	Humidify the air with a cold-water vaporizer.	Moisturized air enhances breathing.	
	Assess for signs of respiratory tract infection.	The client is at high risk for respiratory infection.	

Nursing Diagnosis 3 *Ineffective Coping related to terminal illness as evidenced by inability to communicate effectively with family members and to accept their help*

PLANNING/GOALS	NURSING INTERVENTIONS	RATIONALE	EVALUATION
Mrs. O'Riley will express her feelings openly.	Consult Mrs. O'Riley on all aspects of care, giving adequate information. Provide opportunities to express feelings. Acknowledge feelings and let Mrs. O'Riley know that crying and grieving are beneficial.	Mrs. O'Riley needs to be given as much control as she wishes to have. Letting Mrs. O'Riley express her feelings will validate those feelings—she needs to know her feelings are normal and expected.	Mrs. O'Riley is at ease with herself.

continues

| | Listen for clues indicating unfinished business that needs attention. Encourage the process of life review. | There may be something in Mrs. O'Riley's past that needs to be resolved before she can successfully cope with the business of dying. Life review is a process of reflection and pondering of one's past and accepting one's life as having had value and meaning. |
| Mrs. O'Riley will maintain a satisfying relationship with her family. | Encourage family visits. Provide privacy. | Families need privacy in order to feel free to express their emotions. |

CASE STUDY

Mrs. Jason, a 76-year-old with a history of heart failure, has been hospitalized twice within the last year and was critically ill both times. Both times, she was discharged to her home. A home health nurse and a nursing assistant make intermittent visits to monitor her condition and to help with her activities of daily living. Her husband manages the household chores. Mrs. Jason's condition is deteriorating, the shortness of breath becoming more severe. Her energy level is easily depleted, and she is having increasing difficulty getting out of bed. The family is concerned because Mrs. Jason does not have any advance directives. Any attempt to bring up the subject is met with avoidance and a change of subject.

The following questions will guide your development of a nursing care plan for the case study.

1. List the clinical manifestations you would expect Mrs. Jason to experience.
2. Identify four nursing diagnoses to utilize in planning her care.
3. Describe several nursing interventions for implementing palliative care.
4. Describe appropriate interactions with the family to ease their concerns.
5. Cite reasons that Mrs. Jason and her family might benefit from hospice services.

SUMMARY

- Loss is a universal response experienced when someone (or something) of value is no longer available.
- Grief is a psychological response to loss characterized by deep mental anguish and sorrow. Grieving people experience various stages of grief.
- The difference between normal and pathological grief is the inability of the individual to adapt to life without the loved one.
- There are five psychological stages involved in the dying process: denial, anger, bargaining, depression, and acceptance.

- Complicated grief is associated with traumatic death such as by accident, homicide, or suicide.
- Each person dies a unique death.
- Hospice care offers clients an alternative to hospitalization when aggressive medical treatment is no longer an option.
- After death, the nurse focuses on supporting the family and caring for the deceased body.
- Nurses must care for themselves in order to provide quality, compassionate care to the dying person and family.

Review Questions

1. Susan, age 11 years, was left with a distant relative 2 weeks ago. Her parents have not returned or called. Susan is experiencing a:

   a. physical loss.
   b. situational loss.
   c. maturational loss.
   d. anticipational loss.

2. Knowing that a loved one is terminally ill allows family members to begin the grieving process. This is called:

   a. complicated grief.
   b. anticipatory grief.
   c. dysfunctional grief.
   d. disenfranchised grief.

3. A defining characteristic of the NANDA nursing diagnosis *Anticipatory Grieving* is:

   a. prolonged denial or depression.
   b. unsuccessful adaptation to loss.
   c. social isolation or withdrawal from others.
   d. an expression of distress at potential loss.

4. Nursing interventions for a client who has experienced a loss are based on an understanding of:

   a. the degree of the client's depression.
   b. the anger expressed by the client.
   c. the significance of the loss to the client.
   d. the number of support groups available for the loss experienced by the client.

5. The purpose of the Patient Self-Determination Act is to:

   a. serve as an order for "do not resuscitate."
   b. designate a guardian for an incompetent client.
   c. provide a means, instead of a will, to designate what is to be done with a person's property, money, and personal possessions.
   d. provide a legal means for individuals to state those circumstances under which life-sustaining treatment should or should not be provided to them.

6. One of the major goals of hospice care is:

   a. freedom from pain and other symptoms.
   b. free care for all dying clients and their families.
   c. to cure the client using very aggressive medical treatment.
   d. to transfer all dying clients to the hospital when death is imminent.

7. Signs of impending death include:

   a. flushed skin.
   b. slower pulse rate.
   c. increased blood pressure.
   d. Cheyne-Stokes respirations.

8. The nurse must use caution when removing tape from a body because of:

   a. liver mortis.
   b. rigor mortis.
   c. algor mortis.
   d. rimas mortis.

Critical Thinking Questions

1. Find a classmate from a cultural background different from yours. How does your perception of death differ from that of your classmate?

2. Thompson (1994) asks, "Can we afford to leave death in the hands of science, or should we use the benefits of science to provide the dying with a nurturing spiritual environment that feeds the spirit while sustaining the body?" What is your response to this question? What are some ways nurses can promote a "nurturing spiritual environment"?

WEB FLASH!

- What key terms related to loss and death might you search for on the Internet (for instance grief, bereavement)?
- Is there a listing on the Internet of books, videos, or other media on self-care for caregivers to the terminally ill? Are these resources available in your local library?
- What sites can you find that offer information on hospice care?
- Search the Web for "Symptoms of terminal illness"; what can you find?

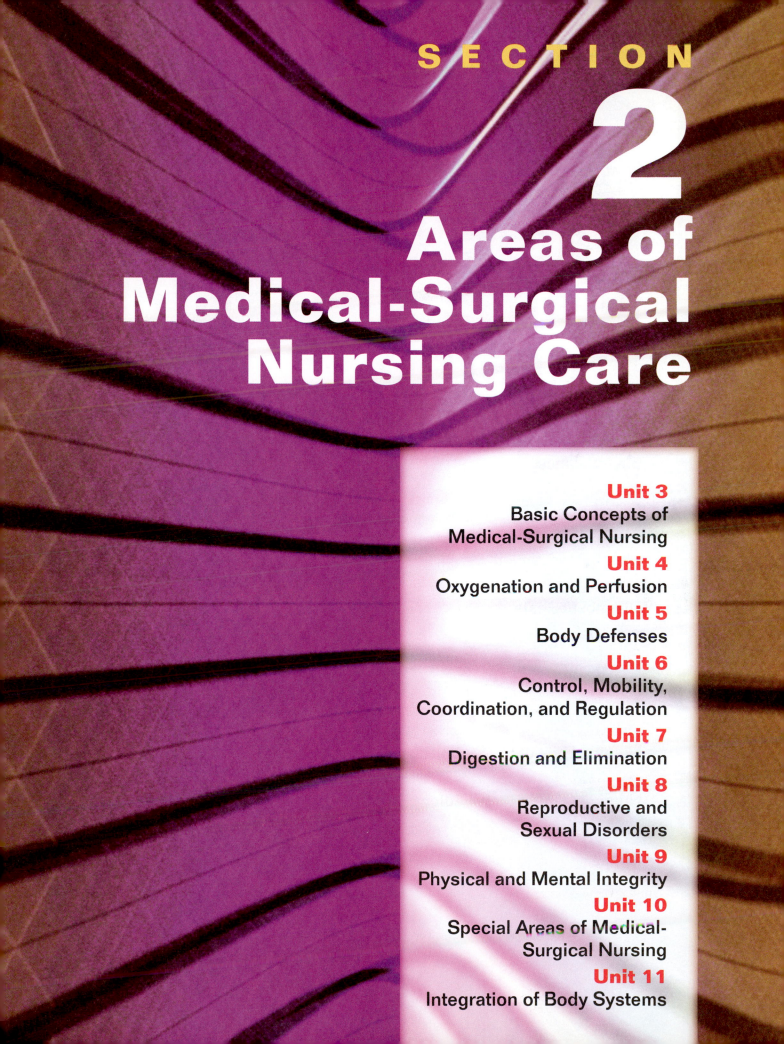

SECTION 2

Areas of Medical-Surgical Nursing Care

UNIT
3
Basic Concepts of Medical-Surgical Nursing

FLUID, ELECTROLYTE, AND ACID–BASE BALANCE

MAKING THE CONNECTION

Refer to the following chapters to increase your understanding of fluid, electrolyte, and acid–base balance:

- **Chapter 12, Health Assessment**
- **Chapter 17, Nursing Care of the Oncology Client**
- **Chapter 18, Nursing Care of the Client: Respiratory System**
- **Chapter 19, Nursing Care of the Client: Cardiovascular System**
- **Chapter 20, Nursing Care of the Client: Hematologic and Lymphatic Systems**

- **Chapter 27, Nursing Care of the Client: Endocrine System**
- **Chapter 28, Nursing Care of the Client: Gastrointestinal System**
- **Chapter 29, Nursing Care of the Client: Urinary System**

LEARNING OBJECTIVES

Upon completion of this chapter, you should be able to:
- *Define key terms.*
- *Discuss the importance of pH regulation in the body.*
- *Describe the three buffer systems of the body.*
- *Describe and give examples in the body of diffusion, osmosis, and filtration.*
- *Name the fluid compartments, the fluids contained in them, and the function of those fluids.*
- *Describe the way the kidneys work to maintain fluid and electrolyte balance.*
- *Describe the way the lungs work to maintain pH in the body.*
- *Detail causes, assessment data, nursing interventions, and criteria for evaluating effectiveness of care for clients with a nursing diagnosis of* Fluid Volume Deficit *or* Fluid Volume Excess.
- *Detail causes, assessment data, nursing diagnoses, nursing interventions, and criteria for evaluating the effectiveness of nursing care for clients with sodium, potassium, calcium, and magnesium imbalances.*
- *Relate principles of nursing management for clients receiving fluids and electrolytes via oral supplements, intravenous solutions, enteral feedings, and total parenteral nutrition.*
- *Differentiate the causes, assessment data, and nursing management of metabolic and respiratory acidosis and alkalosis.*
- *Use the nursing process to plan care for a client experiencing a fluid, electrolyte, and/or acid–base imbalance.*

KEY TERMS

acid	crenation
acidosis	decomposition
alkalosis	dehydration
anion	dialysis
arterial blood gases	diffusion
atom	edema
base	electrolyte
buffer	element
cation	extracellular fluid
compound	filtration

INTRODUCTION

The external environment within which we live undergoes continual changes, both small and large. For example, the daily and seasonal temperatures may fluctuate over a wide range. The light intensity may be bright on sunny days and less so on cloudy days. The humidity may be either high or low. These are just a few of the many factors that may change constantly in the external environment. Our bodies must continually adjust to such changes in the external environment. In order for life to continue, however, our internal environment—the one inside our bodies—must remain relatively constant, varying only slightly within narrow ranges. This internal environment consists of the various body fluids such as the fluid inside cells, the blood, tissue fluids that bathe the cells, and other fluids. Constant maintenance of the internal environment within very narrow limits—in equilibrium—is termed **homeostasis**.

HOMEOSTASIS

Homeostasis is an ongoing process; that is, the body simply does not reach a state of equilibrium and remain there. Small changes constantly occur in response to the physiologic processes. As a result, changes occur in the internal environment. The body must therefore continuously make subtle adjustments to maintain the constancy of the internal environment within a range of normal values.

Homeostasis is accomplished by various physiologic processes and the coordinated activities of the organ systems. Some examples are as follows:

- The gastrointestinal (GI) system changes large, complex molecules of ingested food to simpler, less-complex molecules that can be utilized by the cells of the body to produce the energy necessary for life.
- The respiratory system supplies the cells with the constant source of oxygen required to release the energy from the products of digestion.
- The respiratory system also eliminates carbon dioxide, the waste product produced by the cells as a result of energy production.
- The blood acts as a transport mechanism, carrying the products of digestion along with hormones and oxygen to the cells, where these substances are utilized.
- The blood also transports carbon dioxide from the energy-releasing processes of the cells to the lungs, where it will be eliminated.
- All of the activities of the various organ systems are integrated and coordinated through the nervous system and the endocrine system.

When the body loses the ability to maintain homeostasis, and the internal environment changes, the physiologic processes can be interrupted or changed, leading to disease, disorder, or death. In essence, then, maintaining homeostasis is essential to life. Because the processes of homeostasis involve many chemical and physical processes, it is necessary to examine some of these before studying homeostasis in more detail.

CHEMICAL ORGANIZATION

The human body is highly organized. This organization exists in increasing levels of complexity. Most basic is the chemical level. To understand the higher levels of organization, it is necessary to know something about basic chemical and physical principles.

Elements

The cell consists of living matter. **Matter** is anything that occupies space and possesses mass. All matter has certain physical properties such as color, odor, hardness, and density. Matter also has extensive properties such as size, shape, and weight. Matter is composed of basic substances called **elements**. Elements are made of tiny units called atoms. Atoms of each element are alike. Different elements have different kinds of atoms. Presently, 108 elements are recognized. Some examples are iron, gold, carbon, hydrogen, oxygen, nitrogen, and copper. Many of the elements occur in the human body in varying amounts. Some are present in large amounts, and others are found in only trace amounts. The four elements oxygen, carbon, hydrogen and nitrogen constitute more than 95% of the total body weight of the elements. Some of the elements and their function in the body are presented in Table 10–1.

Atoms

An **atom** is the smallest unit of chemical structure, and no chemical change can alter it. Atoms are made

Table 10–1 ELEMENTS OCCURRING IN THE HUMAN BODY

ELEMENT	APPROXIMATE % OF BODY WEIGHT	FUNCTION
Major Elements		
Oxygen	65.0	Found in both organic and inorganic compounds; as a gas, is necessary in metabolizing glucose and other chemical compounds into energy
Carbon	18.5	Found in all organic compounds such as carbohydrates, protein, lipids, and nucleic acids; necessary for cellular respiration
Hydrogen	9.5	Found in many organic and inorganic compounds; in ionic form, involved in pH; component of water; necessary for life
Nitrogen	3.2	Important in proteins, which are the body building blocks, an energy source, and a component of hormones
Calcium	1.5	Important element in bone and tooth composition; involved in nerve conduction, muscle contraction, and blood clotting
Phosphorus	1.0	Found in bones, teeth, the high-energy carrying compound adenosine triphosphatase (ATP), some proteins, and nucleic acid
Potassium	0.4	Major electrolyte in intracellular fluid; important in muscle contraction and transmission of nerve impulses; activates enzymes; influences cellular osmotic pressure; involved in kidney function and acid–base balance
Sulfur	0.3	Found in some proteins, nucleic acids, and some vitamins and hormones
Sodium	0.2	Constitutes major electrolyte in extracellular fluid; important in osmoregulation and acid–base balance; necessary for nerve transmission and muscle contraction
Chlorine	0.2	Found in extracellular fluid; important in water balance, acid–base balance, and production of hydrochloric acid in the stomach
Magnesium	0.1	Important to muscle and nerve function and bone formation and in some coenzymes
Essential Trace Elements		
Present in the human body in minimal amounts, constituting approximately 0.1% of body weight; have known functions		
Cobalt		Important component of vitamin B_{12}
Copper		Necessary for formation of hemoglobin and for bone development
Chromium		A cofactor involved with enzymes for fat, cholesterol, and glucose metabolism
Flourine		Gives hardness to teeth and bones
Iodine		Necessary for synthesis of thyroid hormone
Iron		Necessary for transportation of oxygen by hemoglobin
Manganese		Necessary in activating some enzymes
Selenium		Acts with vitamin E as an antioxidant; component of teeth
Zinc		Found in some enzymes; needed for protein metabolism and carbon dioxide transport
Other Trace Elements		
Have probable, but as yet undetected, functions		
Aluminum Nickel Arsenic Tin Boron Silicon Cadmium Vanadium		

up of three basic particles: protons, neutrons, and electrons. Protons and neutrons are similar in size, but whereas protons have a positive electrical charge, neutrons have no charge. Together, they form the nucleus of the atom. Because the protons have a positive charge and the neutrons are neutral, the nucleus of an atom has a positive charge. The electrons have a negative charge and move in an orbit around the nucleus. There are as many electrons as protons, rendering the overall atom neutral. The number of protons in an atom is called its atomic number. The simplest element is hydrogen. It has an atomic number of 1. One proton with a positive charge forms the nucleus, and one electron moves in an orbit around the nucleus. Hydro-

gen atoms may or may not have a neutron. A hydrogen atom is illustrated in Figure 10-1.

Depending on the element, other atoms may have more than one proton and one electron shell and may have neutrons. The number of protons and neutrons in the nucleus is approximately equal to the atomic weight. Thus, hydrogen has an atomic weight of 1.

Isotopes

The number of protons in the nucleus is the same for all atoms of a given element, but the number of neutrons may vary in atoms of the same element. For instance, all hydrogen atoms have one proton and one electron. However, whereas some hydrogen atoms

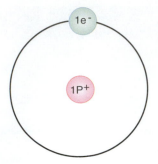

Figure 10-1 Hydrogen Atom Showing Positively Charged Proton in the Nucleus and Negatively Charged Electron in Orbit

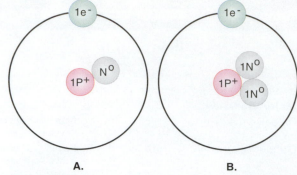

Figure 10-2 Isotopes of Hydrogen: A. Deuteridium has one positively charged proton and one neutron in the nucleus and one electron in orbit; B. Tritium has one positively charged proton and two neutrons in the nucleus and one electron in orbit.

have one neutron in the nucleus, others have two (Figure 10-2). Atoms of the same element that have different atomic weights (i.e., have a different number of neutrons) are called **isotopes**. All of the isotopes of a given element react chemically in the same way.

Some isotopes, called radioactive isotopes, have an unstable nucleus, which decomposes and gives off energy in the form of radiation. This radiation can be in the form of alpha, beta, or gamma rays. All are damaging to cells. Alpha radiation is the least harmful, and gamma radiation is the most harmful. Iodine, oxygen, and cobalt are examples of elements having radioactive isotopes. Some of the radioactive isotopes are useful as biological markers and can be used to track metabolic pathways of food. Others such as iodine[131] can be injected in the body and used to track the circulation of blood. Still others such as cobalt[60] are used in cancer treatment.

Molecules and Compounds

Atoms of the same element can unite with each other to form a **molecule**. For example, atoms of hydrogen unite to form a hydrogen molecule. This can be expressed in a chemical equation using the chemical symbol for hydrogen:

$$H + H \rightarrow H_2$$

In this reaction, the atoms on the left are the reactants; the arrow is read as "yield"; and the last symbol is the product—a molecule of hydrogen. A chemical equation uses the chemical symbols of elements and shows the ratios by which they combine. Because atoms of elements always combine in the same ratio under similar conditions, it is possible to predict the nature of a chemical change.

When atoms of two or more different elements combine (react) they form a **compound**. For example, if one atom of sodium (Na) and one atom of chlorine (Cl) react, they form a molecule of the compound called sodium chloride. This is expressed in the following equation:

$$Na + Cl \rightarrow NaCl$$

Compounds can be divided into two groups. Those without carbon are inorganic compounds, and those with carbon are organic compounds. By using chemical equations, chemical changes, called chemical reactions, can be shown. Sometimes, different substances are combined in no specific way, and the components do not have a definite ratio every time. For instance, water, sugar, and table salt mixed without being measured will yield different results depending on the ratio of each substance. Such a combination is called a **mixture**. Its composition may vary each time the components are mixed.

Chemical reactions occur whenever atoms join together or separate. They join together by forming bonds, and they separate by breaking bonds. Either way, new combinations result. When two or more atoms (reactants) bond and form a more complex molecular product, the reaction is called **synthesis**. A sample equation would be as follows:

$$2H + O \rightarrow H_2O$$
hydrogen and oxygen yields water

When the bonding between the atoms in a molecule is broken and simpler products are formed, the reaction is called **decomposition**. If a molecule of sodium chloride is decomposed it forms sodium and chlorine. This can be expressed as follows:

$$NaCl \rightarrow Na + Cl$$
sodium chloride yields sodium and chloride

(decomposition)

It is important to understand that when synthesis occurs, energy is tied up in the bonds formed during the reaction. When decomposition occurs, energy is released. In the cells of the body, these kinds of chemical reactions are repeatedly occurring: Molecules form and decompose. Body cells can utilize these reactions to form energy sources and to free energy to drive the various metabolic processes of the cells.

Ions

When some compounds are placed in water, they decompose, or ionize. The result is an **ion**, an atom bearing an electrical charge. An ion with a positive charge is called a **cation**; an ion with a negative charge is termed an **anion**. For example, sodium chloride in water dissociates to form sodium ions bearing a positive charge and chloride ions bearing a negative charge (Figure 10-3). Because the atoms in this combination are charged, they will conduct electricity. The reaction can be shown as follows:

$$NaCl \rightarrow Na^+ + Cl^-$$

sodium chloride yields sodium and chloride
(cation)   (anion)

A compound that dissociates into ions in water is called an **electrolyte**. Many electrolytes are extremely important in body chemistry; some of these are listed in Table 10–2.

WATER

Water constitutes approximately 60% of the total body weight of an adult and is involved in many of the physical and physiological processes of the body. Because water is so integral to the body's processes, fluctuations in the amount of water in the body can have harmful or even fatal consequences.

Water is the major component of blood. Approximately 92% of the body's organic and inorganic compounds dissolve in this water into less-complex molecules and atoms and then are transported throughout the body. Necessary substances such as oxygen and nutrients from the GI system are carried to the cells, where they are utilized. Cellular waste products such as carbon dioxide, urea, and excessive minerals are carried by water to sites of elimination: carbon dioxide to the lungs, urea and minerals to the kidneys.

Solute
(the thing being dissolved)

Solvent
(does the dissolving)

Electrolyte solution
(result of the dissolving process)

Figure 10-3 Dissociation of Electrolytes

Table 10–2 IMPORTANT ELECTROLYTES IN BODY FLUIDS

FORMULA	CHEMICAL NAME
$NaCl$	Sodium chloride
Na_2SO_4	Sodium sulfate
Na_2HPO_4	Disodium phosphate
$NaHCO_3$	Sodium bicarbonate
$MgCl$	Magnesium chloride
$CaCl_2$	Calcium chloride
KCl	Potassium chloride

PROFESSIONAL TIP

Body Water and Body Size
The amount of body water is inversely proportional to body size. The smaller the body, the higher the water content:

Embryo:	97%
Infant:	77%
Child:	60% to 77%
Adult:	60%
Elders:	45% to 50%

Body water diminishment in elderly persons is related to tissue loss.

Water also absorbs heat resulting from muscle contractions and distributes this heat over the body. Water in the form of perspiration released from sweat glands in the skin can cool the body by evaporation. Water also can break apart the bonds in large molecules such as starches to form smaller molecules in the digestive process. This type of reaction is called *hydration.*

GASES

Two important gases in the body are oxygen (O_2) and carbon dioxide (CO_2). Because these elements are gases, their molecules are free and can move swiftly in all directions. Oxygen enters the body through the lungs and is transported by the red blood cells throughout the body to the cells. The cells use oxygen in the release of energy from glucose and other molecules. This energy is needed by the cells to carry out their activities. As a result of the energy-releasing processes, carbon dioxide is produced by the cells and transported in the blood to the lungs, where it is eliminated.

ACIDS, BASES, SALTS, AND PH

Other chemical substances important for life are acids, bases, and salts; pH is the measure of acid and base strength.

Acids

An **acid** is any substance that in solution yields hydrogen ions bearing a positive charge. As an example, hydrochloric acid (HCl) in water dissociates as shown following:

$$HCl \rightarrow H^+ + Cl^-$$
hydrochloric acid yields hydrogen and chlorine

The hydrogen ion characterizes this as an acid. Important acids in the body are hydrochloric acid, produced in the stomach, and carbonic acid, formed when the carbon dioxide released from cells reacts with some of the water in the extracellular fluid (all body fluids except for those contained within the cells).

Bases

A **base** is a substance that when dissociated produces ions that will combine with hydrogen ions. For example, when sodium hydroxide dissociates in water, it forms a sodium ion bearing a positive charge and a hydroxyl ion bearing a negative charge as shown following:

$$NaOH \rightarrow Na^+ + OH^-$$
sodium hydroxide yields sodium and hydroxyl

The hydroxyl ion is capable of combining with a hydrogen ion to form water. Sodium bicarbonate is an example of a base found in the body.

Salts

A **salt** is formed when an acid and a base react with each other. Salts result from the neutralization of an acid by a base, as illustrated by the following reaction:

$$HCl + NaOH \rightarrow H_2O + NaCl$$
hydrochloric and   sodium   yields water and sodium
acid   hydroxide   chloride

The hydrochloric acid reacts with the sodium hydroxide to form a molecule of water and a molecule of a salt—sodium chloride. When salts are placed in water, they dissociate into a cation and an anion. For instance, in water, the sodium chloride would dissociate into Na^+ and Cl^-. One reason salts are of great biological importance is that many of the compounds that dissociate into ions in living cells are salts. For example, sodium and chlorine ions are present in great amounts in body fluids. Many other salts occur in lesser amounts.

pH

Acid and bases are classified as either strong or weak by the number of hydrogen ions or hydroxyl ions they produce when they dissociate. Strong acids release many hydrogen ions; weak acids release relatively few. The same is true of hydroxyl ions in strong and weak bases. The acidity or alkalinity of a solution is determined by the concentration of hydrogen ions in the solution. Potential hydrogen (pH) indicates the hydrogen ion concentration in a solution, expressed as a number from 0 to 14. A solution with a pH of 7 is neutral, that is, it is neither an acid or a base. A solution with a pH greater than 7 is a base, or alkaline. A solution with a pH below 7 is an acid. The higher above 7 the pH, the more alkaline the solution; the lower below 7 the pH, the more acid the solution. pH is of great biological importance. The human body can tolerate only very slight changes in pH. For example, the pH of human blood ranges from 7.35 to 7.45. Blood pH above or below this range can cause severe or even fatal physiological problems.

Although small amounts of acids may enter the body through food intake, the greatest source of acids—and thus H^+ ions—is cellular metabolism, resulting in products including lactic acid, phosphoric acid, pyruvic acid, and many fatty acids. When blood pH falls below 7.35 as a result of an elevated concentration of H^+ ions, **acidosis** occurs. Rarely does blood pH fall to 7 or become acidic, because death will usually occur first. As acidosis increases, the central nervous system (CNS) becomes involved, and the client may become unconscious. The heartbeat may become weak and irregular, and blood pressure may decrease or even disappear.

When blood pH increases above 7.45, **alkalosis** occurs. Alkalosis is a condition characterized by an excessive loss of hydrogen ions. This happens less often than does acidosis. Symptoms of alkalosis include a heightened state of nervous system activity, resulting in spasmodic muscle contractions, convulsions, and even death.

BUFFERS

Buffers are substances that attempt to maintain pH range, or H^+ ion concentration, in the presence of added acids or bases. Buffers usually occur in pairs in the body fluids. They act to keep the pH of body fluids within normal range. If body fluids become acidic, buffers in the body fluids combine with the excess hydrogen ions and restore normal pH. Likewise, if the body fluids become alkaline, other buffers in the blood combine with the strong bases, converting them to weak bases and restoring normal pH.

Three important buffer systems occur in body fluids: the bicarbonate buffer system, the phosphate buffer system, and the protein buffer system. Because a change in pH of one fluid may bring corresponding changes in the pH of other fluids, an interplay between buffer systems acts to maintain the body's pH. The buffer systems react quickly to prevent excessive changes in the hydrogen ion concentration.

Bicarbonate Buffer System

The bicarbonate buffer system is found in both the extracellular and intracellular fluids and is the body's primary buffer system. It has two components: carbonic acid (H_2CO_3) and sodium bicarbonate ($NaHCO_3$). When a strong acid such as hydrochloric acid is added to this buffer system, the acid will react with the sodium bicarbonate and form a weaker acid (carbonic acid) and a salt (sodium chloride).

HCl	+	$NaHCO_3$	→	H_2CO_3	+	NaCl
hydrochloric acid	and	sodium bicarbonate	yields	carbonic acid	and	sodium chloride

The strong acid is converted into a weak acid, and the pH is raised toward normal.

If a strong base such as sodium hydroxide is added to this buffer system, the carbonic acid will react with it to form a weak base (sodium bicarbonate) and water.

NaOH	+	H_2CO_3	→	$NaHCO_3$	+	H_2O
sodium hydroxide	and	carbonic acid	yields	sodium bicarbonate	and	water

The strong base, which initially raised the pH, is converted to a weak base, which will lower the pH toward normal. It is vital to note that hydrochloric acid and sodium hydroxide are substances not normally added to the blood. They are used here only as good examples of the way buffers work. This buffer system normally buffers organic acids found in body fluids.

In the body, bicarbonate helps to stabilize pH by combining reversibly with hydrogen ions. Most of the body's bicarbonate is produced in red blood cells, where the enzyme carbonic anhydrase accelerates the conversion of carbon dioxide to carbonic acid. The production of bicarbonate is illustrated in the following reversible equation:

CO_2	+	H_2O	↔	H_2CO_3	↔	H^+	+	HCO_3^-
carbon dioxide		water		carbonic acid		hydrogen		bicarbonate

When the hydrogen ion concentration increases in the extracellular (outside of the cell) space, the reaction shifts toward the left. A decreased concentration of hydrogen ions drives the reaction to the right.

Phosphate Buffer System

The phosphate buffer system is involved in regulating the pH of intracellular fluid and the fluid of the kidney tubules. It has two phosphate compounds: sodium monohydrogen phosphate ($NaHPO_4$) and sodium dihydrogen phosphate (NaH_2PO_4). In the presence of a strong acid such as hydrochloric acid, the sodium monohydrogen phosphate reacts with the acid to form a weak acid (sodium dihydrogen phosphate) and a salt (sodium chloride), thus raising the pH.

HCl	+	$NaHPO_4$	→	NaH_2PO_4	+	NaCl
hydrochloric acid	and	sodium monohydrogen phosphate	yields	sodium dihydrogen phosphate	and	sodium chloride

When sodium dihydrogen phosphate encounters a strong base such as sodium hydroxide, a weak base (sodium monohydrogen phosphate) and water are formed.

NaOH	+	NaH_2PO_4	→	$NaHPO_4$	+	H_2O
sodium hydroxide	and	sodium dihydrogen phosphate	yields	sodium monohydrogen phosphate	and	water

Protein Buffers

Proteins are complex substances formed when amino acids bond. Each amino acid contains a carboxyl group (COOH) and an amino group (NH_2). The carboxyl group can ionize and release hydrogen, thus acting as an acid. The amino group can accept hydrogen, thus acting as a base. This ability allows proteins to act as a buffer system. The protein buffer system is found inside cells, especially in the hemoglobin of red blood cells, where the proteins can act to maintain the pH inside the cell. They are also found in the plasma.

SUBSTANCE MOVEMENT

Substances must be able to both enter and leave cells. For example, oxygen and various end products of digestion must enter a cell through the cell membrane for use by the cell. Waste products from cellular processes must be eliminated from the cell. Various ions must also both enter and leave cells. Everything that enters and leaves the cell must pass through the cell membrane. Thus, the cell membrane serves not only as an envelope around the cell, but also as a gatekeeper, regulating which substances can enter and leave the cell. The cell membrane is a very thin and delicate, but complex and living, elastic covering around each cell. It consists of an inner and outer layer of phospholipids in which protein molecules are embedded. Many small channels pass through the membrane. These channels allow some water molecules and some water-soluble substances to pass through the membrane. The ability of a membrane to permit substances to pass through it is called **permeability**. Because a cell membrane allows passage of only certain substances, it is called a selective permeable membrane, or **semipermeable membrane**.

Some substances can pass through the cell membrane without energy expenditure on the part of the cell. This is called passive transport. The passage of other substances requires an expenditure of energy by the cell. This is called active transport.

Passive Transport

There are several types of passive transport: diffusion, osmosis, and filtration.

Diffusion

Diffusion is the tendency of molecules of either gases, liquids, or solids to move from a region of higher molecular concentration to a region of lower molecular concentration until an equilibrium is reached. This movement is due to the kinetic energy in molecules. Kinetic energy causes the molecules to move constantly, colliding with one another and knocking each other about, thus causing them to move farther apart. An example is a drop of black ink placed in a glass of water; over a period of time, the glass of water will turn a uniform black color because of diffusion, as shown in Figure 10-4.

In the body, oxygen moves by diffusion from the lungs to the bloodstream because the oxygen concentration is higher in the lungs and lower in the blood. Carbon dioxide moves by diffusion from the bloodstream, where the concentration of carbon dioxide is higher, to the lungs, for elimination. The size of the channels in the cell membrane can prevent large molecules from passing through the membrane. Some substances, such as glucose molecules, combine with carrier molecules, which carry them into the interior of the cell, where they are released.

The term **dialysis** is used when diffusion is employed to separate molecules out of a solution by passing them through a semipermeable membrane. Dialysis is the process used in the artificial kidney. Blood from a client is circulated through a long, coiled tube. Small, toxic waste molecules such as urea leave the blood and pass through the pores of the tubing by diffusion and out into the fluid surrounding the tubing. The blood, thus cleaned, is then returned to the body.

Osmosis

Osmosis is the diffusion of water through a semipermeable membrane from a region of higher water concentration to a region of lower water concentration. In a solution undergoing osmosis, only the water (solvent) molecules move through the membrane; the dissolved molecules do not (Figure 10-5).

If a cell, having both a membrane that will not allow sodium chloride to pass through and a molecular con-

centration of 10% sodium chloride, were placed in a container with a 5% sodium chloride solution, the cell would contain 10% sodium chloride and 90% water, and the 5% solution in which it was placed would contain 5% dissolved sodium chloride and 95% water. There would be more water outside than inside the cell; thus, water would pass through the membrane into the cell. Because the cell membrane is elastic, the cell would increase in size as a result of the water accumulation within it facilitated by the process of osmosis. The pressure exerted against the cell membrane by the water inside the cell is called **osmotic pressure**.

A solution that has the same molecular concentration as does the cell is called an **isotonic solution**. It neither increases nor decreases the size of the cell. A solution that has a lower molecular concentration than does the cell is called a **hypotonic solution**. Placing cells in a hypotonic solution causes them to swell, possibly to the point of eventual rupture. The rupture of red blood cells due to osmosis is called **hemolysis**. As red blood cells swell, the hemoglobin contained within passes to the outside of the cell and into the solution surrounding the cell, rendering the blood cells no longer capable of carrying oxygen. A solution that has a higher molecular concentration than does the cell is called a **hypertonic solution**. When placed in such a solution, water leaves the cell, and the cell decreases in size. In the case of red blood cells, they shrivel and become wrinkled. This shrinkage, called **crenation**, leaves the cells incapable of functioning.

In persons who have lost large volumes of blood, it is sometimes necessary to administer additional fluids to maintain blood pressure. Generally, normal saline can be used. This 0.9% sodium chloride solution has approximately the same osmotic concentration as does blood. Because it is isotonic, it will not damage the cells. Figure 10-6 shows osmosis in cells with different solution concentrations.

Figure 10-4 Diffusion is the spreading of particles from an area of greater concentration to an area of lesser concentration. Dye put into a beaker of water gradually spreads throughout the water.

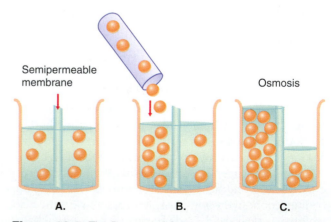

Semipermeable membrane

Osmosis

A.   B.   C.

Figure 10-5 The Process of Osmosis (*Adapted from* Fundamentals of Nursing: Standards & Practice, *by S. DeLaune and P. Ladner, 1998, Albany, NY: Delmar. Copyright 1998 by Delmar. Adapted with permission.*)

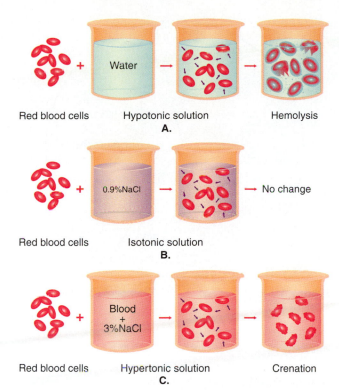

Figure 10-6 Osmosis is the movement of water through a membrane from an area of lower concentration to one of higher concentration. A. In a hypotonic solution, the water moves into the cells, causing them to swell and burst. B. In an isotonic solution, cells are normal in size and shape because the same amount of water is entering and leaving the cells. C. In a hypertonic solution, cells are losing water because water moves from an area of lower concentration (inside the cell) to an area of higher concentration (outside the cell).

Filtration

In **filtration**, fluids and the substances dissolved in them are forced through cell membranes by hydrostatic pressure. **Hydrostatic pressure** is the pressure that the fluid exerts against the membrane. The molecules passing through the membrane are determined by the size of the pores in the membrane. Tissue fluids are formed by filtration. As blood passes through the capillaries, hydrostatic pressure exerted by the pumping action of the heart causes some of the liquid fraction of the blood (but not the cells) to pass out of the capillaries, resulting in the formation of the tissue fluid (Figure 10-7). As the blood circulates through the capillaries of the kidneys, the hydrostatic pressure of the blood causes many materials to leave the blood through the filtration process. These materials pass into the tubules of the kidneys, where the toxic waste products are removed to form urine. The urine is then eliminated from the body.

Active Transport

In the processes discussed thus far, the movement of molecules depends on the concentration of mole-

cules or on pressure. In other words, the cells do not have to expend energy to move the molecules in or out of the cell. In active transport, the cell must use energy to move the molecules. For instance, in the body, sodium ions are in higher concentration in the fluids surrounding the cell than inside the cell. Though some sodium ions can diffuse into the cell, the cell actively transports them through the membrane to the outside. Active transport is accomplished by means of carrier molecules, which can latch onto specific molecules and transport them in or out of the cell. This process requires an expenditure of cellular energy (Figure 10-8). Examples of important ions transported by this process are calcium, sodium, potassium, and magnesium.

FLUID AND ELECTROLYTE BALANCE

Human life is suspended in a saline solution having a salt concentration of 0.9%. This solution, which both surrounds the cells and is contained within them, constitutes the body fluids. The water and electrolytes composing these body fluids come from ingested water and nutrients, and from the water that results from metabolism.

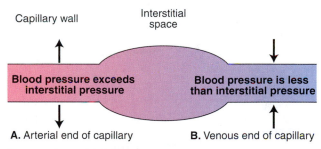

Figure 10-7 Filtration: A. Pressure in the arteriole is greater than interstitial (between the cells) pressure, causing fluid with dissolved substances to move out of capillaries. B. Pressure in venules is less than interstitial fluid pressure, causing fluid and waste products to move back into the capillaries.

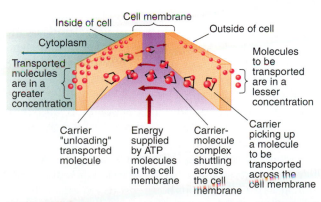

Figure 10-8 Active Transport of Molecules from an Area of Lesser Concentration to an Area of Greater Concentration

For life to continue and the cells to properly function, the body fluids must remain fairly constant with regard to the amount of water and the specific electrolytes of which they are composed. Water is essential because it is the basic component of all the body fluids. Water is involved in many of the metabolic processes in the body and is a by–product of some of these reactions. The various electrolytes all have essential roles in cellular physiological processes. If some of either is lost, it must be replaced, and if either water or an electrolyte is in excess, it must be removed. Maintaining the consistency of this fluid environment is homeostasis.

For cells to survive and carry out their multitude of physiologic functions, they need both a continuing source of water, nutrients, and oxygen and a mechanism to remove cellular wastes. These physiologic processes affect the amount of water, the pH, and the ions both inside and outside the cells. A balance must be maintained between the components of the fluids inside and outside the cell. Because the ions are dissolved in water, these two components are tied together: Anything affecting the amount of water in the body will affect the ion concentration.

Body Fluids

Much of the body weight of an average adult is due to the water in the body fluids surrounding the cells and contained within them. The fluid around the cells cushions them and serves as the medium of exchange. Everything that enters or leaves the cells must pass through this fluid layer.

There are two kinds of body fluids. They can be thought of as being contained within two separate containers, called compartments. The **intracellular fluid** (ICF) compartment contains all of the water and ions inside the cells. By far the largest amount of water in the body, approximately 65%, is found within this compartment.

The extracellular fluid compartment contains the remaining body fluids, called **extracellular fluid** (ECF), or fluid outside the cells. These can be further subdivided into interstitial, intravascular, and other fluids. **Interstitial fluid** is the fluid in the tissue spaces around each cell. The **intravascular fluid** is the plasma in the blood vessels and the lymph in the lymphatic system (Figure 10-9). There are also small amounts of other specialized body fluids such as synovial fluid, cerebrospinal fluid, serous fluid, aqueous and vitreous humor, and the endolymph and perilymph. The proportions of extracellular fluid and intracellular fluid vary with age.

Generally speaking, the major ions in the extracellular fluid are sodium (Na^+), chloride (Cl^-), and bicarbonate (HCO_3^-), although other ions do occur. In the intracellular fluid, the major ions are potassium (K^+), phosphate (PO_4^{--}), and magnesium (Mg^{++}), with lesser

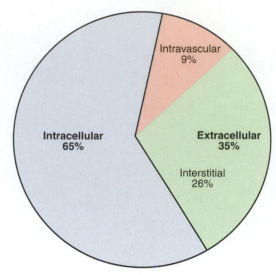

Figure 10-9 Body Fluid Compartments of an Adult

amounts of other ions present. There are also large numbers of protein molecules bearing a negative charge.

Exchange between the Extracellular and Intracellular Fluids

Water and ions moving between the extracellular and intracellular fluids must first pass through the selectively permeable cell membrane. This movement is governed primarily by osmosis. Diffusion and active transport also play a role.

The difference in the ion concentration inside the cell and outside the cell is due primarily to the cell's ability to pump some ions inside and pump others out. If the intracellular fluid becomes hypertonic to the extracellular fluid, water from the extracellular fluid will move by osmosis into the cell to restore the balance, and vice versa.

A fluid balance also occurs between the interstitial fluid and the plasma. This balance is regulated primarily by hydrostatic pressure (blood pressure) and osmotic pressure. When the circulating blood passes from the arterioles into the capillaries, the pressure in the capillaries is higher than that in the interstitial fluid. This forces some of the water from the plasma out of the capillaries and into the interstitial fluid. Due to osmotic pressure, some of the water in the interstitial fluid is forced back into the capillaries in the area where they join the venules. Some water is also returned to the bloodstream through the lymphatic system. If the amount of interstitial fluid returned to the circulatory system lessens and the fluid accumulates in the tissue spaces, the tissues become swollen. This condition is called **edema**. A number of conditions can cause edema, including kidney or liver disease and heart disorders. Many of these conditions can have serious consequences.

When more water is lost from the body than is replaced, **dehydration** occurs. Among the various causes of dehydration are water deprivation, excessive urine production, profuse sweating, diarrhea, and extended periods of vomiting. As water is lost, the amount of water in the interstitial fluid decreases. Water then moves from the cells to the tissue spaces by osmosis, causing an electrolyte imbalance. Circulatory impairment occurs, which in turn affects the kidney's ability to function normally. This condition is corrected by supplying water and the appropriate electrolytes.

Regulators of Fluid and Electrolyte Balance

There must be a balance in the amounts of fluids and electrolytes consumed and lost daily. Under typical conditions, the average adult loses some water through the skin, lungs, and GI tract and loses the largest amount of water through urine production. This can amount to a per-day fluid loss of approximately 2500 mL, depending on conditions.

Skin

In the average adult, an estimated water loss of 300 to 400 mL per day occurs by diffusion through the skin. Because the person is not aware of this water loss, it is called *insensible loss*. Water is also lost through the skin by perspiration. The total amount of water lost through perspiration varies depending on environmental factors and body temperature.

Lungs

In the average adult, an estimated insensible water loss of 300 to 400 mL per day occurs with expired air, which is saturated with water vapor. This amount varies with the rate and depth of respirations.

Gastrointestinal Tract

Although a large amount of fluid—approximately 8,000 mL per day in the average adult—is secreted into the gastrointestinal tract, almost all of this fluid is reabsorbed by the body. In adults, approximately 200 mL of water is lost per day in feces. Severe diarrhea can cause a fluid and electrolyte deficit because the GI fluids contain a large amount of electrolytes.

Kidneys

The kidneys play a major role in maintaining fluid balance by excreting 1,200 to 1,500 mL of water per day in the average adult. The excretion of water by healthy kidneys is proportional to the fluid ingested and the amount of waste or solutes excreted.

When an extracellular fluid volume deficit occurs, hormones play a key role in restoring the extracellular fluid volume. The release of the following hormones into circulation causes the kidneys to conserve water:

- Antidiuretic hormone (ADH): released by the posterior pituitary gland; acts on the distal tubules of the kidneys to reabsorb water
- Aldosterone: produced in the adrenal cortex; causes the reabsoption of sodium from the renal tubules, leading to water retention in the extracellular fluid, thereby increasing its volume
- Renin: released by the juxtaglomerular cells of the kidneys; promotes vasoconstriction and the release of aldosterone

The interaction of these hormones with regard to renal functions serves as the body's compensatory mechanism to maintain homeostasis.

Sodium is the main electrolyte that promotes the retention of water. An intravascular water deficit causes the renal tubules to reabsorb more sodium into circulation. Because water molecules go with the sodium ions, the intravascular water deficit is corrected by this action of the renal tubules.

Fluid and Food Intake

Fluids must be replaced in the amounts lost. The primary source of fluid replacement is water consumption. Approximately 60% may be obtained in this way, with an additional 30% being obtained from foods and 8% to 10% being a product of metabolism (metabolic water) for a total of 2,500 mL. Figure 10-10 illustrates fluid balance.

Figure 10-10 Water Balance

Thirst

Water consumption usually occurs in response to the sensation of thirst. This mechanism is poorly understood. It is generally believed to be brought about by the loss of body fluids, which in turn causes a dryness in the mouth and the thirst sensation. Replacing the lost fluids by water consumption causes the sensation to diminish. The thirst mechanism appears to be regulated by the hypothalamus in the brain.

Dehydration is one of the most common and most serious fluid imbalances that can result from poor monitoring of fluid intake. One nursing goal is to ensure that all clients understand both the role that water plays in health and the way to maintain adequate hydration.

DISTURBANCES IN ELECTROLYTE BALANCE

In health, normal homeostatic mechanisms function to maintain electrolyte balance. In illness, one or more of the regulating mechanisms may be affected, or an imbalance may become too great for the body to correct without treatment. Electrolytes are measured by laboratory analysis of a blood sample.

Sodium

Sodium (Na^+) is the major electrolyte in extracellular fluid. It regulates fluid balance through osmotic pressure that results from water following sodium in the body. Sodium stimulates conduction of nerve impulses and helps maintain neuromuscular activity. Excretion occurs primarily via the kidneys. The normal serum sodium for an adult is 136 to 145 mEq/L.

Hyponatremia

A subnormal serum sodium value (< 136 mEq/L) indicates hyponatremia. The cause is either a sodium deficit or a water excess. A hypo-osmotic state exists: The water moves out of the vascular space, into the interstitial space, and then into the intracellular space, causing edema. Hyponatremia may be caused by prolonged vomiting, diarrhea, or gastric or intestinal suctioning.

Hypernatremia

A serum sodium level of > 145 mEq/L indicates hypernatremia. Excess sodium or a loss of water causes a rise in the extracellular osmotic pressure and pulls water out of the cells and into the extracellular space.

Potassium

Potassium (K^+) is the major electrolyte in intracellular fluid. Its concentration inside cells is approximately 150 mEq/L. The normal value range of extracellular (serum) potassium is narrow: 3.5 to 5.0 mEq/L. Consequently, the slightest changes can dramatically affect physiological functions. Potassium maintains normal

PROFESSIONAL TIP

Hypokalemia

Hypokalemia can cause cardiac arrest when:

- The potassium level is < 2.5 mEq/L.
- The client is taking digitalis (a drug that strengthens the contraction of the myocardium and slows down the heart rate). *Hypokalemia enhances the action of digitalis, causing toxicity.*

nerve and muscle activity, especially of the heart, and osmotic pressure within the cells. It also assists in the cellular metabolism of carbohydrates and proteins. The kidneys prefer to retain sodium and excrete potassium, even when both electrolytes are depleted. When potassium is lost from cells, sodium and hydrogen move into the cells. This aids in regulating acid–base balance. Intracellular potassium deficit may coexist with an excess of extracellular potassium.

Hypokalemia

A serum potassium level < 3.5 mEq/L indicates hypokalemia. Excessive loss of gastric fluids and the use of diuretics can place the client at risk for hypokalemia and an acid–base imbalance (metabolic alkalosis). Potassium-wasting diuretics, such as furosemide (Lasix) or chlorothiazide (Diuril) can cause hypokalemia.

Safety: Potassium Chloride

- Use IV route only when hypokalemia is life threatening or when oral replacement is not feasible
- Always dilute potassium chloride in a large amount of IV solution
- Never administer more than 10 mEq/L of IV potassium chloride (KCl) per hour; the normal dose of IV KCl is 20 to 40 mEq/L infused over an 8-hour period
- Never give KCl intramuscularly (IM) or as an IV bolus; potentially fatal hyperkalemia may result
- Monitor the IV site frequently for early signs of infiltration, as potassium is caustic to the tissues

Hyperkalemia

A serum potassium level > 5.0 mEq/L indicates hyperkalemia. Clients with renal disease develop hyperkalemia, because potassium cannot be excreted adequately by the kidneys. Extensive trauma causes potassium to be released from the cells and enter the bloodstream, leading to hyperkalemia. Hyperkalemia inhibits the action of digitalis. This condition is much more critical than is hypokalemia.

PROFESSIONAL TIP

Serum Calcium

Approximately 50% of serum calcium is bound to protein. Correlate the serum calcium level with the serum albumin level when evaluating laboratory results. *Any change in serum protein will result in a change in the total serum calcium.*

CLIENT TEACHING

Calcium and Vitamin D

Vitamin D is necessary for the absorption of calcium from the GI tract. Clients who do not get adequate exposure to the sun or who use sunscreen (which is needed to prevent skin cancer) may not make enough vitamin D to support adequate calcium absorption. Advise these clients to consult their physicians regarding a vitamin D supplement.

Calcium

Calcium (Ca^{++}) plays an essential role in bone and teeth integrity, blood clotting, muscle functioning, and nerve impulse transmission. Vitamin D is required for absorption of calcium from the GI tract. Only 1% of the body's calcium is found in the blood plasma (serum). Normally, 50% of the serum calcium is ionized (physiologically active), with the remaining 50% being bound to protein. Free, ionized calcium is needed for cell membrane permeability. The calcium that is bound to plasma protein cannot pass through the capillary wall and, therefore, cannot leave the intravascular compartment. The normal ionized serum calcium range for an adult is 4.5 to 5.6 mEq/L. Total serum calcium concentration measures both the ionized calcium and the calcium bound to albumin. The normal value range of total serum calcium concentration for an adult is 9.0 to 10.5 mg/dL, with values for the older adult being slightly lower.

Hypocalcemia

Hypocalcemia is indicated by a total serum calcium concentration of < 9.0 mg/dL or an ionized serum calcium level of < 4.5 mEq/L. An ionized serum calcium level of < 3.0 mEq/L is related to tetany. Alkalosis, elevated serum albumin, and the rapid administration of citrated blood increase the activity of calcium binders, thereby decreasing the amount of free calcium.

Hypercalcemia

A total serum calcium level of > 10.5 mg/dL or an ionized serum calcium level of > 5.6 mEq/L indicates hypercalcemia. Generally, three separate evaluations of either total serum calcium or ionized serum calcium are performed before a diagnosis of hypercalcemia is made. Often, hypercalcemia is a symptom of an underlying disease such as metastatic bone tumors, Paget's disease, acromegaly, and hyperparathyroidism, which all increase bone reabsorption and, thereby, foster the release of calcium into circulating blood. Calcium-containing antacids and excess calcium from the diet may also cause hypercalcemia.

Magnesium

Most magnesium (Mg^{++}) is found in intracellular fluid and in combination with calcium and phosphorus in bone, muscle, and soft tissue. Blood serum contains only approximately 1%. Magnesium plays an important role as a coenzyme, in the metabolism of carbohydrates and proteins, and as a mediator, in neuromuscular activity. It is the only cation that is found in higher concentration in cererospinal fluid than in extracellular fluid. When a magnesium deficiency develops, the body conserves magnesium at the expense of excreting potassium. A close relationship exists between magnesium, calcium, and potassium in the intracellular fluid: A low level of one results in low levels of the other two. The normal serum magnesium level for an adult is 1.5 to 2.5 mEq/L.

Hypomagnesemia

A serum magnesium level of < 1.5 mEq/L indicates hypomagnesemia, which most commonly results from chronic alcoholism. Increased renal excretion is associated with prolonged diuretic therapy or use of gentamicin (Garamycin), cyclosporin (Sandimmune), or cisplatin (Platinol).

Hypermagnesemia

A serum magnesium level of > 2.5 mEq/L indicates hypermagnesemia. This condition rarely occurs if kidney function is normal. An increased magnesium level is associated with uncontrolled diabetes (ketoacidosis), renal failure, and ingestion of magnesium antacids (Maalox, Mylanta) or laxatives (milk of magnesia [MOM], magnesium citrate [Citromal]).

PROFESSIONAL TIP

Hypercalcemic Crisis

A rapid increase in the extracellular level of calcium (above 8 to 9 mEq/L) can trigger a hypercalcemic crisis (coma and cardiac arrest). To prevent a hypercalcemic crisis, provide adequate hydration and administer loop diuretics, phosphate, or both, as prescribed by the physician.

PROFESSIONAL TIP

Hyperalimentation

Total parenteral nutrition (TPN) provided continuously (hyperalimentation) and without a magnesium supplement can cause hypomagnesemia.

Safety: Magnesium Level

When the serum magnesium level reaches 10 to 15 mEq/L, respiratory paralysis may occur.

Phosphate

Phosphate (PO_4^{--}) is the main intracellular anion. It appears as phosphorus in the serum, where the normal value range is 1.7 to 2.6 mEq/L. Phosphorus is critical for normal cell functioning. Most phosphorus is found combined with calcium in teeth and bones. Phosphate and calcium exist in an inverse relationship; that is, as one increases the other decreases.

Hypophosphatemia

A client with a serum phosphorus level < 1.7 mEq/L has hypophosphatemia. Rarely does this condition result from decreased dietary intake. More commonly, is stems from respiratory alkalosis. Intense, prolonged hyperventilation can cause severe hypophosphatemia.

Hyperphosphatemia

A client with a serum phosphorus level > 2.6 mEq/L has hyperphosphatemia. This condition most commonly results from renal failure with resultant decreased renal phosphorus excretion. Excessive use of phosphate-containing laxatives or phosphate enemas may cause hyperphosphatemia.

Chloride

Chloride (Cl^-) is the major anion in extracellular fluid. Chloride functions in combination with sodium to maintain osmotic pressure. It also assists in maintaining acid–base balance. When the carbon dioxide level increases, bicarbonate shifts from the intracellular compartment to the extracellular compartment. Chloride, in an effort to maintain homeostasis, then moves

PROFESSIONAL TIP

Hyperphosphatemia

A client with hyperphosphatemia generally remains asymptomatic unless hypocalcemia results, in which case the client may describe both tingling sensations around the mouth and in the fingertips and muscle cramps.

into the intracellular compartment. The kidneys selectively excrete chloride or bicarbonate ions depending on the acid–base balance. The normal serum chloride range is 95 to 106 mEq/L.

Hypochloremia

A serum chloride level < 95 mEq/L indicates hypochloremia. Excess losses of chloride may result from prolonged diarrhea or diaphoresis. Loss of hydrochloric acid related to vomiting, gastric suctioning, or gastric surgery may cause hypochloremia.

Hyperchloremia

A serum chloride level > 106 mEq/L indicates hyperchloremia, which usually occurs in conjunction with dehydration, hypernatremia, or metabolic acidosis.

ACID–BASE BALANCE

As described earlier, the body maintains a normal pH within the relatively narrow range of 7.35 to 7.45. Body pH is maintained by the buffer systems, the respiratory system, and the kidneys. A pH below 7.35 is termed acidosis, and a pH above 7.45 is termed alkalosis. Either of these conditions can be brought about by respiratory or metabolic changes.

Regulators of Acid–Base Balance

The body has three main control systems that regulate acid–base balance to counter acidosis or alkalosis: the buffer systems, respirations, and renal control of hydrogen ion concentration. These systems vary in their reaction times in regulating and restoring balance to the hydrogen ion concentration.

Buffer Systems

The buffer systems—bicarbonate, phosphate, and protein—were previously discussed. They react quickly to prevent excessive changes in the hydrogen ion concentration.

Respiratory Regulation of Acid–Base Balance

The respiratory system helps to maintain acid–base balance by controlling the content of carbon dioxide in extracellular fluid. The *rate of metabolism* determines the formation of carbon dioxide. Various intracellular metabolic processes continuously form carbon dioxide in the body. The carbon in foods is **oxidized** (joined with oxygen) to form carbon dioxide.

It takes the respiratory regulatory mechanism several minutes to respond to changes in the carbon dioxide concentration of extracellular fluid. With the increase of carbon dioxide in extracellular fluid, respiration increases in rate and depth so that more carbon dioxide is exhaled. As the respiratory system removes carbon dioxide, less carbon dioxide is present in the blood to combine with water to form carbonic acid. Likewise, if the blood level of carbon dioxide is low, respirations decrease to maintain a normal ratio between carbonic acid and basic bicarbonate.

Renal Control of Hydrogen Ion Concentration

The kidneys control extracellular fluid pH by eliminating either hydrogen ions or bicarbonate ions from body fluids. If the bicarbonate concentration in the extracellular fluid is greater than normal, the kidneys excrete more bicarbonate ions, making the urine more alkaline. Conversely, if more hydrogen ions are excreted in the urine, the urine becomes more acidic. The renal mechanism for regulating acid–base balance cannot readjust the pH within seconds, as can the extracellular fluid buffer system, nor within minutes, as can the respiratory compensatory mechanism; but it can function over a period of several hours or days to correct acid–base imbalance.

Diagnostic and Laboratory Data

The biochemical indicators of acid–base balance are assessed by measuring the **arterial blood gases** (ABGs). The arterial blood gas test measures the levels of oxygen and carbon dioxide in arterial blood. The test assesses pH, partial pressure of oxygen (PO_2 or PaO_2), partial pressure of carbon dioxide (PCO_2 or $PaCO_2$), saturation of oxygen (SaO_2), and bicarbonate (HCO_3). pH has already been discussed.

The PO_2 or PaO_2 expresses the amount of oxygen that can combine with hemoglobin to form oxyhemoglobin, the form in which oxygen is transported through the body. At sea level, the normal range is 80 to 100 millimeters of mercury (mm Hg). The rate at which the oxygen/hemoglobin reaction occurs is influenced by pH. The rate decreases as the pH value decreases.

The PCO_2 or $PaCO_2$ in the blood is a reflection of the efficiency of gaseous exchange in the lungs. At sea level, the normal range is 35 to 45 mm Hg. If the alveoli are obstructed or damaged by disease, carbon dioxide cannot be eliminated and will combine with water to form carbonic acid, which in turn causes acidosis. Conversely, in a person who is hyperventilating, too much carbon dioxide is eliminated, which may trigger alkalosis.

The SaO_2 is the percent of oxygen that combines with hemoglobin in the blood. The normal range is

95% to 100% saturation. This value along with the PO_2 and hemoglobin levels indicates the degree to which the tissues are receiving oxygen. Oxygen saturation can also be measured with a pulse oximeter, a non-invasive technique.

Determining the amount of bicarbonate (HCO_3) in the blood is important because, along with carbonic acid, bicarbonate is a major buffer in the blood. The two substances occur in a ratio of 20 parts bicarbonate to 1 part carbonic acid. Regardless of the carbonic acid and bicarbonate values, the pH of the blood will remain in the normal range as long as the ratio remains 20:1. The normal range for HCO_3 at sea level is 24 to 28 mEq/L. The carbonic acid level is always 3% of the PCO_2 level.

DISTURBANCES IN ACID–BASE BALANCE

The acid–base imbalances are respiratory acidosis and alkalosis and metabolic acidosis and alkalosis. In determining whether the acid–base imbalance is caused by a respiratory or a metabolic alteration, the key indicators are bicarbonate and carbonic acid levels (Figure 10–11). Table 10–3 lists those changes in laboratory values that indicate the various acid–base imbalances.

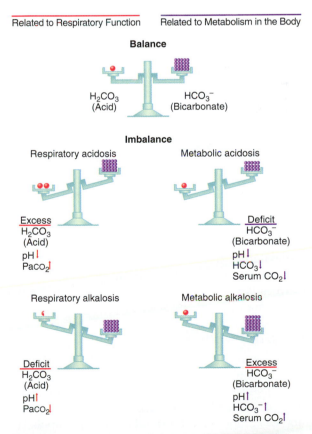

Figure 10-11 Acid–Base Balance and Imbalance (*Adapted from* Fundamentals of Nursing: Standards & Practice, *by* S. DeLaune and P. Ladner, 1998, Albany, NY: Delmar. Copyright 1998 by Delmar. Adapted with permission.)

PROFESSIONAL TIP

Pulse Oximeter Reading

Warming a client's cold hand will provide more accurate results from a pulse oximeter.

Table 10–3 LABORATORY VALUES IN ACID–BASE IMBALANCES

SITUATION	PH	PCO₂	HCO₃
Normal parameters	7.35 to 7.45	35 to 45 mm Hg	24 to 28 mEq/L
Respiratory acidosis			
Acute	< 7.35	> 45 mm Hg	Normal
Chronic	< 7.35	> 45 mm Hg	> 28 mEq/L
Respiratory alkalosis	> 7.45	< 35 mm Hg	Normal
Metabolic acidosis	< 7.35	Normal	< 24 mEq/L
Metabolic alkalosis	> 7.45	Normal	> 28 mEq/L

PROFESSIONAL TIP

Electrolyte Shift

Metabolic acidosis causes an electrolyte shift: Hydrogen and sodium ions move into the cells, and potassium moves into the extracellular fluid. Hyperkalemia may cause ventricular fibrillation and death.

Respiratory Acidosis

When carbon dioxide is not eliminated by the lungs as fast as it is produced by cellular metabolism, the amount of carbon dioxide increases in the blood. It then reacts with water and forms excess hydrogen ions, as shown in the following reaction:

$$CO_2 + H_2O \rightarrow H^+ + HCO_3$$

Respiratory acidosis is characterized by an increased hydrogen ion concentration (a blood pH below 7.35), an increased PCO_2 level (greater than 45 mm Hg), and an excess of carbonic acid. It is caused by hypoventilation or any condition that depresses ventilation. When the respiratory rate and the amount of oxygen supplied to the lungs suddenly lessen, acute respiratory acidosis can occur. This condition can be life threatening, and it must be recognized and corrected quickly. Chronic respiratory acidosis occurs when the respiratory rate is continually depressed.

Clients with respiratory acidosis experience neurological changes resulting from the acidity of the cerebrospinal fluid and brain cells. Hypoventilation causes **hypoxemia** (decreased oxygen in the blood), which in turn causes further neurological impairment. Hyperkalemia may accompany acidosis.

Respiratory Alkalosis

Respiratory alkalosis is characterized by a decreased hydrogen ion concentration (a blood pH above 7.45) and a below normal PCO_2 level (lower than 35 mm Hg). It is caused by hyperventilation (excessive exhalation of carbon dioxide) resulting in hypocapnia (decreased arterial carbon dioxide concentration). As the breathing rate increases, the amount of carbon dioxide in the blood decreases. This in turn increases the pH of the blood.

Hyperventilation can be triggered by anxiety, fear, pain, fever, rapid mechanical ventilation, and hypoxia at high altitudes. This condition is usually self-correcting. As the breathing returns to normal, the carbon dioxide level in the blood increases, and the normal pH is restored. Other causes of hyperventilation, which involves overstimulation of the respiratory center, include salicylate poisoning, brain tumors, meningitis, encephalitis, and pulmonary embolus.

Metabolic Acidosis

Metabolic acidosis is characterized by an increase in hydrogen ion concentration (blood pH below 7.35) or a decrease in bicarbonate concentration. Such a change may be brought about by kidney disease when the mechanism to excrete excess hydrogen ions is compromised. Diarrhea, diabetes mellitus, and, sometimes, diuretics may also be responsible. The lungs eliminate more carbon dioxide but are usually ineffective in decreasing acids. The kidneys try to increase the pH and the excretion of hydrogen by exchanging sodium ions for hydrogen ions. Metabolic acidosis is most common in individuals with kidney disease or diabetes mellitus.

Metabolic Alkalosis

Metabolic alkalosis is characterized by a loss of acid from the body or a gain in base (increased level of bicarbonate). Blood pH is above 7.45. A gain in base may result from excessive ingestion of antacids and milk. These substances neutralize acids, resulting in alkalosis and hypercalcemia. Excessive oral or parenteral administration of sodium bicarbonate or other alkaline salts (e.g., sodium or potassium acetate, lactate, or citrate) increases the amount of base in extracellular fluid. Loss of gastric fluids from vomiting or suctioning may result in metabolic alkalosis.

The respiratory and renal compensatory mechanisms respond to an increased bicarbonate/carbonic acid ratio. The rate and depth of respirations decreases in an effort to retain carbon dioxide. To counter the pH imbalance of metabolic alkalosis, the arterial carbon dioxide concentration rises, creating respiratory acidosis.

A normal serum potassium level is a prerequisite for renal compensation. In alkalosis, potassium ions enter

PROFESSIONAL TIP

Metabolic Alkalosis

The following clinical conditions can place clients at risk for metabolic alkalosis:

- Vomiting and nasogastric suctioning or lavage cause a loss of hydrochloric acid and chloride. With the loss of the hydrogen and chloride ions, bicarbonate ions are absorbed, unneutralized, into the bloodstream, and the pH of the extracellular fluid rises (alkalosis).
- Diarrhea and steroid or diuretic therapy can cause excessive loss of potassium, chloride, and other electrolytes. The potassium deficit causes the kidneys to exchange hydrogen ions (instead of potassium ions) for sodium ions, which promotes the loss of hydrogen, thereby increasing bicarbonate level.

the cells in exchange for hydrogen ions, causing hypokalemia. Hypokalemia further potentiates metabolic alkalosis because the kidneys conserve hydrogen ions by excreting potassium ions in exchange for sodium ions. When hypokalemia is present, the kidneys cannot function as a compensatory mechanism; they continue to excrete hydrogen, and bicarbonate excess continues.

NURSING PROCESS

The nursing process assists the nurse in planning client care.

Assessment

Assessment data are used to identify clients who have potential or actual alterations in fluid volume. Electrolyte and acid–base imbalances are identified primarily with laboratory data, while fluid balances are identified primarily with the health history and physical examination.

Health History

The nursing history should elicit data in the following areas:

- Lifestyle (sociocultural and economic factors, stress, exercise)
- Dietary intake (recent changes in the amount and types of fluid and food, increased thirst)
- Weight (sudden gain or loss)
- Fluid output (recent changes in the frequency or amount of urine output)
- Gastrointestinal disturbances (prolonged vomiting, diarrhea, anorexia, ulcer, hemmorrhage)
- Fever and diaphoresis
- Burns, trauma, draining wounds

- Disease conditions that can upset homeostasis (renal disease, endocrine disorders, neural malfunction, pulmonary disease)
- Therapeutic programs that can produce imbalances (special diets, medications, chemotherapy, IV fluid or TPN administration, gastric or intestinal suction)

Physical Examination

Because fluid alterations may affect any body system, the nurse performs a complete physical examination and identifies all abnormalities.

Daily Weight Changes in the body's total fluid volume are reflected in body weight. For instance, each liter (1,000 mL) of fluid gained or lost is equivalent to 1 kilogram (2.2 lb) of weight.

Vital Signs Measurement of vital signs provides the nurse with information regarding the client's fluid, electrolyte, and acid–base statuses and the body's compensatory response for maintaining balance. An elevated temperature places the client at risk for dehydration related to an increased loss of body fluid.

Changes in the pulse rate, strength, and rhythm are indicative of fluid alterations. Fluid volume alterations may cause the following pulse changes:

- Fluid volume deficit: increased pulse rate and weak pulse volume
- Fluid volume excess: increased pulse volume and third heart sound

Respiratory changes are assessed by inspecting the movement of the chest wall, counting the respiratory rate, and ascultating the lungs. Changes in the rate and depth may cause respiratory acid–base imbalances or may be indicative of a compensatory response to metabolic acidosis or alkalosis, as previously discussed.

Blood pressure measurements can be used to assess the degree of fluid volume deficit. Fluid volume deficit can lower the blood pressure. A narrow pulse pressure (lower than 20 mm Hg) may indicate fluid volume deficit that occurs with severe hypovolemia.

Intake and Output The client's I&O should be measured and recorded for a 24-hour period to assess for an actual or potential imbalance. A minimum intake of 1,500 mL is essential in balancing urinary output and the body's insensible water loss. Intake includes all liquids taken by mouth (e.g., ice cream, soup, gelatin, juice, and water) and liquids administered through tube feedings (nasogastric or jejunostomy) and parenterally (IV fluids and blood or its components). Output includes urine, diarrhea, vomitus, and drainage from tubes such as gastric suction or surgical drains.

Safety: Fluid Measurements

To protect both the nurse and the client from transfer of microorganisms, Standard Precautions are always instituted during fluid administration and output measurement.

Thirst The most common indicator of fluid volume deficit is thirst. With a decrease in extracellular fluid volume or an increase in plasma osmolality, the hypothalamus triggers a thirst response.

Food Intake The intake of food also contributes to maintaining extracellular fluid volume. One-third of the body's fluid needs are met with ingested food. Food also provides the body with necessary electrolytes.

Skin Edema and skin turgor are two important indicators related to fluid, electrolyte, and acid–base balances.

Edema Edema is the main symptom of fluid volume excess. Edema may be localized (confined to a specific area) or generalized (occurring throughout the body's tissue). Localized edema is characterized by taut, smooth, shiny, pale skin. The body may retain 5 to 10 pounds of fluid before edema is noticeable (Bulechek & McCloskey, 1999). The dependent body parts—sacrum, back, and legs—should be assessed for peripheral edema. Pitting edema is rated on a four-point scale, as follows:

+0: no pitting

+1, 0 to ¼ inch pitting (mild)

+2: ¼ to ½ inch pitting (moderate)

+3: ½ to 1 inch pitting (severe)

+4: greater than 1 inch pitting (severe)

Turgor Skin **turgor** refers to the normal resiliency of the skin, a reflection of hydration status. When the skin is pinched and released, it springs back to a normal position because of the outward pressure exerted by the cells and interstitial fluid. To measure the client's skin turgor, the nurse uses the thumb and forefinger to grasp and raise and then release a small section of the client's skin. Dehydration is the main cause of decreased skin turgor, which manifests as lax skin that returns slowly to the normal position. Increased skin turgor, which occurs in conjunction with edema, manifests as smooth, taut, shiny skin that cannot be grasped and raised.

Buccal (Oral) Cavity The nurse should inspect the buccal cavity. With fluid volume deficit, saliva decreases, causing sticky, dry mucous membranes and dry, cracked lips. The tongue displays longitudinal furrows.

GERONTOLOGICAL CONSIDERATIONS

Skin Turgor in Elderly Clients

With aging, the skin loses elasticity, resulting in reduced skin turgor. Assess the tongue for creases or furrows to monitor dehydration in elderly clients (Hogstel, 1994).

Eyes The nurse should inspect the eyes for sunkenness, dry conjunctiva, and decreased or absent tearing all signs of fluid volume deficit. Puffy eyelids (periorbital edema, or papilledema) are characteristic of fluid volume excess. The client may also have a history of blurred vision.

Jugular and Hand Veins Circulatory volume is assessed by measuring venous filling of the jugular and hand veins. The nurse places the client in a low Fowler's position and then:

1. Palpates the jugular (neck) veins. Fluid volume excess causes a distention in the jugular veins (Figure 10-12).
2. Places the client's hand below heart level and palpates the hand veins. Fluid volume deficit causes decreased venous filling (flat hand veins).

Neuromuscular System Fluid and electrolyte imbalances may cause neuromuscular alterations. The muscles lose their tone and become soft and flabby, and reflexes diminish. Calcium and magnesium imbalances cause an increase in neuromuscular irritability. To assess for neuromuscular irritability, the tests for Chvostek's sign and Trousseau's sign are performed. Other neurological signs of fluid, electrolyte, and acid–base imbalances include inability to concentrate, confusion, and emotional lability.

Diagnostic and Laboratory Data

Laboratory tests can reveal imbalances before clinical symptoms are evident in the client. However, unless clients are having the tests for some other reason, symptoms are detected first.

Hemoglobin and Hematocrit Indices Hematocrit (Hct) is affected by changes in plasma volume. For instance, with severe dehydration and hypovolemic shock, hematocrit increases. Conversely, overhydration decreases hematocrit. The hemoglobin (Hgb) level decreases in the event of severe hemorrhage.

Osmolality **Osmolality** is a measurement of the total concentration of dissolved particles (solutes) per kilogram of water. Osmolality measurements are per-

Figure 10-12 Client Position When Assessing Jugular Vein Distention

formed on both serum and urine samples to determine alterations in fluid and electrolyte balance. Osmolality can also be explained in relation to the specific gravity of body fluids. Specific gravity expresses the weight of the solution when compared to an equal volume of distilled water. The osmolality of a solution can be estimated by the specific gravity.

Serum Osmolality Serum osmolality is a measurement of the total concentration of dissolved particles per kilogram of water in serum, recorded in milliosmoles per kilogram (mOsm/kg). The particles measured in serum osmolality include electrolyte ions, such as sodium and potassium, and electrically inactive substances dissolved in serum, such as glucose and urea. Water and sodium are the main entities that control the osmolality of body fluids. Serum sodium is responsible for 85% to 90% of the serum osmolality (McFarland & Grant, 1994).

The normal range of serum osmolality is 280 to 295 mOsm/Kg (Noe & Rock, 1994). The value increases with dehydration and decreases with water excess.

In clinical practice, the terms *osmolality* and **osmolarity** (the concentration of solutes per liter of cellular fluid) are often used interchangeably to refer to the concentration of body fluid. However, these terms actually have different meanings, in that *osmolality* refers to the concentration of solutes in the total body water rather than in cellular fluid. The appropriate term to use in conjunction with IV fluid therapy is *osmolarity* (Bulechek & McCloskey, 1999).

Urine Osmolality Urine osmolality is a measurement of the total concentration of dissolved particles per kilogram of water in urine. The particles measured in urine osmolality come from nitrogenous waste (creatinine, urea, and uric acid), with urea being predominant. Urine osmolality varies greatly with diet and fluid intake and reflects the ability of the kidney to adjust the concentration of urine in order to maintain fluid balance. The dehydrated client with normal kidney function will have elevated urine osmolality, whereas the client with shock, hyperglycemia, hemoconcentration, or acidosis will have elevations in both urine and serum osmolalities.

Urine pH The measurement of urine pH reveals the hydrogen ion concentration in the urine, indicating the urine's acidity or alkalinity. When the kidney buffering system is compensating for either metabolic acidosis or alkalosis, the pH of the urine should be within normal range (4.6 to 8.0). This is considered a sign of normal function. However, when the renal compensatory function fails to respond to the blood pH, the urine pH will either increase, with acidosis, or decrease, with alkalosis.

Serum Albumin Albumin is synthesized in the liver from amino acids. Serum albumin plays an important role in fluid and electrolyte balance by maintaining the colloid osmotic pressure of blood, which in turn prevents fluid accumulation (edema) in the tissues. However, serum albumin has a half-life of 21 days and fluctuates according to the level of hydration. Therefore, it is not a good indicator of acute protein depletion. Clinically, this blood test is used to measure prolonged protein depletion, which occurs in chronic malnutrition.

Nursing Diagnosis

NANDA (2001) identifies the primary nursing diagnoses for clients with fluid imbalances as *Excess Fluid Volume, Deficient Fluid Volume,* and *Risk For Deficient Fluid Volume.* Numerous secondary nursing diagnoses may also apply.

Excess Fluid Volume

Excess Fluid Volume exists when the client has edema and increased interstitial and intravascular fluid retention. Fluid volume excess is related to excess fluid in either the tissues of the extremities (peripheral edema) or the lung tissues (pulmonary edema). Factors that put the client at risk for fluid volume excess are:

- Excessive fluid intake (e.g., IV therapy, sodium);
- Excessive loss or decreased intake of protein (chronic diarrhea, burns, kidney disease, malnutrition);
- Compromised regulatory mechanisms (kidney failure);
- Decreased intravascular movement (impaired myocardial contractility);
- Lymphatic obstruction (cancer, surgical removal of lymph nodes, obesity);
- Medications (steroid excess); and
- Allergic reactions.

Assessment findings in the client with fluid volume excess include acute weight gain; decreased serum osmolality (lower than 275 mOsm/Kg), protein and albumin, blood urea nitrogen (BUN), Hgb, Hct; increased central venous pressure (greater than 12 to 15 cm H_2O); and signs and symptoms of edema. The clinical manifestations of edema are relative to the area of involvement, either pulmonary or peripheral (Table 10–4).

PROFESSIONAL TIP

Urine Osmolality

Urine osmolality is a more accurate indicator of hydration than is the specific gravity of urine. Some medications and the presence of protein and glucose solutes in the urine can give a false high specific gravity reading.

Table 10–4 CLINICAL MANIFESTATIONS OF EDEMA	
PULMONARY EDEMA	**PERIPHERAL EDEMA**
Constant cough	Pitting edema in extremities
Dyspnea	Edematous area: tight, smooth
Engorged neck and hand veins	Shiny, pale, cool skin
Moist rales in lungs	Puffy eyelids
Bounding pulse	Weight gain

From Fundamentals of Nursing: Standards & Practice, *by S. DeLaune and P. Ladner, 1998, Albany, NY: Delmar. Copyright 1998 by Delmar. Reprinted with permission.*

Deficient Fluid Volume

Deficient Fluid Volume exists when the client experiences vascular, interstitial, or intracellular dehydration. The degree of dehydration is classified as mild, marked, severe, or fatal on the basis of the percentage of body weight lost. The multiple causes of fluid volume deficit include:

- Excessive fluid loss resulting from diaphoresis, vomiting, diarrhea, hemorrhage, burns, ascites, wound drainage, indwelling tubes, or suction;
- Diabetes insipidus;
- Diabetes mellitus;
- Addison's disease (adrenal insufficiency);
- Gastrointestinal fistula or draining abscess; and
- Intestinal obstruction.

Assessment findings in the client with fluid volume deficit include thirst and weight loss of an amount consistent with the degree of dehydration. Marked dehydration manifests as dry mucous membranes and skin; poor skin turgor; low-grade temperature elevation; tachycardia; respirations of 28 or greater; decreased (10 to 15 mm Hg) systolic blood pressure; slowed venous filling; decreased urine output (fewer than 25

 PROFESSIONAL TIP

Loss of Gastric Juices

Clients who lose excessive amounts of gastric juices, either through vomiting or suctioning, are prone to not only fluid volume deficit, but also metabolic alkalosis, hypokalemia, and hyponatremia. Gastric juices contain hydrochloric acid, pepsinogen, potassium, and sodium.

mL/hr); concentrated urine; elevated Hct, Hgb, and BUN; and acidic blood pH (less than 7.4).

Severe dehydration is characterized by the symptoms of marked dehydration plus a flushing of the skin. Systolic blood pressure continues to drop (to 60 mm Hg or below), and behavioral changes (restlessness, irritability, disorientation, and delirium) occur. The signs of fatal dehydration are anuria and coma leading to death.

Risk for Deficient Fluid Volume

Risk for Deficient Fluid Volume exists when the client is at risk of developing vascular, interstitial, or intracellular dehydration resulting from active or regulatory loss of body water in excess of needs. The multiple factors that can place the client at risk for fluid volume deficit were listed previously.

Other Nursing Diagnoses

In clients with a fluid imbalance, the relationship between the primary nursing diagnoses previously discussed and the secondary nursing diagnoses is reciprocal: The primary nursing diagnoses influence and are influenced by the secondary nursing diagnoses. Some commonly identified secondary nursing diagnoses include.

- *Impaired Gas Exchange*
- *Decreased Cardiac Output*
- *Ineffective Breathing Pattern*
- *Anxiety*
- *Disturbed Thought Processes*
- *Risk for Injury*
- *Risk for Infection*
- *Impaired Oral Mucous Membrane*
- *Deficient Knowledge (specify)*

Planning/Outcome Identification

Holistic nursing care for clients experiencing a fluid imbalance requires that the nurse, in collaboration with each client, identify specific goals for each nursing diagnosis. These goals should be individualized to reflect the client's capabilities and limitations and should be appropriate to the diagnosis and the assessment data.

During the planning phase, the nurse also selects and prioritizes nursing interventions to support the client's achievement of expected outcomes based on the goals. For example, if vomiting and diarrhea along with a 5% weight loss and dry mucous membranes led to a nursing diagnosis of *Deficient Fluid Volume,* the goals might include relief from vomiting and diarrhea and achievement of the proper balance of intake and output.

Expected outcomes for the client with a fluid imbalance are not only specific to the primary diagnosis, but also must be relative to the interventions. For example, an expected outcome for clients receiving IV therapy might be: "IV site remains free of erythema, edema, and purulent drainage" (because these clients are at risk for infection). Achievement of the goals and the client's expected outcomes indicates resolution of the problem.

Implementation

The nurse has a responsibility to collaborate with and advocate for clients to ensure receipt of care that is appropriate, ethical, and based on practice standards. The data obtained from the history serve as the basis for formulating expected outcomes and selecting nursing interventions appropriate to the client's natural patterns as revealed in their history.

The rationale for interventions related to alterations in either fluid, electrolyte, or acid–base balance is based on the goal of maintaining homeostasis and regulating and maintaining essential fluids and nutrients. Clients' adaptive capabilities are kept in mind when selecting interventions based on the clients' perceptions of their support systems, strengths, and options.

Bulechek and McCloskey (1999) address the importance of the nursing interventions relative to fluid therapy by identifying the nurse's responsibilities to:

- Understand the client's metabolic needs and make judgments concerning the outcomes of therapy,
- Perform frequent assessment and monitoring to recognize the adverse effects of fluid and electrolyte therapy and prevent complications, and
- Prevent the rapid depletion of the body's protein and energy reserves.

The nursing activities relative to assessment and implementation often require the same measurements: for example, weight and vital signs. Common interventions that promote attainment of expected outcomes relative to restoring and maintaining homeostasis are discussed following.

Monitor Daily Weight

Daily weight is one of the main indicators of fluid and electrolyte balance. The nurse is responsible for the accurate measurement and recording of the client's daily weight. The physician uses this data along with other clinical findings to determine fluid therapy for the client.

Measure Vital Signs

The frequency with which vital signs are measured depends on the client's acuity level and clinical situation. For example, the vital signs of the typical postoperative client might be taken every 15 minutes until stable, whereas vital signs should be monitored continuously for the client experiencing shock or hemorrhage. Vital sign measurements and other clinical data are used to determine the type and amount of fluid therapy.

PROFESSIONAL TIP

"Strict" I&O

- "Strict" I&O measurement usually involves accounting for incontinent urine, emesis, and diaphoresis and might require weighing soiled bed linens.
- *Gloves should always be worn when handling soiled linen.*

Measure Intake and Output

Intake and output measurements are initiated to monitor the client's fluid status over a 24-hour period. Agency policy relative to I&O may vary with regard to:

- Time frames for charting (e.g., every 8 hours versus every 12 hours),
- Time at which the 24-hour totals are calculated, and
- Definition of "strict" I&O.

 Safety: Removing Gloves Before Charting
To prevent the transfer of microorganisms when the I&O form is removed from the client's room, remove gloves and wash hands before recording the amount of drainage on the form.

The nurse should review the client's 24-hour I&O calculations to evaluate fluid status. Intake should exceed output by 500 mL to offset insensible fluid loss. Intake and output and daily weight are critical components of intervention, because these measurements are also used to evaluate the effectiveness of diuretic or rehydration therapy.

COMMUNITY/HOME HEALTH CARE

Considerations for Measuring I&O

- Elicit client and family member input when selecting household items to be used for intake measurement
- Provide containers for measuring output, adapting the urinary container to home facilities, and teach client and family about proper washing and storage
- Teach handwashing technique
- Provide written instructions on what is to be measured
- Provide sufficient I&O forms to last between the nurse's visits
- Identify the parameters for evaluating a discrepancy between the intake and the output and for notifying the nurse or physician

Securing an accurate I&O requires the full support of the client and family. The client and family members should be taught the way to measure and record the I&O.

Provide Oral Hygiene

The nurse is responsible for providing oral hygiene to promote both client comfort and the integrity of the buccal cavity. The frequency of oral hygiene depends on the condition of the client's buccal cavity and the type of fluid imbalance. A client who is dehydrated or permitted no oral fluids for more than 24 hours may have decreased or absent salivation, coated tongue, and furrows on the tongue. Such clients are at risk for developing oral diseases such as stomatitis, oral lesions or ulcers, and gingivitis.

Initiate Oral Fluid Therapy

Oral fluids may be totally restricted—a situation commonly referred to as *nothing by mouth* (NPO, which is from the Latin *non per os*)—or they may be restricted or forced, depending on the client's clinical situation.

Nothing by Mouth Clients are placed on NPO status as prescribed by the physician. On the basis of agency policy and clarification from the physician, the client may be allowed small amounts of ice chips when designated NPO. Common clinical situations that may require NPO status include the need to:

- Avoid aspiration in unconscious, perioperative, and preprocedural clients who will receive anesthesia or conscious sedation;
- Rest and heal the GI tract in clients with severe vomiting or diarrhea or a GI disorder (inflammation or obstruction);
- Prevent the further loss of gastric juices in clients on nasogastric suctioning.

Clients designated NPO should receive oral hygiene every 1 to 2 hours or as needed for comfort and to prevent alterations of the mucous membranes.

Restricted Fluids Fluid intake is commonly restricted in the treatment of fluid volume excess related to heart and renal failure. Intake may be restricted to 200 mL in a 24-hour period. Client and family teaching and collaboration are the main nursing interventions in implementing this measure.

PROFESSIONAL TIP

Mouthwashes
Avoid using mouthwashes with alcohol or glycerin, and swabs with lemon or glycerin. Although they may feel refreshing, these ingredients dry the mucous membranes.

PROFESSIONAL TIP

Temperature of Fluids
Advise clients to drink room-temperature fluids. Hot or cold fluids may increase peristalsis and abdominal cramping.

The way fluids are limited should be determined in collaboration with the client. For example:

- Half of the allowed fluid might be divided between breakfast and lunch and
- The remaining half might be divided between the evening meal and before bedtime, unless the client must be awakened during the night for medication.

Forced Fluids "Forcing" or encouraging the intake of oral fluids, mainly water, is sometimes done when treating clients who are at risk for dehydration or who have renal and urinary problems (kidney stones). Compliance is obtained through client education and honoring client preference relative to timing and the type of liquids. A client might, for example, be requested to consume 2,000 mL over a 24-hour period. If the client is intimidated at hearing this amount, which may sound very large, the nurse might explain that the number of glasses to which this volume equates is only eight. This would roughly translate into one glass every 2 hours. The nurse could also tell the client that ice, gelatin, soups, and ice cream all count as liquid.

Maintain Tube Feeding

When the client cannot ingest oral fluids but has a normal GI tract, fluids and nutrients can be administered through a feeding tube as prescribed by a physician.

Monitor Intravenous Therapy

When fluid loss is severe or the client cannot tolerate oral or tube feedings, fluid volume is replaced parenterally through the IV route. **Intravenous** (IV) **therapy** is the administration of fluids, electrolytes, nutrients, or medications by the venous route. The physician prescribes IV therapy to treat or prevent fluid, electrolyte, or nutritional imbalances. The nurse has specific responsibilities relative to IV therapy. Specifically, the nurse must:

PROFESSIONAL TIP

Fluid Replacement
Fluid replacement is based on weight loss. A 2.2 pound (1 kg) weight loss is equivalent to 1 liter (1,000 mL) of fluid loss.

- Know why the therapy is prescribed;
- Document client understanding;
- Select the appropriate equipment according to agency policy;
- Obtain the correct solution as prescribed;
- Assess the client for allergies relative to tape, iodine, ointment, or antibiotic preparations to be used for skin preparation of the venipuncture site;
- Administer the fluid at the prescribed rate;
- Observe for signs of **infiltration** (seepage of the fluid into the interstitial tissue as a result of accidental dislodgement of the needle from the vein) and other complications that are fluid specific; and
- Document in the client's medical record the implementation of the prescribed IV therapy.

Evaluation

Evaluation is an ongoing process for clients with fluid, electrolyte, or acid–base imbalances. When evaluating whether the time frames and expected outcomes are realistic (such as whether the intake and output are within 200 to 300 mL of each other), the focus should be on the client's responses. The client's vital signs should be within normal limits. The IV infusion rate should be accurately calculated and reassessed throughout therapy to maintain the client's hydration. The IV site should remain free from erythema, edema, and purulent drainage. The nursing care plan should be modified as necessary to support the client's expected outcomes.

SAMPLE NURSING CARE PLAN

THE CLIENT WITH EXCESS FLUID VOLUME

When brought to the emergency department by his granddaughter, Mr. Gomez, a 68-year-old widower, stated, "I can't breathe." Mr. Gomez has a history of hypertension and heart disease, and he is obese. The practitioner ordered a stat chest x-ray, CBC, and electrolytes, which revealed pulmonary congestion (x-ray), decreased Hct, and decreased Hgb. The physical assessment results were as follows: Wt 162; TPR 97.6, 98, 30 (labored); BP 186/114; shortness of breath, crackles; constant cough; pitting edema (ankles); and engorged neck veins. Mr. Gomez stated, "I thought I could stop taking the heart medication and eat what I wanted when I felt good again."

Nursing Diagnosis 1 *Excess Fluid Volume related to a compromised regulatory mechanism as evidenced by edema, shortness of breath, crackles, decreased Hgb and Hct, and jugular vein distention*

PLANNING/GOALS	NURSING INTERVENTIONS	RATIONALE	EVALUATION
Mr. Gomez will have a balanced I&O for 2 days.	Measure and document hourly I&O; restrict fluids as ordered	Monitors fluid status	Output for the first 3 hours was 2,020 mL; on day two, I&O was indicative of fluid balance.
	Administer diuretics as ordered and document response	Increases excretion of fluids and electrolytes	
Mr. Gomez will identify a specific amount of weight to lose over the next 6 months.	Weigh daily at the same time, with the same scale, and with Mr. Gomez wearing the same clothing	Allows weight to be compared from one day to another	Mr. Gomez identified the need to lose 30 pounds over the next 6 months.
	Discuss with Mr. Gomez the need for weight loss	Allows Mr. Gomez to voice his thoughts about weight loss and provides an avenue to determine number of pounds to be lost	

continues

Mr. Gomez will show normal hydration status prior to discharge.	Measure and document vital signs every hour until shortness of breath subsides, then every 2 hours	Monitors Mr. Gomez's response to therapy	Mr. Gomez demonstrated normal hydration status, as shown by normal levels of Hct and Hgb; BP 156/92; normal breath sounds; and absence of shortness of breath, jugular engorgement, and peripheral edema.
	Hourly assess heart sounds; breath sounds; rate, rhythm, and depth of respirations; and the position Mr. Gomez takes to relieve the shortness of breath	Provides information for use in modifying the plan of care	

Nursing Diagnosis 2 *Deficient Knowledge related to information misinterpretation as evidenced by Mr. Gomez's statement "I thought I could stop taking the heart medication and eat what I wanted when I felt good again."*

PLANNING/GOALS	NURSING INTERVENTIONS	RATIONALE	EVALUATION
Mr. Gomez will demonstrate an understanding of the causes of fluid excess and the role of heart medications, foods, and exercise in assisting with weight reduction.	Assess Mr. Gomez's knowledge of hypertension; decreased cardiac output; digitalis; the effects of a large abdominal girth on breathing; and foods low in sodium, fats, and carbohydrates.	Provides a basis for educating Mr. Gomez about causes, aggravating and alleviating factors, and effects of fluid excess	Mr. Gomez was unable to verbalize understanding of the way that weight, high-sodium diet, and failure to take his heart medications caused the fluid excess. He was referred to home health for client teaching.

SUMMARY

- Homeostasis is the maintenance of the body's internal environment within a narrow range of normal values. It is an ongoing process, with changes constantly occurring in the body.
- Many chemical and physical processes are necessary for homeostasis.
- Ions are electrically charged atoms.
- Compounds that ionize in water are called electrolytes.
- The normal range of blood pH is 7.35 to 7.45. A decrease or increase beyond this range can cause severe or even fatal physiologic problems.
- The bicarbonate buffer system works to regulate pH in both intracellular and extracellular fluids.
- The phosphate buffer system works to regulate the pH of intracellular fluid and fluid in kidney tubules.

- Protein buffers work to regulate pH inside cells, especially red blood cells.
- Substances move in and out of cells by the passive transport methods of diffusion, osmosis, and filtration and by active transport.
- The kidneys regulate fluid and electrolyte balance.
- Sodium is the main electrolyte that promotes the retention of water.
- The slightest decrease or increase in electrolyte levels can cause serious, adverse, or life-threatening effects on physiologic functions.
- Hospitalized clients, especially elderly clients, are at risk for developing dehydration.
- Clients receiving IV therapy require constant monitoring for complications.

CASE STUDY

Mrs. Meisenbach is a 75-year-old woman with diabetes who has been experiencing flu-like symptoms of vomiting and diarrhea for 5 days. She lives alone and does not like to cook. When she got up this morning, she felt weak and dizzy. She called 911 to take her to the clinic. The emergency medical technicians called the practitioner en route, and Mrs. Meisenbach was taken directly to the infusion center, where 1,000 mL of lactated Ringer's solution was started. Later, she was given Gatorade to drink.

Assessment data revealed:

- *Marked thirst*
- *Temperature 99°F*
- *BP 94/74, Resp. 30*
- *Wt 157 lb (loss from 165)*
- *Dry mucous membranes*
- *Apical pulse 108/min*
- *Increased Hct, Hgb, and BUN*

The following questions will guide your development of a nursing care plan for the case study.

1. What other data would you collect?
2. What is the primary nursing diagnosis for Mrs. Meisenbach?
3. What goals would be appropriate for this nursing diagnosis?
4. Identify the nursing interventions and rationale to meet the goals.
5. Ascertain the fluid intake replacement needed. Include the IV and oral fluids.
6. On the basis of the intake, what should have been her output prior to discharge?

Review Questions

1. The basic unit of an element is:
   a. an atom.
   b. the nucleus.
   c. an electron.
   d. small groups of atoms called molecules.

2. The phosphate buffer system is involved in regulating the pH of the:
   a. carbonic acid in the lungs.
   b. carbon dioxide in the lungs.
   c. bicarbonate ions in the lungs.
   d. intracellular fluid and the fluid in the kidney tubules.

3. Diffusion is:
   a. the movement of molecules from a region of high concentration to a region of low concentration.
   b. the movement of molecules from a region of low concentration to a region of high concentration.
   c. the movement of a liquid from a region of high concentration through a membrane to a region of low concentration.
   d. the movement of a liquid from a region of low concentration through a membrane to a region of high concentration.

4. When gas is exchanged in the lungs:
   a. carbon dioxide concentration is equal in the alveoli and lungs.
   b. oxygen concentration is higher in the alveoli than in the blood.
   c. oxygen concentration is higher in the blood than in the alveoli.
   d. carbon dioxide has a higher concentration in the alveoli than in the blood.

5. When blood flows into a capillary bed, the pressure of the blood is:
   a. high in the venule.
   b. low in the arteriole.
   c. high in the arteriole.
   d. low but increases to high.

6. Acidosis and alkalosis are identified by changes in the pH. Which of the following statements is true?

   a. A pH above 7.45 is called acidosis.
   b. A pH above 7.45 is called alkalosis.
   c. A pH increase caused by an increase of bicarbonate in the blood is metabolic acidosis.
   d. A pH decrease caused by an accumulation of carbonic acid results in respiratory alkalosis.

7. The maximum amount of IV potassium chloride that can be infused per hour is:

   a. 5 mEq.
   b. 10 mEq.
   c. 15 mEq.
   d. 20 mEq.

Critical Thinking Questions

1. A client has been vomiting for 3 days and is unable to keep anything down. Besides fluid volume deficit, what other alterations would you expect to find?

2. Because half of serum calcium is bound to another solute in the blood, which other serum level must be considered when monitoring the serum level of calcium?

 WEB FLASH!

- Visit the Intravenous Nurses Society site for standards for IV therapy; certification information; and education.
- Look on the Web for information about IV therapy.

IV THERAPY

MAKING THE CONNECTION

Refer to the following chapters to increase your understanding of IV therapy:

- **Chapter 3, Legal Responsibilities**
- **Chapter 13, Diagnostic Tests**
- **Chapter 20, Nursing Care of the Client: Hematologic and Lymphatic Systems**
- **Chapter 25, Nursing Care of the Client: Neurological System**
- **Chapter 28, Nursing Care of the Client: Gastrointestinal System**

LEARNING OBJECTIVES

Upon completion of this chapter, you should be able to:
- *Define key terms.*
- *Discuss principles of safe IV administration.*
- *Calculate the drip rate for IVs.*
- *Demonstrate starting an IV.*
- *Describe the process for the safe administration of blood.*

KEY TERMS

angiocatheter
butterfly needle
drug incompatibility
flashback
flow rate
hypervolemia
implantable port
infiltration
intracath
intravenous (IV) therapy
IV push (bolus)
phlebitis
piggyback
vesicant

INTRODUCTION

Intravenous (IV) therapy requires the collaborative efforts of many health care providers. IVs may be prescribed by a physician, dentist, or other authorized prescriber such as advanced practice registered nurses as determined by individual state licensing bodies. Pharmacists often prepare and dispense the solutions. Nurses are responsible for administering IV therapy.

IV therapy administration requires specialized knowledge, judgment, and nursing skills. The focus of this chapter is to assist the student in applying knowledge of IV therapy and in acquiring skills in the safe administration of IV therapy.

IV therapy is the administration of fluids, electrolytes, nutrients, or medications by the venous route. It requires parenteral fluids (solutions) and special equipment: administration set, IV pole, filter, regulators to control IV flow rate, and an established venous route.

PARENTERAL FLUIDS

The nurse should confirm the type and amount of IV solution by reading the physician's order in the client's medical record. Intravenous solutions are sterile and are packaged in plastic bags or glass containers. Solutions that are incompatible with plastic are dispensed in glass containers.

Plastic IV solution bags collapse under atmospheric pressure to allow the solution to enter the infusion set. Plastic solution bags are packaged with an outer plastic bag, which should remain intact until the nurse prepares the solution for administration. When the plastic solution bag is removed from its outer wrapper, the solution bag should be dry. If the solution bag is wet, the nurse should not use the solution. The moisture on the bag indicates that the integrity of the bag has been compromised and that the solution cannot be considered sterile. The bag should be returned to the dispensing department that issued the solution. Glass containers are discussed in the section on equipment.

The three types of parenteral fluids are classified based on the tonicity of the fluid relative to normal blood plasma. A solution may be hypotonic, isotonic, or hypertonic. The type of solution is prescribed on the basis of the client's diagnosis and the goal of therapy. The desired effect of the solution is determined as follows:

- Hypotonic fluid: lowers the osmotic pressure and causes fluid to move into the cells. If fluid is infused beyond the client's tolerance, water intoxication may result.
- Isotonic fluid: increases only extracellular fluid volume. If fluid is infused beyond the client's tolerance, cardiac overload may result.
- Hypertonic fluid: increases the osmotic pressure of the blood plasma, drawing fluid from the cells. If fluid is infused beyond the client's tolerance, cellular dehydration may result (Bulechek & McCloskey, 2000).

Common intravenous solutions are shown in Table 11–1.

Table 11–1 COMMON INTRAVENOUS SOLUTIONS

TONICITY	SOLUTION	CONTENTS (MEQ/L)	CLINICAL IMPLICATIONS
Hypotonic	Sodium chloride 0.45%	77 Na^+, 77 Cl^-	Daily maintenance of body fluid and establishment of renal function.
Isotonic	Dextrose 2.5% in 0.45% saline	77 Na^+, 77 Cl^-	Promotes renal function and urine output.
	Dextrose 5% in 0.2% saline	77 Na^+, 77 Cl^-	Daily maintenance of body fluids when less Na^+ and Cl^- are required.
	Dextrose 5% in water (D_5W)	38 Na^+, 38 Cl^-	Promotes rehydration and elimination; may cause urinary Na^+ loss; good vehicle for K^+.
	Ringer's lactate	130 Na^+, 4 K^+, Ca^{2+}, 109 Cl^-, 28 lactate	Resembles the normal composition of blood serum and plasma; K^+ level below body's daily requirement.
	Normal saline (NS), 0.9%	154 Na^+, 154 Cl^-	Restores sodium chloride deficit and extracellular fluid volume.
	Dextran 40 10% in NS (0.9%) or D_5W		A colloidal solution used to increase plasma volume of clients in early shock; *it should not be given to severly dehydrated clients and clients with renal disease, thrombocytopenia, or active hemorrhaging.*
	Dextran 70% in NS		A long-lived (20 hours) plasma volume expander; used to treat shock or impending shock due to hemorrhage, surgery, or burns. *It can prolong bleeding and coats the RBCs (draw type and crossmatch prior to administering).*
Hypertonic	Dextrose 5% in 0.45% saline	77 Na^+, 77 Cl^-	Daily maintenance of body fluid and nutrition; treatment of FVD.
	Dextrose 5% in saline 0.9%	154 Na^+, 154 Cl^-	Fluid replacement of sodium, chloride, and calories (170).
	Dextrose 10% in saline 0.9%	154 Na^+, 154 Cl^-	Fluid replacement of sodium, chloride, and calories (340).
	Dextrose 5% in lactated Ringer's	130 Na^+, 4 K^+, 3 Ca^{2+}, 109 Cl^-, 28 lactate	Resembles the normal composition of blood serum and plasma; K^+ level below body's daily requirement; caloric value 180.
	Hyperosmolar saline 3% and 5% NaCl	856 Na^+, 865 Cl^-	Treatment of hyponatremia; raises the Na osmolarity of the blood, and reduces intracellular fluid excess.
	Ionosol B with dextrose 5%	57 Na^+, 25 K^+, 49 Cl^-, 25 lact., 5 Mg^{2+}, 7 PO^{4-}	Treatment of polyionic parenteral replacement caused by vomiting-induced alkalosis, diabetic acidosis, fluid loss from burns, and postoperative FVD.

From Fluids and Electrolytes With Clinical Applications *(6th ed.), by J. L. Kee & B. J. Paulanka, 1999, Albany, NY: Delmar.*

EQUIPMENT

Intravenous equipment is sterile, disposable, and prepackaged with user instructions. The user instructions are usually placed on the outside of the package and include a schematic that labels the parts, allowing the user to read the package before opening. The syringe tip and port require sterile technique during handling because they are in direct contact with fluids to be infused into the bloodstream.

The administration (infusion) set includes the plastic tubing used to infuse solutions. It contains an insertion spike with a protective cap, a drip chamber, tubing with a slide clamp and regulating (roller) clamp, a rubber injection port, and a protective cap over the needle adapter (Figure 11-1). The protective caps keep both ends of the infusion set sterile and are removed only just before use. The insertion spike is inserted into the port of the IV solution container.

Infusion sets can be vented or nonvented. The nonvented type is used with plastic bags of IV solutions and vented bottles. The vented set is used for glass containers that are not vented (Figure 11-2).

The drip chamber is calibrated to allow a predictable amount of fluid to be delivered. There are two types of drip chambers: a macrodrip, which delivers 10 to 20 drops per milliliter of solution, and a microdrip, which delivers 60 drops per milliliter. The drip rate, which is indicated on the package, varies with the manufacturer.

The IV tubing has a roller clamp that is used to compress the plastic tubing to control the rate of flow. The end of the IV tubing contains a needle adapter that attaches to the sterile injection device inserted into the client's vein. Extension tubing may be used to lengthen the primary tubing or to provide additional Y-injection ports for the administration of additional solutions.

Intravenous Filters

Intravenous filters remove from the solution particulate matter that may cause irritation and **phlebitis** (inflammation in the wall of a vein without clot formation). Intravenous filters come in various sizes; the finer the filter, the greater is the degree of solution filtration. Although studies have shown that IV filters reduce the risk of bacteremia and phlebitis as much as 40%, some agencies do not use IV filters because of cost. Many IV catheters contain an in-line filter. If the catheter has an in-line filter, it is not necessary to add a filter to the tubing.

Needles and Catheters

Needles and catheters provide access to the venous system. A variety of devices is available in different sizes to complement the age of the client and the type and duration of the therapy (Figure 11-3). The larger the number, the smaller the lumen of the needle or catheter.

Butterfly (scalp vein or wing-tipped) **needles** are short, beveled needles with plastic flaps attached to the shaft. The flaps (which are flexible) are held tightly together to facilitate ease of insertion and then are flattened against the skin to prevent dislodgment during infusion. These needles are commonly used for short-term or intermittent therapy and for infants and children.

There are several types of catheters used to access peripheral veins. During insertion, some of these catheters are threaded over a needle, and others are threaded

Figure 11-1 Sample Basic Administration Set

- 10 drops/mL
- Slide clamp
- Regulating clamp
- Injection site
- Luer-Lok adapter
- Lever lock cannula

Figure 11-2 Sample Vented Administration Set

- Vented
- 10 drops/mL
- Check valve
- Injection site
- Slide clamp
- Regulating clamp
- Injection site
- Slide clamp
- Injection site
- Luer-Lok adapter

GERONTOLOGICAL CONSIDERATIONS

Selecting Needle Gauge

Consider the client's age and body size and the type of solution to be administered when selecting the gauge of the needle or catheter.

- Teenagers and adults, 22 or 20 gauge
- Elderly, 22 or 24 gauge

inside a needle. **Intracath** is a term used to refer to a plastic tube inserted into a vein. An **angiocatheter** (angiocath, for short) is a type of intracath with a metal stylet to pierce the skin and vein, after which the plastic catheter is threaded into the vein and the metal stylet is removed, leaving only the plastic catheter in the vein.

Peripheral Intravenous and Heparin Locks

Peripheral intravenous (PI) and heparin locks are devices that establish a venous route as a precautionary measure for clients whose condition may change rapidly or who may require intermittent infusion therapy. A butterfly needle or peripheral catheter is inserted into a vein and the hub is capped with a lock port, also called a Luer-Lok. The patency of the device is maintained with the injection of either normal saline or heparin (an anticoagulant drug) in accord with the agency's protocol.

Needle-Free System

Safety is a concern with IV therapy. Accidental needlestick injuries and puncture wounds with conta-

minated devices increase the employee's risk for infectious diseases such as AIDS, hepatitis (B and C), and other viral, rickettsial, bacterial, fungal, and parasitic infections. Most health care agencies now use totally needle-free IV systems (Figure 11-4) to decrease the risk of employee injuries.

Vascular Access Devices

Vascular access devices (VADs) include various catheters, cannulas, and infusion ports that allow for long-term IV therapy or repeated access to the central venous system. The kind of VAD used depends on the client's diagnosis and the type and length of treatment. Central venous catheters (CVCs) are inserted by a physician.

Another type of VAD is an **implantable port** (a device made of a radiopaque silicone catheter and a plastic or stainless steel injection port with a self-sealing silicone-rubber septum). *Only nurses who have been specially trained are allowed to access an implanted port because of the risk of infiltration into the tissue if needle placement is incorrect.*

PREPARING AN INTRAVENOUS SOLUTION

To prepare an IV solution, the nurse should first read the agency's protocol and gather the necessary equipment. Because IV equipment and solutions are sterile, the expiration date on the package should be checked before use. The solution can be prepared at the nurses' work area or in the client's room.

The nurse will prepare and apply a time strip to the IV solution bag to facilitate monitoring of the infusion rate as prescribed by the physician (Figure 11-5). The IV tubing is tagged with the date and time to indicate when the tubing replacement is necessary. Intravenous

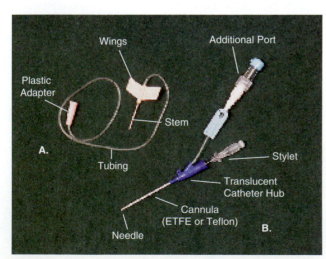

Figure 11-3 Peripheral IV Devices: A. Butterfly; B. Angiocatheter

Figure 11-4 Needle-Free System

PROFESSIONAL TIP

Inserting a CVC

When assisting with the insertion of a long-line central catheter, observe the client for symptoms of a pneumothorax: sudden shortness of breath or sharp chest pain; increased anxiety; a weak, rapid pulse; hypotension; pallor or cyanosis. These symptoms indicate accidental puncture of the pleural membrane.

tubing is changed every 24 to 48 hours according to agency policy. The nurse initials the time strip and the IV tubing tag.

 Safety: Marking an IV Bag
Do not use a felt-tip pen to mark an IV bag. The ink from the pen can leak through the plastic and contaminate the solution. Instead, mark a sticker or piece of tape, then affix this to the bag.

INITIATING IV THERAPY

When initiating IV therapy, the nurse should first consider the type of fluid to be infused and then assess for a venipuncture site. Ellenberger (1999) suggests that the smallest gauge and shortest needle appropriate be

selected (22 gauge for maintenance fluids and routine antibiotics, 20 gauge or larger for blood products).

When assessing a client for potential sites, the nurse should consider age, body size, activity, clinical status and impairments, and skin condition. Generally, it is best to begin with the hand and advance up the arm if new sites are needed. Figure 11-6 illustrates common peripheral sites for initiating IV therapy. Venipuncture site contraindications are:

- Signs of infection, infiltration, or thrombosis
- Affected arm of a postmastectomy client

Figure 11-5 Applying a Time Strip to the IV Container

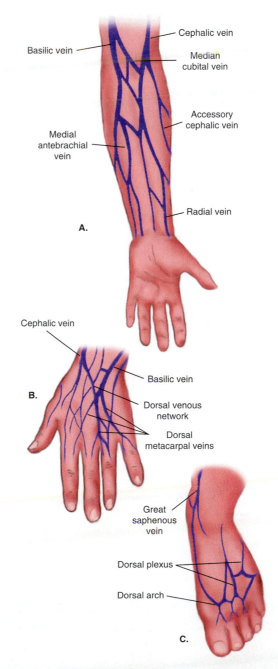

Figure 11-6 Peripheral Veins Used in Intravenous Therapy: A. Forearm; B. Dorsum of the hand; C. Dorsal plexus of the foot

- Arm with a functioning arteriovenous fistula (dialysis)
- Affected arm of a paralyzed client
- Any arm that has circulatory or neurological impairments

Locating a Vein

With the client's arm extended on a firm surface, place a tourniquet on the arm, tight enough to impede venous flow yet loose enough that a radial pulse can still be palpated. Next, use the index and middle fingers of the nondominant hand to palpate a vein. It should feel soft and resilient and not have a pulse. If no vein can be seen or felt, a warm, moist compress may be applied for 10 to 20 minutes, the area may be massaged toward the heart, or the client may open and close the fist (Ellenberger, 1999).

GERONTOLOGICAL CONSIDERATIONS

Locating a Vein

For clients who are elderly or have fragile veins, eliminate the tourniquet or apply it very loosely if a vein can be palpated.

Placing the Needle

With hands washed and gloved, prepare the selected site according to agency policy. Without touching the prepared site, stabilize the vein by placing your thumb beside the vein and pulling down. Hold the needle at a 10- to 30-degree angle, bevel up to puncture the skin, then the angle is lessened to prevent puncturing the back of the vein (Ellenberger, 1999). Secure the needle in place according to agency policy.

 Safety: Prepping Skin for Venipuncture
When prepping the client's skin for a venipuncture, cleanse the skin with Betadine and wait for it to dry. Do not apply alcohol after the skin has been prepped with Betadine. If these substances are combined, they form a toxic material that may be absorbed through the skin.

PROFESSIONAL TIP

Venipuncture
Standard Precautions must be followed when performing a venipuncture.

ADMINISTERING IV THERAPY

Once the solution has been prepared for administration, the nurse calculates the rate and explains the procedure to the client. Fluid administration can be continuous, ongoing over a 24-hour period, or intermittent, 1,000 mL ordered once in a 24-hour period. Although fluids may be continuous, the type of fluids can alternate over a 24-hour period. For example, an order might be *add 40 mEq of KCl to first bag of 1,000 mL of normal saline.*

Intravenous medications may be **piggybacked**, connected to an existing IV to infuse concurrently. Intravenous solutions and medications that have been refrigerated should be warmed to room temperature before administration (usually for 30 minutes) to increase the client's comfort.

Regulating IV Solution Flow Rate

The flow rate for IV solutions can be regulated by calculating the drops per minute and adjusting the drip rate to that number or by the use of volume controllers and pumps.

Calculating Flow Rate

The **flow rate** is the volume of fluid to infuse over a set period of time as prescribed by the physician. The physician will identify the amount to infuse per time period such as: 125 mL per hour or 1,000 mL over an 8-hour period. The hourly infusion rate is calculated as follows:

$$\frac{\text{Total volume}}{\text{Number of hours to infuse}} = \text{mL/hour infusion rate}$$

For example, if 1,000 mL is to be infused over 8 hours:

$$\frac{1,000}{8} = 125 \text{ mL/hour}$$

Calculate the actual infusion rate (drops per minute) as follows:

$$\frac{\text{Total fluid volume}}{\text{Total time (minutes)}} \times \text{Drop factor} = \text{Drops per minute}$$

For example, if 1,000 mL is to be infused over 8 hours with a tubing drop factor of 10 drops per milliliter:

$$\frac{1,000 \text{ mL}}{8 \ (60) \text{ min}} \times 10 \text{ drops/mL} = \frac{10,000 \text{ drops}}{480 \text{ min}} = 20.8, \text{ or } 21, \text{ drops/min}$$

Another way to calculate the actual infusion rate is to use the hourly infusion rate; for the first example:

$$\frac{125 \text{ mL} \times 10 \text{ drops/mL}}{60 \text{ min}} = 20.8 \text{ or } 21 \text{ drops/min}$$

Volume Controllers and Pumps

Controllers are devices that depend on gravity to maintain a preselected flow without adding pressure to IV systems to overcome resistance (for example, Dial-a-Flo or Buretrol). Resistance may develop from the use of a large catheter in a small vein, infusion of a viscous solution, high venous pressure, or a decrease in the height of the container from the IV site. Resistance may cause a decrease in the flow and sound the controller alarm. Volumetric controllers permit flow rates to be set in milliliters per hour.

Pumps are devices that maintain preselected volume delivery by adding pressure to the system when needed. They do not depend on gravity. Pumps may be used for viscous fluids and when large volumes must be delivered in a short period of time. Pumps have maximum pressure limits that, when reached, sound an alarm. Clients are at a greater risk for complications when a drug or solution is administered under high pressure.

MANAGING IV THERAPY

Intravenous therapy requires frequent client monitoring by the nurse to ensure an accurate flow rate and other critical nursing actions. These other actions include ensuring client comfort and positioning; checking the IV solution to ensure that the solution, amount, and timing are correct; monitoring expiration dates of the IV system (tubing, venipuncture site, dressing) and changing as necessary; and being aware of safety factors.

The nurse must coordinate client care with the maintenance of IV lines. Clients with IV therapy usually require assistance with hygienic measures, including changing the gown. Changing IV tubing when doing site care to decrease the number of times the access device is manipulated will thereby decrease the risk for infiltration and phlebitis. Peripherally inserted devices are changed every 72 hours as directed by the Centers for Disease Control and Prevention (CDC) guidelines.

Hypervolemia

Hypervolemia (increased circulating fluid volume) may result from rapid IV infusion of solutions. This causes cardiac overload, which may lead to pulmonary edema and cardiac failure. The infusion rate must be monitored hourly to prevent this complication.

If a solution infuses at a rate greater than prescribed, the rate must be decreased to *keep vein open* (KVO) and the physician notified immediately. The nurse must report the amount and type of solution that is infused over the exact time period and the client's response.

Infiltration

Infiltration (seepage of foreign substances into the interstitial tissue, causing swelling and discomfort) may

PROFESSIONAL TIP

Setting Volume to Be Infused

When setting the volume to be infused (e.g., 1,000 mL), set the volume to be infused slightly lower (e.g., 950 mL) so that the alarm will go off before the fluids are completely gone. This practice gives time to have the next bag of fluid ready when all 1,000 mL has be absorbed. Having the extra time is especially helpful when dealing with refrigerated fluids that must be warmed to room temperature before being administered. If you will be off duty when the volume will be absorbed and the alarm is set to go off early, tell the oncoming nurse during report.

result from inserting the wrong type of device, using the wrong-gauge needle, dislodgment of the device from the vein, or pressure on the vein. Administration of a drug or solution under high pressure by a pump may also cause infiltration or vein irritation. The client usually complains of discomfort at the IV site. The nurse should inspect the site by palpating for swelling, and feel the temperature of the skin (coolness and paleness of skin are indications of infiltration).

The nurse should also confirm that the needle is still in the vein by pinching the IV tubing. This action should cause **flashback** (blood will rush into the tubing if the needle is still in the vein). If flashback does not occur, the injection port nearest the device should be aspirated. The needle or catheter should be discontinued if it cannot be aspirated and a sterile dressing applied to the puncture site.

After the IV has been removed, the puncture site may ooze or bleed (especially in clients receiving anticoagulants). If oozing or bleeding occurs, pressure is

PROFESSIONAL TIP

Catheter Sepsis

If a client complains of chills and fever, check the length of time that this IV solution has been hanging and the needle or catheter has been in place. Assess the client's vital signs, and assess for other symptoms of pyrogenic reactions, such as backache, headache, malaise, nausea, and vomiting. Unexplained fever may be related to catheter sepsis. Pulse rate increases, and temperature is usually above 100°F if IV-related sepsis occurs. Stop the infusion, notify the physician, and obtain blood specimens if ordered.

applied and a sterile dressing reapplied until it stops. The degree of edema must be accurately assessed and documented.

Clients may be injured by infiltration. If the IV site becomes grossly infiltrated, the edema in the soft tissue may cause a nerve compression injury with permanent loss of function to the extremity. If a **vesicant** (solution capable of causing tissue injury or destruction when it escapes into surrounding tissue) infiltrates, it may cause significant tissue loss with permanent disfigurement and loss of function (Hadaway, 1999).

Phlebitis

Phlebitis may result from either mechanical or chemical trauma. Mechanical trauma may be caused by inserting a device with too large a gauge, using a vein that is too small or fragile, or leaving the device in place for too long. Chemical trauma may result from infusing too rapidly or from an acidic solution, hypertonic solution, a solution that contains electrolytes (especially potassium and magnesium), or other medications.

Phlebitis may be a precursor of sepsis. Client descriptions of tenderness are usually the first indication of an inflammation. The IV site must be inspected for changes in skin color and temperature (a reddened area or a pink or red stripe along the vein, warmth, and swelling are indications of phlebitis).

If phlebitis is present, the IV infusion must be discontinued. Before removing and discarding the venous device, the nurse should check the agency's protocol to see whether the tip of the device is to be cultured. If so, it must be sent to the laboratory for a culture and sensitivity test. After removing the device, a sterile dressing should be applied to the site and wet, warm compresses to the affected area. Documentation in the nurse's notes must reflect the time, symptoms, and nursing interventions.

Intravenous Dressing Change

Intravenous dressing changes require the use of Standard Precautions and aseptic technique. Institutional protocol and the type of intravenous access device and dressing determine the frequency of care. Persistent drainage at the IV site may require dressing changes more frequently or may necessitate changing the IV site.

INTRAVENOUS DRUG THERAPY

The intravenous (IV) route is used when a rapid drug effect is desired or when the medication is irritating to tissue. Intravenous administration provides immediate release of medication into the bloodstream; conse-

quently it can be dangerous. Intravenous medications are administered by one of the following methods:

- Intravenous fluid container
- Volume-control administration set
- Intermittent infusion by piggyback or partial fill
- Intravenous push (IVP or bolus)

Adding Drugs to an Intravenous Fluid Container

When administering IV medications, regardless of the method used, the nurse should assess the patency of the infusion system and the condition of the injection site for signs of complications such as infiltration and phlebitis. Some IV medications or solutions with high or low pH or high osmolarity are irritating to veins and can cause phlebitis.

Before administering any IV medication, the nurse should note the client's allergies, drug or solution incompatibilities, the amount and type of diluent needed to mix the medication, and the client's general condition to establish a baseline for administering medication. The nurse should check for drug compatibilities of drug additives before injecting a medication into an infusion bag. **Drug incompatibilities** cause an undesired chemical or physical reaction between a drug and a solution, between two drugs, or between a drug and the container or tubing. For example, diazapam (Valium) and chlordiazepoxide hydrochloride (Librium) must not come into contact with a saline solution; insulin should not be added to an infusion bag because the insulin adheres to the inside of the solution bag.

Adding Drugs to a Volume-Control Administration Set

A volume-control set is used to administer small volumes of IV solution. These devices have various names as determined by the manufacturer, such as Soluset, Metriset, VoluTrol, or Buretrol. To administer a drug by this method, the nurse should:

- Withdraw the prescribed amount of medication into a syringe that is to be injected into the volume-control set.
- Cleanse the injection port of a partially filled volume-control set with an alcohol swab.
- Inject the prepared medication into the port of the volume-control set.
- Gently mix the solution in the volume-control chamber.

After injecting the medication into the volume-control chamber, the nurse should check the infusion rate and adjust as necessary to the prescribed rate of infusion.

Administering Medications by Intermittent Infusion

A common method of administering IV medications is by using a secondary, or partial-fill additive bag, often referred to as an IV piggyback (IVPB). A secondary line is a complete IV set (fluid container and tubing with either a microdrip or a macrodrip system) connected to a Y-port of a primary line. The primary line maintains venous access. The IVPB is used for medication administration (Figure 11-7). When the IVPB medication is incompatible with the primary IV solution, the nurse must flush the primary IV tubing with normal saline before and after administering the medication.

Intermittent Infusion Devices

When the client requires only the administration of IV medications without the infusion of solutions, an intermittent infusion device is attached to a peripheral needle or catheter in the client's vein. This device is commonly referred to as a heparin or saline lock (Figure 11-8) depending on the agency's policy regarding the device's maintenance. A lock provides continuous access to venous circulation, eliminating the need for a continuous IV, and it increases the client's mobility.

The device can be used to infuse intermittent IVPB or IV push (also called bolus) medications, or it can be converted to a primary IV. An **IV push (bolus)** is a method of administering a large dose of medication in a relatively short time, usually 1 to 30 minutes. A major consideration for inserting a heparin lock device is that it provides venous access in case of an emergency. Lock devices are routinely used with cardiac clients.

Administering IV Push Medications

The method of medication administration by IV push (bolus) injection is determined by the type of IV system. For example, an IV push medication can be injected into a saline or a heparin lock (Figure 11-9) or into a continuous infusion line. When giving an IV push medication into a continuous infusion line, the nurse must stop the fluids in the primary line by pinching the IV tubing closed while injecting the drug (Figure 11-10). This technique is safe and prevents the nurse from having to recalculate the drip rate of the primary infusion line.

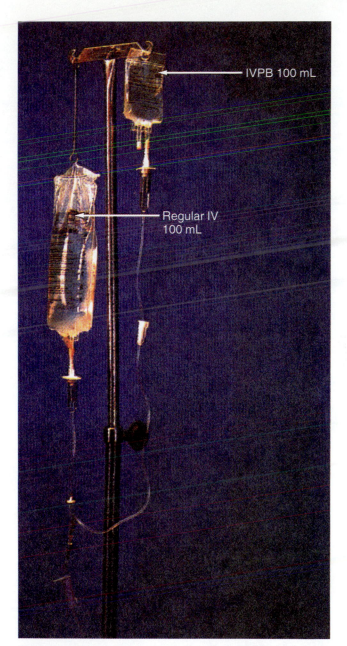

Figure 11-7 Intravenous with Piggyback (IVPB)

Figure 11-8 Heparin-Locking Device

Figure 11-9 Injecting an IV Push (Bolus) Medication into a Peripheral Saline Lock

Figure 11-10 Injecting an IV Push (Bolus) Medication into a Primary Infusion Line. The IV tubing must be pinched closed first.

DOCUMENTATION

When IV therapy is begun, the date, time, venipuncture site, number of attempts made, amount and type of fluid, and equipment used are to be documented. Each time the insertion site, venipuncture device, or IV tubing is changed, the reason for the change must be documented (e.g. routine, infiltration). The condition of the insertion site and the fluid type, amount, and flow rate are documented each shift and at intervals specified by agency policy. Any complications are precisely documented along with the nurse's actions.

BLOOD TRANSFUSION

The purpose of a blood transfusion is to replace blood loss (deficit) with whole blood or blood components. On the basis of the client's unique needs, the physician determines the type of transfusion to administer, either whole blood or a component of whole blood.

Whole Blood and Blood Products

Clients with a demonstrated deficiency in either whole blood or a specific component of blood are given a blood transfusion. Whole blood contains red blood cells (RBCs) and plasma components of blood. It is used when the client needs all the components of blood to restore blood volume after severe hemorrhage and to restore the capacity of the blood to carry oxygen.

When the physician prescribes the administration of whole blood or a blood product, the client's blood is typed and crossmatched. Check with the family for donors if time and the client's condition permit. The blood is stored in the blood bank after typing and crossmatching.

COMMUNITY/HOME HEALTH CARE

Blood Temperature

Blood is transported to the client in a container that maintains proper storage temperature for 6 hours. Because the container does not have thermometers and alarms, it is not considered "monitored" storage, and the blood cannot be returned to inventory if the transfusion is canceled (Fitzpatrick & Fitzpatrick, 1997).

Although whole blood has a refrigerated shelf life of 35 days, platelets must be administered within 3 days after they have been extracted from whole blood. If the RBCs and plasma are frozen, their shelf life can be extended up to 3 years (Kee & Paulanka, 1999).

Initial Assessment and Preparation

The nurse must perform an initial assessment before administering blood. The nurse should:

- Verify that the client has signed a blood administration consent form and that this consent matches what the physician has prescribed.
- Verify whether the client has an 18- or a 19-gauge needle or catheter in a vein. The viscosity of whole blood usually requires this gauge needle or catheter to prevent damage to the red blood cells. If blood is to be infused quickly, a 14- or 15-gauge device must be used.
- Ensure patency of the existing IV site.
- Establish baseline data for vital signs, especially temperature, and assess skin for eruptions or rashes.
- Check client's blood type against the label on the whole blood or blood component before administration, to ensure compatibility.
- Assess the client's age and state of nutrition.

GERONTOLOGICAL CONSIDERATIONS

Initial Assessment

If elderly clients are at risk for circulatory overload, notify the blood bank to divide the 500-mL bag of blood into two 250-mL bags or discuss with the physician other alternatives, such as packed RBCs rather than whole blood.

Scheduled IV medications should be infused before blood administration. This sequence prevents a reaction to a medication while blood is infusing. If a reaction were to occur, the nurse would not be able to discern whether the medication or the blood was causing the reaction.

Administering Whole Blood or a Blood Component

The agency's blood protocol may require that a licensed person sign a form to release the blood from the blood bank and that a blood product be checked by two licensed personnel before infusion. The following information must be on the blood bag label and verified for accuracy: the client's name and identification number, ABO group and Rh factor, donor number, type of product ordered by the practitioner, and expiration date.

Blood should be administered within 30 minutes after it has been received from the bank, to maintain RBC integrity and to decrease the chance of infection. Whole blood should not go unrefrigerated for more than 4 hours. Room temperature will cause RBC lysis, releasing potassium and causing hyperkalemia.

Safety Measures

The client should be observed for the initial 15 minutes for a transfusion reaction. Vital signs are usually taken every 15 minutes for the first hour, then every hour while the blood is transfusing.

Safety: Blood Transfusion Incompatibilities

Only normal saline should be used with a blood product. Blood transfusions are incompatible with dextrose and with Ringer's solution.

There are three basic types of transfusion reactions: allergic, febrile, and hemolytic. Other complications

PROFESSIONAL TIP

Transfusion Reaction

The severity of a transfusion reaction is relative to its onset. Severe reactions may occur shortly after the blood starts to infuse. At the first sign of a reaction, stop the blood infusion immediately.

Table 11–2 NURSING ACTIONS FOR BLOOD REACTIONS	
IMMEDIATE NURSING ACTION	**OTHER MEASURES**
• Stop transfusion. • Keep vein open with normal saline. • Notify the physician.	• Monitor client's vital signs every 15 minutes for 4 hours or until stable. • Monitor I&O. • Send IV tubing and bag of blood back to the blood bank. • Obtain a blood and urine specimen. • Label specimen "Blood Transfusion Reaction." • Process a transfusion reaction report.

include sepsis, hypervolemia, and hypothermia. An allergic reaction may be mild or severe, depending on the cause. Hemolytic reactions may be immediate or delayed up to 96 hours, depending on the cause of the reaction. The classic symptoms of a reaction and sepsis are fever and chills.

The nursing actions for all types of reactions and complications are given in Table 11–2.

SUMMARY

- The nurse is responsible for checking that IV solutions are not outdated and the containers are intact.
- Common peripheral veins used in IV therapy are the forearm, dorsum of hand, and dorsal plexus of the foot.
- Accurate calculation of the flow rate is a nursing responsibility.
- Medications may be added to IV solutions or administered directly by IV.
- Clients receiving IV therapy or a blood transfusion must be monitored frequently.
- The nurse must always carefully monitor client reactions to medications and ensure that clients are appropriately educated as to the actions, side effects, and contraindications of all medications they are receiving.
- Clients receiving intravenous therapy or blood transfusions require constant monitoring for complications.

SAMPLE NURSING CARE PLAN

Mrs. Saegart, a thin, 80-year-old woman, is receiving IV therapy in her left arm.

Nursing Diagnosis 1 *Risk for Imbalanced Fluid Volume related to risk factor of infusion rate too rapid.*

PLANNING/GOALS	NURSING INTERVENTIONS	RATIONALE	EVALUATION
Mrs. Saegart's IV will infuse at the appropriate rate.	Calculate drip rate based on physician's orders.	Obtains proper drip rate.	Mrs. Saegart's IV is infusing at appropriate rate.
	Set the drip rate according to calculations.	Fluid will infuse at proper rate.	
	Attach time strip to solution container.	Provides a visual check on infusion rate.	
	Monitor drip rate and fluid level relative to time strip every 30 minutes.	Prevents fluid volume excess from rapid infusion.	

Nursing Diagnosis 2 *Risk for Injury related to external biological risk factor of infiltration.*

PLANNING/GOALS	NURSING INTERVENTIONS	RATIONALE	EVALUATION
Mrs. Saegart's IV will not become infiltrated.	Adequately anchor IV needle or catheter.	Helps prevent infiltration.	Mrs. Saegart's IV shows no signs of infiltration.
	Explain to Mrs. Saegart to be careful with her left arm.	Client can help to keep the IV in the vein.	
	Monitor IV site hourly for infiltration.	Prevents severe injury from infiltration.	

Review Questions

1. The gauge of the needle or catheter used for IV fluid therapy should be:
   a. the smallest available.
   b. ordered by the physician.
   c. decided upon based on the client's preference.
   d. chosen based on the client's age, body size, and type of solution.

2. Mrs. Mohr had a right mastectomy this A.M. The IV in her left hand has infiltrated and must be restarted. The best site to restart the IV would be the:
   a. left hand.
   b. right hand.
   c. left forearm.
   d. right forearm.

CASE STUDY

Mr. Biro is an 80-year-old, thin client admitted because of dehydration. The skin on his arm stays in a peak when skin turgor is assessed. The physician's orders include initiating IV therapy of 1,000 mL 5% D5W, to infuse over an 8-hour period.

The following questions will guide your development of a nursing care plan for the case study.

1. What gauge needle should be used?
2. Which site should be assessed first for the infusion?
3. What would be the drip rate for this infusion using tubing with a drop factor of 10 drops/mL?
4. What other assessments would you make about Mr. Biro?
5. Which nursing diagnosis and goal might be appropriate for Mr. Biro?
6. What nursing interventions might help Mr. Biro meet the goal?

3. Rapid infusion of IV fluids may result in:
   a. polyvolemia.
   b. hypovolemia.
   c. hypervolemia.
   d. oligovolemia.

4. Standard Precautions are required with:
   a. venipuncture.
   b. IM injections.
   c. oral medications.
   d. nasal instillation.

5. An intravenous solution of sodium chloride (0.45%) is:
   a. isotonic.
   b. iso-osmolar.
   c. hypertonic.
   d. hypotonic.

6. A client receiving a blood transfusion tells the nurse, who is taking the first set of 15-minute vital signs, that she is cold (chills) and her chest hurts. The first thing the nurse should do is:
   a. get a warm blanket.
   b. stop the transfusion.
   c. call the blood bank to come and check the blood.
   d. stay with the client and talk quietly to her help her relax.

Critical Thinking Questions

1. You discover that a similar but incorrect drug (not the drug ordered) is being given IV to a client. What is the first thing you should do? What is your next course of action? How do you feel about the nurse who made the medication error but did not recognize it?

2. How can the different transfusion reactions be differentiated?

WEB FLASH!

- Visit the Web for sites related to IV therapy. What type of information is available?
- Are there any organizations on the Web related to IV therapy?

HEALTH ASSESSMENT

MAKING THE CONNECTION

Refer to the following chapters to increase your understanding of health assessment:

- Chapter 5, Communication
- Chapter 6, Cultural Diversity and Nursing
- Chapter 9, Loss, Grief, and Death
- Chapter 10, Fluid, Electrolyte, and Acid-Base Balance
- Chapter 16, Nursing Care of the Surgical Client
- Chapter 17, Nursing Care of the Oncology Client
- Chapter 18, Nursing Care of the Client: Respiratory System
- Chapter 19, Nursing Care of the Client: Cardiovascular System
- Chapter 20, Nursing Care of the Client: Hematologic and Lymphatic Systems
- Chapter 21, Nursing Care of the Client: Integumentary System
- Chapter 22, Nursing Care of the Client: Immune System
- Chapter 24, Nursing Care of the Client: Musculoskeletal System
- Chapter 25, Nursing Care of the Client: Neurological System
- Chapter 27, Nursing Care of the Client: Endocrine System
- Chapter 28, Nursing Care of the Client: Gastrointestinal System
- Chapter 29, Nursing Care of the Client: Urinary System
- Chapter 30, Nursing Care of the Client: Female Reproductive System
- Chapter 31, Nursing Care of the Client: Male Reproductive System
- Chapter 32, Nursing Care of the Client: Sexually Transmitted Diseases
- Chapter 35, Nursing Care of the Older Client

LEARNING OBJECTIVES

Upon completion of this chapter, you should be able to:
- *Define key terms.*
- *Identify the components of functional health patterns.*
- *Utilize the framework of functional health to facilitate a holistic assessment process.*
- *Analyze the components of the head-to-toe assessment.*
- *Incorporate the four assessment techniques within the head-to-toe assessment.*
- *Utilize the head-to-toe assessment in clinical situations.*

KEY TERMS

adventitious breath sound	dyspnea
affect	eupnea
auscultation	health history
borborygmi	hyperventilation
bradycardia	hypoventilation
bradypnea	inspection
bronchial sound	orthostatic hypotension
bronchovesicular sound	palpation
crackle	percussion
cyanosis	pleural friction rub
	pulse amplitude
	pulse deficit

KEY TERMS continued

pulse rate
pulse rhythm
review of systems
sibilant wheeze
Snellen chart

sonorous wheeze
stridor
tachycardia
tachypnea
vesicular sound

INTRODUCTION

Within the scope of the nursing profession, a complete nursing assessment is necessary to analyze each client's needs in a holistic manner. Nursing assessment includes both physical and psychosocial aspects to evaluate a client's condition. A nurse demonstrates caring, respect, and concern for each client when doing a nursing assessment.

A thorough nursing assessment includes both a health history and a physical examination. To perform a health history, the nurse interviews the client to identify how the client adjusts to or lives within the environment. This data is subjective data, or information based on client self-report. During the physical examination the nurse collects objective data, which includes observations made by the nurse while utilizing the assessment techniques of inspection, palpation,

percussion, and auscultation. Other sources of objective data are laboratory tests, x-rays, and measurements of the client's vital signs, height, and weight.

The health history and the physical examination assist the nurse in focusing on the client as a whole. The initial nursing assessment generally occurs within 8 hours of a client's admission to a health care facility, and continues throughout the stay. In a physician's office or health care clinic, the nursing assessment would be completed immediately. Most institutions have a standard asessment form (Figure 12-1).

Usually a health history is completed prior to the physical examination. However, in emergency situations or when performing care in a health care facility after the initial admitting assessment, it will be necessary to incorporate history-taking within the physical examination. When incorporating a health history within the head-to-toe assessment, the nurse must remember to incorporate questions about the client's habits or usual patterns along with the physical data collected in the head-to-toe assessment. Functional assessment is best done within the framework of the physical assessment since the environment in which each client resides and participates becomes a part of the physical assessment. The functional assessment brings the environment in which the client lives and the physical needs of that client together to establish a holistic picture.

Figure 12-1 Patient Admission Data Base (*Courtesy of Christus Spohn Health System, Corpus Christi, TX*)

continues

RN ASSESSMENT: DATE:_____ TIME:_____ SIGNATURE:_____, RN

INSTRUCTION:
1. Complete physical assessment
2. Identify problems/nursing diagnosis for each system as appropriate
3. Prioritize Problems
4. Enter problems for problem list in computer

SYSTEMS	YES	NO	COMMENTS	PROBLEMS
NEUROLOGICAL				
L.O.C.				□ Thought processes, alteration in
• Alert				
• Drowsy				□ Coping, ineffective
• Comatose				
• Disoriented				□ Communication, impaired
• Cooperative				
• Agitated				
EYES				□ Injury potential
• Pearl				
• Vision Normal				□ Vision, impaired
• Prosthesis				
MOUTH				□ Sensory, perception
• Moist				
• Lesions				□ Other
• Teeth				
• Other				
EARS				
• Responds to normal voice tone				
• Drainage				
SPEECH				
• Clear				
• Slurred				
• Hoarse / raspy				
• Aphasic				
RESPIRATORY				
RESPIRATIONS				□ Airway clearance, ineffective
• Rate				
• Labored				□ Breathing pattern, ineffective
BREATH SOUNDS				□ Gas exchange, impaired
• Clear				
• Wheezes				□ IF PROBLEM IDENTIFIED SEND
• Rales / Rhonchi				RESPIRATORY CONSULT
COUGH				
• Present				□ Other
• Sputum				
MUSCLE / SKELETAL				
EXTREMITIES				□ Self Care deficit
• Moves all on command				□ Mobility impaired, physical
WEAKNESS (specify)				□ Activity intolerance comfort, alterations in
RA____ LA____				
RL____ LL____				ACUTE □
• Edema				CHRONIC □
• Normal ambulation				□ Tissue perfusion, alterations in
• Prosthesis (specify)				

27053183.F10 02/12/99

SYSTEMS				PROBLEM
CARDIOVASCULAR				
Apical Rate				
Rhythm (circle one)				
Regular				
Irregular				□ Tissue perfusion alterations in
On Cardiac Monitor:	Yes	No		
If Yes: Rhythm_____				□ Comfort, alterations in pain:
Peripheral Pulses:	Right	Left		
Carotid	□	□		
Radial	□	□		
Popliteal	□	□		
Femoral	□	□		ACUTE □
Pedal	□	□		CHRONIC □
	YES	NO	COMMENTS	
Pacemaker				Post Operative □
Peripheral Edema				
Chest Pain				Other □
Jugular Vein Distention				
Extremity Discoloration				
Rt. Arm/Hand				
Lt. Arm/Hand				
Rt. Leg/Foot				
Lt. Leg/Foot				
GENITOURINARY				
VOIDING				□ Urinary Elimination, alterations in pattern
• Normal				
• Frequency				
• Burning				
Decreased Force of urinary stream				□ Urinary Retention
INCONTINENCE:				
• Stress				
• Nocturia				□ Incontinence, Total
UROSTOMY				
DIALYSIS				
If Yes: Hemo				□ Incontinence, Stress
Peritoneal				
Routine schedule				
Date of last Dialysis				□ Comfort, alterations in
Catheter insertion Date				
Date of last menstrual period				ACUTE □ CHRONIC □

GASTROINTESTINAL				PROBLEM
ABDOMEN	YES	NO	COMMENT	Bowel elimination alterations in
• Soft				
• Distended				□ Diarrhea
• Tenderness				□ Constipation
ELIMINATION				□ Incontinence,
• Bowel Sounds				□ Comfort, altered pain
• Diarrhea				
• Constipation				ACUTE □
• Incontinence				CHRONIC □
• Ostomy				
Last B.M. Date:				

SAFETY ASSESSMENT

	MEDICATIONS
□ (5) Age greater than 60	
□ (5) History of previous falls	□ (5) Diuretics
□ (3) From nursing home	□ (5) Laxatives / G.I. preps
□ (3) Has had sitter / companion at home	□ (3) Antihypertensives
	□ (3) Antiseizures
STATUS: MENTAL/PHYSICAL	□ (3) Sedative / hypnotics
□ (5) Confused / Judgement Impaired	□ (3) Analgesics
□ (5) Sensory impairment	□ (3) Antipsychotics / antidepressants
□ (5) Combative/Aggressive	
□ (5) "Sundowners" Syndrome	
□ (5) Noncompliance/uncooperativeness	
□ (5) Paralysis / amputee	□ LEVEL 1 (0-17)
□ (5) Weakness / debilitation	□ LEVEL 2 (18-24)
□ (5) Urgent/frequent elimination needs	□ LEVEL 3 (25 or greater)
TOTAL	

□ Safety precautions implemented   □ Patient/family instructed
□ Restraints per protocol   □ Color coded band on

NUTRITIONAL SCREENING

indicate as appropriate for patient   Previous diet_____
□ (8) TPN/Parental Nutrition
□ (8) Tube Feeding
□ (2) Unplanned weight loss or gain > 20 lbs in 3 months
   □ Referral to S.S. screen for neglect/abuse?
□ (1) Loss of appetite/Eats less than 50% of meal
□ (1) Nausea, vomiting or diarrhea
□ (1) Difficulty chewing
□ (1) Difficulty swallowing
*Diagnosis of:
□ (2) Heart disease, hypertension, CHF, gestational diabetic, hepatic or renal failure, diabetic, anemia, cancer other than ENT, geriatric surgery
□ (5) AIDS, malnutrition, DKA, decubitus ulcer, septic condition requiring ICU, burn patient, ENT cancer
□ (1) modified diet; NPO for 48 hrs.
□ (1) age > 65 years
*LAB VALUES: Albumin   Glucose   Hgb
   □ (2) 2.5 - 3.0   □ (1) <60 or   □ (1) male < 13
   □ (2) < 2.5   □ > 300   □ (1) female < 11

High Risk - 8 pts or >   □ SEND NUTRITION SCREEN
Moderate Risk - 5-7 pts   CONSULT WITH TOTAL SCORE OF 5 OR ABOVE AND IDENTIFY
Low Risk - 0-4 pts   SCORE OF PATIENT IN ORDER   TOTAL SCORE

INTEGUMENTARY	YES	NO	COMMENT	PROBLEM
SKIN				□ Other:
• Color Normal				
• Warm, dry				□ Tissue perfusion, alterations in
• Turgor good				
• Bruises, abrasions, lacerations, Color, Size, Location			□ Referral to Social Service (screen for neglect / abuse)	□ Skin integrity impairment of: actual
• Poor hygiene				
• Rash, lesions				□ Skin integrity impairment of: potential
• Scars				
• Dressing				
• Pressure points intact				□ Tissue integrity, comfort, alterations in pain
• coccyx				
• heels				
• elbows				ACUTE □
• hips				
• ankles				CHRONIC □
• cast edges				
• Other				WOUND CARE □
• E-Z graph				
• Vascular access				

Type_____ Insertion Date:_____
Site:_____ Purpose_____

SKIN BREAKDOWN POTENTIAL CHECKLIST

_____ (1) Fair: Major underlying disease, controlled
_____ (2) Poor: Uncontrolled underlying disease
MENTAL STATUS
_____ (1) Lethargic: Listless
_____ (2) Confused: Inappropriate communication
_____ (4) Comatose: Unresponsive
MOBILITY / ACTIVITY
_____ (2) Minor Deficit: Some limitation in movement   Needs assistance w / ADL's
_____ (4) Major Deficit: Movement requires assistance
_____ (6) Immobile: No voluntary movement
INCONTINENCE
_____ (1) Mild: Stress incontinence, 1 BM / day
_____ (4) Frequent: No bladder control, BMs > 2-4 /day
_____ (6) Total: No bladder control, frequent / continuous BM
NUTRITION
_____ (2) Fair: Intake < body requirements, eats 75% or less
_____ (3) Poor: Eats 50% or less, started on TPN or tube feeding
_____ (4) Compromised: No intake, dehydrated
SKIN INTEGRITY
_____ (2) Fair: Single stage I or II
_____ (4) Poor: More than one break in skin integrity
_____ TOTAL SCORE OF 8 OR ABOVE, ENTER SKIN INTEGRITY POTENTIAL ON   PCP PROBLEM LIST, INITIATE PREVENTATIVE ADL's

PATIENT / SIGNIFICANT OTHER PARTICIPATION IN ADMISSION PROCESS

1. Answered question   Yes_____   No_____   3. Family/significant other present   Yes_____   No_____
2. Volunteered information   Yes_____   No_____   4. Plan of care reviewed with: Patient_____ Family / Significant other_____
5. Comments:

2705318-4.F10

Figure 12-1 *continued*

HEALTH HISTORY

A primary focus of the data collection interview is the health history. The **health history** is a review of the client's functional health patterns prior to the current contact with a health care agency. While the medical history concentrates on symptoms and the progression of disease, the nursing health history focuses on the client's functional health patterns, responses to changes in health status, and alterations in lifestyle. The health history is also used in developing the plan of care and formulating nursing interventions.

Demographic Information

Personal data including name, address, date of birth, gender, religion, race/ethnic origin, occupation, and type of health plan/insurance should be included. Factors that are derived from this information may be useful in helping to foster understanding of a client's perspective.

Reason for Seeking Health Care

The client's reason for seeking health care should be described in the client's own words. For example, the statement "fell off four-foot ladder and landed on right shoulder; unable to move right arm" is the client's actual report of the event that precipitated his or her need for health care. The client's perspective is important because it explains what is significant about the event from the client's point of view. It is also important to determine the time of the onset of symptoms as well as a complete symptom analysis.

Perception of Health Status

Perception of health status refers to the client's opinion of his or her general health. It may be useful to ask clients to rate their health on a scale of 1 to 10 (with 10 being ideal and 1 being poor), together with the client's rationale for their rating score. For example, the nurse may record a statement such as the following to represent the client's perception of health: "Rates health a 7 on a scale of 1 (poor) to 10 (ideal) because he must take medication regularly in order to maintain mobility, but the medication sometimes upsets his stomach."

Previous Illnesses, Hospitalizations, and Surgeries

The history and timing of any previous experiences with illness, surgery, or hospitalization are helpful in order to assess recurrent conditions and to anticipate responses to illness, since prior experiences often have an impact on current responses.

Client/Family Medical History

The nurse needs to determine any family history of acute and chronic illnesses that tend to be familial. Health history forms will frequently include checklists of various illnesses that the nurse can use as the basis of the questions about this aspect. The client should be instructed that family history refers to blood relatives. It is also helpful to indicate the relative's relationship to the client (e.g., mother, father, sister).

Immunizations/Exposure to Communicable Diseases

Any history of childhood or other communicable diseases should be noted. In addition, a record of current immunizations should be obtained. This is particularly important with children; however, records of immunizations for tetanus, influenza, and hepatitis B can also be important for adults. If the client has traveled out of the country, the time frame should be indicated in order to determine incubation periods for relevant diseases. The client should also be asked about potential exposure to communicable diseases such as tuberculosis or human immunodeficiency virus (HIV).

Allergies

Any drug, food, or environmental allergies should be noted in the health history. In addition to the name of the allergen, the type of reaction to the substance should be noted. For example, a client may report that he or she developed a rash or became short of breath after taking penicillin. This reaction should be recorded. Clients may report an "allergy" to a medication because they developed an upset stomach after ingesting it, which the nurse will recognize as a side effect that would not preclude administration of the drug in the future.

Safety: Assessment for Allergies

It is essential that the nurse explore possible allergies prior to administering any medications. Allergic reactions can be life-threatening and can occur even with very low dosages of medications. A client's sensitivity to a drug can also change over time, resulting in severe reactions even though the client has successfully taken the drug during prior illnesses or experienced only mild reactions to the drug in the past.

Current Medications

All medications currently taken, both prescription and over-the-counter, should be recorded by name, frequency, and dosage. Clients should be reminded that this information should include medications such as birth control pills, laxatives, nonprescription pain relief medications, herbal remedies, and vitamin and mineral supplements.

PROFESSIONAL TIP

Expired Medications
Remind clients to check all medications for expiration dates prior to use.

Developmental Level

Knowledge of developmental level is essential for considering appropriate norms of behavior and for appraising the achievement of relevant developmental tasks. Any recognized theory of growth and development can be applied in order to determine if clients are functioning within the parameters expected for their age group. For example, if the nurse uses Erikson's stages of psychosocial development, validation of an adult client's attainment of the developmental task of generativity versus stagnation can be made by the nurse's statement, such as "client prefers to spend time with his family; very involved in children's school activities."

Psychosocial History

Psychosocial history refers to assessment of dimensions such as self-concept and self-esteem as well as usual sources of stress and the client's ability to cope. Sources of support for clients in crisis, such as family, significant others, religion, or support groups, should be explored.

Sociocultural History

In exploring the client's sociocultural history, it is important to inquire about the home environment, family situation, and client's role in the family. For example, the client could be the parent of three children and the sole provider in a single-parent family. The responsibilities of the client are important data through which the nurse can determine the impact of changes in health status and thus plan the most beneficial care for the client. Patterns related to caffeine and alcohol intake and use of tobacco or recreational drugs should also be explored.

Alternative/Complementary Therapy Use

Lazar and O'Conner (1997) report that 70% of clients using alternative/complementary therapies as well as conventional medicine do not report using these therapies to their healthcare providers. Simple open-ended questions such as "Do you do anything to improve your health?" may provide important information. If an alternative/complementary therapy is mentioned, the nurse might ask if this is something the client would consider using (Hodge & Ullrich, 1999).

Activities of Daily Living

The activities of daily living is a description of the client's lifestyle and capacity for self-care and is useful both as baseline information and as a source of insight into usual health behaviors. This baseline should include information on nutritional intake and eating habits, elimination patterns, rest/sleep patterns, and activity/exercise.

Review of Systems

The **review of systems** (ROS) is a brief account from the client of any recent signs or symptoms associated with any of the body systems. This can most effectively be obtained as the physical examination is being performed. The review of systems relies on subjective information provided by the client rather than on the nurse's own physical examination. When a symptom is encountered, either while eliciting the health history or during the physical examination of the client, the nurse should obtain as much information as possible about the symptom. Relevant data include:

- *Location:* The area of the body in which the symptom (such as pain) is felt.
- *Character:* The quality of the feeling or sensation (e.g., sharp, dull, stabbing).
- *Intensity:* The severity or quantity of the feeling or sensation and its interference with functional abilities. The sensation can be rated on a scale of 1 (very little) to 10 (very intense).
- *Timing:* The onset, duration, frequency, and precipitating factors of the symptom.
- *Aggravating/alleviating factors:* The activities or actions that make the symptom worse or better.

PHYSICAL EXAMINATION

The physical examination is performed in all health care settings (home, outpatient facilities, extended care institutions, and acute care facilities) for all age groups to gather comprehensive, pertinent assessment data. The physical examination provides a complete picture of the client's physiological functioning. When combined with a health and psychosocial assessment, it forms a database to direct decision making. The examination should be performed according to the agency's policy. Policy may vary from one agency to another.

The physical examination is done in a sequential, head-to-toe fashion to ensure a thorough assessment of each system. This method not only prevents the nurse from forgetting to examine an area, it also decreases the number of times the nurse and the client have to change positions.

The nurse performs the physical or the head-to-toe assessment by using specific assessment techniques. These techniques include: inspection, palpation, percussion, and auscultation.

Inspection

Inspection consists of a thorough visual observation of the client. This visual assessment gives the nurse a description of the body's outward response to its internal functioning. Inspection of the skin, for example, can assist the nurse in identifying signs of a fever through the client's flushed facial cheeks. The skin can also be an indicator of a decreased oxygen supply when **cyanosis**, a bluish or dark purple coloration, is noted in the client's lips, skin, or nail beds. Sharing observations with the client during inspection enhances the holistic data collected. For example, when the nurse mentions the observation of visible scars, the client may discuss previous surgeries or hospitalizations. Instruments such as a penlight and otoscope are often used to enhance visualization.

Effective inspection requires adequate lighting and exposure of the body parts being observed. Beginning nurses often feel self-conscious or embarrassed using the technique of inspection; however, most become comfortable with the technique over time. Nurses must also be sensitive to the client's feelings of embarrassment with the use of inspection and respond to this situation by discussing the technique with the client and using measures such as draping in order to increase the client's comfort level.

Palpation

In **palpation**, the nurse uses the sense of touch to assess texture, temperature, moisture, organ location and size, vibrations, pulsations, swelling, masses, and tenderness. The nurse's finger pads are placed flat against the client's skin, exerting slight pressure for light palpation, as seen in Figure 12-2. Assessment of the kidneys, liver, spleen, bowel, and fundal height may be accomplished through deep palpation, in which more pressure is exerted. Pulses are also palpated. The abdomen is palpated for distention, softness, firmness, rigidity, or tenderness.

Figure 12-2 Light Palpation

Palpation requires a calm, gentle approach and is used systematically, with light palpation preceding deep palpation and palpation of tender areas performed last.

 Safety: Palpation
Deep palpation is a technique requiring significant expertise and should not be employed by beginning nursing students without supervision.

Percussion

Percussion uses short, tapping strokes on the surface of the skin to create vibrations of underlying organs. It is used for assessing the density of structures or determining the location and size of organs in the body. The nurse uses the fingertips to tap the client's body to produce sounds and vibrations. The nurse places the middle finger of the nondominant hand on the client's skin in the area to be percussed, then taps lightly with the middle finger of the dominant hand on the distal phalanx of the middle finger positioned on the body surface (Figure 12-3). The nurse taps twice in one place before moving to a new area. Percussion should not be painful to the client. If it is painful, the percussion should be discontinued and the response documented.

Percussion is a skill that requires much practice to master, and it is important to be familiar with the sounds produced when percussion is used. Table 12–1 describes the various percussion tones.

Auscultation

Auscultation involves listening to sounds in the body that are created by movement of air or fluid. Areas most often auscultated include the lungs, heart, abdomen, and blood vessels. Although direct auscultation is sometimes possible, a stethoscope is usually employed in order to channel the sound (Figure 12-4).

HEAD-TO-TOE ASSESSMENT

Prior to beginning the examination, the nurse should keep in mind some important concepts to be utilized throughout the examination. The client's privacy should be respected by pulling the curtain, closing the door, and providing appropriate draping of the

Figure 12-3 Percussion

Figure 12-4 Auscultation

client. When possible, distracting noises such as radio or television and people talking should be eliminated. Assessment should be performed under natural light because fluorescent light can change the color tones of the skin. All procedures should be explained to the client and confidentiality of data acquired during the examination maintained.

Table 12–1 DESCRIPTION OF PERCUSSION TONES

TONE	INTENSITY	PITCH	DURATION	QUALITY	NORMAL LOCATION
Dullness	Medium	High	Medium	Thudlike	Liver
Flatness	Soft	High	Short	Extreme dullness	Muscle
Hyperresonance	Very loud	Very low	Long	Booming	Child's lung
Resonance	Loud	Low	Long	Hollow	Peripheral lung
Tympany	Loud	High	Medium	Drumlike	Stomach

Infection Control: Standard Precautions
Remember to utilize standard precautions when in contact with any body fluids by using gloves, gown, or mask when appropriate.

The nurse should position the client to ensure accessibility to the body part being assessed. Figure 12-5 presents the positions used in conducting a physical examination.

Sitting

To examine head, neck, back, posterior thorax and lungs, anterior thorax and lungs, breast, axillae, heart, extremities.

Client can expand lungs; nurse can inspect symmetry. *Institute risk precautions for elderly and debilitated clients.*

Dorsal recumbent

To examine head, neck, anterior thorax and lungs, breast, axillae, heart.

Client comfortable; increases abdominal muscle tension. *Contraindicated in abdominal assessment.*

Prone

To examine posterior thorax and lungs, hip

Assessment of hip extension. *Contraindicated in clients with cardiopulmonary alterations.*

Supine

To examine head, neck, anterior thorax and lungs, breasts, axillae, heart, abdomen, extremities.

Client relaxed; decreases abdominal muscle tension; nurse can palpate all peripheral pulses. *Contraindicated in clients with cardiopulmonary alterations.*

Sims'

To examine rectum and vagina.

Relaxes rectal muscles. Painful for clients with joint deformities.

Knee-chest

To examine rectum

Maximal rectal exposure. *Contraindicated in clients with respiratory alterations.*

Lithotomy

To examine female genitalia, rectum, genital tract.

Maximal genitalia exposure; embarrassing and uncomfortable for client. *Contraindicated in clients with joint disorders.*

Figure 12-5 Various Positions for Physical Examination (*Adapted from* Health Assessment and Physical Examination (*2nd ed.*), by M.E.Z. Estes, 2002, Albany, NY: Delmar. Copyright 2002 by Delmar. Adapted with permission.)

The primary purpose of draping the client is to prevent unnecessary exposure during the examination. Feelings of embarrassment elicit tension and restlessness and will decrease the client's ability to cooperate. The drapes also prevent the client from being chilled.

General Survey

The nurse's introduction to the client is an important first step at the start of a complete head-to-toe assessment. It is important for the nurse to identify herself and to express intent for the care of the client and the time frame involved. During this introductory time, it is appropriate for the nurse to utilize inspection to make a general assessment of the client. This overview is the first impression the nurse will have of the client and is the beginning point of the head-to-toe assessment. It includes such aspects as the general state of health and any signs of distress, such as pain or breathing difficulties. It also includes observations regarding the client's awareness of the surroundings, body type and posture, facial expressions, and mood.

The nurse should document the general survey data in an organized fashion to portray a clinical picture of the client. Certain clients such as the elderly, disabled, and abused will require special consideration during the physical examination.

Elderly

When nurses assess elderly clients, it is important to know the normal changes that result from aging. Aging may reduce the body's resistance to illness, tolerance of stress, and the ability to recuperate from illness. The nurse should make sure the client understands and can follow instructions, and allow extra time if the client has difficulty changing positions quickly.

Disabled Clients

When assessing disabled clients, nurses should adapt

GERONTOLOGICAL CONSIDERATIONS

The Older Client
- All senses are less acute.
- Endorphin level rises with age, which decreases awareness of painful events.
- Temperature normal range is 96°F to 98.9°F.
- Strength and endurance decline.
- Height decreases.
- Digestive and urinary functions slow down.
- Older clients are prone to constipation and nocturia.
- Respirations are slowed.
- Older clients are prone to fatigue, dizziness, and falls (Andresen, 1998).

CULTURAL CONSIDERATIONS

Cultural Values and Assessment
Cleanliness is highly valued by mainstream American society. However, in some cultures, a daily bath is not perceived as necessary or desirable. In fact, some cultures do not define natural body odors as offensive. It is important to consider the client in the context of cultural beliefs before labeling a client. Think of the terms *dirty, unkempt,* or *foul-smelling*. These value-laden terms can certainly cloud the assessment process and subsequently the care provided to a client.

their interactions to the client's ability; for example, a hearing-impaired client should be given a written questionnaire. An intellectually impaired client might require simple, direct sentences and questions or use of pictures. It is best to determine the client's ability to participate before conducting the examination. To allay the disabled client's fears and anxiety, a family member may be allowed to remain with the client during the examination. The nurse should ascertain the client's level of independence and feelings about the disability.

Abused Clients

Nurses must be observant for signs of abuse, especially in the elderly. The symptoms may be psychological as well as physical; for example, refusal to be touched, inability to maintain eye contact, or unwillingness to talk about bruises, burns, or other injuries may indicate abuse. Bruises or lacerations most typically appear on breasts, buttocks, thighs, or genitalia. The nurse should also inspect for healed scarring or burns. The nurse must know state laws and agency policies for reporting possible abuse.

Vital Signs

Once the nurse has established rapport with the client through introductions, measurement of vital signs is the next step in a head-to-toe assessment. Vital signs are the "signs of life" of an individual. They provide a way of connecting the external inspection of each client with the internal functioning of the client's organs. When checking vital signs, the nurse obtains the temperature, pulse, respirations, and blood pressure of the client. See Table 12–2 for normal values and variations. Equipment used for vital sign measurement is shown in Figure 12-6.

Temperature

When assessing the client's temperature (T), the nurse can use an electronic, chemical, or mercury thermometer. Body temperature can be taken by 5 routes: oral, rectal, axillary, skin, or tympanic membrane. The

Thermometer

Oral   Slim tip

Rectal   Stubby, pear-shaped tip

Disposable (chemical), single-use   Thin strips of plastic with chemically impregnated dots that change color to reflect temperature

Electronic   Battery-powered display unit with a sensitive probe (blue for oral and red for rectal) covered with a disposable plastic sheath for individual use

Tympanic   Battery-powered display unit with disposable probe covers.

Stethoscope

Acoustical   Closed cylinder that prevents dissipation of sound waves and amplifies the sound through a diaphragm. Flat-disc diaphragm transmits high-pitched sounds, and the bell-shaped diaphragm transmits low-pitched sounds.

Ultrasound (Doppler)   Battery-operated headset with earpieces attached to a volume-controlled audio unit and ultrasound transducer that detects movement of red blood cells through a vessel.

Sphygmomanometer

Mercury manometer   Wall or portable unit that contains a mercury-filled glass column, calibrated in millimeters; the mercury rises and falls in response to pressure created when the cuff is inflated. *(Courtesy of Omron Health Care)*

Aneroid manometer   Portable unit with a glass-enclosed gauge containing a needle to register millimeter calibration and a metal bellows within the gauge that expands and collapses in response to pressure variations from the inflated cuff.

Figure 12-6 Equipment Used for Vital Sign Assessment *(From Fundamentals of Nursing: Standards and Practice, by S. DeLaune & P. Ladner, 1998, Albany, NY: Delmar. Copyright 1998 by Delmar. Reprinted with permission.)*

Table 12–2 VITAL SIGNS AND VARIATIONS

VITAL SIGN	NORMAL READING		VARIATIONS
Temperature	Axillary Tympanic Oral Rectal	36.5°C or 97.6°F 37°C or 98.6°F 37°C or 98.6°F 37.5°C or 99.6°F	<36°C or 96.8°F Hypothermia > 38°C or 100.4°F Pyrexia
Pulse	60–100 beats/min.		< 60 Bradycardia > 100 Tachycardia
Respirations	16–20 resp./min.		< 16 Bradypnea > 20 Tachypnea
Blood Pressure	90/60–140/90		< 90/60 Hypotension > 140/90 Hypertension

route is chosen depending upon the client's age and physical condition. Factors such as age, gender, physical activity, and environment can affect a person's temperature. Consumption of hot or cold food or beverage and smoking 15 to 30 minutes before taking an oral temperature can also affect the result.

Pulse

Pulse assessment is the measurement of a pressure pulsation created when the heart contracts and ejects blood into the aorta. Assessment of pulse characteristics provides clinical data regarding the heart's pumping action and the adequacy of peripheral artery blood flow.

There are multiple pulse points (Figure 12-7). The most accessible peripheral pulses are the radial and carotid sites. Because the body shunts blood to the brain whenever a cardiac emergency such as hemorrhage occurs, the carotid site should always be used to assess the pulse in these situations. Pulse point assessments are described in Table 12–3.

Assessment of the client's pulse (P) includes the rate, rhythm, and amplitude.

Pulse rate is an indirect measurement of cardiac output obtained by counting the number of peripheral pulse waves over a pulse point. A normal pulse rate for adults is between 60 and 100 beats per minute. **Bradycardia** is a heart rate less than 60 beats per minute in an adult. **Tachycardia** is a heart rate in excess of 100 beats per minute in an adult.

Pulse rhythm is the regularity of the heartbeat. It describes how evenly the heart is beating: regular (the beats are evenly spaced) or irregular (the beats are not evenly spaced). Dysrhythmia (arrhythmia) is an irregular rhythm caused by an early, late, or missed heartbeat.

Pulse amplitude is a measurement of the strength or force exerted by the ejected blood against the arterial wall with each contraction. It is described as normal

PROFESSIONAL TIP

Temperature Conversion

To convert Fahrenheit to Celsius (centigrade):

(Temperature °F – 32) × ⅝ = °C

Example:

98.6°F – 32 = 66.6 × ⅝ = 37°C

To convert Celsius to Fahrenheit:

⅝ × temperature°C + 32 = °F

Example:

⅝ × 40°C = 72 + 32 = 104°F

Figure 12-7 Pulse Points

Table 12–3 PULSE POINT ASSESSMENT

PULSE POINT	ASSESSMENT CRITERIA
Temporal: over temporal bone, superior and lateral to eye	Accessible; used routinely for infants and when radial is inaccessible
Carotid: bilateral, under lower jaw in neck along medial edge of sterno-cleidomastoid muscle	Accessible; used routinely for infants and during shock or cardiac arrest when other peripheral pulses are too weak to palpate; also used to assess cranial circulation
Apical: left midclavicular line at fourth to fifth intercostal space	Used to auscultate heart sounds and assess apical-radial deficit
Brachial: inner aspect between groove of biceps and triceps muscles at antecubital fossa	Used in cardiac arrest for infants, to assess lower arm circulation, and to auscultate blood pressure
Radial: inner aspect of forearm on thumb side of wrist	Accessible; used routinely in adults to assess character of peripheral pulse
Ulnar: outer aspect of forearm on finger side of wrist	Used to assess circulation to ulnar side of hand and to perform the Allen's test
Femoral: in groin, below inguinal ligament (midpoint between symphysis pubis and anterosuperior iliac spine)	Used to assess circulation to legs and during cardiac arrest
Popliteal: behind knee, at center in popliteal fossa	Used to assess circulation to legs and to auscultate leg blood pressure
Posterior tibial: inner aspect of ankle between Achilles tendon and tibia (below medial malleolus)	Used to assess circulation to feet
Dorsalis pedis: over instep, midpoint between extension tendons of great and second toe	Used to assess circulation to feet

From Fundamentals of Nursing: Standards and Practice, by S. DeLaune & P. Ladner, 1998, Albany, NY: Delmar. Copyright 1998 by Delmar. Reprinted with permission.

PROFESSIONAL TIP

Carotid Pulse Assessment

When assessing a carotid pulse, apply light pressure to only one carotid artery to avoid disruption of cerebral blood flow. Then assess the other one.

During the pulse assessment, the nurse should integrate questions about endurance, fatigue, and any possible episodes of palpitations, "feeling the heart beating," over the chest area.

Respirations

Respiratory assessment is the measurement of the breathing pattern. Assessment of respirations provides clinical data regarding the pH of arterial blood. Normal breathing is slightly observable, effortless, quiet, automatic, and regular. It can be assessed by observing chest wall expansion and bilateral symmetrical movement of the thorax. Another method the nurse can use to assess breathing is to place the back of the hand next to the client's nose and mouth to feel the expired air.

Assessment of external respirations (R) should include specific characteristics of respirations as well as the use of any type of oxygen equipment. Each respiration includes one complete inhalation (breathing in) and exhalation (breathing out) by the client. When identifying the characteristics of respirations, the rate, depth, and rhythm of each breath should be determined.

Eupnea refers to easy respirations with a rate of breaths per minute that is age-appropriate. **Bradypnea** is a respiratory rate of 10 or fewer breaths per minute. **Hypoventilation** is characterized by shallow respirations. **Tachypnea** is a respiratory rate greater than 24 breaths per minute. **Hyperventilation** is characterized by deep, rapid respirations. **Dyspnea** refers to difficulty in breathing as observed by labored or forced respirations through the use of accessory muscles in the chest and neck. Dyspneic clients are acutely aware of their respirations and complain of shortness of breath.

PROFESSIONAL TIP

Positioning for Dyspneic Clients

Dyspneic clients should never be placed flat in bed; maintain them in a semi-Fowler's or Fowler's position. To facilitate maximal lung expansion, place the client in a forward-leaning position over a padded, raised overbed table with arms and head resting on the table.

(full, easily palpable), weak (thready and usually rapid), or strong (bounding).

Usual assessment of the radial pulse occurs for 30 seconds and the number of beats is doubled for documentation. If the pulse rhythm is irregular, assessment must occur for 60 seconds. In addition, the nurse must assess for a **pulse deficit** (condition in which the apical pulse rate is greater than the radial pulse rate). A pulse deficit results from the ejection of a volume of blood that is too small to initiate a peripheral pulse wave.

It is also important to observe for nasal flaring and the use of accessory muscles for breathing as evidenced by sternal, costal, and subclavicular retractions. The nurse should be aware that children and males typically utilize abdominal muscles to breathe, whereas women use thoracic muscles (Fuller & Shaller-Ayers, 1999). If a client is receiving oxygen, the route and flow rate must be identified.

During the assessment of respirations, the nurse may determine functional ability by asking about any periods of shortness of breath, any difficulty in breathing with increased exercise, or problems following through with activities of daily living.

Blood Pressure

After checking a client's respirations, the nurse assesses the client's blood pressure (BP). The most common site for indirect blood pressure measurement is the client's arm over the brachial artery.

When pressure measurements in the upper extremities are not accessible, the popliteal artery, located behind the knee, becomes the site of choice. The nurse can also assess the blood pressure in other sites, such as the radial artery in the forearm and the posterior tibial or dorsalis pedis artery in the lower leg. The extremity should be at the level of the heart when blood pressure is measured. Because it is difficult to auscultate sounds over the radial, tibial, and dorsalis pedis arteries, these sites are usually palpated to obtain a systolic reading.

A person's blood pressure is the result of the interaction of cardiac output and peripheral resistance, and will be dependent on the speed with which the arterial blood flows, the volume of blood supplied, and the elasticity of the walls of the artery. The force exerted by the blood against the wall of the artery as the heart contracts and relaxes is called the *arterial pressure*. When the ventricles contract and blood is forced into the aorta and pulmonary arteries, the systolic arterial pressure is measured. This is the first sound heard. When the heart is in the filling or relaxed stage, the

COMMUNITY/HOME HEALTH CARE

Electronic Sphygmomanometers

Electronic sphygmomanometers are used by clients for self-measurements. A stethoscope is not required because the device electronically inflates and deflates the cuff while simultaneously reading and displaying the systolic and diastolic pressures. The electronic device is useful for clients who must monitor their own pressure at home. However, it must be recalibrated routinely to ensure an accurate reading.

force is described as the *diastolic blood pressure*. This is when the last sound is heard. The difference between the systolic and diastolic blood pressures is called the *pulse pressure*. A pulse pressure is usually between 30 and 40 mm Hg.

An accurate reading also requires the correct width of the blood pressure cuff as determined by the circumference of the client's extremity. The bladder cuff must encircle the width and length of the site. According to the American Heart Association (1987), the bladder width should be approximately 40% of the circumference or 20% wider than the diameter of the midpoint of the extremity. To measure the width of the bladder, the nurse should place the cuff lengthwise on the client's extremity and extend the width to cover 40% of the extremity's circumference (Figure 12-8). Table 12–4 recommends bladder sizes based on different arm circumferences. A falsely elevated reading will result if the bladder is too narrow, and a falsely low reading will result if it is too wide.

This is an appropriate time to ask if the client ever becomes lightheaded or dizzy when moving from a reclining position to a sitting or standing position. This may occur as a result of an abnormally low blood pressure caused by the inability of the peripheral blood

PROFESSIONAL TIP

Contraindications for Brachial Artery Blood Pressure Measurement

When the client has any of the following, *do not* measure blood pressure on the involved side:
- Venous access devices, such as an intravenous infusion or arteriovenous fistula for renal dialysis
- Surgery involving the breast, axilla, shoulder, arm, or hand
- Injury or disease to the shoulder, arm, or hand, such as trauma, burns, or application of a cast or bandage

Figure 12-8 Measure width of arm by holding cuff against client's upper arm.

Table 12–4 GUIDELINES FOR SPHYGMOMANOMETER CUFF SELECTION		
MIDPOINT* ARM CIRCUMFERENCE**	**BLADDER CUFF WIDTH****	**LENGTH****
24–32 (average adult)	13	24
32–42 (large adult)	17	32

*Distance between the acromion and olecranon processes.
**Measurement in centimeters (cm).

Adapted from Fundamentals of Nursing: Standards and Practice, *by S. DeLaune & P. Ladner, 1998, Albany, NY: Delmar. Copyright 1998 by Delmar. Adapted with permission.*

vessels to compensate quickly for the change in position and is referred to as **orthostatic hypotension**.

Height and Weight Measurement

Measuring height and weight is as important as assessing the client's vital signs. Routine measurement provides data related to growth and development in infants and children and signals the possible onset of alterations that may indicate illness in all age groups. The client's height and weight are routinely taken on admission to acute care facilities and on visits to physicians' offices, clinics, and in other health care settings.

Height

A scale for measuring height, calibrated in either inches or centimeters, is usually attached to a standing weight scale. This type of scale is used for measuring the height of children and adults. The nurse should ask the client to stand erect on the scale's platform. The metal rod attached to the back of the scale should be extended to gently rest on the top of the client's head, and the measurement should be read at eye level.

Weight

When a client has an order for "daily weight," the weight should be obtained at the same time of day on the same scale, with the client wearing the same type of clothing.

Infection Control: Measuring Weight
When standing on a scale, the client should wear some type of light foot covering, such as socks or disposable operating room slippers, to prevent the transmission of infection and to enhance comfort.

Head and Neck Assessment

The nurse will assess the head and neck and determine the client's mental and neurological status, and the client's overall **affect** (outward expression of mood or emotion).

Hair and Scalp

The hair and scalp of a client should be inspected. The hair distribution, quantity, texture, and color should be noted. The scalp should be smooth and free of any debris or infestations.

Eyes

The eyes should be examined to determine if they are symmetrical. The nurse should look at the eyebrows and eyelids to determine if there is any drooping, which may be a sign of muscle weakness or neurological impairment. The color of the sclera and conjunctiva, as well as the presence of any drainage, should be noted.

The pupils should be assessed to determine their size, shape, and reaction to light. This is accomplished by darkening the room and asking the client to gaze into the distance. The nurse will move a light in from the side and notice if the pupil constricts; this is called the *direct light reflex*. The pupil size in millimeters both before and after the light response (Figure 12-9) is noted. Accommodation is tested by asking the client to focus on an object in the distance; this will dilate the pupils. The client is then asked move his or her gaze to a near object such as a pen or finger held approximately 3 inches from the nose. The pupils should constrict as they focus on the near object and the eyes will converge or move in toward midline. This normal response is documented as PERRLA or Pupils Equal, Round, Reactive to Light and Accommodation.

The nurse should determine if the client utilizes glasses and for what reason, and ask if any eye problems such as blurry vision, diplopia (double vision), or difficulty seeing at night are being experienced.

The assessment of visual acuity is a simple, noninvasive procedure that is performed with the use of a **Snellen chart** (a chart that contains various-sized letters with standardized numbers at the end of each line of letters). The standardized numbers (called the denominator) indicate the degree of visual acuity when the client is able to read that line of letters at a distance of 20 feet.

Nose

The nose should be symmetrical, midline, and in proportion to other features. Any deformity, inflammation,

Figure 12-9 Scale Used to Measure Pupil Size, in Millimeters

or prior trauma should be noted. The patency of the nostrils can be tested by asking the client to sniff inward while closing off each nostril. The nurse should ask the client if the following are ever experienced: nosebleeds, dryness, or decrease in sense of smell.

Lips and Mouth

The lips and mucous membranes of the mouth are observed for color, symmetry, moisture, or lesions. If the client has dentures or partial plates, the nurse should ask them to be removed for a more thorough inspection of the mouth. Unusual breath odors should be noted. The oral mucosa can be inspected by inserting a tongue depressor between the teeth and the cheek. The mucous membranes and gums should be pink, moist, smooth, and free of lesions. Inspection of the tongue assists in determining the client's hydration. The tongue should be pink with a slightly rough texture. During the examination the nurse can determine if the client is able to enunciate words appropriately and if there have been any voice changes such as hoarseness. Usual dental hygiene practices should be discussed and the client's history of tobacco usage obtained.

Neck

The neck should be assessed to determine if there is full range of motion. The accessory neck muscles should be symmetrical. As the client moves the head, any enlargement of the lymph nodes or thyroid gland should be noted. The nurse should observe for any pulsations in the neck. The carotid pulsation is seen just below the angle of the jaw. Normally there are no other visible pulsations while the client is in the sitting position.

Mental and Neurological Status and Affect

All head-to-toe assessments must incorporate an assessment of the client's mental and neurological status and affect. A client's mental status includes identification of the level of orientation to person, place, and time. Also included within the mental status is the client's responsiveness to the environment. When assessing for responsiveness, the client's ability to follow directions and to respond appropriately to comments and to his or her name when called is observed.

Neurological assessment of the client focuses on the following: level of consciousness (LOC), pupil response, hand grasps, and foot pushes. Each of these assessments will be discussed in the area of the head-to-toe assessment in which it will be observed. The level of consciousness is the client's degree of wakefulness. For example, a client who is alert is fully awake with eyes open and responds to environmental stimuli. The client who is less awake will be drowsy and slow in response to environmental stimuli.

PROFESSIONAL TIP

Common Abnormal Breath Odors

- Acetone breath ("fruity" smell) is common in malnourished or diabetic clients with ketoacidosis.
- Musty smell is caused by the breakdown of nitrogen and presence of liver disease.
- Ammonia smell occurs during the end stage of renal failure from a buildup of urea.

When documenting the client's affect, words such as *pleasant, happy, cooperative, uncooperative, angry, depressed,* or *hostile* should not be used. Instead, the description of affect should focus specifically upon the behaviors exhibited by the client such as facial expression and verbal and nonverbal behaviors. In doing this, the nurse not only maintains the accuracy of the conversation or the behaviors observed, but also maintains the legal appropriateness of the assessment.

Skin Assessment

Assessment of the skin should be performed as each area of the body is assessed. The color of the skin as well as its moisture or dryness should be noted. The nurse should inspect and palpate the client's skin, assessing temperature, turgor, edema, and integrity. Palpation of the skin with the dorsal aspect of the hand on the right and left sides of the body provides a comparison of the client's skin temperature. The client should also be asked if any pain or discomfort in relation to the skin and/or mucous membranes has occurred. Identification of the skin's turgor is best accomplished by pinching the skin of the anterior chest and observing the speed of return of the skin to its previous position. If the skin stays pinched during assessment, it may indicate dehydration, and further assessment should occur.

Palpate dependent areas (sacrum, legs, ankles, feet) for edema. Firmly apply pressure with a finger for 5 seconds. The degree of edema is based on the depth of indentation in centimeters:

1+	equals an indentation of 1 cm or less
2+	equals an indentation of 2 cm
3+	equals an indentation of 3 cm
4+	equals an indentation of 4 cm
5+	equals an indentation of 5 cm or more

The location, size, distribution, and appearance of skin lesions throughout the body should be determined. Documentation of any breaks in or changes in the skin integrity is an important aspect of nursing assessment. Scratches, bruises, skin tears, cuts, and scars from previous injuries or surgeries are examples of skin characteristics that should be noted. The general

CULTURAL CONSIDERATIONS

Skin Color

- The darker the client's skin, the more difficult it is to assess changes in color.
- Establish a baseline skin color by observing the least pigmented skin surfaces, which include the volar surfaces of the forearms, the palms of the hands, the soles of the feet, the abdomen, and the buttocks. There should be an underlying red tone in these areas. Absence of this red tone may indicate pallor.
- Oral hyperpigmentation often is found in dark-skinned persons. If the hard palate is not hyper-pigmented, it has a yellow discoloration in the presence of jaundice.
- The lips may be used to assess jaundice and cyanosis, and the sclera may be used to assess jaundice if a baseline color has been established for each.
- The conjunctiva reflect color changes of cyanosis or pallor.
- Nail beds can be used to note how quickly the color returns after pressure has been released from the free edge of the nail, regardless of the nail bed color.

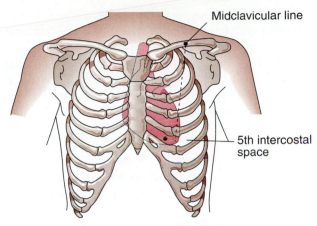

Figure 12-10 Assessing the Apical Pulse

hygiene of the skin should be noted, and the client asked about usual skin care routines.

Thoracic Assessment

During thoracic assessment, the nurse will determine the condition of the client's cardiovascular and respiratory systems along with assessment of the breasts.

Cardiovascular Status

Assessment of the client's cardiovascular status by the LP/VN focuses specifically on listening to the apical pulse, identifying heart tones, and checking the nail beds. The apical pulse is determined by using auscultation and palpation. To assess the apical pulse, the nurse must palpate over the apex of the heart at the fourth or fifth left intercostal space at the midclavicular line. A slight, short duration tap against the fingers will be felt, and this is where the apical pulse will be auscultated (Figure 12-10). Listening to the apical pulse is the most accurate assessment of the heart rate, and should occur for 60 seconds. The apical pulse is assessed first with the diaphragm of the stethoscope for the regularity or irregularity of its rhythm. Second, the bell of the stethoscope is used to differentiate the loudness or tones of the heart. Along with the apical pulse, the other pulse points may be assessed now or when the extremities are asessed.

To assess blood perfusion of peripheral vessels and skin, the nurse should note changes in skin temperature, color, and sensation, and changes in the pulses. Feeling the toes for warmth and color provides important information relative to peripheral circulation and tissue perfusion. Because the position of the extremities can affect the skin temperature and appearance, extremities must always be assessed at heart level and at normal room and body temperature. Peripheral pulses should be compared bilaterally, and changes in strength and quality should be noted (Bosley, 1995).

The focus of the functional assessment includes personal habits contributing to or preventing cardiovascular disease. The nurse should determine the client's personal exercise habits and elicit information regarding past chest pain or shortness of breath. The client should describe any pain, its location, duration, precipitating factors, and what is done to alleviate the pain. The nurse should also ask if the client has ever fainted or felt dizzy. Any lower leg swelling and its cause should also be noted.

Respiratory Status

Breath sound assessment is performed after determination of the apical pulse rate. Respiratory auscultation reveals the presence of normal and abnormal breath sounds. During auscultation, the client should be instructed to breathe only through the mouth because mouth breathing decreases air turbulence that could interfere with an accurate assessment.

There are three distinct types of normal breath sounds with their own unique pitch, intensity, quality, location, and relative duration in the inspiratory and expiratory phases of respiration:

- **Bronchial sounds:** loud and high-pitched sounds with a hollow quality heard longer on expiration than inspiration from air moving through the trachea
- **Bronchovesicular sounds:** medium-pitched and blowing sounds heard equally on inspiration and expiration from air moving through the large airways,

posteriorly between the scapula and anteriorly over bronchioles lateral to the sternum at the first and second intercostal spaces

- **Vesicular sounds:** soft, breezy, and low-pitched sounds heard longer on inspiration than expiration that result from air moving through the smaller airways over the lung's periphery, with the exception of the scapular area

Breath sounds that are not normal are described as either abnormal or **adventitious breath sounds**. Adventitious breath sounds include sibilant wheeze (formerly wheeze), sonorous wheeze (formerly rhonchi), fine and coarse crackle (formerly rales), pleural friction rub, and stridor. **Sibilant wheezes** are high-pitched, whistling sounds heard during inhalation and exhalation. A **sonorous wheeze** is a low-pitched snoring sound that is louder on exhalation. Coughing may alter the sound if caused by mucous. **Crackles** are popping sounds heard on inhalation or exhalation, not cleared by coughing. A **pleural friction rub** is a low-pitched grating sound on inhalation and exhalation. **Stridor** is a high-pitched, harsh sound heard on inspiration when the trachea or larynx is obstructed. Breath sounds of the anterior, posterior, and lateral chest wall must be assessed for normal as well as adventitious breath sounds. Adventitious breath sounds must be monitored on a consistent basis. The lungs are assessed from side to side so the two sides can be compared as shown in Figure 12-11.

The functional assessment information to be obtained when assessing the respiratory status of the client includes any difficulty breathing or the presence of a cough. The client should be asked if the cough is nonproductive or productive, and to describe the secretions produced. Terms used to describe secretions expectorated would be *thick, thin, yellow, green*. The client's occupational or home environment may affect breathing patterns; exposure to dust, chemicals, vapors, tobacco, smoke, or paint fumes, and irritants such as asbestos should be noted.

Wounds, Scars, Drains, Tubes, Dressings

When assessing the thorax, the nurse should note any type of wounds, scars, drains, tubes, or dressings the client may have. Assessment of these must include the location, size, and amount of drainage or discharge, and if present, signs of inflammation.

Breasts

Assessment of the breast tissue should be done for both male and female clients. The nurse can begin by inspecting the breasts for size and symmetry. It is common to have a slight difference in size of breasts. Any obvious masses, dimpling (a depression in the surface skin), or inflammation should be noted. The skin nor-

mally is smooth and even in color. The nurse should determine if the nipples and areola are symmetrical in size, shape, and color, and note any discharge from the nipples.

Any abnormal area should be palpated for size, consistency, mobility, tenderness, and location of the lesion. Another area to include in breast assessment is the axillary lymph nodes that drain the breasts. The nurse should palpate the axilla for enlarged or inflamed lymph nodes, ask if there is any tenderness, and also determine if and when the client performs self-breast exams. The nurse can note if the client has had mammography and when the last x-ray was taken.

Abdominal Assessment

During abdominal assessment, the nurse determines the status of the client's gastrointestinal and genitourinary systems. The nurse should also note any type of wounds, scars, drains, tubes, dressings, or ostomies the client may have. Assessment of these must include the location, size, and amount of drainage or discharge, and if present, any signs of inflammation.

Gastrointestinal Status

The abdomen is first inspected for rashes and scars. The nurse should determine if the abdomen is flat, rounded, or distended, and should observe the abdomen for symmetry and visible signs of peristalsis or pulsations. If the abdomen is distended, the client should be asked questions pertaining to bowel movements and urinary status.

Auscultation is the second component of the abdominal assessment of a client's bowel status. A "bubbly-gurgly" sound, caused by peristalsis and movement of the intestinal contents, can be heard by placing the stethoscope on each quadrant of the abdomen and listening for approximately 1 minute. These sounds should be present in all four quadrants of the abdomen, beginning in the right lower quadrant (RLQ) and moving clockwise around the four quadrants as

PROFESSIONAL TIP

Assessment of the Abdomen

Although the usual sequence for implementing assessment techniques is inspection, palpation, percussion, and auscultation, assessment of the abdomen entails a different sequence. Because palpation can affect sounds heard on auscultation, the sequence for abdominal assessment is as follows:

- Inspection
- Auscultation
- Percussion
- Palpation

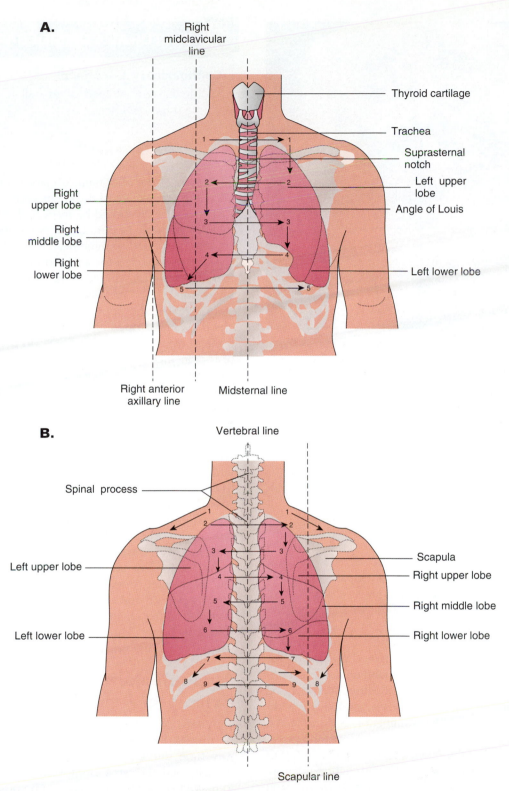

A.

Right midclavicular line

Thyroid cartilage

Trachea

Suprasternal notch

Left upper lobe

Angle of Louis

Right upper lobe

Right middle lobe

Right lower lobe

Left lower lobe

Right anterior axillary line

Midsternal line

B.

Vertebral line

Spinal process

Left upper lobe

Scapula

Right upper lobe

Right middle lobe

Left lower lobe

Right lower lobe

Scapular line

Figure 12-11 Symmetrical Assessment of Breath Sounds: A. Anterior; B. Posterior

shown in Figure 12-12. When approximately 5 to 20 bowel sounds are heard per minute, or 1 at least every 5 to 15 seconds, the bowel sounds are considered active.

The absence of bowel sounds during 1 minute of auscultation in each quadrant is documented as absent bowel sounds. Bowel sounds of less than 5 "bubbly-gurgly" sounds per minute are described as hypoactive, while an excess of 20 or more bowel sounds per minute is defined as hyperactive. High-pitched, loud, rushing sounds heard with or without a stethoscope are termed **borborygmi**. This is caused by the passage of gas through the liquid contents of the intestine.

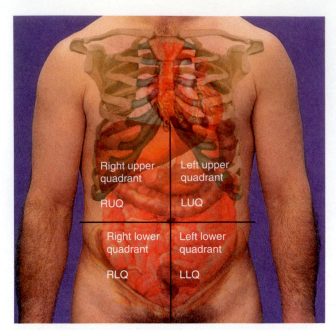

Figure 12-12 The Four Quadrants of the Abdomen (*From Health Assessment and Physical Examination, 2nd ed., by M.E.Z. Estes, 2002, Albany, NY: Delmar. Copyright 2002 by Delmar. Reprinted with permission.*)

Percussion of the abdomen should occur in all four quadrants. The predominant abdominal percussion sound is tympany caused by percussing over the air-filled stomach and intestines.

Light palpation of the abdomen is done to assess for muscle tone, masses, pulsations, or any signs of tenderness or discomfort. Abdominal muscles may be palpated and should feel relaxed on light palpation, not tightly contracted or spastic. If the client is anxious, muscle contraction may be evident. Palpation of a separation of the rectus abdominous muscle may be felt, especially in clients who are obese or pregnant. The rectus abdominous muscle includes two large, midline muscles that extend from the xiphoid process to the symphysis pubis, and can be palpated midline as the client raises his or her head. Rebound tenderness, indicating possible inflammation of the appendix, may be elicited by depressing the abdomen and quickly withdrawing the fingers. This examination is done at the end of the abdominal assessment because of the possibility of increasing the client's level of pain. If any of the abdominal organs can be felt with light palpation, it is abnormal and should be reported to the nursing supervisor. After assessment of bowel sounds, the nurse should question the client about diet, usual bowel patterns, appetite, weight changes, indigestion, heartburn, nausea, pain, and use of enemas or laxatives.

Genitourinary Status

Assessment of the client's urinary and reproductive status is accomplished mainly by inspection and use of interview skills. Genitourinary assessment includes ex-

CULTURAL CONSIDERATIONS

Genitourinary Assessment
Middle Eastern women often will remain veiled during this assessment.

amination of the abdomen, urinary meatus and genitalia, and assessment of the client's urine.

The abdomen should be inspected for any enlargement or fullness. In the normal adult, the abdomen is smooth, flat, and symmetrical. The urinary meatus should be inspected for any abnormalities such as inflammation and discharge, which may signal a urethral infection.

In females, the appearance of the genitalia (labia, clitoris, vaginal opening) should be observed. Questions to ask the client that focus on the reproductive history include: pregnancies, use of birth control, menstrual cycle history, present sexual activity, use of protection during intercourse, date of the last Pap test, and determination of how any present illness has or will affect sexual activity.

In males, assessment of the genitalia includes inspection of the penis, urethral meatus, foreskin (if uncircumcized), and scrotum. Questions to ask the client that focus on the reproductive history include: present sexual activity, use of protection during intercourse, and also how the present illness has or will affect sexual activity. The nurse should determine if the client performs testicular self-examinations.

Any lesions or ulcerations that may indicate sexually transmitted disease should be noted. The usual voiding pattern and any recent changes should be determined if the client has had any history of urinary tract infections, kidney stones, change in the urinary stream, or painful urination or nocturia.

Musculoskeletal and Extremity Assessment

Symmetry and strength of major muscle groups can be assessed throughout the head-to-toe assessment. Any time during the assessment when the client is repositioned, the range of movement the client utilizes to make that position change can be observed. Asking the client to walk across the room and noting the client's movements and stance when sitting up in bed are observations made to assess gross motor movement and posture. Assessment of the client's handshake gives an estimate of muscle strength. Palpating muscles lightly determines swelling, tone, or any specific changes in shape of the muscles.

Hand grasps and foot pushes assess the strength and equality of the client's extremities. Upper extremity strength is assessed by having the client grasp the nurse's index and middle fingers of each hand. The grasp should be equal in both hands. Foot pushes assess the lower extremities. The nurse's hands should be placed on the soles of the client's feet. The client is asked to push both feet against the nurse's hands. The push should be equal in both feet. Asking the client to touch the tip of her nose with a finger and then the tip of the nurse's finger as it is moved to different locations tests the client's coordination skills.

Strength and symmetry of some of the major muscle groups can be assessed by watching gait and postural movements. Any aids to ambulation must be noted. Symmetrical examination of muscles should occur in pairs, first one extremity and then the other; equality of size, contour, tone, and strength should be assessed.

The skin of the lower extremities should be carefully assessed to determine color changes, loss of feeling or hair, change in temperature within the extremity and from one extremity to the other, and presence of vari-cose veins, ulcers, and edema. The nurse should determine if the client experiences any leg pain or cramps.

The nurse should ask the client if muscle weakness is experienced or if difficulty or pain when walking or performing routine daily activities occurs. The functional assessment should also include asking the client about routine activities such as cooking, shopping, exercise, yard work, and hobbies. Tolerance limitations can be observed by assessing for stiffness, crepitus, or fatigue during ambulation. Safe and appropriate performance of functions essential for home life and activities of daily living must be determined.

SUMMARY

- Psychosocial needs of clients are identified within the scope of a functional assessment.
- The health history and the physical examination used together present a holistic view of client needs.

CASE STUDY

Tom Turner, age 40, has been admitted to the hospital with pneumonia. He has never been hospitalized before. His wife and three children are at home. Because his wife has just given birth to their third child, Tom's wife cannot drive the other two children to school. Tom provides the sole income for the family, and he has only three more sick days to use at work before he will be off without pay.

Tom's vital signs are BP 120/72, P 100, R 34, T 100.6°F. His breath sounds show sonorous wheezes throughout, cleared by coughing. His cough is frequent and productive of foamy, cloudy, yellow secretions. His apical pulse is 102 and regular, but distant heart tones were noted. The abdomen is firm and distended with hypoactive bowel sounds noted in all four quadrants. He moves all extremities slowly but per self and with purpose.

Tom is oriented to person, place, and time. His pupils are PERRLA. Hand grips are strong and equal bilaterally, as are foot pushes. He speaks only when spoken to, and his eye contact with staff is minimal. Whenever his wife visits, his voice raises and his heart rate increases about 2–5 beats. At one point, Tom stated, "How much more of this can we take?" Tom's wife mentions that their church would love to help, but Tom refuses to take charity. Tom states, "Any income for this family has to come from me."

Other added information acquired during the assessment includes the fact that Tom has a history of drinking 1 to 2 beers daily, and has not performed testicular self-exams. He eats and drinks what he likes, and he states he really "hates seafood." Usually he bathes daily in the early morning and helps to bathe two of their children each evening. He works 9–5:30 P.M., five days per week, and also some Saturday mornings. Tom pays all of the household bills, and is the sole decision maker of the family.

The following questions will guide your development of a nursing care plan for the case study.

1. List the functional assessment data collected from Mr. Turner that identify psychosocial concerns.

2. What are two possible reasons for identifying the added information about Mr. Turner in the last paragraph?

3. Write two nursing diagnoses that are supported by the health history and physical assessments documented about Mr. Turner.

4. Write goals and nursing interventions for each nursing diagnosis.

- Introduction of the nurse at the beginning of a physical assessment enhances the ability to accomplish the complete assessment.
- Collection of vital signs is the foundation to each head-to-toe assessment and includes: temperature, pulse, respirations, and blood pressure.
- Assessment of a client's mental and neurological status is performed when the nurse obtains information about the client's level of consciousness, pupil response, as well as hand grip and foot push capabilities.
- When describing a client's affect, the nurse must utilize terms that are descriptive of the specific behavior observed, not the nurse's judgment about the behavior.
- Assessing the cardiovascular status of each client includes palpation of specific pulse points.
- Auscultation of lung fields assists in collection of data regarding the breath sounds of the client.
- An abdominal assessment includes use of inspection, auscultation, percussion, and palpation within the four quadrants of the abdomen to establish bowel status and function.
- Through observation of client gait and overall range of movement, the nurse is able to obtain some knowledge of the symmetry and strength of muscles.
- During the assessment of wounds, drains, dressings, and other external devices, the nurse must maintain accurate documentation of the amount of drainage, color, or other changes.

Review Questions

1. Jim's apical pulse is 102. He states to the nurse that he can feel his heart pounding. Which of the following charting terms would accurately describe Jim's statement of concern regarding his heart rate?

   a. bradycardia
   b. changing of rhythm
   c. palpitation
   d. tachycardia

2. Mrs. Jones is 54 years old. While performing the assessment overview, Mrs. Jones states, "I just get so lightheaded when I first get up in the morning." Mrs. Jones most likely has:

   a. cyanosis.
   b. hypertension.
   c. orthostatic hypertension.
   d. orthostatic hypotension.

3. During the physical head-to-toe assessment of the client, the nurse checks the pulse and blood pressure. Which of the four assessment techniques did the nurse utilize?

   a. auscultation, palpation, and inspection
   b. auscultation, percussion, and inspection
   c. auscultation and palpation
   d. palpation and inspection

4. Upon admission to your unit, the client verbalizes an increased pain in her left leg. What would be the pertinent assessment information to collect about this client?

   a. listen to the client's bowel sounds.
   b. check circulation in the right leg.
   c. assess both of the client's legs.
   d. ask the client about her current diet.

5. Which of the pulses should be palpated when assessing circulation to the lower extremities?

   a. dorsalis pedis
   b. femoral
   c. temporal
   d. popliteal

6. How often a nurse assesses a client's vital signs depends upon the:

   a. availability of personnel.
   b. doctor's orders.
   c. nurse's discretion.
   d. client's condition.

7. The nurse checks the radial pulse for 30 seconds and multiplies by 2. She notices an irregularity in the beat. What is the next action the nurse should take?

   a. check the radial pulse for 60 seconds.
   b. listen to the apical pulse for 60 seconds.
   c. listen to the apical for 30 seconds and multiply by 2.
   d. continue with the rest of the assessment.

Critical Thinking Questions

1. How do you feel about performing a complete physical assessment on a client?

2. How do you feel when you receive a complete physical assessment?

WEB FLASH!

- Search the Internet for information regarding physical examination (assessment). What type of information is available?
- Are there any organizations on the Internet that focus on physical examination (assessment)? Are they specific by age group (elderly)?

CHAPTER 13

DIAGNOSTIC TESTS

MAKING THE CONNECTION

Refer to the following chapters to increase your understanding of diagnostic tests:

- **Chapter 8, Alternative/Complementary Therapies**
- **Chapter 12, Health Assessment**
- **Chapter 15, Anesthesia**

LEARNING OBJECTIVES

Upon completion of this chapter, you should be able to:

- *Define key terms.*
- *Discuss the relevant client teaching guidelines for the care of the client before, during, and after diagnostic testing.*
- *Describe the common specimen collection methods.*
- *Describe common invasive and noninvasive diagnostic procedures.*
- *Discuss nursing responsibilities for the common diagnostic procedures.*

KEY TERMS

agglutination	aspiration
agglutinin	bacteremia
agglutinogen	barium
analyte	biopsy
aneurysm	cation
angiography	central line
anion	computed
antibody	tomography
antigen	conscious sedation
arteriography	contrast medium
ascites	culture

cytology	Papanicolaou test
electrocardiogram	paracentesis
electroencephalogram	phlebotomist
electrolyte	pneumothorax
endoscopy	port-a-cath
enzyme	radiography
fluoroscopy	sensitivity
hematuria	stable
invasive	stress test
ketone	thoracentesis
lipoprotein	transducer
lumbar puncture	trocar
magnetic resonance	type and cross-
imaging	match
necrosis	ultrasound
noninvasive	urobilinogen
occult blood	venipuncture
oliguria	void

INTRODUCTION

Health care providers use the findings from a thorough history and physical examination to determine the need for diagnostic testing. The client's history and presenting symptoms determine those diagnostic procedures that are necessary to formulate a medical diagnosis and course of treatment. The challenge of cost-effective health care pushes practitioners to rely on basic assessment and to be selective with regard to expensive diagnostic tests. To reflect the emphasis on cost containment, the nurse's role has changed from doing for the client to teaching clients to do for themselves. The role of the nurse is to teach the client, family, and significant others about the procedures involved in diagnostic testing, the steps to be taken in preparation for the specific test(s) in question, and the care that will follow the procedure. Although the primary focus is on teaching, the nurse may assist in performing various noninvasive and invasive procedures. Nurses must be aware of the implications of diagnostic testing so as to deliver appropriate nursing care to the client.

To understand the nature of diagnostic tests, nurses must review anatomy and physiology. Knowing the anatomic and physiologic functions of the body will assist nurses in relating certain diagnostic tests to specific disease processes and in understanding the meaning of test results.

This chapter discusses common diagnostic tests. The terms *test* and *procedure* are used interchangeably throughout the chapter. The term *practitioner* is used in this chapter to refer to either the physician or an advanced practice registered nurse. Most state boards of nursing allow advanced practice registered nurses to order and perform certain diagnostic tests.

DIAGNOSTIC TESTING

Diagnostic tests are either noninvasive or invasive. **Noninvasive** means that the body is not entered with any type of instrument; the skin and other body tissues, organs, and cavities remain intact. **Invasive** means that the body's tissues, organs, or cavities are accessed through some type of procedure making use of instruments.

Nursing Care of the Client

Diagnostic testing is a critical element of assessment. In collaboration with feedback from the client, assessment data are used to formulate nursing diagnoses, a plan of care, and outcome measures. Ongoing client assessment and evaluation of the client's expected outcomes require the incorporation of diagnostic findings.

 Safety: Diagnostic Testing
To protect your health and safety, as well as that of other health care providers and the client, use Standard Precautions whenever performing invasive or noninvasive procedures.

Preparing the Client for Diagnostic Testing

The nurse plays a key role in scheduling and preparing the client for diagnostic testing. When tests are not scheduled correctly, not only is the client inconve-

Figure 13-1 Preparing a Client for Diagnostic Testing

nienced, but interventions may be delayed, which may place the client's health at risk. The institution is also at risk to lose money. Table 13–1 outlines a sample protocol of the nursing care to prepare a client for diagnostic testing.

During the assessment of the client, the nurse must ensure that the client is wearing an identification band and understands those things to be done. It is also the nurse's responsibility to see that needed consent forms have been signed (Figure 13-1).

Other key nursing measures in ensuring client safety are to establish baseline vital signs, identify known allergies, and assess the effectiveness of teaching. In ambulatory and outpatient centers, the nurse might have only one opportunity to assess and record vital signs. It is important for the nurse to confirm that the vital signs are normal values *for the client*. To accurately assess the client's response to anesthetic agents and the procedure performed, the nurse must compare the vital signs taken during and after the procedure to those obtained before as baseline data.

The client must be made aware of those things to expect during the procedure. Such teaching can both increase the level of cooperation and decrease the degree of anxiety. The client's family should also be informed of what will happen during the procedure and approximately how long the procedure should last. Nurses must also know the institution's specific protocols and procedures, because these are not standardized in all practice settings.

Care of the Client during Diagnostic Testing

Although client care must be individualized according to the specific procedure, general guidelines for client care during a procedure are outlined in Table 13–2. Protocols are used to assist the nurse with client care.

Standard Precautions are initiated when exposure to body fluids presents a threat to the safety of the caregiver or client. Protective barriers, such as gloves and a gown, should be used during invasive procedures.

Table 13–1 PROTOCOL: PREPARING THE CLIENT FOR DIAGNOSTIC TESTING

Purpose	To increase the reliability of the test by providing client teaching on the reason the test is being performed, those things the client can expect during the test, and the outcomes and side effects of the test
	To decrease the client's anxiety about the test and the associated risks
Supportive Data	Increase the client's knowledge, thereby promoting cooperation and enhancing the quality of the testing
	Decrease the time required to perform the tests, thereby increasing cost effectiveness
	Prevent delays by ensuring proper physical preparation
Assessment	Ensure that the client is wearing an identification band
	Review the medical record for allergies and previous adverse reactions to dyes and other contrast media; a signed consent form; and the recorded findings of diagnostic tests relative to the procedure
	Assess for the presence, location, and characteristics of physical and communicative limitations or pre-existing conditions
	Monitor the client's knowledge of both the reasons for the test and those things to expect during and after testing
	Monitor vital signs of the client who is scheduled for invasive testing, to establish baseline data
	Assess client outcome measures relative to the practitioner's preferences for preprocedure preparations
	Monitor level of hydration and weakness for clients who are designated nothing by mouth (NPO)
Report to Practitioner	Notify practitioner of allergy, previous adverse reaction, or suspected adverse reaction following the administration of drugs
	Notify practitioner of any client or family concerns not alleviated by discussions with nurse
Interventions	Clarify with practitioner whether regularly scheduled medications are to be administered
	Implement NPO status, as determined by the type of test
	Administer cathartics or laxatives as denoted by the test's protocol; instruct clients who are weak to call for assistance to the bathroom
	Teach relaxation techniques, such as deep breathing and imagery
	Establish intravenous (IV) access if necessary for the procedure
Evaluation	Evaluate the client's knowledge of those things to expect
	Evaluate the client's anxiety level
	Evaluate the client's level of safety and comfort
Client Teaching	Discuss the following with the client and family, as appropriate to the specific test:
	• The reason for the test and those things to expect
	• An estimation of how long the test will take
	• Specifics of NPO status, including amount of water to drink if oral medication is to be taken
	• Cathartics or laxative: amount, frequency
	• Sputum: cough deeply, do not clear throat
	• Urine: voided, clean-catch specimen; timing of collection
	• Removal of objects (e.g., jewelry or hair clips) that will obscure x-ray film
	• Contrast medium:
	Barium: taste, consistency, after effects (lightly colored stools for 24 to 72 hours; possibly, obstruction/impaction)
	Iodine: metallic taste, delayed allergic reaction (itching, rashes, hives, wheezing and breathing difficulties)
	• Positioning during the test
	• Positioning posttest (e.g., immobilize limb after angiography)
	• Posttest (encourage fluid intake if not contraindicated)
Documentation	Record in the client's medical record:
	• Practitioner notification of allergies or suspected adverse reaction to contrast media
	• Presence, location, and characteristics of symptoms
	• Teaching and the client's response to teaching
	• Responses to interventions (client outcomes)

Table 13–2 PROTOCOL: CARE OF THE CLIENT DURING DIAGNOSTIC TESTING

Purpose	To increase cooperation and participation by allaying the client's anxiety To provide the maximum level of safety and comfort during a procedure
Supportive Data	Encourage relaxation of the muscles and thus facilitation of instrumentation by increasing the client's participation and comfort Ensure both efficient use of time during the test and reliable results from the test with proper preparation of the client
Assessment	Check the client's identification band to ensure the correct client Review the medical record for allergies Assess the client's reaction to the preprocedure sedatives administered prior to the induction of anesthesia during the procedure Assess airway maintenance and gag reflex, if a local anesthetic is sprayed into the client's throat Assess vital signs throughout the procedure and compare to baseline data Assess the client's ability to maintain and tolerate the prescribed position Assess the client's comfort level to ensure the effectiveness of the anesthetic agent Assess for related symptoms indicating complications specific to the procedure (e.g., accidental perforation of an organ)
Report to Practitioner	Notify the practitioner of any client concerns or questions not answered in discussions with the nurse Notify the practitioner of any family members present and their location during the procedure Notify the practitioner when the client is positioned properly and the anesthetic agent has been administered to the client
Interventions	Institute Standard Precautions or appropriate aseptic technique for the specific test Report to all personnel involved in the test any known client allergies Place the client in the correct position, drape, and monitor to ensure that breathing is not compromised Remain with the client during induction and maintenance of anesthesia If the procedure requires the administration of a dye, ensure that the client is not allergic to the dye; if the client has not received the dye before, perform the skin allergy test according to the manufacturer's instructions that accompany the medication Maintain the client's airway and keep resuscitative equipment available Assist the client to relax during insertion of the instrument by telling the client to breathe through the mouth and to concentrate on relaxing the involved muscles Explain what the practitioner is doing so that the client knows what to expect Label and handle the specimen according to the type of materials obtained and the testing to be done Report to the practitioner any symptoms of complications Secure client transport from the diagnostic area Posttest in the diagnostic area: • Assist the client to a comfortable, safe position • Provide oral hygiene and water to clients who were designated NPO for the test, if they are alert and able to swallow • Remain with the client awaiting transport to another area
Evaluation	Evaluate the client's ventilatory status and tolerance to the procedure Evaluate the client's need for assistance Evaluate the client's understanding of what was performed during the procedure Evaluate the client's understanding of findings identified during the procedure Evaluate the client's knowledge of what to expect after the procedure
Client Teaching	Discuss the following with the client and family, as appropriate to the specific test: • Those things that occurred during the procedure • Questions and concerns of the client or family member • Those things to expect during the immediate recovery phase • Those things to report to the nurse during the immediate recovery phase
Documentation	Record in the client's medical record: • Person who performed the procedure • Reason for the procedure • Type of anesthesic, dye, or other medications administered • Type of specimen obtained and where it was delivered • Vital signs and other assessment data such as client's tolerance of the procedure or pain/discomfort level • Any symptoms of complications • Person who transported the client to another area (designate the names of persons who provided transport and the destination)

The nurse is responsible for labeling any specimen with the client's name and room number (for hospitalized clients), and the date, time, and source of the specimen. Some specimens may need to be taken immediately to the laboratory or placed on ice (e.g., arterial blood gases [ABGs]).

Ongoing assessment of the client's status is required during the procedure. The patency of the client's airway should be continuously assessed, as it may be compromised by the client's position, by anesthesia, or by the procedure itself. During an invasive procedure, the nurse also must monitor for signs and symptoms of accidental perforation of an organ (e.g., sudden changes in vital signs).

The nurse has the following additional responsibilities:

- Preparing the procedure room (e.g., ensuring adequate lighting)
- Gathering and charging for supplies to be used during the procedure
- Testing the equipment to ensure it is functional and safe
- Securing proper containers for specimen collection

Practitioners usually have preference cards within the diagnostic testing area that specify the type of equipment to be used, the position in which to place the client, and the type of sedative or anesthesic agent to be used.

Some diagnostic tests are performed with the registered nurse administering IV sedation, also called conscious sedation. **Conscious sedation** is a minimally depressed level of consciousness during which the client retains the ability to maintain a continuously patent airway and respond appropriately to physical stimulation or verbal commands (Somerson, Husted, & Sicilia, 1995). The nurse managing conscious sedation is usually functioning in an expanded role that requires additional education and demonstrated ability beyond that afforded by basic education.

Care of the Client after Diagnostic Testing

Postprocedure nursing care is directed toward restoring the client's prediagnostic level of functioning (Table 13–3). Nursing assessment and interventions are based mainly on the nature of the test and whether the client received anesthesia.

The client is monitored closely for signs of respiratory distress and bleeding. Some diagnostic procedures require that vital signs be measured every 15 minutes for the first hour, and then at gradually longer intervals until the client is **stable** (alert and with vital signs within the client's normal range).

Some diagnostic tests require the use of medications that are excreted through the kidneys. The client's in-take and output (I&O) is monitored by the nurses for 24 hours. The client is taught to monitor I&O and to report **hematuria** (presence of blood in the urine).

Safety: Radioactive Iodine and Urine Collection
Clients receiving radioactive iodine must have their urine collected and properly discarded in a special container, according to agency policy for handling radioactive medical wastes.

When clients are discharged after diagnostic testing, they should receive written instructions. Most agencies have discharge forms on which the nurse documents teaching regarding medications, dietary and activity restrictions, and signs and symptoms to be reported immediately to the practitioner. Clients may also need to have follow-up appointments made for them.

LABORATORY TESTS

Common laboratory studies are usually simple measurements to determine the amount or number of **analytes** (i.e., measured substances) present in a specimen. Laboratory tests are ordered by the practitioner to:

- Detect and quantify the risk of future disease,
- Establish or exclude diagnoses,
- Assess the severity of the disease process and formulate a prognosis,
- Guide the selection of interventions,
- Monitor the progress of the disorder, or
- Monitor the effectiveness of the treatment.

Specimen Collection

The scheduling and sequencing of laboratory tests are important functions of the nurse. All tests requiring **venipuncture** (the use of a needle to puncture a vein to aspirate blood) are grouped together so that the client is subjected to only one venipuncture. Fasting laboratory and radiological studies are scheduled on the same day so that the client is required to fast for only 1 day. Appropriate scheduling increases the client's comfort level and satisfaction.

PROFESSIONAL TIP

Documentation of Specimen-Collection Difficulties
Document on the laboratory requisition slip and in the nurses' notes any difficulty experienced during collection of a specimen. Such problems may indicate adverse effects related to the nature of the test and thus must be reported and treated immediately.

Table 13–3 PROTOCOL: CARE OF THE CLIENT AFTER DIAGNOSTIC TESTING

Purpose	To restore the client's prediagnostic level of functioning by providing care and teaching relative to both those things the client can expect after a test and the outcomes or side effects of the test
Supportive Data	Decrease client anxiety by increasing the client's participation and knowledge of expected outcome measures after a diagnostic test
	Through proper postprocedure care and client teaching, alert the client to those signs and symptoms that must to be reported to the practitioner
Assessment	Check the identification band and call the client by name
	Assess the client closely for signs of airway distress, adverse reactions to anesthesic or other medications, and other signs that may indicate accidental perforation of an organ
	Assess for bleeding those areas where a biopsy was performed
	Assess the client's color and skin temperature
	Assess vascular access lines or other invasive monitoring devices
	Assess the client's ability to expel air, if air was instilled during a gastrointestinal test
	Assess the client's knowledge of those things to expect during the recovery phase
Report to Practitioner	Notify the practitioner of any signs of respiratory distress, bleeding, or changes in vital signs; adverse reactions to anesthetic, sedative, or dye; and other signs of complications
	Notify the practitioner of any client or family concerns or questions not answered in discussions with the nurse
	Notify the practitioner when any results are obtained from the diagnostic test
	Notify the practitioner when the client is fully alert and recovered (for an order to discharge)
Interventions	Implement the practitioner's orders regarding the postprocedure care of the client
	Institute Standard Precautions or surgical asepsis as appropriate to the client's care needs
	Position the client for comfort and accessibility so as to facilitate performance of nursing measures
	Monitor vital signs according to the frequency required for the specific test
	Observe the insertion site for hematoma or blood loss; replace pressure dressing, as needed
	Monitor the client's urinary output and drainage from other devices
	Enforce activity restrictions appropriate to the test
	Schedule client appointments as directed by the practitioner
Evaluation	Evaluate the client's respiratory status, especially if an anesthetic agent was used
	Evaluate the client's tolerance of oral liquids
	Evaluate the client's understanding of the procedural findings of when the practitioner expects to receive written results
	Evaluate the client's knowledge of those things to expect after discharge
Client Teaching	Based on client assessment and evaluation of knowledge, teach the client or family about the following: • Dietary or activity restrictions • Signs and symptoms that should be reported immediately to the practitioner • Medications
Documentation	Record in the client's medical record on the appropriate forms: • Assessment data, nursing interventions, and achievement of expected outcomes • Client or family teaching and demonstrated level of understanding • Written instructions given to the client or family members

Accuracy in laboratory testing requires that:

- The practitioner's order be transcribed onto the correct requisition form,
- All requested information be written on the form (e.g., the client's full name and medical number),
- Pertinent data that could influence the test's results, such as medications taken, be included,
- Collection of the specimen from the correct client be confirmed by checking the identification band, and
- Laboratory results be placed in the correct medical record.

Venipuncture

Venipuncture can be performed by various members of the health care team. Although laboratories employ **phlebotomists** (individuals who perform venipuncture) to collect blood specimens, the nurse must know how to perform venipuncture, because nurses routinely perform venipuncture in the home, long-term care settings, and hospital critical care units.

Venipuncture can be performed by using either a sterile needle and syringe or a vacuum tube holder with a sterile two-ended needle. Test tubes are used to collect blood specimens. Test tubes have different colored stoppers to indicate the type of additive in the test tube. Collection tubes are universally color coded as follows:

- Red: no additive
- Lavender: ethylenediaminotetraacetic acid (EDTA)
- Light blue: sodium citrate
- Green: sodium heparin
- Gray: potassium oxalate
- Black: sodium oxalate

Arterial Puncture

Assessment of ABGs reveals the ability of the lungs to exchange gases by measuring the partial pressures of oxygen (PaO_2) and carbon dioxide ($PaCO_2$) and evaluates the potential of hydrogen (pH) of arterial blood. Blood gases are ordered to evaluate:

- Oxygenation,
- Ventilation and the effectiveness of respiratory therapy, and
- Acid–base balance in the blood.

Arterial blood samples are drawn from a peripheral artery (e.g., radial or femoral) or from an arterial line. The arterial blood sample is collected in a 5 mL heparinized syringe. To prevent clotting, the syringe is then rotated to mix the blood with the heparin. The blood sample is then placed on ice to reduce the rate of oxygen metabolism.

In some agencies, it is within the scope of nursing practice to perform radial artery puncture; however, femoral artery puncture is usually performed only by an advanced practitioner, because of the associated increased risk of hemorrhage. Although it is not common practice for student nurses to draw ABG samples, students often assist with the procedure and care for the client after the procedure.

Regardless of who performs the arterial puncture, the nurse is responsible for assessing the client for symptoms of postpuncture bleeding or occlusion. Direct pressure must be applied to the puncture site until all bleeding has stopped (for a minimum of 5 minutes). Symptoms of impaired circulation include the following:

CLIENT TEACHING

Postarterial Puncture

The client should *immediately* notify the nurse if any pain or numbness occurs in the arm or leg after an arterial puncture. These symptoms indicate impaired circulation.

- Numbness and tingling
- Bluish color
- Absence of a peripheral pulse

Capillary Puncture

Skin punctures are performed when small quantities of capillary blood are needed for analysis or when the client has poor veins. Capillary puncture is also commonly performed for blood glucose analysis. Figure 13-2 illustrates a capillary puncture of a fingertip.

Central Lines

Blood samples can also be collected from central lines. A **central line** refers to a venous catheter inserted into the superior vena cava through the subclavian or internal or external jugular vein. Central lines are used in the treatment of alterations in fluid or electrolyte balance, such as severe dehydration due to vomiting. Insertion is necessary when a peripheral route cannot be obtained. Central lines can be used for treatment and to withdraw blood for analysis.

The first sample of blood drawn from the central line cannot be used for diagnostic testing; it must be discarded, with the volume of discard being directly related to the dead space (catheter size) (Laxson & Titler, 1994). The agency's protocol should indicate the volume to discard relative to the type and size of catheter.

The care of central lines requires strict sterile technique. The practitioner must write an order to allow a blood sample to be obtained from a central line.

PROFESSIONAL TIP

Arterial Blood Gases

To ensure an accurate determination of the client's actual blood gases, ABGs should not be drawn within 30 minutes after any respiratory treatment.

Puncture site

Figure 13-2 Capillary Puncture of Fingertip

PROFESSIONAL TIP

Common Sites for Capillary Puncture
- Inner aspect of a palmar fingertip is the most commonly used site
- Earlobe is used when the client is in shock or the extremities are edematous

COMMUNITY/HOME HEALTH CARE

Central Line

Clients receiving prolonged therapy in the home environment usually have a central line in place. Because one of the primary complications of central venous catheter insertion is infection, the nurse must be alert for signs of infection (e.g., fever).

Implanted Port

Some clients have a **port-a-cath** (a port that has been implanted under the skin) over the third or fourth rib. The port has a catheter that is inserted into the superior vena cava or right atrium through the subclavian or internal jugular vein. The implanted port is used for the same purpose as is a central line. Blood can be withdrawn for sampling by accessing the port while using strict sterile technique. Accessing a port should be performed only by a nurse who has the education to be able to properly do so. Students are not usually taught how to access an implanted port.

Urine Collection

Urine can be collected for various studies. The type of testing determines the method of collection. The different methods of urine collection are as follows:

- Random collection (routine analysis)
- Timed collection (24-hour urine)
- Collection from a closed urinary drainage system
- Sterile specimen (catheterized)
- Clean-voided specimen

Client teaching depends on the client's age and the method of collection. The method of collection should be written on the laboratory requisition.

Safety: Standard Precautions and Urine Collection

All urine collection requires the use of Standard Precautions to prevent the transmission of microorganisms among nurses, clients, and other health care providers. All specimen containers should be sealed in a biohazard bag prior to transport to the laboratory.

Random Collection The practitioner usually writes the order for a UA (routine urine analysis), which is also called a random collection. The specimen can be collected at any time using a clean cup. The container does not have to be sterile. The specimen should be taken immediately to the laboratory to prevent both bacteria growth and changes in the urine's analytes.

Timed Collection Timed collection is done over a 24-hour period. The urine is collected in a plastic gal-

lon container that contains preservative(s), some of which are caustic.

For a timed collection, the client is told to **void** (eliminate urine) and discard the specimen at the beginning of the collection. Timing for a 24-hour urine collection begins after the first voiding has been discarded. For example, if the client voids at 1000 hours (24-hour [military] time), that urine should be discarded, but all other urine specimens until 1000 hours the following day saved. The client can void throughout the test into a clean container, then pour the urine into the collection bottle. Toilet tissue should not be dropped into the container used to catch the urine. The collection container should be refrigerated or kept on ice throughout the 24 hours to retard bacterial growth and stabilize the analytes.

Collection from a Closed-Drainage System

A sterile specimen can be collected from a client with an indwelling Foley catheter and closed drainage system. A sterile specimen is used for urine culture. The urine specimen should *not* be obtained from the drainage bag, because the analytes in the urine drainage bag change, leading to inaccurate results, and bacteria grows quickly in the drainage bag. The catheter's closed drainage tubing has an aspiration port that is used for sterile specimen collection.

Sterile Specimen Sometimes a sterile urine specimen is required when the client does not have an indwelling catheter and closed drainage system. In such cases, the client is catheterized. A small amount of urine is allowed to run out of the catheter into a basin, then the urine is allowed to run into a sterile specimen bottle.

COMMUNITY/HOME HEALTH CARE

Urine Collection in the Home

Clients in the home should place the urine container in a reclosable ("zipper") plastic bag and refrigerate until delivering to a laboratory. Doing so prevents bacteria growth and promotes accuracy of results.

Clean-Voided Specimen Clean-voided (clean-catch, or midstream) specimen collection is done to secure a specimen uncontaminated by skin flora. Different aseptic techniques are used for women and men. The female client is instructed to cleanse from the front to the back and then void into the specimen bottle; the male client is instructed to cleanse from the tip of the penis downward and then void into the specimen bottle.

Stool Collection

The nurse should first explain to the client the reason for collection of the stool specimen. The client can then be instructed to defecate into a clean bed pan or container, discarding used tissue in the toilet. Stools can be collected for a one-time defecation or over 24, 48, or 72 hours. If stools are to be collected over a prolonged period of time, all must be placed into a container and refrigerated. Once all stools have been collected, the container should be labeled with the client's name, the date and time, and the test to be performed on the specimen. All stool specimens are placed in a biohazard bag before being transported to the laboratory.

Safety: Collecting Stool from a Client with Hepatitis

When collecting a stool specimen from a client with hepatitis, write on the requisition form that the client has hepatitis. Doing so alerts laboratory personnel to be especially careful when handling the specimen.

Specific Tests

Many tests can be performed on the blood. Tests specific to the hematological system are described in Table 13–4.

Type and Crossmatch

A **type and crossmatch** is a laboratory test that identifies the client's blood type and determines the compatibility of blood between a potential donor and recipient (client). There are four basic blood types: A, B, AB, and O. The blood types are determined by the presence or absence of A or B antigens. **Antigens** are substances, usually proteins, that cause the formation of and react specifically with antibodies. **Antibodies** are immunoglobulins produced by the body in response to bacteria, viruses, or other antigenic substances. Type A and type B are antigens that are classified as **agglutinogens**, or substances that cause **agglutination** (clumping of RBCs). **Agglutinins** are specific kinds of antibodies whose interaction with antigens manifests as agglutination.

Blood types are also designated as either positive or negative, depending on the presence or absence of the Rh factor. The Rh factor is an antigen that may be found on the RBC. The designation *Rh positive* means

the antigen is present; *Rh negative* means the antigen is absent. An individual's blood type and Rh are determined genetically.

Crossmatch determines the compatibility of the donor's blood with that of the recipient. In the laboratory, a sample of the recipient's blood is mixed with the blood of a possible donor. If the blood sample is compatible, the mixed sample does not agglutinate.

Blood Chemistry

Blood chemistry tests are often grouped together into profiles, or panels, requiring one requisition and a single venous specimen. Tests performed include glucose, electrolytes, enzymes, lipids, creatinine, and protein values. Other tests that may be performed on a blood specimen are listed in Table 13–5.

Blood Glucose Blood for glucose measurement is obtained by either skin puncture or venipuncture; glucose is measured as either fasting (FBS) or nonfasting (usually 2 hours postprandial) blood sugar. This test is used to screen for diabetes mellitus. If the results are abnormal, the practitioner may order a glucose tolerance test, the most accurate test for diagnosing hypoglycemia and hyperglycemia (diabetes mellitus).

Serum Electrolytes An **electrolyte** is a substance that, when in solution, separates into ions and conducts electricity. Some electrolytes act on the cell membrane, allowing for the transmission of electrochemical impulses in nerve and muscle fibers. Other electrolytes determine the activity of different enzymatically catalyzed reactions necessary for cellular metabolism (Guyton & Hall, 1996).

Cations are ions that have a positive charge, such as sodium (Na^+), potassium (K^+), calcium (Ca^{++}), and magnesium (Mg^{++}). **Anions** are ions that have a negative charge, including chloride (Cl^-), bicarbonate (HCO_3^-), and phosphate (HPO_4^{--}).

Blood Enzymes **Enzymes** are globular proteins produced in the body that catalyze chemical reactions within the cells by promoting the oxidative reactions and synthesis of various chemicals, such as lipids, glycogen, and adenosine triphosphate (ATP). Enzyme tests play a key role in diagnosing the degree of tissue damage, mainly to the myocardium and, to a lesser degree, to the brain.

Elevations in plasma levels of intracellular enzymes occur in the presence of myocardial **necrosis** (tissue death as the result of disease or injury). Enzymes are released into the bloodstream in proportion to the degree of cellular damage. The enzymes are not used as single diagnostic values in determining a diagnosis but, rather, are reviewed in relation to other diagnostic studies.

Blood Lipids An elevated serum lipid level is one of the controllable contributing risk factors to CHD. **Lipoproteins** (blood lipids bound to protein) are measured along with cholesterol.

Table 13–4 TESTS SPECIFIC TO THE HEMATOLOGIC SYSTEM

TEST	EXPLANATION/NORMAL VALUES	NURSING RESPONSIBILITIES
Red blood cells (RBCs)	Number of RBCs per mm³ of blood. May be low in clients with rheumatoid arthritis. Clients living in high altitudes may have an elevated RBC level. Normal: Male: 4.6–5.9 million/mm³ Female: 4.2–5.4 million/mm³	The client is not required to fast for the test.
White blood cells (WBCs)	Number of WBCs per mm³ of blood. Elevation is associated with infectious processes. Normal: 4300–10,800 mm³	The client is not required to fast for the test. Exercise, stress, last month of pregnancy, labor, previous splenectomy, and eating may increase level and alter differential values. Note medications taken that may affect test; aspirin, heparin, and steroids may increase WBC level, whereas antibiotics and diuretics may decrease WBC level.
Differential count Neutrophils Segs (mature neutrophils) Bands (immature neutrophils)	Percentage of types of WBCs in 1 mm of blood. Increase in bacterial infections and trauma. Normal: Segs: 50%–65% Bands: 0%–5%	The client is not required to fast for the test.
Eosinophils	Increased in allergic reactions or parasitic infestation. Normal: 1%–3%	Corticosteroid therapy causes a decreased level.
Basophils	Increased in allergic reactions and during healing periods. Normal: 0.4%–1.0%	Steroids cause a decreased level.
Lymphocytes	Increased in viral infections and other diseases, such as pertussis and tuberculosis (TB). Decreased in acquired immunodeficiency syndrome (AIDS). Normal: 25%–35%	Steroids cause a decreased level.
Monocytes	Increased in chronic diseases, such as malaria, TB, Rocky Mountain spotted fever. May be low in clients with rheumatoid arthritis. Normal: 4%–6%	
Hemoglobin (Hgb)	Measures the oxygen-carrying capacity of the blood. Normal: Male: 14–18 g/dL Female: 12–16 g/dL Critical value: < 5 g/dL	The client is not required to fast for the test. Sample may be drawn from a finger of a child or the heel of an infant.
Hemoglobin electrophoresis	Detects abnormal forms of hemoglobin. Performed after positive sickle cell test. If the hemoglobin electrophoresis is negative, the client has the sickle cell trait. If the hemoglobin electrophoresis is positive, the client has sickle cell anemia. Normal: Hgb S: 0% Hgb F: < 2% Hgb Ca: 0%	If the client has had a blood transfusion within the last 12 weeks, the results of the test may be altered.
Hematocrit (Hct)	Measures the percentage of blood cells in a volume of blood. Clients living in high altitudes may have an increased level. Normal: Male: 42%–52% Female: 37%–47% Critical value: < 15%	The client is not required to fast for the test.

continues

Table 13–4 TESTS SPECIFIC TO THE HEMATOLOGIC SYSTEM *continued*

TEST	EXPLANATION/NORMAL VALUES	NURSING RESPONSIBILITIES
Platelet count	Measures the number of platelets per cubic milliliter of blood. Normal: 150,000–400,000/mm^3 Critical level: < 50,000 and > 1 million/mm^3	Instruct the client that strenuous exercise and oral contraceptives increase platelet level. Instruct the client that aspirin, acetaminophen, and sulfonamides decrease platelet level. If the client has a low platelet count, maintain digital pressure to the puncture site.
Bleeding time	Measures the length of time for a platelet plug to occlude a small puncture wound. Normal: 1–9 minutes (Ivy method) Critical value: > 12 minutes	Notify the laboratory if the client is taking aspirin, anticoagulants, or other medications that may affect the clotting process.
Prothrombin time (PT, protime)	Measures the effectiveness of several blood-clotting factors. Normal: 11–12.5 seconds INR: 2.0–3.0 In the presence of anticoagulant therapy, the values should be 1½–2 times the normal value. Critical value: > 20 seconds In the presence of anticoagulant therapy, the critical value should be > 3 times the normal critical value.	Ensure that the blood specimen is drawn before the daily dose of warfarin (Coumadin) is administered. Instruct the client that alcohol intake may increase PT and that a diet high in fat may decrease PT. Note those medications taken that may affect results; salicylates, sulfonamides, and methyldopa (Aldomet), as these may increase PT, whereas digitalis and oral contraceptives decrease the level. Instruct the client not to take any medication without notifying the physician, as medications may affect the PT level.
International normalized ratio (INR)	Normal: 2–3 (2.5–3.5 for the client with a mechanical prosthetic heart valve). The INR is more accurate than PT in monitoring warfarin (Coumadin) therapy.	The daily warfarin (Coumadin) dose should be given after blood has been drawn for the INR.

Partial thromboplastin time (PTT), also called activated partial thromboplastin time (APTT)	Normal:
	    PTT: 60–70 sec
	    APTT: 30–40 sec
	
	In the presence of anticoagulant therapy, the normal value is 1.5–2.5 times the control value.
	
	Critical value:
	    APTT: > 70 seconds
	    PTT: > 100 seconds
		If the client is receiving intermittent heparin doses, schedule the APTT to be drawn 30–60 minutes before the next heparin dose.
		
		If heparin is given continuously, the blood specimen can be drawn at any time.
		
		If APTT is greater than 100 seconds, the client is at risk for bleeding, and the physician is notified.
		
		The antidote for heparin is protamine sulfate.
		
		Note whether the client is taking antihistamines, vitamin C, or salicylates, as these prolong PTT time.

D dimer test (fragment D dimer, fibrin degradation fragment)	Measures a fibrin split product that is released when a clot breaks. Confirms the diagnosis of disseminated intravascular coagulation (DIC). Normal: negative for D-dimer fragments	Note whether the client is on thrombolytic therapy, as the results of this test would be increased from negative to positive.

Table 13–5 ADDITIONAL TESTS PERFORMED ON BLOOD SPECIMEN

TEST	EXPLANATION/NORMAL VALUES	NURSING RESPONSIBILITIES
Acid phosphatase	Acid phosphatase is an enzyme found in highest concentrations in the prostate gland. An elevated level is seen in clients with prostatic cancer that has metastasized to other body parts. If tumors are treated successfully, the level will decrease. A rising level may indicate a poor prognosis. Normal: 0.11–0.60 U/L	Tell the client that no food or drink restrictions are associated with this test. Apply pressure to the venipuncture site. Observe the site for bleeding.

continues

Table 13–5 ADDITIONAL TESTS PERFORMED ON BLOOD SPECIMEN *continued*

TEST	EXPLANATION/NORMAL VALUES	NURSING RESPONSIBILITIES
Adrenocorticotropic hormone (ACTH), corticotropin	Determines the function of the anterior pituitary. Because of diurnal variation, specimens should be drawn in both morning and evening. Normal: A.M.: 15–100 pg/mL, or 10–80 ng/L P.M.: < 50 pg/mL, or < 50 ng/L	Emotional or physical stress or recent radio-isotope scans can interfere with test results. Drugs that may increase ACTH level include corticosteroids, estrogens, ethanol, and spironolactone. Explain the procedure to the client. This is especially important to decrease the client's stress level. Evaluate the client for increased stress level. Initiate NPO status after midnight. The blood specimen must be drawn with a heparinized syringe, chilled by placing the specimen on ice, and immediately transported to the lab.
ACTH stimulation test, cortisol stimulation test, cosyntropin test	Monitors plasma cortisol level to indicate adrenal gland response to ACTH. Normal: Rapid: ↑ 7 µg/dL above baseline 24 hours: > 40 µg/dL 3 days: > 40 µg/dL	Note those medications taken that may affect results: cortisone, estrogens, hydrocortisone, and spironolactone may increase plasma cortisol level. Explain the procedure to the client. Initiate NPO status after midnight. For all tests, obtain baseline serum cortisol level. Rapid test: Administer IV injection of cosyntropin over 2 minutes. Draw blood specimen at 30 and 60 minutes after injection. 24-hour test: Start an IV infusion of cosyntropin in 1 liter normal saline and run at 2 U/h for 24 hours. Draw plasma cortisol level after 24 hours. 3-day test: Administer 25 units cosyntropin IV over 8 hours for 2 or 3 days. At the end of 3 days, draw plasma cortisol level.
Alanine aminotransferase (ALT, formerly serum glutamic pyruvic transiminase [SGRT])	ALT is an enzyme released in response to liver injury. Normal: 5–35 U/L	Note those medications taken that affect results: many medications may increase level, including antibiotics, narcotics, oral contraceptives, and many others.
Albumin	Albumin, a protein formed by the liver, is responsible for maintaining colloidal osmotic pressure. Indicates how well the liver is functioning. Normal: 3.5–5.0 g/dL	Note those medications taken that may affect results; steroids and hormones such as insulin, and growth hormones may increase level, whereas oral contraceptives and liver toxic drugs may decrease level.
Alkaline phosphatase	Alkaline phosphatase is an enzyme found in many tissues. The highest concentrations are found in the liver, biliary tract, and bone. Detection is important for determining possible liver and bone cancers. Normal: 30–85 ImU/mL	Fasting may be required. Apply pressure to the venipuncture site. Observe the site for bleeding.
Alpha-fetoprotein	Test for tumor marker; elevated in nonseminomatous testicular cancer. Performed between 16 and 18 weeks of pregnancy. A high level is suggestive of neural tube defects, whereas a low level may suggest Down syndrome. Normal: 0.9 ng/mL	Apply pressure to site and watch for bleeding or hematoma. First sample must be drawn between 15–20 weeks of gestation.
Amylase	Amylase is an enzyme secreted by the pancreas. Elevation indicates pancreatitis. Normal: 56–190 IU/L	Note those medications taken that affect test results; steroids, aspirin, alcohol, some narcotics, some diuretics, and other drugs may increase level, whereas citrate, glucose, and oxalates may decrease level.
Antidiuretic hormone (ADH), vasopressin	Determines the production of ADH by the posterior pituitary. Normal: 1–5 pg/mL, or < 1.5 ng/L	Explain the procedure to the client. The blood specimen should be collected in a plastic, not glass, container.

continues

Table 13–5 ADDITIONAL TESTS PERFORMED ON BLOOD SPECIMEN *continued*

TEST	EXPLANATION/NORMAL VALUES	NURSING RESPONSIBILITIES
Antidiuretic hormone (ADH), vasopressin (*continued*)		Note those medications taken that may interfere with test results. Drugs that elevate ADH level include acetaminophen, barbiturates, cholinergic agents, estrogen, nicotine, oral hypoglycemic agents, some diuretics such as thiazides, and tricyclic antidepressants. Drugs that decrease ADH level include alcohol, beta-adrenergic agents, morphine antagonists, and phenytoin (Dilantin). Client should fast for 12 hours before the test. Evaluate the client for high level of physical or emotional stress.
Antinuclear antibodies (ANAs)	ANA attack cell nuclei. The result is positive in 95% of clients with systemic lupus erythematosis. Levels are low in clients with mononucleosis, rheumatic fever, and liver diseases. Normal: negative	Fasting is not required. Hydralazine (Apresoline) and procainamide (Pronestyl) may increase level. A radioactive scan in the past week may alter results; inform the lab, if applicable.
Antistreptolysin O (ASO)	High titer indicates presence of *beta-hemolytic streptococcus*, which may cause rheumatic fever or acute glomerulonephritis. Upper limit of normal varies with age, season, and geographic area. Normal: Adult: < 1 : 100 12–19 years: < 1 : 200 2–5 years: < 1 : 100	There are no food or fluid restrictions. Antibiotics decrease ASO level. Check urine output if ASO is elevated. Urine output of less than 600 mL/24 h is associated with acute glomerulonephritis.
Antithyroid microsomal antibody, antimicrosomal antibody, microsomal antibody, thyroid autoantibody, thyroid antimicrosomal antibody	Used to detect thyroid microsomal antibodies found in clients with Hashimoto's thyroiditis. Normal: titer < 1 : 100	Explain the procedure to the client.
Aspartate aminotransferase (AST, formerly serum glutamic oxaloacetic transiminase [SGOT])	AST is an enzyme that indicates inflammation of heart, liver, skeletal muscle, pancreas, or kidneys. Normal: Male: 7–21 U/L Female: 6–18 U/L	Avoid intramuscular (IM) injections; record date and time of any injections. Avoid hemolysis. Withhold medications that affect results, for 12 hours if possible; several medications, such as antihypertensives, cholinergic agents, anticoagulants, digitalis, and others, may increase level, as may exercise.
Arterial blood gases (ABGs)	Direct measurement of the pH, PaO_2, and $PaCO_2$, and calculated measurement of HCO_3^- and SaO_2 from samples of arterial blood. pH = expresses the acidity or alkalinity of the blood. PaO_2 = partial pressure of oxygen in the blood. $PaCO_2$ = partial pressure of carbon dioxide in the blood. SaO_2 = arterial oxygen saturation. HCO_3^- = bicarbonate ion concentration in the blood. The oxygen content of the blood expressed as a percentage of the oxygen carrying capacity of the blood. Normal: pH: 7.35–7.45 PaO_2: 80–100 mm Hg $PaCO_2$: 35–45 mm Hg HCO_3^-: 22–26 mEq SaO_2: > 95% (at sea level)	Explain that an arterial sample of blood is required. Arterial punctures cause more discomfort than venous. Instruct the client not to move. Assess the adequacy of collateral circulation. The blood sample is drawn in a syringe containing heparin. After the specimen has been obtained, rotate the syringe to mix the blood and heparin. The blood sample is placed on ice and taken immediately to the lab. Apply pressure to the arterial site for 3 to 5 minutes or 15 minutes if client is on an anticoagulant. Assess site for bleeding.

continues

Table 13–5 ADDITIONAL TESTS PERFORMED ON BLOOD SPECIMEN *continued*

TEST	EXPLANATION/NORMAL VALUES	NURSING RESPONSIBILITIES
Bilirubin	Measures bilirubin in the blood. Indicates how well the liver is functioning. Normal: 0.1–1.0 mg/dL	Note those medications taken that affect results; steroids, antibiotics, oral hypoglycemics, narcotics, as well as others may cause increased level, whereas barbiturates, caffeine, penicillins, and salicylates may cause decreased level. Fasting may be required. Do not shake the tube; protect the tube from light.
Blood glucose, fasting blood sugar, (FBS)	Measures blood level of glucose (serum values). Results depend on method used by laboratory. Normal: 70–115 mg/dL Diabetic: ≥ 126 mg/dL Critical values: > 400 mg/dL < 50 mg/dL	Client must fast (except for water) for 6–8 hours before test. Withhold insulin or oral antidiabetic medications until blood is drawn. Be certain client receives medications and meal after fasting specimen drawn. Cortisone, thiazide, and loop diuretics cause increase.
2 hour post prandial glucose (2h PPG) or 2 hour post prandial blood sugar (2h PPBS)	Measures blood glucose 2 hours after a meal. Normal: 70–140 mg/dL Diabetic: > 140 mg/dL	Instruct the client to eat entire meal and then to not eat anything else until blood is drawn. Notify the laboratory of the time meal was completed.
Blood urea nitrogen (BUN)	Measures urea, end product of protein metabolism. Normal: 5–25 mg/dL	Initiate NPO status 8 hours prior to test, if possible. Note the client's hydration status. Note those medications taken that may affect results, including phenothiazines, nephrotoxic drugs, diuretics (hydrochlorthiazide [Hydro-Diuril], ethacrynic acid [Edecrin], furosemide [Lasix]); antibiotics (bacitracin, gentamicin, kanamycin, methicillin, neomycin); antihypertensives (methyldopa [Aldomet], guanethidine [Ismelin]), sulfonamides, propranolol, morphine, lithium, carbonate, salicylates.
CA-15-3	CA-15-3 (cancer antigen) is a tumor marker for monitoring breast cancer. Because benign breast or ovarian disease can also cause elevations, it has limited use in diagnosis. Normal: < 22 U/mL	Fasting is not required. Apply pressure to the venipuncture site. Observe the site for bleeding.
CA-19-9	CA-19-9 (cancer antigen) is a tumor marker used primarily in the diagnosis of pancreatic carcinoma. Normal: < 37 U/mL	Fasting is not required. Apply pressure to the venipuncture site. Observe the site for bleeding.
CA-125	CA-125 (cancer antigen) is a tumor marker especially helpful in making the diagnosis of ovarian cancer. Normal: 0–35 U/mL	Fasting is not required. Apply pressure to the venipuncture site. Observe the site for bleeding.

Calcitonin, HCT, thyrocalcitonin	Determines thyroid and parathyroid activity. Also used as a tumor marker to detect thyroid cancer and several other cancers.
	Normal: basal
	  Male: ≤ 19 pg/mL, or ≤ 19 ng/L
	  Female: ≤ 14 pg/mL, or ≤ 14 ng/L
		Note those medications taken that may increase calcitonin level, including calcium, cholecystokinin, epinephrine, glucagon, pentagastrin, and oral contraceptives.
		Explain the procedure to the client.
		The client should fast overnight but may have water.

Carcinoembryonic antigen (CEA, carcinoembryonic antigen)	CEA was thought to be a specific indicator of the presence of colorectal cancer, but has been found in clients with a variety of carcinomas. It is especially useful in monitoring treatment response in breast and gastrointestinal cancers and is occasionally the first sign of tumor recurrence. Normal: < 5 ng/mL	Fasting is not required. Apply pressure to the venipuncture site. Observe the site for bleeding. Note whether the client smokes or has a disease that will alter results, such as hepatitis, cirrhosis, or colitis.

continues

Table 13–5 ADDITIONAL TESTS PERFORMED ON BLOOD SPECIMEN *continued*

TEST	EXPLANATION/NORMAL VALUES	NURSING RESPONSIBILITIES
Cardiac enzymes	Indicates possible tissue damage if elevated.	Neither fasting nor NPO status is necessary.

Serum AST	Normal:
	  Male: 7–21 U/L
	  Female: 6–18 U/L
		Pattern of elevated levels of AST, CPK, and LDH is indicative of myocardial infarction (MI).

Creatine kinase CPK (CK)	Normal:
	  Male: 55–170 U/L
	  Female: 30–135 U/L
		CPK is the first enzyme elevated after MI, and peaks within the first 24 hours.

CK isoenzymes	Present in skeletal muscle, brain, lungs, and heart muscle. Normal:	Elevation of an isoenzyme indicates damage to tissue in a specific organ; CK-MB is specific for myocardial cells.
CK-MM (muscle) CK-BB (brain) CK-MB (heart)	95%–100% 0%–1% < 3%–4% (> 5% in MI)	
Lactic dehydrogenase (LDH)	Normal: 70–180 mg/dL, or 95–200 U/L	LDH_1 value greater than LDH_2 value is indicative of an acute MI. LDH_5 is elevated with congestive heart failure (CHF).

LDH isoenzymes
  LDH_1 (heart and erythrocytes)
  LDH_2 (reticuloendothelial system)
  LDH_3 (lungs and other tissues)
  LDH_4 (kidney, placenta, pancreas)
  LDH_5 (liver and striated muscles)
	
	*17.5%–28.3%
	*30.4%–36.4%
	*18.8%–26.0%
	*9.2%–16.5%
	*5.3%–13.4%	

Cardiac troponin	A protein found only in cardiac muscle. Protein is released when the muscle is injured or dead. Elevated level within 3 hours and remains elevated 7 to 14 days. Often used in the ED. Normal: <0.1 ng/mL	Explain to client that blood sample is needed.
CD4 T-cell count	Predictor of HIV progression; baseline taken after positive HIV test. Normal: 500–1000/mm³ Critical value: < 200/mm³	Explain the meaning of the test. Provide follow-up explanation of test results.
Cholesterol (lipid profile)	Lipid necessary for steroid, bile, and cell membrane production. Normal: < 200 mg/dL (total)	Have client fast 12 to 14 hours prior to test. No alcohol 24 hours prior to test. Diet intake 2 weeks prior to test will affect results. Note those medications taken that may affect results; steroids, phenytoin, diuretics, and others may elevate level, whereas MAO inhibitors, some antibiotics, lovastatin, and others may decrease level. If elevated, increased risk of coronary artery disease (CAD), hypertension, and MI.
High density lipoprotein (HDL) Low density lipoprotein (LDL) Very low density lipoprotein (VLDL) Triglycerides	Normal: 30–70 mg/dL Normal: 60–160 mg/dL Normal: 25%–50% Normal: 40–150 mg/dL	 Elevated level in CAD; level increases when LDL level increases.

Complement assay (total complement, C3 and C4)	Decreased levels in autoimmune diseases due to depletion of complement by antibody–antigen complexes.
	Normal:
	  C3: Male: 80–180 mg/dL
	      Female: 76–120 mg/dL
	  C4: 15–45 mg/dL
		Fasting is not required.

Coombs' test (direct antiglobulin test)	Detects whether immunoglobulins are attached to RBCs. Normal: negative	Note whether the client is taking ampicillin (Unasyn), captopril (Capoten), indomethacin (Indocin), or insulin, as these cause false-positive results.

*% of total LDH

continues

Table 13–5 ADDITIONAL TESTS PERFORMED ON BLOOD SPECIMEN *continued*

TEST	EXPLANATION/NORMAL VALUES	NURSING RESPONSIBILITIES
Cortisol, hydrocortisone	Determines adrenal cortex function. There is normally a diurnal variation, with higher level around 6 to 8 A.M. and lowest levels around midnight. Normal: 8 A.M.: 6–28 μg/dL, or 170–625 nmol/L 4 P.M.: 2–12 μg/dL, or 80–413 nmol/L	Note whether the client has been under physical or emotional stress as either can artificially elevate plasma cortisol level. Likewise, recent use of radioisotopes can interfere with test results. Note those medications taken that may affect results. Drugs that may increase plasma cortisol level include estrogen, oral contraceptives, and spironolactone (Aldactone). Drugs that may decrease plasma cortisol level include androgens and phenytoin (Dilantin) Explain the procedure to the client. Two specimens are drawn—one at 8 A.M. and another at 4 P.M. Assess the client for physical or emotional stress and report to the physician. Indicate times of collection on laboratory requisitions.
C-reactive protein test (CRP)	An abnormal protein appears in the blood of clients with an acute inflammatory process. Used to monitor the progress of clients with autoimmune disorders such as rheumatoid arthritis. Negative except in pregnancy. More sensitive than erythrocyte sedimentation rate (ESR).	Some labs may require clients to fast, except for water, for 4 to 12 hours prior. Note those mediations that may affect results: nonsteroidal anti-inflammatory drugs (NSAIDs), steroids, and salicylates may decrease level, whereas oral contraceptives and intrauterine devices (IUDs) may increase level. Inform laboratory, if applicable.
Dexamethasone suppression test (DST), prolonged/rapid DST, cortisol suppression test (ACTH suppression test)	Monitors plasma cortisol level to measure adrenal gland function. Normal: nearly 0 cortisol level	Stress can interfere with test results. Note those medications taken that may affect results, including barbiturates, estrogens, oral contraceptives, phenytoin (Dilantin) spironolactone, steroids, and tetracyclines. Explain the procedure to the client. Weigh the client for baseline weight. Rapid test: Administer dexamethasone 1 mg orally at 11 P.M. with milk or antacid. Administer sedative, if ordered. At 8 A.M. before client rises, draw plasma cortisol level. Overnight 8-mg dexamethasone suppression test: If no cortisol suppression occurs, repeat test using 8 mg dexamethasone. If there is still no cortisol suppression, a prolonged test over 6 days involving six 24-hour urine collections should be done.
Electrolytes	Determines blood electrolyte levels. First four are the most commonly measured.	Sodium and potassium are necessary for cardiac electrical conduction.
Sodium (Na⁺)	Measures level of serum sodium. Function in the body: Major electrolyte in extracellular fluid, regulates fluid balance, stimulates conduction of nerve impulses, helps maintain neuromuscular activity. Normal: 135–145 mEq/L	There are no food or fluid restrictions.
Potassium (K⁺)	Measures level of serum potassium. Function in the body: Major electrolyte in intracellular fluid, maintains normal nerve and muscle activity, assists in cellular metabolism of carbohydrates and proteins Normal: 3.5–5.0 mEq/L	There are no food or fluid restrictions. If the client has hypokalemia or hyperkalemia, evaluate the client for cardiac dysrhythmias.
Chloride (Cl⁻)	Measures level of serum chloride Function in the body: Major electrolyte in extracellular fluid, functions in combination with sodium to maintain osmotic pressure, assists in maintaining acid–base balance Normal: 100–110 mEq/L	There are no food or fluid restrictions.

continues

Table 13–5 ADDITIONAL TESTS PERFORMED ON BLOOD SPECIMEN *continued*

TEST	EXPLANATION/NORMAL VALUES	NURSING RESPONSIBILITIES
Electrolytes *(continued)*		
Calcium, total/ionized Ca^{++}	Indicates parathyroid gland function and calcium metabolism. Because ionized calcium is un-affected by serum albumin, it can give more accurate results; however, most laboratories do not have the equipment to perform the test. Normal: 　Total: 9.0–10.5 mg/dL, or 2.25–2.75 nmol/L 　Ionized: 4.5–5.6 ng/dL, or 1.05–1.30 nmol/L	Note those medications taken that may affect results. Drugs that may increase serum calcium level include calcium salts, hydralazine, lithium, thiazide diuretics, parathyroid hormone (PTH), thyroid hormone, and vitamin D. Drugs that may decrease serum calcium level include acetazolamide, anticonvulsants, aspara-ginase, aspirin, calcitonin, cisplatin, cortico-steroids, heparin, laxatives, loop diuretics, magnesium salts, and oral contraceptives. Vitamin D and excessive milk ingestion can also interfere with test results. Explain the procedure to the client. Fasting is not required for serum calcium, but might be required if other blood chemistry tests are to be drawn.
Magnesium (Mg^{++})	Measures level of serum magnesium Function in the body: 　Combines with calcium and phosphorous in intracellular bone tissue, essential for neuro-muscular contraction, synthesis of protein, and body temperature regulation Normal: 1.5–2.5 mEq/L	There are no food or fluid restrictions.
Phosphate (PO_4^{--})	Measures level of serum phosphate Function in the body: 　An essential intracellular electrolyte, exists in an inverse relationship with calcium Normal: 1.8–2.6 mEq/L	Initiate NPO status after midnight. Intravenous fluids containing glucose are sometimes discontinued several hours before the test.
Bicarbonate (HCO_3^-) (total carbon dioxide content or carbon dioxide capacity)	Always in a 20 : 1 ratio with carbonic acid. Normal: 24–30 mEq/L	There are no food or fluid restrictions. Loss of gastric contents is the most common reason for increased level.
ELISA	Screening test used to indicate the presence of HIV Normal: negative	Inform the client that if the first ELISA test is positive, a second ELISA will be drawn before confirmation is done with Western blot. Provide pretest counseling. Obtain informed consent. Provide or arrange for post-test counseling.
Erythrocyte sedimentation rate (ESR or sed rate test)	Measures, in mm, RBC descent in a normal saline solution after 1 hour. Level is increased in inflammatory, infectious, necrotic, or cancerous conditions, due to increased protein content in plasma. Used to monitor the course of therapy for clients with autoimmune diseases, such as rheumatoid arthritis. Normal: 　Male: 1–13 mm/h 　Female: 1–20 mm/h	The test should be performed within 3 hours after the blood is drawn. Menstruation or pregnancy may increase level. Ethanbutal, quinine, aspirin, cortisone, and prednisone may alter results.
Folic acid (Folate level)	Measures folic acid level in the blood. Normal: 5–20 ug/mL, or 14–34 mmol/L	Fasting is not required. Instruct the client not to drink any alcoholic beverages before the test. The test is drawn before folic acid medications are administered. Note whether the client is taking phenytoin (Dilantin), primidone (Mysoline), methotrexate, antimalarial agents, or oral contraceptives, as these cause decreased level.

continues

Table 13–5 ADDITIONAL TESTS PERFORMED ON BLOOD SPECIMEN *continued*

TEST	EXPLANATION/NORMAL VALUES	NURSING RESPONSIBILITIES

Follicle-stimulating hormone (FSH)	Determines anterior pituitary function. Usually measured with luteinizing hormone level.
	
	Normal: varies with phase of menstrual cycle
	    Follicular: 5–20 mU/mL
	    Midcycle peak: 15–30 mU/mL
	    Luteal: 5–15 mU/mL
	    Postmenopause: 50–100 mU/mL
	    Male: 5–20 mU/mL
		Note whether client is taking estrogen or progesterone, as these may decrease FSH level. Recent use of radioisotopes can also interfere with test results.
		
		Explain the procedure to the client.
		
		Indicate on the laboratory requisition the date of the last menstrual period (LMP) or that the client is postmenopausal. Indicate use of estrogen or progesterone on laboratory requisition.
		
		The client should be relaxed and recumbent for 30 minutes before the test.

Gamma-glutamyl transpeptidase (GGT or GGTP)	Enzyme that detects liver cell dysfunction.
	Normal:
	    Female, < 45 years: 5–27 U/L
	    Female, > 45 years; male: 8–38 U/L
		The client must fast for 8 hours prior to test.
		
		Note those medications taken that interfere with results; alcohol, dilantin, and phenobarbital may elevate results, whereas oral contraceptives and clofibrate may decrease results.

Globulin	Key for antibody production. Indicates how well the liver is functioning. Normal: 2.3–3.3 g/dL	Note those medications taken that affect results (see albumin).
Glucose tolerance test (GTT)	Evaluates blood and urine glucose 30 minutes before, and 1, 2, 3, and 4 hours after a standard glucose load. Normal: blood glucose ≤ 140 mg/dL within 2 h. urine negative for glucose Diabetic: blood glucose 200 mg/dL or greater, 2 hr after a load of 75 g anhydrous glucose	The client must fast (except for water) for 6–8 hours prior to the test. Withhold drugs that interfere with results. After administration of glucose load, withhold all food. The client should drink water, however. Collect urine specimens at hourly periods. Administer meal and medications after test is completed.

Glycosylated hemoglobin (GHb)	Measures glycohemoglobin, evaluating average blood glucose level over 120 days.
	Normal: 4%–8%
	    Good control: 7.5% or less
	    Fair control: 7.6%–8.9%
	    Poor control: ≥ 9% or more
		Fasting is not required.
		Blood can be drawn at any time.

Growth hormone (GH), human growth hormone (HGH), somatotropin hormone (SH)	Determines the function of the anterior pituitary, although other tests such as the growth stimulation test are more accurate.
	Normal:
	    Males: < 5 ng/mL, or < 5 µg/L
	    Female: < 10 ng/mL, or < 10 µg/L
		The client should fast but may have water.
		
		Random measurement of growth hormone is not adequate because the hormone is not secreted constantly.
		
		A radioactive scan within the week; stress; exercise; or decreased blood glucose level can interfere with test results.
		
		Drugs that may increase GH level include amphetamines, arginine, dopamine, estrogens, glucagon, histamine, insulin, levodopa, methyldopa, and nicotinic acid.
		
		Drugs that may decrease GH levels include corticosteroids and phenothiazines.
		
		Explain the procedure to the client.
		
		The client should be well rested and not emotionally or physically stressed.
		
		Additional blood specimens should be obtained during sleeping hours.
		
		Additional information for the laboratory requisition includes fasting time, time of specimen collection, and the client's recent activity.
		
		Because GH half-life is only 20–25 minutes, the specimen should be taken to the laboratory immediately.

continues

Table 13–5 ADDITIONAL TESTS PERFORMED ON BLOOD SPECIMEN *continued*

TEST	EXPLANATION/NORMAL VALUES	NURSING RESPONSIBILITIES
GH stimulation test, GH provocation test, insulin tolerance test (ITT), arginine test	Indicates growth hormone deficiency Normal: > 10 ng/mL, or 10 µg/L	This test is not to be done on a client with epilepsy, cerebrovascular disease, MI, or decreased basal plasma cortisol levels. Explain the procedure to the client and parents. Initiate NPO status after midnight, except for water. To prevent multiple puncture, a heparin lock should be inserted. Baseline GH, cortisol, and glucose levels are done. An injection of insulin or arginine is given. Blood specimens for growth hormone are drawn at 0, 60, and 90 minutes after injection. Blood glucose level is monitored every 15 to 30 minutes. Blood glucose must drop to 40 mg/dL for effectiveness. Monitor client for signs and symptoms of hypoglycemia. This test takes approximately 2 hours. Although the test can be performed by a nurse, a physician should be readily available. If vigorous exercise is used instead of medication, the client should run or stair-climb for 20 minutes. Blood specimens are drawn at 0, 20, and 40 minutes. At the conclusion of the test, the client is given cookies and punch or IV glucose. Blood specimens should be taken to the laboratory immediately after being drawn.
Hepatitis B surface antigen (HB$_s$AG)	A positive result indicates presence of hepatitis or that the person is a carrier. Normal: negative	

Human chorionic gonadotropin (hCG)	Test for tumor marker; elevated in germ cell testicular cancer.
	
	Normal:
	    Male: 0
	    Female, pregnant: < 5.0 mIU/mL
	    Female, abnormal pregnancy or choriocarcinoma: > 25 mIU/mL
		Apply pressure to the site and observe for bleeding or hematoma.

Human leukocyte antigen DW4 (HLA-DW4)	Positive (present in 50% of clients with rheumatoid arthritis. Normal: negative	Fasting is not required.
Lupus erythematosus test (LE prep)	Positive in 70%–80% of clients with systemic lupus erythematosus. May be positive in clients with rheumatoid arthritis. Used to diagnose and monitor the course of treatment for clients with systemic lupus erythematosus. Normal: negative	Fasting is not required. May be ordered daily for 3 days. Note whether the client is taking Apresoline, Pronestyl, oral contraceptives, quinidine, penicillin, Aldomet, tetracycline, isoniazid, or reserpine, as these may cause false-positive results.

Luteinizing hormone (LH) assay	Determines anterior pituitary function. It can be used to determine whether ovulation has occurred. Can also determine whether gonadal insufficiency is primary or secondary.
	
	Normal:
	    Males: 7–24 mU/mL
	    Females: 6–30 mU/mL
		Note whether the client is taking estrogen or progesterone, as these may decrease LH level. Recent use of radioisotopes can also interfere with test results.
		
		Explain the procedure to the client.
		
		Indicate on the laboratory requisition the date of the LMP or that the client is postmenopausal.

Parathyroid hormone (PTH), parathormone	Measures the quantity of PTH to determine hyperparathyroidism or whether hypercalcemia is caused by parathyroid glands. Normal: < 2,000 pg/mL	Recent use of radioisotope can interfere with test results. Explain the procedure to the client. Initiate NPO status after midnight, except for water. Obtain morning blood specimen and indicate time of collection.

continues

Table 13–5 ADDITIONAL TESTS PERFORMED ON BLOOD SPECIMEN *continued*

TEST	EXPLANATION/NORMAL VALUES	NURSING RESPONSIBILITIES
Phosphorus	Determines the level of phosphorus in the blood. Normal: 3.0–4.5 ng/dL, or 0.97–1.45 nmol/L	Laxatives or enemas containing sodium phosphate can increase serum phosphorus level. Note those medications taken that may affect results. Drugs that may increase serum phosphorus level include methicillin and excessive vitamin D. Recent carbohydrate ingestion including IV administration causes decreased serum phosphorus level, as do antacids and mannitol. Explain the procedure to the client. Initiate NPO status after midnight. Discontinue IV fluids containing glucose for several hours before test, if possible.

Plasma renin assay, plasma renin activity (PRA)	Measures the amount of renin and is used as a screening procedure to detect essential or renal hypertension. When combined with plasma aldosterone level, determines adrenal cortex activity.
	Normal:
	  Upright position, sodium depleted or restricted diet:
	    20–39 years: 2.9–24 ng/mL/h
	    > 40 years: 2.9–10.8 ng/mL/h
	  Upright position, sodium repleted or normal diet:
	    20–39 years: 0.1–4.3 ng/mL/h
	    > 40 years: 0.1–3.0 ng/mL/h
		Pregnancy, salt intake, or licorice ingestion can interfere with test results. Time of day (early in the day), a low-salt diet, or an upright position increases renin value.
		Note those medications taken that may interfere with test results, including antihypertensives, diuretics, estrogens, oral contraceptives, and vasodilators.
		Explain the procedure to the client. The client should maintain a normal diet with sodium restricted to 3 grams per day for 3 days before the test. Drugs and licorice should be discontinued for 2 to 4 weeks before the test. The client should stand or sit upright for 2 hours before blood is drawn. Client position, dietary status, time of day, and drugs should be recorded on the laboratory requisition. Blood specimen should be placed in ice and taken immediately to the laboratory. After blood specimen is obtained, the client may resume a normal diet and restart medications.

Polymerase chain reaction (PCR)	Detects HIV-specific DNA (virus). Normal: negative	Explain the meaning of the test. Provide follow-up explanation of test results.
Progesterone assay	Determines ovulation and function of corpus luteum. Adrenal tumors can elevate level. Normal, midcycle: 300–2,400 ng/dL	Recent use of radioisotopes or hemolysis resulting from rough handling of blood specimen can interfere with test results. Note those medications taken that may interfere with test results, including estrogen and progesterone. Explain the procedure to the client. Indicate the date of LMP on the laboratory requisition.

Prolactin level (PRL)	Determines anterior pituitary secretion. Among the problems indicated by an elevated level are pituitary tumors or primary hypothyroidism.
	Normal:
	  Female, or male: 0–20 ng/mL
	  Pregnant: 20–400 ng/mL
		Note those medications taken that may affect results. Drugs that may increase prolactin level include phenothiazines, oral contraceptives, reserpine, opiates, verapamil, histamine antagonists, monoamine oxidase (MAO) inhibitors, and antihistamines. Drugs that may decrease prolactin level include ergot alkaloid derivatives, clonidine, levodopa, and dopamine.
		Explain the procedure to the client.
		The blood specimen should be obtained in the morning and placed on ice if not taken immediately to the laboratory

Prostate-specific antigen (PSA)	PSA is an antigen detected in all males; level increases with prostatic cancer. It is more sensitive and specific than the acid phosphatase. Normal: < 4 ng/mL	Fasting is not required. Apply pressure to the venipuncture site. Observe the site for bleeding.

continues

Table 13–5 ADDITIONAL TESTS PERFORMED ON BLOOD SPECIMEN *continued*

TEST	EXPLANATION/NORMAL VALUES	NURSING RESPONSIBILITIES
Rheumatoid factor (RF)	Abnormal protein in serum of approximately 80% of clients with rheumatoid arthritis. Formed as a result of the reaction of IgM to an abnormal IgG. Also elevated in clients with other autoimmune diseases such as systemic lupus erythematosus. Normal: < 60 IU/mL	Fasting is preferred.
Schilling test	Determines vitamin B_{12} absorption by the intestine. Differentiates between pernicious anemia and gastrointestinal malabsorption problems. Normal: 8%–40% of the radioactive vitamin B_{12} is excreted in the urine within 24 hours.	Collect the urine for a 24- to 48-hour period. Laxatives are not given during the test, as they decrease the absorption of vitamin B_{12}.
Serum acid phosphatase (prostatic)	Serum measurement of prostatic acid phosphatase, elevated in malignancy; because it detects cancer in the later stages, no longer commonly used. Normal: 0.0–0.8 U/L	Apply pressure to the site. Observe the site for bleeding or hematoma.
Serum alkaline phosphatase	Serum measurement of alkaline phosphates, elevated in malignancy. Normal: 30–120 U/L	Apply pressure to the site. Observe the site for bleeding or hematoma.

Serum creatinine	Specific indicator of renal disease.
	
	Normal:
	  Male: 0.6–1.5 mg/dL
	  Female: 0.6–1.1 mg/dL
		Note those medications taken that may affect results, including amphotericin B, cephalosporins (cepfazolin [Ancef], cephalothin [Keflin]), methicillin, ascorbic acid, barbiturates, lithium carbonate, methyldopa (Aldomet), triamterene (Dyrenium).

Sickledex (sickle-cell test)	Screening test to determine the presence of Hgb S. Normal: no Hgb S If results are positive, a hemoglobin electrophoresis test is done.	There are no food or fluid restrictions. Note on the laboratory requisition whether the client had a blood transfusion in the past 3 to 4 months.
Thyroid-stimulating hormone (TSH), thyrotropin	Determines thyroid function as well as monitors exogenous thyroid replacement. Normal: 2–10 μU/mL, or 2–10 mU/L	Recent use of radioisotopes may affect test results. Severe illness may decrease TSH level. Note those medications taken that may affect results. Drugs that may increase TSH level include antithyroid drugs, lithium, potassium iodide, and TSH injection. Drugs that may decrease TSH level include aspirin, dopamine, heparin, steroids, and T_3. Explain the procedure to the client. The client should be relaxed and recumbent for 30 minutes before the test.
TSH stimulation test	Differentiates between primary and secondary hypothyroidism. Normal: none given	Explain the procedure to the client. Obtain baseline level of radioactive iodine intake or serum T_4. Administer 5–10 units of TSH intramuscularly for 3 days. Repeat radioactive iodine intake or T_4 as indicated for comparison studies.
Thyrotropin-releasing hormone (TRH) test, thyrotropin-releasing factor (TRF) test	Assesses the responsiveness of the anterior pituitary by its secretion of TSH in response to an IV injection of TRH. Also tests the function of the thyroid gland. Normal: undetectable to 15 μU/mL	Pregnancy may increase TSH response to TRH. Note those medications taken that may modify TSH response, including antithyroid drugs, aspirin, corticosteroids, estrogens, levodopa, and T_4. Explain the procedure to the client. Any thyroid preparations should be discontinued for 3–4 weeks before the test.

continues

Table 13–5 ADDITIONAL TESTS PERFORMED ON BLOOD SPECIMEN *continued*

TEST	EXPLANATION/NORMAL VALUES	NURSING RESPONSIBILITIES
Triiodothyronine (T_3) radio-immunoassay (T_3 by RIA)	Determines thyroid gland function Normal: 110–230 ng/dL, or 1.2–1.5 nmol/L	Radioisotope administration may interfere with test results. Pregnancy increases T_3 results. Note those medications taken that may affect results. Drugs that may increase T_3 level include: estrogen, methadone, and oral contraceptives. Drugs that may decrease T_4 level include anabolic steroids, androgens, phenytoin (Dilantin), propranolol (Inderal), reserpine, and salicylates (high dose). Explain the procedure to the client. Determine whether exogenous T_3 is being taken. With physician's approval, withhold those drugs that would interfere with test results.
Triiodothyronine (T_3) serum free	Measures the amount of free T_3 that actually enters the cells and is active in metabolism. A true indicator of thyroid activity. Can be used to diagnose thyroid status in pregnant females or clients on drugs that can interfere with results of other tests. Normal: 0.2–0.6 ng/dL	Explain the procedure to the client. Blood specimens for T_3 and T_4 uptake must be obtained to calculate T_3.
Thyroxine (T_4) Screen	Directly measures the amount of T_4 present. Normal: radioimmunoassay: 5–12 µg/dL, or 65–155 nmol/L	X-ray iodinated contrast studies may increase T_4 levels. Pregnancy will increase T_4 level. Note those medications taken that may affect results. Drugs that may increase T_4 level include clofibrate, estrogens, heroin, methadone, and oral contraceptives. Drugs that may decrease T_4 level include anabolic steroids, androgens, antithyroid drugs, lithium, phenytoin (Dilantin), and propranolol (Inderal). Explain the procedure to the client. Evaluate the client's drug history. If needed, instruct the client to stop exogenous T_4 medications for 1 month prior to test.
Thyroxine index free, FTI, FT_4 Index	Measures the amount of free T_4 that actually enters the cells and is active in metabolism. A true indicator of thyroid activity. Can be used to diagnose thyroid status in pregnant females or clients on drugs that can interfere with results of other tests. Normal: 0.8–2.4 ng/dL, or 10–31 pmol/L	Recent radionuclear scans can interfere with test results. Explain the procedure to the client. Blood specimens for T_4 and T_3 uptake must be obtained to calculate T_4.
Total iron-binding capacity (TIBC)	Determines the ability of iron to bind to a protein called transferrin. Normal: 250–420 ug/dL, or 45–73 umol/L	If possible, initiate NPO status 8 hours prior to the test. A recent blood transfusion or a diet high in iron may affect test results. Note whether the client is taking oral contraceptives, as these increase TIBC level.

Triglycerides	Form of fat produced in the liver.
	Normal:
	  Male: 40–160 mg/dL
	  Female: 35–135 mg/dL
		Instruct the client to fast for 12–14 hours prior to the test, and to have no alcohol for 24 hours before. Dietary intake for 2 weeks prior to the test affects results.

Total protein	Total measure of albumin and globulin. Normal: 6.4–8.3 g/dL	Note medications taken that affect results (see Albumin, this table). Instruct the client to avoid eating foods high in fat for 24 hours before the test.

Uric acid (serum, urine)	Elevated in gout.
	Normal, serum:
	  Male: 2.1–8.5 mg/dL
	  Female: 2.0–6.6 mg/dL
		There are no food or drink restrictions. Note those medications and other substances taken that may affect results, including ascorbic acid, diuretics, levadopa, allopurinol, and Coumadin.

continues

Table 13–5 ADDITIONAL TESTS PERFORMED ON BLOOD SPECIMEN *continued*

TEST	EXPLANATION/NORMAL VALUES	NURSING RESPONSIBILITIES
Uric acid (serum, urine) (*continued*)	Normal, urine: 250–750 mg/24 h	Label container with client's name and date/times of collection. Note those medications and other substances taken that may affect results, including corticosteroids and cytotoxic agents.
VDRL (Venereal Disease Research Laboratories), RPR (rapid plasma reagin), FTA-ABS (fluorescent treponemal antibody-absorption test), Reiter test, fluorescent antibody Treponema pallidum immobilization (TPI) test (performed only at Centers for Disease Control [CDC] in Atlanta)	Blood tests for presence of syphilis. Normal: negative or nonreactive	Explain the test to the client, including amount of blood to be drawn.
Western blot	Confirmatory test for the presence of antibodies to HIV. Normal: negative	Provide pretest counseling. Obtain informed consent. Provide or arrange post-test counseling.

Urine Tests

Urinalysis is performed to assist in the diagnosis of various conditions. Urine specimens are obtained to measure substances such as amylase, catecholamines, chloride, and certain hormones. Substances not normally found in the urine include RBCs, white blood cells (WBCs), protein, glucose, ketones, and casts. Tests often performed on a urine specimen are found in Table 13–6.

Urine pH

The pH is governed by the hydrogen ion concentration in the urine. Disorders such as diabetes mellitus, dehydration, diarrhea, emphysema, and starvation make the urine acidic. Chronic renal failure, renal tubular acidosis, urinary tract infections, and salicylate poisoning cause the urine to be alkaline.

Specific Gravity

Specific gravity measures the number of solutes in a solution. Urea and uric acid (the by–products of nitrogen metabolism) have the greatest influence on the specific gravity of urine. A urinometer and cylinder are used to measure specific gravity (Figure 13-3). The urinometer has a specific gravity scale and a weighted mercury bulb. A fresh urine specimen is poured into the cylinder, then the urinometer is twirled into the cylinder. When the urinometer stops spinning, the urinometer is read at eye level.

Figure 13-3 Urinometer measures specific gravity.

PROFESSIONAL TIP

Drugs and Laboratory Tests

Note drugs the client is taking when those drugs may influence the results of laboratory tests.

PROFESSIONAL TIP

Testing for Blood Lipid Level

To allow for the proper balance between the vascular and extravascular compartment and ensure valid test results, the blood should always be drawn after the client has been sitting quietly for 5 minutes.

Specific gravity increases with conditions that increase fluid loss from the body. Decreases in specific gravity result from renal disease. When the amount of urine increases and the specific gravity decreases, there is an absence of the antidiuretic hormone (ADH), usually triggered by diabetes insipidus (a disorder of the posterior pituitary gland).

Urine Glucose

When the blood level of glucose exceeds the renal threshold (180 mg/dL), glucose spills into the urine. Many agents are available for measuring the glucose content of urine, although these agents are not as accurate as is measuring the blood glucose level.

Urine Ketones

Ketones, products of incomplete fat metabolism, are completely metabolized by the liver under normal conditions. The most common cause of ketonuria (excessive ketones in the urine) is diabetes.

Urine Cells and Casts

Normally, the urine is free of blood cells and casts. When the renal system is impaired, as in cases of renal damage or failure, nephritis, and urinary stones or infections, the following can occur:

Table 13–6 TESTS PERFORMED ON URINE

TEST	EXPLANATION/NORMAL VALUES	NURSING RESPONSIBILITIES
Urinalysis		Explain the procedure and purpose to the client and assist with specimen collection, if needed.
Color	Clear amber	Ensure that specimen is taken to the laboratory in a timely manner.
Odor	Pleasantly aromatic until left standing; offensive and unpleasant in kidney infection.	
pH	4.6–8.0	
Specific gravity	1.005–1.030	
Glucose	Negative	
Acetone (ketone)	Negative	
Casts	Rare	
Albumin (protein)	Negative	
RBCs	2–3/HPF	
WBCs	4–5/HPF	
Bilirubin	Negative	
Bacteria	Negative	

Aldosterone Assay	A blood test or 24-hour urine collection to evaluate the adrenal cortex, especially for tumors. The 24-hour urine is more reliable, but the blood specimen is more convenient.
	
	Normal, blood:
	  Supine: 3–10 ng/dL, or 0.08–0.30 nmol/L
	  Upright:
	    Male: 6–22 ng/dL, or 0.17–0.61 nmol/L
	    Female: 5–30 ng/dL, or 0.14–0.80 nmol/L
	Normal, urine: 2–80 μg/24 h, or 5.5–72.0 nmol/24 h
		Strenuous exercise and stress can increase aldosterone level.
		
		Excessive licorice ingestion can decrease aldosterone level.
		
		Posture, dietary sodium, and pregnancy can interfere with test results.
		
		Note those medications taken that may affect results. Drugs that may increase aldosterone level include diazoxide, hydralazine, and nitroprusside. Drugs that may decrease aldosterone level include fludrocortisone and propranolol (Inderal).
		
		Explain the procedure to the client. The client should follow a normal diet with 3 grams of sodium/day and no licorice for at least 2 weeks before the test. Medications should be stopped for at least 2 weeks before the test, if possible.
		
		Blood: Blood should be drawn before the client gets out of bed. A second blood specimen might be obtained 4 hours later. Indicate on laboratory requisition time and client position. Transport blood specimen on ice to the laboratory.

continues

Table 13–6 TESTS PERFORMED ON URINE *continued*

TEST	EXPLANATION/NORMAL VALUES	NURSING RESPONSIBILITIES
Aldosterone Assay (*continued*)		24-hour urine: Initiate 24-hour urine collection after discarding first specimen. Post signs with times of collection. Each voiding does not have to be measured. Instruct the client not to contaminate urine with feces or toilet tissue. Force fluids unless medically contraindicated. Collection must be preserved and refrigerated. Indicate times of collection and any drugs that might interfere with results on laboratory requisition. Send collection to laboratory immediately upon conclusion.
Bence Jones Protein	Bence Jones proteins are immunoglobulins typically found in the urine of clients with multiple myeloma. They may also be associated with tumor metastases to the bone and chronic lymphocytic leukemia. Normal: no Bence Jones proteins present in urine.	Instruct the client to collect an early morning urine specimen of at least 50 mL. Instruct the client not to contaminate specimen with toilet paper or stool.
Creatinine clearance	Normal: Male: 95–135 mL/min Female: 85–125 mL/min Minimum: 10 mL/min to maintain life	Instruct the client about the 24-hour urine test. Encourage hourly water intake. Keep urine on ice or in special refrigerator. Drugs that affect results include phenacetin, anabolic steroids, thiazides, ascorbic acid, levodopa, methyldopa (Aldomet), phenolsulfonphthalein (PSP) (test).
17-hydroxycorticosteroids (17-OHCS)	24-hour urine test that measures adrenal cortex function. Normal: Male: 4.5–10.0 mg/24 h Female: 2.5–10.0 mg/24 h	Emotional or physical stress or licorice ingestion may increase adrenal activity. Note those medications taken that may affect results. Drugs that may increase 17-OHCS level include acetazolamide, chloral hydrate, chlorpromazine, colchicine, erythromycin, meprobamate, paraldehyde, quinidine, quinine, and spironolactone. Drugs that may decrease 17-OHCS level include estrogens, oral contraceptives, phenothiazines, and reserpine. Explain the procedure to the client. Initiate 24-hour urine collection after discarding first specimen. Post signs with times of collection. Each voiding does not have to be measured. Instruct the client not to contaminate urine with feces or toilet tissue. Force fluids unless medically contraindicated. Collection must be refrigerated. Indicate on laboratory requisition times of collection and any drugs that might interfere with results. Send collection to laboratory immediately upon conclusion.
17-ketosteroids (17-KS)	24-hour urine test that measures adrenal cortex function. Normal: Male: 7–25 mg/24 h, or 24–88 μmol/24 h Female: 4–15 mg/24 h, or 14–52 μmol/24 h	Stress may increase adrenal activity. Note medications taken that may affect results. Drugs that increase 17-KS level include antibiotics, chloramphenicol, chlorpromazine, dexamethasone, meprobamate, phenothiazines, quinidine, secobarbital, and spironolactone. Drugs that may decrease 17-KS level include estrogen, oral contraceptives, probenecid, promazine, reserpine, salicylates (prolonged use), and thiazide diuretics. Explain the procedure to the client. With physician's approval, withhold all drugs for several days before test. Monitor client for stress and report to physician. Initiate 24-hour urine collection after discarding first specimen. Post signs with times of collection. Each voiding does not have to be measured. Instruct the client not to contaminate urine with feces or toilet tissue. Force fluids

continues

Table 13–6   TESTS PERFORMED ON URINE *continued*

TEST	EXPLANATION/NORMAL VALUES	NURSING RESPONSIBILITIES
17-ketosteroids (17-KS) (*continued*)		unless medically contraindicated. Collection must be preserved and refrigerated. Indicate on laboratory requisition times of collection and any drugs that might interfere with results. Send collection to laboratory immediately upon conclusion.
Urine cortisol, hydrocortisone	24-hour urine test that measures adrenal cortex function. Normal: 10–100 µg/24 h, or 27–276 nmol/24 h	Pregnancy or stress increases cortisol level. Recent radioisotope scans can interfere with test result. Note medications taken that may interfere with test result, including oral contraceptives and spironolactone. Explain the procedure to the client. Assess for stress and report to physician. Initiate 24-hour urine collection after discarding first specimen. Post signs with times of collection. Each voiding does not have to be measured. Instruct the client not to contaminate urine with feces or toilet tissue. Force fluids unless medically contraindicated. Collection must be preserved and refrigerated. Indicate on laboratory requisition times of collection and any drugs that might interfere with results. Send collection to laboratory immediately upon conclusion.

Vanillylmandelic acid (VMA) and catecholamines (epinephrine, norepinephrine, metanephrine, normetanephrine, dopamine)	24-hour urine test that diagnoses pheochromocytoma and other adrenal tumors.
	Normal:
	  VMA: 2–7 mg/24 h, or 10–35 µmol/24 h
	  Epinephrine: 0.5–20.0 µg/24 h, or < 275 nmol/24 h
	  Norepinephrine: 15–80 µg/24 h
	  Metanephrine: 24–96 µg/24 h
	  Normetanephrine: 75–375 µg/24 h
	  Dopamine: 65–400 µg/24 h
		Certain foods (e.g., tea, coffee, cocoa, vanilla, chocolate), vigorous exercise, stress, or starvation may increase VMA level.
		
		Uremia, alkaline urine, or iodinated contrast dyes may falsely decrease VMA level.
		
		Note those medications taken that may affect results. Drugs that may increase VMA level include caffeine, epinephrine, levodopa, lithium, and nitroglycerine. Drugs that may decrease VMA level include clonidine, disulfiram (Antabuse), guanethidine, imipramine, MAO inhibitors, phenothiazines, and reserpine. Drugs that may increase catecholamine level include ethyl alcohol, aminophylline, caffeine, chloral hydrate, clonidine (chronic therapy), contrast media (iodine containing), disulfiram (Antabuse), epinephrine, erythromycin, insulin, methenamine, methyldopa, nicotinic acid (large doses), nitroglycerin, quinidine, riboflavin, and tetracyclines. Drugs that may decrease catecholamine level include guanethidine, reserpine, and salicylates.
		
		Explain the procedure to the client. The client should be on a VMA-restricted diet for 2–3 days before the test. Items restricted include coffee, tea, bananas, chocolate, cocoa, licorice, citrus fruit, anything with vanilla, and aspirin. Client should not take antihypertensive drugs before the test.
		
		Initiate 24-hour urine collection after discarding first specimen. Post signs with times of collection. Each voiding does not have to be measured. Instruct the client not to contaminate urine with feces or toilet tissue. Collection may need to be preserved (consult laboratory) and is to be refrigerated. Indicate times of collection and any drugs that might interfere with results.

- Bleeding, resulting in RBCs in the urine
- Accumulation of epithelial cells accompanied by cast formation
- WBCs in the urine, which indicate infection

Stool Tests

Stool specimens are collected for examination of both normal substances (such as urobilinogen) and blood, bacteria, and parasites (Table 13–7).

Urobilinogen

Urobilinogen is a colorless derivative of bilirubin formed by the normal bacterial action of intestinal flora on bilirubin. It increases in the presence of severe hemolysis and decreases in the presence of most biliary obstructions.

Occult Blood

Occult blood is invisible on inspection; it is blood in the stool that can be detected only with a microscope or by chemical means. In the gastrointestinal tract, the digestive process acts on blood, making it occult. Random sampling for occult blood is done to diagnose gastrointestinal bleeding, ulcers, and malignant tumors.

To decrease the possibility of a false-positive result when occult blood is to be used to confirm suspicions of a gastrointestinal disorder, the client is placed on a 3-day diet free of meat, poultry, and fish. Common drugs that can cause a false-positive test for occult blood are salicylate, steroids, and indomethacin.

Parasites

The gastrointestinal tract can harbor parasites and their eggs (ova). Whereas some of these parasites are harmless, others cause clinical symptoms. With the exception of pinworms (which can enter the body through both the oral and anal routes), most common parasites enter the body through the mouth when contaminated water or food is ingested.

PROFESSIONAL TIP

Cultures

All culture tests should be performed before initiating antibiotic therapy so as to identify the type of pathogen and its sensitivity to specific antibiotics.

Culture and Sensitivity Tests

Culture refers to the growing of microorganisms to identify the pathogen. Culture and **sensitivity** (C&S) tests are performed to identify both the nature of the invading organism and its susceptibility to commonly used antibiotics. Sensitivity allows the practitioner to select the appropriate antibiotic therapy. All C&S specimens should be taken immediately to the laboratory.

Blood Culture

Bacteremia is bacteria in the blood. The blood culture should be obtained while the client is experiencing chills and fever. A series of three venipuncture collections are performed using strict sterile technique. The needle should be changed after the specimen is collected and before injecting the blood sample into the test tube.

Throat (Swab) Culture

The throat normally hosts many organisms. Throat cultures serve to isolate and identify such pathogens as beta-hemolytic streptococci, *Staphylococcus aureus,* meningococci, gonococci, *Bordetella pertussis,* and *Corynebacterium diphtheria.* A throat swab is commonly done to identify streptococcal infections, which, if left untreated, can cause rheumatic fever or glomerulonephritis.

To obtain a throat swab, the nurse uses a wooden blade to depress the tongue and swabs the white patches, exudate, or ulcerations of the throat using a

Table 13–7 TESTS PERFORMED ON STOOL

TEST	EXPLANATION/NORMAL VALUES	NURSING RESPONSIBILITIES
Stool occult blood (guaiac) Fecal occult blood test (FOBT) Hemocult	Fecal occult blood screening studies may be utilized as possible indicators of colorectal cancer. Normal: negative for blood	Place a smear of stool on a card. Medications such as anticoagulants, aspirin, iron preparations, NSAIDs, and steroids may cause a false-positive result, whereas vitamin C may cause a false negative. Red meat should not be ingested for 3 days prior to the test. Wear gloves when obtaining and handling the specimen.
Stool O & P (ova & parasite)	A positive result indicates infection. Normal: negative	Place the stool specimen in a container and take warm to the laboratory.

sterile applicator. The applicator should not touch any other parts of the mouth. Once the swab is obtained, the applicator should be placed in a sterile container.

Sputum Culture

Sputum tests performed include culture, smear, and cytology. Sputum is created by the mucous glands and goblet cells of the tracheobronchial tree and is raised by coughing. Sputum is sterile until it reaches the throat and mouth, where it comes in contact with normal flora. To yield a more accurate identification of pulmonary organisms, sputum can be obtained by tracheobronchial suctioning and transtracheal aspiration.

In addition to the same organism(s) found in a culture, a sputum smear identifies eosinophils, epithelial cells, and other substances. Smears are helpful in diagnosing asthma (eosinophils) and fungal infections. The specimen must be refrigerated if it cannot be taken immediately to the laboratory.

Sputum **cytology** (the study of cells) is performed to diagnose cancer of the lungs. The specimen should be collected early in the morning and after a deep cough.

Urine Culture

Urinary C&S tests are performed whenever a urinary tract infection is suspected.

Stool Culture

Stool C&S is performed to identify bacterial infections. If the client has diarrhea, a rectal swab can be taken and used as a specimen. Fecal material must be visible on the swab in order for the laboratory to perform the test.

Papanicolaou Test

The **Papanicolaou test** (a smear method of examining stained exfoliative cells), commonly called a Pap smear, is performed to evaluate the cellular maturity, metabolic activity, and morphological variations of cervical tissue. Papanicolaou testing can also be done on specimens from other organs, such as bronchial aspirations and gastric secretions.

RADIOLOGICAL STUDIES

Radiography (the study of film exposed to x-rays or gamma rays through the action of ionizing radiation) is used by the practitioner to study internal organ structure. When used in conjunction with a **contrast medium** (a radiopaque substance that facilitates roentgen imaging of the body's internal structures), **fluoroscopy** (immediate, serial images of the body's structure and function) reveals the motion of organs. X-rays are valuable to the practitioner in either formu-

CLIENT TEACHING

Pap Smear

Advise female clients to prepare for a Pap smear by:

- Avoiding intercourse, douches, and vaginal creams for 24 hours before the test and
- Informing the practitioners if they are menstruating, as the test will need to be delayed.

Cervical Pap smear testing is recommended every 2 to 3 years after the onset of sexual activity. Annual testing is indicated for those women who:

- Are over 40 years of age,
- Have a family history of cervical cancer, and/or
- Previously had a positive Pap smear.

lating a diagnosis or helping to determine the necessity for other studies (e.g., a lung lesion requiring biopsy to differentiate between a benign or malignant tumor).

Certain radiological tests require a contrast medium that might interfere with other diagnostic studies. Barium and iodine are commonly used contrast media. Laboratory blood samples measuring thyroid function should be drawn before initiating an intravenous pyelogram (IVP), where radioactive iodine dye is administered. If the client needs both an IVP and a barium enema, the IVP is performed first because the barium is likely to decrease visualization of the kidneys. Commonly performed radiological studies are described in Table 13–8.

Safety: X-rays

- Prior to scheduling x-rays, question the client about the possibility of pregnancy, asthma, and allergic reactions to contrast media (iodine) as well as to other foods and drugs.
- If the client has not previously received iodine, note this on the requisition to indicate that allergic status is unknown.

PROFESSIONAL TIP

Contrast Media

Carefully monitor those clients who are scheduled for dye injection studies and have a history of allergies to any foods or drugs (particularly fish or iodine), because such allergies may predispose these clients to allergic reactions to contrast media.

Table 13–8 RADIOLOGIC STUDIES

TEST	EXPLANATION/NORMAL VALUES	NURSING RESPONSIBILITIES
Radiograph (x-ray)	Most common diagnostic study. Identifies traumatic disorders, i.e., fractures, dislocations, tumors, bone disorders, joint deformities, bone density, and changes in bone relationships. Performed by a technician.	Explain the procedure to the client. Prepare the client as ordered. No specific post procedure care is required. Administer an analgesic, especially for the arthritic client.
Abdominal x-rays	Determines diaphragm position and gas and fluid distribution in the abdomen.	No preparation is required.
Adrenal angiography, Adrenal arteriogram	Study of adrenal glands and arterial system after injection of radiopaque dye to detect benign or malignant tumors or hyperplasia of the adrenal glands. Normal: no growth or enlargement	Assess for allergy to shellfish or iodine; arteriosclerosis; pregnancy; or blood disorders, as they preclude the test. Explain the procedure to the client. Assess for allergies. Informed and written consent must be obtained before the procedure. Note whether client has been taking anticoagulants. Initiate NPO status after midnight. Mark peripheral pulses with a pen before the procedure. Inform the client that a warm flush may be felt when the dye is injected. Observe the puncture site. Monitor vital signs. Monitor peripheral pulses, color, and temperature of extremities. Institute bed rest for 12–24 hours. Apply cold compresses to puncture site, if needed. Force fluids to prevent possible dehydration from the dye.
Adrenal venography	Involves insertion of a catheter through the femoral vein and into the adrenal vein to withdraw a blood specimen to detect the function of each adrenal gland. A contrast dye is injected to visualize size and position of the adrenal glands. Normal: no growth or enlargement	Explain the procedure to the client. Assess for allergies. Obtain informed and written consent. Inform the client that a burning sensation may be experienced when the dye is injected. Although this study involves the venous system, monitor vital signs and injection site as well as pulses, temperature, and color of extremities.
Arthrogram (-graphy)	Visualization of a joint. Radiopaque dye or air is injected into the joint cavity to outline soft tissue, usually on knee/shoulder joints. Local anesthetic and sterile technique are used. Performed by a physician; takes approximately 30 minutes.	Explain the procedure to the client. Obtain informed consent. Client wears an elastic bandage for several days; check for edema. Administer a mild analgesic for pain. Monitor for increased pain. Neither fasting nor sedation is required.
Barium enema	An enema of barium is given while x-rays are taken of the large intestine.	Initiate NPO status the night before. Administer the ordered medication to clean the bowel. Observe the results of the laxatives, and inform the x-ray department if there have been no results. After the test, force oral fluids and administer a cleansing enema, as ordered. Document status of abdomen and stools.
Barium swallow	The client drinks a glass of barium while x-rays are taken of the esophagus and cardiac sphincter.	Initiate NPO status the evening before. Explain the procedure and the time frame for results. Encourage the client to drink fluids and eat fiber after the test. A laxative is sometimes given after the test. The client should be instructed that bowel movements will be white for 1–2 days. During the test, the client will be tilted on the x-ray table in various positions. There may be repeated pictures taken at ½-hour intervals as the barium moves through the bowel. Document the client's tolerance of the procedure and passage of the barium. Because the procedure can be lengthy, encourage the client to take reading material.
Cardiac catheterization (cardiac angiogram, coronary arteriogram)	A catheter is passed into the right and/or left side of the heart to determine oxygen level, cardiac output, and pressure within the heart chambers.	Assess the client for allergy to iodine or shellfish. The client is to fast for 6 hours prior to the test, but medications can be taken with sips of water. Inform the client of the possibility of feeling warm or flushed during the test.

continues

Table 13–8 RADIOLOGIC STUDIES continued

TEST	EXPLANATION/NORMAL VALUES	NURSING RESPONSIBILITIES
Cardiac catheterization (*continued*)		After the procedure, assess the peripheral pulses every 15 minutes for 2–4 hours, or according to physician's orders. Assess color, temperature, and pulse in the extremity below the catheter insertion site. Instruct the client to keep the involved extremity straight for 6–8 hours.
Chest x-ray	Provides a two-dimensional image of the lungs without using contrast media. Used to detect the presence of fluid within the interstitial lung tissue or the alveoli; tumors or foreign bodies; and the presence and size of a pneumothorax. The size of the heart can also be determined by chest x-ray.	Explain the test to the client. If appropriate, inquire whether the client may be pregnant, to prevent exposure of the fetus to x-ray. The client is generally required to stand for various views; if the client is unable to stand, views may be obtained with the client in a sitting position, or a portable x-ray may be obtained. Instruct the client to inspire deeply and hold the breath. Instruct the client to remove all metal objects from the chest and neck area and to don a hospital gown that does not have snap closures.
Conduitogram	Radiopaque dye is injected through a catheter into either the conduit or a piece of ileum to assess by means of x-ray the length and emptying ability of the conduit as well as the presence of stricture or obstruction.	A conduit is a connection between the bladder or pouch and the outside of the body. Explain the procedure to the client. Assess the client for allergies to iodine-based dye.
Fistula gram	Radiopaque dye or barium is given to drink, and x-rays are taken as the dye or barium passes through the gastrointestinal tract. The dye shows the location of the fistula and how it is connected to the gastrointestinal tract.	Initiate NPO status as ordered. Explain the procedure and the time frame for the results and identify the person who will give the client the results.
Fluoresce in angiography	Following IV injection of sodium fluorescein, rapid-sequence photographs of the fundus are taken with a special camera. Visualization of microvascular structures of the retina and choroid are enhanced, allowing evaluation of the entire retinal vascular bed.	Instill eye drops to dilate the pupils. Start an IV so the sodium fluorescein can be injected. Remove the IV following completion of the test. Inform the client that skin and urine may be yellow for 24–48 hours.
Gallbladder series	X-ray visualization of the gallbladder.	Administer dye tablets the evening before the test. Provide a low-fat or fat-free meal the evening before. Initiate NPO status except for water after taking the dye.
Hysterosalpingogram	Radiopaque dye is instilled through the cervix. Used to diagnose uterine cavity and tubal abnormalities. Performed as a part of an infertility workup.	Explain the procedure and prepare the client in the lithotomy position. The test is done in the radiology department. Inquire about allergies to iodine or other dyes. Assist the physician.
Intravenous pyelogram (IVP)	Infusion of radiopaque dye into a vein, allowing visualization of the urinary system. The renal pelvis, ureters, and bladder can be seen.	Explain the procedure to the client. Explain that client will experience a warm feeling during dye injection. Ask the client about allergy to iodine or shellfish. Serve a light supper, then initiate NPO status overnight. Administer a laxative or enema. Schedule test before barium studies. Post-test, observe for untoward reaction to dye. Encourage fluids for 24 hours to eliminate dye.
Kidney-ureter-bladder x-ray (KUB)	Shows abnormalities such as calculi, tumors, or changes in anatomic position.	Explain the procedure to the client. No preparation is required.
Long bone x-rays	Serial x-rays of the long bones to determine bone growth.	Explain the procedure to the client. Instruct the client to keep extremities still while the x-ray is being taken. Shield ovaries, testes, or pregnant uterus. Remove all metallic objects from area being x-rayed.

continues

Table 13–8 RADIOLOGIC STUDIES *continued*

TEST	EXPLANATION/NORMAL VALUES	NURSING RESPONSIBILITIES
Lymphangiogram	A contrast dye is injected into the lymph vessels in the hands or feet to examine the lymph vessels and nodes. Used to stage lymphomas and evaluate the effectiveness of chemotherapy and radiation therapy. Normal: Normal-sized lymph nodes with no malignant cells	The dye remains in the lymph nodes for 6 months to 1 year, so disease progress can be evaluated with an x-ray. Obtain informed consent. Inform the client that if a blue-colored dye is used, the skin and urine may have a bluish discoloration. Assess the client's breath sounds after the procedure, as lipoid pneumonia is a possible complication if the dye gets into the thoracic duct.
Mammography	Used to diagnose benign and malignant disorders of the breast.	Explain the procedure to the client. The breast will be compressed, possibly causing discomfort for several seconds. Explain that it is important to have a baseline mammogram done between the ages of 35 and 40 and a breast examination done by a physician or nurse practitioner every 3–4 years. For women ages 40–49, a mammogram should be performed every 1–2 years; for those over 50, an annual mammogram is recommended along with an annual breast examination by physician or nurse practitioner.
Myelogram	X-ray of spinal subarachnoid space following injection of an opaque medium.	Follow nursing responsibilities for lumbar puncture in Table 27-14. Inform the client that the table may be tilted during the procedure. Obtain informed consent according to facility guidelines. Withhold the meal prior to procedure. Administer a light sedative, if ordered. Postprocedure care is determined by the type of medium used; follow physician's orders for activity and fluids.
Pouchogram	Installation of radiopaque dye into the Kock or Indiana pouch. Done with the continent ostomies to determine the state of healing and size of the pouch created.	Assess the client for allergy to iodine. Explain the procedure to the client.
Pulmonary angiography	Assesses the arterial circulation of the lungs. Most often used to detect pulmonary emboli.	Explain the procedure to the client. Assess for allergy to iodine or shellfish. Inform the client that an arterial puncture is required, usually of the femoral artery, and that injection of the dye may cause a flushing or warm sensation due to vasodilation. After the study, assess the arterial puncture site frequently for evidence of bleeding. Assess vital signs and respiratory status. The client may be required to lie flat for up to 6 hours if the femoral artery is used for access. Obtain informed consent per facility policy.
Renal angiography	A catheter is inserted into the femoral artery and threaded into the renal artery. Dye is injected to show blood vessels in the kidney.	Initiate NPO status; administer enema. Assess client for allergy to iodine or shellfish. Check vital signs and peripheral pulses. Institute post-test bedrest, with leg straight. Monitor vital signs, peripheral pulses, urine output, and puncture site.
Voiding cystourethrography	The bladder is filled with dye, and x-rays are taken to observe bladder filling and emptying. Detects structural abnormalities of the bladder and urethra and reflux into the ureters.	Administer enema. Insert a Foley catheter and inject dye into bladder while x-rays are taken. Remove catheter and ask the client to void while more x-rays are taken. Allow the client to express feelings, as this test may be embarrassing.

continues

Table 13–8 RADIOLOGIC STUDIES *continued*

TEST	EXPLANATION/NORMAL VALUES	NURSING RESPONSIBILITIES
Computed tomography (CT) scan	Provides a three-dimensional cross sectional view of tissues. Computer-constructed picture interprets densities of various tissues. Most useful for viewing tumors in the chest, abdominal cavity, and brain.	Explain the procedure to the client. Obtain informed consent. Remove wigs and hairpins and clips for head CT. Initiate NPO status 8 hours prior to scan. Assess for iodine allergy. Observe for signs of anaphylaxis, if dye is used. Check for claustrophobia. Inform the client that the test will take approximately 45 minutes to 1 hour. The client must lie still on a hard, flat table and will be put through a large machine. Because barium will interfere with the test, schedule tests using barium either after or 4 or more days before the scan.
Cardiac positron emission tomography (PET) scan	Radioactive tracers are injected intravenously prior to the test. Nuclear imaging is used to confirm tissue that has adequate blood supply and tissue that has become impaired due to a lack of blood.	Instruct the client not to have caffeine for 18 hours and not to smoke for 4 hours prior to the test. Initiate NPO status from 10 P.M. the evening before the test, except for medications and water. Obtain informed written consent. Encourage the client to drink fluids after the procedure to facilitate faster excretion of the radioactive material.
Orbital CT scan	Allows visualization of abnormalities not readily seen on standard x-rays, delineating size, position, and relationship to adjoining structures. The orbital CT is a series of images reconstructed by a computer and displayed as anatomic slices on an oscilloscope. It identifies space-occupying lesions earlier and more accurately than do other x-ray techniques. It also provides three-dimensional images of orbital structures, especially the ocular muscles and optic nerve. Enhancement with a contrast agent may help define ocular tissue and circulation abnormalities.	Explain the test and the procedure to the client: that the client is positioned on an x-ray table; that the head of the table is moved into the scanner; that the scanner rotates during the test and may make loud, crackling sounds; that if an IV contrast agent is required, the client may feel flushed and warm or experience a transient headache; and that salty taste, nausea, and vomiting may occur following injection of the IV contrast dye. Reassure the client that the reaction is common and she may signal the technician if she is unable to tolerate the test.

Chest X-Ray

The most common radiological study is the noninvasive, noncontrasted chest x-ray. Radiographic projections of chest x-ray films are taken from various views (Figure 13-4), because the practitioner needs multiple views of the chest to assess the entire lung field. To prepare for a chest x-ray, the client should remove all clothing from the waist up and don a gown. The client should also remove all metal objects (jewelry), as metal will appear on the x-ray film, thereby obscuring visualization of parts of the chest. Pregnant women are advised against x-rays; however if x-ray is absolutely necessary, the woman should be draped with a lead apron to protect the fetus.

Computed Tomography

Computed tomography (CT) is the radiological scanning of the body. X-ray beams and radiation detectors transmit data to a computer that transcribes the data into quantitative measurement and multidimensional images of the internal structures. Figure 13-5 illustrates the sagittal, transverse, and coronal planes used in CT scanning.

The procedure requires the client's informed consent. Because the client will be positioned on the scanning table and told to remain motionless, the client's cooperation is essential during the CT scanning. The nurse should prepare the client by providing an explanation and pictures of what to expect.

Safety: Contrast Media

If a contrast medium is used, observe the client for indicators of allergic reaction to the dye, such as respiratory distress, urticaria, hives, nausea, vomiting, decreased production of urine (**oliguria**), and decreased blood pressure.

PROFESSIONAL TIP

Computed Tomography

Assess the client's ability to relax, and review imagery relaxation. Sedation can be administered with an order from the practitioner.

PA chest x-rays travel from posterior to anterior

A.P. chest x-rays travel from anterior to posterior

Posteroanterior (PA) projection

Anteroposterior (AP) projection

Lateral (Lat.) position

Left posterior oblique (LPO) position

Figure 13-4 Radiographic Projection Positions

Sagittal

Transverse

Coronal

Figure 13-5 Computed Tomography

Barium Studies

Barium (a chalky white contrast medium) is a preparation that permits roentgenographic visualization of the internal structures of the digestive tract. The results of barium studies can reveal congenital abnormalities, lesions, spasm, reflux, stricture, obstruction, inflammation, ulceration, varices, and fistula.

Angiography

Angiography allows visualization of the vascular structures through the use of fluoroscopy in conjunction with a contrast medium. The test reveals the blood flow to the heart, lungs, brain, kidneys, and lower extremities. It is also useful in diagnosing an **aneurysm** (weakness in the wall of a blood vessel).

Arteriography

Arteriography is the radiographic study of the vascular system following injection of a radiopaque dye through a catheter. The practitioner uses fluoroscopy to thread the catheter through a peripheral artery and into the area to be studied, such as the aorta or the cerebral, coronary, pulmonary, renal, iliac, femoral, or popliteal artery. The client is placed on a cardiac monitor. Dye is injected through the vascular catheter, and a rapid sequence of films is taken to visualize the vasculature.

Dye Injection Studies

Iodine is a common dye used in radiographic studies. Iodine injection might cause the client to experience the following temporary symptoms: shortness of breath; nausea; and a warm to hot flushed sensation. Most dye injections studies are invasive and thus require written consent.

ULTRASONOGRAPHY

An **ultrasound,** also called an echogram or sonogram, is a noninvasive procedure that uses high-frequency sound waves to visualize deep body structures. To ensure accuracy, this procedure should be scheduled before any studies requiring the use of a contrast medium or air, because the contrast medium would reflect the sound waves differently than body structures do. The client is instructed to lie still during the procedure.

Ultrasound is used to evaluate the brain, thyroid gland, heart, vascular structures, abdominal aorta, spleen, liver, gallbladder, pancreas, and pelvis. An ultrasound is commonly done during pregnancy to evaluate the size of the fetus and placenta. A full bladder is needed to ensure visualization.

To increase the contact between the skin and the **transducer** (instrument that converts electrical energy to sound waves), a coupling agent (lubricant) is placed on the surface of the body area to be studied. The transducer emits waves that travel through the body tissue and are reflected back to the transducer and recorded. The varying density of body tissues deflects the waves into a differentiated pattern on an oscilloscope. Photographs can be taken of the sound wave pattern on the oscilloscope. Table 13–9 describes some ultrasound tests.

Table 13–9 ULTRASOUND TESTS

TEST	EXPLANATION/NORMAL VALUES	NURSING RESPONSIBILITIES
Ultrasound	High-frequency ultrasound waves are sent into the body, and echoes are recorded as they strike tissues of different densities, producing an image or photograph. Useful in distinguishing between cystic and solid masses. Most often used to assess the pelvis, heart, and abdomen. Diagnostic for cysts, tumors, pregnancy, fetal gestational age, and multiple gestation.	Explain the procedure to the client. Most ultrasound tests require no special preparation: Pelvic sonogram: Instruct the client to have a full bladder. Abdominal sonogram: Initiate NPO status at bedtime; prepare bowel as directed. Gallbladder sonogram: Initiate NPO status for 12 hours and institute a fat-free diet the evening before the test. Vaginal sonogram: Client does not need to have a full bladder.
Doppler ultrasound	Determines patency of veins and arteries in conditions such as arterial occlusive disease, arteriosclerotic disease, or Raynaud's disease. Normal: audible "swishing" sound of the Doppler when placed over vessel A Doppler unit with blood pressure cuffs can measure the pulse volume of arteries and veins. An AB index is obtained by dividing the blood pressure reading in the ankle by the blood pressure reading in the arm (brachial artery). This is known as the ankle-to-brachial arterial blood pressure. There should be a less than 20 mm Hg difference between the pressure in the lower extremity as compared to the pressure in the upper extremity. Normal, AB index: 0.85 or greater	Inform the client that the procedure is painless. Remove clothing from the extremity being evaluated. Instruct the client not to smoke for 30 minutes prior to the test, because nicotine causes vasoconstriction of the vessels. Remove conductive or acoustic gel from the skin after the test is completed.
Echocardiogram	An ultrasound of the heart to determine hypertrophies, cardiomyopathies, or congenital defects. Very helpful in diagnosing valve abnormalities and pericardial effusion.	Explain the procedure to the client and assure the client that there is no discomfort during the procedure, although some pressure may be felt on the chest wall from the transducer.
Thyroid ultrasound	Detects the size, shape, and position of the thyroid gland.	Explain the procedure to the client: that the client will lie supine, with the neck hyperextended; that breathing or swallowing will not be affected by the sound transducer; that a liberal amount of lubricating gel will be placed on the neck for the transducer; and that a series of photos will be taken over a 15-minute period. Assist the client in removing the lubricant.
Transrectal bladder ultrasound	Produces an image of the prostate or bladder and surrounding tissue.	Explain the procedure to the client.

Table 13–10 MAGNETIC RESONANCE IMAGING

TEST	EXPLANATION/NORMAL VALUES	NURSING RESPONSIBILITIES
Magnetic resonance imaging (MRI)	Uses magnetic field and radio waves to detect edema, hemorrhage, blood flow, infarcts, tumors, infections, aneurysms, demyelinating disease, muscular disease, skeletal abnormalities, intervertebral disk problems, and causes of spinal cord compression. Provides greater tissue discrimination than do chest x-ray or CT scans. Performed by qualified technologist. Takes approximately 1 hour.	Assess the client for the presence of metal objects within the body (i.e., shrapnel, cochlear implants, pacemakers). Explain the procedure to the client: that the client will be required to lie still for up to 20 minutes at a time; that the client will be placed within a scanning tunnel; that sedation may be required if the client has claustrophobic tendencies; that the magnet will make a loud thumping noise as images are obtained (provide earplugs as necessary). As the test may require up to 2 hours to perform, have the client void prior to entering the scanning tunnel. Obtain informed written consent, per facility policy.

MAGNETIC RESONANCE IMAGING

Magnetic resonance imaging (MRI) uses radiowaves and a strong magnetic field to make continuous cross-sectional images of the body. A noniodine IV paramagnetic contrast agent may be used during the study. The study reveals lesions and changes in the body's organs, tissues, and vascular and skeletal structures (Table 13–10).

RADIOACTIVE STUDIES

Radionuclide imaging (nuclear scanning) uses radionuclides (or radiopharmaceuticals) to image the morphological and functional changes in the body's structure. A scintigraphic scanner is placed over the area of study to detect emitted radiation and produce a visual image of the structure on film. Radiopharmaceutical agents are administered by various routes, with consideration given to time delays of absorption. The results reveal congenital abnormalities, lesions, skeletal changes, infections, and glandular and organ enlargement (Table 13–11).

Table 13–11 RADIOACTIVE STUDIES

TEST	EXPLANATION/NORMAL VALUES	NURSING RESPONSIBILITIES
Scan (radioisotope test)	A radioactive substance or isotope is taken up by the part of the body being examined. Organ sites most frequently studied are the liver, spleen, lungs, heart, urinary tract, thyroid, and brain. The radioactive substance is given orally or intravenously by nuclear medicine personnel.	Explain the procedure to the client: that the client must lie still for 30–60 minutes and that the machine makes clicking noise at times. For liver, spleen, lung, thyroid, and brain scans, no special preparation is required. For a heart scan, initiate NPO status the evening before. For a kidney scan, hydrate as ordered.
Brain scan	A radioactive agent is injected into a vein and allowed to circulate to the brain; the brain is then scanned in successive layers and a picture composite of the structures developed. Useful in identifying structural lesions, whether vascular or tumors.	No food or fluid restrictions. The test takes approximately 2 hours. Obtain informed consent according to facility guidelines. Explain that the client may experience a hot feeling when dye is injected. Assess for allergies, especially to iodine or shellfish. Administer a light sedative, if ordered.
Radioactive iodine uptake, (RAIU), iodine uptake test, ^{131}I uptake	Uses oral radioactive iodine to determine thyroid function by the thyroid's ability to trap and retain iodine. Normal: 2 hours: 4%–12% absorbed 6 hours: 6%–15% absorbed 24 hours: 8%–30% absorbed	The client who is allergic to iodine or shellfish or is pregnant should not have the test. Exogenous iodine preparations or recent x-ray studies using iodinated contrast material will decrease thyroid gland uptake.

continues

Table 13–11 RADIOACTIVE STUDIES *continued*

TEST	EXPLANATION/NORMAL VALUES	NURSING RESPONSIBILITIES
Radioactive iodine uptake, (*continued*)		Note those medications taken that may affect results. Drugs that may increase RAIU level include barbiturates, estrogen, lithium, phenothiazines, and TSH. Drugs that may decrease RAIU level include ACTH, antihistamines, saturated solution of potassium iodine, thyroid drugs, antithyroid drugs, and tolbutamide.
Radionuclide angiography (multiplegated radioisotope scan, multigated acquisition scanning, MUGA)	A radioisotope is injected to evaluate the function of the left ventricle. The ejection fraction (a comparison of the volume of blood pumped by the left ventricle to the total volume of blood left in the ventricle) is measured.	Obtain informed written consent per agency policy.
Renal scan	Uses radioactive material (gallium 67) to show blood flow in the kidneys.	Check policy on disposal of client's urine for first 24 hours. Pregnant nurses should not care for clients undergoing this test because of the associated radiation.
Technetium pyrophosphate scanning	Important in diagnosing acute MIs, with the best accuracy obtained at 48 hours after the client experiences symptoms suggestive of an infarct. A tracer or radioisotope, which is injected intravenously, accumulates in the damaged or infarcted tissue areas, called hot spots.	Instruct the client not to smoke or consume caffeine or alcohol for 3 hours before the test. Inform the client that the test will take 45–60 minutes.
Thyroid scan, thyroid scintiscan	Uses a radioactive substance to visualize the size, shape, position, and function of the thyroid gland. Normal: no growth or enlargement	Assess for allergy to iodine or shellfish and for pregnant. Recent exposure to iodine-containing foods or x-ray iodinated contrast agents can interfere with test results. Drugs that can interfere with test results include cough medicines, multiple vitamins, some oral contraceptives, and thyroid drugs. Explain the procedure to the client. Certain drugs may have to be restricted for weeks before the test. Obtain a history concerning previous contrast x-ray studies, nuclear scans, or intake of thyroid-suppressive or antithyroid drugs. Fasting is usually not required. The scan may be taken 2 hours or 24 hours after oral ingestion of the radioactive substance. The client should be instructed to remove all jewelry, metal objects, and dentures before the scan. The scan takes approximately 30 minutes. Neither isolation nor specific urine precautions are necessary.
Ventilation-perfusion scan	Assesses ventilation and perfusion of the lungs. Most often used to detect the presence of pulmonary emboli.	Assess for allergy to iodine and shellfish. Explain the procedure to the client: that a radioactive contrast media will be introduced via an IV access and inhalation of radioactive gas and that the client will be required to hold the breath for short periods as images are obtained. Obtain informed written consent per facility policy.

ELECTRODIAGNOSTIC STUDIES

Electrodiagnostic tests use devices to measure the electrical activity of the heart, brain, and skeletal muscles. Electrical sensors (electrodes) are placed at certain anatomic points to measure the tone, velocity, and direction of the impulses. The impulses are then transmitted to an oscilloscope or printed on graphic paper. Table 13–12 describes the various electrodiagnostic studies.

Electrocardiography

An **electrocardiogram** (ECG or EKG) is a graphic recording of the heart's electrical activity. The client may be asked not to smoke or drink caffeinated beverages

Table 13–12 ELECTRODIAGNOSTIC STUDIES

TEST	EXPLANATION/NORMAL VALUES	NURSING RESPONSIBILITIES
Electrocardiogram (ECG or EKG)	Electrodes are placed on the skin to record wave patterns of the electrical conduction of the heart. Detects myocardial damage, rhythmic disturbances, and hyperkalemia.	Explain the procedure to the client. Inform the client that the test is painless.
Electroencephalogram (EEG)	Record of electrical activity generated in the brain and obtained through electrodes applied to the scalp or microelectrodes placed in brain tissue during surgery.	Withhold caffeine due to stimulant effect. Serve meal so that blood sugar will not be altered. Explain the procedure to the client: that the test takes approximately 45 minutes to 2 hours; that electrical shock will not occur; that the procedure is painless and that there are no after effects; that the client may be asked to open and close the eyes during the test and that there may be flashing lights or small electrical stimulations.
Electromyography (EMG)	Detects primary muscular disorders. A needle electrode is inserted into the muscle being examined. Measures electrical activity of skeletal muscle at rest and during voluntary muscle contraction.	Explain the procedure to the client. Obtain informed written consent. Instruct the client to refrain from consuming caffeine and smoking for 3 hours before the test. Assure client that the needle will not cause electrocution. Inform the client that there will be temporary discomfort when the needle electrode is inserted. Observe the site for hematoma or inflammation after the test. The procedure takes approximately 1 hour.
Electroretinogram (ERG)	A record of the changes in the retina's electric potential following stimulation by light. Clinically useful in some clients with retinal disease. Performed by placing a contact lens electrode on the anesthetized cornea. The electrical potential recorded on the cornea is identical to the response that would be obtained if the electrodes were placed directly on the surface of the retina.	Explain the test and procedure to the client.
Esophageal motility studies (manometry)	Evaluates muscle contractions and coordination by using a tube with transducers. Used as a diagnostic tool for disorders of the esophagus and lower esophageal sphincter (LES).	Initiate NPO status 6–8 hours prior to the test.
Holter monitor	A portable EKG monitors and records the electrical conduction of the heart for a period of 24 hours. The heart rhythm is compared to client activities.	Instruct the client to engage in normal daily activities and to keep a journal of symptoms experienced in performing these activities.
Stress test	An EKG taken as the client exercises. Evaluates the effects of exercise on the heart. Often, the client is asked to walk on a treadmill, the incline of which is elevated at various times throughout the test. Used frequently on clients who have CAD.	Explain the procedure to the client. Encourage the client to wear good walking shoes during the test.
Thallium test (myocardial perfusion scan)	A radioactive tracer (Thallium^{201}) is injected and accumulates in myocardial tissue that is well perfused. Accumulation is lessened in areas of myocardial tissue that are not well perfused, areas called "cold spots." The client may be asked to perform exercise, such as riding a bike, during the test to evaluate the perfusion of myocardial tissue during exercise.	Instruct the client to refrain from eating and drinking for 3 hours prior to the test.

for 24 hours before the test, as nicotine and caffeine can affect heart rate.

Electrodes are applied to the chest wall and extremities. A lubricating gel applied to the electrodes increases the conduction of electrical activity between the skin and electrodes. The client is instructed to lie still during the pain-free test. The test can reveal abnormal transmission of impulses and electrical position of the heart's axis.

A portable cardiac monitor (Holter monitor) is a device that records the heart's electrical activity. It produces a continuous recording over a specified time (e.g., 24 hours). The portable unit allows the client to ambulate and perform regular activities. Clients are instructed to maintain a log of those activities that result in the heart beating faster or irregularly. The practitioner reviews the ECG tracing in relation to the client's log to determine whether certain activities, such as walking, are associated with abnormal transmission of impulses.

Stress Test

A **stress test** measures the client's cardiovascular fitness. It demonstrates the ability of the myocardium to respond to increased oxygen requirements (the result of exercise) by increasing the blood flow to the coronary arteries.

The client is connected to an ECG machine and asked to walk on a treadmill. Continuous ECG recordings are made of the client's heart response (rate, electrical activity, and cardiac recovery time) to frequent changes in the treadmill's speed and slope. The test is stopped immediately if the client experiences any symptoms of decreased cardiac output (chest pain, dyspnea, fatigue, or ischemic changes revealed by the ECG monitor).

Thallium Test

Thallium[201] is a radioactive isotope that emits gamma rays and closely resembles potassium. Although a radioactive study, the thallium test is discussed here because it is often performed in conjunction with an ECG. Thallium is rapidly absorbed by normal myocardial tissue but is slowly absorbed by areas with poor blood flow and damaged cells. During the test, thallium is administered intravenously and the scanner detects the radiation and makes a visual image. The light areas on the image represent heavy isotope uptake (normal myocardial tissue), whereas the dark areas represent poor isotope uptake (poor blood flow and damaged cells).

There are two types of thallium test: resting imaging and stress imaging. Resting imaging can detect a myocardial infarction within its first few hours. Stress imaging (thallium stress test) is performed while the client is on a treadmill and being monitored with an ECG. At peak stress, the IV thallium is injected. Scan-

ning is performed 3 to 5 minutes postinjection and again in 2 to 3 hours. The test is stopped immediately if the client becomes symptomatic for ischemia.

Electroencephalography

An **electroencephalogram** (EEG) is the graphic recording of the brain's electrical activity. During the procedure, electrodes are placed on the client's scalp. The electrodes transmit impulses from the brain to an EEG machine. The machine amplifies the brain's impulses and makes a recording of the waves on strips of paper. An EEG can reveal not only the presence of a seizure disorder or intracranial lesion, but also the type. The absence of the brain's electrical activity is used to confirm death.

ENDOSCOPY

Endoscopy is the visualization of a body organ or cavity through a scope. An endoscope (a metal or fiberoptic tube) is inserted directly into the body structure to be studied (Figure 13-6). A light and, in some studies, a camera at the end of the scope allow the practitioner to assess, via direct visualization or television picture, for lesions and structural problems. The endoscope has an opening at the distant tip that allows the practitioner to administer an anesthetic agent and to lavage, suction, and biopsy tissue. Common endoscopic procedures are listed in Table 13–13.

After the procedure, the nurse must monitor vital signs, observe for bleeding, and assess for procedural risks (e.g., return of the gag and swallowing reflexes following a bronchoscopy performed under local anesthesia).

ASPIRATION/BIOPSY

Aspiration is performed to withdraw fluid that has abnormally collected or to obtain a specimen. To min-

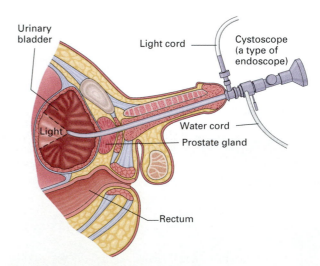

Figure 13-6 Cystoscope

Table 13–13 ENDOSCOPIC PROCEDURES

TEST	EXPLANATION/NORMAL VALUES	NURSING RESPONSIBILITIES
Endoscopy	Permits visual examination of internal structures of the body using specially designed instruments. The observation may be done through a natural body opening or through a small incision. A biopsy of suspicious areas may then be done for further study.	Explain the procedure to the client. Initiate NPO status 8–10 hours before test, except for sigmoidoscopy, before which a liquid diet should be followed for several days prior to the examination. Administer a laxative and then a cleansing enema.
Arthroscopy	Endoscopic procedure for direct visualization of a joint. Done in an operating room under sterile conditions and local or general anesthesia.	Perform frequent neurovascular checks. Elevate the client's leg. Apply compression dressing. Administer analgesic for discomfort.
Bronchoscopy	Direct visual examination of the bronchi through a fiber optic scope. Used to remove foreign bodies, for aggressive pulmonary cleansing, and to obtain sputum and tissue specimens.	Explain the procedure to the client: that the client must be NPO for at least 6 hours prior to the test; that, if ordered, preprocedure sedation is administered; that an IV access will be obtained and sedation given during the procedure via this route. Following the procedure, frequently assess vital signs and respiratory status. Assess the client for unusual amounts of bleeding. Inform the client that sputum may be blood tinged initially following the procedure. Maintain the client in a side-lying position until the gag reflex returns. Withhold all food and fluids until the client is fully awake and has a gag reflex. Obtain written informed consent per facility policy.
Colonoscopy	Examination of the rectum, colon, cecum, and ileocecal valve.	Initiate sedation. Cleanse the bowel. Offer only clear liquids after cleansing. Initiate NPO status for 6–8 hours prior to the test. Inform the client that flatulence and cramping will be experienced after the test.
Cystoscopy	A cystoscope is passed through the urethra and into the bladder to examine the interior of the bladder for inflammation, stones, tumors, or congenital abnormalities. A biopsy may be performed, and small stones may be removed. Ureteral catheters may be inserted to obtain urine from each kidney. May require topical, spinal or general anaesthesia.	Explain the procedure to the client. Obtain informed written consent. Check vital signs. Instruct in deep breathing, if general anesthesia is to be used. Allow a full liquid diet if topical anesthetic is to be used. Monitor I&O.
Endoscopic retrograde cholangiopancreatogram (ERCP)	Examination of the common bile duct (CBD) and biliary and pancreatic systems following injection of dye. Sphincterotomy, stone crushing, and stone removal can be done.	Initiate sedation. X-ray is used in conjunction. Initiate NPO status 6–8 hours prior to examination. Schedule PT, PTT, and bleeding time tests prior to this examination. Inform the client that the test can last up to 2 hours.
Esophagogastro-duodenoscopy (EGD)	Examination of the esophagus, stomach, and duodenum. Biopsies can be taken, and dilations done.	Initiate sedation. Initiate NPO status 6–8 hours prior to the examination.
Flexible sigmoidoscopy	Examination of the sigmoid colon and rectum.	Sedation is optional. Administer enemas prior to examination. Inform the client to expect some flatulence and cramping after the examination.
Laparoscopy	Examination of the internal pelvic structures by direct visualization with a laparoscope. Usually performed under general anesthesia. Diagnostic for pelvic disorders and infertility problems.	Explain the procedure to the client. Prepare the client, conduct pre- and postoperative assessment, and institute interventions. Provide discharge instructions on activity and follow-up.

imize client discomfort when the skin is pierced by the needle, a local anesthetic is administered in the area to be studied.

A stylet with an outer, hollow-bore needle is used to pierce the skin. Once the needle is in place, the stylet is withdrawn, leaving only the outer needle to aspirate the fluid. A **biopsy** (excision of a small amount of tissue) can be obtained during aspiration or in conjunction with other diagnostic tests (e.g., bronchoscopy). Table 13–14 outlines various aspiration/biopsy procedures.

Table 13–14 ASPIRATION/BIOPSY PROCEDURES

TEST	EXPLANATION/NORMAL VALUES	NURSING RESPONSIBILITIES
Aspiration Procedures		
Arthrocentesis	Procedure to obtain fluid from a joint using strict sterile technique. The knee is anesthetized, the sterile needle is inserted into joint space, and synovial fluid is aspirated. Used to diagnose infections, crystal-induced arthritis, and synovitis, and to inject anti-inflammatory medications. Performed by physician. Takes approximately 10 minutes.	Explain the procedure to the client. Obtain informed consent. Assess site for edema, pain. The client should fast if possible. Apply pressure dressing and ice.
Bone marrow aspiration	Evaluates how well the bone marrow is producing RBCs, WBCs, and platelets. Normal: adequate numbers of RBCs, WBCs, and platelets.	Inform the client that pressure will be felt when the physician aspirates the bone marrow. Assess the site for bleeding after the procedure is completed. Institute bed rest for at least 30 minutes after the test.
Gastric analysis, tube and tubeless test	Determines the amount of hydrochloric (HCl) acid in the stomach. If no HCl acid is present, that indicates parietal cells are malfunctioning. Parietal cells secrete the intrinsic factor that is essential for vitamin B_{12} absorption. Used to diagnose pernicious anemia. Normal tube test: Basal acid output: 2–5 mEq/h Maximal acid output 10–20 mEq/h Normal, tubeless test: presence of dye in urine (usually blue or blue-green in color)	If the client is having the tube test, initiate NPO status after midnight and instruct the client not to smoke prior to the test. Inform the client that a nasogastric tube is inserted prior to the test so that gastric contents can be aspirated after the administration of pentagastrin. If the client is having the tubeless test, inform the client of the possibility of a blue or blue-green discoloration of urine. Note any medications taken that affect results; antacids, anticholinergics, and cimetidine (Tagamet) decrease HCl level, whereas adrenergic-blocking agents, cholinergics, steroids, and alcohol elevate HCl level.
Lumbar puncture (LP)	A needle is inserted into the subarachnoid space to measure CSF pressure and/or to obtain a specimen. Normal pressure: 60–180 mm water pressure Normal specific gravity: 1.007 Normal glucose: 60–80 mg/100 mL Normal complete blood count (CBC): 0 Normal WBC: 0–5 cells/mm^3	Obtain informed written consent. Have the client empty the bowel and bladder prior to procedure. Position the client in the dorsal recumbent position on the side of bed of physician's choice. Place the hips at the edge of the bed, client's back to the physician. Assist in setting up a sterile field and pouring solutions, if not included in the tray. Assist the client to maintain the position. Postprocedure, deliver the specimen to the lab for testing, keep the client flat in bed for 3–24 hours or as ordered by physician; encourage fluid intake to replace fluids lost; and monitor vital and neurological signs.
Peritoneal aspiration	Fluid is withdrawn from the abdominal cavity by inserting a needle into the abdomen. The specimen in analyzed for infection or bleeding.	Have the client empty the bladder prior to the procedure. Prepare the abdomen by scrubbing it with a surgical prep solution and draping it with a sterile drape. Post procedure, dress the site with a sterile dressing and monitor the site for further drainage. Assess vital signs one time post procedure.
Perciardiocentesis	Fluid is removed from the pericardial sac for analysis or to relieve pressure.	Inform the client that the procedure will be done under a local anesthetic and that pressure may be felt when the needle is inserted. Position the client in the semi-Fowler's position during the procedure and attach to an EKG monitor. Postprocedure, take vital signs every 15 minutes and monitor EKG rhythm.
Thoracentesis	Removal of fluid for diagnostic purposes. May also obtain biopsy, instill medications, and remove fluid for client comfort and safety.	Explain the procedure to the client. Obtain informed consent. Position the client in an upright sitting position, leaning forward.

continues

Table 13–14 ASPIRATION/BIOPSY PROCEDURES *continued*

TEST	EXPLANATION/NORMAL VALUES	NURSING RESPONSIBILITIES
Thoracentesis (*continued*)		Have client rest the arms on an overbed table to facilitate this position. Explain to the client that the area will be anesthetized prior to the procedure. Instruct the client to hold as still as possible during the insertion of the thoracentesis needle. Assist the physician during the procedure. Deliver the specimen to the laboratory as soon as possible. Observe the thoracentesis site for bleeding following the procedure. Assess breath sounds before and after the procedure. Report absent breath sounds immediately.
Biopsy procedures	Removal of sample tissue for microscopic study. Tissue may be quickly frozen or placed in formalin before it is chemically stained and thinly sliced for analysis. Frozen section analysis takes only a few minutes and is often completed while a client is still in surgery. The full biopsy analysis takes 24–48 hours to complete but is the most accurate means of establishing a cancer diagnosis. Tissue biopsy is essential to confirming the type of cancer, the amount of lymph node involvement, and whether the cancer was successfully removed.	Explain the procedure to the client. Follow the physician's orders and/or agency protocol for client preparation. Obtain informed written consent.
Breast biopsy	Performed with or without local or general anesthesia and by aspiration, needle biopsy, excision, or incision. Tissue or fluid is obtained and sent to pathology for examination and identification of abnormal cells. New method of obtaining breast biopsies may be done with the stereotactic mammography studies.	Explain the procedure to the client. Have the client undress down to the waist. Cleanse the biopsy region and shave the area, if needed. Drape the breast and adjacent skin. Provide emotional support prior to, during, and following the procedure. Monitor vital signs. Apply a sterile dressing or bandage. Instruct the client in post-biopsy wound care.
Cardiac biopsy	Done during a cardiac catheterization. The tissue sample is taken from the apex or septum to determine toxicity related to drugs; inflammation; or rejection of a transplanted heart.	Preparation is the same as for Cardiac Catheterization (refer back to Table 27-8). After the procedure, observe the client for symptoms of a perforation, such as chest pain, decreased blood pressure, or dyspnea.
Endometrial biopsy	Obtained with special biopsy instruments and used to diagnose endometrial tissue abnormalities.	Explain the procedure to the client. Prepare the tissue preservation agent and label and send the sample to pathology. Assist the client in relaxing during the procedure, to offset the discomfort/cramping she may experience.
Liver biopsy	Obtained by inserting a needle into the liver. May be done with ultrasound or CT scan to guide needle placement. Evaluates cirrhosis, cancer, and hepatitis.	Schedule H&H, PT, PTT, and platelet tests prior to the procedure. Instruct the client to refrain from using NSAIDs including aspirin for 1 week prior to the procedure. Prepare the site by scrubbing it with a surgical prep solution and draping with a sterile towel. Monitor for signs of hemorrhage post procedure by frequently monitoring vital signs and pain. Have the client lie on the right side. Support the biopsy site with a towel or bath blanket for 2 hours. Monitor the site for ecchymosis.
Prostatic biopsy	Removal of a small piece of tissue for microscopic examination.	Monitor for and educate the client about signs and symptoms of hemorrhage, infection, and post-procedure pain.
Testicular biopsy	Determines presence of sperm and rules out vas deferens obstruction.	Monitor for and educate the client about signs and symptoms of infection or hemorrhage.
Thyroid biopsy	Excision of thyroid tissue for histological examination after noninvasive tests prove abnormal or inconclusive. Can be obtained through needle biopsy or open surgical biopsy under general anesthesia.	Explain the procedure to the client. Obtain informed written consent. Assess for allergies. Have coagulation blood studies done. Assess for bleeding and respiratory and swallowing difficulties after the test. To prevent undue strain on the biopsy site, instruct the client to put both hands behind the neck when sitting up. Warn the client that a sore throat is possible after the biopsy.

Bone Marrow Aspiration/Biopsy

The sternum and iliac crest are common sites for bone marrow puncture. During a bone marrow puncture, a fluid specimen (aspiration) or a core of marrow cells (biopsy) can be obtained. Both tests are commonly done concurrently to obtain the best possible marrow specimen. The test can reveal anemias; cancers such as leukemia, multiple myeloma, or Hodgkin's disease; or the client's response to chemotherapy.

Client positioning is determined by the site to be used, supine for the sternum and side lying for the iliac crest. The site is prepped to decrease the skin's normal flora in the area to be punctured. The nurse should explain to the client that pressure may be experienced as the specimen is withdrawn. The client should not move when the specimen is being withdrawn, as a sudden movement may dislodge the needle.

After the procedure, the client should be kept on bed rest for 1 hour. The nurse should monitor vital signs to assess for bleeding (rapid pulse rate, low blood pressure), and the client instructed to report to the practitioner any bleeding or signs of inflammation.

Paracentesis

Paracentesis is the aspiration of fluid from the abdominal cavity. This test can be diagnostic, therapeutic, or both. With end-stage liver or renal disease, for instance, **ascites** (an accumulation of fluid in the abdomen) occurs. Pressure caused by the ascites can interfere with breathing and gastrointestinal functioning. Aspiration in this instance is therapeutic. If a culture specimen is taken, it is also diagnostic.

The client should be instructed to void and the nurse should weigh the client before the procedure. The client should be placed in a high-Fowler's position in a chair or sitting on the side of the bed. The skin is prepped, anesthetized, and punctured with a **trocar** (a sharply pointed surgical instrument contained in a cannula). The trocar is held perpendicular to the abdominal wall and advanced into the peritoneal cavity. When fluid appears, the trocar is removed, leaving the inner catheter in place to drain the fluid. The client's vital signs are observed for changes resulting from the rapid removal of fluid.

After the procedure, a sterile dressing is applied to the puncture site, and the client monitored for changes in vital signs and electrolytes. The nurse should instruct the client to record the color, amount, and consistency of drainage on the dressing after discharge.

Thoracentesis

Thoracentesis is the aspiration of fluids from the pleural cavity. The pleural cavity normally contains a small amount of fluid to lubricate the lining between the lungs and pleura. Infection, inflammation, and trauma may cause an increased production of fluid, which can impair ventilation.

To facilitate access to the rib cage, the client should be positioned with the arms crossed and resting on a bedside table (Figure 13-7). The nurse should instruct the client not to cough during insertion of the trocar. The practitioner selects, preps, and anesthetizes the puncture site. The trocar is usually inserted into the intercostal space at the location of maximum dullness to percussion. The site should be above the ninth rib posteriorly and above the seventh rib laterally.

During the procedure the client must be carefully monitored for symptoms of a **pneumothorax** (collection of air or gas in the pleural space, causing the lungs to collapse), such as dyspnea, pallor, tachycardia, vertigo, and chest pain. After the procedure, the nurse assesses for signs of cardiopulmonary changes and a mediastinum shift, as indicated by bloody sputum and changes in vital signs.

Cerebrospinal Fluid Aspiration

Lumbar puncture ("spinal tap") is the aspiration of cerebrospinal fluid (CSF) from the subarachnoid space. The specimen is examined for organisms, blood, and tumor cells. A spinal tap is also performed:

- To obtain a pressure measurement when blockage is suspected,
- During a myelogram, or

Figure 13-7 Client Position for Thoracentesis

- To instill medications (anesthetics, antibiotics, or chemotherapeutic agents).

The client assumes a lateral recumbent position, with the craniospinal axis parallel to the floor, the flat of the back perpendicular to the procedure table. The client should assume a flexed knee–chest position to bow the back, thereby separating the vertebrae. Most clients require assistance in maintaining this position throughout the procedure. To do so, the nurse stands facing the client and places one hand across the client's shoulder blades and the other hand over the client's buttocks.

The practitioner selects, preps, and anesthetizes the puncture site (usually interspace L3–L4, L4–L5, or L5–S1). The needle and stylet are inserted into the midsagittal space and advanced through the longitudinal subarachnoid space (Figure 13-8).

Once in the subarachnoid space, the stylet is removed, leaving the needle in place. An initial CSF pressure reading is taken. If the pressure reading is greater than 200 mm H_2O or falls quickly, only 1 or 2 mL of CSF is withdrawn for analysis. If the pressure is less than 200 mm H_2O, an adequate specimen is withdrawn slowly.

After the pressure reading is taken, the stopcock is turned to allow the CSF to slowly flow into a sterile test tube. A sterile cap is placed on the test tube, and the sample is taken to the laboratory for analysis. Rapid withdrawal of CSF can cause a transient postural headache. The client's cardiorespiratory status is monitored throughout the procedure (Noe & Rock, 1994).

OTHER TESTS

Other diagnostic tests are described in Table 13–15.

Dura Mater
Subarachnoid Space
L4
L5

L_4 L_5 Space

Figure 13-8 Lumbar puncture: Position of client and insertion of the needle into the subarachnoid space are shown.

PROFESSIONAL TIP

CSF Pressure

The client should remain relaxed and quiet during the initial pressure reading, because straining increases CSF pressure.

After the procedure, pressure is applied to the puncture site, followed by a sterile bandage to prevent leakage of CSF. The client's neurological and cardiorespiratory statuses are then assessed. A postural headache is the most common complication of a lumbar puncture.

Table 13–15 OTHER TESTS		
TEST	**EXPLANATION/NORMAL VALUES**	**NURSING RESPONSIBILITIES**
Arterial plethysmography (pulse volume recorder)	Determines arteriosclerotic disease in the upper extremities and occlusive disease in the lower extremities. Done by applying three blood pressure cuffs to an extremity. The cuffs are connected to a pulse volume recorder, which records the amplitude of each pulse wave. If there is a decrease in the amplitude of the pulse wave, an occlusion is in the artery proximal to the cuff. A decrease of 20 mm Hg of pressure indicates arterial occlusion. The test is not as reliable as arteriography but also does not have the risks associated with an arteriogram. Normal: normal arterial pulse waves	Explain to the client that the test is painless. Instruct the client to lie still during the test. Instruct the client not to smoke for 30 minutes prior to the test. Instruct the client to remove clothing from the extremity on which the test is to be done.

continues

Table 13–15 OTHER TESTS *continued*

TEST	EXPLANATION/NORMAL VALUES	NURSING RESPONSIBILITIES
Audiometric testing	Evaluates both bone and air conduction and determines the degree of hearing loss. The client wears headphones, through which a series of tones is delivered at different frequencies. The client signals to the audiologist when the tones are audible. The results are recorded on an audiogram. The client is kept in a sound proof booth during the test.	Explain the procedure and its purpose to the client. Ensure that the client is not claustrophobic.
Brainstem auditory-evoked response (ErA and BAER)	Detects hearing dysfunctions of the central nervous system and cochlear nerve (cranial nerve VII). Valuable for testing comatose clients, clients with neurological damage, and children. An altered appearance of the brainstem waveforms or a delay or loss of a waveform indicates an abnormality including a possible cochlear lesion or acoustic neuroma.	Explain the procedure and its purpose to the client particularly that the client will be in a darkened room and will have both electrodes attached to the head and earphones in place.
Caloric test	Assesses alteration in vestibular function. The client is placed in a supine or Fowler's position and each ear is irrigated with cold and then warm water. A decreased response or failure to respond within 3 minutes indicates that an abnormality may be present. Most commonly done on comatose clients. A punctured eardrum or Meniere's disease may contraindicate the test. Normal: vertigo, nystagmus, nausea, vomiting, and unsteady gait.	Explain the procedure and its purpose to the client. Tell the client that nystagmus, vertigo, nausea, vomiting, and an unsteady gait represent a normal response. Stay with the client and have an emesis basin and tissues available.
Color vision tests	Most common color vision tests use pseudoisochromatic (seemingly the same color) plates comprising patterns of dots of the primary colors superimposed on backgrounds of randomly mixed colors. A client with normal vision can identify the patterns; a client with a color deficiency cannot distinguish between pattern and background.	Explain the test and procedure to the client.
Colposcopy	Direct visualization of the vagina and cervix through a high-powered microscope. Acetic acid or other solution is applied to the tissue to dehydrate the cells for improved visualization. Used to diagnose cervical dysplasia or carcinoma in situ of the cervix. Biopsies may be obtained as needed.	Explain the procedure and prepare the client in the dorsal lithotomy position. Assist with the procedure. Prepare biopsy specimens for pathological examination.
Culture and sensitivity (C&S)	Determines presence of microorganism and identifies the antibiotic that will kill or inhibit growth of microorganism. Drainage from infected lesions is obtained with a sterile swab and is incubated in order to identify the causative organism and to determine antibiotic sensitivity. Normal: negative for microorganism growth.	Ensure that the specimen has been obtained before initiating antibiotic therapy. Specimens should be taken to the laboratory within 30 minutes of being obtained.
Cytology	The study of cells and fluids obtained from various organs by scrapings, brushings, or needle aspiration. Cytologic smears, such as the Pap smear, are routinely done to study cells from the female genital tract. A cytological smear showing evidence of malignancy is followed by a biopsy to facilitate a more comprehensive diagnosis.	Explain the procedure to be used for obtaining cells and fluids for study. Follow agency protocol for client preparation.
Dark field examination of wart scrapings	Microscopic examination to differentiate genital warts from syphilis condylomata.	Take a careful client history. Examine the genital area carefully and provide scalpel and slide, if specimen is to be obtained. Explain the procedure thoroughly to the client.
Dilatation and curettage (D&C)	Surgical scraping of the endometrial lining, performed under general, epidural, or paracervical anesthesia and on an outpatient basis. Diagnostic or therapeutic for uterine bleeding disorders.	Explain the procedure to the client. Perform pre- and postoperative assessment and provide care. Provide discharge instructions related to activities and follow-up appointments..

continues

Table 13–15 OTHER TESTS *continued*

TEST	EXPLANATION/NORMAL VALUES	NURSING RESPONSIBILITIES
Dynamic infusion cavernosometry and cavernosography (DICC)	Group of diagnostic tests that measure neuro-vascular events of penile erection.	Perform baseline assessment, monitor during the procedure, and assess for postoperative complications; advise the client of possible discomfort related to the injection. Explain the procedure to the client. Assess for allergies. If preferred by the laboratory, initiate NPO status after midnight. Restrict iodine and thyroid preparations a week before test. Inform the client that radioactive iodine may be given orally or intravenously. Withhold food for 45 to 60 minutes after the iodine is given. Provide the client with a list of times to report to radiology. Tell the client that he will lie supine for test, which takes about 30 minutes, and that neither isolation nor specific urine precautions are necessary.
Huhner test (post-coital test)	Performed in the office. The couple has intercourse 2 hours before the appointment. A sample of secretions is removed from the vagina and placed on a microscopic slide. The sperm are observed for number and motility in the cervical mucous. Normal: a minimum of 20 sperm per field that demonstrate good motility	Explain the procedure to the client and schedule it near client's normal ovulation. Prepare the client in the lithotomy position. Assist the physician or nurse practitioner with the procedure. Perform microscopic observations as directed.
Nocturnal tumescence penile monitoring	Various devices are attached to the penis at night to monitor swelling (tumescence).	Explain to the client that the test will require application of a device to the penis and that the device is to be worn while sleeping. Show the client the device and explain how to apply it.
Ophthalmoscopic examination	Examination of the fundus (posterior eye) using an ophthalmoscope. Magnifies vascular and nerve tissue of the fundus, including the optic disk, retinal vessels, macula, and retina. Used to diagnose diseases of the eye and aberrations in the refractive mechanism.	Explain the test and procedure to the client.
Otoscopic examination	Visual examination of the ear canal using an otoscope. The examiner looks for signs of inflammation, discharge, or foreign bodies. The tympanic membrane is normally pearly gray. The position and color of the membrane are noted as is any unusual appearance.	Explain the procedure and its purpose to the client. The ear should be clear of cerumen. Tilt the head away from the examiner and pull the earlobe up, back, and out to straighten the auditory canal. In children, pull the earlobe down and out to straighten the canal.
Papanicolaou (Pap) smear	Cells are obtained from the external and internal cervical canal. Used to diagnose cervical dysplasia or cancer.	Explain the procedure. Have client empty bladder and undress. Position client in dorsal lithotomy position. Help client relax during procedure. Prepare microscopic slides for pathology. Instruct the client on the importance of having an annual Pap smear.
Past-point testing	Measures the ability or inability to accurately place a finger on some part of the body, usually the client's or examiner's face and fingers. For example, the examiner will instruct the client to close her eyes and touch her nose, then, with eyes open, touch the examiner's nose or the examiner's index finger.	Explain the test and procedure to the client. Explain that it is painless and represents a helpful measure of vestibular function (coordination).
Patch testing	Allergens within occlusive patches are applied to normal skin (usually the upper back) for 48 hours. If the client is allergic to a specific allergen, an erythematous skin reaction will occur.	Clean and dry the skin where the patches are to be applied. Tell the client that the patches must be left in place for the full 48 hours.
Pelvic examination (recommended annually for women over 18 through menopause)	Performed by a physician or nurse practitioner. The external and internal pelvic structures are visualized, the pelvic organs are palpated via bi-manual examination, and the cervix is examined via a speculum. A Pap smear and rectovaginal exam are also performed, and cultures and wet smears may be obtained.	Explain the procedures to the client; prepare the client by having her void and undress; position the client on the examination table in a dorsal lithotomy position; help the client to relax during the examination, prepare slides and culture medium; obtain other supplies; and assist with the procedure.

continues

Table 13–15 OTHER TESTS *continued*

TEST	EXPLANATION/NORMAL VALUES	NURSING RESPONSIBILITIES
Prostatic smears	Microscopic examination of prostatic secretions obtained via rectal massage performed by a physician.	Explain to the client that to obtain the specimen, the prostate must be massaged via the rectum and that this will cause some discomfort.
Pulmonary function tests (PFTs)	A group of studies used to evaluate ventilatory function. Measurements are obtained directly via spirometer or calculated from the results of spirometer measurements. Bronchodilators may be used during the study. Measurements included are: Tidal volume: the amount of air inhaled and exhaled during a normal respiration. Inspiratory reserve volume: the amount of air inspired at the end of a normal inspiration. Expiratory reserve volume: the amount of air expired following a normal expiration. Residual volume: the amount of air left in lungs after maximal expiration. Vital capacity: the total volume of air that can be expired after maximal inspiration. Total lung capacity: the total volume of air in the lungs when maximally inflated. Inspiratory capacity: the maximum amount of air that can be inspired after normal expiration. Forced vital capacity: the capacity of air exhaled forcefully and rapidly following maximal inspiration. Minute volume: the amount of air breathed per minute.	Explain the procedure to the client, PFTs should not be done within 1–2 hours after a meal. After the test, monitor respiratory status. Advise the client to avoid activity and to rest following the test, as fatigue may result.
Pulse oximetry	A noninvasive procedure. A transdermal clip is placed on a finger or earlobe to detect the arterial oxygen saturation (SaO_2). Normal: > 95% (at sea level)	Explain the procedure to the client. Assess peripheral circulation, as this may alter results. Place the sensor on the earlobe, fingertip, or pinna of the ear. Keep the sensor intact until a consistent reading is obtained. Observe and record readings. Report to the physician measurements below 95%.
Rinne test (tuning fork)	Detects loss of hearing in one or both ears. Tuning fork is struck and placed against the mastoid bone to measure the sound conduction through the bone. The tuning fork is then placed beside and parallel to the ear to test conduction through the air. If the sound is louder when the tines are placed beside the ear, hearing is normal or the hearing loss is sensorineural. If the sound is louder when conducted through the bone, the hearing loss is conductive.	Explain the procedure and its purpose to the client.
Romberg test	Assesses vestibular (balance) function. The client stands with the eyes closed, arms extended in front, and feet together. Normal: slight swaying.	Explain the procedure and its purpose to the client. Stand close and reassure the client that someone will catch him if he begins to fall.
Schiller test	Performed during colposcopy. An iodine solution is applied to the cells of the cervix. Abnormal cells turn white or yellow. Aids in visualization of abnormal tissue and indicates areas for biopsy. Normal: cells turn brown	Explain the reason for the application of the solution. Assist with the biopsy procedure as necessary. Label tissue specimens and send to histology.
Segmented bacteriologic localization cultures	The first 5–10 mL of urine is collected, the next 200 mL is discarded, then 5–10 mL is collected midstream. The prostate is then massaged until prostatic secretions can be collected. Finally, 5–10 mL urine is collected before the bladder is emptied. Four samples are needed in sterile culture tubes.	Ensure that the client is well hydrated and has a full bladder.
Semen analysis	Determines the presence, number, and motility of sperm.	Teach the client about proper collection of sperm.

continues

Table 13–15 OTHER TESTS *continued*

TEST	EXPLANATION/NORMAL VALUES	NURSING RESPONSIBILITIES
Skin scrapings	A lesion is scraped with an oiled scalpel blade. The cells are then examined under a microscope. Used to diagnose fungal lesions.	Explain the procedure and its purpose to the client.
Slit-lamp examination	The cornea is examined with the aid of a slit lamp. A slit-like beam facilitates visualization of the layers of the cornea and lens, facilitating evaluation of the thickness of these structures and the location of disease processes. Useful in detecting and evaluating abnormalities of anterior segment tissues and structures. May reveal disorders such as iritis, corneal abrasions, conjunctivitis, and lens opacities (cataracts).	Explain the procedure and its purpose to the client.
Speech audiometry (Spondee threshold)	Evaluates ability to hear and understand the spoken word. A series of two-syllable words commonly recognized by their vowel sounds (like *toothbrush* and *baseball*) are delivered through earphones. When the client correctly repeats the word, the sound intensity is recorded in decibels. The test is normally conducted in a soundproof booth.	Explain the procedure and its purpose to the client. Ensure that the client is not claustrophobic.
Sputum analysis	Sputum samples are examined for the presence of bacteria, fungi, molds, yeasts, and malignant cells. Appropriate antibiotic therapy is determined via C&S studies.	Explain the procedure and its purpose to the client. Obtain specimens early in the morning to prevent contamination via ingested food or fluids. Instruct the client to breathe deeply and cough, so as to facilitate collection of a specimen originating from the lower respiratory tract. If necessary, pulmonary suctioning may be used to induce such a specimen. Instruct the client to expectorate sputum into the appropriate container. Deliver specimens to the laboratory as soon as possible.
Tonometry	Used to measure intraocular pressure and to aid in the diagnosis and follow-up evaluation of glaucoma. Two types of tonometric devices are used for assessment: applanation and indentation. An applanation tonometer is the most accurate and commonly used device and measures the force (delineated by the reading on the tension dial on the tonometer) required to flatten a small, standard area of the cornea. An indentation tonometer measures the deformation of the globe in response to a standard weight placed on the cornea. Before use of either apparatus, the eyes are anesthetized with a local ophthalmic solution, such as benoxinate with fluorescein or tetracaine, so that the pressure from the tonometer will not be felt. Normal: 12–22 mm Hg	Explain the procedure and its purpose to the client. Explain to the client that this test measures the pressure within the eyes and that although the test requires the client's eyes to be anesthetized, the anesthesia will wear off shortly after the examination is complete. Reassure the client that the procedure is painless.
Typanometry	Measures the movement of the eardrum in response to air pressure in the ear canal. Evaluates the presence of fluid in the middle ear and is commonly used to evaluate otitis media in children or adults.	Explain the procedure and its purpose to the client. Inform the client a small burst of air is introduced through the otoscope, which may produce an uncomfortable sensation.
Tzanck smear	Fluid from the base of a vesicle is applied to a glass slide, stained, and examined under a microscope. Used to diagnose herpes zoster, herpes simplex, varicella, or pemphigus. Normal: negative	Describe to the client how the laboratory technician will obtain the specimen and that although the procedure will likely not be painful, the client must remain still to prevent injury. Provide scalpel blade, glass slide, and stain for collection.
Urethra pressure profile (UPP)	Assesses functional urethral length and general competency of the urethra and sphincter, either at rest or during coughing, straining, or voiding. Functional profile length is the length from bladder outlet to the point in the urethra where urethral	Explain the procedure and its purpose to the client: that it is often performed when the bladder is empty and the client is at rest; that it may be performed simultaneously with CMG; and that the client may be asked to cough or

continues

Table 13–15 OTHER TESTS continued

TEST	EXPLANATION/NORMAL VALUES	NURSING RESPONSIBILITIES
Urethra pressure profile (UPP) (continued)	pressure equals intravesical pressure. Used to diagnose stress or overflow incontinence or urethral obstruction. Normal: Male: bladder outlet through membranous urethra Female: bladder outlet through mid-urethra	void. Provide privacy, as the test can be embarrassing.
Uroflowmetry	Noninvasive assessment of urination. An electronic device connected to a funneled commode calculates the rate of urine flow, volume voided, and time taken to void.	Explain the procedure and its purpose to the client. Instruct the client to void as usual, leaving client alone to do so, if possible.
Venous plethysmography (cuff pressure test)	Assists in determining patency of veins. Two blood pressure cuffs are placed on the extremity, one proximally (occlusion cuff) and one distally (recording cuff). The cuffs are attached to pulse volume recorders. The occlusion cuff is inflated to 50 mm Hg pressure to occlude the venous flow of blood; the recording cuff is inflated to 10 mm Hg pressure. The pulse volumes are recorded and then the occlusion cuff is rapidly deflated. The pulse volume of the extremity should return to the preocclusion volume within 1 second if there is no occlusion in the venous system. A delay in the return of volume pressure is indicative of a thrombus. Normal: return of volume pressure to preocclusion value within 1 second after deflation of occlusion cuff The test is often done in conjunction with a doppler ultrasound. The test is not as reliable as a venogram.	Nursing responsibilities are the same as for Arterial Plethysmography (see beginning of table).
Visual acuity	Used to test distant and near visual acuity and to identify refractive errors in vision. Distant visual acuity is measured with a standardized visual acuity chart, e.g., a Snellen chart. Near visual acuity is measured with a Jaeger card (a card with print in graded sizes). Visual acuity is recorded as a fraction, with the numerator representing the distance to the chart and the denominator representing the distance at which a normal eye can read the line. Thus, the larger the denominator, the poorer the client's visual acuity. For example, if the client's vision is normal, results are expressed as 20/20, which means that the smallest symbol one can identify at 20 feet is the same symbol the normal eye can identify from the same distance.	Explain the procedure and its purpose to the client. Have the client stand the specified distance from the eye chart, usually 10 feet. Instruct the client to first cover one eye and then the other. If the client wears glasses, perform the test first with the client's glasses on and then with the client's glasses off.
Weber test (tuning fork)	Detects loss of hearing in one or both ears. Tuning fork is struck and the handle is placed in the middle of the forehead. Clients with normal hearing or bilateral deafness will hear or not hear the sound equally in both ears. Clients with unilateral hearing loss will hear the sound only in the unaffected ear.	Explain the procedure and its purpose to the client.
Wood's light examination	Skin and hair are examined under ultraviolet light (black light) in a darkened room. Used to diagnose fungal infections (tinea) of hair and skin.	Explain the procedure and its purpose to the client. Reassure the client that the rays are not harmful.

SUMMARY

- Most invasive procedures require that the client give informed consent.
- Nurses prepare clients for diagnostic testing by ensuring client understanding and compliance with preprocedural requirements.
- Clients, families, and significant others must be involved in the testing process. The nurse must advise them of the estimated time required to perform the procedure.
- To help offset the discomfort and anxiety experienced during procedures, the nurse teaches the client how to perform relaxation techniques such as imagery.
- After a diagnostic test, the nurse provides care and teaches the client those things to expect, including the outcomes or side effects of the test.
- The role of the nurse in diagnostic testing is to facilitate the scheduling of diagnostic tests, perform client teaching, perform or assist with procedures, and assess clients for adverse responses to procedures.
- Nurses should schedule diagnostic procedures to promote both client comfort and cost containment.
- Standard Precautions are used when obtaining a specimen for diagnostic examination or when assisting with an invasive procedure.
- Before the procedure, the nurse is responsible for obtaining baseline vital signs and assessing the client's preparation for testing.
- After the procedure, the nurse assesses the client for secondary procedural complications and performs any necessary nursing interventions.

Review Questions

1. Scheduling and sequencing of laboratory tests are important functions of the:

    a. nurse.
    b. physician.
    c. phlebotomist.
    d. laboratory supervisor.

2. The most commonly used site for capillary puncture in neonates and infants is the:

    a. heel.
    b. toetip.
    c. earlobe.
    d. fingertip.

3. When collecting a 24-hour urine specimen, the nurse knows:

    a. to put a large bottle at the client's bedside.
    b. the collection begins at the time of the first discarded voiding.

    c. that the client must urinate at a specific start time.
    d. to teach the client how to void in the large collection bottle.

4. The nurse knows that glucose spills into the urine when the blood glucose level exceeds the renal threshold of:

    a. 120 mg/mL.
    b. 140 mg/mL.
    c. 160 mg/mL.
    d. 180 mg/mL.

5. Occult blood may be found in which type of specimen?

    a. Blood
    b. Stool
    c. Urine
    d. Sputum

6. When scheduling a series of tests, the nurse knows to schedule:

    a. a barium enema before an upper GI.
    b. an ultrasound after all other tests.
    c. an upper GI before a gallbladder x-ray.
    d. a gallbladder x-ray before any barium studies.

7. A test that combines a radioactive scan with an electrodiagnostic study is a:

    a. MUGA.
    b. brain scan.
    c. thallium stress test.
    d. radioactive iodine uptake test.

Critical Thinking Questions

1. If a client's blood type is AB positive, what are the possible blood types of the client's parents? Can the client receive Rh-negative blood? Explain your answer.

2. The physician orders gallbladder x-rays, a barium swallow, an upper GI, and a barium enema. In which order should these tests be scheduled? Why?

 WEB FLASH!

- Search the Web for "diagnostic tests." How many sites can you find? What type of information is available?
- Search the Web for the specific diagnostic tests discussed in this chapter. How many tests have sites devoted to them? Is the information for health professionals or the general public?

PAIN MANAGEMENT

MAKING THE CONNECTION

Refer to the following chapters to increase your understanding of pain management:

- **Chapter 5, Communication**
- **Chapter 6, Cultural Diversity and Nursing**
- **Chapter 8, Alternative/Complementary Therapies**
- **Chapter 9, Loss, Grief, and Death**
- **Chapter 16, Nursing Care of the Surgical Client**
- **Chapter 17, Nursing Care of the Oncology Client**

LEARNING OBJECTIVES

Upon completion of this chapter, you should be able to:
- *Define key terms.*
- *Identify the four components of pain conduction.*
- *Discuss the gate control theory of pain.*
- *Describe the types of pain.*
- *List three guidelines that should be included in a thorough pain assessment.*
- *Identify three general principles of pain management.*
- *List the nurse's responsibilities in administration of analgesics.*
- *Identify site of action of both nonopioid and opioid analgesics.*
- *Describe three examples of nonpharmacological measures for pain relief.*
- *Discuss nursing interventions that promote comfort.*

INTRODUCTION

Pain is a phenomenon that crosses all specialties of nursing. No matter the setting a nurse practices in, including neonatal intensive care, intraoperative, home care, or clinics, the nurse will be exposed to challenges in pain management. While other health care team members address pain management with clients, it is the nurse who spends the most time with the client experiencing pain. For example, in an acute care setting,

KEY TERMS

acupuncture	myofascial pain
acute pain	syndromes
adjuvant medication	neuralgia
afferent pain pathway	nociceptor
analgesia	noxious stimulus
analgesic	pain
ceiling effect	pain threshold
chronic acute pain	pain tolerance
chronic nonmalignant	patient-controlled-
pain	analgesia
chronic pain	perception
colic	phantom limb pain
cryotherapy	progressive muscle
cutaneous pain	relaxation
distraction	recurrent acute pain
efferent pain pathway	referred pain
endorphin	reframing
epidural analgesia	relaxation technique
gate control pain	somatic pain
theory	tolerance
hypnosis	transcutaneous
intrathecal analgesia	electrical nerve
ischemic pain	stimulation
mixed agonist-	transduction
antagonist	transmission
modulation	visceral pain

the physician orders the **analgesics** (substances that relieve pain) for the client, but may only spend 10 to 15 minutes each day with that client. The nurses are the ones who are present 24 hours a day, administer the medications, assess the client's response, and report the response to the physician. It is for this reason the nurse is often called the "backbone" or "cornerstone" of pain management. The nurse's role can be pivotal in relieving the client's pain.

Studies have documented undertreatment of pain of all types and in all age groups (Liebeskind & Melzack, 1987). In one such study, the researchers interviewed medical and surgical clients, finding that 58% had experienced excruciating pain in the previous 72 hours. Fifty-five percent of these clients could not recall a nurse asking about their pain (Donovan, Dillon, & McGuire, 1987). Another study examined pain management in metastatic cancer clients in an outpatient setting. Forty-two percent of the clients with pain were not given adequate analgesic therapy (Cleeland, Gonin, Hatfield, Edmonson, Blum, Stewart, & Pandya, 1994).

It is generally thought that this undertreatment of pain is partially due to the lack of knowledge in both physicians and nurses. It is, therefore, important for the nurse to understand not only the psychological and physiological components that add up to the pain experience, but also the wide range of interventions available to provide relief. Another reason for undertreatment may be the health care workers' own biases regarding pain. Consequently, nurses should also recognize their own responses to pain and how they respond to others' expressions of pain.

The experience of pain is a factor that can have a significant impact on a client's health. It is a personal experience that can affect all other aspects of an individual's health, including physical well-being, mental status, and effectiveness of coping mechanisms. This chapter provides an overview of the complex phenomenon of pain, including: pain definitions, pain physiology, and pain assessment. Strategies to control pain will also be discussed, including pharmacological, noninvasive, and invasive techniques.

DEFINITIONS OF PAIN

The phenomenon of pain is evidenced in ancient history with references being made as far back as the Babylonian clay tablets. Aristotle (4th century B.C.) described pain as an emotion, being the opposite of pleasure. While emotions certainly play an important role in pain perception, we now know there is much more to the experience than the feelings involved.

In the Middle Ages, pain was viewed with religious connotations. Pain was seen as God's punishment for sins, or as evidence that an individual was possessed by demons. This definition of pain is still embraced by some clients, who might tell the nurse that the suffer-

ing is their "cross to bear." Pain relief may not be the goal for those individuals who believe in this definition of pain. Spiritual counseling may need to be implemented before this person is willing to work toward relief.

Currently, the most widely accepted definition of **pain** is that developed by the International Association for the Study of Pain (IASP). This organization defines pain as "an unpleasant sensory and emotional experience associated with actual or potential tissue damage or described in terms of such damage" (Merskey & Bogduk, 1994). This definition incorporates both the sensory and emotional components of pain. It also acknowledges that evidence of actual tissue damage is not required in order for the pain to be considered real.

Many pain experts emphasize the subjective nature of pain. Unlike a blood pressure or a blood glucose measurement, the intensity of discomfort the client is feeling cannot be measured with an instrument. McCaffery and Pasero (1999) say it best by defining pain as "whatever the person experiencing it says it is, existing whenever [he or she] says it does." This philosophy is emphasized in professional pain management guidelines. For example, the Agency for Health Care Policy and Research (AHCPR) now called Agency for Healthcare Research and Quality (AHRQ) (1994) guideline for cancer pain states, "Health professionals should ask about pain, and the patient's self-report should be the primary source of assessment." "Guidelines are still published under the old name." The American Pain Society (APS) also stresses the importance of self-report: "Pain is always subjective. . . . The clinician must accept the patient's report of pain" (1999).

Though pain has had many definitions throughout humankind's history, research in pain physiology has shown that pain is a complex phenomenon. Pain is often difficult for clients to describe and nurses to understand; yet it is among the most common complaints that cause individuals to seek health care. Until recently, pain was viewed as a symptom that required diagnosis and treatment of the underlying cause. It is now clear that pain itself can be detrimental to the health and healing of clients. McCaffery and Pasero (1999) write that pain control, not just relief from pain once it occurs, must be recognized as a priority in the care of clients in all settings.

NATURE OF PAIN

A major function of the pain experience is to signal ongoing or potential tissue damage (Schecter, Berde, & Yaster, 1993), as is seen in the pain of cancer and chronic illness. Pain can also be a protective mechanism to prevent further injury, as is seen in clients who guard or protect an injured body part. The sensation of pain as the warning of potential tissue damage may be absent in people with hereditary sensory neuro pathies, congenital nerve or spinal cord abnormalities, diabetic neuropathy, multiple sclerosis, leprosy, alcoholism, and nerve or spinal cord injury (Brand & Yancey, 1993).

COMMON MYTHS ABOUT PAIN

Because pain is subjective (dependent on the client's perception) and cannot be objectively measured by another individual through a laboratory test or diagnostic data, pain is often misunderstood and misjudged. A client's report of level of pain will vary on the basis of cultural and experiential backgrounds, and the nurse's interpretations of a client's pain will be filtered through the nurse's own biases and expectations. Misalignment of the nurse's view and the client's perception of pain can often lead to undermedication and unnecessary suffering on the client's part. Some common myths related to pain are discussed in Table 14–1.

TYPES OF PAIN

Pain can be qualified or described in two basic ways: by its cause or origin and by its description or nature. Pain categorized by its origin is either cutaneous, somatic, or visceral. Pain categorized by its nature is either acute or chronic.

Pain Categorized by Origin

Cutaneous pain is caused by stimulation of the cutaneous nerve endings in the skin and results in a well-localized "burning" or "prickling" sensation; getting a knot in the hair that is pulled out during combing may cause cutaneous pain. **Somatic pain** is nonlocalized and originates in support structures such as tendons, ligaments, and nerves; jamming a knee or finger will result in somatic pain. **Visceral pain** is discomfort in the internal organs and is less localized and more slowly transmitted than cutaneous pain. Visceral pain is often difficult to assess because the location may not be directly related to the cause. Pain originating from the abdominal organs is often called **referred pain** because the sensation of pain is not felt in the organ itself but instead is perceived at the spot where the organs were located during fetal development (Figure 14–1).

Pain Categorized by Nature

It is important to understand the difference between acute and chronic pain, as they each present a different clinical picture.

Acute Pain

Acute pain is most frequently identified by its sudden onset and relatively short duration, mild to severe intensity, and a steady decrease in intensity over a period of days to weeks. Some forms of acute pain may have a slower onset. Once the **noxious stimulus** (underlying pathology) is resolved, the unpleasant sensation usually disappears (Stevens, 1994) (see Table 14–2). It can usually be associated with a specific injury, condition, or disease that has caused tissue damage. Acute pain should diminish as healing occurs. Everyone has experienced acute pain, for example:

Table 14–1 COMMON MYTHS ABOUT PAIN	
MYTH	**FACT**
• The nurse is the best judge of a client's pain.	• Pain is a subjective experience; only the client can judge the level and severity of pain.
• If pain is ignored, it will go away.	• Pain is a real experience that is appropriately treated with nursing and medical intervention.
• Clients should not take any measures to relieve their pain until the pain is unbearable.	• Pain control and relief measures are effective in lowering the pain level, which will help clients function more normally and comfortably.
• Most complaints of pain are purely psychological (e.g., "it's all in your head"); only "real" pain manifests in obvious physical signs such as moaning or grimacing.	• Most clients report honestly on their perception of pain, both physical and emotional, and need effective intervention and teaching; physical responses to pain vary greatly depending on experience and cultural norms, and visible expressions of pain are not always reliable indicators of its severity.
• Clients taking pain medications will become addicted to the drug.	• Addiction is unlikely when analgesics are carefully administered and closely monitored.
• Clients with severe tissue damage will experience significant pain; those with lesser damage will feel less pain.	• Individuals' perceptions of pain are subjective; the extent of tissue damage is not necessarily proportional to the extent of pain experienced.
• Clients ask for pain medication when they need it.	• Many clients do not ask for medication because they are afraid of side effects, do not want to bother the nurse, have cultural norms and beliefs against it, or believe pain is inevitable and untreatable.

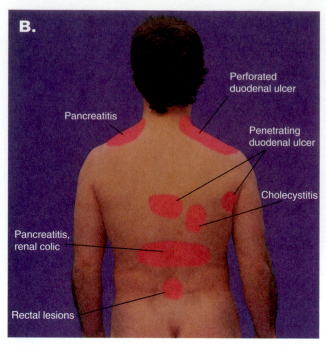

Figure 14-1 Areas of Referred Pain: A. Anterior view; B. Posterior view

Table 14–2 **ACUTE VERSUS CHRONIC PAIN**		
	ACUTE	**CHRONIC**
Time Span	Less than 6 months	More than 6 months
Location	Localized, associated with a specific injury, condition, or disease	Difficult to pinpoint
Characteristics	Often described as sharp, diminishes as healing occurs	Often described as dull, diffuse, and aching
Physiologic Signs	• Elevated heart rate • Elevated BP • Elevated respirations • May be diaphoretic • Dilated pupils	• Normal vital signs • Normal pupils • No diaphoresis • May have loss of weight
Behavioral Signs	• Crying and moaning • Rubbing site • Guarding • Frowning • Grimacing • Complains of pain	• Physical immobility • Hopelessness • Listlessness • Loss of libido • Exhaustion and fatigue • Complains of pain only when asked

headaches, toothaches, needle sticks, burns, skinned knees, muscle pain, childbirth, postoperative pain, fractures, and a sprained ankle. The client will describe the pain as highly localized and is usually able to pinpoint the hurt. Acute pain is often described as sharp, although if the pain is deep, it may be described as dull and aching. Accompanying signs will be those of the activation of the sympathetic nervous system, that is, the fight-or-flight response. Therefore, the client will exhibit elevated heart rate, respiratory rate, and blood pressure. The client may become diaphoretic and have dilated pupils. These signs resemble those of anxiety, which often accompanies acute pain. Behaviors may include crying and moaning, rubbing the site of pain, guarding, frowning, and grimacing. The client will often verbally complain of the discomfort.

Recurrent acute pain is identified by repetitive painful episodes that may recur over a prolonged period or throughout the client's lifetime. These painful episodes alternate with pain-free intervals. Examples of recurrent pain often seen in children include recurrent abdominal, chest, or limb pain that occurs in 5% to 10% of school-age children; headaches; and sickle cell pain crises with vaso-occlusion that leads to ischemia or infarction (Schecter, et al., 1993). Examples of recurrent pain experienced by adults include migraine headaches, sickle cell pain crises, and the pain of angina pectoris due to hypoxia of the myocardium.

Chronic Pain

Chronic pain is generally identified as long-term (lasting 6 months or longer), persistent, nearly constant, or recurrent pain that produces significant negative changes in the client's life. Unlike acute pain, chronic pain may last long after the pathology is resolved. Although severe chronic persistent pain is experienced by some infants, children, and adolescents, it is much more common in the adult population (Schecter et al., 1993). More than 30% of all persons in the U.S. experience chronic pain, with the most common chronic pain in adults being back pain (Vasudevan, 1993).

Chronic acute pain occurs almost daily over a long period, has the potential for lasting months or years, and has a high probability of ending. Severe burn injuries and cancer are examples of pathophysiology that leads to chronic acute pain, which may last for long periods before the condition is cured or controlled. In some cases, the pain ends only with the death of the client, as in the case of those terminally ill with cancer (McCaffery & Pasero, 1999). This type of pain is also known as *progressive pain.*

Chronic nonmalignant pain, also called *chronic benign pain,* occurs almost daily and lasts for at least 6 months, with intensity ranging from mild to severe. McCaffery and Pasero (1999) identify three critical characteristics of chronic nonmalignant pain in that it:

- is due to non–life-threatening causes.
- is not responsive to currently available methods of pain relief.
- may continue for the remainder of the client's life.

Examples of pathophysiology leading to chronic nonmalignant pain include:

- Many forms of **neuralgia** (paroxysmal pain that extends along the course of one or more nerves)
- Low back pain
- Rheumatoid arthritis
- Ankylosing spondylitis
- **Phantom limb pain** (a form of neuropathic pain that occurs after amputation with pain sensations referred to an area in the missing portion of the limb)
- **Myofascial pain syndromes** (a group of muscle disorders characterized by pain, muscle spasm, tenderness, stiffness, and limited motion)

When chronic nonmalignant pain is severe enough to disable the client, it is identified as *chronic intractable nonmalignant pain syndrome.*

The signs and symptoms of chronic pain can look very different from those of acute pain. The body cannot tolerate the sympathetic nervous system signs for such a long period of time and, therefore, adapts. The vital signs will often be normal, with no accompanying pupil dilatation or perspiration. Lack of these signs may prompt some health care workers to question the client's description of pain.

The signs and symptoms of chronic pain, such as hopelessness, listlessness, and loss of libido and weight, are similar to those of depression. The client will often complain of exhaustion and fatigue. Behaviors include no complaints of pain unless asked and physical inactivity or immobility that can lead to functional disability. The crying, moaning, guarding, and grimacing that most clinicians associate with pain are absent. Treatment of chronic pain is more complex than that of acute pain. Chronic pain is viewed by pain experts as a disease state, rather than a symptom (Bonica, 1990). Management includes identifying the cause of pain, recognizing emotional and environmental factors that may be contributing to the pain, and rehabilitation to improve the client's functional abilities.

PURPOSE OF PAIN

Pain serves an important purpose as a protective mechanism. For example, if a person touches a hot stove, the pain signal will cause the person to pull the hand away immediately. The skin would be seriously burned if this did not happen. Pain not only protects, but it prompts clients to seek out medical care.

Pain is also useful as a diagnostic tool. Characteristics of the pain, such as the quality and duration, can give important clues in determining a client's medical diagnosis. For example, in acute appendicitis, the clinician looks for rebound tenderness (the pain increases when pressure is released) when palpating the abdomen. This particular type of pain helps to confirm the diagnosis of appendicitis rather than other gastrointestinal disorders.

PHYSIOLOGY OF PAIN

There are two known endogenous (developing within) analgesia systems in humans: the opioid system and the nonopioid system. The opioid system is best known and is mediated by a family of chemicals known as **endorphins** (endogenous neuropeptides that have morphinelike effects). The nonopioid system is mediated by monoamine substances such as norepinephrine and serotonin.

When pain occurs, sensory input from injured tissue causes peripheral **nociceptors** (receptive neurons for painful sensations) and central nervous system (CNS) pain pathways to enhance subsequent responses to pain stimuli (Dubner, 1991). Thus, long-lasting changes in cells within the spinal cord **afferent** (ascending) and **efferent** (descending) **pain pathways** may occur after a brief noxious stimulus.

Physiological responses (such as elevated blood pressure, pulse rate, and respiratory rate; dilated pupils; pallor; and perspiration) to even a brief acute pain episode will begin showing adaptation within a short period, possibly minutes to a few hours. Physiologically, the body cannot sustain the extreme stress response for other than short periods of time. The body conserves its resources by physiological adaptation: returning to normal or near normal blood pressure, pulse rate, and respiratory rate; normal pupil size, and dry skin with little evidence of poor perfusion, *even in the face of continuing pain of the same intensity.*

Stimulation of Pain

The specific action of pain varies depending on the type of pain. In cutaneous pain, cutaneous nerve transmissions travel through a reflex arc from the nerve ending (point of pain) to the brain at a speed of approximately 300 feet per second, with a reflex response causing an almost immediate reaction. This explains why, when a hot stove is touched, the person's hand jerks back *before* there is conscious awareness that damage is occurring (Figure 14-2). After a hot stove is touched, a sensory nerve ending in the skin of the finger initiates nerve transmission that travels through the dorsal root ganglion to the dorsal horn in the gray matter of the spinal cord. From there, the impulse travels though an interneuron that synapses with a motor neuron, which exits the spinal cord at the same level. This motor neuron, and the stimulation of the muscle it innervates, is responsible for the swift movement of the hand away from the hot stove.

In the case of the hot stove, the sensory neuron synapses not only with an interneuron but also with an afferent sensory neuron. The impulse travels up the spinal cord to the thalamus, where a final synapse conducts the impulse to the cortex of the brain. Once the signal reaches the cortex and is interpreted by the brain, the information is available on a conscious level. It is then that the person becomes aware of the intensity, location, and quality of pain. This information is interpreted in light of previous experience, adding the affective component to the pain experience. Efferent or descending motor neuron response is conducted from the brain through the spinal cord, where it synapses with a motor neuron that exits the spinal cord and innervates the muscle.

In visceral pain, transmission of pain impulses is slower and less localized than in cutaneous pain. The internal organs (including the gastrointestinal tract) have a minimal number of nociceptors, which explains why visceral pain is poorly localized and is felt as a dull aching or throbbing sensation. However, internal

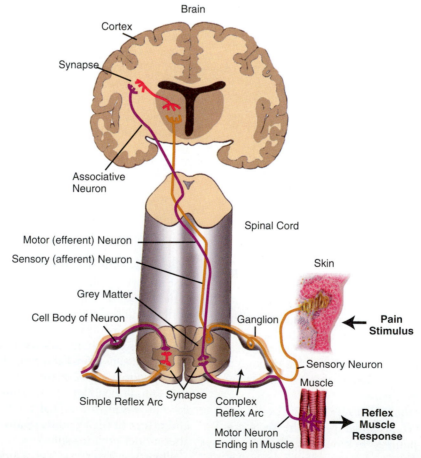

Figure 14-2 Reflex Arcs *(From* Fundamentals of Nursing: Standards and Practice, *by S. DeLaune and P. Ladner, 1998, Albany, NY: Delmar. Copyright 1998 by Delmar. Reprinted with permission.)*

PROFESSIONAL TIP

Sensation of Pain

It takes 0.2 grams of pressure per square millimeter for the cornea of the eye to feel pain, as opposed to 20 grams on the forearm, 200 grams on the sole of the foot, and 300 grams on the fingertips (Brand & Yancey, 1993).

organs have extreme sensitivity to distension. The cramping pain of **colic** (acute abdominal pain), for example, results when:

- Flatus or constipation causes distension of the stomach or intestines
- There is hyperperistalsis, as in gastroenteritis
- Something tries to pass through an opening that is too small

The physiology of **ischemic pain**, or pain occurring when the blood supply of an area is restricted or cut off completely, also differs from that of cutaneous pain. The restriction of blood flow causes inadequate oxygenation of the tissue supplied by those vessels, as well as inadequate metabolic waste product removal. Ischemic pain has the most rapid onset in an active muscle and a much slower onset in a passive muscle. Examples of ischemic pain are muscle cramps, sickle cell pain crisis, angina pectoris, and myocardial infarction. When ischemic pain occurs in a muscle that continues to work, a muscle spasm (cramp) is the outcome. If the blood supply to the heart is severely restricted or completely cut off and is not restored quickly, a myocardial infarction will occur.

Safety: Ischemic Pain

Supplemental oxygen and pain medication must be administered quickly to clients with ischemic pain to minimize oxygen deprivation and prevent infarction (tissue death).

In acute pain episodes, substances released from injured tissue lead to stress hormone responses in the client. This causes an increased metabolic rate, enhanced breakdown of body tissue, impaired immune function, increased blood clotting, and water retention. It triggers the fight-or-flight reaction leading to tachycardia and negative emotions.

The Gate Control Theory

Theories of pain transmission and interpretation attempt to describe and explain the pain experience. Early pain theorists focused on the neuroanatomical and neurophysiological mechanisms while failing to consider the psychological, social, cultural, and developmental factors involved (Stevens, 1994).

In 1965, Melzack and Wall proposed the **gate control pain theory**, which was the first to recognize that the psychological aspects of pain are as important as the physiological aspects. The gate control theory combines cognitive, sensory, and emotional components—in addition to the physiological aspects—and proposes that they can act on a gate control system to block the individual's perception of pain. The basic premise of this theory is that transmission of potentially painful nerve impulses to the cortex is modulated by a gating mechanism in the spinal cord and by CNS activity. As a result, the level of conscious awareness of painful sensation is altered.

The theory suggests that nerve fibers that contribute to pain transmission converge at a site in the dorsal horn of the spinal cord. This site is thought to act as a gating mechanism that determines which impulses will be blocked and which will be transmitted to the thalamus. The image of a gate can be useful in teaching clients and their families about pain relief measures. If the "gate" is closed, the signal is stopped before it reaches the brain, where **perception** (being aware of) of pain occurs. If the gate is open, the signal will continue on through the spinothalamic tract to the cortex, and the client will feel the pain. Whether the gate is opened or closed is influenced by the impulses from peripheral nerves (the sensory components) and nerve signals that descend from the brain (motivational-affective and cognitive components). For example, stimulation of some types of peripheral nerves by cutaneous stimulation such as massage can close the gate, whereas stimulation of the nociceptors will open the gate.

If a person is anxious, the gate can be opened by signals sent from the brain down to the mechanism in the dorsal horn of the spinal cord. On the other hand, if the person has had positive experiences with pain control in the past, the cognitive influence can send signals down to the gating mechanism and close it. The gate theory offered a great benefit by suggesting new approaches to relieving both acute and chronic pain. Pain could be relieved by blocking the transmission of pain impulses to the brain by both physical modalities and by altering the individual's thought processes, emotions, or other behaviors.

Conduction of Pain Impulses

Conduction of pain impulses refers to the physiologic processes that occur from the initiation of the pain signal to the realization of pain by the individual. There are four processes involved in the conduction of this signal. The first of these, **transduction**, is the step where a noxious stimulus triggers electrical activity in the endings of afferent nerve fibers (nociceptors). Once the signal is triggered, **transmission** occurs. The impulse travels from the receiving nociceptors to the spinal cord. Projection neurons then carry the message to the thalamus, and the message continues to the somatosensory cortex. This is where the third step, perception of pain, occurs. It is here that neural messages are converted into the subjective experience. The fourth process, **modulation**, is a central nervous system pathway that selectively inhibits pain transmission by sending blocking signals back down to the dorsal horn of the spinal cord.

FACTORS AFFECTING THE PAIN EXPERIENCE

McCaffery and Pasero (1999) point out that *the client is the only authority about the existence and nature of his or her pain.* Many factors account for the differences in clients' individual responses to pain, including age, previous experience with pain, drug abuse, and cultural norms.

Age

Age can greatly influence a client's perception of the pain experience. Clients may continue pain behaviors they learned as children and may also be reluctant to admit pain or seek medical care because of fear of the unknown or fear of the impact that treatment may have on their lifestyle. Older adults may often ignore their pain, viewing it as an unavoidable consequence of aging; family and health care members may inadvertently support this stereotype and be less than responsive to an older client's complaints of pain.

Previous Experience with Pain

Clients' previous exposures to pain will often influence their reactions. Coping mechanisms that were used in the past may affect clients' judgments about how the pain will affect their lives and what measures are within their control to successfully manage the pain on their own. Client teaching about pain expectations and management methods can often allay client fears and lead to more successful pain management, especially in those clients who do not have previous pain experience or who have memories of a previous devastating pain experience that they do not wish to repeat.

GERONTOLOGICAL CONSIDERATIONS

Elders and Pain

Older clients often are resigned to living with pain believing that nothing can be done. Pain often is not reported by older clients for fear of being labeled a "bother" or "complainer." The nurse should convey empathy and encourage the client to request pain relief as needed.

Drug Abuse

According to Compton (1999), a drug abuser is likely to be *less* tolerant of pain than someone who does not use drugs. Drug abuse may cause changes in the central nervous system that result in an exaggerated neurophysiologic response to painful stimuli. To keep a drug abuser comfortable, withdrawal must be prevented.

Cultural Norms

Cultural diversity in pain responses can easily lead to problems in pain management. Laboratory studies on subjects of various cultures found no significant difference among the groups in the level of intensity at which pain becomes appreciable or perceptible. However, the same studies showed that the subjects differed significantly in the level of intensity or duration of pain the client was willing to endure. Expression of pain is also governed by cultural values. In some cultures, tolerance to pain, and therefore "suffering in silence," is expected; in others, full expression of pain may include animated physical and emotional responses. The nurse must be careful not to equate the level of expression of pain with the level of actual pain experienced, but to instead consider cultural and other influences that affect the expression of pain.

JCAHO STANDARDS

New pain management standards were included in the 2000–2001 standards of the Joint Commission on Accreditation of Healthcare Organizations (JCAHO). They will first be scored for compliance in 2001.

The health care organizations will be expected to:

- Recognize the right of patients to appropriate assessment and management of pain;
- Assess the existence and, if so, the nature and intensity of pain in all patients;
- Record the results of the assessment in a way that facilitates regular reassessment and follow up;
- Determine and assure staff competency in pain assessment and management and address pain assessment and management in the orientation of all new staff;
- Establish policies and procedures which support the appropriate prescription or ordering of effective pain medications;
- Educate patients and their families about effective pain management; and
- Address patient needs for symptom management in the discharge planning process (JCAHO, 1999).

NURSING PROCESS

The nursing process will provide the correct framework for managing a client's pain.

Assessment

Assessment of the client's pain is a crucial function of the nurse. During the assessment process, nurses need to be aware of their own values and expectations about pain behaviors. Just as the client's experience and cultural background help determine how pain is demonstrated, nurses' cultures and experiences help determine which pain behaviors are viewed as acceptable. Nurses need to be aware of these values and avoid biases when assessing client pain and planning client care. Once a self-assessment about pain has been conducted, the nurse is ready to assess the client.

Pain assessment tools are the single most effective method of identifying the presence and intensity of pain in clients. *These tools must be used, and the results must be believed.* Figure 14-3 shows the Initial Pain Assessment Tool developed by McCaffery and Beebe and found in AHCPR's acute pain management guideline (AHCPR, 1992). This tool is particularly effective when clients have complex pain problems because it as-

sesses location, intensity, quality, precipitating and alleviating factors, and how the pain affects function and quality of life. Once this tool is completed, another less detailed tool can be used for ongoing monitoring of the client's pain level.

Subjective Data

Gathering subjective information regarding the client's pain is the first step in pain assessment. The nurse should determine a client's pain threshold and pain tolerance level. **Pain threshold** is the level of intensity at which a person feels pain. It will vary with each individual and with each different type of pain. **Pain tolerance** is the level of intensity or duration of pain the client is willing or able to endure.

The client's description of the pain should cover several qualifiers, including its location, onset and duration, quality, intensity, aggravating factors (variables that worsen the pain, such as exercise, certain foods, or stress), alleviating factors (measures the client can

Figure 14-3 Initial Pain Assessment Tool (*From* Pain: Clinical Manual for Nursing Practice, *by M. McCaffery and A. Beebe, 1989, St. Louis, MO: Mosby. Copyright 1989 by Mosby. Reprinted with permission.)

PROFESSIONAL TIP

Location of Pain

During intershift report on a postoperative client recovering from abdominal surgery, the nurse reported that the client had stated she had pain and had been medicated with IM Demerol. When greeting her client, the nurse asked the client about the pain she had experienced during the night. The client replied, "Oh, it is fine now, I only had a headache." The night nurse had assumed the client's pain was in her surgical site and chose the medication accordingly. The headache probably could have been relieved with a milder medication. All reports of pain must be thoroughly asessed prior to any interventions being implemented.

CLIENT TEACHING

Pain at Night

- It is common for pain to be worse at night when there are fewer distractions. Knowing that this is normal can be reassuring because the client may attribute the increased pain to complications.

take that lessen the effect of the pain, such as lying down, avoiding certain foods, or taking medication), associated manifestations (factors that often accompany the pain, such as nausea, constipation, or dizziness), and what pain means to the client.

Whenever subjective and objective data conflict, the subjective reports of pain are to be considered the primary source.

Location The client can point to the location of the pain on the client's own body or locate it on a body diagram on a pain assessment tool. The client should be asked if there is more than one site of pain; if the pain radiates, and if so to where; and ask if the pain is deep or superficial.

Onset and Duration The nurse should ask the client how long the pain has existed; what, if anything, triggers its onset; and if there are any patterns to the pain; for example, whether it is worse at certain times of the day or night.

Quality The nurse should ask the client what the pain feels like, and record the words used to describe the pain. Clients may use sensory-type words, such as "pricking," "radiating," "burning," or "throbbing." However, some clients use words that have an affective connotation, such as "fearful," "sickening," or "punishing." Other words used may be evaluative, such as "miserable" or "unbearable." The quality of pain provides information that may be useful in diagnosing the cause of the pain. For example, pain described as "burning" or "freezing" is usually neuropathic in origin.

Intensity The client may have difficulty in judging the intensity of pain. However, it is important to obtain an estimate of the severity of the pain. This information allows the clinician to evaluate the effectiveness of pain relief measures tried by comparing intensity before and after the interventions.

Pain intensity scales are an effective method for clients to rate the intensity of their pain (Figure 14-4).

The simple descriptive pain-intensity scale and the visual analog scale (VAS) are best used by showing the scale to the client and asking the client to point to the spot on the scale that corresponds to the present pain. The pain scale most frequently used with adolescent and adult clients is the verbal 0 to 10 scale. No equipment or supplies are needed, and it requires only enough time to ask one question: "On a scale of 0 to 10, with 0 being no pain at all and 10 being the worst pain you could ever have, how much do you hurt right now?" If there are multiple painful areas, this question can be asked regarding each area.

Although developed for use with children, the FACES Pain Rating Scale (Figure 14-5) can be used effectively with clients when a language barrier exists. A translator should be used initially to explain what the faces represent.

Aggravating and Alleviating Factors The nurse should question the client about what makes the pain worse and what makes the pain better, including

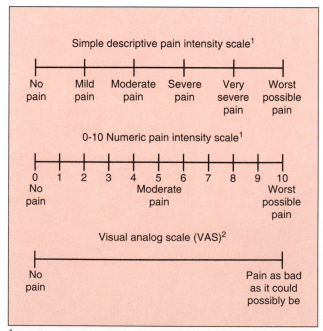

[1] If used as a graphic rating scale, a 10-cm baseline is recommended.
[2] A 10-cm baseline is recommended for VAS scales.

Figure 14-4 Pain Intensity Scales: Three Commonly Used Self-Report Intensity Scales *(Courtesy of Agency for Health Care Policy and Research, 1992.)*

0	1	2	3	4	5
No hurt	Hurts little bit	Hurts little more	Hurts even more	Hurts whole lot	Hurts worst

Figure 14-5 Wong/Baker FACES Pain Rating Scale (*From Wong, D. L., Hockenberry-Eaton, M., Wilson, D., Winkelstein, M. L., Ahmann, E., DiVito-Thomas, P. A.: Whaley and Wong's Nursing Care of Infants and Children, ed. 6, St. Louis, 1999. Mosby, p. 1153. Copyrighted by Mosby. Reprinted by permission.*)

behaviors or activities that influence the pain. This information provides input into developing the plan of care for the client in pain. If there are specific activities that relieve the pain, the nurse can incorporate them into the care plan. Being aware of activities that increase the pain can allow for interventions that may prevent the pain. For example, if physical therapy exercises trigger an increase in pain, the nurse can administer an analgesic as ordered prior to treatment.

Associated Manifestations The initial pain assessment should include the impact of pain on the activities of daily living. Pain may cause changes in sleep patterns or the ability to work and carry out the many roles in a client's life. Pain may affect appetite, mood, sexual functioning, or the ability to participate in recreational activities. If pain is interfering with daily life, the client's quality of life can be greatly affected.

Pain is fatiguing. It requires a significant amount of energy to deal with pain. The longer a person suffers from pain, the greater the level of fatigue. Although there is no conscious awareness of pain during sleep, there may be a dream-state awareness (McCaffery & Pasero, 1999). The stress response (which can be seen even in clients under general anesthesia) continues, and the body physiologically pays the price. Clients also wake up with considerably more pain than they had going to sleep, thereby requiring even more intervention (pharmacologic and nonpharmacologic) to reduce the pain.

Meaning of Pain Due to the motivational-affective components of the pain experience, the meaning of pain can have a great impact on how the client perceives the pain. A frequently cited classic study on this phenomenon was conducted by Beecher (1956), who compared the pain perceived by soldiers wounded in battle to pain perceived by civilians with similar surgical wounds. He found that only 32% of the soldiers required narcotics for pain relief, whereas 85% of the civilians needed the narcotics. This was interpreted that for the soldiers, the wound represented a ticket away from the battlefield, while for the civilians, the surgical wound was a depressing event.

The nurse should explore with the client what implications the pain may have for the individual. Does it mean that the client's cancer is metastasizing? Or that the client's condition is worsening? All of these interpretations may influence the pain experience for the client.

Objective Data

As discussed when addressing acute versus chronic pain, the objective data often presents a different picture depending on the type of pain the client is experiencing.

Physiologic Acute pain activates the sympathetic nervous system, and the client may exhibit the following: elevated heart rate, elevated respiratory rate, elevated blood pressure, diaphoresis, pallor, muscle tension, and dilated pupils. These signs resemble those of anxiety, which often accompanies acute pain. The signs and symptoms of chronic pain show adaption, and, therefore, are different from those of acute pain, with vital signs being normal and no accompanying pupil dilation or perspiration.

Behavioral Acute pain behaviors may include crying and moaning, rubbing the site of pain, restlessness, a distorted posture, clenched fists, guarding the painful area, frowning, and grimacing. The client usually speaks of the discomfort and may be restless or afraid to move.

The client in chronic pain may demonstrate behaviors similar to those of depression such as hopelessness, listlessness, and loss of libido and weight. Chronic pain also often leads to physical inactivity or immobility, which can lead to functional disability.

Clients' behavioral adaptation may yield no report of pain unless questioned specifically. **Distraction** (focusing attention on stimuli other than pain) may also be used by clients. McCaffery and Pasero (1999) recognize that clients often minimize the pain behaviors they are able to control for a number of reasons including:

PROFESSIONAL TIP

Assessing the Effect of Pain on Sleep

Questioning clients about the effect pain has on their sleep habits will help clarify the intensity of the pain and its effect on the clients' patterns of daily living. The nurse should ask the client whether the pain:

- Prevents the client from falling asleep
- Makes finding a comfortable sleeping position difficult
- Wakes the client from a sound sleep
- Keeps the client from falling back asleep once awakened
- Leaves the client feeling tired and unrefreshed after a sleeping session

- To be a "good" client and avoid making demands
- To maintain a positive self-image by not becoming a "sissy"
- By using distraction as a method of making pain more bearable (young children are particularly adept at this)
- Exhaustion

Occasionally, there is a discrepancy between pain behaviors observed by the nurse (objective data) and the client's self-report of pain. Client pain behaviors (AHCPR, 1992) include splinting of the painful area, distorted posture, impaired mobility, insomnia, anxiety, attention seeking, and depression. Discrepancies between behaviors and the client's self-report can be due to good coping skills (e.g., relaxation techniques or distraction), stoicism, anxiety, or cultural differences in expected pain behaviors. Whenever these discrepancies occur, they should be addressed with the client, and the pain management plan must be renegotiated accordingly.

Ongoing Assessment

The initial assessment obtains a baseline of information regarding the client's pain. Subsequent assessments provide information regarding the effectiveness of the interventions. Physiologic and behavioral signs, and most important, the client's subjective pain ratings of the intensity will all help the health care team determine whether the interventions should be continued or changed. Pain assessments should be performed to coincide with when the intervention should be providing the most relief. For example, the onset of intravenous morphine is rapid, peaking approximately 20 minutes after administration. If the client has not obtained relief by 20 minutes, the intravenous morphine was ineffective, and the plan of care would need to be changed.

CULTURAL CONSIDERATIONS

Perception of Pain

Culture determines the way persons derive meaning from their lives and also determines appropriate behaviors. One's cultural upbringing teaches behaviors, including those that are exhibited when in pain. People from different cultures use different types of words to describe pain (for example, in sensory or emotional terms). These differences should not be ignored, but the nurse also needs to be careful not to prejudge a client based on cultural background or ethnicity. Due to the unique experience of pain, the person will exhibit individualized behaviors even though they are influenced by cultural upbringing.

Recording Pain Assessment Findings

No matter which pain assessment tool is chosen, it will be of little effect unless the pain rating and related information are recorded in a manner easily understood by the health care team. Figure 14-6 is a flow sheet (McCaffery & Beebe, 1989) that is an excellent record in an acute care setting. It provides one place to document the majority of information used to make pain management decisions, including pain rating, vital signs, analgesic administered, and level of arousal.

Nursing Diagnoses

The two primary nursing diagnoses used to describe pain are *Acute Pain* and *Chronic Pain*. According to the North American Nursing Diagnosis Association (NANDA, 2001), *Acute Pain* is defined as "an unpleasant sensory and emotional experience arising from actual or potential tissue damage or described in terms of such damage . . . [with] sudden or slow onset of any intensity from mild to severe, with an anticipated or predictable end and a duration of less than 6 months" (p. 129). *Chronic Pain* is defined as *Acute Pain*, with the last phrase replaced by "constant or recurring without an anticipated or predictable end and a duration of greater than 6 months" (p. 130).

Pain may be the etiology (cause) of other problems, for example: *Impaired Physical Mobility*, related to arthritic hip pain. Whether the pain is addressed in the problem statement or the etiology will be determined by the client's primary problem. There are many diagnoses that can be related to the client in pain depending on the effects of the pain:

- *Activity Intolerance*
- *Anxiety*
- *Constipation*
- *Deficient Knowledge*
- *Disturbed Body Image*
- *Disturbed Sleep Pattern*
- *Disturbed Thought Processes*
- *Fatigue*
- *Fear*
- *Hopelessness*
- *Impaired Physical Mobility*
- *Impaired Social Interaction*
- *Ineffective Breathing Pattern*
- *Ineffective Coping*
- *Ineffective Role Performance*
- *Ineffective Therapeutic Regimen Management*
- *Powerlessness*

Planning/Outcome Identification

When planning care for the client experiencing pain, mutual goal setting is of utmost importance. After assessing the client's perception of the problem, the

Patient _____   Date _____
Pain rating scale used* _____
Purpose: To evaluate the safety and effectiveness of the analgesic(s)
Analgesic(s) prescribed: _____

Time	Pain rating	Analgesic	R	P	BP	Level of arousal	Other**	Plan and comments

May be duplicated for use in clinical practice.
*Pain rating: A number of different scales may be used. Indicate which scale is used and use the same scale each time.
**Possibilities for other columns: bowel function, activities, nausea and vomiting, and other pain relief measures. Identify the side effects of greatest concern to patient, family, physician, and nurse.

Figure 14-6 Flow Sheet for Pain Management Documentation (*From* Pain: Clinical Manual for Nursing Practice, *by M. McCaffery and A. Beebe, 1989, St. Louis, MO: Mosby. Copyright 1989 by Mosby. Reprinted with permission.*)

nurse and client can work together in developing realistic outcomes. Both nonpharmacologic and pharmacologic interventions should be considered in planning strategies to return clients to control or to maintain them at desired levels of functioning and pain.

When asking about the client's goal for pain relief, the nurse often has to state, "We can't usually get rid of all your pain, but if we could get it down to a place that it didn't bother you so much, what would that be?" That way the client, the family, and health care professionals involved will all be aware of the goal for pain relief and can adjust the plan of care accordingly.

Often several approaches must be combined for adequate relief to be obtained. No matter which type of intervention is being utilized, there are general principles that apply: individualization, prevention, and utilization of a multidisciplinary approach.

Individualize the Approach

A variety of pain relief measures can be tried in many combinations until the goal of pain relief is reached. This often means some trial-and-error of interventions until the right combination is found. It is important to include measures that the client believes will be effective. The cognitive component of pain perception can have a powerful influence on the effectiveness of interventions. This may mean including folk remedies or nonscientific relief measures. It is important to keep an open mind. This comes with the caution that the nurse needs to avoid those remedies that may harm the client.

Use a Preventive Approach

Pain is much easier to control if it is treated before it gets severe. Interventions should be implemented when pain is mild, or when it is anticipated. For example, medicate a client prior to a painful dressing change or treatment rather than waiting for the pain to occur.

Use a Multidisciplinary Approach

Pain relief is a complex phenomenon requiring input from various members of the health care team. The nurse's role is pivotal in managing a client's pain. The physician also plays a key role, diagnosing and treating the medical cause of the pain, which includes prescribing appropriate medications. In complex cases, other professionals, such as physical therapists, psychologists, social workers, or chaplains may be needed. The multidisciplinary team approach is the most successful way to manage chronic pain and improve the quality of a client's life.

Nursing Interventions

Pharmacologic and nonpharmacologic interventions can both be effective in caring for clients with pain. In some cases of mild pain, nonpharmacologic techniques may be the primary intervention, with medication available as "backup." In cases of moderate to severe pain, nonpharmacologic techniques can be an effective adjunctive, or complementary, treatment.

There are three categories of pain control interventions: (1) pharmacological, (2) noninvasive, and

(3) invasive. Each category will be discussed separately, but these methods are often used in combination.

Pharmacological Interventions

Drug therapy is the mainstay of treatment for pain control. The American Pain Society (1999) and AHCPR (1992, 1994) have published guidelines that provide specific recommendations for the use of drug therapy in pain control. These guidelines were developed by panels of experts who analyzed current research available on pain control and represent concise information that can help nurses, physicians, and other health care workers to effectively administer medications for pain relief.

The World Health Organization (WHO) has made worldwide relief of cancer pain one of their primary goals (1990). In order to help meet this goal, it developed an analgesic ladder to help the clinician determine which analgesic to prescribe (Figure 14-7). Combining analgesics and the use of adjuvant medication provides effective pharmacologic intervention for clients with pain. **Adjuvant medications** are those drugs used to enhance the analgesic efficacy of opioids, to treat concurrent symptoms that exacerbate pain, and to provide independent analgesia for specific types of pain. The ladder recommends that the analgesic, plus or minus an adjuvant, is chosen based on the level of pain the client is experiencing. For mild pain, the ladder recommends a nonopioid. If the pain persists or if the client has moderate pain to begin with, WHO recommends a weak opioid, plus or minus the nonopioid, plus or minus an adjuvant. If pain persists, a strong opioid is used. The *nonopioid should be continued,* and an adjuvant medication should be considered (AHCPR, 1994). This ladder gives health care workers guidelines in determining if the drug regimen is appropriate for the client with cancer pain.

Nurses' Role in Administration of Analgesics The nurse is the health care professional who spends the most time with the client in pain and is the team member who is most often able to assess the effectiveness of pain control interventions. When analgesics are prescribed, the nurse is often given choices of drug, route, and interval. For example, the postop client may have the following orders:

- Morphine 10–15 mg IM or IV q2–4h prn severe pain
- Vicodin i–ii tabs q3–4h prn moderate pain

When this client complains of pain, which analgesic should the nurse administer? Which route? Which dose? How frequently? The nurse in this situation carries a large responsibility in making these decisions. The nurse also has autonomy in making these decisions. The client may not be aware of all the available choices. Each nurse may make a different decision, often based on the nurse's own biases.

Figure 14-7 WHO Analgesic Ladder gives guidelines for choosing analgesic therapy for cancer pain based on the level of pain the client is experiencing. (*Courtesy of World Health Organization, 1990. Used with permission.*)

These choices and autonomy require responsibility on the part of the nurse. McCaffery and Pasero (1999) identify the following as the responsibilities of the nurse in administering analgesics. The nurse must:

- Determine whether or not to give the analgesic, and if more than one is ordered, which one
- Assess the client's response to the analgesic, including assessing the effectiveness in pain relief and occurrence of any side effects
- Report to the physician when a change is needed, including making suggestions for changes based on the nurse's knowledge of the client and pharmacology
- Teach the client and family regarding the use of analgesics

Principles of Administering Analgesics "How an analgesic is used is probably more important than which one is used" (McCaffery & Pasero, 1999). There are principles that should be applied in the administration of analgesics, no matter which one is given.

Establishing and maintaining a therapeutic serum level is important. Figure 14-8 illustrates the peaks and valleys that often occur when analgesics are administered in the traditional prn (as needed) manner. When the dose is administered on an intermittent schedule, a

Figure 14-8 Peaks and Valleys of Analgesic Administration. *(From Pain: Clinical Manual for Nursing Practice, by M. McCaffery and A. Beebe, 1989, St. Louis, MO: Mosby. Copyright 1989 by Mosby. Reprinted with permission.)*

CLIENT TEACHING

Pain Management

Clients and their families must be educated regarding:

- The importance of taking or requesting pain medication before the pain becomes severe and more difficult to control
- The numerous nonpharmacologic approaches that clients can use to augment their pharmacologic pain management
- The individualization of pain management (The client may be taking different medications or different dosages than other individuals.)

larger dose is often required, causing the client to have a peak serum drug level in the sedation range. The client must wait for the return of pain before requesting the next dose of analgesic. Depending on the length of time it takes to obtain the medication and, once taken, to reestablish an adequate blood level, there could be a period of up to an hour or so with inadequate pain control.

Preventive Approach Pain is much easier to control if treated when it is anticipated or at a mild intensity. Once pain becomes severe, the analgesics ordered may not be effective enough to relieve it. Many clinicians still teach their clients to wait to take medication until they are sure they really need it. This practice leads to uncontrolled pain. There are two ways the preventive approach may be implemented:

- ATC (around the clock)—When pain is predictable, for example, the first few days following surgery or with chronic cancer pain, the medication is administered on a scheduled basis. This prevents the peaks and valleys of serum drug level that can lead to oversedation or toxicity and recurrence of pain, respectively. If the analgesics are ordered by the physician to be given PRN, it can still be a nursing measure to administer the drugs ATC, as long as they are given within the time constraints of the order.
- PRN (Latin for *pro re nata,* which means "as required")—Pain cannot always be predictable, therefore PRN dosing may be required. For some clients this may be used in addition to scheduled dosing for "breakthrough" pain (pain that surpasses the level of **analgesia**, or pain relief, that the steady level of analgesics is providing). Examples of this include a cancer client on prolonged-release morphine who needs extra analgesics to participate in activities such as shopping or receiving visitors. Another example would be the orthopedic client who

is receiving regularly scheduled analgesics for postop pain who needs additional pain relief for therapy sessions. In order to implement the preventive approach with PRN dosing, the medications should be given as soon as the pain appears, or when it is anticipated to begin.

Titrate to Effect Due to the unique nature of the pain experience, the analgesic regimen needs to be titrated until the desired effect is achieved. This involves adjusting the following:

- *Dosage*—Some clients may require more or less than the standard dose. There are many factors that may influence the pharmacokinetics in an individual client. The individual's response is assessed and the dosage of the analgesic is regulated accordingly. In clients with chronic cancer pain, opioid analgesics are recommended to be increased until pain relief is obtained or unacceptable side effects occur. This may be done due to the lack of a **ceiling effect** (the dosage beyond which no further analgesia occurs) in pure opioids. The lack of a ceiling effect means there is no limit to the dose that can be given. For example, cancer clients have been known to receive over 1 gram per hour intravenously. Because the dosage is gradually increased, the client develops a **tolerance** (requiring larger and larger doses of an analgesic to achieve the same level of pain relief) to the side effects of the opioid.
- *Interval*—Some clients metabolize the analgesics faster than others. For example, young adults tend to metabolize opioids faster, therefore they may need more frequent doses. Older clients tend to metabolize them slower, therefore they will require a longer interval between doses.
- *Route*—The appropriate route is chosen depending on how rapidly pain relief is required, the client's ability to take medications orally, the client's diag-

nosis, and assessment of the client's response to the current route. Intravenous administration provides the most rapid onset of pain relief. All other routes require a lag time for absorption of the analgesic into the circulation. In postoperative pain, IV is the preferred route for opioids when the oral route is not appropriate. If IV access is not available, sublingual, rectal, or transdermal routes should be considered (AHCPR, 1992).

With cancer pain, the oral route is preferred. If these clients are unable to take oral medications, rectal and transdermal routes are preferred since they are less invasive than other routes (AHCPR, 1994). In addition, tolerance develops at a slower rate with the oral route compared to the more invasive routes.

- *Choice of drug*—If one drug is not providing relief or has unacceptable side effects, another analgesic may be tried.

The key to administering an analgesic is to monitor the client's response to it. This includes assessing the effectiveness of pain relief and the occurrence of side effects.

Classes of Analgesics There are three classes of drugs used for pain relief: (1) nonopioid analgesics; (2) opioid analgesics; and (3) analgesic adjuvants already discussed (WHO, 1986). Nonopioid and opioid analgesics will be addressed separately, as indications and side effects are different for each one.

Nonopioids The medications in this category are useful for a variety of painful conditions, including surgery, trauma, and cancer (American Pain Society, 1992). The indications include mild to moderate pain, and they are used in conjunction with opioids. These drugs differ from opioids in several ways in that they:

- Are subject to the ceiling effect
- Do not produce the effect of tolerance or physical dependence
- Are antipyretic, and should not be given in cases where they may mask an infection

Ketorolac is the only NSAID available in parenteral form and has proven useful in clients on NPO status who would benefit from a NSAID. Even when administered intramuscularly or intravenously, ketorolac produces significant gastric irritation and the potential for gastric bleeding. The most frequent use of ketorolac is orally or intramuscularly in adults, but some pediatric

centers have used it intravenously under strict supervision for a limited course (less than 5 days) in children and adolescents with great success.

Action Action of these drugs is thought to inhibit prostaglandin formation. If prostaglandins are inhibited, the sensory neurons are less likely to receive the pain signal. Thus, this class of analgesics works in the peripheral nervous system.

Opioids The opioid analgesics fall into three classes: pure opioid agonists, partial agonists, and **mixed agonist-antagonists** (a compound that blocks opioid effects on one receptor type while producing opioid effects on a second receptor type). Pure agonists are those that produce a maximal response from cells when they bind to the cells' opioid receptor sites. Morphine (the gold standard against which all other opioids are measured), fentanyl (Duragesic), methadone (Dolophine), hydromorphone hydrochloride (Dilaudid), and codeine are pure agonists. Meperidine (Demerol), although classified as a pure agonist, is not recommended except in clients with a true allergy to all other narcotics, because of its neurotoxicity. Meperidine produces clinical analgesia for only 2.5 to 3.5 hours when given intramuscularly in adults.

Unlike the NSAIDs, pure agonist opioids are not subject to the ceiling effect. As the dosage is increased, there is increasing pain relief.

Action Opioids act in the central nervous system by binding to opiate receptor sites on afferent neurons.

PROFESSIONAL TIP

Types of Nonopioid Drugs

- *Salicylates*—These include aspirin and other salicylate salts. Common side effects of aspirin include gastric disturbances and bleeding due to the antiplatelet effect. Some of the salicylate salts, such as choline magnesium trisalicylate (Trilisate) and salsalate (Salgesic) have fewer gastrointestinal and bleeding effects than aspirin.
- *Acetaminophen*—This is a nonsalicylate that is similar to aspirin in its analgesic action, but has no anti-inflammatory effect. Its mechanism of action for pain relief is not known.
- *NSAIDs*—The effectiveness of these drugs varies, with some being close to the effectiveness of aspirin and acetaminophen, while others are much stronger. Clients tend to vary in response, so once the maximum recommended dose has been tried with ineffective results, it would be worth trying another NSAID. The drugs in this group inhibit platelet aggregation, and are contraindicated in clients with coagulation disorders or on anticoagulation therapy.

PROFESSIONAL TIP

Ketorolac
Ketorolac should not be used in a client with any history of renal dysfunction, gastric irritation, bleeding problems, low platelet count, or allergy to aspirin or other NSAIDs.

GERONTOLOGICAL CONSIDERATIONS

Effects of Meperidine (Demerol)

- In the elderly, most of whom show decreased glomerular filtration rates, there is generally a higher peak and longer duration of action as it takes longer to excrete the opioid as well as its toxic metabolite, normeperidine.

The pain signal is stopped at the spinal cord level, and does not reach the cortex where pain is perceived.

Side Effects The only limiting factor in the use of pure agonist opioids is the degree of side effects, particularly respiratory depression and constipation. Other side effects include pruritus and nausea, but the degree to which they are present from each medication varies among individuals. Clients must be instructed regarding these normal responses to opioids and informed that it does not mean that they are allergic to them. A true allergy to opioids would be indicated by a rash or hives that starts after receiving the opioid, a local histamine release at the site of infusion, or anaphylaxis. Clients also need to know that the pruritus and nausea generally subside after 4 to 5 days of opioid therapy. In the meantime, an antihistamine such as diphenhydramine hydrochloride (Benadryl) or hydroxyzine hydrochloride (Atarax, Vistaril) may be used for pruritus, and an antiemetic such as metoclopromide hydrochloride (Clopra) or trimethobenzamide hydrochloride (Tigan) can be used to treat the nausea.

Almost all medications used to treat side effects have their own side effect of sedation. Thus, there is the possibility of a cumulative effect of severe sedation. These medications must be used with caution and appropriate monitoring until the client's response is determined. Ondansetron hydrochloride (Zofran) is one antiemetic on the market with little, if any, sedative effect. It has recently received Food and Drug Administration (FDA) approval for use with postoperative nausea and has been effective in clients with refractory nausea and vomiting unresponsive to other antiemet-

PROFESSIONAL TIP

Constipation and Opioids

Clients who are expected to require opioid analgesics for more than 1 or 2 days should be administered a stool softener as soon as they are taking fluids orally. While they are still NPO, a glycerin or bisacodyl (Dulcolax) suppository should be administered if the client has not had a bowel movement in 1 or 2 days.

ics. The current cost per dose, close to $100 in many hospitals, limits its use to the extreme nausea associated with cancer chemotherapy or to clients with refractory nausea and vomiting.

Mixed agonist-antagonist opioids are believed to be subject to the ceiling effect for pain relief, as well as a ceiling effect for respiratory depression. Mixed agonist-antagonist opioids activate one opioid receptor type while simultaneously blocking another type. Butorphanol tartrate (Stadol), pentazocine hydrochloride (Talwin), and nalbuphine hydrochloride (Nubain) are the most frequently used in pain management.

Opioid antagonists include naloxone (Narcan) and naltrexone (Trexal), with the most commonly used being naloxone (Narcan). They work by blocking opioid stimulation of receptor sites. Naloxone effectively reverses opioid side effects of sedation, respiratory depression, and nausea *while it completely reverses any pain control.*

Alternative Delivery Systems Opioids are administered in more than just the traditional oral, subcutaneous, intramuscular, intravenous, and rectal routes.

Patient-Controlled Analgesia Patient-controlled analgesia (PCA) is most often delivered by a device that allows the client to control the delivery of intravenous, epidural, or subcutaneous pain medication in a safe, effective manner through a programmable pump (Figure 14-9). This system helps to eliminate the time required for the nurse to draw up the medication, and allows the client to feel some control over the pain. The pump has the safety feature of locking out once a maximum dose has been reached. This prevents the client from overdosing. Requirements for the use of PCA are the cognitive ability to understand how to use the pump and the physical ability to push the button. The PCA has been successfully used with many types of pain and in many settings, including pediatrics and home health.

Oral PCA is relatively new in hospitals and, according to Pasero (2000), is becoming increasingly popular.

Figure 14-9 Client on IV Patient-Controlled Analgesia (PCA)

Client teaching is the key for success. The client must understand how pain, pain medication, and pain relief are related and how to maintain a pain-relief diary. A Velcro®-sealed wrist pouch is applied to the client with one or two doses of the prescribed oral analgesic, even controlled substances, in the pouch. The client notifies the nurse when a dose is taken, so it can be replaced. If the client does not comply with the oral PCA policy, it is discontinued.

Epidural/Intrathecal Analgesia **Epidural analgesia** refers to administering the opioid via a catheter that terminates in the epidural space, the space outside the dura mater that protects the spinal cord. **Intrathecal analgesia** refers to administering the drug directly into the subarachnoid space. These may be administered as a one-time injection by the anesthesiologist, or via a catheter that has been placed. Both of these routes are occasionally referred to as *intraspinal anesthesia*. Because the opioid is delivered close to the site of action, these routes require much lower doses of opioid (usually morphine [Duramorph] or fentanyl [Sublimaze] are used) for pain relief. The incidence of systemic side effects is also much lower with these routes. Duration is longer than systemic routes, for example, the duration of one dose of intrathecal morphine can last 24 hours.

Transdermal Analgesia Another route of opioid administration is the transdermal patch. The only opioid drug currently available via this route is fentanyl (Duragesic). This medication is on an adhesive patch that attaches to the skin. It is available in 25, 50, 75, and 100 mcg/hour dosages. The fentanyl transdermal patch allows slow infusion of the drug through the skin. The fentanyl patch is indicated for continuous pain with high dosage requirements. The advantage of this route is that it is simple to apply and it is effective for 72 hours. The disadvantage is that dosage adjustments are difficult to make due to the slow infusion rate. In addition, side effects may not be reversed as rapidly as when opiates are administered via the oral route.

Local Anesthesia Local anesthetics are effective for pain management in a variety of settings. Topical anesthetics are available for teething, sore throats, den-

GERONTOLOGICAL CONSIDERATIONS

Opioid Analgesia in the Elderly

- Cheyne-Stokes respiratory patterns are not unusual during sleep in the elderly and should not be used as a reason to restrict appropriate opioid pain relief unless accompanied by unacceptable degrees of arterial desaturation (less than 85%).
- The elderly experience a higher peak and longer duration of effect of opioid medications and are more sensitive to sedation and respiratory depressant effects.
- Opioid dose titration must be based on analgesic effects and degree of side effects such as sedation, urinary retention, constipation, respiratory depression, or exacerbation of Parkinson's disease (AHCPR, 1992).

ture pain, laceration repair, and intravenous catheter insertions. One topical anesthetic, EMLA cream, is a mixture of local anesthetics, combining prilocaine and lidocaine (Xylocaine). It produces complete anesthesia for at least 60 minutes when topically applied on intact skin. Another topical anesthetic, TAC, is available for anesthesia during closure of lacerations. It is a combination of tetracaine hydrochloride (Pontocaine) 0.5%, adrenaline (epinephrine) 1:2000, and cocaine 11.8% in a normal saline solution that can be applied directly to the open wound surface in place of local anesthetic infiltration with a needle. This allows pain-free cleansing of the laceration as well as suturing. Because both adrenaline (epinephrine) and cocaine cause vasoconstriction, TAC cannot be used in areas supplied by end-arteriolar blood supply such as digits, the ear, or the nose. It also is contraindicated on burned or abraded skin because this could lead to increased systemic absorption of cocaine and tetracaine, thus placing the client at risk for seizures.

Noninvasive Interventions

Noninvasive relief measures consist of cognitive-behavioral strategies and physical modalities that use cutaneous stimulation. These treatments can be used to supplement pharmacological therapy and other modalities to control pain. Clients and their families can also be instructed to utilize these treatments at home and in inpatient settings.

Cognitive-Behavioral Interventions The cognitive-behavioral interventions influence the cognitive and the motivational-affective components of pain perception. These methods can not only help influence the level of pain, but also help the client gain a sense of self-control.

CLIENT TEACHING

Timed-Release Tablets

Teach clients and families the difference between extended-release and immediate-release tablets. Emphasize that the extended-release tablets become immediate-release if crushed (e.g., for a client who has difficulty swallowing the tablet).

Trusting Nurse–Client Relationship Establishment of a therapeutic relationship is the foundation for effective nursing care of the client experiencing pain. Clients who trust their nurses to be there, to listen, and to act are the clients who are most likely to be comfortable.

Relaxation Relaxation techniques (a variety of methods used to decrease anxiety and muscle tension) result in decreased heart rate and respiratory rate, and decreased muscle tension. These signs and symptoms are opposite of the effects of sympathetic nervous system activation that occurs with acute pain. The body's response to pain is almost "tricked" into reversing itself when relaxation exercises are implemented.

Relaxation exercises help reduce pain by decreasing anxiety and decreasing reflex muscular contraction. There are a wide variety of relaxation techniques, including focused breathing, progressive muscle relaxation, and meditation. Simple techniques should be used during episodes of brief pain (for example, during procedures) or when pain is so severe that the client is unable to concentrate on complicated instructions.

To teach simple relaxation techniques, the nurse can instruct the client to: (1) take a deep breath and hold it; (2) exhale slowly and concentrate on going limp; and (3) start yawning (McCaffery & Pasero, 1999). The yawning triggers a conditioned response in the client, that is, the body associates yawning with relaxation and will relax when the client yawns. The technique can be enhanced if the nurse starts yawning. It is so contagious that even the client compromised by severe pain will usually start yawning with the nurse.

A more complex technique is **progressive muscle relaxation**, a strategy in which muscles are alternately tensed and relaxed. This type of technique is especially useful for clients who do not know what muscle relaxation feels like. By purposely contracting and releasing the muscle groups, the client is able to compare the difference and identify feelings of relaxation. Meditative relaxation techniques are also available, including audiotapes sold in most bookstores.

Relaxation is a learned response. The more frequently the client practices these techniques, the more skilled the body will be in learning to relax. Ideally, the best time to teach the client these methods is when pain is controlled, or before the pain occurs (for example, in the preoperative period).

Reframing Reframing is a technique that teaches clients to monitor their negative thoughts and replace them with ones that are more positive. Teaching a client to view pain by replacing an expression such as, "I can't stand this pain, it's never going away," with one such as, "I've had similar pain before, and it's gotten better," is an example of effective reframing.

Distraction Distraction focuses one's attention on something other than the pain, therefore placing pain on the periphery of awareness (McCaffery & Pasero, 1999). Successful use of distraction does not eliminate the pain; it makes it less troublesome to the client. The main disadvantage of distraction is that as soon as the distractive stimuli stop, the pain returns in full force. For this reason, the most appropriate use of distraction techniques is for the relief of brief, episodic pain. For example, it can be effective for procedural pain or the period of time between administration of an analgesic and the onset of the drug. Examples of distraction include:

- Active listening to recorded music (have the client tap fingers in rhythm to the beat)
- Reciting a poem or rhyme (children do this well)
- Describe a plot of a novel or movie
- Describe a series of pictures

Guided Imagery Guided imagery is using one's imagination to provide a pleasant substitute for the pain. This modality incorporates features of both relaxation and distraction. The client imagines a pleasant experience, such as going to the beach or the mountains. The experience should include use of all five senses in order to fully involve the client in the image.

The images chosen need to be ones that are pleasant for the client. Describing an ocean cruise would not be appropriate for a person who becomes seasick.

Humor The old saying, "Laughter is the best medicine," carries some truth to it. While there is nothing very funny about pain, laughing has been shown to provide pain relief. The act of laughing can cause distraction from the pain, induce relaxation by taking deep breaths and releasing tension, release endorphins, and provide a pleasant substitute for pain. Norman Cousins (1991) relates obtaining 2 hours of pain relief from watching episodes of the Candid Camera television show and Marx Brothers films. The nurse can implement this technique by encouraging the client to watch humorous movies, read funny books,

PROFESSIONAL TIP

Cognitive–Behavioral Interventions

Cognitive–behavioral interventions should be introduced as early as possible so that clients can learn and practice the techniques before experiencing intense pain, which impairs learning.

PROFESSIONAL TIP

Using Distraction

Distraction should never be used as the *only* pain management intervention, but it can be extremely helpful while waiting for other techniques to take effect.

or listen to comedy routines. Because different people see humor in different types of situations, the nurse needs to be sensitive to what the client views as funny.

Biofeedback Biofeedback training is another method that may be helpful for the client in pain, especially one who has difficulty relaxing muscle tension. Biofeedback is a process through which individuals learn to influence their physiological responses to stimuli. Through the use of biofeedback, clients can alter their pain experience.

Cutaneous Stimulation The technique of cutaneous stimulation involves stimulating the skin to control pain. It is theorized that this technique provides relief by stimulating nerve fibers that send signals to the dorsal horn of the spinal cord to "close the gate." The main advantage of these therapies is that many techniques are easy for the nurse to implement, and easy to teach the client and family to perform. They are not usually meant to replace analgesic therapy, but to complement it.

The site chosen on which to apply the skin stimulation will depend on the client's diagnosis, treatments or procedures being performed, and client preference. There are several options to choose from:

- *Site of pain*—Apply stimulation directly to the site.
- *Around the pain*—Apply stimulation in circular motion around the site.
- *Proximal*—Apply between site of pain and the center of the body (McCaffery & Pasero refer to this as "between pain and the brain").
- *Contralateral*—Apply stimulation to the opposite side of the body. (This is effective due to the crossing over of the nerves in the spinal cord.)
- *Acupuncture points*—Stimulation is applied to specific sites defined by Oriental medicine that is based on a system of meridians.
- *Trigger points*—Apply stimulation to areas that cause referred pain, pain felt in a point other than the point of origin.

CLIENT TEACHING

Hot or Cold Applications

Teach the client or family that hot or cold applications:
- Must have at least one layer of towel between the heating or cooling device and the skin
- Should be placed on the skin only for short periods of time
- Should not be applied to tissue that has been exposed to radiation therapy (AHCPR, 1994)

Heat and Cold Application In addition to stimulating nerves that can block pain transmission, superficial heat application serves to increase the circulation to the area, which can promote oxygenation and nutrient delivery to the injured tissues. It can also decrease joint and muscle stiffness. Heat is contraindicated in cases of acute injury because it can increase the initial response of edema. It is also contraindicated in rheumatoid arthritis flare-ups, and over topical applications of mentholated ointments. Heat treatments should be limited to 20- to 30-minute intervals because maximum vasodilatation occurs in that time.

Cryotherapy (cold applications) induces local vasoconstriction and numbness, therefore altering the pain sensations. It is contraindicated in any condition where vasoconstriction might increase symptoms, for example, peripheral vascular disease. For best results, cold therapy should be limited to 20- to 30-minute intervals. Either heat or cold can be used as cutaneous stimulation unless one is specifically contraindicated. Cold often provides faster relief (McCaffery & Pasero, 1999). If the client has used heat or cold before, the nurse should incorporate the modality that the client believes will be the most effective. Combining the two might provide better relief. An example of this would be to apply a hot pack for 4 minutes, followed by an ice pack for 2 minutes, repeated 4 times. In a hospital setting, a physician order is required for this therapy.

Acupressure and Massage One of the first responses to pain is to rub the painful part. Instinctively people seem to understand the pain-relieving aspects of this intervention. In addition to blocking the pain transmission through nerve stimulation, massage can also promote relaxation. Acupressure is a type of massage that consists of continuous pressure on or the rubbing of acupuncture points. It is based on the same principles as acupuncture, but needles are not used. Massage also provides a form of nonverbal communication that can be therapeutic on its own.

Mentholated Rubs Ointments or lotions containing menthol are thought to provide relief by providing a counterirritation to the skin. The menthol gives the client the perception that the temperature of the skin has changed (becoming either warmer or cooler). This alters the sensation of pain or provides a distraction from the pain. Client response varies to mentholated rubs; some gain effective relief, while others have poor results. Their use is contraindicated on broken skin, on mucous membranes, or if pain increases.

Transcutaneous Electrical Nerve Stimulation Transcutaneous electrical nerve stimulation (TENS) is the process of applying a low-voltage electrical current to the skin through cutaneous electrodes. This modality modulates the pain transmission as do other cutaneous stimulation methods but also distracts the client from pain. Research supports the effectiveness of using TENS for the relief of postoperative pain (AHCPR, 1992). It has also been used successfully in many pain syndromes, for example: chronic low back pain, menstrual cramps, temporomandibular joint (TMJ) syndrome, phantom limb pain, and others. It is administered by health professionals especially trained in its use, usually a physical therapist. Other modalities of pain management should *not* be abandoned while a trial of TENS occurs.

Safety: TENS Contraindications
- No electrodes should be placed in the area over or surrounding demand cardiac pacemakers.
- No electrodes can be placed over the uterus of a pregnant woman.

Exercise Exercise is an important treatment for chronic pain because it strengthens weak muscles, helps mobilize joints, and helps restore balance and coordination. Passive range of motion should not be used if it increases pain or discomfort. Immobilization is frequently used for clients with episodes of acute pain or to stabilize fractures; however, prolonged immobilization should be avoided whenever possible because it can lead to muscle atrophy and cardiovascular deconditioning.

Psychotherapy Psychotherapy may be beneficial to many clients, particularly those:

- In whom the pain is difficult to control
- Who are clinically depressed
- Who have a history of psychiatric problems

Some psychotherapists use **hypnosis** (a state of heightened awareness and focused concentration) to help clients alter their perception of pain. Hypnosis can be effective in modifying the pain response, but it should be used only by specially trained professionals.

Positioning The final noninvasive technique is proper positioning and body alignment. Moving the client with the least possible stress on joints and skin will minimize exposure to painful stimuli. This includes supporting joints appropriately and maintaining wrinkle-free sheets.

Invasive Interventions

Invasive interventions are meant to complement behavioral, physical, and pharmacological therapies in those clients who do not obtain relief from those measures alone (AHCPR, 1994). Invasive measures are indicated primarily for chronic cancer pain and in some cases of chronic benign pain. These procedures are usually tried only when noninvasive measures have been attempted first with poor results.

Nerve Block Neural blockade is the process of injecting a local anesthetic or neurolytic agent into the nerve. An anesthetic agent may be injected to act as a diagnostic tool in order to identify the nerves involved in a pain syndrome. A neurolytic agent is a chemical agent that causes destruction of the nerve and, therefore, creates an interruption in the pain signal.

Neurosurgery Neurosurgical measures for pain control include neurostimulation procedures and destructive or ablative procedures. Neurostimulation procedures involve the implantation of electrical stimulation devices that send impulses to different parts of the nervous system. Some of these devices stimulate areas of the brain; others stimulate the spinal cord. Relief is thought to be provided by blocking the afferent fiber input at the spinal cord level, or by stimulating release of endorphins using the body's ability to modulate pain.

Destructive or ablative procedures are used to destroy part of the nervous system that conducts pain. By interrupting the pain signal, it is prevented from reaching the cortex where realization of pain occurs. These procedures are reserved for clients with terminal illness.

Radiation Therapy Radiation can be used as a palliative measure for pain relief in clients with cancer. It can relieve both metastatic pain and pain caused by tumors at the primary cancer site. It enhances other pain management strategies such as analgesic therapy because it is aimed specifically at the cause of the client's pain. When administered for pain relief, the smallest dose of radiation is utilized to minimize the side effects that accompany radiation therapy.

Acupuncture Acupuncture is the insertion of small needles into the skin at selected (or hoku) sites. The specific sites will be chosen after the practitioner takes a detailed history and uses traditional Oriental diagnostic techniques. The needles used for acupuncture have rounded ends that enter the skin without cutting the tissue. The practitioner may twirl or vibrate the needles manually or electrically. It is important that the nurse keep an open mind when the client chooses this therapy, or the client may be reluctant to discuss its use.

The advantages and disadvantages of selected pain therapies are outlined in Table 14–3.

Evaluation

Evaluating the efficacy of the pain management interventions is ongoing, with client input throughout the process. Evaluation focuses primarily on the client's subjective reports. Objective data used to evaluate pain management efficacy include:

- Client's facial expression and posture
- Presence (or absence) of restlessness
- Vital sign monitoring
- Ongoing use of pain assessment tools

Table 14–3 ADVANTAGES AND DISADVANTAGES OF SELECTED PAIN THERAPIES

INTERVENTION	ADVANTAGES	DISADVANTAGES
Relaxation, Imagery, Biofeedback, Distraction, and Reframing	• May decrease pain and anxiety without drug-related side effects. • Can be used as adjuvant therapy with most other modalities. • Can increase client's sense of control. • Most are inexpensive, require no special equipment, and are easily administered.	• Patient must be motivated to use self-management strategies. • Requires professional time to teach interventions.
Psychotherapy, Structured Support, and Hypnosis	• May decrease pain and anxiety for clients who have pain that is difficult to manage. • May increase client's coping skills.	• Requires skilled therapist.
Cutaneous Stimulation (Superficial Heat, Cold, Massage)	• May reduce pain, inflammation, or muscle spasm. • Can be used as adjuvant therapy with most other modalities. • Relatively easy to use. • Can be administered by clients or families. • Relatively low cost.	• Heat may increase bleeding and edema after acute injury. • Cold is contraindicated for use over ischemic tissues.
Transcutaneous Electrical Nerve Stimulation (TENS)	• May provide pain relief without drug-related side effects. • Can be used as adjuvant therapy with most other modalities. • Gives patient sense of control over pain.	• Requires skilled therapist to initiate therapy. • Potential risk of infection, bleeding.
Acupuncture	• May provide pain relief. • Can be used as adjuvant therapy with most other therapies.	• Requires skilled therapist.

Adapted from Agency for Health Care Policy and Research, Clinical Practice Guideline. Acute Pain Management: Operative or Medical Procedures and Trauma, *1992 [AHCPR Publication No. 92-0032], Rockville, MD: Author.*

SAMPLE NURSING CARE PLAN

THE CLIENT WITH CHRONIC PAIN

Sally Jeffries, a 48-year-old woman, injured her back 3 years ago while lifting some boxes of paper at work. Since that time, she has had 4 epidural steroidal injections for the pain associated with 2 ruptured discs. Her pain has been intermittent with some alleviation from the epidural injections. Her last epidural was 3 months ago. She arrives at the clinic stating, "I just don't know how I can go on like this. The pain has been tolerable until last night. I'm hurting so bad!" She is tearful and pacing, saying, "It hurts too much when I sit down." Verbalizes pain is "9" on a 1 to 10 pain intensity scale. Blood pressure is 148/90. Pulse is strong and regular at 92. She has guarded movements.

Nursing Diagnosis 1 *Chronic Pain related to muscle spasm and ruptured discs as evidenced by back injury 3 years ago and client statement "I just don't know how I can go on like this. The pain has been tolerable until last night. I'm hurting so bad!"*

PLANNING/GOALS	NURSING INTERVENTIONS	RATIONALE	EVALUATION
Ms. Jeffries will verbalize a decrease in pain.	Assess Ms. Jeffries's level of pain, determining the intensity at its best and worst.	Determines a baseline for future assessment.	After practicing relaxation techniques,

continues

	Listen to Ms. Jeffries while she discusses the pain; acknowledge the presence of pain.	Acknowledging Ms. Jeffries's pain decreases anxiety by communicating acceptance and validating her perceptions.	Ms. Jeffries rates her pain as a 2 to 3 on the pain intensity scale.
	Discuss reasons why pain may be increased or decreased.	Helps Ms. Jeffries determine a cause-and-effect relationship between pain and specific activities.	
Ms. Jeffries will practice selected noninvasive pain relief measures.	Teach relaxation techniques such as deep breathing, progressive muscle relaxation, and imagery.	Reduces skeletal muscle tension and anxiety, which potentiates the perception of pain.	Ms. Jeffries demonstrates the use of deep breathing and progressive muscle relaxation.
	Teach Ms. Jeffries and her family about treatment approaches (biofeedback, hypnosis, massage therapy, physical therapy, acupuncture, and exercise).	Makes Ms. Jeffries and her family aware of the availability of treatment options.	
	Teach Ms. Jeffries about the use of medication for pain relief. Provide accurate information to reduce fear of addiction.	Lack of knowledge and fear may prohibit Ms. Jeffries from taking analgesic medications as prescribed.	
	Encourage Ms. Jeffries to rest at intervals during the day.	Fatigue increases the perception of pain.	

Nursing Diagnosis 2 *Anxiety related to chronic pain as evidenced by pacing and tears*

PLANNING/GOALS	NURSING INTERVENTIONS	RATIONALE	EVALUATION
Ms. Jeffries will verbalize an increase in psychological and physiological comfort level.	Assess Ms. Jeffries's level of anxiety.	To collect baseline data to be used in measuring a decrease or increase in anxiety level.	After practicing relaxation techniques, Ms. Jeffries rates her pain as a 2 to 3 on the pain intensity scale. She voices concern that the pain will soon come back.
	Encourage Ms. Jeffries to verbalize angry feeling.	Anger is often a component of chronic conditions because of the prolonged sense of powerlessness.	
Ms. Jeffries will demonstrate ability to cope with anxiety as evidenced by normal vital signs and a verbalized reduction in pain intensity.	Speak slowly and calmly.	Avoids escalating Ms. Jeffries's anxiety level and increases the likelihood of her comprehension.	After a relaxation session, her vital signs returned to normal limits. Ms. Jeffries denies feeling angry.

CASE STUDY

Johnny Prince, a 27-year-old male, is admitted to the medical unit diagnosed with hemophilia and septic arthritis in his left ankle. He has a history of epilepsy, arthritis, artificial knee joints (bilateral), and two hip surgeries. Medications taken at home include: factor VIII, phenobarbital 100 mg hs, and Naprosyn 5 mg tid. His chief complaint is swelling and severe pain in his left ankle.

Current RX*: Colace, Milk of Magnesia, ceftriaxone sodium (Rocephin) IV piggy-back, phenobarbital 100 mg qhs, FeSO$_4$, multivitamins, vitamin C, oxacillin (Bactocill), factor VIII 20,000 IVP q12h, hydromorphone HCl (Dilaudid) 8 mg po q8h (hold SBP < 90, resp. < 12), MS 4 mg IVP q4h prn, flurazepam HCl (Dalmane) 30 mg po qhs prn.*

The following questions will guide your development of a nursing care plan for the case study.

1. What will you include in assessing Mr. Prince's pain?

2. What factors in his history will influence his pain perception?

Your pain assessment gives you the following information:
- Location—through center of ankle.
- Intensity—pain at time of assessment is 5 (medicated 30 minutes prior to interview) on scale of 0 to 10; worst is 25, best is 3.
- Quality—describes pain as throbbing at times, a jabbing pain. It hurts worse between 9 and 10 A.M., and 9 and 12 at night. Mainly worse when medicine wears off.
- Effects of pain—only gets 2 or 3 hours of sleep, often dreaming about it. Pain makes him avoid activity, get grumpy and snappy. Concentration turns totally to pain.
- Behaviors—he yells at times, but doesn't like to. He'd prefer to "sweat it out." Also grimaces, grips hands, and tries repositioning.

3. Why did the physician order the analgesics on that schedule?

4. Mr. Prince requests a dose of morphine. The narcotic drawer has the following available in prefilled syringe cartridges: 2 mg per cc, and 8 mg per cc. Which cartridge(s) should the nurse select?

5. Why is the morphine ordered IVP, not IM?

6. Why did the physician order colace and Milk of Magnesia?

7. What are some noninvasive relief measures that might be tried with Mr. Prince?

8. Write two individualized nursing diagnoses and goals for Mr. Prince.

9. What teaching will Mr. Prince need before discharge?

SUMMARY

- *Pain* may be defined as "an unpleasant sensory and emotional experience associated with actual or potential tissue damage," and "whatever the client says it is, existing whenever the client says it does."
- The gate control theory proposes that several processes (sensory, motivational-affective, and cognitive) combine to determine how a person perceives pain.
- Assessment of pain helps establish a baseline of data, and helps to evaluate the effectiveness of interventions.
- Several factors influence the perception of pain, including age, previous experience with pain, and cultural norms.

- The subjective data to gather includes: location of pain, onset and duration, quality, intensity (on a scale of 0 to 10), aggravating and relieving factors, and how pain affects the activities of daily living.
- The three general principles to follow with pain relief measures are: (1) individualize the approach; (2) use a preventive approach; and (3) use a multidisciplinary approach.
- The nurse carries a great deal of autonomy in administering analgesics, which leads to specific responsibilities for which the nurse is accountable.
- Pharmacologic agents can be therapeutic for clients experiencing pain. However, the medications should not be the only interventions used.

- Noninvasive treatments for pain relief are measures that can supplement pharmacological and invasive treatments for pain relief.
- Invasive techniques are interventions used when the noninvasive and pharmacological measures do not provide adequate relief. Methods include nerve blocks, neurosurgery, radiation therapy, and acupuncture.

Review Questions

1. According to McCaffery and Pasero, pain may be defined as:
   a. discomfort resulting from identifiable physiologic or iatrogenic sources.
   b. a syndrome of behavioral and physical manifestations that can be objectively identified by the nurse.
   c. whatever the patient says it is, existing whenever and wherever the patient says it does.
   d. a sensory response to noxious stimuli.

2. Which of the following is a useful tool for assessing the intensity of pain that is easy to use?
   a. The gate control scale
   b. Acute pain monitor
   c. Numeric pain scale
   d. Pressure pain monitor

3. Mr. Levy, 45, has experienced chronic low back pain since a fall 8 years ago. He describes his pain as "a gnawing, constant dull pain" that makes him feel tired. The nurse caring for him recognizes that one of the differences between acute and chronic pain characteristics is:
   a. acute pain is more severe.
   b. chronic pain is often described as dull and is difficult to localize.
   c. chronic back pain is often not real.
   d. acute pain is more diffuse and difficult to describe.

4. Nancy Johnson, 84 years old, is recuperating from a total hip replacement. Morphine, 8 mg IV q4h prn, is prescribed for Ms. Johnson. Her respiratory rate is 18, her pulse rate is 96 beats per minute, and her blood pressure is elevated slightly above her normal level. She is complaining of severe pain, 8 on a scale of 0 to 10. The most appropriate initial nursing intervention is:
   a. question the physician regarding the dosage amount for a client this age.
   b. turn her and then reevaluate her need for opioid analgesia.
   c. administer the medication as ordered.
   d. advise Ms. Johnson to cough and breathe deeply since you are unable to give her anything for pain until her respiratory rate is 20.

5. Ms. Redgrave, 55 years old, is hospitalized with an exacerbation of rheumatoid arthritis. She has a favorite television show she watches every afternoon. She reports feeling comfortable during this show and seldom requests pain medication when she is watching it. The nurse's assessment of this phenomenon is that:
   a. the assessment of pain that prompted hospitalization is inaccurate.
   b. Ms. Redgrave is bored and the boredom usually makes her pain seem worse.
   c. inactivity is the best approach to Ms. Redgrave's pain.
   d. distraction is an effective modifier of the pain experience for Ms. Redgrave.

6. One of the general principles of pain management is:
   a. anticipated or mild pain is easier to relieve than severe pain.
   b. the more experience a person has with pain, the better that person will be able to tolerate it.
   c. no pain, no gain.
   d. the cause of pain must be identified in order to relieve it.

Critical Thinking Questions

1. What are the differences between somatic, cutaneous, visceral, referred, ischemic, acute, and chronic pain?

2. How would you decide which noninvasive technique to use with a client?

 WEB FLASH!

- Search the Internet for the organizations listed in the Resources for this chapter at the end of the book. What kind of information is available for clients, families, and health care professionals?
- Search the word *pain* on the Internet. What information is available?

ANESTHESIA

CHAPTER 15

MAKING THE CONNECTION

Refer to the following chapters to increase your understanding of anesthesia:

- **Chapter 3, Legal Responsibilities**
- **Chapter 10, Fluid, Electrolyte, and Acid–Base Balance**
- **Chapter 14, Pain Management**
- **Chapter 16, Nursing Care of the Surgical Client**

LEARNING OBJECTIVES

Upon completion of this chapter, you should be able to:
- *Define key terms.*
- *Describe the difference between regional and general anesthesia.*
- *List the purposes of sedation.*
- *Describe the effects of sedation or general anesthesia on memory and cognitive function.*
- *Describe the types of monitoring necessary to ensure client safety during sedation.*
- *Describe the signs and symptoms and risks of oversedation.*
- *Describe the dangers involved in aspiration of gastric contents and how gastric aspiration is prevented during anesthesia.*
- *List the medications that are typically given on the day of surgery.*
- *List and describe the different types of regional anesthesia.*
- *Describe the risks involved with regional and general anesthesia.*
- *Describe the residual effects of anesthesia on the client.*
- *List three methods of postoperative pain management and explain briefly how each is administered.*

KEY TERMS

amnesia	general anesthesia
analgesia	orthostatic hypotension
anesthesia	regional anesthesia
anesthesiologist	sedation
anesthetist	synergism

INTRODUCTION

Anesthesia refers to the absence of normal sensation. **Analgesia** refers to pain relief without producing anesthesia. The delivery of general anesthesia for the purpose of preventing pain during surgery began in the United States in the 1800s. When surgeons began using anesthesia routinely, they soon realized the need for someone trained in its administration and turned to the nurses with whom they worked daily. Early nurse anesthetists were trained on the job by the surgeons with whom they worked.

Anesthesia is now a specialty of both nursing and medicine. Experienced registered nurses (RNs) with a baccalaureate degree can become certified registered nurse anesthetists (CRNAs) after completing two or more years of graduate education in nurse anesthesia. In March 2000, the Health Care Financing Administration (HCFA) announced the removal of the federal requirement that a nurse anesthetist must be supervised by a physician when administering anesthesia to Medicare clients (AANA, 2000b).

Today, there are more than 27,000 CRNAs in the United States (AANA, 2000a). Certified registered nurse anesthetists administer 65% of all anesthetics given in the United States every year, often working in groups with anesthesiologists (AANA, 2000a). An **anesthesiologist** is a licensed physician educated and skilled in the delivery of anesthesia who also adds to the knowledge of anesthesia through research or other scholarly pursuits. An **anesthetist** is a qualified RN, dentist, or physician who administers anesthetics.

Prior to administering an anesthetic, the anesthesia provider will assess a client's health status, discuss anesthesia with the client, and plan an anesthetic appropriate for the client and the surgical procedure. The surgical nurse can help prepare clients to talk with their anesthesia providers by encouraging them to ask any questions they have about anesthesia and the care they will receive.

The delivery of an anesthetic is essential to the health and well-being of clients undergoing surgery. Yet, while anesthesia prevents the sensation of what would be extreme pain, it also temporarily eliminates or diminishes the client's ability to control many essential physiologic functions such as respiration, heart rate, and temperature regulation. In addition to ensuring adequate levels of anesthesia throughout a surgical procedure, the anesthesia provider monitors and, when necessary, controls physiologic functions such as respiratory rate and blood pressure. Prior to the end of the surgery, the anesthesia provider administers appropriate medications to ensure that the client is comfortable when emerging from the anesthetic. Pain relief may be accomplished with local anesthetic infiltration, opioid analgesics, or nonopioid analgesics.

PREANESTHETIC PREPARATION

Preparing a client for anesthesia and surgery is a cooperative effort involving the surgeon, the anesthesia provider, and the nursing staff who will care for the client both before and after surgery. The client may be having general (total body) anesthesia, where the control of body functions is temporarily lost; regional anesthesia, where a region of the body is made insensible to pain; or local anesthesia, where only a small area of the body is made insensible to pain.

Oral Intake

Normally, only air should enter the trachea and lungs. The body prevents foreign material from entering the trachea by coughing forcefully when something other than air enters or by tightly closing the vocal cords to prevent entry of the foreign substance. Anyone who has ever been drinking something and had it go down the wrong "pipe" knows how uncomfortable it is and how hard the body works to cough up the foreign substance.

General anesthesia removes a person's ability to guard the airway by coughing or closing the vocal cords. Passive regurgitation of stomach contents into the back of the throat can occur at any time during the delivery of general anesthesia. Aspiration of gastric contents into the lungs can cause significant illness or

CLIENT TEACHING

Oral Intake Prior to Surgery
- Clearly explain to clients those things that they will or will not be allowed to eat or drink before surgery.
- Emphasize the need to exactly follow the instructions related to the time at which eating or drinking must cease before surgery.

death. An important step in preventing aspiration of gastric contents is ensuring that the stomach is as empty as possible. In the past, adults have been instructed not to eat or drink anything for at least 8 hours prior to surgery, and usually nothing past midnight the night before surgery. More recent information, however, strongly indicates that adults need not go without clear liquids for 8 or more hours prior to surgery; 2 hours are sufficient (Crenshaw, 1999). In fact, the amount of liquid in a person's stomach at the time of surgery may actually be decreased if water is taken a couple of hours before surgery. Some anesthesia providers still prefer that their clients not have anything to eat or drink for at least 8 hours prior to surgery; others may allow water up to 2 hours before.

Preoperative Medication

Most scheduled medications that a person receives while in the hospital or takes at home every day will be continued up until the time of surgery. Most oral medications should be given with just enough water to swallow them, even when a client is going to have surgery first thing in the morning. The anesthesia provider will usually write orders to specify how the morning medication should be managed. Cardiovascular medications such as antihypertensives and heart medications are especially important for the client to receive.

Exceptions to the practice of continuing scheduled medications prior to surgery include administration of drugs such as insulin and oral antihyperglycemics, nonsteroidal anti-inflammatory drugs (NSAIDs) like aspirin, and anticoagulants like heparin or coumadin. Because food is being withheld, giving insulin or oral antihyperglycemic drugs is likely to result in a dangerously low blood sugar level. The way insulin and glucose administration is handled will depend on the severity of the client's disease and the preference of the physician and anesthesia provider. Anticoagulants and NSAIDs affect clotting. With some types of surgery, the bleeding caused by aspirin-like drugs or low-dose heparin is more likely. In some cases, no NSAIDs are allowed for 10 days to 2 weeks prior to surgery. In other circumstances, they may be taken right up until surgery. Low-dose heparin or heparinoids may be given preoperatively to prevent postoperative thromboembolism, but higher doses of heparin and any dose of coumadin will almost certainly be stopped prior to surgery to allow the return of normal coagulation time.

Additional medications may be ordered to prepare the client for surgery or anesthesia. Surgeons often order prophylactic antibiotics. The anesthesia provider may order a sedative to help the client sleep the night before surgery or to ease the client's anxiety while waiting for surgery. Opioids like morphine or meperidine (Demerol) may also be used for pain relief or to ease the induction of anesthesia. Some anesthesia providers prefer to give preoperative medications in the operating room to precisely control the medication's effect on the client. This is especially true for very sick clients.

Consent

Consent for anesthesia is usually obtained on the same form as is surgical consent. The anesthesia department may have a separate consent form instead of or in addition to the combined consent. In either case,

PROFESSIONAL TIP

Preanesthetic Care
- Complete preoperative checklist.
- Make sure all preoperative orders are executed, especially those for blood tests, preoperative medications, and blood from the blood bank.
- Check, verify, and document the presence or absence of drug allergies for each client.
- Administer regular daily oral medications with a small sip of water as ordered.
- Remind the client of the importance of following instructions regarding any eating or drinking restrictions.
- Administer preoperative medications as close to the ordered time as possible. Timing can be crucial to achieving the desired effect at the correct time.
- If the client responds abnormally to the preoperative medication, notify the anesthesia department immediately.
- Be sure the client's chart is complete when it goes to the operating room with the client. Recent diagnostic test results are especially important to include; otherwise, surgery may be delayed while these results are sought.
- Make sure the client's consents are in order and included in the chart when the client is transported to surgery.

for an informed consent to be obtained, the anesthetic must be discussed with the client by someone with expert knowledge of anesthesia, usually an anesthesia provider or the surgeon.

SEDATION

Sedation refers to a reduction of stress, excitement, or irritability, and involves some degree of central nervous system (CNS) depression. Sedation is used to decrease awareness of events, relieve anxiety, control the physiologic changes that often accompany anxiety, and ease the induction of general anesthesia. This is welcome news to many clients who fear local or regional anesthesia because they do not want to be awake and see and hear everything during surgery or a diagnostic procedure.

Some drugs are better sedatives than others, although many drugs have sedative properties. Oftentimes, different sedatives given in combination have a greater effect on the client than does any one of the sedatives given alone. This phenomenon is called **synergism**. The synergistic effect that occurs when different sedative drugs are administered together, however, makes respiratory depression and unconsciousness more likely. In general, benzodiazepines (diazepam [Valium] and midazolam hydrochloride [Versed]) are better sedatives than are opioids (morphine and fentanyl [Sublimaze]). Even so, if a client's anxiety is due to pain, an opioid is a better choice of sedative than a benzodiazepine because the opioid will relieve the pain that caused the anxiety.

There is a great deal of variability in the dose of drugs needed to sedate different clients. Whereas many drugs given for specific effects are administered according to a set "mg per kg" dose alone, this is not possible with drugs used for sedation. Sedative medications should be administered based on the client's physical condition, weight, mental state, and the procedure being performed, with close observation of the effects of the drugs on the client.

The amount of sedation required by a client for comfort is always in balance with the amount of stimulation experienced due to pain or anxiety. A client who is only mildly stimulated (i.e., experiencing little anxiety) will be sufficiently sedated with a relatively small dose of sedative medication. A client who is greatly stimulated (i.e., undergoing a painful procedure or very frightened) will require a much larger dose of sedative to be comfortable. Sedation and general anesthesia both involve CNS depression; thus sedation and anesthesia exist on a continuum. As sedation becomes deeper and deeper, it eventually becomes general anesthesia. Sometimes, the line between sedation and general anesthesia is very difficult to distinguish. When sedation becomes general anesthesia, all the risks of general anesthesia are present, including airway obstruction, respiratory arrest, and aspiration of gastric contents. For this reason, all but the lightest sedation should be administered by an anesthetist or another provider skilled and experienced in airway assessment, protection, and management, as well as assessment of oxygenation and ventilation.

Sedation and Monitoring

Sedation is often used to alleviate client anxiety and discomfort during procedures performed under local anesthesia. Properly administered, local anesthetic injection blocks the painful stimulus of small incisions and minor surgical procedures. However, the injections necessary for local anesthetic administration can cause significant discomfort in some people due to tissue irritation caused by the acidity of the local anesthetic solution. Additionally, most clients are uncomfortable knowing that they are undergoing surgery and thus prefer to be less alert during the procedure. Sedation decreases the client's perception of these physical and mental discomforts.

During local anesthesia and sedation, the client must remain conscious and in control of his own airway and breathing reflexes. Oversedation is likely to result in airway obstruction and places the client at risk for aspiration of gastric contents. Because sedatives are CNS depressants and, thus, respiratory depressants, supplemental oxygen should be given to clients during sedation. Monitoring during sedation is done through observation by an individual knowledgeable and experienced in the assessment of respiratory volume and airway patency. Monitoring should also include an electrocardiogram (EKG), blood pressure, pulse rate, respiratory rate, and continuous oxygen saturation monitoring (pulse oximetry). The individual monitoring the client's breathing and vital signs should be devoted to that task to the exclusion of any other duties.

Residual Effects of Sedation

Sedation usually persists beyond the duration of the surgical procedure itself. The length of time it takes to recover from sedation depends on the health of the client, the properties of the drugs used, other drugs the client may be taking, and the amount of sedative drugs administered.

Amnesia (inability to remember things) produced by sedatives commonly lasts longer than the procedure itself, even in clients who appear to be completely recovered. Such clients will probably not remember any instructions given to them during or soon after the procedure. Given that minor procedures and surgery are commonly performed on an outpatient basis, some clients may be discharged prior to regaining the ability to remember verbal instructions. All instructions should thus be given in writing and explained to the person responsible for taking the client home.

If heavy sedation has been used or the procedure ends suddenly, the client may remain significantly sedated after the procedure is over, because the CNS stimulation has ended while the CNS depressant effect of the sedative remains. In such an instance, the client should be closely monitored until the effects of the sedative medications have worn off enough for the client to wake and become oriented.

REGIONAL ANESTHESIA

In **regional anesthesia** a region of the body is temporarily rendered insensible to pain by injection of a local anesthetic. Local anesthetics are a class of drugs that temporarily block the transmission of small electrical impulses through nerves. The duration of anesthesia produced by a local anesthetic depends on the drug used, the amount injected, and into which part of the body the drug is injected. In general, nerves carry either sensory information to the brain or instructions from the brain to muscles, telling them how and when to contract. Both types of nerves can be blocked by local anesthetics. Sensory nerves are highly subspecialized to carry specific types of information to the brain. One type carries information about the pain we experience when stuck with a needle; another carries information about joint position that tells us, without looking, whether our arm is down by our side or elevated over our head. There are many different types of nerves, and not all of them are blocked to the same degree or at the same time when a local anesthetic is injected. The amount of insulation surrounding a nerve fiber, the anatomic location of the fiber, and the diameter of the fiber all influence the ease with which nerve impulses are blocked by local anesthetics.

Types of Regional Anesthesia

There are three types of regional anesthesia: local anesthesia, nerve blocks, and spinal and epidural blocks.

Local Anesthesia

Clinically, the use of local anesthetics to block nerves is identified by different names depending on the amount of local anesthetic used and where it is injected. When a small amount of local anesthetic drug is injected either into the skin and subcutaneous tissues around a cut or at the site of a needle puncture for a central line placement, it is called *local anesthesia*. When a local anesthetic is injected in this way, it is not aimed at a specific nerve, rather it is meant to anesthetize whatever small superficial nerves are in the target area. Local anesthesia is most commonly performed using lidocaine (Xylocaine) and lasts approximately 1 hour. Occasionally, for some types of plastic surgery, this type of anesthesia is used over a large area of the body. When this is the case, longer acting local anesthetics may be used. Local anesthesia is technically easy to administer and presents little risk of bleeding or nerve damage. Because very small amounts of local anesthetics are generally used, the risk of local anesthetic toxicity is also small.

Topical anesthesia, achieved with direct application of a local anesthetic to tissue, may be desired in some situations. The anesthetic may take the form of an ointment, lotion, solution, or spray.

Safety: Preventing Choking and Aspiration

In order to prevent choking and aspiration after the use of an oral anesthetic solution (e.g., viscous lidocaine) or spray, fluids and foods must be withheld until the gag reflex returns.

Nerve Blocks

When a local anesthetic is injected more deeply into the body and/or is directed at a specific nerve or nerves, it is called a *nerve block*. Nerve blocks are often called by the name of the specific nerve or nerves they block. Examples include an ulnar nerve block in the arm or a brachial plexus block of all the nerves in the arm. Nerve blocks are technically more difficult to administer than are local anesthetics, and because the needle is usually directed into deeper structures that are often close to major veins or arteries, involve a variable risk of bleeding or nerve damage. Nerve blocks are often performed using lidocaine (Xylocaine), mepivacaine (Carbocaine), or bupivacaine (Marcaine) and may last from 1 to 12 hours. Larger volumes of drug are needed than are used for local anesthesia, and local anesthetic toxicity is a rare but known complication of these types of blocks.

Spinal and Epidural Blocks

Blocks may also be identified according to where the local anesthetic is injected. One example is an *epidural block,* for which local anesthetic is injected into the epidural space near the spinal cord to anesthetize a number of spinal nerves at once. With *spinal blocks* (also called subarachnoid blocks), the local anesthetic is injected into the cerebrospinal fluid, where it can bathe uninsulated spinal nerves as they exit the spinal cord to the periphery of the body (Figure 15-1).

Spinal and epidural blocks are generally used to anesthetize a significant area of the body. They are capable of safely producing anesthesia sufficient for surgery in the abdomen, pelvis, perineum, or lower extremities. When an epidural block is performed, a catheter is usually inserted into the epidural space, making it possible to inject additional doses of drug. The client must either be sitting in a bent-over position or lying on the side with head and knees as close together as possible. Either position separates the vertebra, making insertion of the needle or catheter possible. Epidural blocks have an added advantage in that by varying the way the anesthetic is used, the block can produce analgesia (pain relief without producing anesthesia), complete anesthesia, and even profound muscular relaxation (needed for some types of surgery). This allows epidural anesthesia to be used not only for surgical procedures, but also for analgesia during labor and for postoperative pain relief.

Spinal blocks are most often performed using lidocaine (Xylocaine) or bupivacaine (Marcaine) and last from 1 to 3 hours. Epidural blocks are most commonly performed using bupivacaine (Marcaine), and the block can be continued as long as local anesthetic is injected through the catheter into the epidural space (Figure 15-2).

Figure 15-1 A. Cross sectional anatomy of the spine. B. Side view of the anatomy of the spine with the tip of an epidural needle placed in the epidural space. C. Side view of the anatomy of the spine with the tip of an epidural catheter placed in the epidural space.

Sacrum

Pelvis   Spinous   Transverse   Vertebra
          process   process

Figure 15-2 Correct positions for performing a spinal block or inserting an epidural catheter in the lumbar area. The assistance of trained personnel is crucial to the proper positioning, reassurance, and safety of the client.

Opioids such as morphine and fentanyl citrate (Sublimaze) may be added to the local anesthetic in either of these blocks to intensify the analgesic or anesthetic effect, or to provide postoperative pain relief after the block has worn off (Liu, Chiu, Carpenter, Mulroy, Allen, Neal, & Pollock, 1995).

One type of complication is peculiar to spinal and epidural regional anesthetics. When cerebrospinal fluid (CSF) leaks out through a hole made in the dural membrane during performance of a subarachnoid block or an accidental dural puncture during the attempted performance of an epidural block, a postdural puncture headache (PDPH) may result. The headache is caused by the loss of CSF from around the brain. The headache is relieved by lying down and returns when the individual sits up or stands. Pain commonly occurs in both the front and the back of the head and is sometimes accompanied by neck and shoulder stiffness. Photophobia or double vision may be present with severe headache. The onset of the headache is usually not immediate and may take 1 to 2 days to become bothersome. Treatment involves adequate hydration to allow the normal production of CSF; analgesics; and bed rest in a supine position. Oral caffeine and sumatriptan succinate (Imitrex) are effective in preventing and treating PDPH in some people. The definitive treatment for significant or persistent PDPH, however, is a procedure called an epidural blood patch, which involves injecting 15 to 20 mL of the client's own blood

into the epidural space. Once the blood clots, it plugs the hole in the dural membrane.

A local anesthetic drug will always block the sympathetic nerves that control the dilation or constriction of blood vessels before it blocks sensory or motor nerves. This results in vascular dilation. With most blocks, the resultant vascular dilation is not sufficient to change blood pressure. With widespread spinal or epidural blocks, however, blood pressure may decrease due to sympathetic nerve block. To prevent this, the anesthesia provider will often infuse an extra volume of intravenous (IV) fluid or administer a vasoconstrictor such as ephedrine before the sympathetic block sets up. Client harm from hypotension is rare.

Spinal and epidural blocks, like other nerve blocks, carry some risk of bleeding (Horlocker, Wedel, Schroeder, Rose, Elliott, McGregor, & Wong, 1995) and nerve damage (Ben-David, Vaida, Collins, Naum, & Gaitini, 1994), but the high degree of expertise that many anesthesia providers have in delivering these blocks minimizes the risk. Only a small dose of local anesthetic is needed for a spinal block, so local anesthetic toxicity is very unlikely. Variable amounts of local anesthetic are used for epidural blocks, and some doses can approach the upper limits of safety. Anesthesia providers are careful to avoid overdoses of local anesthetics when delivering this block, and toxicity is exceedingly rare. If opioids, like morphine, are added to the local anesthetic solution, there is a risk of the drug migrating to the brain and causing respiratory depression, but this risk is small in light of careful dosing and is easily detected in time to prevent client harm.

Residual Effects of Regional Anesthesia

All anesthetics must wear off as the drug responsible for causing the anesthesia is removed from its site of action within the body and is metabolized, and eliminated. Some anesthetic effects wear off faster than others, and important residual effects may not be detected by casual observation. This is especially true of a regional anesthetic because the client may be wide awake and able to carry on a conversation as if nothing has happened. Three common residual effects are discussed following.

Residual Motor Block

A motor block is a temporary condition caused when local anesthetic blocks nerves that carry instructions to skeletal muscles telling them to contract. Motor block results in the inability to move a body part and is usually the last effect to develop and the first to wear off. It results only when the regional block is very dense and complete.

A complete motor block results in a temporary paralysis, with the client being incapable of moving the blocked part despite tremendous effort. In the presence of a complete motor block, there is usually no function in any other type of nerve in the same area. A client experiencing a complete motor block of any part of the body would not likely be released from the recovery area because there would be no evidence that the block was wearing off. Clients experiencing residual (incomplete) motor block may be released from recovery, however; thus any client who has had any type of block involving the legs should never be allowed to get out of bed without assistance until it can be demonstrated that a complete recovery of motor strength in the legs has been regained. Even a small amount of residual motor block greatly increases the possibility that a client will fall.

As a regional block begins to wear off, motor function begins to return first, sensation begins to return next, and sympathetic nervous function returns last. Motor function and sensation can be detected easily by asking the client to move the blocked part or by touching the skin and asking the client whether it feels normal. The return of sympathetic function is more difficult to detect. Because sympathetic nervous function returns last, orthostatic hypotension may still occur even after motor and sensory function have completely returned and the regional block appears to have worn off. To prevent fainting, clients should not be allowed to get out of bed without the presence of a nurse until after they have been able to do so without any dizziness or significant decrease in blood pressure.

Residual Sensory Block

The effects of any regional anesthetic used for surgery is the loss of pain sensation. Normal sensation may not have returned completely upon client discharge from the recovery area. As the regional block wears off, sensation will return gradually. Not all types of sensation return at the same time, however. For example, as sensation begins to return, the client may experience a "pins and needles" feeling in an arm or leg that has been blocked and may feel touch or pressure before recovering complete sensation. Until complete recovery of normal sensation, any blocked areas of the client's body must be frequently checked and carefully protected, as the client may be unaware that a finger or hand, for example, is being pinched or denied blood supply.

Residual Sympathetic Block

The first types of nerve fibers to be blocked when a local anesthetic begins to work, and the last to recover as a local anesthetic wears off, are those responsible for carrying instructions to the muscles that surround blood vessels. When these sympathetic nerves are blocked, veins and arteries dilate, lowering the blood pressure. The venous system has a large capacity, and venous dilation results in the pooling of a large amount of blood. This decreases the amount of blood that returns to the heart, and the blood pressure falls. The amount of blood that pools is greatest in parts of the body that are farthest below the level of the heart. Even in a client who has had a spinal or epidural block and is lying supine, a significant amount of venous pooling occurs, resulting in lower-than-normal blood pressure. If the same client is allowed to sit up, even more venous pooling will occur, less blood will return to the heart, and blood pressure will fall substantially. This phenomenon of having a large drop in blood pressure when sitting up or standing is called **orthostatic hypotension**. Orthostatic signifies that it involves body position, and hypotension means low blood pressure. Clients who have had a spinal or epidural block are more likely to have orthostatic hypotension the higher in the spinal column the level of their block.

GENERAL ANESTHESIA

General anesthesia involves unconsciousness; complete insensibility to pain; amnesia; motionlessness; and muscle relaxation. With general anesthesia, the body also loses the ability to control many important functions, including the abilities to maintain an airway, control vital functions like breathing and heart rate, and regulate temperature. These functions are controlled by the anesthesia provider during administration of general anesthesia.

General anesthesia involves four overlapping stages: induction (going to sleep), maintenance, emergence (waking up), and recovery.

Induction and Airway Management

The induction of general anesthesia is a short but critical period of time during which the client is rendered unconscious, vital functions are controlled, and enough anesthetic drug is introduced into the body to keep the client asleep during surgery. In adults, drugs are usually injected into an IV line to quickly produce unconsciousness, and additional anesthetic is then inhaled.

Immediately after the induction of general anesthesia, the anesthesia provider will usually secure the airway using a cuffed endotracheal tube (ETT). The ETT is usually inserted under direct visualization with the aid of a laryngoscope, an instrument designed to provide visualization and illumination of the trachea, as shown in Figure 15-3. An ETT provides a breathing passage from outside the client to within the client's trachea. The ETT cuff seals the space between the ETT and the trachea, making it difficult, though not impossible, for air to escape from or gastric contents to enter into the lungs. An ETT also offers a dependable way to

Figure 15-3 Placing an Endotracheal Tube in the Trachea with Direct Visualization by Laryngoscopy.

Figure 15-4 A typical anesthesia machine is a complex equipment set. This machine has anesthetic vaporizors and flowmeters to deliver oxygen, nitrous oxide, and air, and also contains a small ventilator and equipment to monitor ventilation, oxygen content of inspired gas, client oxygen saturation, blood pressure, heart rate, and respiration. (*Pictured above is the Ohmeda Excel 210 SE Anesthesia Delivery System equipped with the Hewlett Packard OmniCare Anesthesia Component Monitoring System [A-CMS] and the Anesthesia Gas Module [AGM]. Reprinted with permission of Ohmeda, Inc.*)

provide oxygen and ventilation to the client's lungs. Breaths given through a properly positioned cuffed ETT go directly into the lungs and prevent any gas from entering the stomach.

Maintenance

General anesthesia is maintained with some combination of IV and inhaled drugs. Some of these drugs are used only as general anesthetics, and others are used for other purposes but are also useful as anesthetics. Isoflurane (Forane) is an example of a drug used only for anesthesia. It produces all the components of a general anesthetic by itself. Figure 15-4 shows a client connected to an anesthesia machine by a breathing circuit. Benzodiazepines and opioids (sometimes called narcotics), used for many other purposes, are sometimes used as part of a general anesthetic. Neither produces all the components of a general anesthetic by itself. In healthy clients undergoing simple surgeries, anesthetic drugs may be all that are needed. In critically ill clients and those undergoing complicated types of surgery other drugs may be needed to strengthen heart contraction, control blood pressure, or produce complete paralysis of skeletal muscles.

Skeletal Muscle Relaxation

Some types of surgery require complete relaxation of skeletal muscles. In these cases, the anesthesia provider administers a skeletal muscle relaxant like pancuronium bromide (Pavulon) or vecuronium bromide (Norcuron) to completely paralyze the client. These types of drugs prevent clients from breathing on their own, requiring the anesthesia provider to ventilate clients during surgery. Usually, a mechanical ventilator is used. Paralysis must be eliminated prior to emergence from anesthesia in order for the client to be able to breathe independently again. As soon as the skeletal muscle relaxant has begun to wear off, an anticholinesterase drug such as neostigmine methylsulfate (Prostigmin), or pyridostigmine bromide (Regonol) is used to reverse the remaining paralysis. When the paralyzing effect of an anesthetic muscle relaxant has begun to wear off on its own, the anesthesia provider can administer an anticholinesterase drug to reverse the remaining paralysis. This normally results in a quick return of muscle strength and the ability to breathe.

Inadequate reversal of paralysis may present as anything from total skeletal muscle paralysis to the inability of the client to cough and clear the airway. Typically, a client with partial paralysis has uncoordinated large muscle movements and is weak. If only small levels of paralysis remain, the client may complain of difficulty swallowing or difficulty breathing deeply. Any detectable paralysis in a postoperative client should immediately be brought to the attention of the anesthesia service for evaluation. If the client is having difficulty breathing, basic life support should be provided until the arrival of an anesthesia provider.

Emergence

Emergence from general anesthesia occurs when anesthetic drugs are allowed to wear off. The anesthesia provider must carefully control the timing and amount of anesthetic drug given in order for the client to emerge from general anesthesia at the desired time. This takes experience and a detailed understanding of both the drugs used and the client's response to those drugs. The initial phase of emergence is usually quite quick, allowing the client to awaken enough to respond to verbal directions and maintain an airway. After this time, the client's breathing tube can usually be removed, and the client can be taken to the post-anesthesia care unit (recovery room). If, for some reason, the client must be left on a ventilator and with a breathing tube in place, the anesthesia provider may take the client to an intensive care unit asleep instead of waking the client up from the anesthetic.

Recovery

Recovery from general anesthesia is not complete simply because the client has regained consciousness. The client may not remember what has happened for minutes or even hours after having received an anesthetic. The ability to think clearly often takes longer to return, with some residual thinking difficulty persisting for several days or even weeks. Inhalation anesthetics are eliminated from the body through the lungs, and very small amounts of anesthetic are still being exhaled for several weeks. Many anesthetic drugs are stored in body fat and released back into the bloodstream very slowly after anesthetic administration has ended. The speed of this release depends on the amount of anesthetic given during the surgery, the length of the surgery, and how deeply the client is breathing.

Oxygenation and Ventilation

Almost all anesthetics are respiratory depressants. Benzodiazepines, opioids, and inhalation anesthetic agents have significant respiratory depressant effects. Any one of these drugs may be used in a dose that causes apnea, or lack of respirations for more than 10 seconds, during a general anesthesia. When used in combination their effect on respiration is at least additive. When the rate or depth of respirations decrease,

GERONTOLOGICAL CONSIDERATIONS

Oxygenation and Ventilation in the Elderly Client

- Impaired mobility allows secretions to pool in the lungs. Therefore, elderly clients must be monitored more closely, and secretions suctioned.
- Most anesthetic agents cause decreased respiratory rate and decreased tidal volume, putting elderly clients at greater risk for hypoventilation.

the elimination of carbon dioxide is retarded, and carbon dioxide builds up in the blood and in the lungs. The buildup of carbon dioxide actually blocks the entry of oxygen into the bloodstream and makes it harder to keep the client adequately oxygenated. Oxygen saturation is monitored by pulse oximetry. Even small amounts of supplemental oxygen given to a client whose rate or depth of breathing is decreased adds significantly to the amount of oxygen in the bloodstream. This is the most important reason that oxygen is given to even healthy clients when they are recovering from general anesthesia.

Heart Rate and Blood Pressure

Few direct effects on heart rate (HR) and blood pressure (BP) regulation are seen during recovery from general anesthesia. Some anesthetic techniques that are heavily based on opioids, like fentanyl (Sublimaze) or sufentanil citrate (Sufenta), can cause a slow HR; but as long as BP is maintained, no specific treatment is necessary. Although most general anesthetics are myocardial depressants, the depressive effects of current agents are mild, especially after anesthetic administration is ended. Some individuals become sympathetically activated during the initial period after regaining consciousness. This occurs most commonly in clients with cardiac or vascular disease (hypertension, coronary artery disease, or peripheral vascular occlusive disease). If the increase in HR or BP is a danger to the client, it can usually be successfully treated using a combined alpha and beta blocker like labetalol hydrochloride (Normodyne) or a calcium channel blocker such as nifedipine (Procardia).

Most HR and BP changes seen during recovery result from factors related indirectly to the anesthetic. Both HR and BP increase due to sympathetic stimulation. Pain, hypoxia, and fear can all result in sympathetic stimulation with an increase in HR and BP. Pain results when inadequate analgesia has been provided as the client emerges from anesthesia. An opioid such as morphine or meperidine (Demerol) will relieve the pain. The residual effects of anesthesia on respiratory centers or airway muscles in the throat may result in hypoventilation or airway obstruction. Provision of supplemental oxygen, proper airway management, and mechanical ventilation, if necessary, will ensure adequate oxygenation. Discovering and addressing the source of the client's fear often reduces the anxiety. When the causes of sympathetic stimulation are addressed, HR and BP should normalize.

Temperature Regulation and Shivering

With general anesthesia, the body loses its natural ability to regulate temperature. General anesthetic agents dilate the blood vessels close to the surface of the body, exposing the client's warm blood to the cool exterior. During anesthetization, the client is mostly uncovered in a cold operating room, and the area of the body to be operated on is cleaned with cold solutions. After this is done, the client's insulating covering (skin and subcutaneous fat) is cut open to expose the warm interior of the body and allow its heat to escape. Room temperature intravenous fluids are infused into the veins, and the client breathes cool gases. Surgical clients lose a great amount of heat at a time when the body is least able to respond to warm the tissues. Hypothermia adds to the CNS depression resulting from any residual anesthetics. Surface warming with a forced-air warming blanket is an effective way to increase the temperature of a client recovering from general anesthesia; cloth blankets or heating lamps may also be useful. Forced-air warming blankets are also used to prevent or limit the development of hypothermia intraoperatively. Figure 15-5 shows use of a forced-air warming blanket.

All potent inhalation agents are associated with shivering during emergence from general anesthesia when the blood level of the anesthetic agent is very low. This phenomenon was first associated with halothane and was thus called the "halothane shakes"; but it can occur following the administration of any inhalation anesthetic. The cause of the shivering is not clear but does not appear to be related to the client's body temperature. (Of course, postoperative clients also shiver when they are cold.) The key to eliminating shivering postoperatively is to ensure client warmth and encourage deep breathing so that the anesthetic is eliminated as quickly as possible.

Fluid Balance

Surgical procedures and the injuries that necessitate them have major effects on the body's distribution of fluid. Appropriate care during anesthesia sometimes necessitates the delivery of a large volume of IV fluid. This IV fluid does not stay in the vascular system long, moving out of the vascular space to replace losses from the interstitial and intracellular spaces.

Trauma, whether due to an accidental injury or a surgical incision, results in fluid losses or shifts in three general areas as follows: direct blood loss, evaporation through the surgical wound, and fluid shifts. Large volumes of fluid can be lost to the air through the surgical wound, especially during abdominal procedures. A major abdominal procedure, for example, can result in the loss of up to 10 cc/kg/hour of fluid by evaporation.

POSTOPERATIVE PAIN MANAGEMENT

Pain has many causes. Postoperative pain results from tissue injury, release of local and hormonal substances, inflammation, mental outlook, and, perhaps, neural hyperexcitability related to excessive noxious input.

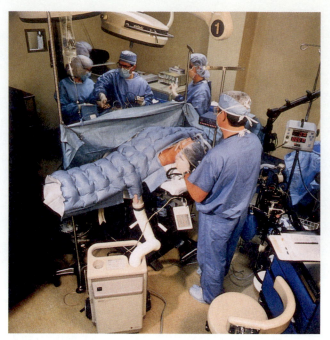

Figure 15-5 A forced-air warming blanket applied to the upper abdomen, chest, and arms of a client during surgery. The unit on the floor to the left of the anesthesia provider (foreground) is the heating unit, which contains a fan that pushes warm air through the hose and into the blanket much like a furnace pushes warm air through heating ducts and into a house. Warm air exits hundreds of pinholes on the surface of the blanket and next to the client. (*Courtesy of Mallinckrodt Medical, Inc.*)

As such, baseline postoperative pain, pain from pressure placed on an incision, and pain from client movement may each respond best to different pain relieving strategies.

The amount of medication needed to relieve pain depends on the intensity and type of pain, the size of the client, and the client's age. The dose requirement for most opioids is dramatically lower for clients who are elderly as compared to younger clients. An 89-year-old needs 50% less opioid analgesic than does a 20-year-old (Scott & Stanski, 1987).

Patient-Controlled Analgesia

Patient-controlled analgesia (PCA) allows clients to self-administer pain medication by pushing a button when they experience pain. After an IV catheter is in place, a client-controlled analgesia pump is connected "piggyback" to the IV line. The pump is programmed to deliver a predetermined dose of morphine or meperidine (Demerol) when the client pushes a button. It will not, however, deliver unlimited amounts. A set time must pass between each successive dose, and when the total dose of opioid delivered in any hour reaches a preset limit, the pump will not deliver any more medicine until the next hour. This is referred to as lockout.

CLIENT TEACHING

Patient-Controlled Analgesia (PCA)
- Only the client should push the button to administer more analgesic.
- The client should not ask visitors to push the button.

Properly programmed, PCA allows the client a great deal of control over when pain medicine is received, which is likely to help decrease anxiety. Patient-controlled analgesia also results in a shorter interval between the need for pain medicine and its administration; better pain relief than that obtained with intermittent IM injections; and a reduction in nursing time necessary for the delivery of pain medicine. It does not, however, decrease the need for client assessment while the PCA machine is in use.

Regional Analgesia

Regional analgesia and anesthesia have many applications in the relief of postoperative pain. Regional anesthetics do not cease working when the surgery ends and provide pain relief for a variable period of time afterwards. The duration of postoperative pain relief can be extended by continuing the infusion of pain medication into the epidural space or by adding opioids to either epidural or spinal anesthetics.

Local Anesthetics

Local anesthetics, either alone or in combination with opioids, can be administered into the epidural space at low concentrations that do not cause complete anesthesia. This type of pain relief is most commonly used for women in labor who receive epidural analgesia. Local anesthetic in low concentrations is a powerful analgesic. If local anesthetic is administered in a way to relieve pain in the lower extremities, clients are usually confined to bed, because even dilute concentrations of local anesthetic may affect the strength of leg muscles enough to increase the risk of falling. Clients receiving analgesia via an epidural block should be watched carefully to ensure that they do not develop pressure necrosis in the blocked areas. Local anesthetic pain relief can occasionally do such an effective job of relieving pain that the client may be unaware that pressure necrosis is occurring.

Opioids

The spinal cord has receptors for opioids, and when opioids are added to a spinal or epidural anesthetic, they provide pain relief even after the anesthetic block has worn off. Morphine added to a spinal or epidural anesthetic can provide hours of postoperative pain relief, often enough so that no other pain medication is needed; it may even provide better pain relief than do IM injections or intravenous PCA. Opioids may be added to spinal or epidural anesthetics as a single dose or be infused into the epidural space postoperatively. Although spinal and epidural morphine provide excellent pain relief, they may also produce significant respiratory depression. Respiratory depression is exceedingly rare in association with properly dosed epidural or spinal fentanyl (Sublimaze). Fortunately, the respiratory depression following spinal or epidural morphine administration is rarely rapid in onset. With current client selection and dosing protocols, life-threatening respiratory depression is a rare event. When it does occur, it can be detected long before it causes harm, by observing the client frequently, noting respiratory rate and depth, and periodically measuring oxygen saturation by pulse oximetry.

PROFESSIONAL TIP

Postanesthetic Care
- Immediately report to the anesthesia provider or surgeon any breathing difficulty.
- Immediately report to the surgeon or the anesthesia department a fall in the client's BP or increase in HR.
- Verify client's ability to stand or walk with normal motor strength and coordination and without any dizziness while in your direct care before allowing the client to get up without assistance.
- Do not allow clients to rub their eyes. Clients who are still drowsy may try to rub out protective eye moisturizer and, in the process, cause painful corneal abrasions.
- Observe clients immediately for bladder distention. Both regional and general anesthesia can sometimes cause temporary urinary retention.
- If clients have an epidural catheter for postoperative pain management, ensure that they change positions from time to time to prevent pressure necrosis. Do not allow the lateral aspect of the leg to rest on the side rails.
- Report to the anesthesia department as soon as possible any headache that gets worse when the client sits up or stands.
- Before giving discharge instructions, verify that the client's ability to remember instructions has returned. Always share discharge instructions with the individual responsible for taking the client home and provide the client with a written copy of the instructions.

CASE STUDY

Mrs. Pinkerton is in the recovery room following outpatient surgery. She received a general anesthetic and is now awake, breathing deeply, and talking to the staff. She has received meperidine (Demerol) intravenously and is quite comfortable. Before being discharged home from the surgery center, Mrs. Pinkerton rests in an easy chair in the transitional recovery area. The nurse taking care of her notices that she asks questions about things that have already been discussed and has even asked one question three times.

The following questions will guide your development of a nursing care plan for the case study.

1. After making these observations what nursing diagnoses and goals might the nurse identify for Mrs. Pinkerton?

2. List the nursing interventions to be performed in caring for Mrs. Pinkerton.

3. Identify teaching approaches.

SUMMARY

- In addition to ensuring an adequate level of anesthesia throughout a surgical procedure, the anesthesia provider monitors and controls physiologic functions.

- Some anesthesia providers prefer that clients not have anything to eat or drink for at least 8 hours prior to surgery. Others allow water up to 2 hours before surgery.

- Most scheduled medications that a client takes every day will be continued up to and including the morning of surgery.

- Sedation depresses brain activity, decreasing awareness, reducing anxiety, and easing the induction of general anesthesia.

- Oversedation results in respiratory depression, which can cause airway obstruction, and places the client at risk for aspiration of gastric contents.

- Regional anesthesia by the injection of a local anesthetic temporarily renders a "region" of the body insensible to pain.

- General anesthesia produces unconsciousness, complete insensibility to pain, amnesia, motionlessness, and muscle relaxation.

- A person is unlikely to remember what has happened for minutes to hours after sedation or a general anesthetic.

- Intravenous patient-controlled analgesia (PCA) allows clients to self-administer pain medication by pushing a button on the PCA machine. Limits are programmed into the machine to prevent overdose.

- Local anesthetics, alone or in combination with opioids, can be injected into the epidural space at low concentrations to provide postoperative analgesia.

- Spinal and epidural morphine can produce dangerous respiratory depression. This can be detected by frequent observations of the client's respiratory rate and depth and by periodic measurement of oxygen saturation via pulse oximetry.

Review Questions

1. Who is qualified to explain anesthesia and its risks and benefits in a manner sufficient to secure an informed consent from a client or legal guardian?

   a. a medical–surgical staff nurse
   b. an anesthesia provider or surgeon
   c. an operating room nurse
   d. a nursing supervisor

2. Why are clients at risk for aspiration of gastric contents into the lungs when receiving a general anesthetic?

   a. General anesthesia causes stomach distention.
   b. General anesthesia eliminates protective airway reflexes.
   c. Gastric peristalsis is reversed during general anesthesia.
   d. Vomiting normally occurs during general anesthesia.

3. What is the most dangerous result of oversedation?

   a. lack of response to verbal directions
   b. longer recovery time and resultant delayed discharge
   c. prolonged amnesia
   d. inability to breathe adequately

4. What is a sign that a client has a postdural puncture headache following a spinal or epidural regional block?

   a. The headache subsides after intake of plenty of liquids.

   b. The headache begins after the surgical procedure.

   c. The headache worsens when the client sits up or stands.

   d. The client is confused in addition to having a headache.

5. In addition to keeping the client unconscious, preventing the sensation of pain, and relaxing muscles to hold the client still and allow for surgical exposure, what does an anesthesia provider do to ensure a safe anesthetic?

   a. controls vital functions like breathing and heart rate

   b. records the amount of anesthetic drug used

   c. monitors the length of surgery

   d. administers prophylactic antibiotics

6. How long after cessation of a general anesthetic might it be before the client can think as clearly as before the client received the anesthetic?

   a. before being discharged from the recovery room

   b. within 2 hours

   c. six hours

   d. several days

7. What effect might a spinal or epidural anesthetic block still have after normal sensation and motor function have returned?

   a. decrease in pulse rate when the client is lying in bed

   b. decrease in blood pressure when the client stands up

   c. inhibition of protective airway reflexes

   d. sore muscles

Critical Thinking Questions

1. Why is physical assessment important relative to anesthesia?

2. Why must clients be monitored very closely after receiving an anesthetic?

WEB FLASH!

- What organizations are identified from which a person could get information about anesthesia?
- How many types of anesthesia can you find discussed on the Web?

NURSING CARE OF THE SURGICAL CLIENT

MAKING THE CONNECTION

Refer to the following chapters to increase your understanding of perioperative nursing:

- Chapter 3, Legal Responsibilities
- Chapter 4, Ethical Responsibilities
- Chapter 5, Communication
- Chapter 6, Cultural Diversity and Nursing
- Chapter 10, Fluid, Electrolyte, and Acid–Base Balance
- Chapter 12, Health Assessment
- Chapter 14, Pain Management

- Chapter 15, Anesthesia
- Chapter 18, Nursing Care of the Client: Respiratory System
- Chapter 19, Nursing Care of the Client: Cardiovascular System
- Chapter 21, Nursing Care of the Client: Integumentary System

LEARNING OBJECTIVES

Upon completion of this chapter, you should be able to:
- *Define key terms.*
- *List risk factors to be identified in a preoperative nursing assessment.*
- *List information to include in a general teaching plan for a preoperative client.*
- *Identify common nursing care for the preoperative, intraoperative, and postoperative phases.*
- *Identify members of the surgical team and describe their functions.*
- *Describe the principles of asepsis and their application to nursing practice.*
- *Identify nursing interventions to prevent or treat postoperative complications.*
- *Identify information needed by the postoperative client prior to discharge.*
- *Discuss the physiologic changes of aging that may affect the elderly client's response to surgery.*

KEY TERMS

Aldrete Score	intraoperative phase
ambulatory surgery	perioperative
asepsis	postoperative phase
aseptic technique	preoperative phase
circulating nurse	scrub nurse
dehiscence	sterile
evisceration	sterile conscience
first assistant	sterile field
informed consent	surgery

INTRODUCTION

Surgery refers to the treatment of injury, disease, or deformity through invasive operative methods. Surgery is a unique experience, with no two clients responding alike to similar operations. Even the same client may respond differently to two separate surgical situations or to the same surgery performed at a later time. Each client has a unique socioeconomic background and fills different family and community roles. Regardless of background or roles, however, surgery is a major stressor for all clients. To a client, there is no such thing as minor surgery; anxiety and fear are normal. Surgery, even when planned well in advance, is a stressor that produces both psychological (anxiety, fear) and physiologic (neuroendocrine) stress reactions. Surgery is a stressful experience because it involves entry into the human body and is sometimes a threat to life itself.

Surgeries are classified as minor (presenting little risk to life) or major (possibly involving risk to life) and may be performed for a variety of reasons. Table 16–1 lists indications for surgery.

The term **perioperative** encompasses the preoperative (before surgery), intraoperative (during surgery), and postoperative (after surgery) phases of surgery. Each phase refers to a particular time during the surgical experience, and each requires a wide range of specific nursing behaviors and functions. Perioperative nursing has one continuous goal: to provide a standard of excellence in the care of the client before, during, and after surgery. Perioperative nursing is client oriented; therefore, the nursing activities must be geared to meet the client's psychosocial needs as well as immediate physical needs.

Surgical intervention is a distinctive event for clients. Individuals face this particular event with their own values. Every client not only has specific expectations of the surgical experience, but also has distinct hopes for the outcome of the surgery. The nurse must take an active part in the entire perioperative process in order to ensure quality and continuity of client care.

PREOPERATIVE PHASE

The **preoperative phase** is that time during the surgical experience that begins with the client's decision to have surgery and ends with the transfer of the client to the operating table.

The outcome of surgical treatment is tremendously enhanced by accurate preoperative nursing assessment and careful preoperative preparation. The client must be assessed by the nurse both physiologically and psychologically. Assessment of the client involves the integration of factors relating to the client's illness, physical condition, related medical conditions, and current surgical diagnosis. Regardless of how minor the surgical procedure, a thorough health history is essential and should be available to the perioperative team throughout the client's surgical experience.

The psychological well-being of the client may have an impact on the surgical outcome. The surgical client is at risk for anxiety related to the surgical experience and the outcome of surgery. Fear and anxiety can affect the client's ability to cope with the proposed plan of care. Anxiety is a normal adaptive response to the stress of surgery. Because individuals differ in their perceptions of the meaning of surgery, the degree of anxiety and fear experienced will vary. If fear and anxiety become excessive, however, these emotions can interfere with recovery by magnifying the normal physiologic stress response. The nurse, by assessing and being aware of the fears and anxieties of the surgical client, can provide support and information so that stress does not become overwhelming. The most common fears related to surgery are as follows:

- Fear of the unknown
- Fear of pain and discomfort
- Fear of mutilation and disfigurement
- Fear of anesthesia
- Fear of disruption of life patterns
    Separation from family/significant others
    Sexuality
    Financial
    Permanent/temporary limitations
- Fear of death/not waking up
- Fear of not being in control

Fear of the unknown is the most prevalent fear prior to surgery and is the fear that the nurse can most easily help control through client education and preoperative teaching.

Preoperative Physiologic Assessment

Physiologic assessment should include a physical examination and a review of the client's laboratory values and diagnostic studies. Laboratory and diagnostic studies may be divided into those that are routine and those that are done specifically to evaluate the client's primary disease process or coexisting condition. The following summarizes common preoperative laboratory tests:

Table 16–1 INDICATIONS FOR SURGERY

TYPE OF SURGERY	PURPOSE	EXAMPLE
Diagnostic	Determine cause of symptoms	Biopsy
		Exploratory laparotomy
Curative	Remove a diseased body part or replace a body part to restore function	Colecystectomy
		Total knee arthroplasty
Palliative	Relieve symptoms without curing disease	Tumor resection associated with cancer
Restorative	Strengthen a weakened area	Herniorrhaphy
Cosmetic	Improve appearance	Face lift
	Change shape	Mammoplasty

- Hemoglobin and hematocrit (Hgb and Hct)
- White blood cell count (WBC)
- Blood typing and cross matching (screening)
- Serum electrolytes
- Prothrombin time (PT) and partial thromboplastin time (PTT)
- Bilirubin
- Liver enzymes: alanine aminotransferase (ALT) and aspartate aminotransferase (AST)
- Urinalysis
- Blood urea nitrogen (BUN) and creatinine

Although it is common practice to obtain a chest x-ray for many clients admitted to the hospital, this study is increasingly omitted for healthy children and healthy adults under the age of 40 years in whom the physical examination is normal and there is no reason to suspect pulmonary or cardiac disease. Additional radiographic or fluoroscopic examinations, sonograms, radioisotopic scans, magnetic resonance imaging, and computerized tomography scans give useful information as to the nature of the disease process and its anatomic location and extent. Any organ that is undergoing major surgery should be adequately evaluated with these techniques prior to the operation.

Electrocardiograms (EKGs) are routinely performed in middle-age and elderly clients undergoing surgery, because of the prevalence of ischemic heart disease in these age groups. It is also of value to have a baseline study for comparison should subsequent EKGs be needed.

Preoperative testing may be done several days be-fore the date of surgery. The type and amount of screening will depend on the age and condition of the client, the nature of the surgery, and the surgeon's preference. Surgeons (doctors who perform surgery) are coming under increasing economic pressure to minimize routine testing procedures. The current trend is based on cost versus benefits, moving away from extensive testing in the absence of indicative/warranting data from the health history and physical examination.

The nurse's role in preoperative testing is to ensure that the tests are ordered and performed and that the results are placed in the client's chart. Abnormal results are reported to the physician immediately.

The physiologic nursing assessment is completed prior to surgery. Preoperative assessment can take place in the surgeon's office, in the hospital during hospitalization, or in the hospital or ambulatory surgery unit on the day of surgery. The nurse collects client health data by interviewing the client, the family, significant others, and health care providers. Data collection can also be accomplished through review of the client's records; assessment; and/or consultation. Assessment is essential to establishing nursing diagnoses and predicting outcomes (Association of Operating Room Nurses [AORN], 1995a). When performing the nursing assessment, the nurse screens the client for risks that may contribute to complications in the perioperative period. Table 16–2 lists risk factors and possible complications of each. The nurse's role in the preoperative phase ensures client safety, understanding, and compliance with health care treatment.

Table 16–2 VARIABLES AFFECTING SURGICAL STATUS

VARIABLE	RELATED RISK FACTORS	POSSIBLE COMPLICATIONS	
Age	Old age	• Decreased metabolism and elimination of anesthetics and medications • Hypothermia • Hypervolemia • Hypovolemia and shock • Deep vein thrombosis, thrombophlebitis, pulmonary embolus • Decreased urinary output/renal function • Urinary incontinence/retention	• Urinary tract infections • Poor or delayed wound healing • Pressure sores • Atelectasis/pneumonia • Constipation/fecal impaction • Infection • Physical injury (falls or joint overextension)
Nutritional status	Malnutrition	• Fluid and electrolyte imbalance • Delayed wound healing • Wound infection	• Poor tolerance to anesthetics • Bleeding/hemorrhage
	Obesity	• Retention of anesthetics and medications • Wound infection • Delayed wound healing	• Deep vein thrombosis, thrombophlebitis, pulmonary embolus • Atelectasis • Pneumonia

continues

Table 16–2 *continued*

VARIABLE	RELATED RISK FACTORS	POSSIBLE COMPLICATIONS	
Fluid and electrolyte status	Deficits and excesses of fluids and electrolytes	• Anorexia, nausea, vomiting • Diarrhea and cramps • Constipation • Paralytic ileus • Hypotension • Hypertension • Edema (including pulmonary edema) • Confusion • Lethargy • Tetany • Weakness	• Parathesias • Paralysis • Restlessness • Delusions and hallucinations • Seizures • Laryngospasm • Respiratory arrest • Tachycardia • Dysrhythmias • Cardiac arrest • Renal failure
Respiratory status	Acute respiratory infections History of chronic respiratory diseases/ smoking	• Bronchospasm • Laryngospasm • Hypoxemia • Atelectasis • Pneumonia	• Atelectasis • Pneumonia
Cardiovascular status	History of preexisting cardiac disease	• Dysrhythmias • Hypotension/syncope • Myocardial infarction • Congestive heart failure	• Cardiac arrest • Stroke • Shock • Deep vein thrombosis, thrombophlebitis, or pulmonary embolism
Renal and hepatic status	History of pre-existing renal or hepatic diseases	• Fluid and electrolyte imbalances • Bleeding/hemorrhage • Infection	• Impaired wound healing • Hyperglycemia/hypoglycemia • Decreased metabolism and elimination of anesthetics and medications
Neurological, musculoskeletal, and integumentary status	Surgical positioning or prolonged immobility	• Pressure alopecia • Pressure point compression • Pressure sores • Nerve injury to axillary neurovascular bundle, subclavian neurovascular bundle, brachial plexus, and facial, peroneal, radial, and ulnar nerves • Neck pain, lower back pain, joint damage	• Postural hypotension • Eye abrasion • Ear compression • Atelectasis on dependent side • Air embolism • Facial and airway edema
Endocrine and immunological status	Diabetes Immunocompromised	• Fluid and electrolyte imbalances • Deep vein thrombosis, thrombophlebitis, and pulmonary embolism • Infection of respiratory and urinary tract • Infection • Respiratory infections	• Neurogenic bladder • Impaired wound healing • Hyperglycemia/hypoglycemia • Ketoacidosis • Pressure sores • Impaired wound healing
Medications	Chemical dependency	• Increased or decreased effectiveness of anesthetic agents, narcotics, and/or sedatives	• Drug interactions • Symptoms of withdrawal (hallucinations, disorientation, convulsions)

Age

Surgery can be performed on individuals of any age, although persons at both extremes of age (infants and elders) may be at greater risk for complications. Infants can easily become dehydrated or fluid over-loaded and suffer resultant electrolyte imbalances. Because their metabolic rate is two to three times that of an adult, infants can have formula up to 6 hours before surgery, and breastfed infants may be nursed up to 4 hours before surgery. Infants may then have clear liquids for up to 2 hours before surgery.

Body temperature regulation and the renal, immune, and respiratory systems are different in infants than in adults. Renal function in the infant is comparatively less efficient due to a lower glomerular filtration rate and less efficient renal tubular function (Atkinson & Fortunato, 1996). This may lead to retention of anesthesia and medications and to fluid overload. Due to a comparatively larger ratio of body surface area to body mass, infants are also more prone to hypothermia when placed in a cool environment or when large areas of their body surface is exposed. Further, an immature immune system renders the infant more susceptible to infections. Because of a smaller and less developed anatomic structure and enlarged tongue and lymphoid tissue, the infant is also more prone to respiratory obstruction. The nursing process and nursing care must be tailored to meet the unique needs of the infant client.

Elderly clients experience many physiologic changes associated with aging and are more likely to have degenerative disease in many organs. Elders are more likely to become dehydrated and are thus less able to adapt to fluid loss during surgery. The elderly client is also more sensitive to central nervous system depressants used during the perioperative period. However, even elderly clients can favorably tolerate extensive surgery when carefully assessed and managed.

Nutritional Status

Nutritional assessment includes evaluation of individual deficiencies or excesses that can place the client at greater risk for complications during surgery. Surgery increases the body's need for nutrients necessary for tissue healing and resistance to infection.

Nutritional deficiencies place the client at higher risk for fluid and electrolyte imbalance, delayed wound healing, and wound infections. The malnourished individual may have diminished stores of carbohydrates and fats; in such an instance, proteins are utilized for energy instead of tissue building and restoration. In addition to carbohydrates and fats, vitamins B complex and C are also significant, because these vitamins are essential to healing. Poor nutritional status can also adversely affect liver and kidney function, leaving the client with a poor tolerance for anesthetic agents and a tendency for bleeding.

GERONTOLOGICAL CONSIDERATIONS

Surgery in the Elderly Client

Morbidity and mortality rates for surgical clients over the age of 90 years are much higher than for those age 70 to 75 years (Hogstel, 1994). Elderly clients do not tolerate emergency or long, complicated surgery as well as do younger clients because of a lesser ability to adapt to physical and psychological stress.

Nutritional excesses or obesity increase the risk for respiratory, cardiovascular, and gastrointestinal complications. Obesity makes access to the surgical site more difficult, which prolongs surgical time and increases the amount of anesthetic agents required. Because inhalation anesthetics are absorbed and stored by adipose tissue and released postoperatively, recovery time from anesthesia is slower in the overweight client. Adipose tissue is less vascular and more difficult to suture, which predisposes the client to wound infection, delayed wound healing, and increased incidence of wound complications including postoperative incisional hernias. Failure to exercise and ambulate increases the chances of decreased respiratory function accompanied by atelectasis and pneumonia, and also may lead to decreased wound healing and an increased risk of thrombus formation. Often, obese clients also have other chronic conditions, such as hypertension or diabetes mellitus, that increase the likelihood of surgical complications. In some surgical situations, such as joint replacement, surgery may be delayed until nutritional status improves and the client loses weight.

Fluid and Electrolyte Status

Dehydration and hypovolemia, with correlating electrolyte disturbances, predispose a client to complications during and after surgery. Both may be caused by diarrhea, excessive nasogastric suctioning, inadequate oral intake, vomiting, and/or bleeding. As outlined in Table 16–2, the complications of fluid and electrolyte imbalances are numerous and varied, ranging from minor (delayed recovery) to major (death). Changes in fluid and electrolyte balance affect cellular metabolism, renal function, and oxygen concentration in the circulation. Nursing care focuses on administering parenteral fluids or blood products as prescribed, keeping a detailed intake and output record, and evaluating results of laboratory studies.

Respiratory Status

Respiratory assessment should include detection of acute and chronic problems. Because acute respiratory

CLIENT TEACHING

Postoperative Deep Breathing, Incentive Spirometry, Coughing, and Turning

Activity	Description	Instruction
Deep breathing	• Mode of breathing during which the diaphragm expands fully, allowing expansion of the thorax, upper abdomen, and alveoli as air enters and followed by abdominal and diaphragmatic contraction during expansion	• Sit in semi-Fowler's position with hands placed over lower ribs and upper abdomen • Inhale deeply through the mouth and nose • Hold the breath for 5 seconds • Exhale fully through mouth and nose • Repeat 15 times with short rest periods as needed • Perform twice daily
Incentive spirometry (Figure 16-1)	• Method of using a commercial cylinder that measures deep breaths, with a float that rises during inhalation	• Sit as upright as possible • Seal lips around mouthpiece • Inhale and watch float rise • Hold deep breath for 5 seconds • Remove mouthpiece and exhale slowly • Repeat 10 to 12 times per hour • Cough after the last breath
Coughing (Figure 16-2)	• Method of moving lung secretions from smaller airways to larger airways	• Sit as upright as possible • Splint incision with hands or pillow • Inhale deeply using deep breathing technique • Cough several times until it feels as if no air is left in the lungs • May continue with another deep inhalation followed by one or two strong coughs • Repeat one time per hour
Turning	• Method of alternating position from back to either side to promote circulation, lung expansion and drainage, and relief from pressure areas	• Change position every 1 to 2 hours (assistance and support pillows may be required)

Figure 16-1 Using an Incentive Spirometer

Figure 16-2 Splinting to Cough

infections may lead to bronchospasms or laryngospasms, surgery for clients with these conditions may be delayed or contraindicated. Chronic respiratory problems, such as asthma and chronic obstructive pulmonary disease, impair the client's gas exchange and increase the risk associated with inhalation anesthetic agents. Clients with chronic respiratory problems are more likely to develop atelectasis and pneumonia.

Respiratory assessment as performed by the nurse includes assessing breath sounds and color of the skin and mucous membranes. It also involves assessing for shortness of breath (dyspnea), clubbed fingers, and coughing. In addition to a chest x-ray, arterial blood gases or an oxygen saturation baseline may be ordered. Restriction of smoking should be encouraged at least 4 to 6 weeks before a scheduled surgery, when possible. All clients, and especially those clients who smoke and have chronic lung disease, should be taught deep breathing, use of incentive spirometry, coughing, and preoperative turning.

Cardiovascular Status

Cardiovascular assessment focuses on diseases that would require close observation by the nurse and make necessary the avoidance of sudden changes of position, overhydration with intravenous fluids, and prolonged immobilization. Examples of such diseases include angina, recent myocardial infarction or cardiac surgery, hemophilia, hypertension, and congestive heart failure. Clients with a history of cardiac disease are prone to developing complications such as dysrhythmias, hypotension, myocardial infarction, congestive heart failure, cardiac arrest, stroke, shock, deep vein thrombosis, thrombophlebitis, or pulmonary embolism.

The nurse also assesses for anxiety; elevated blood pressure; slow, rapid, or irregular pulse; chest pain; edema; coolness or cyanosis/discoloration of extremities; weakness; and shortness of breath (dyspnea). All clients must be taught postoperative leg exercises to prevent thrombophlebitis (Figure 16-3 and the accompanying display). The goal of nursing care is to improve the client's cardiovascular condition to the highest degree possible by promoting rest alternated with activity; encouraging a low-sodium and low-cholesterol diet; administering heart medications; and judiciously administering parenteral fluids and recording intake and output.

Renal and Hepatic Status

Because many medications and anesthetic agents are detoxified by the liver and excreted by the kidneys, renal and hepatic sufficiency constitute a major concern. Renal disease affects fluid and electrolyte balance and protein equilibrium. Liver disease may be accompanied by bleeding tendencies or carbohydrate, fat, and amino acid imbalances that impair wound healing and increase the risk of infection. The nurse assesses for symptoms of urinary frequency, dysuria, and anuria, and records the color and amount of the urine. The nurse also assesses for a history of bleeding tendencies, easy bruising, nosebleeds, and use of anticoagulants. The most commonly ordered preoperative tests to assess renal function are urinalysis, blood urea nitrogen (BUN), and creatinine. The most common liver tests are prothrombin time (PT), partial thromboplastin time (PTT), bilirubin, and the liver enzymes alanine aminotransferase (ALT) and aspartate aminotransferase

---

PROFESSIONAL TIP

Client's Psychological Condition

The client "who fears dying while under anesthesia runs a greater risk of cardiac arrest on the operating table than [do] clients with known cardiac disease" (Atkinson & Fortunato, 1996).

- The psychological condition of the client can have a stronger influence than does the physical condition.
- Encourage clients to express their feelings and fears about receiving anesthetic and having surgery.
- Observe the client for nonverbal clues indicative of anxiety.
- To reduce client anxiety, explain to the client what will be happening throughout the surgical experience.

Figure 16-3 Leg Exercises: A. Lift leg and circle ankle, first to the right and then to the left. Repeat three times; relax. Repeat with other leg. B. With heels on the bed, push toes of both feet toward the foot of the bed until the calf muscles tighten; relax. Pull toes up toward chin until calf muscles tighten; relax feet.

CLIENT TEACHING

Postoperative Leg Exercises

Activity	Instructions
Leg lifts	1. While lying on back or in a semi-sitting position, bend the leg and raise it 2. Hold for count of five. 3. Lower leg to the bed. 4. Repeat five times then proceed to other leg. Perform every hour.
Dorsiflexion and hyperextension of ankles	1. Flex ankles and raise toes toward head, stretching posterior calf 2. Hold for count of two. 3. Relax. 4. Repeat five times then proceed to other foot. Perform every hour.
Foot circles	1. Point the toe and raise the leg slightly off the bed. 2. Use the great toe to trace a circle in the air, first to the right and then to the left. 3. Repeat five times then proceed to other foot. Perform every hour.

(AST). Nursing care focuses on administering fluids and adequate nutrition, monitoring fluid intake and output, and evaluating results of laboratory tests.

Neurological, Musculoskeletal, and Integumentary Status

The nurse assesses the client's overall mental status including level of consciousness; orientation to person, place, and time; and the ability to understand and follow instructions. The nurse assesses the condition of the skin, including turgor; and notes any rashes, bruises, lesions, or previous incisions. Client mobility and sensation are also assessed through observation of both range of motion and ability to ambulate and through client statements. The nurse notes any abnormalities, injuries, or previous surgery and assesses the risk for falls. The presence of internal or external prostheses or implants such as pacemakers, heart valves, or joint prosthesis is also noted, because the presence of these may necessitate preoperative antibiotics.

Thin clients, clients undergoing long surgical procedures or vascular procedures, and elderly clients are the most vulnerable to neurological, musculoskeletal, or integumentary injuries. Some underlying disease processes, such as edema, infection, cancer, osteoporosis, arthritic joints, or neck or back problems, also

place a client at higher risk for injury. Clients who are malnourished, anemic, obese, hypovolemic, paralyzed, or diabetic are also prone to skin breakdown. Information gathered about the neurological, musculoskeletal, and integumentary systems is used for preparation of the surgical site, for surgical positioning, and as a comparative basis for postoperative assessments and complication screening. Table 16–2 lists potential complications of surgical positioning and prolonged immobility after surgery.

Endocrine and Immunological Status

Clients with diabetes who are undergoing surgery require special consideration. They should be scheduled as early in the morning as possible, and a fasting glucose should be drawn immediately prior to surgery. Surgery is a stressor, and stress raises the serum glucose level in the client with diabetes. Thus, the morning dose of insulin may need to be adjusted.

When anesthetized during surgery, the diabetic client exhibits very few symptoms of glucose imbalance. Serum glucose must therefore be checked frequently during surgery, usually by the anesthesia provider. Stability is attained by the administration of insulin, glucose, or both. Besides hyperglycemia and hypoglycemia, a diabetic client is more prone to fluid and electrolyte imbalances; infection including respiratory and urinary tract infections; neurogenic bladder; impaired wound healing; ketoacidosis; deep vein thrombosis; thrombophlebitis; and pulmonary embolism.

Because the immunological system protects the client from infections, the immunocompromised surgical client is very prone to infection. Clients receiving steroids or chemotherapy, or who have systemic lupus erythematosus, Addison's disease, or acquired immunodeficiency syndrome (AIDS) are considered to be immunocompromised. The immune response in these clients is weakened or deficient, resulting in an increased incidence of infection. Because surgery breaks the integrity of the skin and the normal inflammatory response is suppressed, wound healing may be impaired. Strict adherence to aseptic technique, covered later in this chapter, is thus even more imperative. Prevention of infection is crucial in these clients. The role of the nurse is to communicate the presence of potential immunosuppression to other health care team members involved in the client's care, and to help prevent infection by practicing aseptic technique.

Medications

Knowledge of the client's use of drugs for recreational or therapeutic purposes is essential to preoperative assessment. The history of medication usage by the client should include type and frequency of use for over-the-counter, prescription, and street drugs. The use of certain drugs can affect the client's reaction to anesthetic agents and surgery (Table 16–3). Some drugs in-

Table 16–3 MEDICATION CLASSIFI-CATIONS AND POSSIBLE EFFECTS WITH ANESTHETIC AGENTS AND SURGERY

CLASSIFICATION	POSSIBLE EFFECTS
Antibiotics	• Respiratory paralysis when combined with certain muscle relaxants
Anticoagulants	• Hemorrhage
Anti-Parkinson drugs	• Increase hypotensive effects of anesthetic agents
Diuretics	• Electrolyte imbalance
Hypoglycemics	• Hypoglycemia or hyperglycemia
Monoamine oxidase (MAO) inhibitors	• Hypertensive crisis when combined with certain anesthetics
Steroids	• Cardiovascular collapse if abruptly withdrawn • Impaired physiologic response to stress • Delayed wound healing • Increased risk of infection
Street drugs and alcohol abuse	• Tolerance to narcotics
Tranquilizers	• Potentiation of narcotics and barbiturates

PROFESSIONAL TIP

Questions To Assess Psychosocial Status
- Why are you having surgery?
- When did this problem start?
- What do you think caused this problem?
- Has this caused any problems in your relationships with others?
- Has your problem prevented you from working?
- Are you able to take care of your own needs?
- Are you experiencing any discomfort or pain?
- What are you expecting from this surgery?
- Is there anything that you do not understand regarding your surgery?
- Are you worried about anything?
- Will someone be available to assist you when you return home?

knowledge level and ability to understand. The data collected are incorporated into nursing care throughout the perioperative experience.

Cultural beliefs can influence a client's perception of surgery. For example, some cultures believe that surgery is a "final effort" performed only when all other possible treatments have been of no avail. Furthermore, surgeries that cause changes in the appearance of the body can alter body image and self-esteem; the client may worry about being sexually attractive or active after surgery.

Clients should be provided the opportunity to express their spiritual values and beliefs. Many clients wish to see a member of the clergy before having surgery.

Surgical Consent

An **informed consent** is a legal form signed by the client and witnessed by another person that grants permission to the client's physician to perform the procedure described by the physician. An informed consent is needed whenever:

- Anesthesia is used,
- The procedure is considered invasive,
- The procedure is nonsurgical but has more than a slight risk of complications (such as with an arteriogram), or
- Radiation or cobalt therapy is used.

Informed consent protects both the client (against unauthorized procedures) and the physician and the health care institution and its employees (against claims that an unauthorized procedure was performed). Although the ultimate responsibility for obtaining the informed consent lies with the physician, it is often the nurse who obtains and witnesses the client's signature

crease surgical risks; these medications usually are temporarily discontinued when a client goes to surgery. Other medications, such as heart or hypoglycemic medications may still be given even though the client is to undergo surgery; the surgeon or anesthesia provider will write specific orders in such instances. Dosages of medications may also be adjusted during the perioperative period.

Chronic alcohol use increases surgical risk because it is often accompanied by impaired nutrition and liver disease. Postoperatively, the client may exhibit delirium tremens or acute withdrawal syndrome. Furthermore, pain medication may be less effective.

Psychosocial Health Assessment

The psychosocial health status of the client is also assessed. The nurse elicits the client's perceptions of surgery and the expected outcome. The nurse also ascertains the client's coping mechanisms and the client's

CULTURAL CONSIDERATIONS

Impending Surgery
- Special religious rites may be desired by the client before surgery.
- Some clients may not want to receive blood transfusions or other treatments.
- All client beliefs must be respected.

and ensures that the client signs the consent form voluntarily and is alert and comprehending of the action.

Most hospitals use a standard preprinted form. The information written by the health care personnel must be specific to the individual client. The client's signature on the consent form indicates the information has been read and is correct. The client has the right to refuse treatment even after the consent has been signed. When this occurs, the nurse must inform the physician immediately of the client's decision.

Preoperative Teaching

The client about to undergo surgery is at high risk for knowledge deficit related to preoperative procedures and protocols and to postoperative expectations. Preoperative teaching is the giving of information to the client prior to a surgical procedure. The potential benefits of preoperative teaching include reduced anxiety and more rapid recovery with fewer complications and shorter hospitalization. Reduction in anxiety has a secondary benefit: The client usually requires less medication for pain. The purpose of preoperative teaching is to (1) answer questions and concerns about surgery; (2) ascertain the client's present knowledge of the intended surgery; (3) ascertain the need or desire for additional information; and (4) provide information in a manner most conducive to learning.

One-on-one sessions constitute the most personal method of instruction. The nurse should also try to include the family or significant other when possible. The level of learning increases when more than one teaching medium is used. For example, using materials such as videotapes, charts, tours, anatomic models, pictures, and brochures reinforces both visual and auditory learning. Demonstration followed by return demonstration is helpful. Written instructions serve as a reference for later use. Instructions should be simple, using terms the client can understand. Any unfamiliar words or concepts should be thoroughly explained.

Clients are often interested in any information that describes the sights, sounds, tastes, feelings, odors, and temperature of what they are about to experience. For example, the feeling of relaxation from preoperative medications; the sounds of instruments or equip-

ment in the operating room (OR); the pressure from the automatic blood pressure cuff; the warmth or coolness of skin-preparation solutions; or the brightness of the operating room lights are all sensations the client may experience. Analogies or stories of real or fictitious situations of sensory experiences help the client understand concepts being presented. The teaching methods used by the nurse strongly influence the client's degree of learning and retention of information.

Preoperative teaching should begin as soon as surgery is agreed upon. Instructions given over the phone and/or mailed to the client during the time leading up to surgery are beneficial. Just prior to surgery, a brief review with additional information tailored to the needs of the client may be given. The client should be given an opportunity to ask questions.

Information should always be targeted to the client's needs. Teaching plans should be tailored according to the client's level of knowledge and anxiety. Mild to moderate anxiety actually heightens a person's alertness and motivates learning. Mildly anxious clients should receive the most complete instructions. Moderately anxious clients should receive less information but more attention to specific areas of concern. Severely anxious clients should receive only basic information but should be encouraged to verbalize their concerns. Clients in a state of panic are unable to learn; in such cases no instruction shall be given, and the surgeon should be notified.

Physical Preparation

Extremely close attention must be given to identifying the proper client both verbally and by reading the identification name band. The nurse then begins the important task of verifying the operative procedure. This must be completed through client statements, surgeon verification, and the signed surgical consent form. Particular attention should be given to differentiating between right and left operative sites.

In order to lessen the chance of infection, special care is given to the preparation of the operative site. To reduce the number of microorganisms on the skin, the operative site is thoroughly cleansed with an antiseptic soap such as povidone-iodine. Typically, the operative site is not shaved; but if shaving is to be performed, it is done in the operating room immediately prior to surgery. To reduce the number of bacteria in the gastrointestinal tract for gastrointestinal, peritoneal, perianal, or pelvic surgery, an enema is ordered. Enemas prevent contamination of the peritoneal area by fecal content passed during surgery. The reduction in colon size related to the loss of bulk also helps prevent colon injury and increases visualization of the operative site. Enemas are usually given the night before surgery. If the enema is to be done at home, the client must be given detailed instructions. Many types of surgery require special preparations. The specific pro-

CLIENT TEACHING

Preoperative Teaching

- Introduce self
    Identify role in client's care
- Determine client's knowledge level and need or desire for additional information
- Explain the routine for the day of surgery
    Restricted food or fluid intake
    Intravenous fluids
    Premedication
    Time of surgery
    Anticipated length of surgery
    Transportation to the operating room
    Special skin preparations
    Type of surgical incision (Figure 16-4)
- Familiarize the client with the operating room environment
    Operating room lights and table
    Accessory equipment
    Monitoring equipment
    Anesthesia induction
- Include significant others
    Time to arrive at the hospital
    Location of surgical waiting area
    What to expect when client returns to the unit
- Explain postanesthesia care unit (PACU)
    Location of recovery room
    Purpose of recovery room
    Routine of postanesthesia care
- Identify anticipated dressings, drains, catheters, casts, etc.
- Demonstrate and evaluate client's proficiency with:
    Coughing and deep breathing exercises
    Turning
    Incentive spirometry
    Extremity exercises
    Any special transfer procedures or aids required after surgery
- Describe pain management strategies appropriate for the specific surgical procedure

Figure 16-4 Common Surgical Incisions: A. Sternal split; B. Oblique subcostal; C. Upper vertical midline; D. Thoraco-abdominal; E. McBurney; F. Lower vertical midline; G. Pfannenstiel

The nurse checks the client's vital signs including blood pressure, temperature, pulse and respirations. Due to anxiety, some changes in vital signs are normal. If marked differences exist from the baseline data, however, the surgeon must be notified.

The nurse assists the client in putting on a hospital gown, hair cap, and, if ordered, antiembolic hose. Institutional policy requires that jewelry be removed; however wedding rings may be taped on and left in place. Hairpins, wigs, and prostheses must also be removed. The nurse is responsible for recording the disposition of any personal items removed for surgery. If policy requires, nail polish (from at least one nail, if dark polish) is removed so that oxygen saturation may be read via pulse oximetry, although some pulse oximeters may be able to read oxygen saturation through nail polish. Makeup is also removed so that skin color can be observed.

Allergies to medication, food, and chemicals (including contrast agents) are verified, as are previous blood reactions. The nurse must differentiate between a medication intolerance and a true allergic reaction. With a medication intolerance, the client may suffer side effects that are unpleasant. For example, many clients experience nausea when given meperidine (Demerol), although unpleasant, this is not a drug allergy. A true allergy produces a skin reaction or anaphylactic reaction, where the client experiences cardiorespiratory reactions that may be life threatening, such as hypotension and pulmonary edema. A client with multiple food allergies is also prone to hypersensitivities to medications. When allergies are identified, the client's chart is marked accordingly, and an allergy wrist band is applied. By being aware of and alerting other team members to the client's allergies, client safety and comfort are maintained.

tocol for each surgical procedure is available from the health care facility or the physician.

Safety: Iodine Allergy

- Each client must be asked about allergy to iodine.

- If a client is allergic to iodine, document the allergy on the client's record and inform the surgeon and OR personnel so that an iodine-free solution can be used for skin preparation and for other procedures for which iodine is routinely used.

PROFESSIONAL TIP

Implementing NPO Status

- Explain reasons for NPO status to the client
- Remove any food and water from the client's overbed table and nightstand
- Mark the client's door and bed with an NPO sign
- Mark the client's Kardex and other nursing information sources
- Notify the dietary department

GERONTOLOGICAL CONSIDERATIONS

Preparation for Surgery

The elder client may have:

- Increased risk of complications including infection
- Increased incidence of coexisting conditions
- Unpredictable response to medications and anesthetics
- Greater need for support from family and significant other
- Increased skin and bone fragility
- Nutritional and financial deficiencies
- Impaired vision and hearing
- Impaired or slowed thought processes and cognitive abilities
- Fear of death, loss of independence, and change in lifestyle

The nurse verifies the NPO (nothing by mouth) status of the client for the amount of time specified by the surgeon's order. Restricting oral intake reduces the possibility of aspiration pneumonia. If surgery takes place in the afternoon, the client may have a clear liquid breakfast if ordered by the surgeon. Careful client instruction is required because surgery may need to be postponed if the client consumes food or fluid.

In addition to the previously outlined preparations, dentures and bridgework are removed to prevent loss, damage, and possible dislodgement and airway obstruction during the surgery. The nurse also ensures that the client has an empty bladder by allowing time for the client to void prior to transfer to surgery.

The nurse should identify any sensory deficits in the client and communicate this information to other health care team members. Glasses, contact lenses, and hearing aids are usually removed to prevent loss or damage; if policy allows, however, it is best to leave these items in place so that the client is better able to see and hear. The nurse would then be responsible for communicating the presence of these aids to other health care team members.

The surgeon or anesthesiologist (a doctor trained in providing anesthesia) may order preoperative medication. Table 16–4 lists medications that may be given alone or in combination to elicit the desired effects. The nurse gives the medication by the prescribed route (intramuscular, intravenous, or oral) at the specified time (typically 1 hour prior to surgery). Preoperative medications may be ordered "on call," this means that the nurse is notified by a member of the surgical team when the preoperative medication needs to be given. Prior to administering the medication, the nurse should ask the client to void. After administering the preoperative medication, the nurse should raise the side rails of the gurney or bed, put the bed in the lowest position, and instruct the client not to get up without assistance.

When the surgical team is ready, the client is transported on a gurney by a member of the OR team, typically an orderly. The client is always transported feet first and with the side rails up to ensure safety and minimize the likelihood of dizziness and nausea. If on

a clinical nursing unit, the client may be taken to a preoperative holding area first (Figure 16-5). The nurse instructs the family or significant others where to wait.

The information collected as part of preoperative preparation is documented in the client record, usually on a preoperative checklist. Figure 16-6 illustrates a typical preoperative checklist. This checklist is completed prior to the client leaving the clinical unit or upon the client's admission to ambulatory surgery. The nurse must also verbally communicate to other health care members any necessary information collected.

INTRAOPERATIVE PHASE

The **intraoperative phase** is the time during the surgical experience that begins when the client is transferred to the operating room table and ends when the client is admitted to the postanesthesia care unit (PACU).

Figure 16-5 The holding area is used for clients who are waiting to have surgery.

Table 16–4 PREOPERATIVE MEDICATIONS: COMMON CLASSIFICATIONS, EXAMPLES, AND DESIRED EFFECTS

CLASSIFICATION	EXAMPLE	DESIRED EFFECTS
Tranquilizers	diazepam (Valium) lorazepam (Ativan)	Reduce anxiety Decrease motor activity Promote rapid induction of anesthesia
Sedatives	phenobarbitol sodium (Luminal sodium) secobarbital (Seconal) midazolam hydrochloride (Versed)	Promote sleep Decrease anxiety Reduce amount of anesthesia required
Narcotics	morphine sulfate meperidine (Demerol)	Reduce pain Relax the client Reduce anxiety
Vagolytic agents (anticholinergics)	atropine sulfate scopolamine hydrobromide glycopyrrolate (Robinul)	Reduce tracheobronchial secretions Drying of mucous membranes Interrupt vagal stimulation Produce sedative and amnesia effects
Antinausea agents	droperidol (Inapsine) promethazine hydrochloride (Phenergan)	Reduce nausea Prevent vomiting Provide mild relaxation
H_2 receptor antagonists	cimetidine (Tagamet) ranitidine hydrochloride (Zantac) famotidine (Pepcid)	Decrease gastric secretions

Physical Description of the Operating Room Environment

For the purposes of preventing wound infections, the surgical suite is environmentally controlled. Personnel restriction and geographic isolation from other areas of the hospital or clinic constitute part of this control. Constant filtered airflow and positive air pressure in the operating rooms also aid in environmental control. Furthermore, clean areas and contaminated areas are separated within the suite. Finally, equipment and supplies needed for each client are centralized in the surgical suite so that members of the surgical team do not have to leave the area.

Operating rooms vary in size depending on the amount of equipment needed for each particular type of operation, with open-heart surgery operating rooms usually being the largest. Supplies and furniture are limited to prevent dust collection and are usually made of stainless steel to withstand corrosive disinfectants. Furniture and equipment are easily movable on wheels. In addition to general illumination from ceiling lights, the operative site is illuminated by overhead operating lights. Figure 16-7 shows a typical operating room. The temperature of the room can be adjusted but usually is maintained at a cool 66°F to 68°F. This range provides comfort for the surgical team (the members of which are wearing gowns, gloves, and masks under hot lights), and for the client (who is beneath layers of sterile drapes). This atmospheric temperature also provides an unfavorable environment for bacterial incubation and growth.

The client entering the operating room is confronted with an environment that is most likely unfamiliar. The operating room is cold. The surgical team members dress in characteristic surgical scrubs, and have their hair covered by caps and their faces covered by surgical masks, making them appear impersonal and distant. Furthermore, the sounds of equipment being prepared can be unfamiliar and alarming. Finally, the terminology used in conversations among OR personnel may be foreign. These elements in combination with the sight of ominous overhead lights and the feel of the hard operating room table may serve to increase the client's fear, anxiety, and feelings of powerlessness.

Members of the Surgical Team

The surgical team is a group of hospital personnel assigned to successfully see a client through an operative procedure. At no other time during hospitalization will the ratio of personnel to client be higher than when the client is undergoing surgery. The surgical team includes **sterile** (without microorganisms) team members: the surgeon, the **first assistant** (a physician or RN who assists the surgeon in performing hemostasis, tissue

Figure 16-6 Sample Preoperative Checklist (*Courtesy Spohn Health System, Corpus Christi, TX*)

Figure 16-7 A Typical Operating Room and Proper Surgical Attire (*Photo courtesy of the U.S. Army*)

retraction, and wound closure), and the **scrub nurse** (an LP/VN, RN, or surgical technologist who, under the direction of the circulating nurse, prepares and

maintains the integrity, safety, and efficiency of the sterile field throughout the operation). Sterile team members scrub their arms and hands, don sterile gowns and gloves, and then perform their duties in the sterile field. The **sterile field** is that area surrounding the client and the surgical site that is free from all microorganisms. It is created by using sterile drapes to drape the work area and the client. Nonsterile team members include the anesthesia provider (an anesthesiologist or anesthetist) and **circulating nurse** (an RN responsible for management of personnel, equipment, supplies, environment, and communication throughout a surgical procedure). The nonsterile team members perform their duties outside of the sterile field. Each team member has a clearly defined role and duties. Clear communication among team members and coordination of their activities improve the chances of the most favorable outcome for the client. Table 16–5 provides descriptions of surgical team members and their duties.

Table 16–5 MEMBERS OF THE SURGICAL TEAM: QUALIFICATIONS AND RESPONSIBILITIES

TYPE OF TEAM MEMBER	NAME OF TEAM MEMBER	TYPICAL QUALIFICATIONS AND RESPONSIBILITIES
Sterile team members	Surgeon	• May be a doctor of medicine (MD) or osteopathy (DO); oral surgeon; or podiatrist who is specially trained and qualified • Has completed a residency program approved by the American Board of Surgery and may or may not be board certified • Identifies need for surgery • Determines and plans appropriate treatment • Discusses surgical risks, benefits, possible complications, and treatment alternatives with the client • Obtains informed consent • Performs the surgery
	First assistant	• May be an associate physician in practice, referring physician, or surgical resident • May be a registered nurse first assistant (RNFA) who has been approved by the Association of Operating Room Nurses (AORN) and endorsed by the American College of Surgeons • Assists the surgeon • Retracts tissue and aids in the removal of blood and fluids at the operative site • Assists with hemostasis and wound closure
	Second or third assistants	• May be a qualified registered nurse, licensed practical/vocational nurse, or surgical technologist who is qualified by way of training or experience • Usually holds retractors
	Scrub nurse	• May be a registered nurse, licensed practical/vocational nurse, or surgical technologist • Provides services under the direction of the circulating nurse • Opens sterile supplies • Assists in gowning and gloving other sterile team members • Prepares instrument tables • Maintains integrity, safety, and efficiency of sterile field • Assists with sterile draping of client's operative site • Passes instruments, sutures, and the like to the surgeon • Performs instrument, sponge, and sharp counts • Aids in cleaning room after procedure

continues

Table 16–5 *continued*		
TYPE OF TEAM MEMBER	**NAME OF TEAM MEMBER**	**TYPICAL QUALIFICATIONS AND RESPONSIBILITIES**
Nonsterile team members	Anesthesiologist or anesthetist	• Anesthesiologist: may be a doctor of medicine (MD) who has completed a 2-year residency in anesthesia and is preferably board certified by the American Board of Anesthesiology; may also be a doctor of osteopathy (DO) who specializes in anesthesia • Anesthetist: may be a qualified registered nurse, a dentist, or an MD who administers anesthetics • Certified registered nurse anesthetist (CRNA): a registered nurse with critical care nursing experience who has completed an accredited program of nurse anesthesia and has passed a certifying examination • Assesses client during a preoperative visit • Chooses, induces, and maintains anesthesia • Monitors oxygenation and gas exchange • Manages untoward effects of anesthesia during surgery and postoperatively • Monitors and maintains fluid and electrolyte balance
	Circulating nurse	• Always a registered nurse • Responsible and accountable for all activities during a surgical procedure • Manages personnel, equipment, supplies, the environment, and communication throughout the operation • Arranges furniture and equipment in room • Opens sterile supplies • Ties gowns of sterile team members • Attends to needs and supplies of sterile team members • Identifies and assesses client • Brings client to operating room and transfers to operating room table • Applies and assists in insertion of monitoring devices • Assists anesthesiologist in the induction of anesthesia • Positions client for surgery • Performs designated surgical skin preparation • Assists with sterile draping and setup of sterile field around operative site • Monitors sterile technique of surgical team • Collects, labels, and distributes specimens • Completes intraoperative record • Monitors blood and fluid loss • Counts sponges, instruments, and sharps with scrub nurse and reports results to surgeon • Communicates with surgical team members and others such as client's family, pathologist • Applies dressings • Assists in transferring client to cart and, possibly, in transporting client to postanesthesia care unit • Aids in cleaning room after procedure

Asepsis

Prevention of infection is the responsibility of the entire surgical team. The environment of the surgical client contains both pathogenic (disease producing) and nonpathogenic microorganisms. When the skin, a prime barrier to infection, is broken, as during surgery, the susceptibility of the client to a bacterial invasion increases. Bacteria carried by dust or nose and throat droplets are easily transported by air currents. When unnecessary activity occurs in the room, such as when a team member pulls off his mask for any reason, the environment of the operating room is affected, and a wound can easily be invaded by undesirable microorganisms.

Asepsis is the absence of pathogenic microorganisms. **Aseptic technique** is a collection of principles used to control and/or prevent the transfer of pathogenic microorganisms from sources within (endogenous) and outside (exogenous) the client. For example, scrubbed persons wear sterile gowns and gloves; sterile drapes are used to create a sterile field; items used in a sterile field are sterilized; and those working within a sterile field maintain the integrity of the sterile field. Aseptic technique is applicable to other nursing functions such as changing dressings, inserting a foley catheter, or preparing for an obstetrical delivery. Thus, the practice of aseptic technique is not confined to the OR, but applies to other clinical nursing units and other procedures as well.

The practice of aseptic technique requires the development of **sterile conscience**, an individual's personal sense of honesty and integrity with regard to adherence to the principles of aseptic technique. Aseptic technique must be strictly followed. Doing so requires constant assessment and monitoring of self and others. It is sometimes easier or less expensive for surgical team members to overlook an infraction of aseptic technique rather than to correct that infraction. This must *never* be allowed. Compromising the principles of aseptic technique may increase the likelihood of infection and, thus, harm to the client.

Surgical Hand Scrub

An item is considered sterile when all microorganisms are removed. The skin, however, cannot be sterilized. For this reason, the sterile team members wear gloves as barriers between the sterile field and the skin. Because accidental tearing or puncturing of the surgical glove and resultant introduction of microorganisms into the surgical wound are possible, however, the sterile team members must take measures to lower the number of microorganisms on their hands and arms. The surgical hand scrub, performed before gowning and gloving, removes soil and transient (not always present and easily removed) microorganisms from the hands and forearms. The antimicrobial soap used lowers the count of resident (almost always present and not easily removed) microorganisms and continues to prevent sudden bacterial rebound or regrowth after the scrub is completed. The surgical scrub thus reduces the possibility of transmission of microorganisms from the surgical team to the client.

Watches, rings, and bracelets are removed before the surgical hand scrub. Fingernails must be short, clean, and healthy. Artificial nails cannot be worn, although unchipped fingernail polish that has been applied within the last 4 days may be worn (AORN, 1995b). The hands and forearms should be free of breaks in skin integrity.

To perform the surgical scrub, an antimicrobial soap, usually iodophor or chlorhexidine, is applied to moistened hands and arms, making a lather. The subungual (under the nails) areas are cleaned first. A sterile brush with the same antimicrobial soap is then used to scrub all four sides of each finger, the hands, and the forearms for a minimum of 5 minutes or for the time designated by the institutional policy. Hands are always held higher than the elbows, allowing the fluid to run from the cleanest area (the fingers and hands) to the dirtiest area (the forearms and elbows).

Surgical Skin Preparation

Like the skin of the surgical team members, the skin surface at the client's incision site also cannot be sterilized. As with the surgical hand scrub, the goal of surgical skin preparation at the client's incision site is to lower the number of microorganisms on and near the incision site, thereby reducing the possibility of postoperative wound infections from microorganisms on the client's own skin. Surgical skin preparation removes soil and transient microorganisms from the incision site. The antimicrobial soap used lowers the count of resident microorganisms and continues to prevent sudden bacterial rebound after the scrub is completed.

Typically, the client is asked to shower or to wash the operative site either before arriving at the surgical facility or immediately prior to surgery. The client is then transferred to the operating room. After general anesthesia induction or regional block completion or before local infiltration of the operative site, the circulating nurse performs the surgical skin preparation. Using aseptic technique, the circulating nurse scrubs the area with an antimicrobial soap. Typically the soap used is povidone iodine (containing iodine) or chlorhexidine, thus, potential allergies to iodine must be verified. The circulating nurse scrubs a generous area surrounding the operative site to allow for extension of the surgical incision if the need arises. The scrub is completed in an ever-widening circular motion from the incision site, which is considered clean, to the periphery, which is considered dirty (Figure 16-8). Once the periphery is reached, the same sponge is never brought back toward the center of the area. The concept of cleansing from the center (incision site) to the periphery also applies to skin preparation for other procedures such as intravenous (IV) insertion, chest tube

Operative site

Figure 16-8 Skin Preparation at Operative Site

insertion, thoracentesis, or subclavian catheter placement. Surgical skin preparation lasts 5 to 10 minutes. After the scrub is completed, the area is blotted dry with sterile towels. An antiseptic solution, often also iodine based, is then applied in the same manner.

Intraoperative Nursing Care

The success of nursing care in the operating room is measured by client outcomes. The AORN has established client outcome standards for evaluating perioperative clients upon completion of surgery. These outcomes state that the client is to be free from infection and injury related to positioning, foreign objects, or chemical, physical, and electrical hazards. In addition, skin integrity and fluid and electrolyte balance are to be maintained. Consequently, nursing care in the operating room strives to provide these standards to all clients undergoing surgery.

Although the responsibilities of the circulating nurse and scrub nurse may seem to be a series of tasks or duties, these same tasks and duties provide quality nursing care to the client. The nurse planning for surgery is involved in selection of equipment and supplies, room preparation, and formation of the sterile field prior to the delivery of actual nursing care. There are six areas of risk that nurses are responsible for managing.

1. *Clients undergoing surgery are at Risk for Infection related to the invasive procedure undertaken and the exposure to pathogens from the environment, personnel, and client.* Some clients are at a higher risk for developing nosocomial infections. Clients undergoing surgery lasting longer than 2 hours or surgeries of the abdomen or thorax are more prone to infection. Poor nutritional status, the presence of an underlying disease process, obesity, and smoking or substance abuse also place a client at higher risk for infection. In addition, the very young (under 1 year of age) and those who are elderly (over 65 years of age) are at increased risk. Regardless of risk factors, nursing care for all clients requires strict aseptic technique to prevent nosocomial surgical wound infections.

2. *Clients undergoing surgery are at Risk for Injury related to positioning during surgery.* Positional injuries may include postural hypotension, pressure alopecia, lower back or neck pain, facial and airway edema, eye abrasion, ear compression, joint damage, and nerve injury to the brachial plexus, suprascapular nerve, subclavian neurovascular bundle, axillary neurovascular bundle, or peroneal, radial, or ulnar nerve. The client's position during surgery is usually determined by the surgical approach, the surgeon's preference, and individual considerations. The ideal surgical position

does not interfere with respiration and circulation, and should not cause pressure on any nerve. Proper positioning provides access to the operative site and allows easy access for the administration of anesthesia. Proper body alignment to prevent postoperative discomfort is maintained as much as possible.

Because positioning usually occurs after initiation of anesthesia, the client is never moved without the anesthesia provider's guidance. The circulating nurse ensures availability of positioning devices and adequate personnel for lifting or turning.

3. *The client is at Risk for Injury related to retention of foreign objects inadvertently left in the wound.* The placement of some foreign objects is deliberate and recorded. For example, vascular replacement grafts or orthopedic implants are designed to be left in the surgical wound as part of the surgical procedure. A wound occasionally may be packed with gauze or sponges for a physiological purpose such as hemostasis. Retention of a foreign object inadvertently left in the wound, however, constitutes a significant risk. Nursing interventions to prevent this type of injury include using only x-ray detectable sponges on the operative field and counting sponges, instruments, and sharps according to institutional policy. The circulating nurse both reports the results of the various counts to the surgeon and documents the counts on the operative record.

4. *The client undergoing surgery is at Risk for Injury related to chemical, physical, and electrical hazards.* Clients are exposed to numerous chemicals used to clean the environment, prepare the skin, and sterilize instruments. Because anesthetized clients do not have the reflexes to protect themselves, bodily injury is more likely to occur during positioning, transfers, or falls. Physical hazards may also include the use of both ionizing (x-ray) and nonionizing (laser) radiation, when the surgical procedure warrants their use. The majority of equipment used during surgery requires electricity, thus exposing the client to electrical hazards. A frequently used piece of equipment is the electrical surgical unit (ESU), or cautery, which stops bleeding through electrical coagulation of blood vessels.

Safety: Electrical Equipment
- Electrical equipment must be plugged into grounded outlets.
- Electrical equipment must be regularly checked by a bioelectronic technician.
- A grounding pad must be placed under the client and in direct contact with the client's skin.

Nursing care focuses on minimizing and documenting the exposure to these hazards. Skin integrity is assessed prior to and after completion of the surgical procedure. Allergies to antimicrobial soaps are verified. Pooling of preparation solutions beneath the client is prevented. Institutional protocols are followed for radiation and laser safety. In addition, after surgery the area around the dressing site is cleansed to remove any residual antibacterial soap and antiseptic solution. Equipment is set up, checked prior to use, and operated according to the manufacturers' recommendations.

5. *The client undergoing surgery is at Risk for Impaired Tissue Integrity related to positioning, electrical hazards, and chemical hazards.* Nursing actions are geared toward ensuring no bruising, areas of skin breakdown, reddened areas, discolored skin, open skin lesions, excoriation, or itching after surgery. Nursing care to prevent skin breakdown is similar to that prevent injury related to positioning and chemical, physical, or electrical hazards.

6. *The client undergoing surgery is at Risk for Deficient Fluid Volume related to abnormal blood loss and NPO status.* The goal of nursing care is to maintain fluid and electrolyte balance. Application of hemodynamic monitoring devices by the circulating nurse and anesthesia provider allows the physiologic monitoring of fluid and electrolyte parameters. Intravenous patency is protected and maintained. Nursing care is aimed at monitoring and replacing fluid loss. The circulating nurse accomplishes this by assisting the anesthesia provider in estimating blood loss as evidenced in sponges and suctioning and monitoring urine output. Intravenous fluids and blood products are administered according to the anesthesia provider's instructions. Fluid and electrolyte values and vital signs should be consistent with preoperative measurements.

After completion of surgery, the circulating nurse applies and secures the dressing. When the anesthesia provider is ready, the client is transferred to a stretcher or a gurney. The unconscious or semiconscious client is placed in a side-lying or semiprone position unless contraindicated by the surgical procedure. If the client is supine, the client's head is turned to the side in case the client vomits. The client is then taken to the PACU, accompanied by the anesthesia provider and another surgical team member.

POSTOPERATIVE PHASE

The **postoperative phase** is the time during the surgical experience that begins with the end of the surgical procedure and lasts until the client is discharged not just from the hospital or institution, but from medical care by the surgeon. Upon transfer from the operating room, the client usually goes to the PACU (Figure 16-9). All clients who receive general anesthesia, spinal anesthesia, or regional anesthesia are admitted to the PACU. Occasionally, clients who have undergone surgery with local anesthesia or no anesthesia or who have received only IV sedation are placed in the PACU for a short period to be monitored closely until their conditions stabilize. The PACU is usually located next to the operating room. Typically, it is one large room with individual units for clients along the perimeter of the room. Each of these units has an oxygen delivery system, suction, various other supplies, and cardiac, respiratory, and blood pressure monitoring devices. Curtains can be pulled to provide privacy if needed, but an open view allows continual assessment of all clients.

Postoperative Nursing Care

The postanesthesia care nurse is an RN specially trained in caring for immediate postoperative clients. The goal of postanesthesia nursing care is to promote recovery from anesthesia and the immediate effects of surgery. The postanesthesia nurse has knowledge and skill in recognizing and treating anesthetic and surgical complications very quickly. The postanesthesia nurse is empathetic and is able to assess and manage pain for the client who may not be able to express himself.

Upon the client's arrival in the PACU, the anesthesia provider verbally reviews the client's anesthesia and operative procedure with the postanesthesia nurse. The postanesthesia nurse begins the following nursing assessment and care in the immediate postoperative period:

- Time of arrival in recovery room
- Patency of airway
- Respirations

Figure 16-9 Postanesthesia Care Unit (PACU)

- Presence of artificial airway devices
  Oral airway
  Nasopharyngeal airway
  Endotracheal airway
- Oxygen saturation
- Need for supplemental oxygen
  Mode of administration
  Flow rate
- Breath sounds
- Color of skin, nail beds, and lips
- Presence of cardiac dysrhythmias
- Other vital signs
  Blood pressure, pulse
- Skin condition (moist or dry, warm or cool) and skin temperature
- Initiate Aldrete Score
- Intravenous infusion
  Type of solution
  Amount in bottle or bag
  Flow rate
  Appearance and location of IV site
- Dressings
  Amount and character of drainage
- Drains and tubes
  Intactness and function
  Connection to drainage and/or suction
  Amount and character of drainage
- Level of consciousness
- Activity level
- Other assessments according to surgical procedure
- Pain

The postanesthesia nurse notes the client's arrival time to the unit and immediately begins to assess the patency of the airway by placing a hand above the client's nose and mouth to feel exhalation. The quality and quantity of respirations are then immediately observed, as is the presence of an artificial airway. The client is attached to a pulse oximeter, and breath sounds are auscultated. The color and condition of the skin are noted as part of the respiratory assessment. Peripheral cyanosis may be an indication of hypothermia rather than respiratory distress. Thus, correlating with the "A-B-Cs" of *a*irway, *b*reathing, and *c*irculation, the respiratory system is assessed first.

Because the vast majority of clients admitted are in an unconscious state and have received muscle relaxants during surgery, respiratory exchange is often affected. Snoring, stridor, labored chest movement, sternal retractions, cyanosis, and apnea are all signs of respiratory distress. Respiratory distress is the gravest of all complications because respiratory crisis and subsequent death can occur in a matter of minutes if distress is not observed and treated quickly. In the event of any signs of respiratory distress, the postanesthesia nurse must be alert to the possibility of respiratory arrest and be ready to initiate cardiopulmonary resuscitation. There

are seven areas of risk that postoperative nurses are responsible for managing:

1. *The postoperative client is at Risk for Ineffective Airway Clearance.* Respiratory complications can occur with any anesthetized client. Often airway obstruction occurs from the tongue falling backward over the pharynx. Nursing interventions include manually lifting the jaw forward to raise the tongue from the pharynx and open the airway (Figure 16-10). Because of airway obstruction, clients will often arrive in the PACU with an artificial airway inserted (Figure 16-11).

   Laryngospasm is the spastic contraction of the larynx that effectively causes airway obstruction. It is often caused by larynx irritation from the ET tube or may be a side effect of some anesthetic gases. Laryngospasm is most likely to occur after removal of the ET tube and when the client develops an acute inspiratory stridor with sternal retractions. The postanesthesia nurse starts oxygen via a mask, reassures the client, and immediately notifies the anesthesia provider.

2. *The postoperative client is at Risk for Ineffective Breathing Pattern.* Hypoventilation is most likely due to the depressant effects of anesthesia. In hypoventilation, oxygen and carbon dioxide are not exchanging adequately in the alveoli of the lung. Additional oxygen is provided to the client, as needed, through the oral airway or a nasal catheter or mask, if indicated. The client's oxygen saturation is monitored via a pulse oximeter (Figure 16-12). It is desirable to maintain oxygen satu-

A.

B.

Figure 16-10 A. An Obstructed Airway (tongue against pharynx); B. Manual Jaw Lift (anterior displacement) ration above 90%, with the aid of additional oxygen, if necessary. Pallor, hypotension, tachycardia, and respiratory distress are other indications for oxygen administration. Oxygen may be provided prophylactically to clients who have undergone prolonged or traumatic surgery.

3. *The postoperative client is at Risk for Aspiration.* With certain anesthesias, the client temporarily loses the gag and cough reflexes necessary to protect the lungs, increasing the risk of aspiration of stomach contents, oral secretions, bloody secretions, and foreign bodies into the lungs. Aspiration later causes pneumonia and atelectasis. The post-anesthesia nurse intervenes by having suction ready and using it frequently to prevent aspiration. Anti-

emetics are given as needed to prevent nausea and vomiting. Coughing and deep breathing are initiated as soon as the client is able to follow directions. If not contraindicated, the client may be positioned on the side to prevent aspiration. When the client must be supine, the head is turned to the side so that any secretions will drain out of the mouth.

4. *The postoperative client is at Risk for Decreased Cardiac Output.* The cardiovascular system is assessed next, according to the A-B-Cs of airway, breathing, and circulation. The client is attached to an EKG monitor. Then blood pressure and pulse are taken and, along with respirations, are reported to the anesthesia provider, if still present in the PACU. If a client does not already have a skin thermometer or other means of obtaining temperature, one is applied and the temperature noted. Skin condition is observed for the presence of diaphoresis. The initial Aldrete Score is then determined.

The **Aldrete Score**, also known as the Post-anesthetic Recovery Score, is used in PACUs to objectively assess the physical status of clients recovering from anesthesia, and serves as a basis for discharge from the PACU (Table 16–6). The Aldrete Score was recently adapted to also assess the readiness of clients for discharge from ambulatory surgery. The first five indexes are used for discharge from the PACU. Clients are assessed at the time of admission to the PACU and every 15 minutes until discharge. The first five indexes include assessing activity, respiration, consciousness, circulation, and color (oxygen saturation). Each of the five indexes is scored from 0 to 2, according to the degree of functional disturbance. The score is expressed as a total score, with 10 being the maximum. Typically, a minimum score of 8 is required for discharge from the PACU.

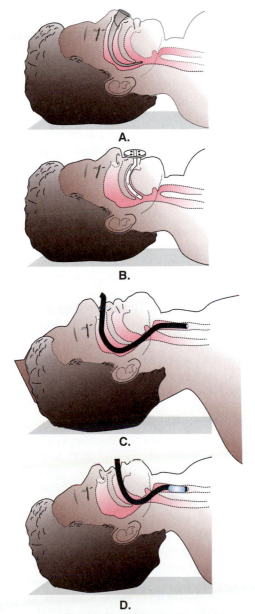

Figure 16-11 Four Types of Artificial Airways: A. Nasal trumpet; B. Oral airway; C. Nasal endotracheal tube; and D. Oral endotracheal tube with cuff inflated

Figure 16-12 Client with Pulse Oximeter on Finger

Table 16–6 ALDRETE SCORE/ POSTANESTHETIC RECOVERY SCORE

Activity	Able to move 4 extremities voluntarily or on command	2
	Able to move 2 extremities voluntarily or on command	1
	Able to move 0 extremities voluntarily or on command	0
Respiration	Able to breathe deeply and cough freely	2
	Dyspnea or limited breathing	1
	Apneic	0
Conscious-ness	Fully awake	2
	Arousable on calling	1
	Not responding	0
Circulation	B/P ± 20% of preanesthetic level	2
	B/P ± 20% to 50% of preanesthetic level	1
	B/P ± 50% of preanesthetic level	0
Color	Normal	2
	Pale, dusky, blotchy, jaundiced, other	1
	Cyanotic	0

Additional Assessments: Aldrete Score/Postanesthetic Recovery Score for Clients Having Anesthesia on an Ambulatory Basis

Dressing	Dry and clean	2
	Wet but stationary or marked	1
	Growing area of wetness	0
Pain	Pain free	2
	Mild pain handled by oral medication	1
	Severe pain requiring parenteral medication	0
Ambulation	Able to stand up and walk straight	2
	Vertigo when erect	1
	Dizziness when supine	0
Fasting/ feeding	Able to drink fluids	2
	Nauseated	1
	Nausea and vomiting	0
Urine output	Has voided	2
	Unable to void but comfortable	1
	Unable to void and uncomfortable	0

Courtesy J. Antonio Aldrete, M.D., M.S., Defuniak Springs, FL.

As complete as the Aldrete Score may seem, it does not consider some problems that may warrant either continued stay in the PACU or admission to a critical care unit. Cardiac dysrhythmias that do not affect blood pressure, bleeding at the incision site, uncontrollable severe pain, and persistent nausea and vomiting may be present even if the client has an Aldrete Score of 10. Any such problems indicate a need to stay in the PACU or to be transferred to a critical care unit until the problem is resolved.

Hypotension is frequently encountered during the immediate postoperative period. Hypotension can be caused by blood loss, residual effects of anesthesia, narcotics or tranquilizers, position changes, and even pain. If hypotension is due to the residual effects of anesthesia, the effects are usually mild, and the client's blood pressure gradually returns to the preoperative level. Narcotics may potentiate the effects of residual anesthesia and may contribute to hypotension. Sympathetic nerve blockages in the spinal cord that occur during spinal and epidural blocks may result in arterial dilation and decreased venous return, producing hypotension. Whereas mild to moderate pain may cause an increase in blood pressure, severe pain may cause hypotension resulting from the release of norepinephrine, which, in turn, decreases heart rate and cardiac output. Hypotension may even have existed preoperatively.

The cardiovascular assessment includes comparing the present blood pressure to the preoperative blood pressure and to the blood pressures during surgery. In addition to reduced blood pressure, the postanesthesia nurse assesses other symptoms of hypotension, such as pallor, clammy skin, diaphoresis, rapid weak pulse, rapid shallow respirations, and restlessness. An imperceptible blood pressure and weak pulse are reported to the surgeon and anesthesia provider immediately. Oxygen is begun, the intravenous rate is increased, and the client is placed in the Trendelenburg position while evidence of bleeding is sought. If blood pressure is low but all other signs are normal, the client is watched closely until the client has a chance to awaken; he may be merely depressed from anesthesia. If pulse is slow (under 50 and not comparable to the preoperative range) or irregular but other signs are normal, the anesthesia provider should be notified. Again, in the event of cardiac arrest, the postanesthesia nurse is ready to initiate cardiopulmonary resuscitation.

5. *The postoperative client is at risk for Deficient Fluid Volume.* Blood loss usually ranges from 100 mL to 500 mL in an average surgery. Blood transfusions are usually not given unless more than one unit of blood is needed and blood loss is greater than 500

mL. Hypovolemic shock usually does not occur until the client has lost more than 1.5 L to 2.0 L of blood, or 20% to 25% of the blood volume (Lewis, Collier, & Heitkemper 1996).

Fluid intake and output are assessed. The amounts and types of IV solutions hanging are identified, as are any added medications. The IV fluids are infused according to the surgeon's order and are run at a specified rate. The IV site is assessed for patency, redness, and swelling. The client is restrained as necessary to maintain patency of the IV site. All other infusions and irrigations are also assessed.

The postanesthesia nurse checks dressings and/or peripads for any evidence of bloody drainage and notes the amount so that any subsequent appearance of blood may be accurately evaluated. All drainage tubes are then connected, and the type of drain and the drainage amount are recorded according to physicians' orders. Table 16–7 outlines common types of drains placed in surgery. Urinary output is also monitored. Scanty urinary drainage (less than 50 cc/hour or as ordered) is noted and reported to the surgeon.

Surgical drains are placed so that the wound can drain freely of blood clots, body fluids, pus, and necrotic material that otherwise would collect in the wound and provide a rich medium for bacterial growth. Figure 16-13 illustrates common drainage devices. All drains are inserted at the operative site and exit through the incision or a separate stab wound adjacent to the incision. The type of drain is chosen according to the location of wound, size of wound, and type of drainage anticipated. The use of drains decreases pain and infection while aiding wound healing. However, if the wound is draining, the skin is not closed, and a pathway exists for the entrance of microorganisms. Drain sites can thus also be a source of infection.

Potential complications of drains include hemorrhage, sepsis, drain loss, and bowel herniation. Thus, nursing care of all drains includes assessing the color, character, and odor of drainage, ensuring the patency of the drain (making sure there are no kinks in the tubing), and ensuring that the drain does not accidentally become dislodged. Table 16–8 lists additional nursing care according to surgical procedure.

Hypertension may also be assessed in the postoperative period. Because the client may have preexisting hypertension, blood pressure is compared to the client's normal and admitting blood pressure. Hypertension can be due to pain, the anesthesia or medication used, or restlessness or apprehension. Increased intracranial pressure, increased or rapid fluid intake, hypoxia, and fighting the artificial airway may also increase blood pressure. The postanesthesia nurse uses judgment and then proceeds to treat the probable cause by medicating for pain, slowing the IV rate, removing the artificial airway, administering oxygen, or raising the head of the bed. If these measures fail or if blood pressure is dangerously high, the surgeon or anesthesia provider is notified.

6. *The postoperative client is at Risk for Disturbed Sensory/Perception.* The next system to be assessed, therefore, is the neurological system. In the Aldrete Score, level of consciousness and activity level are assessed. With regard to level of consciousness, the client is typically labeled as able to answer questions clearly, demonstrates arousal only when called, or unresponsive to verbal stimulation. The neurological assessment does not include orientation to person, place, and time. A surgical client is usually oriented to person. Due to the amnesic effects of some medications, however, the client may be oriented to the facility yet may not be oriented to the specific area of the facility even after being told. Because the postoperative client loses the ability to track time while undergoing some types of anesthesia and has no way of knowing how long the surgical procedure has taken, the client may be oriented to year and month but is rarely oriented to the specific time of the day. For these reasons, assessing orientation to person, place, and time is not part of the neurological assessment. Level of consciousness affects the ability to breathe, maintain oxygen saturation without assistance, and move on command.

Part of the neurological assessment involves assessing the activity level, or the ability to move extremities voluntarily. The ability to move extremities on command indicates voluntary movement. Hearing is the first sensation to return to the client after having been anesthetized. Clients in the PACU are asked to squeeze the postanesthesia

A. B.

C.

Figure 16-13 Common Drainage Devices: A. Penrose drains; B. Hemovac; C. Jackson-Pratt

Table 16–7 DESCRIPTION, USES, AND NURSING CARE OF COMMON DRAINAGE DEVICES PLACED DURING SURGERY

TYPE	EXAMPLE	DESCRIPTION	USES	NURSING CARE
Passive	Penrose	A single-lumen, soft latex tube that works with gravity directly from the surgical incision	To remove drainage when more than a minimal amount of drainage is expected	• Inspect dressing • Check underneath client to ensure drainage has not leaked from the side of the dressing • Always keep a dressing over drain • Check safety pin through end of drain
	T-tube	A single-lumen tube shaped like a T and made of latex	Used after common bile duct exploration to drain bile from the duct as suture lines heal and swelling decreases	• Attach to a drainage bottle or to a T-tube bag
Active	Hemovac Jackson Pratt J-Vac Relia Vac Surgivac	Closed wound drainage system with drain and reservoir having self-suction when reservoir is compressed	Used after multiple types of procedures; provides continuous gentle suction of the operative site to increase drainage of serosanguinous fluid and collapse tissue to facilitate healing	• Assess the drainage system as appropriate to client's condition for: 1. Continued drainage 2. Maintained decompression 3. Air-tight tubings 4. Need for emptying • To reactivate suction, wash hands and wear gloves and eye/face protection • Empty reservoirs every 8 hours, when drainage nears the full line, or as ordered by the physician
Passive or active	Davol Sump Axiom Sump	Large, multilumen tube with a larger main port for drainage and/or suction and with smaller side port(s) for irrigation and/or air venting to help prevent tissue from being suctioned against catheter and damaged	To drain intra-abdominal fluids from abscesses, cysts, or hematomas	• Use one of the smaller or sump ports for continuous irrigation • Calculate intake and output carefully with irrigations • Place impervious pads underneath client • Change dressings frequently when saturated • Attach to catheter drainage bag if not attached to suction • Do not plug sump ports
	Chest tube ThoraKlex Pleure Vac	Large single-lumen drain attached to closed water-seal drainage system	To drain fluid or air from pleural cavity	• Assess breath sounds and respirations, including depth, rate, symmetry of chest expansion, color of mucous membranes, and presence of crepitus with suction off or tubing clamped • If present, assess amount and type of suction • Ensure that connections are tight and sealed with tape • Keep chest tube drainage reservoir lower than client's chest • Observe for air leaks in air leak indicator or drainage chamber of drainage reservoir • Place petroleum jelly gauze nearby for quick access should the tube become dislodged • Measure drainage at least every 8 hours (more frequently if in a critical care unit or client's condition warrants it) • Clamp or milk the chest tube only if ordered by surgeon • Notify surgeon if drainage is greater than 100 cc/hour • Change drainage system when ⅔ full

Table 16-8 ADDITIONAL NURSING CARE ACCORDING TO CLASSIFICATION OR TYPE OF SURGICAL PROCEDURE

CLASSIFICATION OR TYPE OF SURGICAL PROCEDURE	NURSING CARE
Orthopedic	• Expose wet casts to the air. • Check surgeon's orders for positioning of client; operated extremities typically are elevated. • Check for digital warmth, color, mobility, circulaton (pulses), and sensation in affected extremity.
Urologic	• Attach all catheters to drainage. • Closely monitor continuous irrigation to ensure that flow in and flow out are equal; if obstructed, the bladder could rupture. • Increase or decrease irrigation flow rate according to amount of bleeding. • Assess for chills or elevated pulse, possibly indicative of hemolysis or bacterial infection. • Assess abdomen for signs of distension and rigidity and report, especially if client complains.
Oral	• Suction frequently and carefully around sutures. • Observe breathing; ensure that drainage or packing does not obstruct airway. • Apply ice bag, when ordered. • Remove dental packs as ordered and assess every 15 minutes for further bleeding.
Eye, ears, nose, & throat (EENT)	*Eye surgery* • Assess for facial paralysis • Minimize head movement, coughing, vomiting, and restlessness. *Ear surgery* • Assess edema and tracheal patency (listening for stridor and observing for restlessness). *Nose surgery* • Maintain open airway; suction orally; and apply ice. *Tonsillectomy* • Place on side to facilitate drainage: elevate head of bed; have suction available; and observe closely for bleeding, vomiting, and obstruction.
Neurologic	• Assess level of consciousness; be alert to drowsiness, slurred speech, disorientation, or irritability that differs from that exhibited in the preoperative state. • Observe for pupil changes: inequality, constriction, and nonreactivity to light. • Assess for respiratory changes such as snoring, retraction of cheeks and trachea, shallowness, and slowed rate. • Monitor blood pressure and pulse; an elevated blood pressure coupled with a lowered pulse leads to shock. • Observe extremity movement for weakness, paralysis, and rigidity; observe for unilateral drooping of facial features. • Use caution when medicating. *Laminectomy or discectomy* • Move only as ordered. • Assess sensation, circulation, and motion of extremities distal to incision site. *Craniotomy* • Position as ordered. • Complete a neurological check. • Use Trendelenburg position only with permission of the surgeon.
Vascular (all grafts, carotid endarterectomy, femoral-popliteal bypass)	• Assess color, sensation, warmth, and mobility of extremity. • Observe presence and strength of pedal and post-tibial pulses. • Complete a neurological check for carotid endarterectomy. • Frequently check all dressings and the area directly beneath the client.
Thoracic	• Closely observe chest tube for patency, amount of bleeding, and air leaks. Tape all connections. Mark drainage container upon client's admission and discharge. Assess fluctuation of drainage in tubing. Attach suction as ordered. • Observe respirations closely with regard to color change, restlessness, apprehension, dyspnea, or mediastinal shift.

continues

CLASSIFICATION OR TYPE OF SURGICAL PROCEDURE	NURSING CARE
	• Elevate head of bed 30°, unless contraindicated.
	• Encourage coughing and deep breathing.
	• Use caution in administering narcotics, especially morphine sulfate, as client cannot afford respiratory depression.
Pneumonectomy	• Do not turn on nonoperative side. Alternately turn from back to operated side.
Lobectomy and resection	• May turn client to either side.
Gynecologic	• Assess vaginal drainage.

Table 16–8 *continued*

nurse's hands and to plantarflex and dorsiflex the feet. Due to a regional block or previous condition, however, the client may be unable to move more than two extremities.

7. *The postoperative client is at Risk for Injury and for Disturbed Thought Processes.* Some clients are in a state of delirium, wherein uncontrollable physical movements occur. Thus, all clients are restrained: The side rails are put up, the stretcher safety strap is applied across the torso, and the stretcher wheel brakes are locked. Clients showing signs of restlessness may need additional physical restraint. Safety is the utmost concern, but when placing restraints, the postanesthesia nurse must first determine that the restlessness is related to the state of anesthesia rather than pain or anoxia.

Continuing Nursing Care in the PACU

After the client has been admitted and assessed in PACU, the postanesthesia nurse checks the surgeon's and the anesthesia provider's orders and initiates any therapy designated for the PACU. All stat IV or intramuscular (IM) medications are given, and inhalation therapy and specific equipment are initiated as ordered. The clinical unit is notified of any specialized equipment that will be needed in the client's room.

Narcotics are given in the PACU in reduced amounts and according to the client's state of consciousness, vital signs, and the type of anesthesia administered during surgery. A typical dosage is one-half or less of a regular dose, which may be repeated in ½ hour if the client continues to experience pain. Some anesthesia providers write specific orders for the administration of narcotics during the client's stay in the PACU. Clients who are medicated typically stay in the PACU for at least ½ hour after administration of the first dose and

for 15 minutes after administration of the second dose. The postanesthesia nurse considers the client's need for medication and dosage based on the length of time it takes to arouse the client, the type of anesthetic agent used during surgery, the type of surgery performed, and the client's general condition, vital signs, and age.

The postanesthesia nurse charts on a separate nursing record for the PACU. Anything unusual must be adequately documented. If vital signs are in the normal range, the postanesthesia nurse checks them every 15 minutes. If vital signs are unstable, they are checked every 5 minutes or as often as necessary until stable. If vital signs fail to stabilize, the surgeon and anesthesia provider are notified. The surgical site is checked at least every 30 minutes. If any initial bleeding has not subsided, the surgeon is notified. Routine checks are continued until the client is discharged from the PACU.

The Aldrete Score is assessed every 15 minutes, as is skin temperature. Temperature may be checked with a thermometer if there is any question. If temperature is abnormal, the surgeon and/or anesthesia provider is notified. A significantly elevated temperature can be indicative of malignant hyperthermia, a potentially fatal complication of some anesthetics in sensitive individuals that is characterized by a hypermetabolic crisis.

The postanesthesia nurse determines whether the client meets the criteria for discharge from the PACU. Typically, the client's vital signs must be stable and within the client's normal limits. The Aldrete Score must be 8 to 10. If 7 or less, a surgeon's or anesthesia provider's order is required for discharge. Also prior to client discharge, the dressing must be checked, changed, or reinforced according to orders. All other parameters are reassessed and charted. Institutional protocol dictates minimum stay in the PACU. Adults are typically kept in the PACU for a minimum of 1 hour, except outpatients, who go to ambulatory surgery when they are awake and when postmedication time has been fulfilled. Children are typically kept in the PACU until they are awake, stable, and have an Aldrete Score of 8 to 10. When criteria for discharge are met, the postanesthesia nurse calls the clinical unit or ambulatory surgery unit and reports the client's name, vitals, surgery, and any other pertinent information. The client is then transferred to the appropriate unit.

Later Postoperative Nursing Care

Prior to the client's arrival in the clinical unit, the nurse has prepared for the client. The linen has been changed, the bed clothing folded down, and the room cleared of clutter. Special required equipment, as directed by the postanesthesia nurse, has been gathered. An emesis basin and tissue are available. The nurse is ready to assess the client in an organized manner, focusing on the body system affected by surgery.

Upon the client's arrival in the clinical unit, the nurse assists in the transfer of the client to the bed. Nursing assessment and care of the client upon admission to the clinical unit includes the following:

- Time of arrival in unit
- Transfer from cart to bed
   Place bed in lowest, locked position, with side rails up
   Place client in position of comfort, or as ordered
- Vital signs including airway assessment and breath sounds
- Color of skin, nail beds, and lips
- Skin condition (moist or dry, warm or cool)
- Level of consciousness
- Activity level
- Intravenous infusion
   Type of solution
   Amount in bottle or bag
   Flow rate
   Appearance and location of IV site
- Dressings
   Amount and character of drainage
- Drains and tubes
   Intactness and function
   Connection to drainage and/or suction
   Amount and character of drainage
- Urinary output
   Need to void or time of voiding
   Presence of patency and catheter; output/hour
- Pain
   Last dose of analgesia
   Current pain location, intensity, quality
- Compare assessment with PACU report
- Call light within reach
   Reorient client to usage
- Location of family or significant others
- Postoperative orders

A brief assessment including vital signs is completed every 15 minutes for 1 hour; every ½ hour for 2 hours; and every hour for 4 hours, or as prescribed by physician. The possibilities of postanesthetic complications continue, but as time passes, different postsurgical complications may develop; the nurse is responsible for managing these.

1. *The client is at Risk for Ineffective Airway Clearance caused by atelectasis and hypostatic pneumonia.* Respiratory complications can still occur with any anesthetized client. As in the PACU, the postoperative client is at high risk for ineffective airway clearance, ineffective breathing patterns, and aspiration. Now, however, nursing measures are directed toward preventing ineffective airway clearance caused by atelectasis and hypostatic pneumonia, both of which usually occur within the first 48 hours postoperatively. In postoperative atelectasis, the bronchioles of the lungs become plugged with mucus so that air cannot reach the alveoli. The alveoli then collapse. The client develops dyspnea, fever, tachypnea, tachycardia, and cyanosis. In postoperative hypostatic pneumonia, stagnant mucus promotes the growth of bacteria, and atelectasis then develops into a secondary infection. To prevent these complications, the client is actively encouraged by the nurse to cough, deep breathe (with and without incentive spirometry), and turn as instructed preoperatively. In addition, the client is encouraged to sit up and ambulate as soon and as often as possible. The nurse must ensure adequate pain relief measures so that mobility is well tolerated.

2. *The client is at Risk for Peripheral Neurovascular Dysfunction, Excess/deficient Fluid Volume, and Activity Intolerance.* The client continues to be at high risk for decreased cardiac output and fluid volume deficit; but as the postoperative period progresses, the client becomes at risk for additional complications. The nurse implements measures to prevent deep vein thrombosis; thrombophlebitis; pulmonary embolism; complications of fluid overload; fluid deficit; hypokalemia; and syncope.

The stress response to surgery; inactivity; pressure related to body position; obesity; and injury to pelvic veins during surgery may contribute to the formation of deep vein thrombosis, thrombophlebitis, or pulmonary embolism. These complications may appear immediately following surgery or 1 to 2 weeks later. The nurse routinely assesses for a positive Homan's sign and for warm, tender, reddened, hardened areas in the calves. To assess for Homan's sign, the client is asked to forcefully dorsiflex the foot. If pain is felt in the calf of the leg, it is considered a positive finding for Homan's sign; if no pain is felt, it is considered a negative finding. A positive finding for Homan's sign may indicate thrombophlebitis and should be reported to the surgeon. Deep vein thrombosis and thrombophlebitis may lead to a pulmonary embolus, although there may be no warning of pulmonary embolism. When pulmonary embolism occurs, the client may experience dyspnea, chest pain, cyanosis, cough, hemoptysis, tachycardia, and fever coupled with an elevated white blood cell count. If the embolism is large enough, shock may develop rapidly. Pulmonary embolism may be fatal.

To prevent the formation of deep vein thrombosis, thrombophlebitis, and pulmonary embolism, the nurse should encourage the client to ambulate to the extent that the client is able. When in bed, the client should perform postoperative leg exercises each hour. Antiembolism stockings are usually ordered, as is a sequential compression device, which is a sleeve applied to the legs to simulate walking by repetitive pumping. The sleeves and antiembolism stockings should be removed every day so that the skin can be cleansed. It is very important to note that antiembolism stockings and the sequential compression device are not substitutes for leg exercises. Leg exercises must still be performed.

When it is ordered, the nurse also administers low-dose heparin therapy to hemostatically stable clients who are more than 40 years of age and have undergone pelvic, abdominal, or thoracic surgery. Heparin is usually given subcutaneously every 12 hours until discharge. If the drug is administered at low dosage and if preoperative prothrombin time, partial thromboplastin time, and platelet count were within the normal range, no laboratory test is necessary to determine the drug's effect. This regimen is followed and ordered at the discretion of the surgeon.

The nurse measures intake and output and monitors laboratory findings (e.g., electrolytes, hematocrit, hemoglobin, and serum osmolality) and signs and symptoms of hemorrhage by assessing vital signs, skin color and condition, dressings, drains, and tubes, as in the PACU.

Clients often experience syncope when changing from a lying position to a sitting or standing position. The nurse can prevent syncope by assisting the client to change positions slowly, proceeding in steps and allowing time for the client's internal equilibrium to adjust. The nurse checks the radial pulse frequently and asks the client for subjective statements of dizziness or nausea. If syncope occurs during ambulation, the nurse can ask for assistance in obtaining a wheelchair for the client, use a nearby chair, or lower the client to the floor until the client recovers. Although frightening for the client, syncope is not physiologically threatening unless the client is injured in a fall.

3. *The client may be at Risk for Imbalanced Nutrition: Less than Body Requirements related to nausea and vomiting, hiccoughs, abdominal distension, constipation, and NPO status.* Gastrointestinal complications become more prevalent after immediate postoperative recovery. The client also may experience pain related to hiccoughs and slowed gastrointestinal function.

Nausea and vomiting are caused by anesthetic agents, narcotics, hypotension, and the manipulation of the bowel during surgery. Handling of the bowel during pelvic and abdominal surgery causes peristalsis to stop or severely slow. Bowel function normally returns 2 to 5 days following surgery. If bowel inactivity persists, a paralytic ileus may develop. As bowel function resumes, the nurse continues to assess the client for bowel sounds and, if a nasogastric tube is present, a reduction in drainage. As peristalsis returns in a discontinuous fashion, the client may experience distention along with flatulence and gas pains. After bowel sounds resume in all quadrants, the client may be removed from NPO status according to the surgeon's orders. The nurse also provides good oral hygiene when the client is designated NPO and administers antiemetics as needed for nausea and vomiting.

Hiccoughs are caused by irritation of the phrenic nerve. Impulses then cause the diaphragm to contract rhythmically and violently. Abdominal distention, gastric distention, and the presence of a nasogastric tube are common causes, but electrolyte and acid–base disturbances, intestinal obstruction, and intra-abdominal bleeding may also initiate hiccoughs. The nurse may need to notify the surgeon when hiccoughs are prolonged.

Gas pains and signs and symptoms of abdominal distention may be minimized by early and frequent ambulation and resumption of oral intake. Gas pains might also be helped by frequently repositioning the client to encourage movement of air through the intestines. As air rises and peristalsis moves from right to left, the client can be moved from lying on the left side (where air will rise on the right), to lying supine, to lying on the right side (where air will rise on the left). If the client can tolerate it and there are no contraindications, lying prone with the head turned to the side places pressure on the abdomen, forcing air to rise and move out through the rectum. Other nursing care measures to relieve abdominal distention might include irrigation of the nasogastric tube, if present. Irrigating the nasogastric tube may also relieve hiccoughs.

Constipation is a major source of discomfort for the client. Analgesics combined with decreased activity and NPO status are very constipating. Oral fluids and activity should be encouraged. If ordered, the medical regimen of stool softeners and suppositories may be indicated.

4. *The client is at Risk for developing Urinary Retention related to anesthesia, immobility, and pain. The client is also at Risk for Infection related to Foley catheter placement.* The quantity and quality of urine are more directly related to cardiac output and the perfusion of the kidneys than to anesthesia, immobility, and pain; although a stress response following surgery causes the body to retain fluids for 24 to 48 hours following surgery. Urine output should be at least 30 cc per hour if a catheter is in place. The catheter must be assessed for patency. If not catheterized, the client should void at least 200 cc at the first postoperative voiding. Most clients void within 6 to 8 hours after surgery. However, urinary retention occurs frequently in the postoperative period, especially following abdominal or pelvic surgery. Anesthesia depresses the urge to void. Narcotics, vagolytic agents (anticholinergics), and spinal anesthesia also interfere with the ability to initiate voiding. The nurse can facilitate voiding by encouraging fluid intake and assisting the client to void in an anatomically correct position depending on the client's condition. Privacy, running water, indirect bladder pressure (placing a firm hand over the bladder), and warm water over the perineum may also encourage voiding.

   If the client has not voided, the nurse should palpate, inspect, and percuss the bladder. Often, the surgeon orders a Foley catheter to be inserted if the client has not voided after 8 to 10 hours.

5. *The client may become at Risk for Disturbed Sensory Perception related to anesthesia, narcotics, change of environment, fluid and electrolyte imbalances, sleep deprivation, hypoxia, and sensory deprivation or overload. The client may also experience Acute Pain related to the surgical incision; Hypothermia related to anesthesia and surgical environment; and Hyperthermia related to infection.* Alterations in neurological function vary and may manifest as pain, fever, or delirium. Assessing the level of consciousness is a priority. A change in level of consciousness may be the first indication of a stroke and/or increased intracranial pressure. Determining the level of consciousness may be difficult, especially in the elderly client or at night, when clients may be groggy from being awakened. Often, thoughts will clear if the client is given the opportunity to thoroughly awaken. Encouraging the presence of loved ones, offering explanations, and listening to the client may decrease sensory perceptual alterations. Encouraging previous sleep patterns, providing uninterrupted sleep, and alternating rest and activity may also be beneficial.

Pain assessment is essential. Subjective data regarding pain location, intensity on a scale of 0 to 10, quality, and duration as well as factors contributing to pain are assessed and recorded. Objective data such as grimacing and crying are also recorded. Analgesics are usually ordered to be administered via patient-controlled analgesia (PCA) or epidural analgesia or intravenously, intramuscularly, or orally, all on a prn (as needed) basis. The client must be encouraged to ask for the medication before the pain becomes severe. The nurse should offer medication before activity or painful procedures such as wound irrigation. The nurse must attend to analgesic requests promptly. Ensuring comfort encourages the client's full participation in coughing, deep breathing, turning, and ambulation.

Hypothermia is common in the first few hours following surgery. The nurse can offer blankets as needed. Because of the normal inflammatory response, temperature may later elevate to a low-grade fever. If temperature rises higher than 101°F, the surgeon must be notified. Atelectasis and dehydration may cause elevated temperature (higher than 101°F) in the first 24 to 48 hours following surgery. After 48 hours, temperature higher than 101°F may be indicative of a wound, respiratory, or urinary tract infection; thrombophlebitis; or pulmonary embolism.

The nurse's primary role is to prevent infection by using aseptic technique. Once a fever has occurred, the nurse follows orders to ascertain the cause of the elevation by taking urine, wound, blood, or sputum cultures. The nurse also administers antipyretics as ordered. Providing light covers and clothing, performing frequent linen changes, offering cool washcloths, and ensuring a cool environment are nursing measures that may increase comfort.

6. *The surgical client is at Risk for Impaired Skin Integrity and Infection related to surgical incision.* The nurse generally does not remove the primary dressing without an order to do so. Bleeding may be monitored by circling the drainage on the dressing and then reassessing later to ascertain whether the drainage area has increased in size. The dressing may also be reinforced with additional absorbent dressings as needed. In some institutions, the nurse may change the dressing as necessary after the first dressing change. Dressings may not be necessary if there is no drainage or drains, but this is usually the surgeon's preference.

Drainage on dressings and in drains typically changes from sanguineous to serosanguineous to serous over several hours to several days, depending on the type of surgery. The amount should also decrease over the same time period. Purulent, odorous drainage may be a sign of infection. A sudden increase in drainage may be a sign of impending wound separation. The surgeon should always be notified of any excessive or abnormal drainage.

All wounds heal by primary, secondary, or tertiary intention. In primary intention, the wound layers are sutured together and have no gaping edges. The wound generally heals in 8 to 10 days, but may take up to 3 months. There is minimal scar formation. Most surgical wounds are of this type.

In secondary intention, the wound heals by filling in with granulation tissue and by contracting where the skin edges are not approximated. This method is used for ulcers when there is not enough tissue to approximate the edges or for infected wounds when drainage is desirable. Wounds healing by secondary intention are assessed according to the presence of granulation tissue having a red, granular appearance. Wound healing is slow, possibly taking many months or years. Thus, wound healing by primary intention is preferable.

In tertiary intention, the approximation of tissue edges is delayed. This allows an infection to drain or an area of extensive tissue removal to begin healing. The edges of the wound are closed 4 to 6 days later. Because areas of granulation tissue are brought together at this time, the scar is usually much wider (Figure 16-14).

Wound dehiscence and evisceration are serious complications of wound healing. **Dehiscence** occurs when the wound edges separate. **Evisceration** occurs when the wound separates completely and the viscera protrude from the wound (Figure 16-15). Both are more likely to occur 7 to 10 days following surgery and are preceded by a sudden spillage of serosanguinous drainage. Dehiscence and evisceration are more likely to occur in the very elderly client, the malnourished client, the client with an infection, or the client with abdominal distention who is straining severely. If evisceration occurs, the viscera should be immediately covered with sterile saline dressings and the surgeon notified of the wound disruption.

When dressings are changed, the surgical incision is cleansed to remove debris and bacteria from the incision. The choice of cleansing agent depends on the physician's prescription as well as institutional protocol. It is recommended that isotonic solutions such as normal saline or lactated ringers be used.

The major principles to keep in mind when cleansing a surgical incision are:

- Use Standard Precautions at all times.
- Use a sterile swab or gauze and work from the clean area out toward the dirtier area. Begin over the incision line and swab downward from top to bottom. Change the swab and proceed

Figure 16-14 Wound Healing: A. Primary intention; B. Secondary intention; and C. Tertiary intention

again on either side of the incision, using a new swab each time (Figure 16-16).

The surface closures, staples, or sutures must be removed as the incision heals. Continuous sutures are made with one thread and tied at the beginning and end of the suture line. Intermittent sutures are each tied individually. In blanket continuous sutures, the single thread is grounded again in the last suture exit (Figure 16-17).

A.   **B.**

Figure 16-15 A. Dehiscence; B. Evisceration

The incisional dressing keeps the incision clean and protects it from physical trauma and bacterial invasion. Generally, the same kind of dressing can be put on as was taken off. As the incision heals and drainage lessens, a small, thinner dressing can usually be applied. Bandages and binders may be applied over the incision dressing to secure, immobilize, or support a body part; to hold the dressing in place; or to prevent or minimize swelling of a body part. Bandages are long rolls of material, such as gauze, webbing, or muslin, designed to be wrapped around body parts. Figure 16-18 illustrates several different methods of bandaging. Binders are bandages made for specific body parts, usually the abdomen, perineal area, or arm (sling) (Figure 16-19). Abdominal binders support the abdomen and are used following abdominal surgery or childbirth. Perineal binders, called T-binders, are used to hold pads or dressings in the perineal area. Because of the urination and defecation needs of clients, T-binders must be changed regularly. A sling is a cloth support for an injured arm; it wraps around the back of the neck to maintain the arm in a set position.

During dressing changes and after the dressing has been removed, the surgical wound is assessed for the skin edge approximation, edema, and bleeding. The skin edges may be slightly reddened and swollen from the normal inflammatory response. Possible signs of a wound infection include increased suture tension, warmth, erythema, drainage, odor, pain, and induration around the incision site. The nurse can enhance wound healing by promoting nutrition, discouraging smoking, and performing proper wound cleansing. The practice of aseptic technique cannot be emphasized enough in preventing nosocomial infections in a surgical incision.

7. *Clients are at risk for anxiety or ineffective individual coping related to disturbance in body image, change in lifestyle, financial strain, or a poor*

Figure 16-16 Use a clean, sterile swab for each stroke when cleansing a surgical incision. A. Gently clean the incision, then each side alternately. B. Gently wipe swab outward, away from the incision. C. Clean around a drain site in a circular motion.

Figure 16-17 Selected Suturing Methods: A. Continuous; B. Intermittent; and C. Blanket continuous

Figure 16-18 Common Bandaging Methods: A. Circular turns are wrapped around a body part several times to anchor the bandage or supply support. B. Spiral turns begin with a circular turn then proceed up the body part, with each turn covering two-thirds the width of the preceding turn. C. Spiral reverse turns begin with a circular turn. The bandage is then reversed, or twisted, once each turn to accommodate a limb that gets larger as the bandaging progresses. D. Figure-eight turns crisscross in the shape of a figure eight and are used on a joint that requires movement. E. Recurrent turns are anchored with circular turns, follow a back-and-forth motion, and are completed with circular turns; they are used to cover a fingertip, head, or amputated stump.

COMMUNITY/HOME HEALTH CARE

Dressing Wounds

- Because of early discharge, clients are often sent home with incisions that need dressing changes.
- Ascertain the client's support system, including caregivers, the home environment, and available resources.
- Teach the client and/or home caregiver the correct method of changing the dressing.
- Have the client and/or home caregiver actually change the dressing before the client is discharged.
- Provide a list of signs and symptoms of complications of wound healing.
- At times, a referral for home care nursing is necessary.

Figure 16-19 Common Binders: A. Abdominal; B. T-binders; female and male; and C. Arm sling

prognosis. Many clients undergo a psychological adjustment to surgery. Taking time to talk and listen to the client as well as offering simple explanations and reassurances may be all the support the client needs to combat anxiety.

As the client recovers and is discharged from the hospital, the client is at risk for knowledge deficit related to home care. Ideally, the client has been instructed routinely about home care since admission. Adequate teaching about home care results in a quicker recovery, fewer complications, and greater independence.

AMBULATORY SURGERY

Ambulatory surgery is defined as surgical care performed under general, regional, or local anesthesia and involving fewer than 24 hours of hospitalization. Other names for ambulatory surgery include same-day, one-day, outpatient, in and out, or short-stay surgery.

A trend in health care is to promote a philosophy of wellness. Clients are encouraged to accept more personal responsibility for their state of health. In the past, the message sent to clients was that the client is sick, and the medical community will provide all care. Today, ambulatory surgery clients are being sent a totally different message: that the postoperative client is not sick and, except for a few minor limitations, can often resume normal daily activities soon after undergoing anesthesia and surgery.

Ambulatory surgery provides the longest period of time for the client to receive skilled postoperative care or monitoring without being formally admitted to the hospital. The practice of ambulatory surgery attempts to overcome the risk of premature dismissal while at the same time meeting fiscal requirements. The emphasis on cost containment coupled with government reductions in Medicare and Medicaid payments has further promoted the concept of ambulatory surgery.

To further reduce health care costs, few clients are admitted to the hospital prior to the day of surgery. Most surgical clients are processed through the ambulatory surgery unit. These clients are called "day of surgery" or "A.M. admit" clients. Necessary laboratory work, radiology tests, or other examinations are completed on an outpatient basis prior to the day of surgery. Even clients undergoing extensive surgeries such as open-heart surgery (a coronary artery bypass), craniotomy, or total joint replacement, can be admitted the day of surgery. Then, after discharge from the perioperative suite, the client may either be admitted to the hospital as an inpatient or may be sent home from the ambulatory surgery unit.

In addition to fiscal considerations, the growth of ambulatory surgery can also be traced to technological advances. Clients now require shorter recovery periods due to new procedural technology, such as laporoscopic

COMMUNITY/HOME HEALTH CARE

Postoperative Care

For proper home care, the client and family must be given information about the following topics:

- Medication regimen
- Diet
- Activity restrictions
- Follow-up appointments
- Wound care
- Special instructions

The specifics for each topic will vary with each client and will depend on the surgical procedure and the client's age and physical condition.

PROFESSIONAL TIP

Ambulatory Surgery

- Precertification documents are approved before the preadmission visit.
- Preadmission diagnostic tests, preoperative nursing assessment, and initial teaching are usually performed the day before the scheduled surgery.
- On the day of surgery, care is focused on the immediate needs of the client.

cholecystectomy. The introduction of shorter-acting anesthetic agents also decreases the immediate postoperative recovery time, facilitating the client's ability to function independently upon discharge from the ambulatory surgery setting.

The benefits of ambulatory surgery are many. Ambulatory surgery decreases cost to the client, institution, insurance carriers, and governmental agencies. Because clients are hospitalized for such a short period of time, the risk of acquiring a nosocomial infection during the perioperative period is also decreased. The client experiences less disruption to personal life and less psychological distress related to hospitalization. With ambulatory surgery, the client especially benefits from early postoperative ambulation.

Ambulatory surgery is performed in several different settings. Hospital-based integrated facilities are formal ambulatory surgery programs incorporated into existing inpatient surgery programs. Clients are cared for preoperatively and postoperatively in the ambulatory surgery unit, but are mixed with inpatients on the operating room schedule. This type of facility also allows preoperative processing of day-of-surgery clients. Hospital-affiliated facilities consist of a separate department with designated preoperative, intraoperative, and postoperative areas. Such a facility may be located within the hospital, adjacent to the hospital, or at a satellite location. Free-standing facilities are independently owned and operated and are not affiliated with a hospital or medical center. In the past, physicians generally owned such facilities, but today the trend is for health care corporations to own these facilities. Some doctors' offices also have facilities for performing minor ambulatory surgery.

The Aldrete Score has been modified for use with clients having anesthesia on an ambulatory basis. Five assessments were added to the Aldrete Score for this purpose (Table 16–6). Attainment of these criteria indicates that clients should be able to care for themselves at home and accomplish activities of daily living independently and safely. The points are totaled at regular intervals (usually every ½ hour), and clients may be discharged home when their total score is 18 or higher.

ELDERLY CLIENTS UNDERGOING SURGERY

Elderly clients (over 65 years of age) are at risk for developing complications from surgery or anesthesia. Unfortunately, because an increased incidence of disease correlates with increasing age, more elderly clients require surgery than does any other age group. As the percentage of elderly persons in the whole population rises, the number of surgeries on elders will also rise. Because of the complex needs of the elderly client undergoing surgery, the nurse must be knowledgeable in promoting health and rehabilitation in the elderly client.

Surgery is a stressor. Because of depleted energy sources, the elderly client may not have sufficient resilience to react defensively to this stressor. The risk of complications from surgery further rises in elderly clients who have one or more chronic diseases. In these clients, surgery then can be the source of a downward spiraling effect toward debilitation or possibly death.

Elderly clients vary in their abilities to respond to the stress of surgery. Physiologic changes related to the aging process may inhibit the elderly client from readily coping with surgery. The number of physiologic changes in the very elderly client (over 80 years of age) is markedly greater than that in those in their 60s and 70s. Breathing capacity, renal blood flow, cardiac output, and conduction velocity of the nervous system all diminish. Table 16–9 lists the physiologic changes in the elderly client along with correlating nursing interventions for postoperative care. Aging affects all body systems, and the nurse must be familiar with these changes and the interventions geared toward each to prevent and detect complications of surgery.

Table 16–9 PHYSIOLOGIC CHANGES OF AGING AND RELATED POSTOPERATIVE NURSING INTERVENTIONS

BODY SYSTEM	CHANGES	NURSING INTERVENTIONS
Cardiovascular	• Decreased elasticity of the vascular system • Decreased cardiac output • Decreased peripheral circulation	• Closely monitor vital signs and peripheral pulses • Encourage early ambulation • Use antiembolism stockings • Monitor intake and output, including blood loss • Monitor preoperative response to activity and compare to postoperative response
Respiratory	• Decreased vital capacity • Decreased alveolar volume • Decreased movement of cilia	• Closely monitor respirations • Auscultate breath sounds frequently • Encourage coughing and deep breathing • Turn frequently • Monitor oxygen saturation
Urinary	• Decreased glomerular filtration rate • Decreased bladder muscle tone • Weakened perineal muscles	• Monitor intake and output every 1 to 2 hours • Assist frequently with toileting • Monitor fluid and electrolyte status
Gastrointestinal	• Decreased gastric and intestinal motility • Altered digestion and absorption • Decreased food consumption	• Assess for obesity and malnutrition • Encourage fluids and activity • Encourage high-protein foods and supplements • Assist with meals as needed • Provide companionship during mealtime
Immunological	• Decreased level of gamma globulin • Decreased plasma proteins	• Follow strict aseptic technique • Monitor temperature • Assess incision site
Neurological	• Decreased conduction velocity • Decreased visual acuity • Loss of hearing • Decreased sensation	• Allow use of glasses and hearing aids • Orient to environment • Provide for safe environment • Repeat information as needed • Use medications sparingly • Provide written instructions • Allow for extra education time
Integumentary	• Lack of elasticity • Loss of collagen • Decreased subcutaneous fat	• To prevent shearing forces on skin when positioning client, lift rather than slide client • Pad bony prominences • Use tape that is easy to remove • Use warm prepping solutions, irrigating solutions, and IV solutions intraoperatively • Provide extra blankets • Ensure warm room temperature • Turn frequently • Encourage early ambulation

In the cardiovascular system, the elderly client experiences decreased elasticity of the blood vessels and decreased pumping action of the heart, resulting in less blood reaching the peripheral circulation. Ultimately, blood flow is slower, and less blood reaches vital organs such as the brain, heart, lungs, liver, and kidneys. In the older adult, decreased blood flow to vital organs delays elimination of anesthetics and medications through the lungs, liver, and kidneys. Decreased elasticity of the blood vessels does not allow vasoconstriction and vasodilation to compensate for hypovolemia and hypervolemia; thus the elderly client is more prone to hypotension and shock or, conversely, fluid overload. Slower blood flow combined with an increased incidence of atherosclerosis, the presence of other cardiovascular diseases, and decreased mobility increases the elderly client's risk for developing deep vein thrombosis, thrombophlebitis, and accompanying pulmonary embolism. Decreased blood flow to vital organs may also cause confusion, decreased urinary output, and drug retention or overdose. Decreased peripheral circulation may contribute to poor or delayed wound healing as well. The effects of aging on the cardiovascular system increase the likelihood of multiple surgical complications in the elderly client.

As with the cardiovascular system, the respiratory system in elderly clients demonstrates less elasticity, and expansion of the chest wall and lungs is adversely affected. As a result, elderly clients are unable to exhale fully, causing increased air retention in the lung (residual lung volume) and decreased ability to forcefully exhale air (forced expiratory volume). The amount of air inhaled and exhaled (vital capacity) also decreases. Less air reaches the alveoli, causing decreased alveolar volume. Decreased vital capacity and alveolar volume result in reduced exchange of carbon dioxide and oxygen in the lungs. The cilia lining the passageways of the lungs do not move as efficiently, resulting in a decreased cough reflex in the elderly client. All of these changes may lead to atelectasis, pneumonia, and postoperative confusion.

The urinary system is affected by age as well. Kidney function deteriorates as blood flow to the kidneys decreases. Waste products are not excreted as quickly and urine output decreases. Reduced blood flow also decreases the glomerular filtration rate. Decreased bladder muscle tone results in urinary retention, and weakened perineal muscles can lead to urinary incontinence. The effects of aging also increase the likelihood of renal failure.

A combination of age-related changes in renal and liver function, related to decreased perfusion rate, results in slower drug metabolism. To prevent side effects of postoperative analgesics, the elderly client may need either a reduced dosage, given less frequently, or smaller, more frequent doses. Decreased peripheral circulation may reduce or delay the absorption of intramuscular analgesics. Oral analgesics may also be poorly absorbed due to decreased gastrointestinal motility and decreased mesenteric blood flow. Intravenous analgesia may be preferred for the elderly client to provide careful dosing according to individual response and need.

In the gastrointestinal system, decreased gastric and intestinal motility result in constipation and fecal impaction. Decreased activity stemming from loss of muscle strength and range of motion further contributes to constipation. Because elderly clients are often less mobile after surgery, constipation and fecal impaction are very common.

The nutritional status of the elderly client prior to surgery may also have a profound effect on wound healing, susceptibility to infection, degree of postoperative recovery, and length of hospital stay (Talabiska, 1995). Nutritional status can be affected by the presence of a chronic illness, resulting in the client expending more energy to maintain metabolism and activities of daily living. Dementia, depression, and altered mental status may also affect nutritional status. Because the elderly client may take multiple medications, drug–food interactions are common. Food consumption, gastric motility, and digestion and absorption all decrease. The financial situation and social status of the elderly client may also affect nutritional status, as may poorly fitting dentures and decreased sense of taste. The nutritional status of the elderly client must be carefully assessed both preoperatively and postoperatively to facilitate optimal recovery from surgery.

Elderly clients are prone to infections such as wound infections, pneumonia, and urinary tract infections. Delayed wound healing, including wound dehiscence or evisceration, are also common in the elderly client. Changes in the metabolism and the immune system of the elderly client may contribute to these effects. The levels of gamma globulin and plasma proteins fall, causing inadequate inflammatory responses. Fewer killer T-cells and a decreased response to foreign proteins render the body less able to protect itself from pathogenic microorganisms. An increased production of leukocytes and an elevated temperature for 48 hours postoperatively is a normal inflammatory response. If temperature elevates markedly and continues longer than 48 hours, however, an infectious process may be occurring. In the elderly client, a reduction in the basal metabolic rate results in a lower normal temperature. Thus, fever in the elderly client is even more significant.

The conduction velocity of the nervous system diminishes in the elderly client, slowing movements and impairing equilibrium. These and other sensory changes increase the risk of injury in the elderly surgical client. Dimished vision, hearing, and sensation contribute to falls, burns, and other injuries. Overstimulation and the lack of a familiar environment often cause confusion, another factor in injury. Chronic conditions that limit mobility, such as arthritis or previous stroke, may also contribute to the incidence of injury. The physiologic changes in the nervous system may lead to integumentary complications as mobility and sensation decrease.

Due to lack of elasticity and loss of collagen, the skin of the elderly client is often dry, flaky, and itchy. It thins and is easily bruised and abraded. Lack of subcutaneous fat and decreased circulation render the older adult prone to hypothermia and pressure sores.

The elderly client has a lifetime of experiences that affects the response to surgery. A lifetime of watching family and friends experience surgery, illness, and death particularly influences personal reactions to impending surgery. Due to the variation in such experiences, each client reacts differently to similar situations. Simply talking with the client to provide information or listening to the client's fears helps the client prepare for upcoming surgery.

Third-party reimbursement policies often require elderly clients to undergo surgical procedures on an outpatient basis. Because many elderly clients have neurological deficits and other chronic disease processes, the elderly outpatient poses a particular challenge

CASE STUDY

Mr. Glen Stone, a 74-year-old retired schoolteacher who is married and the father of four and the grand-father of sixteen, weighs 275 lbs. He has undergone a right hemicolectomy, wherein the right side of his colon was removed because of cancer. He has a history of smoking, but has no other health problems. The surgery was uncomplicated, and he is in the PACU. He has a midline incision with a Penrose drain; a stab wound with a Jackson Pratt drain is adjacent to the incision. He also has a nasogastric tube attached to low intermittent suction. He is alert and oriented, and he can move all four extremities. His blood pressure is normal for him in comparison to his preoperative levels. He is breathing regularly and easily at a rate of 16 breaths per minute, and his skin color is normal. His oxygen saturation, however, is 86% with additional oxygen being given via mask.

The following questions will guide your development of a nursing care plan for the case study.

1. What risk factors for developing postoperative complications can you identify for Mr. Stone?
2. What is his Aldrete Score at this point?
3. What nursing measures can you institute to promote oxygenation?
4. What type of drainage is expected from the incision and the drains during the first 1 to 2 days?
5. What nursing observations can be made and reported to indicate to the surgeon that the nasogastric tube can be removed?
6. What nursing measures can be implemented to prevent deep vein thrombosis, thrombophlebitis, and pulmonary embolism?
7. Write and prioritize three individualized nursing diagnoses and goals for Mr. Stone.
8. What information will Mr. Stone need prior to discharge?

to the nurse. Additional postoperative self-care deficits may result from the surgical procedure and the effects of anesthesia. Elderly clients often live alone and lack the support systems necessary for home care. In order to provide realistic discharge planning, the nurse must assess the ability of the client, family, and friends to provide care at home.

SUMMARY

- Surgery is a major stressor for all clients. Anxiety and fear are normal. Fear of the unknown is both the most prevalent fear prior to surgery and the fear easiest for the nurse to help the client overcome.
- The outcome of surgical treatment is tremendously enhanced by accurate preoperative nursing assessment and careful preoperative preparation. Information gathered through preoperative assessment and risk screening is later used for preparation of the surgical site, for surgical positioning, and as a comparative basis for postoperative assessments and complication screening.
- The teaching methods used by the nurse strongly influence the degree of learning and the retention of information.
- Aseptic technique is a collection of principles used to control and/or prevent the transfer of micro-

organisms from sources within (endogenous) and outside (exogenous) the client. These principles are practiced in all clinical nursing units. The sterile conscience governs personal behavior with regard to adherence to aseptic technique.

- Nursing care in the operating room focuses on the safety and protection of the client.
- Postoperative nursing assessments are completed in an organized manner, focusing first on the priorities of airway, breathing, and circulation, and then on the body system affected by surgery.
- The nurse can help prevent the formation of deep vein thrombosis, thrombophlebitis, and pulmonary embolism through encouraging early ambulation and postoperative leg exercises and by providing antiembolism stockings and/or sequential stockings, if ordered.
- Ambulatory surgery is defined as surgical care performed under general, regional, or local anesthesia and involving fewer than 24 hours of hospitalization. Cost containment, governmental changes, and technological advances have all promoted the concept of ambulatory surgery.
- Because of the physiologic changes and complex needs of the elderly client undergoing surgery, the nurse must be knowledgeable in promoting health and rehabilitation in the elderly surgical client.

Review Questions

1. When performing client teaching, the nurse does which one of the following?
    a. assesses barriers to learning
    b. completes teaching in a single time frame
    c. provides information in one mode of learning
    d. allows little time for questions

2. Client education is:
    a. completed when time allows.
    b. started when discharge is scheduled.
    c. always more beneficial when completed in a structured group setting.
    d. directed toward the client's family when the client is unable to learn.

3. The role of the nurse in obtaining consent includes which of the following?
    a. judging the quality of the explanation and ascertaining the client's understanding of the consent form
    b. acting as a witness to the signature of the client
    c. administering the preoperative medication before the client signs the consent
    d. ensuring that coercion was used to obtain the client's signature on the consent

4. The use of drains will:
    a. increase postoperative pain.
    b. prevent tissue healing.
    c. increase scarring.
    d. eliminate fluid accumulation.

5. Upon the client's admission to the PACU, the nurse must first:
    a. take the client's blood pressure.
    b. assess the airway.
    c. assess the client's level of consciousness.
    d. check the incision site.

6. The nurse is making a preoperative assessment on a client. Which of these findings is the most important to know for a client who is having general anesthesia?
    a. hearing impaired
    b. a right-leg amputee
    c. color blind
    d. a smoker

7. Which of the following persons is responsible and accountable for all activities during a surgical procedure?
    a. surgeon
    b. anesthesia provider
    c. circulating nurse
    d. scrub nurse

8. The surgical skin preparation will:
    a. sterilize the skin.
    b. cleanse the skin and inhibit bacterial growth.
    c. prevent fingernails from growing.
    d. remove the dermis.

9. The nursing intervention that has the greatest impact on reducing overall surgical risk is:
    a. encouraging activity and early ambulation.
    b. assessing blood pressure.
    c. ensuring adequate nutrition.
    d. monitoring intake and output.

10. Surgical risk increases in the elderly client due to:
    a. type of surgery.
    b. physiologic changes of aging.
    c. exposure to infectious processes.
    d. number of children.

Critical Thinking Questions

1. How can you use a sterile conscience when providing nursing care?

WEB FLASH!

- Research "incision glue" on the Web. What information is available on this topic?
- What sites could a client access for information on a particular surgery (e.g., coronary bypass)?

CHAPTER 17

NURSING CARE OF THE ONCOLOGY CLIENT

MAKING THE CONNECTION

Refer to the following chapters to increase your understanding of oncology nursing:

- Chapter 4, Ethical Responsibilities
- Chapter 9, Loss, Grief, and Death
- Chapter 13, Diagnostic Tests
- Chapter 14, Pain Management
- Chapter 16, Nursing Care of the Surgical Client
- Chapter 20, Nursing Care of the Client: Hematologic and Lymphatic Systems

- Chapter 21, Nursing Care of the Client: Integumentary System
- Chapter 22, Nursing Care of the Client: Immune System
- Chapter 30, Nursing Care of the Client: Female Reproductive System
- Chapter 31, Nursing Care of the Client: Male Reproductive System
- Chapter 35, Nursing Care of the Older Client

LEARNING OBJECTIVES

Upon completion of this chapter, you should be able to:
- *Define key terms.*
- *Explain how the behavior of cancer cells differs from that of normal cells.*
- *Describe the role of the nurse in cancer detection.*
- *Discuss three medical treatments for cancer.*
- *Describe four complications that can occur in advanced cancer.*
- *Discuss ways the licensed practical/vocational nurse can aid the client in coping with cancer.*

KEY TERMS

alopecia	leukemia
anorexia	lymphoma
antineoplastic	malignant
benign	metastasis
biologic response modifier	neoplasm
cachexia	oncology
cancer	palliative
carcinogen	radiotherapy
carcinoma	reconstructive
chemotherapy	sarcoma
curative	stomatitis
differentiation	tumor marker
extravasation	vesicant

INTRODUCTION

Cancer is a disease resulting from the uncontrolled growth of cells, which causes malignant cellular tumors. One in three Americans will develop some type of cancer during their lifetime. Cancer is the second leading cause of death in the United States and can develop in individuals of any race, gender, age, socioeconomic status, or culture. It is not a single disease but, rather, a group of more than 200 different diseases that can attack any tissue or organ of the body.

According to the American Cancer Society (ACS), in the 1930s fewer than one in five cancer clients was alive 5 years after diagnosis. In the 1940s one in four survived 5 years. Today, 59% of people diagnosed with cancer will be alive in 5 years (American Cancer Society, 2000). Survival rates are influenced by the type of cancer, the progression of the disease at diagnosis, and the client's response to the treatment.

INCIDENCE

In the United States, men have a 1 in 2 lifetime risk of developing cancer while women have a risk of 1 in 3 (ACS, 2000). Incidence and mortality rates are usually higher for African Americans than for Anglo Americans. The incidence of cancer is higher in the elderly population than in any other age group. In men, the most common cancers are prostate, lung, and colorectal; in women, they are breast, colorectal, lung, and uterine cancer (Figure 17-1).

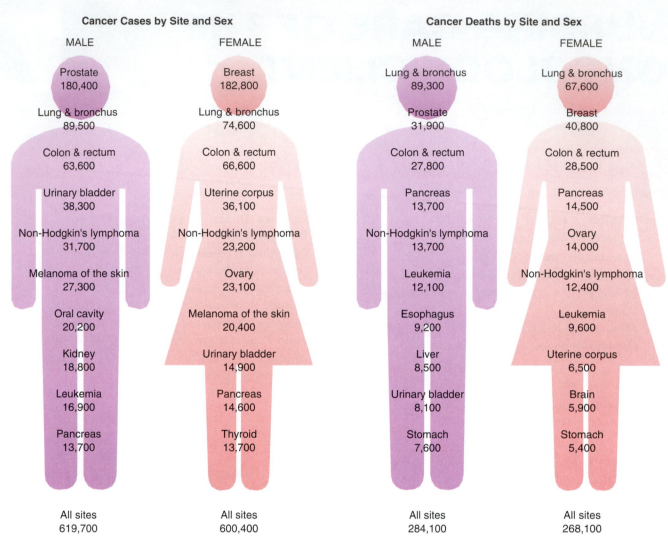

Cancer Cases by Site and Sex

MALE

- Prostate 180,400
- Lung & bronchus 89,500
- Colon & rectum 63,600
- Urinary bladder 38,300
- Non-Hodgkin's lymphoma 31,700
- Melanoma of the skin 27,300
- Oral cavity 20,200
- Kidney 18,800
- Leukemia 16,900
- Pancreas 13,700

All sites 619,700

FEMALE

- Breast 182,800
- Lung & bronchus 74,600
- Colon & rectum 66,600
- Uterine corpus 36,100
- Non-Hodgkin's lymphoma 23,200
- Ovary 23,100
- Melanoma of the skin 20,400
- Urinary bladder 14,900
- Pancreas 14,600
- Thyroid 13,700

All sites 600,400

Cancer Deaths by Site and Sex

MALE

- Lung & bronchus 89,300
- Prostate 31,900
- Colon & rectum 27,800
- Pancreas 13,700
- Non-Hodgkin's lymphoma 13,700
- Leukemia 12,100
- Esophagus 9,200
- Liver 8,500
- Urinary bladder 8,100
- Stomach 7,600

All sites 284,100

FEMALE

- Lung & bronchus 67,600
- Breast 40,800
- Colon & rectum 28,500
- Pancreas 14,500
- Ovary 14,000
- Non-Hodgkin's lymphoma 12,400
- Leukemia 9,600
- Uterine corpus 6,500
- Brain 5,900
- Stomach 5,400

All sites 268,100

*Excluding basal and squamous cell skin cancer and in situ carcinomas except urinary bladder.

Figure 17-1 Leading Sites of New Cancer Cases and Deaths—2000 Estimates (*Reprinted from American Cancer Society Cancer Facts and Figures, 1999*)

The ACS estimates that 1,220,100 new cancer cases were diagnosed in the United States in 2000. Not included in this estimate are basal- and squamous-cell skin cancers and noninvasive cancers except for urinary bladder cancer. Approximately 1.3 million cases of highly curable basal- and squamous-cell skin cancers were estimated to be diagnosed in 2000 (ACS, 2000).

In 2000, approximately 173,000 cancer deaths were estimated to be caused by tobacco, with an additional 19,000 cancer deaths related to excessive alcohol use. Up to one-third of the 522,200 cancer deaths estimated for 2000 are related to nutrition and other lifestyle factors and could be prevented (ACS, 2000).

PATHOPHYSIOLOGY

Cancer is a disease characterized by neoplasia, an uncontrolled growth of abnormal cells. Unlike normal cells, which reproduce in an orderly manner and grow for a purpose, cancer cells develop rapidly, undiscriminatingly, and serve no useful function as they grow at the expense of healthy tissue. **Neoplasms**, or any abnormal growth of new tissue, can be found in any body tissue. Neoplasms may be **benign** (not progressive, and thus, favorable for recovery) or **malignant** (becoming progressively worse and often resulting in death).

Benign neoplasms are not cancerous and are usually harmless. They grow slowly, are encapsulated and well-defined, and do not spread to neighboring tissues. Unless their location interferes with vital functions, benign neoplasms are associated with a favorable prognosis.

Malignant neoplasms form irregularly-shaped masses with fingerlike projections. They usually multiply quickly and spread to distant body parts through the bloodstream or the lymph system. This process is called **metastasis**. Patterns of metastasis will differ depending on the type of cancer.

Cancers are usually named according to the site of the primary tumor or to the type of tissue involved. There are four main classifications of cancer according to tissue type:

- **lymphomas** (cancers occurring in infection-fighting organs, such as lymphatic tissue)
- **leukemias** (cancers occurring in blood-forming organs, such as the spleen, and in bone marrow)
- **sarcomas** (cancers occurring in connective tissue, such as bone)
- **carcinomas** (cancers occurring in epithelial tissue, such as the skin)

The exact mechanism that causes cancer is unknown, but most authorities believe that cancer develops from a combination of factors rather than from a single factor. Environmental, genetic, and viral factors have been implicated in the development of cancer. Chemical substances that initiate or promote the development of cancer are known as **carcinogens**. These agents are thought to alter the DNA in the cell nucleus.

RISK FACTORS

A number of risk factors, such as environmental, lifestyle, genetic, and viral, may increase an individual's chances of developing cancer. These factors are discussed following.

Environmental Factors

The first environmental carcinogen was discovered in 1760 when Percival Pott noted that chimney sweeps had a very high rate of what is now known to be scrotal cancer because they were exposed to cancer-causing oils in the soot that was rubbed into their clothing. Since that time, hundreds of chemical carcinogens have been identified.

Many individuals come into contact with cancer-causing agents through occupational exposure. Many industrial chemicals, such as asbestos or vinyl chlorides, have been found to be carcinogenic. For workers who handle these chemicals, the risk of developing cancers is greatly increased if occupational exposure is combined with cigarette smoking. Tobacco may act synergistically with other substances to promote cancer development. Occupational exposure to coal tar, creosote, arsenic compounds, or radium constitutes a risk factor for development of skin cancer. The effects of carcinogenic agents are usually dose dependent. The larger the dose or the longer the duration of exposure, the greater the risk of cancer development. It is estimated that 80% of all cancers may be associated with environmental exposures and might be prevented if exposure is avoided. For those likely to be exposed to chemical carcinogens at work, safety standards and levels of exposure have been established by the Occupational Safety and Health Administration (OSHA).

In 1993, the U.S. Environmental Protection Agency (EPA) declared secondhand smoke a human carcinogen. Approximately 3,000 nonsmoking adults die each year of lung cancer from breathing secondhand smoke (ACS, 1998).

Lifestyle Factors

Other agents include exposures determined by individual lifestyle choices such as the use of tobacco, sun exposure, alcohol consumption, and diet. Tobacco accounts for nearly one in three deaths in the United States (ACS, 2000). Tobacco use includes cigarettes, cigars, pipes, and smokeless forms (snuff and chewing tobacco). The same carcinogens are found in all forms of tobacco, causing cancer of the oral cavity, esophagus, pharynx, and larynx. When tobacco is smoked, it can also cause cancer of the lung, pancreas, uterus, cervix, kidney, and bladder.

Overexposure to the sun's ultraviolet rays over long periods of time is the cause of many skin cancers. The most serious form of skin cancer is melanoma. The ACS (2000) estimates 47,700 newly diagnosed cases of melanoma in 2000. Other factors predisposing a person to skin cancer are family history, multiple nevi, and atypical nevi.

Heavy alcohol consumption has also been implicated in mouth, throat, esophageal, and liver cancers. Alcohol is hypothesized to cause 5% of cancer deaths. Alcohol and tobacco used together greatly increase the risk of oral and esophageal cancers. The combined effect of alcohol and tobacco is greater than the sum of their individual effects (ACS, 2000). The association between alcohol consumption and breast cancer has also been noted in some studies. Despite the epidemiological evidence linking alcohol to cancer, the exact carcinogen in alcohol is yet to be determined. Table 17–1 lists some risk factors for cancer.

Although findings from studies of the link between cancer and diet are controversial, current research suggests an increase in dietary fiber may help prevent colon cancer (Hansen, 1995). Some studies have suggested that obesity is a significant risk factor for breast, colon, endometrial, and prostate cancers. Studies have also shown that diets high in salt-cured, smoked, and nitrite-cured foods increase an individual's risk for

Table 17–1 RISK FACTORS FOR CANCER	
Breast Cancer	• Family history (immediate female relatives) • High-fat diet • Obesity • Early menarche • Late menopause • Long-term estrogen therapy • First child after age 30
Cervical Cancer	• Multiple sexual partners • Exposure to genital herpes • Exposure to human papillomavirus • Smoking
Colorectal Cancer	• Family history (immediate relatives) • Low-fiber diet • History of rectal polyps
Esophageal Cancer	• Heavy alcohol consumption • Smoking
Lung Cancer	• Smoking • Asbestos exposure • Air pollution • Tuberculosis
Skin Cancer	• Extensive exposure to ultraviolet sunlight • Fair complexion • Work with coal, tar, pitch, or creosote
Stomach Cancer	• Family history • Diet heavy in smoked, pickled, or salted foods
Testicular Cancer	• Undescended testicles • Consumption of hormones by mother during pregnancy
Prostate Cancer	• Increasing age • Family history • Diet high in animal fat

Genetic Factors

Some families have a high incidence of certain types of cancer. Breast cancer, for example, occurs more frequently in women whose mothers, grandmothers, or sisters have had the disease. Leukemia and cancers of the colon, stomach, prostate, lung, and ovary, may also run in families. Therefore, relatives of persons with these cancers should be carefully monitored.

Viral Factors

Although viruses have been linked to a number of cancers, their exact role is unclear. It has been theorized that they incorporate themselves into the genetic structure of the cell. Herpes simplex II virus and some of the human papillomaviruses that are transmitted sexually are known to predispose women to cervical cancer. Reducing the number of sexual partners can reduce the risk of contracting these viruses.

DETECTION

When cancer does develop, the earlier it is detected the more likely it is to be controlled. In some cases, diagnosis can be made before symptoms become apparent. Cancer is usually found by the affected individual, who notices a warning sign, or a health care provider

CLIENT TEACHING

Dietary Guidelines To Reduce the Risk of Cancer

• Choose most foods from plant sources.
 – Eat five or more servings of fruits and vegetables each day, especially green and dark-yellow vegetables and those in the cabbage family.
 – Consume other foods from plant sources including breads, cereals, pastas, beans (legumes), and soy products.

• Limit intake of high-fat foods, particularly from animal sources.
 – Choose foods low in fat.
 – Limit consumption of meats, especially red meats and high-fat meats.

• Be physically active and achieve and maintain a healthy weight.
 – Physical activity can help by balancing caloric intake with energy expenditures or by other mechanisms.

• Limit or eliminate consumption of alcoholic beverages.

(ACS, 2000)

cancer of the stomach and esophagus. Food substances that may reduce cancer risk include cruciferous vegetables (cabbage, broccoli, cauliflower, brussels sprouts, kohlrabi); possibly vitamins A, E, and C; and selenium. Some foods have been found to contain carcinogens in the forms of additives or as byproducts of storage. On the basis of current knowledge, the ACS has offered dietary guidelines to reduce cancer risk (see Client Teaching).

CLIENT TEACHING

Lifestyle Guidelines to Reduce the Risk of Cancer

- Do not smoke or use tobacco in any form.
- Avoid overexposure to the sun.
- Eat a healthy diet.
- Get plenty of exercise.
- Have a physical examination on a routine basis, including a mammogram, Pap smear, testicular, and colon examinations.
- Get plenty of sleep (6 to 8 hours per night).
- Keep weight within normal limits.
- Practice regular self-examinations and see your physician if any changes are noted.
- Know and follow health and safety rules at the workplace.

during a checkup. A cancer checkup is recommended every 3 years for persons ages 20 to 39 years and annually for those ages 40 years and over. Risk assessment is the first step in cancer prevention. The cancer examination should include both a medical history of exposures to environmental agents and a comprehensive family history.

If cancer is suspected, diagnostic studies are ordered. The diagnostic studies performed depend on the suspected primary or metastatic site of the cancer and include laboratory studies or blood tests, radiologic studies, endoscopy, cytology, and biopsy. Nurses must be able to give brief descriptions of such tests as well as assist in client preparation.

Although no one blood test can confirm a cancer diagnosis, some malignancies do alter the chemical composition of the blood. Specialized laboratory tests have been developed to detect **tumor markers**, substances such as specific proteins, antigens, genes, hormones, or enzymes that are found in the serum and indicate the possible presence of malignancy. Tumor markers are not 100% accurate, as benign processes can also cause elevations; they are, however, useful in monitoring response to treatment or detecting a relapse.

COMMON DIAGNOSTIC TESTS

Commonly used diagnostic tests for clients who present with symptoms of cancer are listed in Table 17–2. See Chapter 13, Diagnostic Tests, for explanation/normal values and nursing responsibilities related to each test.

STAGING OF TUMORS

Staging determines the extent of the spread of cancer. The TNM classification proposed by the American Joint Commission on Cancer is one of the most frequently used systems. The *T* refers to the anatomical size of the primary tumor; *N*, the extent of lymph node involvement; and *M*, the presence or absence of metastasis (Table 17–3). Use of this internationally recognized staging system for tumors ensures a reliable comparison of clients in many different hospitals. Staging is important because it influences decisions about treatment modalities and helps predict overall prognosis.

GRADING OF TUMORS

Normal body cells have individual characteristics that allow them to perform different body functions. This process is called **differentiation**. Tumor cells that retain many of the identifiable tissue characteristics of the original cell are termed *well differentiated*. Tumor cells having little similarity to the tissue of origin are termed *undifferentiated*. Tumor grading is based primarily on the degree of differentiation of malignant cells. Grading evaluates tumor cells in comparison to normal cells. Pathologists indicate tumor cell grades by using the Roman numerals I through IV; the higher the grade, the higher the number and the worse the prognosis. Thus, a grade I tumor is the most differentiated, and a grade IV tumor is the most undifferentiated (or least differentiated). Tumors containing poorly differentiated cells are more aggressive in growth and

Table 17–2 COMMON DIAGNOSTIC TESTS FOR CANCER DETECTION

Laboratory Tests
- Acid phosphatase
- Alkaline phosphatase
- Bence Jones protein
- CA-15-3
- CA-19-9
- CA-125
- CEA (carcinoembryonic antigen)
- PSA (prostate-specific antigen)
- Stool for occult blood (Guaiac)
- Serum calcitonin

Radiologic Studies
- X-ray studies
- Computerized axial tomography (CT scan or CAT scan)
- Magnetic resonance imaging (MRI)
- Scans (radioisotope test)
- Ultrasound

Invasive Diagnostic Techniques
- Endoscopy
- Cytology
- Biopsy

Table 17–3 STAGING OF TUMORS: TNM CLASSIFICATION

STAGE	TUMOR	LYMPH NODE	METASTASIS
I	< 2 cm diameter Mobile Often superficial Confined to organ of origin	No involvement	No evidence
II	2 to 5 cm diameter Not as mobile Extension into adjacent tissue	Palpable, mobile > 2 to 3 cm diameter Firmer than normal	No evidence
III a	> 5 cm diameter Not mobile Regional involvement	No involvement	No evidence
III b	< 2 to > 5 cm diameter Mobile or not mobile Localized or extended	> 2 to 3 cm diameter Firmer than normal	No evidence
IV a	> 10 cm diameter Extension into another organ; major arteries, veins, or nerves; or bone	No involvement or > 2 to 3 cm diameter Firmer than normal	No evidence
IV b	No evidence to > 10 cm diameter	3 to 5 cm diameter Partially mobile Firm to hard; or > 5 cm diameter Extended and fixed to bone, large blood vessels, skin, or nerves	No evidence
IV c	No evidence to > 10 cm diameter	No evidence to > 10 cm diameter Fixed and destructive Extension to second or distant stations	Solitary or multiple

may display uncharacteristic behaviors, leading to a poorer prognosis. Grading criteria vary for different neoplasms.

TREATMENT MODALITIES

After cancer is diagnosed, staged, and graded, a medical treatment plan is developed. The most common treatment methods used today are surgery, radiation therapy, and **chemotherapy** (use of drugs to treat illness); biotherapy and bone marrow transplantation may also be used. These methods may be used alone or in combination.

Surgery

Surgery is the oldest form of cancer treatment and remains the most common method of treatment today. Surgery can be classified as curative, palliative, or reconstructive.

The goal of **curative** surgery is to heal or restore to health; this involves excising all of the tumor, the involved surrounding tissue, and the regional lymph nodes. Surgery most often has curative results when performed in the early stages of such diseases as cervical, breast, or skin cancer. The first commonly used surgical procedure for treating cancer was the radical mastectomy for breast cancer, which removed the breast, the lymph nodes from the axilla, and the pectoral muscles. This radical approach to operable tumors is no longer routinely used because results are just as good with less radical surgery combined with radiation and/or chemotherapy.

Because 70% of clients unfortunately show evidence of metastasis at diagnosis, cure is not always possible, and **palliative** surgery may be necessary. This surgery is effective in relieving symptoms in more advanced stages of cancer, although it does not alter the course of the disease. It is usually performed in an attempt to relieve complications such as obstructions or to surgically interrupt nerve pathways for intractable pain. It may also be used to insert special access devices or to place tubes for enteral nutrition.

Reconstructive surgery may follow curative or radical surgery. The goal is to reestablish function or rebuild for a better cosmetic effect. Reconstructive surgery to areas such as the head, neck, breast, and extremities can minimize deformity. The surgery may be completed all at once or done in stages.

Radiation Therapy

Radiation therapy is the second most common method of treating cancer. Radiation therapy, or **radiotherapy**, uses high-energy ionizing radiation to kill cancer. Ionizing radiation has the ability to penetrate tissue cells and deposit energy within them. This intense energy causes breakage in chromosomes within the cell, thus preventing the ability of the cell to replicate. Cell death may occur hours, days, or even years after treatment, depending on the rate of mitosis.

The goal of radiation therapy is to eradicate malignant cells without causing harm to healthy tissues. Some cells are more sensitive to radiation than others. Better vascularized, better oxygenated cells and those that divide rapidly are the most sensitive.

It is estimated that radiation therapy is used to treat more than one-half of all people with cancer, at some point during their illnesses. It may be used alone or as an adjunct to other therapies. As a single treatment modality, it is most often used when the disease is localized. Preoperative radiation is frequently used to reduce the tumor mass before surgery. Postoperative radiation therapy is frequently used to decrease the risk of local recurrence following surgery. Some chemotherapeutic drugs increase the sensitivity of cancer cells to radiation and thus are used together with radiation. Radiation therapy can be classified as curative or palliative. It is frequently used to alleviate symptoms of metastasis, such as pain.

There are two types of radiation therapy: external radiation and internal radiation.

PROFESSIONAL TIP

Drug To Enhance Radiation's Effect

The drug diamine metronidazole may enhance radiation's effects on cancer by 500 times. If clinical trials demonstrate this degree of effectiveness, radiation dose could be reduced by 60% to 70%, thereby resulting in fewer side effects from radiation. ("Researchers Say New Drug," 1998)

CLIENT TEACHING

External Radiation
- Do not wash off the skin markings used to designate reference points for treatment.
- Client is alone in the room during treatment.
- Client must lie absolutely still.
- Treatment typically lasts 1 to 3 minutes.
- Treatment is usually painless.

External Radiation

External radiation, or teletherapy, is performed with special equipment that can deliver high-energy radiation. Treatments are usually administered on an outpatient basis, divided over many days or weeks. Customized shielding blocks may be created to protect healthy tissues, and immobilization devices may be used to maintain the exact position for each treatment. Dyes or tattoos may be used to designate reference points on the skin.

Nursing care should be directed toward client teaching, safety, and carrying out interventions that provide relief from side effects. Undesirable side effects that are most likely to occur include varying degrees of skin reactions and gastrointestinal discomfort such as abdominal cramping, diarrhea, loss of appetite, and fatigue. Treatments have a cumulative effect and may thus produce symptoms after the therapy has been completed.

Internal Radiation

Internal radiation delivers radioactive isotopes directly within the body. Clients treated with internal sources of radiation can be a source of radioactivity. Isotopes may be introduced into the body by sealed or unsealed sources.

With sealed sources, radioactive elements are encapsulated in special containers such as tubes, wires, needles, seeds, or capsules. These containers are implanted close to the cancer cells in the hope that they will deliver a highly concentrated dose of radiation to the cancer cells. Radioactive implants are commonly used in the treatment of cancers of the tongue, lip, breast, vagina, cervix, endometrium, rectum, bladder, and brain.

Because sources are sealed, body fluids are not radioactive. Personnel caring for clients who have sealed sources must still be familiar with the hazards of radiation, however. Generally, the degree of exposure is dependent on three factors:

- The distance between the individual and the source (Figure 17-2)
- The amount of time an individual is exposed
- The type of shielding provided

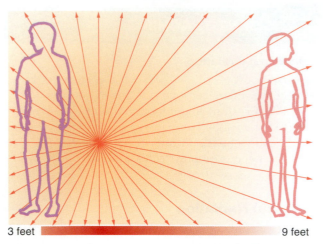

Figure 17-2 Radiation dose decreases with distance. (*Courtesy of the U.S. Nuclear Regulatory Commission*)

Safety: Internal Radiation

Client care should be modified based on the three factors related to the degree of exposure to sealed-source radiation by:

- Preparing everything outside of the room so that as little time as possible is spent close to the client;
- Having several nurses assigned to care for the client so that the time of exposure of each nurse is lessened; and
- Wearing a lead apron or other shielding device, as provided.

Radioactive isotopes can also be placed in suspensions or solutions as unsealed sources of radiation. They may be given orally or parenterally or be instilled into intrapleural or peritoneal spaces.

Some radioactive elements used in unsealed radiation sources are eliminated in body secretions, including urine and stool; thus special precautions should be taken by health care workers to avoid exposure. Agency policies and procedures as well as Standard Precautions must be followed closely. Unsealed sources are not usually radioactive as long as sealed sources are.

Chemotherapy

Chemotherapy may be used to cure, prevent, or relieve cancer symptoms. The term *chemotherapy* means using chemical therapy or drugs to treat illness, especially cancer. Drugs used in chemotherapy are called **antineoplastics** because they inhibit the growth and reproduction of malignant cells. To understand how anticancer drugs work, one must have a basic understanding of the cell cycle.

Almost all anticancer drugs kill cancer cells by affecting DNA synthesis or function, but they vary in how they exert their activity within the cell-cycle. Most chemotherapeutic drugs are classified as cell-cycle specific (CCS) or cell-cycle nonspecific (CCNS).

Cell-cycle specific drugs attack cancer cells when the cells enter a certain phase of reproduction. These agents are most effective against rapidly growing tumors. Many of the drugs are "schedule dependent" because they produce a greater cell kill when given in multiple, repeated doses.

Cell-cycle nonspecific drugs can destroy cancer cells in any phase of the cell cycle and are used for large tumors that have fewer actively dividing cells. These drugs are not schedule dependent, but, rather, dose dependent. This means that the number of cells destroyed is determined by the amount of drug given.

Anticancer agents are cytotoxic (toxic to cells) and destroy both normal and abnormal cells. They are most effective against cells that reproduce rapidly, such as those in bone marrow, gastrointestinal lining, hair follicles, and the ova and sperm. Because cells multiply at their most rapid rate at the beginning of the disease, the drugs work best against cancer in its earliest stages.

Classifications of drugs commonly used in chemotherapy include:

- Alkylating agents (CCNS): act by causing breaks in DNA strands, preventing mitosis.
- Antimetabolites (CCS): block essential enzymes necessary for DNA synthesis or become incorporated into the DNA and RNA so that a false message is transmitted.
- Antibiotics (CCNS): disrupt DNA transcription and inhibit DNA and RNA synthesis. Antitumor antibiotics are not used for infections because they are highly toxic.
- Nitrosureas (CCNS): inhibit DNA and RNA synthesis.
- Vinca alkaloids (CCS): bind to proteins during M phase, causing the cell to lose the ability to divide.
- Hormones (CCNS): alter the environment of the cell by affecting the cell membrane's permeability, thereby reducing tumor growth.
- Antihormones (CCNS): inhibit natural hormones used by hormone-dependent tumors.
- Miscellaneous agents (CCS or CCNS): act by a variety of mechanisms. (For example, L-asparaginase [Elspar] acts by inhibiting protein synthesis.)
- Corticosteroids: reduce inflammation.

Many of these drugs are given in combination with or after radiation or surgery to achieve maximum effect. They are usually given intermittently over an extended period of time. Drug resistance can occur.

The most common routes of administration are oral and intravenous. A few drugs may be given topically, subcutaneously, or intramuscularly. Recently, other methods have been introduced to increase the local concentration of the drug at the tumor site, including intrathecal injection and intracavity instillation. Table 17–4 lists some commonly used drugs.

Careful attention must be given to intravenous administration. Leakage of chemotherapeutic drugs from the vein into the surrounding tissues during infusion is called **extravasation**. Because most of these drugs are irritating to the tissues, extravasation is a potentially serious problem, especially if the drugs being administered are **vesicants**. These agents are so irritating that they can cause blistering and even necrosis. All sites must be monitored carefully. Pain, swelling, redness, and the presence of vesicles are all signs of extravasation. Additional signs include the following:

- Pain or burning at the site or along the vein
- Absent or sluggish blood return
- Redness 6 to 12 hours later
- Swelling
- Diffuse hardening

PROFESSIONAL TIP

Chemotherapy and Protective Equipment

- Because many chemotherapy drugs are carcinogenic, the nurse preparing and administering the chemotherapy must wear protective equipment.
- All personnel involved in any aspect of handling chemotherapeutic agents must receive instructions about the known risks of the drugs, the proper use of protective equipment, the applicable skill procedures, and the policies regarding pregnant personnel.

Table 17–4 DRUGS COMMONLY USED IN CHEMOTHERAPY

Antimetabolites (CCS)
cytarabine (Cytosar)
fluorouracil (Adrucil)
methotrexate (Mexate)
6-mercaptopurine (Purinethol)

Antibiotics (CCNS)
dactinomycin (Cosmegan)*
daunorubicin (Cerubidine)*
doxorubicin hydrochloride (Adriamycin)*
mitomycin (Mutamycin)*
mithramycin (Mithracin)
bleomycin (Blenoxane)

Antihormonal Agents (CCNS)
flutamide (Eulexin)
goserelin acetate (Zoladex)
tamoxifen (Nolvadex)

Vinca Plant Alkaloids (CCS)
vinblastine sulfate (Velban)*
vincristine sulfate (Oncovin)*

Hormones (CCNS)
diethylstilbestrol (DES)
megestrol acetate (Megace)
medroxyprogesterone acetate (Depo-Provera)
testosterone (Histerone, Testoderm)

Nitrosureas (CCNS)
carmustine (BiCNU)
lomustine (CeeNU)

Alkylating Agents (CCNS)
busulfan (Myleran)
chlorambucil (Leukeran)
cisplatin (Platinol)
cyclophosphamide (Cytoxan)
mechlorethamine hydrochloride
  (Mustargen)*
melphalan (Alkeran)
thiotepa (Thiotepa)

Corticosteroids
dexamethasone (Decadron)
hydrocortisone sodium succinate
  (Solu-Cortef)
prednisone (Deltasone)

Miscellaneous Agents
etoposide (VePesid)
L-asparaginase (Elspar)
procarbazine hydrochloride
  (Matulane)

Frequently Used Combinations

CMF±P	cyclophosphamide, methotrexate, 5-fluorouracil, and prednisone
CAMP	cyclophosphamide, doxorubicin (Adriamycin), methotrexate, and procarbazine
CAE	cyclophosphamide, doxorubicin (Adriamycin), and etoposide
CVP	cyclophosphamide, vincristine, and prednisone
FAC	5-fluorouracil, Adriamycin, and Cytoxan
MOPP	mechlorethamine hydrochloride (Mustargen), vincristine (Oncovin), procarbazine, and prednisone

*=vesicant drug

Figure 17-3 Explantable/Implantable Devices: A. Mini-vital port; B. Peripherally inserted central venous catheter (*Courtesy of Cook Incorporated, Bloomington, IN*)

If extravasation does occur, the drug must be stopped immediately and protocols for treatment initiated.

Chemotherapy may also be administered with explantable venous access devices (EVADs) or implantable vascular access devices (IVADs) (Figure 17-3).

Explantable devices are special catheters that may be used for short- or long-term periods. They may be inserted peripherally or centrally into the subclavian or jugular vein, and they terminate in the superior vena cava or right atrium. Long-term central venous catheters are used when a prolonged course of therapy is expected. They are surgically threaded to an exit site in the chest and are sutured in place.

Implantable devices consist of a self-sealing silicone rubber septum enclosed in a metal or plastic port that is attached to a silicone catheter. The port is implanted under the skin. The catheter is surgically threaded subcutaneously into the right atrium. The system is accessed by a needle puncture through the skin and into the port's septum.

Implantable devices are especially useful in clients who have poor quality veins or require multiple venipunctures or long-term therapy. These devices can also be used to administer blood products, total parenteral nutrition, and other medications.

Safety: Chemotherapy and Contamination

- Any personnel handling blood, vomitus, or excreta from clients who have received chemotherapy within the previous 48 hours should wear disposable latex gloves and a disposable gown.
- Place contaminated linen in specially marked laundry bags according to agency procedures.

COMMUNITY/HOME HEALTH CARE

Home Care Following Chemotherapy

Teach clients receiving chemotherapy to monitor the side effects of therapy at home.

- Inspect the skin daily for any signs of rash or dermatitis, which may signal hypersensitivity to a drug.
- Report taste loss and tingling in the face, fingers, or toes, which may signal peripheral neuropathy.
- Report signs of dizziness, headache, confusion, slurred speech, or convulsions, which may be signs of central nervous system (CNS) toxicity.
- Report signs of unusual bleeding or bruising; fever; sore throat; or mouth sores, which may signal developing myelosuppression.
- Report signs of jaundice; yellowing of the eyes; clay-colored stools; or dark urine, which may signal developing hepatic dysfunction.
- Report a continued cough or shortness of breath, which may signal developing pulmonary fibrosis.

Improved infusion techniques, control of symptoms such as nausea and vomiting, and cost-containment restrictions have reduced the length of hospitalizations for clients undergoing chemotherapy. Teaching clients and family members to monitor side effects in the home setting is thus an essential function of the **oncology** (study of tumors) nurse. Some important points to emphasize are outlined in the accompanying display.

Clients should also be advised that lifestyle may need to be adjusted to accommodate the side effects of chemotherapy. Clients should be instructed to pace themselves according to their energy levels and allow time for rest throughout the day. It is also important to inform clients that even between treatments they may not have the same amount of energy as before the initiation of treatment. Whereas many clients do not experience any adverse effects, others experience life-threatening toxicity. Nursing care of the client receiving chemotherapy requires not only a thorough understanding of the drugs used to destroy the cancer,

PROFESSIONAL TIP

Drugs to Eradicate Cancer

A combination of the drugs angiostatin and endostatin cuts off the blood supply to all forms of cancer in mice. Clinical trials in humans are to begin soon (Noonan, 1998).

but also skills in helping clients and families cope with the side effects of the therapy.

Biotherapy

Biotherapy is performed with **biologic response modifiers** (BRMs), which are agents that stimulate the body's natural immune system to control and destroy malignant cells. Most BRMs are still being evaluated in trial studies. Biotherapy is used after surgery, radiation, and chemotherapy have removed the bulk of the tumor. Some agents currently being investigated include interferons, monoclonal antibodies, interleukin-2, tumor necrosis factor, *bacillus Calmette-Guérin* (BCG), and colony-stimulating factors. Side effects are usually less severe than those seen in chemotherapy and may include fever, malaise, myalgia, and headache. Because an anaphylactic reaction can occur, the client must be closely monitored.

Bone Marrow Transplantation

Bone marrow transplantation (BMT) is used for cancers that respond to high doses of chemotherapy or radiation therapy. Treatment involves aspirating and storing a fraction of bone marrow, exposing the client to high-dose drug therapy or total body irradiation, and then reinfusing the bone marrow after the treatment is complete.

The bone marrow used in transplantation can be the client's own marrow (autologous), marrow taken from an identical twin (syngeneic), or marrow taken from a histocompatibly matched donor, preferably a sibling (allogeneic).

According to Otto (1997), the cost of BMT is high. Client expenses may range from $100,000 to $200,000 unless covered or partially covered by insurance. The average length of hospital stay is 35 to 40 days. Complications can be life threatening and include infection, bleeding, gastrointestinal effects, renal insufficiency, veno-occlusive disease (deposits of fibrin obstruct venules of liver), and graft-versus-host disease (new bone marrow cells recognize environment as foreign and try to destroy the host). Clients who undergo autologous BMT do not experience graft-versus-host disease.

SYMPTOM MANAGEMENT

Cancer clients undergoing treatment experience a variety of secondary problems. One of the most important responsibilities of the oncology nurse is to formulate nursing interventions to manage these problems.

Bone Marrow Dysfunction

Cancer treatments kill both malignant cells and normal cells in bone marrow. Blood counts should thus be monitored carefully during and after treatment.

A low white-cell count increases the risk of infec-tion. A decreased neutrophil count (below 500/mm³), is an indicator that special infection prevention measures should be initiated. Scrupulous handwashing is the most effective method of controlling bacterial infection. Personnel should maintain strict asepsis when changing dressings or performing invasive procedures. Clients should avoid contact with anyone who is ill. Antimicrobial soaps should be used for bathing clients. The skin and mucous membranes should be inspected daily for signs of infection. Vital signs should be taken every 4 hours, and the client observed for fever and chilling.

Clients with a platelet count below 50,000/mm³ should be monitored for bleeding. Their skin should be inspected daily for bruises or petechiae. Shaving should be done with an electric razor to minimize the chance of cutting the skin. Stool and urine should be monitored for occult blood. The nurse should observe the client for bleeding from the vagina, rectum, nose, mouth, and venipuncture sites. If bleeding does occur, pressure should be applied to the site for 5 minutes. Any bleeding that does not stop in 5 minutes should be reported. A soft toothbrush may be recommended for oral care. Aspirin or any medication containing acetylsalicylic acid should not be given.

Nutritional Alterations

Blackburn (1998) describes cytokines, substances that are secreted by the tumor in an attempt to cannibalize the body and by the immune system to fight the tumor. Cytokines make the body digest muscle for energy instead of using stored fat for this purpose. This state of malnutrition and protein (muscle) wasting is called **cachexia**. It occurs in conjunction with lung, pancreatic, stomach, bowel, and prostate cancers but rarely with breast cancer.

In some cases, untreated cachexia, rather than the cancer itself, is the cause of death. Untreated cachexia also can decrease the effectiveness of cancer treatments and may increase the side effects of these treatments. Treating cachexia with drugs has met with little success. Some drugs such as megesterol acetate (Megace) improve appetite but do not add muscle mass.

Blackburn (1998) suggests that nurses can help the cachexic client find a registered dietitian who understands cancer cachexia and can identify appetizing foods that are nutrient and calorie dense. Foods that appeal to the client should be eaten anytime. The use of liquid nutritional supplements and a multivitamin is often recommended (Wilkes, 2000).

Hallmarks of malnutrition are a weight loss of 10% or more or a serum albumin level below 3.4 g/dL. Clients unable to maintain sufficient oral intake for long periods of time may be given enteral or total parenteral nutrition (TPN). Nutritional problems associated with cachexia include anorexia, nausea and vomiting,

CLIENT TEACHING

Increasing Nutritional Intake
- Drink 4 ounces of a nutritional supplement before breakfast.
- Eat breakfast (if desired), then take a walk. Doing so will help to build muscle and increase appetite.
- Drink another 4 ounces of nutritional supplement 1 hour before having a lunch consisting of whatever foods are appealing.
- Have another 4 ounces of nutritional supplement at mid-afternoon and at bedtime.
- If not hungry for dinner, take another walk.

altered taste sensation, mucosal inflammation, and dysphagia.

Anorexia

Anorexia, or loss of appetite, is a common complaint among individuals with cancer. It is generally best for these clients to eat small, frequent, high-calorie (carbohydrate and fat-rich) meals. Nurses should try to ascertain the client's likes and dislikes. Highly seasoned foods help increase taste. Clients should be encouraged to eat when they are feeling best. Weight should be monitored weekly.

Nausea and Vomiting

Nausea and vomiting usually occur within 3 to 4 hours after chemotherapy is administered and may last up to 72 hours. According to Held-Warmkessel (1998), antiemetics should be given before chemotherapy and continued afterward as needed (Table 17–5). Small, frequent feedings of complex carbohydrates may be beneficial. Liquids should be given 30 to 60 minutes before meals. Although highly seasoned foods may increase taste, they often also increase nausea and vomiting. Cool, bland foods are more easily tolerated. Foods with strong odors should be avoided. Frequent mouth care can help remove the taste of chemotherapy and thus increase the likelihood of the client's wanting to eat. The client should be monitored for dehydration and electrolyte imbalances.

CLIENT TEACHING

Enhancing Taste Sensation
- Tart food usually enhances taste sensation.
- Many foods taste better if they are cold or at room temperature.
- Using plastic utensils reduces metallic taste.

Table 17–5 COMMONLY USED ANTIEMETICS

prochlorperazine (Compazine)
metoclopramide (Reglan)
trimethobenzamide hydrochloride (Tigan)
ondansetron hydrochloride (Zofron)
lorazepam (Ativan)

Altered Taste Sensation

Taste sensation can be altered because cancer cells release substances that stimulate bitter taste buds, causing a bitter or metallic taste in the mouths of some clients. Some find they no longer enjoy the taste of red meat and others say they have an aversion to sweets.

Mucosal Inflammation

Stomatitis, or inflammation of the mucous membrane of the oral cavity, occurs in one-half of cancer clients receiving treatment. It usually occurs 7 to 14 days after chemotherapy administration and lasts 2 to 3 weeks. To minimize stomatitis, assess for early signs and symptoms such as edema, ulceration, erythema, excessive saliva, and infection. If the client is receiving a chemotherapy drug that is known to cause stomatitis (methotrexate, for example) oral care should be administered at least 4 times a day.

Rough, chewy foods and acidic foods should be avoided. Straws are beneficial because food can be taken in the back of the mouth and swallowed. Popsicles and frozen fruit bars sometimes help numb and lessen pain. Commercial mouthwashes containing alcohol should be avoided. A saline rinse may be helpful after meals. If the client has dentures, they should be removed at night. Viscous Xylocaine rinses can be ordered for pain. Lemon and glycerine swabs should not be used because lemon may be irritating to mouth lesions.

PROFESSIONAL TIP

Mucosal Inflammation
- The condition of the client's mouth provides a clue to the appearance and integrity of other areas of the gastrointestinal tract because mucosal inflammation caused by cancer treatments affects all mucosa.
- Mucositis (inflammation of the mucous membrane) in the esophagus, also called esophagitis, may cause painful swallowing.
- In female clients, mucosal inflammation may be found in the vagina, causing pain, itching, and discharge.

CLIENT TEACHING

Stomatitis
- Use soft bristle toothbrush.
- Avoid flossing if bleeding or discomfort occurs.
- Avoid tobacco products and alcohol because of their drying effects.

Dysphagia

Dysphagia, or difficulty in swallowing, often occurs in clients with esophageal cancers, or in those receiving radiotherapy.

Artificial saliva may be ordered for severe dryness. A softer diet along with nutritional supplements may be prescribed. Dry foods such as toast can scratch the delicate tissues of the throat. Food pureed in a blender may be easier to tolerate. Clients should take plenty of time to chew and swallow.

Pain

Approximately 60% to 90% of all individuals with progressive malignancy will experience pain. The pain may be acute, but it is more likely to be chronic (greater than 3 months in duration). Pain usually does not occur until the advanced stages of the disease. The most common causes of pain are metastatic bone disease, venous or lymphatic obstruction, or nerve compression.

Pain can have profound effects on a cancer client, possibly causing anxiety, depression, and feelings of helplessness in addition to physical discomfort. It can affect the client's sleeping habits, eating patterns, work, family, and social relationships. Ultimately, pain can affect the client's quality of life.

Noninvasive pain-relief techniques may be useful in pain management. They include cutaneous stimulation (heat, cold, massage), transcutaneous electrical nerve stimulation (TENS), relaxation techniques, imagery, and hypnosis. Most of these techniques are inexpensive and easy to perform. They have few side effects and can usually be done in any environment. They also give the client some control over the treatment of pain. Although not every client will respond successfully to these measures, it is worthwhile to attempt them before using invasive techniques.

The federal government has taken steps toward ensuring that cancer pain can be treated. The Agency for Health Care Policy and Research (AHCPR, 1994) has developed Cancer Pain Guidelines for clients, family members, and health care professionals. Some points emphasized by the guidelines include the following:

- Cancer pain can be managed effectively through relatively simple means in up to 90% of cancer clients in the United States. Skin patches, slow-release tablets, and client-controlled pumps are now available to complement standard drugs.
- The mainstay of pain assessment is the client self-report. Because there is no standard test for pain, the nurse must respect the client's report of pain and regard it as the single most reliable indicator. Kohr (1995) recommends using both a verbal assessment measurement tool based on a scale from 0 to 5, where each number represents a precise description of pain; and a pain intensity flow sheet. For example:

  0 no pain
  1 mild pain
  2 moderate pain or discomfort
  3 severe or distressing pain
  4 horrible or incapacitating pain
  5 excruciating or unbearable pain

- The simplest dosage schedules and least invasive pain management modalities should be used first. Nonopioids are the first step in the analgesic ladder. They should be tried first for mild to moderate pain. Because much of cancer pain is due to inflammation, many of the nonopioids used are potent, anti-inflammatory drugs. These drugs are helpful in pain relief because they inhibit the release of prostaglandins, which cause pain, edema, and inflammation.
- Morphine is the most commonly used opioid for moderate to severe pain because it is available in a wide variety of dosage forms, it has well-characterized pharmacokinetics and pharmacodynamics, and it is relatively low in cost. Morphine can be given orally, subcutaneously, intramuscularly, intravenously, rectally, and intraspinally. It can also be given in sustained-release preparations. Because needs vary with cancer pain, there is no limit to the dosing of morphine.
- Health care providers should work to prevent pain in the first place rather than try to treat pain after it has occurred. Analgesics work better when given regularly around the clock before pain becomes severe. A major nursing responsibility is to teach the client to request pain medication before the pain becomes severe. When medication is ordered

PROFESSIONAL TIP

Inadequate Pain Control in the Cancer Client
A major reason given for inadequate pain control in the cancer client is the fear of inducing respiratory depression. This, however, is a rare occurrence in the cancer client.

around the clock, the nurse should not hesitate to wake the client to administer analgesics.

If pain control cannot be achieved with noninvasive techniques or medications, neurosurgical procedures such as nerve blocks may be performed.

Fatigue

Fatigue occurs as a direct result of cancer treatment or because of anemia, chronic pain, stress, depression, insufficient rest, or inadequate nutritional intake. Although the etiology is not well understood, fatigue is often related to the effects of the tumor itself (Greifzu, 1998). Fatigue may contribute to client non-compliance with the treatment regimen.

Frequent rest periods should be provided for the client. The nurse should assess for the presence and pattern of fatigue. Proper planning allows for the client to be active during times when energy levels are higher, which may in turn restore a greater sense of control. The nurse should evaluate factors that increase or decrease fatigue, such as nutritional intake. Blood count should be monitored for anemia.

Alopecia

Alopecia, the thinning or loss of hair, may be induced by chemotherapy or radiation treatments. The extent of hair loss depends on the dose and duration of the therapy. Scalp hair is most commonly affected, but pubic, axillary, and facial hair, even eyebrows and eyelashes, may also be affected. The treatments cause hair loss by interfering with the growth processes in the hair follicle. This results in weakening of the hair shaft, thereby causing the hair to break off at the surface of the scalp. Hair loss usually begins 2 to 3 weeks after the initial treatment. Drug induced alopecia is not permanent. Hair usually begins to grow back within 8 weeks after treatment is completed. The color and consistency of the hair may change.

CLIENT TEACHING

Alopecia, Threat to Body Image

Encourage client to:

- Buy a wig or hairpiece before treatment actually begins so that it will match the client's normal hair;
- Wear hats, scarves, or bandanas to cope with the change in body image due to hair loss; and
- Focus on other positive aspects rather than on just physical appearance.

Odors

Unpleasant odors emanating from the cancer client may be a source of embarrassment. These odors are usually associated with drainage, exudates, or incontinence. Fortunately, meticulous nursing care can eliminate most offending odors. Soiled linens, drainage pads, and dressings should be changed immediately and washed or discarded. The client's skin should be washed gently with soap and warm water. Protective creams may be used if the areas are not receiving radiation. Room deodorizers can be helpful but should be used cautiously as many clients experience nausea when exposed to the odors from room fresheners. Placing a drop of oil of wintergreen or oil of cloves on a cotton ball near the ventilation system can sometimes lend a light freshness to the environment.

Dyspnea

One-half of all clients with terminal cancer experience dyspnea, or difficulty in breathing. Possible causes include fluid development in the chest, infection such as pneumonia, fibrosis due to radiation, and anemia. Lungs should be auscultated every 4 hours. Oxygen may be ordered. Fluid may be drained by an invasive procedure called a thoracentesis. High-Fowler positioning helps maximize ventilation. The nurse should plan care to keep activity to a minimum so as to balance oxygen requirements and oxygen supply. Oxygen status can be monitored with a pulse oximeter. The nurse should report a sustained reading of less than 90%. The nurse should avoid pulling the privacy curtain or shutting the client's door unless absolutely necessary, because either of these actions may reduce air flow and create more anxiety.

Bowel Dysfunctions

Cancer clients frequently exhibit changes in bowel patterns. Constipation, diarrhea and subsequent perineal skin breakdown, and bowel obstructions are common elimination disorders.

Constipation results from decreased motility of the colon. It is frequently caused by chemotherapy, opioid analgesic, or inactivity. Nurses should monitor and record the frequency of the client's bowel movements. Constipation can be an early sign of vincristine toxicity. Fluid consumption may be encouraged and a stool softener given daily. Clients at risk for constipation should be started on a high-fiber diet, with increased intake of bran and prune juice.

Common causes of diarrhea include radiation therapy, chemotherapy, antibiotics, tube feedings, hyperosmolar dietary supplements, stress, and fecal impactions. Clients can develop fluid and electrolyte imbalances from constant diarrhea. If the client is receiving a chemotherapy drug known to cause diarrhea (such as fluorouracil [Adrucil] or doxorubicin hydrochloride

[Adriamycin]), a low-residue and lactose-free diet should be encouraged. The nurse should instruct the client to avoid foods that stimulate the gastrointestinal tract, such as warm liquids and coffee.

Bananas (which are high in potassium) and sports drinks (which contain sodium and potassium) can help replace lost fluids and electrolytes without irritating the gastrointestinal tract.

The perineum should be kept clean and dry after each loose stool. Anal irritations should be treated cautiously with agents such as heat lamps, ointments, and cornstarch, although these may be contraindicated in clients receiving radiation therapy. Signs of fluid and electrolyte imbalances such as thirst, dry mucous membranes, and decreased skin turgor, should be noted. The potassium level should be monitored. The nurse should measure and record the amount, frequency, and characteristics of all client bowel movements. Antidiarrheal medications such as Lomotil or Imodium should be given for every loose stool. Sitz baths will help soothe sore or broken-down tissues.

Bowel obstructions occur more commonly in conjunction with advanced abdominal malignancies and should always be suspected if the client has received radiation or has adhesions from prior surgeries. Symptoms include nausea, vomiting, and abdominal pain. Surgery may be required to relieve the obstruction.

Pathological Fractures

Pathological fractures are a major problem in cancers that metastasize to bone. These cancers weaken the bone to the point that normal activities can cause painful breaks. Thus, limbs should be supported and handled gently and extreme care should be taken when moving clients. Special devices such as splints may be used for extra protection. Weight-bearing restrictions may be ordered.

Ascites

Abdominal cancers may cause ascites, or fluid accumulation in the abdomen. Clients may experience abdominal swelling and difficult breathing. Symptoms may be treated temporarily with an invasive procedure called a paracentesis, wherein a small, plastic tube is advanced through the abdominal wall and excess fluid is withdrawn. Chemotherapy drugs sometimes are instilled in an attempt to prevent the fluid from returning. The nurse should visually assess the abdomen. A protruding abdomen may be indicative of ascites as well as intestinal distention and enlarged organs. Abdominal girth at the umbilicus should be measured daily with a tape measure to monitor changes. The abdomen should then be auscultated in all four quadrants. Gurgling bowel sounds heard every 5 to 15 seconds indicate normal peristalsis. Decreased or absent bowel sounds may indicate peritonitis or paralytic ileus. Fluid accumulation can be confirmed by percussing for shifting dullness. When a large amount of fluid is present, the nurse may see fluid waves. Gentle palpation is used to detect pain and tenderness as well as abdominal masses. The nurse should carefully document any abnormal findings.

The nurse should weigh the client daily to monitor weight gain. Fluid consumption may be restricted. Good skin care, especially to the abdomen, is essential. Fowler positioning helps maximize ventilation. Clients should be observed closely for electrolyte imbalance if large amounts of fluids are withdrawn via paracentesis.

Sexual Alterations

Many chemotherapy drugs can interfere with sexual functioning and reproduction. Premenopausal women may become infertile. Those under age 35 may regain their fertility after therapy is completed. Men may experience impotence, decreased libido, interrupted sperm production, and ejaculation problems. Women may experience vaginal dryness.

The nurse should encourage clients and their partners to express their feelings and concerns to each other and to explore other avenues of sexual expression, such as cuddling, kissing, and stroking. Birth control should be practiced during therapy and for 1 or 2 years after therapy (depending on physician recommendation) to ensure that all chemotherapy drugs have been eliminated and, thus, will have no ill effects on a pregnancy.

MEDICAL EMERGENCIES

Medical emergencies occur in approximately 20% of clients with advanced-stage cancer. Early recognition and treatment can prevent irreversible complications and improve the quality of life. Four complications with which nurses should become familiar are hypercalcemia, spinal cord compression, superior vena cava syndrome, and cardiac tamponade.

HYPERCALCEMIA

Hypercalcemia occurs commonly and can be a potentially fatal complication if not detected early. It is found most often in clients with malignant tumors that have metastasized to bone, such as breast cancer tumors. The condition occurs when the serum calcium level rises higher than 10.5 mg/dL. Hypercalcemia often signals the final stages of cancer (Clayton, 1997).

Early symptoms of hypercalcemia, such as nausea, vomiting, constipation, and weakness, may be overlooked because these are common side effects of many cancer therapies. Later symptoms such as dehydration, renal failure, coma, and cardiac arrest may develop swiftly.

Hypercalcemia is treated aggressively with intravenous normal saline and furosemide (Lasix), which increase calcium excretion. Clients may also be given drugs to decrease bone reabsorption. Serum calcium level should be monitored when Lasix is being administered. Clients should be taught early symptoms of hypercalcemia so that they can recognize a recurrence. These clients are also at increased risk for pathological fractures because calcium has been released from the bones, leaving them very fragile.

SPINAL CORD COMPRESSION

Spinal cord compression can result in permanent paralysis if not treated promptly. Cancer of the lung, breast, and prostate carry the greatest risk of metastasizing to the spinal cord.

The chief symptom of metastasis to the spinal cord is back pain. The discomfort is aggravated by lying down, coughing, or moving, and may be relieved by sitting upright.

Treatment is aimed at reducing tumor size to decrease pressure on the spinal cord. Radiation, surgery, and steroid therapy may be initiated. Pain medications should be given frequently, and clients should be supported carefully during transfers.

SUPERIOR VENA CAVA SYNDROME

Superior vena cava syndrome is a collection of symptoms caused by an obstruction of the superior vena cava. It occurs more frequently in conjunction with lung cancer and lymphomas. Typically, clients experience dyspnea and swelling of the face and neck. Edema in the upper extremities, chest pain, and coughing are other possible symptoms. Central nervous system symptoms such as headache, visual disturbances, and alteration in consciousness rarely occur.

The goal of treatment is to reduce tumor size. Radiation along with diuretics is usually ordered. The nurse should administer oxygen as ordered and provide a calm, restful environment. The client should be encouraged to limit activities and lie in Fowler's position. Respirations should be carefully monitored, and lower extremities should not be elevated, as doing so will increase venous return to an already engorged area.

CARDIAC TAMPONADE

Cardiac tamponade is caused by the formation of pericardial fluid, which reduces cardiac output by compressing the heart. Tumor metastasis to the pericardium is associated with lung cancer, breast cancer, Hodgkin's disease, lymphoma, melanoma, gastrointestinal tumors, and sarcoma. Common symptoms of cardiac tamponade include a rapid, weak pulse; distended neck veins during inspiration; ankle or sacral edema; pleural effusion; ascites; enlarged spleen; lethargy; and altered consciousness.

Treatment is aimed at aspirating the fluid constricting the heart (pericardiocentesis). The nurse should reassure the client, explain the procedure, and administer medication for pain.

PSYCHOSOCIAL ALTERATIONS

Perhaps of all the problems that clients with cancer experience, none is more challenging than the associated psychosocial alterations. The mere diagnosis of cancer invokes fear and misunderstanding. A myriad of emotions may surface initially. These may range from deep depression to denial and total refusal of treatment. Anxiety, sadness, and withdrawal are common. Some clients may feel that the disease is a punishment for some misguided deed. Every client will respond differently to the diagnosis, depending on individual coping mechanisms and support systems.

Research has identified effective and ineffective coping mechanisms. Clients who seek information or share feelings tend to cope more effectively than do those who submit to treatment and procedures without asking questions or who use small talk to avoid discussing threatening issues.

Cancer affects not only the client, but the client's family as well. Responses of family members to the disease will have a significant impact on the client's coping. The client and family must face issues such as loss of control, changes in body image, and financial burdens.

The nurse has several roles in this context. The client needs time and space to adjust to the diagnosis. Nurses should be available to offer support and reassurance. They should answer questions but not bombard the client with information. They may interpret information given by the physician and may help the client formulate questions to ask the physician. The nurse should also encourage the client to express feelings and fears about the illness.

The initial treatment is very frightening for most cancer clients, many of whom have heard the myth that "the treatment is worse than the cure." Nurses can allay anxiety by giving information about the treatment's purpose; adverse reactions; and signs and symptoms to report to the physician. Explaining procedures and answering questions in simple language can help the client and family regain a feeling of some control. Treatment modalities cause many discomforts, but if the client knows what to expect, the distress can generally be handled. Symptom management is critical in preventing lifestyle disruptions.

COMMUNITY/HOME HEALTH CARE

Psychosocial Aspects of Cancer

- Clients may see themselves as burdens to their families.
- Family caregivers may be angry that their own needs must go unmet.
- Family caregivers may feel inadequate with regard to caring for the client.
- Medical equipment such as a hospital bed, commode chair, or wheelchair may need to be brought into the home. These may have an impact on family member state of mind and disposition with regard to the family member with cancer.

Families and clients facing the terminal phase of cancer are confronted with a complex set of problems. The client and family must face separation and impending death. Some families will demand that extraordinary measures be taken to keep the client alive. Some will search for meaning in life and will experience a genuine closeness. Nurses should give the client and family privacy and time to share feelings. Sometimes, the only psychosocial support the client needs is to have someone sitting by the bedside. Touch, especially at times when words are hard to find, can often be the most comforting intervention.

As the client's condition deteriorates, physical needs become more pronounced. The nurse should focus on keeping the client comfortable and free of pain. Hospice care is designed to provide spiritual, emotional, and physical support during the final days of illness. The goal of hospice is to keep the client as comfortable as possible. Pain relief and symptom management are stressed. The focus is shifted from cure to care. Care may be given in an institution, but most hospice care is given in the home. Hospice care is medically managed and nurse coordinated. Members of the hospice team typically include a chaplain, physician, nurse, social worker, physical therapist, and home health aide, as well as various volunteers. The team functions to ensure that the client's plan of care is carried out and that family members receive adequate support. The family is instructed in the area of care to be given. Bereavement counseling is offered to help family members deal with their loss.

▶ NURSING PROCESS

▶ Assessment

▶ Subjective Data

The client interview serves as a forum for ascertaining the client's perception of the illness, treatment, and prognosis; health practices; and health concerns. The client's significant other may also be interviewed to ascertain support systems.

▶ Objective Data

Vital signs are measured, and a head-to-toe assessment is performed. Past hospital records are reviewed along with the current record. Laboratory reports, biopsy results, treatment modalities, and comments from other health care professionals are studied.

Nursing diagnoses for a client with cancer may include the following:

Nursing Diagnoses	Planning/Goals	Nursing Interventions
▶ *Fear related to cancer diagnosis*	The client will express anxieties and fears to family and/or health care providers.	Review the client's previous experience with cancer to ascertain any current misconceptions based on past beliefs.
		Encourage the client to share feelings regarding the diagnosis to facilitate identification of coping strategies.
		Explain hospital routines and focus on the recommended treatment, including its purpose and potential side effects. Accurate descriptions that convey what the client can expect help ease fears associated with the unknown. A calm, reassuring environment can also enhance coping abilities.
▶ *Anticipatory Grieving related to potential loss of body function*	The client will express grief to family and/or health care providers.	Open, honest discussions can help the client cope with the situation. Be aware that mood swings, hostility, and other negative behaviors often occur. Discuss the loss of body function with the client. Ask what the loss of body function means to the client.
		Encourage the client to seek help and support from close family members.

continues

Nursing Diagnoses	Planning/Goals	Nursing Interventions
▶ *Imbalanced Nutrition: Less than body requirements related to side effects of chemotherapy*	The client will maintain body weight.	Encourage the client to eat a high-calorie, nutrient-rich diet. Supplements may be useful. Some clients may benefit from frequent, small meals and snacks. Foods high in protein, such as cheese, fish, and poultry, are also recommended.
		Provide oral hygiene before and after meals so foods will taste better.
		Administer antiemetics approximately 30 minutes before meals. Mints, hard candies, and saltine crackers may help if the client complains of metallic taste.
		Nondietary interventions may include varying the surroundings, using small plates, eating at a table with friends, and minimizing food odors.
		Monitor intake and output along with daily weight to assess nutritional status.
▶ *Risk for Impaired Skin Integrity related to chemotherapy and radiation*	The client will maintain skin integrity.	Assess skin frequently for side effects of cancer therapy. (A reddening or tanning effect may develop with radiation. Skin reactions such as rashes, pruritus, and alopecia develop with chemotherapy.)
		Use lukewarm water and soap to gently wash the client's skin. Skin often becomes sensitive during radiation treatments.
▶ *Risk for Infection related to side effects of chemotherapy*	The client will remain free of infection.	Monitor vital signs at least every shift. White blood count should be monitored and protective isolation should be instituted if the count falls below $500/mm^3$.
		Educate the client, staff, and visitors in all aspects of infection prophylaxis. Thorough handwashing is the most important means of preventing and controlling the transmission of organisms. Because fresh flowers and raw fruits and vegetables can transmit microbes, they should be eliminated. The client should not be exposed to anyone who has an infection or who has been recently vaccinated against or exposed to a communicable disease. Visitors should be limited.
▶ *Risk for Injury related to altered clotting factors secondary to side effects of chemotherapy*	The client will remain free of injury related to bleeding.	Every shift, assess the client for signs of bleeding (petechiae, ecchymoses, hematomas, bleeding gums, epistaxis, tarry stools, hematuria, frank or prolonged bleeding from puncture sites) because transfusions may be indicated.
		Monitor platelet count, which is an indicator of clotting ability. Institute special precautions if the count falls below $50,000/mm^3$.
		Apply pressure to all puncture sites for 3 to 5 minutes. Doing so prevents prolonged bleeding, which can cause damage to underlying tissues such as nerves.
		Instruct the client to use a soft toothbrush or sponge for oral hygiene to prevent damage to oral mucosa, which is particularly susceptible to bleeding. Instruct the client to use an electric razor when shaving.
▶ *Fatigue related to analgesics, anemia, stress, increased metabolism, and chemotherapy*	The client will experience less fatigue.	Plan frequent rest periods for the client to restore energy, and schedule activities when the client has the most energy.
		Monitor nutritional intake, as adequate nutrients are necessary to meet energy needs.
		Recognize that weakness places the client at increased risk for injury. Because fatigue may make activities of daily living difficult to complete, assistance may need to be provided.

Evaluation Each goal must be evaluated to determine how it has been met by the client.

SAMPLE NURSING CARE PLAN

THE CLIENT WITH LUNG CANCER

Mr. Sanez is a 54-year-old carpenter. He is admitted with pain over his left scapula and radiating to his left arm. He describes having dyspnea and admits that he does have a productive cough. He denies any recent weight loss but does acknowledge experiencing extreme fatigue for the last 2 months. Mr. Sanez has been a chronic smoker for 20 years. A chest x-ray reveals an area of density in the left lung. A needle biopsy confirms small-cell lung cancer. A computerized tomography (CT) scan confirms extrathoracic involvement. His physician referred Mr. Sanez to an oncologist for palliative chemotherapy. Mr. Sanez is to receive his first treatment of cisplatin (Platinol) and etoposide (VePesid). Mr. Sanez states that he is not sure about this treatment given that it will not cure him and he does not know how he will keep breathing. He has never before been hospitalized.

Nursing Diagnosis 1 *Anxiety related to unfamiliar surroundings and uncertainty regarding change in health status as evidenced by Mr. Sanez's statement that he does not know how he will keep breathing and the fact that he has never before been hospitalized*

PLANNING/GOALS	NURSING INTERVENTIONS	RATIONALE	EVALUATION
Mr. Sanez will share his feelings regarding his dyspnea.	Ascertain what the physician has told Mr. Sanez and what conclusions Mr. Sanez has reached. Encourage Mr. Sanez to share his feelings concerning cancer.	Accurate description of the treatment regimen can help decrease fear of the unknown. Verbalization can identify the source of any misconception that is serving to increase anxiety.	Mr. Sanez shares his feelings about his diagnosis and treatment regimen.
Mr. Sanez will express less anxiety about being in the hospital.	Maintain frequent contact with Mr. Sanez. Explain the hospital routine and what Mr. Sanez should anticipate in terms of his care.	Maintenance of contact helps to reassure Mr. Sanez that he is not alone. An unfamiliar environment increases anxiety.	Mr. Sanez exhibits less anxiety about the change in his health status and being in the hospital.

Nursing Diagnosis 2 *Impaired Gas Exchange related to decreased lung capacity and increased secretions as evidenced by dyspnea, productive cough, and dense area in left lung*

PLANNING/GOALS	NURSING INTERVENTIONS	RATIONALE	EVALUATION
Mr. Sanez will report less dyspnea with oxygen saturation > 90%.	Monitor pulmonary status by ascultating breath sounds; checking rate, depth, and pattern of respirations; evaluating skin color for cyanosis; and monitoring pulse oximetry.	Provides information regarding pulmonary status changes indicating either improvement or onset of complications.	Adequate ventilation with oxygen saturation > 90% is maintained.
	Position Mr. Sanez in Fowler's position.	Promotes expansion of lungs and respiratory muscles.	

continues

Administer oxygen at prescribed level.	Supplemental oxygen corrects hypoxemia and provides oxygen for metabolic needs.
Administer opioids with caution.	Opioids can depress the respiratory center.
Monitor amount, color, and consistency of sputum.	Changes in sputum suggest infection or change in pulmonary status.
Plan care and treatments within Mr. Sanez's tolerance.	Oxygen demands increase with activity.

Nursing Diagnosis 3 *Acute Pain related to tumor growth and tissue destruction as evidenced by verbal report of pain over left scapula radiating to left arm*

PLANNING/GOALS	NURSING INTERVENTIONS	RATIONALE	EVALUATION
Mr. Sanez will report less pain following pain-relief measures.	Provide routine comfort measures such as repositioning and backrub.	Noninvasive pain-relief techniques may be helpful in pain management.	Mr. Sanez reports less pain; < 4 on a scale of 0 to 10.
	Teach Mr. Sanez to request pain medication prior to onset of severe pain.	To keep pain under control, medication should be administered as soon as pain begins.	
	Have Mr. Sanez rate pain on a scale of 0 to 10 (0 = no pain and 10 = worst pain).	The scale provides a method of evaluating the subjective experience of pain.	
	Teach Mr. Sanez relaxation techniques.	Relaxation may decrease the perception of pain.	
	Document Mr. Sanez's response to the pain-control regimen and adjust as needed.	Ongoing assessment of the effectiveness of pain-relief techniques is essential for optimal comfort.	

Nursing Diagnosis 4 *Fatigue related to chronic pain and dyspnea as evidenced by client's description of dyspnea and extreme fatigue for 2 months*

PLANNING/GOALS	NURSING INTERVENTIONS	RATIONALE	EVALUATION
Mr. Sanez will report feeling less fatigued.	Plan care to allow for rest periods.	Frequent rest periods help conserve energy.	Mr. Santez exhibits less fatigue in light of having frequent rest periods daily.
	Assess for related factors such as nutritional imbalances, lack of sleep, and causes of stress.	Identification of contributing factors may reduce fatigue.	

continues

	Have Mr. Sanez rate fatigue on a scale of 0 to 10 (0 = not tired, 10 = total exhaustion) throughout a 24 hour period.	Identifies peak energy and exhaustion times and plan activities to minimize energy output.	
	Teach energy-conservation strategies such as planning ahead, setting priorities, scheduling rest periods, and resting before a difficult task.	Conserving energy will decrease physical and psychological stress.	

Nursing Diagnosis 5 *Anticipatory Grieving related to loss of body function as evidenced by Mr. Sanez's statement that he does not know how he will keep breathing*

PLANNING/GOALS	NURSING INTERVENTIONS	RATIONALE	EVALUATION
Mr. Sanez will verbalize his loss and develop coping skills as he acknowledges his illness as terminal.	Provide opportunities for Mr. Sanez to express his feelings.	Such information helps the nurse detect Mr. Sanez's coping strategies for moving through the stages of grief.	Mr. Sanez comes to terms with the reality of his diagnosis and prognosis.
	Answer all of Mr. Sanez's questions honestly.	Open, honest discussions can help Mr. Sanez cope with the situation.	
	Encourage Mr. Sanez's participation in his care.	Gives Mr. Sanez a greater sense of control over his life.	
	Encourage family support and visits from friends.	Assures Mr. Sanez that he is not alone and provides time to discuss concerns openly.	
	Utilize appropriate referrals to professionals such as clergy, as needed.	Facilitates the grief process and spiritual care.	

CASE STUDY

Mr. John Dalton is a 70-year-old male with a history of cancer of the prostate, which was treated with palliative hormones and radiation. His admitting diagnosis is adenocarcinoma of the prostate with widespread bone metastasis. Mr. Dalton is married and has one grown daughter, who often helps with his care. His chief complaint is severe back pain. The physician has ordered intrathecal morphine sulfate and aspirin 10 gr for pain relief.

continues

CASE STUDY continued

The following questions will guide your development of a nursing care plan for the case study.

1. List symptoms typically seen in clients diagnosed with prostate cancer.
2. Identify the population most at risk for developing prostate cancer.
3. List three possible risk factors for prostate cancer.
4. Discuss why the physician's orders include aspirin along with morphine sulfate.
5. Discuss why benzodiazepines should not be used for pain relief.
6. List the subjective and objective data the nurse would want to obtain.
7. When you walk into Mr. Dalton's room he greets you with a smile and continues talking and joking with his daughter. While assessing him, you note that his vital signs are normal. You ask him to rate his pain on a scale of 0 to 10. He pauses to think about it, then rates the pain at 8. In the chart, you must record your nursing assessment by circling the appropriate number on the scale. Which number do you think you should circle?
8. Write three individualized nursing diagnoses and goals for Mr. Dalton.
9. Discuss which oncological emergency Mr. Dalton is most likely to develop.

SUMMARY

- Cancer is the second most common cause of death in the United States.
- Most cancers are curable if treated early.
- Benign neoplasms are localized and encapsulated and do not spread.
- Malignant neoplasms spread to neighboring tissues via blood and lymph.
- Biopsy is the most accurate diagnostic test for cancer.
- The most common medical treatments for cancer are surgery, radiation, and chemotherapy. They may be used alone or in combination.
- Surgery is the treatment of choice for early cancers.
- Chemotherapy is the treatment of choice for metastatic cancers. It is also the treatment most responsible for increasing cancer cure rates in recent years.
- Lung cancer is the leading cause of cancer death among men and women. Eighty percent of all cases are related to smoking.
- Quality of life, not quantity of life, is the ultimate goal for clients living with cancer.

Review Questions

1. The nurse carefully monitors the client's intravenous chemotherapy. Which is an early indicator that extravasation may be occurring?
   a. The fluid stops infusing.
   b. Edema is noted at the site.
   c. Blood returns when the bottle is lowered.
   d. Burning occurs at the site.

2. A breast cancer client states that the doctor says he is going to prescribe hormone therapy. Which of the following hormones would probably be ordered?
   a. thyroxin
   b. parathormone
   c. progesterone
   d. testosterone

3. A cancer client develops a low white-cell count. She is placed on neutropenic precautions. Which of the following menu selections would be best?
   a. meat loaf, mashed potatoes, green beans, and fruit gelatin
   b. meat loaf, mashed potatoes, marinated carrots, and a garden salad
   c. meat loaf, mashed potatoes, chef salad, and tapioca
   d. meat loaf, mashed potatoes, green beans, fruit salad, and a cookie

4. As stomatitis develops, which would be best to encourage in the client?
   a. drinking plenty of orange juice
   b. using lemon and glycerine swabs frequently
   c. brushing teeth before and after eating
   d. rinsing with commercial mouthwash as needed

5. Which should be encouraged in clients receiving radiation?

   a. washing and drying the skin carefully and applying lotion
   b. not bathing
   c. not applying deodorants or lotions
   d. washing the skin with soap and applying baby powder

6. The cancer that causes the most deaths each year is:

   a. skin.
   b. lung.
   c. prostate.
   d. colorectal.

Critical Thinking Questions

1. What diagnostic tests should a person have as part of a routine physical to detect cancer?

2. What methods can a person use to detect a tumor in oneself?

3. What is the rationale for each nursing intervention given for the possible nursing diagnoses in this chapter?

WEB FLASH!

- What new treatments for cancer can you find on the Web?
- What resources are available on the Web for cancer clients and their families?

UNIT
4
Oxygenation and Perfusion

NURSING CARE OF THE CLIENT: RESPIRATORY SYSTEM

MAKING THE CONNECTION

Refer to the the following chapters to increase your understanding of the respiratory system:

- **Chapter 12, Health Assessment**
- **Chapter 13, Diagnostic Tests**
- **Chapter 17, Nursing Care of the Oncology Client**
- **Chapter 19, Nursing Care of the Client: Cardiovascular System**
- **Chapter 20, Nursing Care of the Client: Hematologic and Lymphatic Systems**

LEARNING OBJECTIVES

Upon completion of this chapter, you should be able to:
- *Define key terms.*
- *Describe components of a complete respiratory assessment.*
- *Describe assessment of the client with a chest tube.*
- *Identify normal parameters for common respiratory diagnostic studies.*
- *Discuss the etiology, medical–surgical management, and nursing care for clients with respiratory disorders.*
- *Prepare a nursing care plan for a client with a respiratory disorder.*

INTRODUCTION

Respiratory disorders account for millions of the dollars spent in the U.S. health care arena. From loss of time on the job due to the common cold to care for those with chronic respiratory disorders, the cost of respiratory disease is staggering. This chapter explores the various respiratory disorders, with a focus on the nursing process.

KEY TERMS

adventitious breath sound
asthma
atelectasis
audible wheeze
bronchial breath sound
bronchiectasis
bronchitis
bronchovesicular breath sound
caseation
cavitation
chemoreceptor
coarse crackle
diffusion
emphysema
epistaxis
external respiration
fine crackle

hemopneumothorax
hemothorax
internal respiration
liquefaction necrosis
lung stretch receptor
perfusion
pleural effusion
pleural friction rub
pleurisy
pneumonia
pneumothorax
primary tubercle
respiration
sibilant wheeze
sonorous wheeze
status asthmaticus
stridor
surfactant
ventilation
vesicular breath sound

ANATOMY AND PHYSIOLOGY REVIEW

The primary function of the respiratory system is delivery of oxygen to the lungs and removal of carbon dioxide from the lungs.

Thoracic Cavity

The chest cage is a closed compartment bounded on the top by the neck muscles and at the bottom by the diaphragm. The walls of the chest cage are formed by the ribs and intercostal muscles laterally, the thoracic vertebrae posteriorly, and the sternum anteriorly. The inside of the chest cage is called the *thoracic cavity*. Contained within the thoracic cavity are the lungs. The lungs are cone-shaped, porous organs separated from the other chest organs by the mediastinum. The lungs lie free, except for their attachment to the heart

and trachea, and are encased in the pleura, a thin, transparent double-layered serous membrane lining the thoracic cavity. The layers of the pleura are the parietal pleura, which lies adjacent to the chest wall, and the visceral pleura, which adheres to the surface of the lungs. The area between the two pleura is known as the *pleural space*.

The pleural space contains approximately 5 to 20 cubic centimeters of serous fluid (pleural fluid), which allows the layers of the pleura to slide on each other yet hold together. The pressure within the pleural space is less than that of outside air. This difference in pressure creates a suction that prevents the lungs from collapsing on exhalation.

The right lung is larger than the left and is divided into three sections, or lobes: upper, middle, and lower. The left lung is divided into two lobes: upper and lower (Figure 18-1). The upper portion of the lung is

Figure 18-1 Structures of the Respiratory Tract *(Adapted from* Health Assessment & Physical Examination *(2nd ed.), by M. E. Z. Estes, 2002, Albany, NY: Delmar. Copyright 2002 by Delmar. Adapted with permission.)*

referred to as the *apex* (plural, apices). The lower portion is called the *base*. The lungs possess a dual blood supply, bronchial circulation and pulmonary circulation. Bronchial circulation begins with the bronchial artery, which provides the passageways of the lungs with blood to meet nutritional needs. Bronchial circulation terminates when the venous blood enters the pulmonary veins, which slightly dilutes the oxygen content in the pulmonary vein. Pulmonary circulation is the route by which blood is delivered to the alveoli for gas exchange.

Conducting Airways

The conducting airways are tubelike structures that provide a passageway for air as it travels to the lungs. These are the nasal passages, mouth, pharynx, larynx, trachea, bronchi, and bronchioles (refer again to Figure 18-1). The conducting airways are lined with epithelial tissue containing serous glands, mucus-secreting Goblet cells, and hairlike projections called *cilia*. The mucus of the Goblet cells together with the cilia form a mucociliary blanket that serves to protect the respiratory system from invasion by foreign particles. The constant upward motion of the cilia propels the mucociliary blanket toward the pharynx, where any foreign matter may be expectorated.

The nasal passages are the preferred route for air to enter the respiratory tract. In addition to the function of filtering inspired air, the nasal passages are richly supplied with blood vessels that warm and moisten the air. An alternate route for air to enter is the mouth. Breathing through the mouth, however, reduces the ability to filter, warm, and moisten inspired air, because the mouth lacks cilia and abundant blood supply.

Connecting the nasal passages and mouth to the lower parts of the respiratory tract is the pharynx. The pharynx, located behind the oral cavity, serves as a passageway for both inspired air into the larynx and ingested food passing into the digestive system. At the distal portion of the pharynx is the larynx, also known as the voice box.

The larynx is the passageway for air entering and leaving the trachea, and contains the vocal cords. The larynx is composed of four structures: the uppermost thyroid cartilage (Adam's apple), the cricoid cartilage (which lies at the lower edge), the epiglottis (a leaf-shaped structure that covers the larynx during swallowing), and the glottis (the triangular space between the vocal cords when they are relaxed).

The trachea, commonly known as the windpipe, is a tube composed of connective tissue mucosa and smooth muscle supported by C-shaped rings of cartilage, extending into the bronchi. The trachea is 2.0 to 2.5 centimeters in diameter (approximately 1 inch) and 10 to 12 centimeters in length (4 to 6 inches). The trachea terminates by branching into two tubes: the right and left primary bronchi. They are somewhat smaller in diameter than the trachea, and each passes into its respective lung. The point at which the trachea divides is called the carina, which is a cartilaginous ridge between the two bronchi. An abundant nerve supply to the carina provides further protection against entry of foreign matter into the lungs. Stimulation of the carina results in bronchospasm and cough. The primary bronchi accompanied by the pulmonary vessels and nerves enter the lung through a groove called the hilum and then branch into smaller bronchi.

The right bronchus is wider and more vertically positioned than the left. This difference in positioning allows foreign matter to enter the right bronchus more easily than the left. The bronchi are somewhat smaller in diameter than the trachea and each passes into its respective lung. Within the lungs, the bronchi branch off into increasingly smaller diameter tubes until they become the terminal bronchioles. These branch further, forming alveolar ducts that end in numerous saclike, thin-walled structures called the *alveoli*. Collectively the alveoli and the alveolar ducts within resemble a cluster of grapes. The branching makes this portion of the respiratory tract resemble an inverted tree, giving rise to the term *bronchial tree* (see Figure 18-1).

Respiratory Tissues

The respiratory tissues perform the function of gas exchange. These structures are the alveolar ducts and the alveoli. Although each is supplied with a means for gas exchange, the alveoli constitute the primary site of gas exchange. The alveolar ducts are smooth, muscular tubes containing abundant alveolar macrophages to remove foreign particles (e.g., bacteria). The alveoli, into which the alveolar ducts terminate, consist of interconnected spaces with thin walls, or septa, occupied by a network of capillaries called the *alveolar capillary membrane*.

The alveoli contain two specialized types of cells. Type I alveolar cells are flat, squamous, epithelial cells across which gas exchange occurs. Type II alveolar cells produce a phospholipid substance called **surfactant**. Surfactant coats the inner surfaces of the alveoli, which reduces the surface tension of pulmonary fluids, allows gas exchange, and prevents the collapse of the airways. Each lung contains approximately 300 million alveoli. It is estimated that the alveoli of the lungs, if flattened out, would cover a surface area the size of a tennis court.

Respiration

Respiration is a process of gas exchange. This process is necessary to supply cells with oxygen for carrying on metabolism, and to remove the carbon dioxide produced as a waste by-product. There are two types of respiration: external respiration and inter-

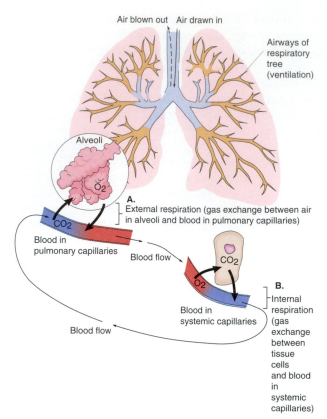

Figure 18-2 A. External Respiration; B. Internal Respiration

Table 18-1 FACTORS AFFECTING VENTILATION, PERFUSION, AND DIFFUSION

Ventilation	Position: Dependent areas receive majority of air.
	Lung volume: Low volume results in shunting air to lung apices.
	Disease: Bronchial constriction and airway collapse decrease ventilation.
Perfusion	Position: Dependent areas receive majority of blood.
	Hypoxia: Results in vasoconstriction and decreased perfusion.
	Blockage: Results in decreased or absent perfusion to distal areas.
Diffusion	Alveolar capillary membrane: Alterations may occur in thickness and permeability of membrane.

nal respiration. **External respiration** is the exchange of gases between the inhaled air, now in the alveoli, and the blood in the pulmonary capillaries. **Internal respiration** is the exchange of gases at the cellular level between tissue cells and blood in systemic capillaries (Figure 18-2). These functions are dependent on the adequacy of ventilation, perfusion, and diffusion. **Ventilation** is the movement of gases into and out of the lung. **Perfusion** refers to the flow of blood through the vessels of a specific organ or body part. Pertaining to the respiratory system, **diffusion** is the movement of gases across the alveolar capillary membrane from areas of high concentration to areas of lower concentration. Factors that affect ventilation, perfusion, and diffusion will affect respiration. These factors are described in Table 18–1.

Neuromuscular Control of Respiration

Unlike the heart muscles, the respiratory muscles must receive continuous neural stimuli to function. Regulation of respiration is integrated by neurons located in the pons and medulla of the brain. The control of respiration is influenced by involuntary (automatic) and voluntary components. Involuntary components include chemoreceptors, lung stretch receptors, and impulses from other sources. **Chemoreceptors** monitor the

levels of carbon dioxide and oxygen and the acidity/alkalinity (pH) of the blood. Normally, chemoreceptors initiate respiration in response to rising levels of carbon dioxide in the blood. With certain chronic pulmonary disorders, such as emphysema, chemoreceptors become more responsive to low levels of oxygen. This becomes significant when administering oxygen to persons whose drive to breathe is dependent on low levels of oxygen in the blood. **Lung stretch receptors** monitor the patterns of breathing and prevent overexpansion of the tissues. Many other sources involuntarily send impulses to the respiratory center. For example, if a person becomes frightened or angry, the respiratory rate increases in response to stimuli from the autonomic nervous system. Voluntary components of respiratory control integrate breathing with acts such as talking and speaking.

The diaphragm acts as the primary muscle of respiration. During inspiration, the diaphragm contracts and flattens out in response to stimuli from the respiratory center, increasing the length of the thoracic cavity. At the same time, the intercostal muscles contract, elevating the ribs and increasing the diameter of the thoracic cavity. The total thoracic space increases, reducing the pressure within the thoracic cavity. The pressure within the thoracic cavity then becomes negative in relation to that of atmospheric pressure, and air moves into the thoracic cavity. Upon expiration, the respiratory center signals the diaphragm and intercostal muscles to relax. The thoracic cavity returns to its original size. Aided by the elastic recoil of the lungs, the decrease in size of the thoracic cavity increases pressure, and air moves out of the lungs.

Gas Exchange

Gas exchange occurs at the alveolar capillary membrane. Venous blood from the right ventricle is pumped into the pulmonary arteries and travels to the alveolar capillary network. Here, blood in the alveolar capillaries is exposed to the inhaled air. Due to the higher concentration of oxygen in the alveoli, oxygen diffuses into the blood within the alveolar capillary network. The majority of oxygen binds to the iron atoms of the hemoglobin molecule in the red blood cells. Approximately 1% to 3% of oxygen dissolves into the blood plasma. The exchange of carbon dioxide also occurs within the alveoli. Most of the carbon dioxide formed as a by-product of cellular metabolism diffuses into the red blood cells. There, due to the presence of carbonic anhydrase, carbon dioxide (CO_2) is hydrated and changed into carbonic acid (H_2CO_3). The carbonic acid dissociates into hydrogen ions (H^+) and bicarbonate ions (HCO_3^-). The hydrogen ions combine with hemoglobin, and the bicarbonate ions enter the blood plasma. Hemoglobin that has been reduced (by removal of the oxygen) combines with approximately 15% to 25% of the carbon dioxide. Within the alveolar capillary network, the carbon dioxide detaches from hemoglobin and diffuses into the alveolar space. Carbon dioxide is removed from the alveolar space when exhalation occurs. The blood within the pulmonary capillary network is now oxygenated and travels to the heart via the pulmonary veins. From this point, oxygenated blood is sent to the body via the aorta and the arterial network (Figure 18-3).

ASSESSMENT

Refer to Chapter 12 for detailed information regarding physical assessment.

To understand the assessment of the respiratory system, the student must be familiar with related terminology, outlined in Table 18–2.

Health History

Nursing assessment begins with a complete history. The client should be questioned regarding allergies, occupation, lifestyle, and health habits such as smoking. The client who smokes must be evaluated for the amount of tobacco smoked daily and length of time the client has smoked. Symptoms such as dyspnea, decreased exercise tolerance, and cough must be explored in depth. Following a complete history, the nurse completes a physical assessment of the client.

Table 18–2 RESPIRATORY TERMS

TERM	DEFINITION
Eupnea	Normal breathing
Apnea	Cessation of breathing, possibly temporary in nature
Dyspnea	Labored or difficult breathing, possibly normal if associated with exercise
Bradypnea	Abnormally slow breathing
Tachypnea	Abnormally rapid breathing
Orthopnea	Discomfort or difficulty with breathing in any but an upright sitting or standing position
Kussmaul's respirations	Abnormal respiratory pattern characterized by irregular periods of increased rate and depth of respiration; most often seen with diabetic ketoacidosis
Biot's respirations	Abnormal respiratory pattern characterized by irregular periods of apnea alternating with short periods of respiration of equal depth; most commonly seen with increased intracranial pressure
Cheyne-Stokes respirations	Abnormal respiratory pattern characterized by initially slow, shallow respirations that increase in rapidity and depth and then gradually decrease until respiration stops for 10 to 60 seconds; pattern then repeats itself in the same manner
Anoxia	Without oxygen
Hypoxia	Lack of adequate oxygen in inspired air such as occurs at high altitude
Hypoxemia	Insufficient amount of oxygen in the blood possibly due to respiratory, cardiovascular, or anemia-related disorders
Cyanosis	Bluish, grayish, or purplish discoloration of the skin due to abnormal amounts of reduced (oxygen-poor) hemoglobin in the blood; not always a reliable indicator of hypoxia
Acrocyanosis	Cyanosis of the fingertips and toes; often due to vasomotor disturbances associated with vasoconstriction
Circumoral cyanosis	Bluish discoloration encircling the mouth
Oxygen saturation	Amount of oxygen combined with hemoglobin

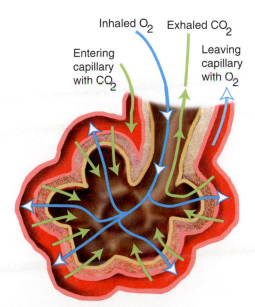

Inhaled O_2

Exhaled CO_2

Entering capillary with CO_2

Leaving capillary with O_2

Figure 18-3 Alveolar Gas Exchange

Inspection

Physical assessment of the respiratory system starts with inspection. The nurse notes the client's color, level of consciousness, and emotional state. Respirations are observed as to their rate, depth, quality, rhythm, and the effort required to breathe. Symmetry of chest wall movement is also noted. The nurse observes for use of accessory muscles to aid breathing. The position the client assumes provides information on respiratory status as individuals having trouble breathing often lean forward.

Palpation and Percussion

The next steps in the respiratory assessment are palpation and percussion. These are normally done by the registered nurse or physician. Through the use of palpation and percussion, areas of varying densities in the lung can be detected. The density of lung tissues changes with disease states such as pneumonia, pneumothorax, and pleural effusion.

Auscultation

Auscultation provides information about respiratory status. The listener assesses breath sounds at each location for the length of a complete inspiration and expiration. Breath sounds are assessed for duration, pitch, and intensity.

Normal Breath Sounds

Under normal circumstances, **bronchial breath sounds** are heard over the sternum. These loud, high-pitched tubular, hollow-like sounds last longer during expiration than during inspiration. When heard in areas other than the sternum, bronchial breath sounds indicate fluid, exudate, or lung tissue compression. **Bronchovesicular breath sounds** are heard over the anterior one-third of the chest near the sternum and also around the scapula posteriorly. Bronchovesicular breath sounds have a medium pitch and intensity with inspiration and expiration being equal in duration. Bronchovesicular breath sounds may be heard in the periphery of the lung when consolidation and fluid are present.

Vesicular breath sounds are heard over the majority of the lungs. These breath sounds are soft and low in pitch. Vesicular breath sounds are best heard during inspiration and may be inaudible during expiration.

Adventitious Breath Sounds

Abnormal breath sounds are called **adventitious breath sounds**. Adventitious breath sounds include: **fine crackles, coarse crackles, sonorous wheezes, sibilant wheezes, pleural friction rub**, and **stridor**. Table 18–3 describes the general characteristics of these adventitious breath sounds.

Table 18–3 CHARACTERISTICS OF ADVENTITIOUS BREATH SOUNDS

BREATH SOUND	RESPIRATORY PHASE	TIMING	DESCRIPTION	CLEAR WITH COUGH	ETIOLOGY	CONDITIONS
Fine crackle	Predominantly inspiration	Discontinuous	Dry, high-pitched crackling and popping of short duration: sounds like hair rolled between fingers when held near ears	Possibly	Air passing through moisture in small airways that suddenly reinflate	Chronic obstructive pulmonary disease (COPD), congestive heart failure (CHF), pneumonia, pulmonary fibrosis, atelectasis
Coarse crackle	Predominantly inspiration	Discontinuous	Moist, low-pitched crackling and gurgling of long duration	Possibly	Air passing through moisture in large airways that suddenly reinflate	Pneumonia, pulmonary edema, bronchitis, atelectasis
Sonorous wheeze	Predominantly expiration	Continuous	Low-pitched snoring	Possibly	Narrowing of large airways or obstruction of bronchus	Asthma, bronchitis, airway edema, tumor, bronchiolar spasm, foreign body obstruction
Sibilant wheeze	Predominantly expiration	Continuous	High-pitched and musical	Possibly	Narrowing of large airways or obstruction of bronchus	Asthma, chronic bronchitis, emphysema, tumor, foreign body obstruction
Pleural friction rub	Inspiration and expiration	Continuous	Creaking, grating	Never	Inflamed parietal and visceral pleura; can occasionally be felt on thoracic wall as two pieces of dry leather rubbing against each other	Pleurisy, tuberculosis, pulmonary infarction, pneumonia, lung abscess
Stridor	Predominantly inspiration	Continuous	Crowing	Never	Partial obstruction of the larynx, trachea	Croup, foreign body obstruction, large airway tumor

Adapted from Health Assessment & Physical Examination *(2nd ed.), by M. E. Z. Estes, 2002, Albany, NY: Delmar. Copyright 2002 by Delmar. Adapted with permission.*

Table 18–4 COMMON DIAGNOSTIC TESTS FOR RESPIRATORY DISORDERS

Laboratory Tests
- Hemoglobin
- Arterial blood gases (ABGs)
- Pulmonary function tests (PFTs)
- Sputum analysis

Radiologic Studies
- Chest x-ray
- Ventilation-perfusion scan
- Computerized axial tomography (CAT scan)
- Pulmonary angiography

Other
- Pulse oximetry
- Bronchoscopy
- Thoracentesis
- Magnetic resonance imaging (MRI)

Table 18–5 ARTERIAL BLOOD GASES: NORMAL VALUES

MEASUREMENT IN BLOOD	NORMAL VALUE
Acidity or alkalinity (pH)	7.3 to 7.45
Partial pressure of oxygen (PaO_2)	80 to 100 mm Hg
Partial pressure of carbon dioxide ($PaCO_2$)	35 to 45 mm Hg
Bicarbonate ion (HCO_3^-)	22 to 26 mm Hg
Arterial oxygen saturation (SaO_2)	95% (at sea level)

COMMON DIAGNOSTIC TESTS

Commonly used diagnostic tests for clients with respiratory disorders are listed in Table 18–4. See Chapter 13, Diagnostic Tests, for explanation/normal values and nursing responsibilities. Table 18–5 lists normal values for arterial blood gases.

INFECTIOUS/INFLAMMATORY DISORDERS

Infectious/inflammatory disorders of the upper respiratory tract, pneumonia, tuberculosis, and pleurisy/pleural effusion are discussed in the sections following.

INFECTIOUS/INFLAMMATORY DISORDERS OF THE UPPER RESPIRATORY TRACT

Infectious and inflammatory disorders of the upper respiratory tract are common and usually self-limiting. Table 18–6 summarizes the various types of disorders associated with infection and inflammation of the upper respiratory tract. Among the causal factors of infectious and inflammatory disorders are various viruses and bacteria such as rhino viruses, influenza viruses, streptococci, and pneumococci. Group A *beta-hemolytic streptococci* infections of the upper respiratory system are associated with serious sequelae such as rheumatic fever. Allergic reactions frequently play a role in the development of sinusitis and pharyngitis. Laryngitis is associated with irritation due to factors such as pollution, smoking, and excessive use of the voice. Breathing cold air decreases local immune responses of the respiratory tract. This fact coupled with closer and prolonged contact with others indoors during the colder months leads to an increased incidence of acute upper respiratory tract inflammatory disorders.

The signs and symptoms that occur with acute upper respiratory tract infection or inflammation are a result of the inflammatory process. Early signs and symptoms include general malaise, low-grade fever, localized redness, and edema of affected tissues. With viral disorders, symptoms such as joint pain are common. Furthermore, the client may complain of nasal or sinus congestion and headache. Drying of the mucous membranes coupled with edema cause local discomfort such as sore throat. Cough and nasal or sinus discharge may occur. Nasal secretions that are thick and purulent indicate bacterial infection.

Table 18–6 UPPER RESPIRATORY TRACT INFECTIONS OR INFLAMMATORY DISORDERS

DISORDER	ETIOLOGY
Rhinitis (coryza, common cold)	Viral
Allergic rhinitis	Exposure to allergens
Sinusitis	Bacterial (streptococci, pneumococci) or viral
Pharyngitis	Bacterial or viral
Tonsillitis	Bacterial (streptococci, most commonly)
Laryngitis	Irritation due to excessive use of voice or exposure to irritants (e.g., cigarette smoke); extension of rhinitis

Medical–Surgical Management

Medical

The majority of clients with acute upper respiratory tract infectious or inflammatory disorders are treated in a clinic or office setting. Unless the disorder becomes chronic or bacterial infection occurs, treatment is symptomatic. When infection is suspected, specimens for culture and sensitivity are obtained, and appropriate antibiotic therapy is initiated.

Surgical

Disorders that develop into chronic conditions (e.g., tonsillitis and sinusitis) may require surgical intervention to remove or drain affected tissues.

Pharmacological

Nonprescription antipyretic, analgesic, anti-inflammatory medications may be used to reduce discomfort, fever, and inflammation. Examples of such medications are acetaminophen (Tylenol), ibuprofen (Advil), and acetylsalicylic acid (aspirin). Antitussives such as dextromethorphan hydrobromide combinations (Comtrex, Dimetane-DM, Rondec-DM) or hydrocodone bitartrate (Hycodan) preparations may be used to suppress cough and allow for rest. To aid in removal of secretions, expectorants such as guaifenesin (Robitussin, Humibid L.A.) are used. Bacterial infections are treated with various antibiotics according to culture and sensitivity studies. Some of the more common antibiotics used are erythromycin base (E-mycin, PCE Disperstab), ampicillin (Omnipen), amoxicillin (Amoxil), cefaclor (Ceclor), and cephalexin monohydrate (Keflex). Comfort measures such as saline gargles may be useful.

Diet

Clear fluids are advocated to liquefy secretions and hydrate dry mucous membranes. Nausea may occur if secretions are swallowed as opposed to expectorated. The client should be encouraged to cough up all secretions and dispose of them in a tissue. With severe coughing, emesis may occur. The client should be encouraged to rest prior to meals and may require an antitussive to reduce coughing.

Activity

Normally, activity does not need to be restricted, but energy level may decrease. The client who is infectious should be encouraged to avoid contact with others. Strenuous activity should be avoided to reduce oxygen requirements and coughing.

▶ NURSING PROCESS

▶ Assessment

▶ Subjective Data

Subjective data include information about present signs and symptoms, onset of symptoms, exposure to allergens or infected individuals, and frequency of the disorder. Common symptoms include sore throat, dyspnea, and headache.

▶ Objective Data

Objective data include fever and inflammation, redness, edema, and drying of the mucous membranes of the oropharynx. Secretions are evaluated for their color, viscosity, amount, and odor, which will help in identifying the specific illness. The client may have hoarseness and a cough. Culture and sensitivity studies may reveal a causative organism and, thus, serve to guide antibiotic therapy. If infection with group A *beta-hemolytic streptococci* is suspected, an ASO (antistreptolysin O) titer may be done to reveal the presence of antibodies formed in reaction to this bacteria. Nonspecific diagnostic studies include elevated white blood cell counts and erythrocyte sedimentation rates.

Nursing diagnoses for a client with an upper respiratory infection or inflammatory disorder may include the following:

Nursing Diagnoses	Planning/Goals	Nursing Interventions
▶ *Deficient Knowledge related to signs and symptoms of respiratory bacterial infection, potential allergens, and antibiotic therapy*	The client will be able to state the signs and symptoms of bacterial infection.	Educate the client regarding signs and symptoms indicating a respiratory bacterial infection, such as purulent or green secretions, fever.
	The client will be able to identify individual potential allergens.	Assist the physician in allergy testing. Teach the client to avoid those things that precipitate an allergic response.
	The client will complete entire course of antibiotic therapy.	Instruct client to complete the entire course of antibiotics.
▶ *Ineffective Airway Clearance related to nasal secretions.*	The client will verbalize a decrease or absence of nasal congestion.	Teach client to blow nose and not "snuffle" secretions back up into nose.

Evaluation Each goal must be evaluated to determine how it has been met by the client.

PNEUMONIA

Pneumonia is inflammation of the bronchioles and alveoli accompanied by consolidation, or solidification of exudate, in the lungs. It can result from bacteria, viruses, mycoplasms, fungi, chemical exposures, or parasite invasions. Pneumonia can also be caused by aspiration, oversedation, or inadequate ventilation. Pneumonia remains a common cause of hospitalization and is often a cause of death, particularly among elderly persons. Under normal circumstances, the alveolar macrophages are able to remove foreign matter. When confronted with overwhelming numbers of virulent microorganisms, however, this protective mechanism fails. The invading organism irritates the walls of the alveoli. In response to this irritation, the alveolar walls secrete exudate (an accumulation of fluid in the pulmonary passageways). Eventually, the alveoli fill with the exudate, resulting in consolidation. The presence of the exudate within the alveoli also interferes with gas exchange.

Risk factors for the development of pneumonia include immobility, depressed cough reflex (due to anesthesia or cerebrovascular accident [CVA]), alterations in respiratory function (e.g., chronic obstructive pulmonary disease [COPD]), advanced age, and numerous other chronic debilitating conditions (e.g., congestive heart failure [CHF], diabetes mellitus). Common bacterial causes of pneumonia are *Streptococcus pneumoniae, Pneumococcus, Staphylococcus aureus, Klebsiella pneumoniae,* and *Pseudomonas aeruginosa.* Chemical pneumonia is due to entry of irritating substances into the pulmonary passageways. A common source of chemical pneumonia is the aspiration of gastric contents. Inhalation of irritating substances can also result in a chemical pneumonia. A common, serious viral source of pneumonia is the *Cytomegalovirus.* The *Cytomegalovirus* affects those clients with compromised immune status, such as those taking immunosuppressant medications or those infected with human immunodeficiency virus (HIV). *Pneumocystis carinii* pneumonia can also occur in the immunosupressed client. The invading organism associated with *Pneumocystis carinii* pneumonia is thought to be a protozoan. The infecting microorganisms that cause pneumonia are spread by airborne droplets or direct contact with infected individuals or carriers. Pneumonia is now classified according to the causative factor rather than the area of the lung affected, as was done in the past. The right middle and lower lobes are affected by pneumonia more frequently than the right upper and left lobes due to the anatomy of the right bronchus and the effects of gravity.

A high fever of sudden onset is often the presenting complaint of the client. The elderly client, however, may be seriously ill and have only a low-grade fever. A productive cough yielding abnormally thick and dis-

colored sputum may be present. Associated respiratory symptoms include dyspnea, coarse crackles, and diminished breath sounds. The majority of clients complain of pleuritic chest pain. This type of pain is stabbing in nature and increases on inspiration. Pain occurs due to irritation of the pleura lying adjacent to the affected alveoli.

In the case of bacterial pneumonia, white blood cell count increases and may go as high as 40,000/mm³. Pneumonia caused by viruses or mycoplasms may produce normal or lowered white blood cell count. Chest x-ray will reveal consolidation in the affected areas. Bacterial pneumonia is likely to produce isolated areas of consolidation on a chest x-ray, while viral and chemical pneumonia appear as more diffuse areas of consolidation. Arterial blood gases (ABGs) may reveal a decrease in PaO_2 or oxygen saturation due to interference with gas exchange. Pulmonary function tests (PFTs) are usually within normal limits unless the client has an underlying pulmonary disorder such as emphysema.

Medical–Surgical Management

Medical

Clearing the airways of exudate and maintaining adequate oxygenation are the goals of treatment for clients with pneumonia. Postural drainage and percussion may be ordered to aid the client in mobilizing secretions (see Figure 18-4). Aerosol or nebulization treatments may also be utilized. Medications are often added to aerosol or nebulization treatments, as discussed in the subsequent section on pharmacological management of pneumonia. The client is encouraged to cough and deep breathe, particularly following respiratory treatments. Incentive spirometry, which measures the amount of air inspired in one inhalation, may be ordered to aid the client when coughing and deep breathing are inadequate (Figure 18-5). If the client is

CLIENT TEACHING

Pneumonia

- Discuss pertinent information about medications being taken
- Instruct in measures to prevent spread of infection (covering the mouth and nose with a tissue when coughing or sneezing)
- Encourage disposal of tissues in a closed paper sack
- Outline individual's specific risk factors (age, chronic respiratory condition, cardiac condition)
- Instruct in methods to prevent future infection (avoiding crowds and obtaining vaccine)

UPPER LOBES
Apical Segment

UPPER LOBES
Anterior Segment

UPPER LOBES
Posterior Segment

LEFT UPPER LOBE
Lingular Segment
Superior/Inferior   14"

RIGHT MIDDLE LOBE
Lateral Segment
Medial Segment   14"

LOWER LOBES
Superior Segment

LOWER LOBES
Anterior Basal
Segment   18"

LOWER LOBES
Lateral Basal
Segment   18"

LOWER LOBES
Posterior Basal
Segment   18"

Figure 18-4 Postural drainage positions facilitate drainage of exudate from the lobes of the lungs and may be used with percussion.

Figure 18-5 An Incentive Spirometer

unable to mobilize secretions, suctioning of the respiratory tract is indicated. When secretions are overwhelming, the physician may perform a bronchoscopy in order to remove them. Intravenous fluids may be utilized to maintain adequate hydration, especially in the presence of fever. Adequate hydration promotes liquefaction of respiratory secretions and thus aids in their removal. Pulse oximetry or ABGs are done to assess the level of oxygenation. Supplemental oxygen is used when oxygenation is inadequate (refer to Figure 18-6 and Table 18–7).

Pharmacological

The treatment of choice for bacterial pneumonia is specific pharmacological therapy. A sputum specimen for culture and sensitivity should be obtained prior to

GERONTOLOGICAL CONSIDERATIONS

Respiratory Status in the Elderly Client
- Respiratory effort increases because muscles atrophy, the diaphragm flattens out, costochondral cartilage calcifies, ligaments and joints stiffen, and intervertebral discs degenerate.
- Alveolar gas exchange diminishes due to a decrease in the lung's elastic recoil, which causes air to be trapped, especially in the lower lobes, for a portion of the respiratory cycle.
- The medulla becomes less sensitive to changes in carbon dioxide and oxygen levels, thereby rendering the respiration triggering mechanism less active.
- Ciliary activity diminishes, thereby increasing susceptibility to infection.
- Cough reflex decreases.
- Aspiration risk increases due to the decrease in the cough reflex.

Figure 18-6 Oxygen Delivery Systems: A. Nasal cannula; B. Simple face mask; C. Reservoir mask; D. Venturi mask

Table 18-7 SUPPLEMENTAL OXYGEN DEVICES AND OXYGEN CONCENTRATIONS PROVIDED

DEVICE	FLOW RATE	OXYGEN CONCENTRATION
Nasal cannula	1 to 6 L/min	20% to 40%
Simple mask	8 to 10 L/min	40% to 60%
Reservoir masks	6 to 10 L/min	60% to 100%
Venturi mask (used to control oxygen concentrations for the COPD patient)	4 to 8 L/min	24% to 40%

initiating antibiotic therapy. After a specimen has been obtained, the physician may start therapy with a broad-spectrum antibiotic. If laboratory data indicate resistant microorganisms, a specific antibiotic will be started. Antiviral agents, such as acyclovir sodium (Zovirax), are utilized for clients with chronic respiratory problems related to viral pneumonia. Prophylactic antibiotic therapy is often utilized for viral pneumonia to prevent a secondary bacterial infection. To promote opening and clearing of the airways, bronchodilators, such as albuterol (Ventolin), and mucolytic agents, such as acetylcysteine (Mucomyst), are administered via aerosol or nebulization by the respiratory therapist

or nurse. Expectorants such as guaifenisin (Robitussin) may be given orally. Cough suppressants and pain relievers, especially those containing narcotics such as codeine sulfate, are administered only with discretion, because they may further inhibit the client's ability to clear the airways.

Diet

The client with pneumonia is encouraged to drink fluids, as doing so aids in the liquefaction of respiratory secretions. Small, frequent, nutritionally balanced meals are preferred. Respiratory treatments that promote coughing should be avoided immediately before and after meals to prevent nausea and vomiting associated with vigorous coughing.

Activity

Bed rest or limited activity for the client with pneumonia promotes optimal tissue oxygenation.

Health Promotion

Pneumococcal vaccine (Pneumovax 23), a vaccine to prevent infection caused by *Streptococcus pneumonia,* should be given to clients at risk of developing pneumonia, such as those with chronic respiratory or cardiac conditions. The vaccine is recommended for all elderly persons.

▶ NURSING PROCESS

▶ Assessment

▶ Subjective Data

Data gathered in the history include the onset, duration, and severity of cough; the color, amount, and odor of sputum, if present; the onset and duration of elevated temperature; and the presence or absence of night sweats.

PROFESSIONAL TIP

Assessment and Respiratory Assistive Devices

When caring for clients with respiratory assistive devices in place, the following must be assessed:

- Oxygen
  - Mode of delivery (e.g., nasal cannula, face mask)
  - Percentage of oxygen that is being delivered (e.g., 25%, 40%)
  - Flow rate of the oxygen (e.g., 2 liters per minute, 4 liters per minute)
  - Humidification provided and oxygen warmed
- Incentive Spirometer
  - Frequency of use
  - Volume achieved
  - Number of times client reaches goal with each use

▶ Objective Data

The client's level of consciousness should be noted. Evidence of dyspnea, orthopnea, tachypnea, and cyanosis may be present. On auscultation of the lung fields, moist crackles or diminished breath sounds are heard. In the event of obstruction of the airways, sibi- lant wheezes occur. Vital signs including temperature are taken prior to and following drug therapy so as to provide information regarding the severity of the ill- ness and the efficacy of treatment. The color, amount, viscosity, and odor of sputum are noted.

Nursing diagnoses for a client with pneumonia may include the following:

Nursing Diagnoses	Planning/Goals	Nursing Interventions
▶ *Ineffective Airway Clearance related to inability to remove airway secretions.*	The client will have clear breath sounds upon ausculta- tion.	Encourage the client to breathe deeply and cough a minimum of every 2 hours.
		Teach use of the incentive spirometer to encourage lung expansion.
		Administer aerosol and nebulizer treatments as ordered.
		Assess breath sounds and respiratory rate prior to and following respiratory procedures to evaluate their effectiveness.
		Encourage fluids to liquefy thickened secretions.
		For clients who are able, assist in sitting up or ambulating three to four times daily.
		For the client who is on bed rest, turn every 2 hours.
		Administer medications as ordered.
		Provide oral care several times a day.
▶ *Impaired Gas Exchange related to inflammatory changes in alveolar capillary membrane*	The client will have an oxy- gen saturation of 92% or greater.	Monitor pulse oximetry and/or ABGs.
		Administer supplemental oxygen as ordered.
▶ *Activity Intolerance related to hypoxia sec- ondary to pneumonia*	The client will be able to complete activities of daily living (ADL) and activity as ordered and without com- plaints of fatigue.	Encourage the client to complete ADL according to ability and the physician's orders.
		To prevent client fatigue, alternate periods of activity and care with periods of rest.

Evaluation Each goal must be evaluated to determine how it has been met by the client.

TUBERCULOSIS

Pulmonary tuberculosis (TB) is an infection of the lung tissue by *Mycobacterium tuberculosis*. Infection by the tubercle bacillus can occur in other parts of the body, but with less frequency. Other parts of the body that may be affected include bones, joints, gastroin- testinal and genitourinary tracts, nervous system, skin, and lymph nodes. In the case of pulmonary tuberculo- sis, the tubercle bacilli are inhaled into the lungs. Whether infection occurs depends on the host's sus- ceptibility, the virulence of the tubercle bacilli, and the number of bacilli inhaled. Tuberculosis is not as highly contagious as once thought. Prolonged exposure to the bacilli is required to produce infection. In addition, per- sons with uncompromised immune systems are able to combat the bacilli and do not develop the disease itself. Those at risk for tuberculosis include persons suffering from malnutrition, those living in crowded conditions, persons with compromised immune status, and health care workers providing care to high-risk individuals.

Once inhaled in sufficient numbers, the tubercle bacilli cause an inflammatory response within the alve- oli of the lung. A small nodule called a **primary tu- bercle**, which contains tubercle bacilli, forms within the lung tissue. In an attempt to isolate these primary tubercles, the body forms a fibrous outer coating around each tubercle. This fibrous surface interferes with the blood and nutritional supplies to the primary tubercle. In time, the interior of the tubercle becomes soft and cheese-like due to decreased perfusion, a process known as **caseation**. At this point, the tubercles may become calcified. The calcified nodule is called a Ghon's tubercle.

Liquefaction necrosis may occur, wherein the tis- sue dies and changes to a liquid or semi-liquid state; this fluid may then be coughed up. A cavity is formed at the site where the primary tubercle liquefied and ruptured. This condition is known as **cavitation** or cavitary disease.

Following the advent of antitubercular medications in the 1950s, the incidence of TB decreased dramatically. In recent years, however, TB has been occurring with increased frequency. In addition, new forms of TB that are resistant to conventional drug therapy have surfaced. Some of the factors that may be responsible for the increase in TB cases are: increased numbers of persons with compromised immune systems (e.g., many AIDS clients suffer from TB); increased mobility of the world's population (persons from areas of high TB incidence moving to areas of low incidence); widespread IV drug abuse; increased numbers of those with poor access to health care; and increased numbers of those living in impoverished conditions.

Symptoms of TB develop gradually following infection. The nurse should suspect TB if the following symptoms are present: low-grade fevers that recur in a specific pattern, persistent cough, hemoptysis, hoarseness, dyspnea on exertion, night sweats, fatigue, and weight loss. Due to the body's attempt to fight the infection, lymph nodes also may be enlarged.

The Mantoux skin test is the preferred method of screening for TB. For the Mantoux test, 0.1cc of purified protein derivative (PPD) of killed tubercle bacilli is injected intradermally in the inner forearm. The test is evaluated by measuring the area of induration (palpable swelling) that occurs 48 and 72 hours following injection. A reddened area with no induration is not considered positive. A positive skin test, however, indicates only that the client has been infected with and developed antibodies against the tubercle bacillus (Table 18–8). It is important for the nurse to educate clients correctly regarding this fact.

The bacteria can remain alive but inactive in the body, often for a lifetime, so a client is given prophylactic treatment, usually isoniazid (INH), for 6 to 12 months. Other medications used against tuberculosis are outlined in Table 18–9. Once antibodies are made and a tuberculin test is positive, the test will thereafter always be positive throughout the individual's lifetime. If INH has not been given and the person later in life is under physical or emotional stress, which weakens the immune system, the bacteria may become active and cause TB disease. However, 9 in 10 persons who have been infected never develop TB disease (Phipps, et al., 1999).

A negative reaction does not rule out the possibility of TB exposure. Individuals at high risk, such as those who are infected with HIV or who have compromised immune status, may have a negative reaction because they are unable to develop antibodies. Immediately following exposure to TB, a skin test may read falsely negative because it can take up to 10 weeks for an infected individual to develop antibodies to react to the killed tubercle bacilli. An additional skin test may be done in 10 to 12 weeks. If the second TB test is positive, the client's history is reviewed for the presence of symptoms suggesting TB, and further evaluation is indicated.

Chest x-ray and sputum specimens are utilized to confirm a diagnosis of TB. Sputum is tested for the presence of acid-fast bacilli, or AFB. The sputum specimen is collected when the client arises in the morning to prevent specimen contamination with ingested food and liquids. In most instances, three specimens collected on consecutive days and testing positive for AFB indicate a positive diagnosis of TB. The TB diagnosis is confirmed if the TB bacilli grow in a culture. Individuals who are unable to produce sputum, including children

Table 18–8 POSITIVE RESULTS OF MANTOUX TUBERCULIN SKIN TEST

CONSIDERED POSITIVE	POPULATION
Induration of 5mm or more	*High-risk groups:* • Persons with HIV infection • Persons in close contact with someone who has infectious TB • Persons who have chest x-rays consistent with old, healed TB • Intravenous drug users whose HIV status is unknown
Induration of 10 mm or more	*Moderate-risk groups:* • Intravenous drug users known to be HIV seronegative • Foreign-born persons from high-prevalence areas (Asia, Africa, Latin America) • Residents of long-term care facilities (prisons, nursing homes, mental institutions) • Medically underserved low-income populations, including high-risk racial or ethnic minority populations (Blacks, Hispanics, Native Americans) • Persons with medical conditions that have been shown to increase the risk of TB, such as silicosis; persons who are 10% or more below ideal body weight; persons receiving high-dose corticosteroid or other immunosuppressive therapy; and persons with some hematologic disorders (leukemias and lymphomas) and other malignancies • Locally identified high-risk populations • Health care workers who provide services to any of the high-risk groups
Induration of 15 mm or more	*Persons having low risk*

From Core Curriculum on Tuberculosis, *1984, Centers for Disease Control and Prevention, Atlanta: U. S. Department of Health and Human Services.*

Table 18–9 TUBERCULOSIS MEDICATIONS

DRUG	MEDICATION PRECAUTIONS AND INFORMATION
First-line Drugs	
ethambutol hydrochloride (Myambutol)	Monthly vision checks are important for acuity and distinction of red and green colors. Take medication with food.
isoniazid (INH) (Laniazid)	Alcohol ingestion interferes with metabolism and may cause hepatitis. Check baseline and monthly hepatic enzymes. Report signs of neuropathy and hepatitis. Have client take pyridoxine (vitamin B_6) to decrease side effects
pyrazinamide (PMS Pyrazinamide)	Take medication with food and drink 2 liters of liquids daily. Check baseline and monthly uric acid and liver enzymes.
rifamate	Drug is a combination of isoniazid and rifampin.
rifampin (Rifadin)	Body secretions (urine, sweat, tears) turn orange while taking the medication.
rifapentine (Priftin)	Drug is as effective as rifampin but taken less frequently. Body secretions (urine, sweat, tears) turn orange. Drug must be given with a least one other tuberculosis drug.
rifater	Drug is a combination of isoniazid, rifampin, and pyrazinamide.
streptomycin sulfate	It is important to have monthly audiograms to check auditory function. Check baseline and monthly renal function.
Second-line Drugs	
cycloserine (Seromycin)	Observe for mental alertness. While taking the medication, monitor renal and liver function, drink 2 to 3 liters of fluid daily, and do not drink alcohol.
ethionamide (Trecator-SC)	Given with other antitubercular drugs to prevent resistant organisms from developing.
kanamycin sulfate (Kantrex)	Drug may cause steatorrhea and electrolyte imbalance.
para-amino-salicylate (Sodium P.A.S.)	Must be taken with other antitubercular drugs; taken with meals.

Figure 18-7 A particulate respirator must be fitted tightly around the nose and face. (*Photo courtesy of Donna Hannum, RN, BSN*)

include placing the client in an isolation room with negative air pressure (where air inflow is controlled through one vent and air outflow is exhausted through another vent directly to the outside and is not recirculated to other rooms.). The doors and windows of the client's room must be kept closed to maintain control of air flow. Furthermore, caregivers should wear N95 particulate respirator masks, as standard isolation masks do not prevent *Mycobacterium tuberculosis* from passing through to the wearer (Figure 18-7).

 Infection Control: Use of a Particulate Respirator

- Follow facility's procedure for fit-testing
- Use the correct size mask
- Put on respirator before entering client's room and remove after leaving client's room
- Ensure that the respirator is free of holes
- Check that the seal between face and respirator is intact
- Discard soiled or damaged respirators

The Centers for Disease Control and Prevention recommend periodic TB skin testing for health care personnel. Health care workers with low risk for developing TB, including those who have contact with fewer than five TB clients per year, should be tested yearly. Health care workers who have had contact with five or more TB clients within the past year should be tested every 6 months. Any health care worker who is exposed to clients in a variety of settings (e.g., ambulance personnel) or who deals with a transitory client population should be tested every 3 months.

 Infection Control: Tuberculosis

- Instruct client to cover mouth and nose when coughing or sneezing
- Double-bag secretions and dispose of them as infectious waste
- Use disposable items for care when possible
- Thoroughly clean and disinfect nondisposable items

and elderly persons, may have stomach contents aspirated for the purpose of AFB testing. Chest x-ray may reveal the presence of primary tubercles in the lung. Areas of calcified lesions and cavitation are also revealed on x-ray.

Medical–Surgical Management

Medical

The majority of clients are treated briefly in the hospital, with long-term treatment continuing at home. In the hospital Airborne Precautions must be followed in addition to Standard Precautions. The precautions

Safety: Caregivers in Health Care Institutions
- Be aware of risks when caring for a client with TB
- Follow Standard Precautions and Airborne Precautions
- Use face and/or eye shield in addition to particulate mask when performing sputum-induction procedure
- Plan care to limit prolonged exposure to client

Surgical

In the past, surgical intervention involving the removal of affected lung tissues was common. With the advent of effective chemotherapy (treatment with drugs), however, surgical intervention is now rarely utilized.

Pharmacological

Active TB is treated with a combination of medications. Three medications—isoniazid (Laniazid, which is most effective), rifampin (Rifadin), and pyrazinamide (Pyrazinamide)—are given for a period of 2 months. Ethambutal hydrochloride (Myambutol) is added to the regimen if drug-resistant TB is in the area. This is followed by a regimen of rifampin and isoniazid for 4 additional months. The combination of three or four drugs is given initially to rapidly decrease the number of active bacilli in the body and to prevent the development of drug-resistant TB. After 3 weeks on medication, the client is usually no longer contagious. Long-term therapy is required because TB bacilli have long periods of metabolic inactivity. Those clients with bone and joint infections, meningitis, or resistant forms of TB must be treated with isoniazid and pyrazinamide for longer periods. Clients who are HIV positive require a 7-month regimen of isoniazid and pyrazinamide; prophylactic treatment with isoniazid is indicated from then on. Ethambutol hydrochloride (Myambutol) and streptomycin sulfate are added to the treatment regimen if the infecting organism is resistant to one of the three medications normally used to treat TB. Infection with a multidrug resistant form of TB requires the use of medications such as kanamycin sulfate (Kantrex), capreomycin sulfate (Capastat Sulfate), and cycloserine (Seromycin). The client is considered noninfectious following three negative AFB sputum specimens. At that point, the client may return to work and other normal activities. Prophylactic treatment of high-risk individuals is recommended to reduce their chances of developing the disease following their exposure.

Taking multiple drugs can be confusing and lead to noncompliance. The development of two new drugs has been valuable. These drugs are Rifater, a combination of isoniazid, rifampin, and pyrazinamide, and Rifamate, a combination of isoniazid and rifampin. Rifapentine was released in June 2000. Although it is as effective as rifampin, it can be taken less frequently.

Diet

The client with TB often also suffers from nutritional deficits. Correction of these deficits is necessary to assist the client in overcoming the disease process. Dietary management is based on the type of deficiency present. A well-balanced diet is encouraged for all clients with TB. Fluids are encouraged to aid in the liquefaction of respiratory secretions.

Activity

Activity is restricted based on the client's tolerance. The client who is severely compromised from a respiratory standpoint may be placed on bed rest. If the client's condition allows, activity should be encouraged, as it promotes lung expansion and aids in the removal of static secretions. The client in isolation

CLIENT TEACHING

Rifampin Side Effects
- Urine, saliva, or tears may turn orange.
- Skin becomes more sensitive to the sun.
- Birth control pills and implants become less effective.
- In the presence of methadone, withdrawal symptoms may occur.

(CDC, 1994b)

COMMUNITY/HOME HEALTH CARE

The Client with Tuberculosis

Advise the client of the following:

- Keep all clinic appointments.
- Continue medications for 6 to 12 months.
- Take all medications exactly as directed.
- After 3 weeks on medication, daily routine (e.g., work, school) may be resumed. Until that time:
  - Put used tissues in a closed paper sack and throw away;
  - Avoid close contact with anyone;
  - Sleep alone in bedroom;
  - Air out bedroom often, using a fan in the window to blow air outside; and
  - Thoroughly clean articles such as eating utensils.

whose condition permits it may ambulate in the hallways, as long as a particulate respirator mask is worn by the client while outside of the room.

Health Promotion

Prevention of TB is by far preferred to treatment of the infection. In areas where the disease remains endemic (seldom in the United States), a vaccine containing attenuated tubercle bacilli, BCG (*bacillus Calmette-Guérin*), may be given. However, the effectiveness of the vaccine has not been proven. One disadvantage of the vaccine is that individuals receiving it will test positive to the tuberculin skin test.

It is currently indicated that any person who has had close contact with a client with TB without practicing appropriate protective measures should be tested. Other measures that decrease the likelihood of TB include adequate nutrition, housing, and health care access, and treatment of individuals who have or are at risk for developing TB.

▶ NURSING PROCESS

▶ Assessment

▶ Subjective Data

The history includes questions about the presence of signs and symptoms of TB, such as night sweats, dyspnea on exertion or at rest in late disease, anorexia, loss of muscle strength, and fatigue. Pleuritic pain occurs when the pleura is involved.

▶ Objective Data

Objective data include weight loss; persistent, low-grade fever; and persistent cough. The cough may be nonproductive early in the disease. Later, the cough is productive and yields thick, purulent sputum. Eventually, hemoptysis (blood spitting) occurs. Auscultation of breath sounds reveals coarse crackles. In the presence of cavitary disease, breath sounds are diminished or absent in the affected areas. Sputum is observed as to amount, color, odor, and consistency.

Nursing diagnoses for a client with TB may include the following:

Nursing Diagnoses	Planning/Goals	Nursing Interventions
▶ *Ineffective Breathing Pattern related to pulmonary infectious process*	The client will have color and respiratory rate within normal limits and will not complain of dyspnea.	Assess the client's color, respiratory rate, and respiratory effort. Auscultate the breath sounds. Obtain sputum specimens for AFB; note the amount, color, and viscosity of the sputum. Plan care activities to allow the client uninterrupted periods of rest. Assist the client in assuming the position that most aids respiratory effort. Administer medications as ordered. Encourage fluids if not otherwise contraindicated.
▶ *Deficient Knowledge related to disease process and its treatment*	The client will verbalize an understanding of the disease process and its treatment.	Teach client and family about the basic pathophysiology of TB, how the infection is contracted, who is at risk of developing an infection, the signs and symptoms of TB infection, and complications that may arise. Present information regarding the actions, side effects, and untoward effects of the drugs being administered. Teach the client signs and symptoms of adverse drug reactions to report to the physician. Emphasize the necessity of long-term therapy to cure TB. Inform the client and family that symptoms decrease and are often gone long before the organism is eliminated from the body.
▶ *Ineffective Individual Therapeutic Regimen Management related to client value system*	The client will continue medication regimen for the prescribed length of time.	Include the client and family in making decisions about the care, when appropriate. Allow the client to be an active participant in care decisions, to increase personal responsibility and accountability. Visits from public health or home care nurses may be necessary to monitor the client for compliance. Explore the reasons for noncompliance with the client and family. Based on information obtained, identify strategies to increase compliance. Refer the client who is unable to afford the cost of medications to agencies such as the local health department for assistance. Begin directly observed therapy if the client continues to be noncompliant. Directly observed therapy involves sending the nurse or another health care worker to the client to administer the medications and verify that they are taken.

Evaluation Each goal must be evaluated to determine how it has been met by the client.

SAMPLE NURSING CARE PLAN

THE CLIENT WITH TUBERCULOSIS

Mr. Stuart is an 87-year-old male admitted to the hospital with a chief complaint of productive cough and fatigue. Four months ago, Mr. Stuart was placed in a long-term care facility due to his inability to care for himself at home following his wife's death 1 year previously. Since admission to the long-term care facility, Mr. Stuart has lost 15 pounds. The nurses at the facility report that Mr. Stuart has experienced progressive fatigue, dyspnea on exertion, cough, night sweats, and anorexia. Initially, his cough was nonproductive, but it is now productive of moderate amounts of thick, purulent sputum that is occasionally streaked with blood. Vital signs are: temperature 99.8°F, pulse 108, respirations 26, and blood pressure 138/86. A TB skin test done at the long-term care facility 1 week ago was evaluated as negative at 6 mm. Sputum specimens for AFB reveal the presence of active tubercle bacilli, and chest x-ray is positive for TB. Auscultation of breath sounds reveals crackles in the right lower half of the lung. Mr. Stuart says, "I don't understand why I can't breathe good and what all this fuss is about."

Nursing Diagnosis 1 *Ineffective Breathing Pattern related to infectious pulmonary process as evidenced by dyspnea on exertion and productive cough*

PLANNING/GOALS	NURSING INTERVENTIONS	RATIONALE	EVALUATION
Mr. Stuart will have respiratory rate, oxygen saturation, and color within normal limits and will not complain of dyspnea.	Initially and periodically assess Mr. Stuart's respiratory status including color, respiratory rate, respiratory effort, oxygen saturation, breath sounds, level of consciousness, cough, and sputum.	The initial assessment provides a database from which the plan of care can be formulated and against which the effectiveness of treatment can be evaluated. Subsequent assessments provide a means of detecting changes in Mr. Stuart's condition, allowing for the evaluation of the effectiveness of interventions and the modification of the care plan.	Mr. Stuart verbalizes a decrease in dyspnea and cough. Mr. Stuart's color, respiratory rate, and oxygen saturation are within normal limits.
	Assist Mr. Stuart in assuming the position which most aids respiratory effort.	An upright, high or semi-Fowler's position allows for greater ease of respiration and lung expansion.	
	Alternate care activities with periods of rest.	Alternating care with periods of rest allows Mr. Stuart to compensate for the increased oxygen demand required by activity.	
	Encourage activity within Mr. Stuart's tolerance and per physician's orders.	Activity promotes expansion of the lungs.	

continues

Encourage fluids.

Fluids promote the liquefaction of respiratory secretions, thus aiding in their removal.

Administer medications for fever as ordered.

Fever increases cellular metabolism, which requires water. Thus, fever that persists can lead to dehydration, which will hinder the removal of respiratory secretions.

Administer oxygen as ordered to maintain an SaO_2 of 95% or greater.

Oxygen saturation of 95% or greater is necessary for optimal cellular function.

Administer antitubercular drugs as ordered.

Antitubercular drugs decrease the number of viable tubercle bacilli and, thus, decrease respiratory secretions.

Nursing Diagnosis 2 *Risk for Infection spread related to viable bacilli in secretions as evidenced by AFB in sputum*

PLANNING/GOALS	NURSING INTERVENTIONS	RATIONALE	EVALUATION
Mr. Stuart will verbalize both those situations that allow for the transmission of the tubercle bacilli and the means to prevent their transmission.	Place Mr. Stuart in a negative air pressure, private room; keep door closed at all times. On the door, place Airborne Precaution signs indicating that Mr. Stuart has an infectious process and asking visitors to see nursing personnel prior to visiting. Instruct visitors to wear N95 respirators when in Mr. Stuart's room, to limit the length of their visits, to avoid intimate contact, such as kissing, with Mr. Stuart, and to wash their hands when leaving the room.	A negative air pressure, private room is required to prevent the transmission of the tubercle bacilli in air that has been circulated into and out of Mr. Stuart's room. Informing the public of the infectious disease process is necessary to prevent inadvertent contact and exposure. The nature of the infection is not revealed publicly to maintain client confidentiality. Visitors are informed of precautions to take to prevent exposure to the tubercle bacilli.	Persons exposed to Mr. Stuart have been tested for TB. Those with TB are being treated. No further unprotected exposures to Mr. Stuart will occur.
	Instruct Mr. Stuart to cover his mouth and nose when coughing and sneezing.	Covering the nose and mouth aids in the containment of the tubercle bacilli.	

continues

Instruct Mr. Stuart to cough up secretions in tissues and to place the tissues in a plastic bag. Dispose of contained secretions as infectious waste.

Containment and proper disposal of infectious secretions aids in preventing the spread of the tubercle bacilli.

Inform the long-term care facility and family/significant others of the positive results of the AFB studies. Instruct those persons who have been exposed to Mr. Stuart to have a TB skin test.

Known exposure to active tubercle bacilli necessitates testing to identify individuals who may have become infected.

Observe Standard Precautions and Airborne Precautions.

Compliance with Standard Precautions and Airborne Precautions decreases the likelihood of transmitting the tubercle bacilli (and other infectious diseases) to staff and other clients.

Wear a fitted N95 respirator when in Mr. Stuart's room.

A fitted N95 respirator is necessary to prevent the inhalation of tubercle bacilli, which are able to pass through a simple surgical mask.

Plan care activities to limit the time spent in close contact with Mr. Stuart.

Prolonged exposure to the tubercle bacilli, even when taking precautions, increases the likelihood of infection.

Nursing Diagnosis 3 *Deficient Knowledge related to disease process and its treatment as evidenced by client statement: "I don't understand why I can't breathe good and what all this fuss is about."*

PLANNING/GOALS	NURSING INTERVENTIONS	RATIONALE	EVALUATION
Mr. Stuart will verbalize an understanding of the disease process and the required medication regimen.	Assess Mr. Stuart's present level of knowledge regarding TB and its treatment.	Provides a database regarding Mr. Stuart's present level of knowledge regarding TB and its treatment. Client education can then be individualized to build and expand on that knowledge base. Misinformation can also be corrected.	Mr. Stuart verbalizes his individual treatment regimen and the purpose of the regimen. Mr. Stuart accurately demonstrates medication administration. Mr. Stuart reports adverse effects of medication to health care personnel to allow for early intervention.

continues

Provide information in small amounts and use a variety of approaches (e.g., verbal, written, video).	Providing information in small amounts increases the likelihood of learning by not overwhelming Mr. Stuart with information. Providing information in a variety of media increases the likelihood of learning by supplying stimuli to the various senses (sight, sound, and touch).
Encourage and allow time for Mr. Stuart to ask questions.	Provides a means for Mr. Stuart to clarify information as well as for the nurse to evaluate learning and to correct misconceptions.
Have Mr. Stuart demonstrate medication administration regimen by setting up a day's dose of medications as ordered.	Demonstration on the part of Mr. Stuart reinforces learning and provides the nurse with a means to evaluate the effectiveness of teaching.
Have Mr. Stuart verbalize signs and symptoms of adverse medication effects that should be reported to the staff of the long-term care facility and/or the physician.	Verbalization provides a means of evaluating the effectiveness of teaching. Mr. Stuart needs to be informed of those signs and symptoms that require further evaluation and follow-up by health care personnel.

PLEURISY/PLEURAL EFFUSION

Pleurisy is a painful condition that arises from inflammation of the pleura, or sac that encases the lung. This pleuritic pain is sharp and stabbing in nature. Pain increases on inspiration as the irritated pleura rub over each other. Inflammation of the pleura occurs with many disorders, such as viral infections, cancer of the lung, trauma, tuberculosis, congestive heart failure, and pulmonary embolism. The inflamed pleura secretes increased amounts of pleural fluid into the pleural cavity, creating a **pleural effusion**. As fluid accumulates within the pleural space, it compresses the lung tissue (Figure 18-8). Collapse, or atelectasis, results if the effusion is left untreated. Those areas of

collapsed lung tissue are unable to take part in gas exchange, thereby decreasing oxygenation. Empyema is a condition wherein the pleural exudate becomes infected.

The primary manifestation of pleurisy is pain on inspiration. Signs and symptoms of pleural effusion depend on the amount of lung tissue compressed and the source of the effusion. With large pleural effusions, the mediastinum (heart, great vessels, and trachea) shifts toward the unaffected side; this can be detected by inspection, and heart sounds will move toward unaffected side. Magnetic resonance imaging (MRI) or computerized tomography (CT) studies are useful in detecting pleural effusions, particularly small ones. A chest x-ray will show pleural effusions of 250 cc of

Figure 18-8 Pleural Effusion

PROFESSIONAL TIP

Assessment of Client with a Chest Tube

- Obtain vital signs as ordered.
- Be alert for dyspnea.
- On an intake and output (I&O) sheet, describe and record amount of drainage.
- Look for loops of tubing containing drainage.
- Monitor water level in the water seal. Fluctuation (called tidaling) should occur with respirations and will stop when lung is reexpanded, tubing is kinked, connections are not tight, or chest tube becomes dislodged.
- Keep chest drainage system below the level of the client's chest.
- Every 2 hours, monitor client's response to coughing and deep breathing.
- If chest tube is accidentally dislodged, cover opening and petrolatum gauze and apply pressure to prevent air from being sucked back into chest.

fluid or more. Culture and sensitivity studies will identify the presence and type of infection, if empyema is suspected. The client with empyema will also have an elevated temperature and white blood cell count.

Medical–Surgical Management

Medical

Treatment of pleurisy is aimed at eliminating the underlying cause, maintaining adequate oxygenation to the tissues, and preventing complications such as atelectasis and pneumonia. Adequacy of oxygenation is evaluated by means of arterial blood gases and/or pulse oximetry. Supplemental oxygen is given to maintain an oxygen saturation of 95% or greater. Respiratory treatments to aid lung expansion such as incentive spirometry are used.

Surgical

Larger pleural effusions require a thoracentesis be performed by the physician to remove accumulated fluid. After the overlying tissues are anesthetized, a large bore needle is placed into the pleural space. Fluid is removed and may be sent to the laboratory for diagnostic purposes (i.e., culture, cytology). If fluid accumulation continues to present a problem, as with empyema, the physician will place a thoracotomy tube into the pleural space to drain fluid continuously. Following administration of local anesthetics, the physician places a large bore catheter into the pleural space. This catheter is attached to an underwater seal drainage device (see Figure 18-9). The underwater seal drainage device prevents the negative pressure within the pleural space from pulling air into the pleural space,

and allows for the drainage of accumulated fluid or air. In addition, most devices also include a chamber to which suction may be applied to assist in the removal of fluid or air from the pleural space. Following insertion of a chest tube, a chest x-ray is done to evaluate its placement and effectiveness.

Figure 18-9 Underwater Seal Chest Drainage Device

Pharmacological

If a pleural effusion is small and does not interfere greatly with respiratory function, diuretics are used to promote removal of fluid from the pleural space. Furosemide (Lasix) and bumetanide (Bumex) may be given for this purpose. If empyema is present, specific therapy is used once the causative agent is identified. Relief of pain is a high priority. Analgesia that also decreases inflammation is preferred. Ketorolac tromethamine (Toradol) and other NSAIDs are often used. Severe pain will require narcotics such as morphine sulfate or meperidine (Demerol). If inflammation is extensive, corticosteroids such as hydrocortisone sodium succinate (Solu-Cortef) may be utilized.

Activity

The client's activity is limited to prevent fatigue. The client on bed rest is placed in a high Fowler's position to assist respirations.

▶ NURSING PROCESS

▶ Assessment

▶ Subjective Data

A nursing history is obtained from the client regarding onset, duration, and severity of symptoms. The client usually describes both chest pain that increases with each inspiration and difficulty breathing.

▶ Objective Data

The client's level of consciousness is assessed, and the client's color, respiratory rate, and effort evaluated. Abnormalities in vital signs are noted. Breath sounds over the areas of involvement are diminished or absent. A pleural friction rub may be audible. Dyspnea, cyanosis, and hypoxia occur proportional to the severity of the condition. If a chest tube is in place, the amount and color of drainage are assessed.

Nursing diagnoses for a client with a pleural effusion may include the following:

Nursing Diagnoses	Planning/Goals	Nursing Interventions
▶ Acute Pain related to inflammation of the pleura	Using a scale of 1 to 10, the client will verbalize a decrease in the level of pain.	Administer pain medications as ordered.
		Assist the client in attaining the position that allows for greatest comfort. Elevate the head of the bed.
		Provide diversional activities.
▶ Impaired Gas Exchange related to compressed lung	The client will maintain an oxygen saturation of 95% or greater and a respiratory rate of 14 to 22 and will have clear breath sounds.	Monitor vital signs and pulse oximetry.
		Provide supplemental oxygen as ordered.
		Encourage the client to breathe deeply or use the incentive spirometer as ordered.
		Administer diuretics and anti-inflammatory medications as ordered.
		Assist the physician with the thoracentesis or the placement of a thoracotomy tube.
		Collect specimen for culture and sensitivity and other studies.
▶ Bathing/Hygiene Self-care Deficit related to mobility restriction	The client will increase self-care activities as mobility increases.	Assist the client with hygiene and self-care needs.
		Encourage participation in self-care activities within the limits of the physician's orders.
▶ Risk for Activity Intolerance related to hypoxia secondary to pleural effusion	The client will increase activity without complaining of fatigue.	Stagger periods of activity with periods of rest.
		To prevent fatigue, plan activities around therapies.

Evaluation Each goal must be evaluated to determine how it has been met by the client.

ACUTE RESPIRATORY TRACT DISORDERS

Acute respiratory tract disorders include atelectasis, pulmonary embolism, pulmonary edema, adult respiratory distress syndrome, and acute respiratory failure.

ATELECTASIS

Atelectasis refers to the collapse of a lung or a portion of a lung. The most common cause of atelectasis is airway obstruction. A bronchiole becomes blocked with secretions, and the alveoli distal to it collapse (Figure 18-10). Airway obstruction of this nature is common after surgery and with immobility problems.

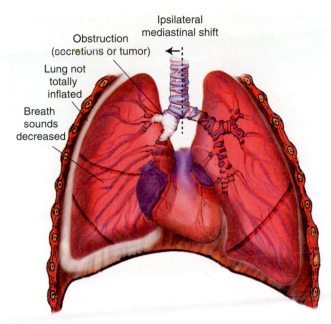

Figure 18-10 Atelectasis (collapsed lung)

Obstruction
(secretions or tumor)

Ipsilateral
mediastinal shift

Lung not
totally
inflated

Breath
sounds
decreased

Anesthesia, pain, narcotics, and immobility can cause hypoventilation and retention of secretions. Hypoventilation can cause atelectasis, and atelectasis increases hypoventilation. Atelectasis also occurs with compression of lung tissue, as is the case with pleural effusion or pneumothorax. An insufficient level of surfactant results in increased recoil properties of the lungs, leading to atelectasis.

Signs of respiratory distress are proportional to the amount of lung tissue involved. When large areas of the lung are involved, orthopnea or cyanosis may develop. Breath sounds are diminished or absent over collapsed areas. Late in the disease process, chest wall movement decreases on the affected side. Oxygenation decreases as demonstrated by ABGs or pulse oximetry. Pulse and respiratory rate increase as the heart and lungs work harder to meet the body's oxygen needs. Trapped secretions are a growth medium for microorganisms. An elevated temperature indicates secondary infection (pneumonia). Chest x-ray studies reveal the areas of collapse. Bronchoscopy (insertion of a bronchoscope through the nasal passages into the trachea) is used to directly visualize the area of obstruction and obtain a specimen for diagnostic purposes.

Medical–Surgical Management

Medical

The physician will order various measures to promote expansion of the lungs. Incentive spirometry and deep breathing and coughing exercises are ordered. Postural drainage along with percussion aids in the removal of any static secretions. If the client is unable to cough up secretions, suctioning of the respiratory tract is performed. Bronchoscopy may be done by the physician to remove secretions and obtain specimens. Arterial blood gases and pulse oximetry are utilized to evaluate the need for supplemental oxygen. Oxygen is administered to maintain an oxygen saturation of 95% or greater.

Surgical

Clients with pneumothorax or pleural effusion as the underlying cause of atelectasis require removal of trapped air or fluid via thoracentesis or placement of a thoracotomy tube (refer to the sections on pleural effusion and pneumothorax). Atelectasis resulting from the growth of a tumor requires treatment of the tumor.

Pharmacological

Adequate pain control aids the client, particularly the surgical client, in being able to breathe deeply and cough. Client-controlled analgesia or a routine schedule of pain medications may be used to provide effective pain management. Aminophylline (Aminophyllin) and other bronchodilators may be used to open the airways. Mucolytic agents such as guaifenisin (Humibid) are used to liquefy respiratory tract secretions. Bronchodilators, such as albuterol sulfate (Ventolin), and mucolytics, such as acetylcysteine (Mucomyst), may also be administered via updraft or nebulizer treatments. The client with an infection requires treatment with an appropriate antibiotic such as ciprofloxacin hydrochloride (Cipro).

Diet

Unless otherwise contraindicated, fluids are encouraged to promote liquefaction of trapped respiratory secretions.

Activity

Activity promotes lung expansion. Immobile clients are turned a minimum of every 2 hours and are assisted in doing range-of-motion exercises. Surgical clients may do leg exercises as well as deep breathing and coughing. Ambulation is recommended if the client's condition allows. If the client is unable to walk, sitting up in a chair is encouraged. To prevent fatigue, rest periods are planned between activities.

▶ NURSING PROCESS

▶ Assessment

▶ Subjective Data

Clients who smoke or those who are immunocompromised or have known chronic respiratory or cardiovascular diseases are at increased risk of developing atelectasis. The client is asked about the onset, duration, and severity of symptoms such as pain, cough, and dyspnea. The client may complain or show signs of air hunger, shortness of breath, fatigue, and anxiety.

▶ Objective Data

The client must be assessed for changes in level of consciousness, an early sign of decreased oxygenation. The client should be periodically evaluated for dyspnea, tachypnea, cyanosis, and restlessness. Vital signs should be measured frequently, with particular attention to respiratory rate and effort. Auscultation reveals diminished or absent breath sounds over the areas of atelectasis. Crackles or sonorous wheezes may be heard if pneumonia develops. Objective indicators of pain such as facial grimacing should be noted, and can be validated by subjective questioning. The effectiveness of the client's cough is assessed. A productive cough is evaluated for amount, color, consistency, and odor of secretions (Table 18–10).

Table 18–10 PATHOLOGIES ASSOCIATED WITH DIFFERENT TYPES OF SPUTUM

SPUTUM	PATHOLOGY
Color	
Mucoid	Tracheobronchitis, asthma
Yellow or green	Bacterial infection
Rust or blood tinged	Pneumonia, pulmonary infarction, TB
Black	Black lung disease
Pink, thin frothy	Pulmonary edema
Odor	
Foul smelling	Anaerobic infection

Adapted from Health Assessment & Physical Examination, *2nd ed., by M. E. Z. Estes, 2002, Albany, NY: Delmar. Copyright 2002 by Delmar. Adapted with permission.*

Nursing diagnoses for a client with atelectasis may include the following:

Nursing Diagnoses	Planning/Goals	Nursing Interventions
▶ *Deficient Knowledge related to the complications of surgery and/or immobility*	The client will verbalize the purpose of deep breathing, coughing, and activity following surgery and will demonstrate deep breathing and coughing.	Teach all preoperative and immobile clients to cough and breathe deeply at least every 2 hours.
		Have the client demonstrate coughing and deep breathing to ensure that learning has occurred.
		Teach the surgical client to splint the surgical incision to minimize discomfort that might occur with coughing and deep breathing.
		Instruct clients at risk for developing atelectasis in the use of incentive spirometry.
		Emphasize the importance of early ambulation and activity to promote lung expansion.
▶ *Impaired Gas Exchange related to decreased alveolar–capillary surface*	The client will have an oxygen saturation of 95% or greater, a respiratory rate of 14 to 22, and clear breath sounds.	Establish a schedule for coughing and deep breathing.
		Encourage clients to ambulate and/or sit up in a chair three to four times daily.
		Turn the immobile client every 2 hours or more frequently.
		Assess the client's vital signs and breath sounds every 4 hours or more frequently as situation warrants.
		Encourage fluids if the client's condition allows.
		Administer respiratory treatments as ordered.
		Administer medications as ordered.
		Assess secretions (sputum) for color, amount, consistency, and odor.
▶ *Risk for Activity Intolerance related to hypoxia secondary to atelectasis*	The client will complete activity without complaints of shortness of breath, dyspnea, or fatigue.	Encourage some activity, such as walking, to promote lung expansion.
		Alternate periods of activity with periods of rest. Avoid client fatigue.
		Provide assistance with ADL as the client's condition requires.
		Place the client in a high or semi-Fowler's position to aid lung expansion.
		Position client on the unaffected side.

Evaluation Each goal must be evaluated to determine how it has been met by the client.

PULMONARY EMBOLISM

Pulmonary embolism develops when a bloodborne substance lodges in a branch of a pulmonary artery and obstructs flow. A common source of pulmonary embolism is a deep vein thrombus. Other sources are air from intravenous infusions; fat from long bone fractures; and amniotic fluid. The size and location of the emboli determine the severity and outcome of the condition.

Pulmonary emboli rarely develop before adulthood. As age increases, the risk for pulmonary embolism becomes greater due to the development of arteriosclerosis and other vascular changes associated with aging. Other factors that increase the risk for pulmonary embolism are heredity, smoking, peripheral vascular disease, diabetes mellitus, and oral contraceptive use.

Emboli interfere with gas exchange to the pulmonary circulation distal to the emboli, resulting in hypoxemia. The client complains of breathlessness and dyspnea. Pulse oximetry or ABGs will demonstrate the degree to which oxygenation has been affected. Obstruction of a main branch of a pulmonary artery can result in lung infarction and necrosis.

All clients at risk for pulmonary embolism should be observed for signs and symptoms of deep vein thrombosis, such as localized calf tenderness or swelling. Measures to prevent thrombus formation should be taken for these individuals. Any signs of thrombophlebitis should be immediately reported to the physician.

Signs and symptoms of pulmonary embolism are abrupt in onset. The client becomes anxious and restless. Sudden, sharp chest pains of a pleuritic nature (worse on inspiration) develop. Dyspnea and cough along with hemoptysis occur. Venous return is diminished, resulting in jugular venous distention. The client becomes diaphoretic. A low-grade fever develops in response to inflammation. A high temperature is indicative of lung infarction. Diagnosis of pulmonary embolism is accomplished by a ventilation/perfusion lung scan. Arterial blood gases show hypoxia and respiratory alkalosis. In severe cases, pulmonary angiography is performed to find the exact location of the clot.

Medical–Surgical Management

Medical

Preventive measures are instituted for the client at risk of developing deep vein thrombosis. Following surgery, antiembolism stockings and early ambulation are indicated. When hypoxia occurs, supplemental oxygen is given to increase oxygenation. The underlying cause of the pulmonary emboli is treated when identified.

Surgical

In severe cases, the physician may elect to remove the clot via an embolectomy. This procedure is usually done at the time of angiography. Clients who experience successive episodes of pulmonary embolism may require a venacaval plication. This surgical procedure involves placing a sieve-like device in the inferior vena cava to catch emboli before they enter the pulmonary circulation (see Figure 19-28 in Chapter 19).

Pharmacological

The client at risk of developing deep vein thrombosis and/or pulmonary embolism may be treated with enoxaparin sodium (Lovenox). Lovenox is often used in the postoperative client to prevent clot formation. After pulmonary emboli have developed, anticoagulation is ordered to prevent the formation of further clots. Heparin (Hep-Lock) is initially used to establish anticoagulation and is administered parenterally by either the intravenous or subcutaneous route. After adequate anticoagulation has been established, warfarin sodium (Coumadin) therapy is initiated. Coumadin is given orally and may be used long term on an outpatient basis. If the clot is large or lies in a branch of a main pulmonary artery, fibrinolytic therapy may be used. Fibrinolytics lyse, or dissolve, the clot versus inhibiting the formation of new clots. Examples of fibrinolytic agents are alteplase (Activase) and streptokinase (Streptase). These agents may be administered intra-arterially at the site of the clot or intravenously to achieve a systemic effect. Narcotic analgesics such as morphine are ordered to control pain.

Diet

To prevent hemoconcentration leading to clot formation, fluids are encouraged. Unless contraindicated,

CLIENT TEACHING

Anticoagulant Therapy (Coumadin)

Stress the importance of the following:

- Follow-up laboratory testing
- Using a soft toothbrush to prevent trauma to the gums (bleeding)
- Inspecting the skin for bruises or petechiae
- Using an electric razor to avoid scratching skin
- Reporting nosebleeds, tarry stool, hematuria, or hematemesis to the physician
- Eating a consistent amount of green, leafy vegetables daily (differing amounts alter anticoagulant effects)
- Avoiding other medications (including aspirin) without approval from physician
- In the female client, monitor menstrual flow for excessive amount

fluids should be encouraged for the client at risk of developing pulmonary embolism.

Activity

To prevent the formation of clots, activity is encouraged. After a clot has formed, however, the client's activity is restricted to prevent the clot from moving and becoming an embolus. Activities such as sitting, crossing the knees, or prolonged bending at the hips are to be avoided, because these promote venous stasis.

▶ NURSING PROCESS

▶ Assessment

▶ Subjective Data

The client's history is obtained to identify potential risk factors for the development of pulmonary emboli. The client is asked about the onset, duration, and severity of symptoms. Shortness of breath, dyspnea, and severe pleuritic chest pain are abrupt in onset. Pain is evaluated as to onset, location, duration, severity, and character.

GERONTOLOGICAL CONSIDERATIONS

Anticoagulant Therapy (Coumadin)
Monitor elderly clients closely, as they are especially sensitive to effects of Coumadin.

▶ Objective Data

Pulse oximetery measurements are monitored. The client's respirations are rapid and shallow. Pallor progressing to cyanosis develops as oxygenation decreases. The client becomes diaphoretic. Increased anxiety or a change in level of consciousness may be the first indication of a pulmonary embolism. The pulse increases in response to anxiety and in an attempt to supply oxygen to the body's cells. Blood pressure may increase or decrease in response to hypoxia, anxiety, and pain. Temperature may elevate in response to inflammation and tissue necrosis. On auscultation, breath sounds may or may not be decreased. The jugular veins are distended.

Nursing diagnoses for a client with pulmonary embolism may include the following:

Nursing Diagnoses	Planning/Goals	Nursing Interventions
▶ Impaired Gas Exchange related to alteration in pulmonary circulation	The client will maintain an oxygen saturation of 95% or greater, have a respiratory rate of 14 to 22, and have color within normal limits.	Assess the client for indications of decreasing oxygenation. Auscultate breath sounds every 4 hours or more often. Assess peripheral pulses and capillary refill. Encourage deep breathing and coughing. Provide supplemental oxygen to maintain oxygen saturation at greater than 95% or as ordered. Administer subcutaneous heparin as ordered. After anticoagulation is established, administer Coumadin as ordered. Encourage fluids, unless contraindicated, to prevent hemoconcentration.
▶ Acute Pain related to decreased perfusion of lung tissue	Using a scale of 1 to 10, the client will indicate decreased pain.	Administer pain medication as ordered. Assist the client in assuming a position of comfort. If possible, place the client in a high Fowler's position to aid respiratory effort.
▶ Risk for Injury related to anticoagulation/ fibrinolytic therapy	The client will be free of abnormal bleeding and maintain hemoglobin and hematocrit within normal limits.	Assess for evidence of bleeding. Monitor lab reports for activated partial thromboplastin time (APTT), international normalized ratio (INR), prothrombin time (PT), and hemoglobin and hematocrit levels. Evaluate blood pressure and pulse for signs of bleeding, i.e., rapid pulse and low blood pressure. Check stool for occult blood. Assess gums for bleeding.

Evaluation Each goal must be evaluated to determine how it has been met by the client.

PULMONARY EDEMA

Acute pulmonary edema is a life-threatening condition characterized by a rapid shift of fluid from plasma into the pulmonary interstitial tissue and the alveoli

(Figure 18-11). As a result, gas exchange is markedly impaired. Pulmonary edema can occur as a result of severe left ventricular failure (i.e., following myocardial infarction), rapid administration of i.v. fluids, inhalation of noxious gases, or opiate or barbiturate overdose.

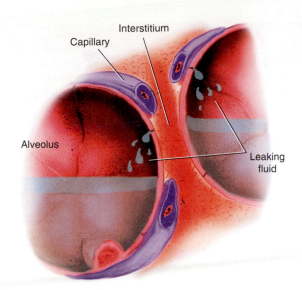

Figure 18-11 Pulmonary Edema

The hallmark of acute pulmonary edema is a cough producing a copious amount of frothy, blood-tinged sputum, often appearing pinkish. The client rapidly becomes dyspneic, orthopneic, and cyanotic. Anxiety ranging from restlessness to panic occurs. Heart and respiratory rate increase. Progressive crackles are heard in the lung fields on auscultation. Initially, fine crackles are present in the posterior bases of the lung. As pulmonary edema progresses, the crackles become increasingly coarser, louder, and more diffuse. Wheezes are heard in the presence of significant airway obstruction by fluid. Left untreated, the client deteriorates rapidly as oxygenation decreases.

Medical–Surgical Management

Medical

The goals of medical management are to remove fluid from the alveoli and pulmonary interstitial space, prevent further influx of fluid, and improve oxygenation. Arterial blood gases and pulse oximetry values are used to assess oxygenation. Oxygen is administered per physician's order when hypoxia is present.

Pharmacological

A diuretic such as furosemide (Lasix) is given to remove fluid, resulting in increased urinary output.

When the pumping force of the left ventricle is impaired, a digitalis preparation, (i.e., digoxin [Lanoxin]) is given to improve the contractile force of the myocardium. To prevent further influx of fluid into the lungs, venous pooling is enhanced. This also decreases the workload on the heart by limiting venous return. Morphine is used to promote vasodilatation and, thus, venous pooling and to relieve anxiety. Bronchodilators such as aminophylline (Aminophyllin) are administered to dilate airways obstructed with fluid.

Diet

To prevent fluid retention, the physician may order a diet restricted in sodium. Intake and output as well as daily weight are measured to monitor fluid balance.

Activity

The client is placed on bed rest to reduce the workload on the heart and lungs. High Fowler's position aids respiratory effort and enhances venous pooling. Activities are increased slowly according to the physician's orders and the client's ability to tolerate activity.

▶ NURSING PROCESS

▶ Assessment

▶ Subjective Data

The nurse needs to be aware of those conditions that predispose the client to pulmonary edema. The client may describe feeling anxious, breathless, and fatigued.

▶ Objective Data

Breath sounds are auscultated for the presence of crackles. Increasingly coarse and diffuse crackles are reported to the physician. The client's level of consciousness, respiratory rate and effort, and color should be assessed. Dyspnea, tachypnea, cyanosis and/or pallor may be present. Oxygenation is assessed via pulse oximetry or ABGs. A productive cough may be present, as may symptoms of CHF, such as rapid weight gain and peripheral edema. Pulse may be rapid and weak. Blood pressure may increase in response to anxiety and decreased oxygenation.

Nursing diagnoses for a client with pulmonary edema may include the following:

Nursing Diagnoses	Planning/Goals	Nursing Interventions
▶ *Impaired Gas Exchange related to fluid in the lung tissue*	The client will maintain an oxygen saturation of 95% or greater and will have respiratory rate and color and blood gases within normal limits and clear breath sounds.	Place the client in high Fowler's or orthopneic position (sitting upright). Continually assess oxygenation with ABG or pulse oximetry measurements and provide supplemental oxygen to maintain an oxygen saturation of 95% or greater or per physician's order.

continues

Nursing Diagnoses	Planning/Goals	Nursing Interventions
		Frequently assess respiratory rate, breath sounds, apical heart rate, and blood pressure. Administer respiratory treatments as ordered.
		Assist the client with activities to reduce the workload on the heart and lungs, and alternate periods of activity with periods of rest to prevent client fatigue. Administer medications as ordered and evaluate the effectiveness of each. Monitor lab reports for electrolyte values.
▶ *Excess Fluid Volume related to altered tissue permeability*	The client's weight will return to normal.	Weigh client daily.
		Monitor I&O.
		Frequently assess the client for peripheral edema.
		Provide the client with a low-salt diet as ordered.
		Administer diuretics per order and evaluate their effectiveness.
		Monitor lab reports for electrolyte values.
		Monitor the rate at which intravenous fluids are given.
		Teach client and family fluid excess symptoms, medication information, and dietary modifications.

Evaluation Each goal must be evaluated to determine how it has been met by the client.

ADULT RESPIRATORY DISTRESS SYNDROME

Adult respiratory distress syndrome (ARDS) is a life-threatening condition characterized by severe dyspnea, hypoxemia, and diffuse pulmonary edema. The condition usually follows a major assault on multiple body systems or severe lung trauma. Underlying causes include trauma, sepsis, coronary artery bypass surgery, major thoracic or vascular surgery, renal failure, severe pulmonary infections, inhalation lung injuries, and acute drug poisoning. Adult respiratory distress syndrome is also called noncardiogenic pulmonary edema, shock lung, progressive pulmonary congestion, or traumatic wet lung. The term *adult respiratory distress syndrome* more accurately describes the pathophysiology underlying this condition.

During the initial assault on the body, the pulmonary capillary membrane is damaged; this allows fluid to leak from the vascular system into the pulmonary interstitial tissue and the alveoli themselves. Gas exchange is severely impaired due to the damage to the pulmonary capillary membrane and the presence of fluid in the alveoli. The surfactant is rendered inactive, resulting in the collapse of the alveoli, further reducing gas exchange. Hypoxemia that is resistant to conventional oxygen therapy then develops.

The client with ARDS is critically ill, as reflected by severe dyspnea, tachypnea, and cyanosis. Arterial blood gases will show PaO_2 less than 70 mm Hg, $PaCO_2$ more than 35 mm Hg, bicarbonate ion less than 22 mEq/L, and initially elevated but steadily decreasing pH. The ABGs and pulse oximetry reveal severe hypoxemia and progressive respiratory and metabolic acidosis. On auscultation, the lung fields are filled with diffuse coarse crackles and sonorous wheezes. The client will have a productive cough yielding blood-tinged sputum. Chest x-ray will show widely scattered infiltrates, often referred to as a "white out."

Medical–Surgical Management

Medical

The client with ARDS is cared for in the intensive care unit. The underlying cause of ARDS is ascertained and treated; until that time, supportive care is given. Mechanical ventilatory support is necessary, with multiple other systems often also being supported. A mechanical ventilator allows the oxygen percentage, pulmonary pressure, and lung volume to be controlled. Oxygenation is monitored with ABGs and pulse oximetry. Respiratory secretions are removed by frequent bronchial suctioning.

Pharmacological

Pharmacological therapy includes high doses of corticosteriods such as hydrocortisone sodium succinate (Solu-Cortef) or methylprednisolone sodium succinate (Solu-Medrol). Furosemide (Lasix) and other diuretics are given to remove fluids and increase urinary output. Aminophylline (Aminophyllin) is administered to open the bronchi. While the client is on the mechanical ventilator, pancuronium bromide (Pavulon) is given to suppress the client's own respiratory effort. Blood pressure can fall dangerously low, and vasopressors such as dopamine hydrochloride (Intropin) may be required to maintain the blood pressure within an acceptable range.

Diet

Total parenteral nutrition (TPN) may be given to the client, especially during the acute phase of the illness. When possible, enteral feedings are preferred.

Activity

The client with ARDS will be on bed rest. Special beds that provide movement and pressure adjustment prevent the complications associated with immobility.

▶ NURSING PROCESS

▶ Assessment

▶ Subjective Data

The client history is typically gathered from family members or significant others, as the client is usually too ill to communicate.

▶ Objective Data

The client's level of consciousness and response to stimuli are assessed, and the client is observed for restlessness and anxiety. Vital signs are measured every 15 minutes or more often if the client is critically ill. Heart rate is increased, and arrhythmias may be present.

PROFESSIONAL TIP

Client on a Mechanical Ventilator

Check the following:
- Type of ventilator (e.g., Servo, Bear)
- FiO_2 setting
- Mode being used (e.g., assist, intermittent mandatory)
- Amount of positive end-expiratory pressure
- Rate and tidal volume
- Peak inspiratory pressure
- Temperature of the humidification
- Alarm set
- Pressure support

Blood pressure is usually low. Respiratory rate, rhythm, and effort are assessed for signs of dyspnea, nasal flaring, cyanosis, tachypnea, and other indications of respiratory distress. Arterial blood gas and pulse oximetry values are assessed to evaluate oxygenation and acid–base balance. Diffuse, coarse crackles and wheezes are heard throughout the lung fields.

Nursing diagnoses for a client with ARDS may include the following:

Nursing Diagnoses	Planning/Goals	Nursing Interventions
▶ *Impaired Gas Exchange related to pulmonary capillary membrane damage*	The client will have an oxygen saturation of 95% or greater, ABGs within normal limits, and respiratory rate and effort within normal limits.	Provide adequate oxygenation and ventilation as ordered. Monitor ABGs and pulse oximetry to evaluate oxygenation and acid–base balance. Assess the client's respiratory rate and effort and auscultate the lungs frequently. Suction the respiratory tract as necessary to remove excess secretions. Provide oral care frequently.
▶ *Anxiety related to the condition and mechanical ventilation*	The client, if able, will verbalize a decrease in anxiety or will exhibit fewer objective signs of anxiety, such as restlessness and facial grimacing.	Describe care and purposes to the client. Allow rest periods between periods of activity to avoid overwhelming the client with stimuli. Plan care to allow for uninterrupted rest. Allow family and significant others to visit and participate in care, as appropriate. Assess the client for signs of sensory overload/deprivation.

Evaluation Each goal must be evaluated to determine how it has been met by the client.

ACUTE RESPIRATORY FAILURE

Acute respiratory failure is not a disease entity in and of itself; rather, the term is used to refer to conditions wherein there is a failure of the respiratory system as a whole. This condition occurs as a result of the client's literally becoming too tired to continue the "work" of breathing. Mechanical ventilatory support is required during the acute phase. Clients with preexisting pulmonary conditions coupled with acute respiratory tract infections are at risk of developing acute respiratory failure.

CHRONIC RESPIRATORY TRACT DISORDERS

Chronic obstructive pulmonary disease (COPD), asthma, chronic bronchitis, emphysema, and bronchiectasis are discussed following.

CHRONIC OBSTRUCTIVE PULMONARY DISEASE

Chronic obstructive pulmonary disease, also called chronic obstructive lung disease (COLD) or chronic airflow limitation (CAL), describes a broad category of respiratory conditions with a variety of etiologic factors. Chronic obstructive pulmonary disease is characterized by chronic airflow limitation. Changes within the lungs lead to a narrowing of the bronchial airways, excessive mucous secretions within the airways, and an increase in the size of the airways distal to the terminal bronchioles (the alveoli) and resultant trapping of air. The conditions most often associated with COPD are: asthma, chronic bronchitis, emphysema, and bronchiectasis.

ASTHMA

Asthma is a condition characterized by intermittent airway obstruction in response to a variety of stimuli. The epithelial lining of the airways responds by becoming inflamed and edematous. Bronchospasm occurs in the smooth muscles of the bronchi and bronchioles. Secretions increase in viscosity. Elastic recoil decreases. All of these changes result in a reduction of the diameter of the airways and in breathing difficulty on inspiration. Over time, the changes may become chronic, and COPD results. Some clients who develop asthma in childhood experience spontaneous recovery.

Asthma may be classified as extrinsic or intrinsic. Extrinsic asthma is caused by substances outside the body that precipitate the asthma response, such as pollen, house dust, or food additives. Intrinsic asthma is diagnosed when no extrinsic factor can be identified

GERONTOLOGICAL CONSIDERATIONS

Asthma and Age

- Asthma attacks usually become more severe and more frequent as the individual ages, and
- Asthma attacks are usually not associated with definite allergens.

and the asthma is the result of internal factors such as emotional stress, exercise, or fatigue. Allergies; environmental factors such as air pollution; heredity; exercise; and psychological factors have been indicated in predisposing an individual to asthma. An asthma attack that does not respond to treatment and persists is known as **status asthmaticus**.

The hallmark of an asthma attack is sudden onset of wheezing, increasing dyspnea, and chest tightness. Mild asthma can usually be controlled by routine medication. Severe asthma attacks usually occur at night and require extra medication. With severe attacks, wheezing may be audible to the unaided ear. Expiratory wheezes are common as air attempts to escape through the narrowed airways. Both inspiratory and expiratory wheezes may be heard. It is important to note that absence of wheezing is not necessarily a positive sign, as it could indicate complete closure of the airway. The respiratory rate rises initially, but as the client tires, the rate may decrease. Nasal flaring and costal and sternal retractions may be present, particularly in the young client. The client uses accessory muscles to assist respiratory effort. Cough occurs as the respiratory secretions become thick and block the airways. Cyanosis and a decrease in oxygen saturation occur. Heart rate elevates, as may blood pressure. The client becomes anxious and may complain of a sense of impending doom. These responses are thought to be caused by a release of catecholamines. Values of ABGs indicate hypoxia and respiratory acidosis. Chest x-ray shows hyperinflation of the lungs. Pulmonary function tests reveal an abnormal flow rate and lung volume. With a severe asthma attack, apnea and sudden death can occur in minutes.

Medical–Surgical Management

Medical

In addition to medications, treatment for asthma may include manipulating known triggers. The client with allergies should avoid specific antigens, such as animal hair, pollens, and dietary factors, that might bring on an attack. Some clients with asthma are aided by control of psychological stressors. Routine physical exercise is beneficial in treating exercise-induced asthma. The client with asthma should be told to avoid other respiratory irritants such as cigarette smoke and air pollution. Clients who develop asthma later in life will develop more symptoms as they age.

Pharmacological

The primary treatment for an acute asthma attack is pharmacological. A combination of medications is used to open the narrowed airways. Medications used to dilate the bronchi include bronchodilators such as aminophylline (Aminophyllin) and terbutaline sulfate (Brethine, Bricanyl); beta agonists such as epinephrine

COMMUNITY/HOME HEALTH CARE

Asthma

- Prohibit smoking in the home, especially if a child has asthma
- Use a humidifier, especially in the bedroom of the person with asthma
- Use fans to circulate air

CLIENT TEACHING

Use of Nebulizer

Advise clients to:
- Keep nebulizer with them at all times,
- Take only two to three whiffs every 4 hours
- Call physician if nebulizer is needed more frequently.

(Primatene Mist) and albuterol sulfate (Ventolin); and anticholinergics such as atropine sulfate and ipratropium bromide (Atrovent). Corticosteroids such as prednisone (Delatsone) are utilized to decrease inflammation. Mucolytic agents such as acetylcysteine (Mucomyst) aid in liquefying secretions. Supplemental oxygen is given when indicated.

Diet

Adequate fluid intake should be maintained to promote liquefaction of secretions.

Activity

The nurse incorporates several rest periods into the day. Relaxation techniques can be used to manage anxiety. The client should not overexert to the point of dyspnea, wheezing, or fatigue. If overexertion occurs, the client sits down and sips warm water. Doing so promotes slower, regular breathing, as well as bronchodilation, and loosens secretions.

▶ NURSING PROCESS

▶ Assessment

▶ Subjective Data

A detailed history is taken regarding exposure to triggering stimuli prior to past asthma attacks. Also ascertained are the onset, duration, and severity of symptoms such as dyspnea.

▶ Objective Data

The effectiveness of ventilation is noted. Wheezes are evaluated as to their duration, location, and the phase of respiration during which they occur (e.g., inspiration). Wheezes heard without the aid of a stethoscope are called **audible wheezes**. Respiratory rate, depth, rhythm and effort; position assumed; and client color are evaluated. Monitoring of pulse oximetry or lab reports of ABG values is done to determine oxygenation and acid–base balance. If sputum is produced, its color, amount, viscosity, and odor are noted.

Nursing diagnoses for a client with asthma may include the following:

Nursing Diagnoses	Planning/Goals	Nursing Interventions
▶ *Inefficient Breathing Pattern related to narrowed airways*	The client will have respiratory rate and color within normal limits, clear breath sounds on auscultation, and ABG or pulse oximetry values within normal limits.	Assist the client in assuming a position that facilitates ventilation. Administer medication as ordered. Assist the client in the use of inhalers and aerosol treatments. Assess oxygenation by ABG or pulse oximetry values, as ordered. Administer supplemental oxygen, as ordered. Frequently assess respiratory rate and effort as well as color as client's condition dictates. Auscultate the lung fields for presence of wheezes. If sputum is produced, note its color, amount, viscosity, and odor. Frequently assess vital signs as client's condition dictates. Unless otherwise contraindicated, encourage fluid intake to promote liquefaction of respiratory secretions.
▶ *Deficient Knowledge related to asthma, asthma treatment, and individual triggers for asthma attacks*	The client will verbalize an understanding of both the pathophysiology and treatment of asthma, including the medications taken and their purposes and side effects. The client will also identify individual triggers and means of avoiding these triggers.	Teach client about the disease process. Teach client and family the purpose, effect, adverse effects, side effects, and use of all prescribed medications, especially inhalers and respiratory aerosol equipment. Assist client in establishing a medication schedule that will facilitate regular and timely taking of medications.

continues

Nursing Diagnoses	Planning/Goals	Nursing Interventions
		Instruct the client to use the inhaler prior to meals to aid in breathing while eating.
		If the client is taking steroids, teach to rinse mouth after using the inhaler so as to prevent fungal infection.
		Encourage exercise because it increases respiratory reserve and improves overall physical condition.
		Assist client in identifying triggering stimuli and ways to avoid them.
		Teach client and family signs and symptoms of asthma attacks and respiratory tract infections.
		Teach client to avoid crowded areas and close contact with persons with infections.
▶ *Anxiety related to perceived threat of dying*	The client will verbalize a decrease in anxiety.	Provide the client with explanations for all care.
		Provide care in a calm, unhurried manner.
		Plan care to allow the client uninterrupted periods of rest.
		Allow the client to make decisions regarding care, if possible.
		Provide the client with opportunities to discuss anxiety with staff, family, or significant others.

Evaluation Each goal must be evaluated to determine how it has been met by the client.

CHRONIC BRONCHITIS

Bronchitis is an inflammation of the bronchial tree accompanied by hypersecretion of mucus. The condition becomes chronic if an individual has an infection with a productive cough at least 3 months a year for two consecutive years. Constant irritation of the bronchi results in hypertrophy of the mucus-secreting glands. The bronchioles fill with exudate, and subsequent infections are common. The alveoli adjacent to the bronchioles eventually become damaged and fibrosed. Environmental factors, especially cigarette smoke, play an important role in the development of chronic bronchitis. Certain individuals may have a hereditary predisposition to developing chronic bronchitis. Exposure to cold, damp air coupled with repeated respiratory infections has been identified as a cause of chronic bronchitis.

The client usually has a history of recurrent respiratory infections, dyspnea, cyanosis, and chronic or recurrent cough yielding copious amounts of sputum. Often, the sputum is purulent or green in color. Over the course of time, the chest wall configuration becomes slightly distended. There are coarse crackles present throughout the lung fields. Breath sounds may be diminished or absent over the periphery of the lung fields. Elevation of pulmonary artery pressure results in increased workload for the right ventricle and in signs and symptoms of right-sided CHF, such as peripheral edema and fatigue. Arterial blood gases reveal increased $PaCO_2$ and decreased PaO_2. The red blood cell count elevates, as do hemoglobin and hematocrit. The increases in the amounts of red blood cells and

hemoglobin represent an attempt by the body to compensate for the lower oxygen level. Chest x-ray shows hyperexpansion of the lungs. When CHF occurs, the chest x-ray also shows an enlarged heart.

Medical–Surgical Management

Medical

The goals of medical treatment are to decrease symptoms of airway irritation, decrease airway obstruction related to secretions and inflammation, prevent infection, maintain oxygenation, and increase the client's exercise tolerance. Respiratory therapy includes the use of updraft (nebulizer) and aerosol treatments along with percussion and postural drainage. Humidification of inspired air helps liquefy secretions. Supplemental oxygen is administered based on ABG or pulse oximetry measurements. The neurological response to breathe becomes altered in some clients with chronic bronchitis so that the stimulus to breathe is initiated when the blood level of oxygen falls instead of when the level of carbon dioxide rises. Consequently, when the level of oxygen in the blood is relatively high in relation to the level of carbon dioxide, the stimulus to breathe is reduced to a dangerous level and further depresses the CNS. When supplemental oxygen is necessary, it should be maintained at the lowest possible flow rate to maintain oxygenation and prevent depression of the client's respiratory drive. The client with chronic bronchitis and congestive heart failure is evaluated for signs of fluid overload. Daily weight, intake, and output are monitored.

Pharmacological

Bronchodilators such as theophylline (Theo-Dur), oxtriphylline (Choledyl), terbutaline sulfate (Brethine), and ipratropium bromide (Atrovent) are given to open the airways. Inhalation or aerosol treatments with bronchodilators such as albuterol (Ventolin) or metaproterenol sulfate (Alupent) are often used in conjunction with oral medications to control symptoms. Prednisone (Meticorten), a corticosteroid, is given as short-term therapy for acute exacerbations. If steroids are required on a long-term basis, they may be given by inhalation to prevent some adverse systemic effects. Examples of inhalation forms of steroids are beclomethasone dipropionate (Beclovent) and triamcinolone acetonide (Azmacort). In addition to agents that open the airways, medications that liquefy respiratory secretions are administered. Acetylcysteine (Mucomyst) may be given by inhalation. Mucolytic medications such as guaifenesin (Humibid LA) may be given orally. If infection occurs, broad spectrum antibiotics such as cephalexin monohydrate (Keflex), cefaclor (Ceclor), erythromycin base (E-Mycin), or penicillin V potassium (Pen-Vee K) are given. Immunization against influenza viruses and *Streptococcus pneumoniae* are recommended.

The client with chronic bronchitis who also suffers from CHF will receive medications to aid the function of the weakened heart. Digoxin (Lanoxin) is given to strengthen the force of the contraction of the heart muscle. Diuretics such as furosemide (Lasix) are given to remove fluid by increasing urinary output. Supplemental potassium chloride (K-Dur, Kay-Ciel elixir) is administered if the client's level of potassium decreases due to the effect of the diuretic.

Diet

The client is encouraged to eat a well-balanced diet. If the client also has CHF, sodium intake is restricted. Unless contraindicated, fluids are encouraged.

Activity

Activity is restricted to decrease the workload on the heart and lungs. With acute exacerbations, the client is placed on bed rest. The level of activity is then slowly increased based on the client's ability to tolerate activity.

Programs consisting of breathing exercises and graded (easy to difficult) exercise regimes are utilized to assist the client in achieving the maximum level of activity tolerance. The client is taught breath-retaining exercises such as coughing techniques, pursed-lip breathing, and diaphragmatic or abdominal breathing. Graded exercise regimens are similar to those used for cardiac rehabilitation, except that the client is monitored from a respiratory standpoint while exercising. The goal is to increase the client's capacity for all ADLs.

▶ NURSING PROCESS

▶ Assessment

▶ Subjective Data

A thorough past medical history is obtained, including informaton about the onset, duration, and severity of symptoms. The client may describe fatigue and difficult breathing.

▶ Objective Data

Changes in level of consciousness or mental status should be noted, as well as the client's color and respiratory rate and effort. The position the client assumes to aid respiratory effort and the use of accessory muscles must be noted. Arterial blood gases or pulse oximetry values are reviewed. Lung fields should be auscultated for crackles and diminished breath sounds. Color, amount, viscosity, and odor of sputum are noted. Specimens are obtained for culture and sensitivity, if indicated. Vital signs must be frequently measured. The pulse may be elevated and irregular. Blood pressure may be elevated or low. An elevated temperature may indicate infection. Assessment of the client for peripheral edema, neck vein distention, and rapid weight gain should be performed.

Nursing diagnoses for a client with chronic bronchitis may include the following:

Nursing Diagnoses	Planning/Goals	Nursing Interventions
▶ *Ineffective Airway Clearance related to thicker and increased amounts of respiratory secretions*	The client's color, respiratory rate, and ABG values will be within normal limits.	Frequently assess level of consciousness, mental status, vital signs, respiratory effort, and color.
		Auscultate breath sounds at least every 4 hours.
		Obtain sputum specimens as ordered, and assess sputum for amount, viscosity, color, and odor.
		Assist the client in assuming the position that most aids respiratory effort, usually an upright position.

continues

Nursing Diagnoses	Planning/Goals	Nursing Interventions
		Administer oxygen and respiratory treatments as ordered and assess their effectiveness.
		Evaluate the results of diagnostic and laboratory tests (ABGs) and notify the physician of abnormalities.
		Alternate care with periods of uninterrupted rest.
		Administer antibiotics and bronchodilators as ordered.
		Provide the client with a well-balanced diet.
		Unless otherwise contraindicated, encourage fluids.
		Assess the client for signs and symptoms of CHF, i.e., fine crackles heard on auscultation, peripheral edema, weight gain, and fatigue.
		Report any signs and symptoms of CHF to the physician.
▶ *Deficient Knowledge related to chronic bronchitis and its treatment and prevention*	The client will verbalize signs and symptoms to report to the physician, safety precautions to take with medication and equipment, medication and respiratory treatment regimen, and techniques for facilitating breathing.	Teach the client to avoid respiratory infections, maintain adequate nutrition, increase fluid intake, and obtain adequate rest.
		Instruct the client in the purpose, expected effects, and side effects of medications.
		Teach the client to administer respiratory treatments and medications prior to eating to aid in breathing.
		If the client is taking steroids, instruct to rinse mouth following administration of inhalers.
		Teach the client to self-administer oxygen.
		Provide information regarding both the use of equipment and safety measures for the equipment.
		Refer the client to an established respiratory rehabilitation program. If such a program is not available, instruct the client in breathing techniques.
		Encourage regular exercise within the client's limitations.
		Encourage the client to obtain immunization against influenza viruses and *Streptococcus pneumoniae*.

Evaluation Each goal must be evaluated to determine how it has been met by the client.

EMPHYSEMA

Emphysema is a complex and destructive lung disease wherein air accumulates in the tissues of the lungs. The airways become fibrotic and lose their elasticity, resulting in narrower lumens. Airflow is impeded as it leaves the lungs (i.e., during expiration). The alveoli distal to these airways become overdistended with trapped air (Figure 18-12). Rupture of the alveolar wall may occur. The alveolar capillary membrane is destroyed, resulting in a loss of available area for gas exchange. Emphysema is the leading cause of respiratory death in the United States. Cigarette smoking is the most common cause of emphysema. Other factors such as air pollution and exposure to occupational respiratory irritants have been identified as contributing to the development of emphysema. Deficiency in alpha-1-antitrypsin is a familial disorder that leads to the development of emphysema. Alpha-1-antitrypsin is an enzyme that inhibits the activity of the enzyme elactase, which breaks down lung tissue.

Emphysema develops slowly over a period of years. The client first notes increasing dyspnea in response to activity. The degree of dyspnea corresponds to the degree of hypoxia, which is usually mild at rest but becomes increasingly severe in response to activity. In advanced stages of the disease, hypoxia is evident even at rest. Sputum produced is scant and mucoid in nature, unless an infection is present. When infection is present, a cough yielding purulent sputum occurs. The client's complexion appears ruddy, or reddish in color. The chest becomes barrel shaped (Figure 31-13) as the chest cage enlarges to accommodate distended lung tissues. The respiratory rate elevates. The expiratory phase of respiration becomes increasingly difficult. Accessory muscles are used to aid respiratory effort. Due to destruction of the alveoli, bronchial breath sounds are heard in the periphery of the lungs. As the disease progresses, breath sounds diminish and eventually disappear over the periphery of the lungs. Arterial blood gases reveal varying degrees of hypoxia depending on the severity of the disease. Hypercapnia, or retention of carbon dioxide, is not as likely as with chronic bronchitis. The extra effort required to breathe increases metabolic need, resulting in weight loss. Chest x-ray reveals hyperinflated lung tissue and a flat-

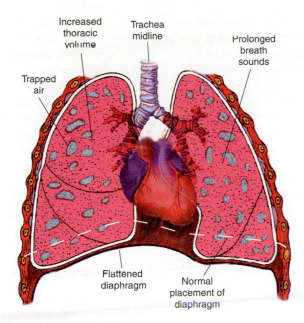

Increased thoracic volume

Trachea midline

Prolonged breath sounds

Trapped air

Flattened diaphragm

Normal placement of diaphragm

Figure 18-12 Emphysema

Figure 18-13 Changes in Chest Configuration and Posture: A. The normal ratio of the anterior posterior diameter to the lateral diameter is 1:2. B. With a barrel chest, the ratio between the diameters is 1:1.

tened diaphragm, which has been displaced by distended lung tissues. Pulmonary function studies reveal a decrease in expiratory volume. Polycythemia and elevation of hemoglobin and hematocrit occur in response to prolonged hypoxia.

Medical–Surgical Management

Medical

The goals of treatment are to prevent further damage to the lung tissues, maintain adequate oxygenation, prevent infection, and improve the client's activity tolerance. The client who smokes should stop or, at least, decrease the number of cigarettes smoked daily. Supplemental oxygen is given to maintain oxygenation. The client with advanced emphysema and severe, chronic hypoxia may be maintained at PaO_2 of 55 to 59 mm Hg and/or oxygen saturation of 90% or greater. As with chronic bronchitis, the client with emphysema is given supplemental oxygen at the lowest possible flow rate, usually 2 to 3 L, to prevent respiratory and CNS depression.

Pharmacological

The client with emphysema receives many of the same medications used to treat chronic bronchitis. To open airways that have become fibrotic, theophylline and similar preparations are used. Steroids may be required for exacerbations. The client with emphysema usually does not need mucolytic agents, unless infection is present. Antibiotics are used to treat and prevent respiratory tract infections. The client should receive immunizations against influenza and *Streptococcus pneumoniae*. The client who smokes may use nicotine polacrilex gum (Nicorette [gum]) or nicotine transdermal system (Nicoderm) to aid in smoking cessation.

Diet

The client with emphysema requires a diet high in carbohydrates to supply the energy necessary for breathing. If a negative nitrogen balance exists due to the client's using muscle tissue to provide energy, a diet high in protein is ordered. Dietary supplements, such as Ensure may be needed to supply the necessary calories and nutrients. Unless contraindicated, fluids are encouraged.

Activity

The client is placed on bed rest. Level of activity is increased based on the client's oxygenation. Oxygen saturation is evaluated periodically as the activity level is increased to determine the effect of activity on oxygenation.

Health Promotion

The client with emphysema benefits from a respiratory rehabilitation program. The client is taught breathing exercises similar to those taught to the client with chronic bronchitis. A graded exercise program is also used for the client with emphysema. Group programs that aid in smoking cessation are useful for the client who smokes.

CULTURAL CONSIDERATIONS

Skin Color
- For a client with highly pigmented skin, establish a baseline skin color
- Observe skin surfaces that have the least amount of pigmentation, such as the palms, the soles of the feet, the abdomen, or the inner aspect of forearms

▶ NURSING PROCESS

▶ Assessment

▶ Subjective Data

Included in the history is information regarding the timing of dyspnea, those factors that exacerbate dyspnea, and those factors that relieve dyspnea.

▶ Objective Data

If cough is present, the client is assessed for other indications of infection, such as elevated white blood cell count and fever. The cough is evaluated as to onset, duration, and severity. Any sputum produced is assessed for color, amount, viscosity, and odor. Vital signs are assessed frequently. An elevated pulse may indicate hypoxia and/or infection. Auscultation of the lungs will reveal the presence of adventitious, diminished, or absent breath sounds. The position the client assumes to aid respiratory effort, and the client's color, respiratory rate and effort, and use of accessory muscles to aid breathing should be noted. Evaluation of the client's nutritional status includes weighing the client and measuring nutrient and caloric intake. The results of laboratory and diagnostic tests should also be reviewed.

Nursing diagnoses for a client with emphysema may include the following:

Nursing Diagnoses	Planning/Goals	Nursing Interventions
▶ *Impaired Gas Exchange related to destruction of the alveoli*	The client's respiratory rate, color, and ABG values will be within normal limits.	Assess the client's level of consciousness and mental status.
		Frequently evaluate the client's respiratory rate, respiratory effort, and color.
		Evaluate oxygenation with ABG and/or pulse oximetry measurement.
		Assess the effect of activity on oxygenation, particularly when activity is being increased.
		Provide supplemental oxygen as ordered.
		Auscultate the lungs and report abnormalities to the physician.
		Assess the client's vital signs: Heart rate and temperature elevations may indicate infection. An elevated pulse can also indicate hypoxia.
		Review the results of diagnostic and laboratory tests and report abnormalities.
		Administer medications and respiratory treatments as ordered.
		Assist the client in assuming the position that offers the most comfort and that most aids respiratory effort.
		Instruct the client in breathing techniques, such as pursed-lip breathing.
▶ *Risk for Activity Intolerance related to hypoxia*	The client will complete activity without experiencing fatigue or dyspnea.	Assist the client with ADL and hygiene needs.
		Plan care and treatments to allow the client uninterrupted periods of rest.
		As activity increases, assess the effects on oxygenation.
		Allow the client to rest prior to and after meals.
▶ *Imbalanced Nutrition: Less than body requirements, related to increased energy requirements to maintain respiration*	The client will achieve or maintain a weight within normal limits for height.	Assess the client's weight and evaluate in relation to the client's height.
		Evaluate the client's diet for nutritional adequacy.
		Review the client's food likes and dislikes.
		Provide a well-balanced diet based on the client's likes and dislikes.
		Provide nutritional supplements as ordered.
		Avoid activities or procedures prior to meals that might reduce appetite (e.g., enemas).
		Administer medications and respiratory treatments prior to meals to aid in breathing.

Evaluation Each goal must be evaluated to determine how it has been met by the client.

BRONCHIECTASIS

Bronchiectasis is chronic dilation of the bronchi. The main causes of this disorder are pulmonary TB infection, chronic upper respiratory tract infections, and complications of other respiratory disorders of childhood, particularly cystic fibrosis. The bronchi become distended and eventually lose their elastic recoil property. The mucociliary blanket's function becomes impaired, and secretions thicken. Secretions accumulate in the bronchi, resulting in a medium for infection. As with chronic bronchitis and emphysema, airflow is hindered, reducing gas exchange.

The client with bronchiectasis complains of a frequent or chronic productive cough. Other complaints include dyspnea, weight loss, and fatigue. Sputum is thick. When infection is present, the sputum is purulent. Crackles, which clear with coughing, are heard scattered throughout the lung fields and are more prominent on the client's arising in the morning. Accessory muscles are used to aid respiration. Over a period of time, right-sided CHF develops, and symptoms such as peripheral edema occur. Arterial blood gases reveal elevated $PaCO_2$, decreased PaO_2, and respiratory acidosis. Sputum analysis reveals whether infection is present, the causative organism, and the organism's resistance or sensitivity to specific antibiotics. Polycythemia and elevated hemoglobin and hematocrit levels are revealed in the complete blood count. Chest x-ray shows slight hyperinflation of lung tissue and, in the presence of CHF, cardiomegaly. Respiratory flow rate decreases, and lung volume increases, as demonstrated by pulmonary function studies. Table 18–11 compares asthma, chronic bronchitis, emphysema, and bronchiectasis.

Table 18–11 SIGNS AND SYMPTOMS OF ASTHMA, CHRONIC BRONCHITIS, EMPHYSEMA, AND BRONCHIECTASIS

	ASTHMA	CHRONIC BRONCHITIS	EMPHYSEMA	BRONCHIECTASIS
History	Intermittent attacks of dyspnea and wheezing	Recurrent respiratory infections, chronic cough	Insidious onset, dyspnea on exertion to dyspnea at rest	Cystic fibrosis, recurrent respiratory infections
Cough	Present during attack	Chronic or recurrent productive cough	Present with infections	Frequent or chronic productive cough
Sputum	Thick	Copious, purulent, green	Scanty mucoid, unless infection present	Thick, tenacious, sometimes purulent secretions
Weight	No weight loss	Slight or no weight loss	Weight loss common	Commonly, weight loss or failure to gain
Appearance	Flushed then cyanotic	Commonly cyanosis ("blue bloater")	Ruddy complexion ("pink puffer")	Clubbing of fingernails
Chest Configuration	Slight overdistention	Slight overdistention	Overdistention prominent ("barrel chest")	Slight overdistention
Breath Sounds	Audible wheezing Prolonged expiration	Coarse crackles	Bronchial breath sounds in peripheral lung fields Diminished or absent in late disease	Crackles
Edema	Infrequent	Peripheral edema common, especially in ankles	Infrequent	Peripheral edema in late disease
Right-sided CHF (Cor Pulmonale)	Infrequent	Frequent	Infrequent	Frequent late in disease
CO Retention (Hypercapnia)	Sometimes	Common	Unlikely	Common in late disease
Hypoxemia	Depends on severity of attack	Possibly severe	Usually mild, especially at rest	Possibly severe in late disease and with infection
Dyspnea	Increases during attack	Progressive	Dyspnea on exertion to dyspnea at rest usually presenting symptom	With respiratory infection and late disease
Accessory Muscles Used for Respiration	Yes	Yes	Yes	Yes
Polycythemia	Uncommon	Late in disease	Yes	In late disease
Respiratory Failure	Possible	Common	Possible	Common

Medical–Surgical Management

Medical

Medical treatment is aimed at removing respiratory secretions, eliminating and preventing infection, and maintaining adequate oxygenation. Percussion and postural drainage are used to aid in the removal of secretions. Aerosol and updraft respiratory treatments may be ordered prior to percussion and drainage. If the client is unable to expectorate secretions, bronchial suctioning is performed. The physician may perform a bronchoscopy to remove especially tenacious and copious secretions. Arterial blood gases and/or pulse oximetry values are evaluated to assess the need for supplemental oxygen. Daily weight and I&O are performed to detect signs of CHF. Pulmonary function studies are performed to evaluate the severity of lung damage. Genetic studies and genetic counseling are indicated for the family and client with cystic fibrosis.

Pharmacological

Acetylcysteine (Mucomyst) and other mucolytic agents are given to promote liquefaction of respiratory secretions. Antibiotics are ordered to treat and prevent infection. The client is immunized against influenza and against *Streptococcus pneumoniae* with the pneumococcal vaccine (Pneumovax 23). Bronchodilators are indicated to open the fibrotic airways. Inflammation is treated with oral steroids such as prednisone (Meticorten), and/or by inhalation with beclomethasone dipropionate (Beclovent). The client with cystic fibrosis is required to take pancreatic enzymes, pancrelipase (Pancrease capsules, Cotazym capsules) to replace those that are missing with this disorder. If CHF occurs, the client is treated with digoxin (Lanoxin), furosemide (Lasix), and potassium supplements, as indicated.

Diet

To provide energy for breathing, the diet should be high in carbohydrates and calories. Protein is supplemented if necessary. Dietary supplements such as En-sure may be required. Fluids are encouraged, unless otherwise contraindicated. Sodium is restricted in the diet of the client with CHF. The diet for the client with cystic fibrosis is restricted in fats.

Activity

During acute exacerbations or in the presence of serious infection, activity is limited. The client is placed on bed rest. Activity is progressively increased depending on the client's tolerance. Respiratory rehabilitation and graded exercise programs are useful in the treatment of bronchiectasis. Regular exercise is encouraged, particularly for the pediatric client with cystic fibrosis.

▸ NURSING PROCESS

▸ Assessment

▸ Subjective Data

When gathering the history, the following information is obtained: history of recent and past respiratory tract infections, history of or exposure to TB or other respiratory infections, and family or client history of cystic fibrosis. The onset, duration, and severity of symptoms such as dyspnea and cough are noted.

▸ Objective Data

The client may display a change in level of consciousness. Dyspnea, tachypnea, and cyanosis may be present. To aid respiratory effort, the client may assume the orthopneic position and use accessory muscles. Heart rate may elevate in response to hypoxia and/or infection. Elevated temperature and purulent sputum indicate infection. Subnormal weight and muscle wasting are seen in the client with chronic disease. Secretions within the airways create crackles heard on auscultation. The results of diagnostic and laboratory data should be evaluated. Signs and symptoms of CHF (e.g., peripheral edema, weight gain) should be noted.

Nursing diagnoses for a client with bronchiectasis may include the following:

Nursing Diagnoses	Planning/Goals	Nursing Interventions
▸ *Ineffective Airway Clearance related to increased and viscous respiratory tract secretions*	The client's breath sounds will be clear and respiratory rate, color, and ABGs will be within normal limits.	Observe the client's level of consciousness, color, respiratory effort, and use of accessory muscles, as well as the position the client assumes to ease respiration.
		Assist the client in assuming the position that most aids respiratory effort.
		Assess vital signs.
		Auscultate the lung fields.
		Alternate care with periods of rest.

continues

Nursing Diagnoses	Planning/Goals	Nursing Interventions
		Evaluate sputum for amount, color, viscosity, and odor.
		Administer medications and respiratory treatments as ordered.
		Obtain ABG or pulse oximetry measurements as ordered.
		Supply supplemental oxygen as indicated.
		Provide the client with prescribed diet, including supplements.
		Unless contraindicated, encourage fluids to aid in the liquefication of secretions.
▶ *Imbalanced Nutrition: Less than Body Requirements, related to increased energy requirements for maintaining respiration*	The client will achieve or maintain a weight within the ideal range for height.	Provide an environment conducive to eating.
		Prior to meals, avoid treatments and therapies that fatigue the client or are painful.
		Assess the client's food likes and dislikes.
		Provide the prescribed diet based on the client's likes and dislikes.
		Prior to meals, administer medications and respiratory therapies that aid breathing.
		Assess the client's weight and compare to the ideal weight for the client's height.
		Assess the client's nutritional intake and evaluate for adequacy.
		Provide dietary supplements as ordered.

Evaluation Each goal must be evaluated to determine how it has been met by the client.

CHEST TRAUMA

Pneumothorax/hemothorax is discussed following.

PNEUMOTHORAX/HEMOTHORAX

Normally, there is no space between the visceral and parietal pleura. They are held together by surface tension. Thus, the pleural space is a closed compartment with a pressure that is negative in comparison to that within the lungs or of the atmosphere. When the integrity of the pleura is interrupted, air from the atmosphere or from the lungs moves between the pleura, creating a space. This condition of accumulated air or gas in the pleural space is known as a **pneumothorax** (Figure 18-14). The lung tissue underlying the pneumothorax is compressed and thus unable to fully expand. If the pneumothorax is large enough, the underlying lung tissue collapses as a result of the compression. A pneumothorax may occur spontaneously following blunt chest trauma, as in a motor vehicle accident; penetrating chest trauma, as in knife or gunshot wounds; or surgery involving the thoracic cavity.

A pneumothorax may be referred to as closed, open, spontaneous, or tension. A closed pneumothorax occurs when there is no communication between the pleura and the external environment. One example of a closed pneumothorax would be that associated with blunt trauma to the chest. In this instance, a broken rib may pierce the pleura and lung, allowing air to enter between the pleura. Conversely, an open pneumothorax exists when there is direct communication between the external environment and the pleural space. A spontaneous pneumothorax occurs without an obvious underlying cause. A tension pneumothorax is a life-threatening condition wherein air enters the pleural space on inspiration but is unable to exit on expiration. The air thus continues to accumulate in the pleural space, compressing the underlying structures.

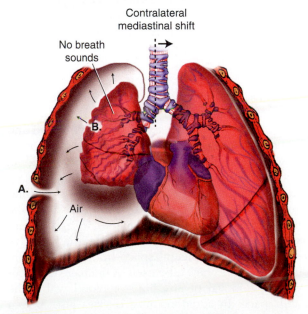

Figure 18-14 Pneumothorax: A. Penetrating wound; B. Ruptured bleb on the lung

If left untreated, a tension pneumothorax will collapse the lung and encroach on the structures on the opposite side. All of the structures within the mediastinum—including the heart, aorta, and vena cava—are affected. Without intervention, tension pneumothorax will result in cardiopulmonary arrest. Tension pneumothorax is often associated with mechanical ventilation. The pressure exerted by the ventilator on compromised lung tissue interrupts the integrity of the pleura. Air continues to enter the pleural space but is unable to exit as mechanical ventilation continues. In the case of a pneumothorax associated with trauma or surgery, bleeding of adjacent vessels into the pleural cavity often occurs. Blood within the pleural space is referred to as a **hemothorax**. When accompanied by air, the condition is called a **hemopneumothorax**.

The severity of injury and the amount of lung tissue affected determine the signs and symptoms the client exhibits. The client with a small pneumothorax may be asymptomatic or may complain of minor dyspnea, whereas the client with a significant pneumothorax may exhibit signs of severe respiratory distress. Dyspnea, tachypnea, orthopnea, and cyanosis may be present. Oxygenation is impaired. Pleuritic pain is common. Breath sounds are absent in the area of the pneumothorax. In the case of a tension pneumothorax, the structures of the mediastinum will shift to the unaffected side as more and more air accumulates in the pleural space. The client with an accompanying hemothorax will exhibit signs and symptoms of shock associated with blood loss.

Medical–Surgical Management

Medical

In order for the affected lung to reexpand, the air and/or blood must be removed from the pleural space. When the blood loss associated with a hemothorax is significant, fluid and blood replacement may be necessary.

Surgical

A thoracotomy tube, or chest tube, is inserted by the physician into the pleural space to drain fluid and air and allow the lung to reexpand. To drain fluid and air, the tube is placed in the midaxillary line at approximately the fifth intercostal space. To drain air alone, the tube is placed in the anterior chest at the midclavicular line and the fourth intercostal space. The thoracotomy tube is connected to an underwater seal drainage device (refer back to Figure 18-9). The underwater seal is necessary to prevent the negative pressure within the pleural space from pulling more air in through the chest tube itself. A drainage chamber allows for removal of any fluid or blood within the pleural space. In addition, most devices also have a chamber to which suction can be applied to assist in the removal of air and fluid from the pleural space.

Following insertion of the chest tube, a chest x-ray is done to confirm proper placement of the tube and to assess reexpansion of the lungs. The underlying cause of the hemopneumothorax then must be treated.

Spontaneous pneumothorax that recurs may require a pleural cortication to prevent further episodes. This surgical procedure involves roughing the adjacent surfaces of the visceral and parietal pleura in the hopes that resulting scar tissue will improve adhesion between the two surfaces. To render emergency treatment for a tension pneumothorax that is severely compromising the function of the heart and lungs, a large bore needle is placed into the anterior chest at the fourth intercostal space. A thoracotomy tube is then inserted until the lung(s) are fully reexpanded and to prevent a recurrence.

Pharmacological

To control pleuritic pain, narcotic analgesics such as morphine sulfate or meperidine (Demerol) are prescribed. Analgesics may be given orally or parenterally depending on the severity of the pain. Prior to insertion of a thoracotomy tube, intravenous narcotics may be given prophylactically. Tissues adjacent to the area of the pneumothorax are injected with local anesthetics prior to insertion of a thoracotomy tube.

Diet

A well-balanced diet with sufficient amounts of protein is encouraged for healing. The client with other injuries and conditions may require TPN or enteral feedings.

Activity

The presence of a pneumothorax or a thoracotomy tube does not in itself call for restricting the client's activity. If hypoxia results from compromised breathing, activity restrictions are necessary. The presence of other injuries or conditions may also necessitate activity restrictions. After the client is adequately oxygenated and stable, activity is encouraged to promote expansion of the lungs.

▸ NURSING PROCESS

▸ Assessment

▸ Subjective Data

Information about the source of the pneumothorax is gathered, and the client asked about previous pneumothoraces, recent chest injury, falls, and severe coughing. The client often describes being very anxious.

▸ Objective Data

The client's level of consciousness and mental status is assessed and the client's color, respiratory effort, and chest wall movement is observed. Chest wall movement is decreased on the affected side. When a large pneumothorax is present, the trachea shifts toward the unaffected side. Dyspnea and cyanosis may occur. The cough is forceful and nonproductive. Respiratory rate and heart rate are elevated. Blood pressure may be elevated due to the presence of pain and anxiety or may be low due to blood loss. Breath sounds are diminished or absent over the affected areas. The location, duration, and severity of pain is noted. Once inserted, chest tubes are assessed for their function, patency, and amount and character of drainage.

Nursing diagnoses for a client with a pneumothorax may include the following:

Nursing Diagnoses	Planning/Goals	Nursing Interventions
▶ *Ineffective Breathing Pattern related to decreased lung expansion*	The client's respiratory rate and color will be within normal limits, and the client will have clear breath sounds in affected area.	Monitor the amount and character of drainage from the chest tube.
		Note any drainage from the chest tube as output.
		Observe fluctuations (tidaling) in the water seal chamber, which indicates that the tube has been placed in the pleural space.
		Investigate the absence of tidaling, as this may indicate that the lung is fully reexpanded or that the tube itself is occluded or kinked.
		Observe for the presence of bubbling in the water seal chamber, which is indicative of an air leak. Assess the connections and chest tube to determine whether leaks are present. If no air leaks are present, notify the physician as to the possibility of an air leak within the client's lungs.
		Encourage the client to cough and deep breathe to prevent further respiratory complications.
▶ *Acute Pain related to pleural space irritation*	The client will verbalize a decrease in pain on a scale of 1 to 10.	Assist the client in assuming the position that most aids respiration. The majority of clients find this to be the orthopneic position.
		Assess vital signs and respiratory status.
		Administer pain medications as ordered.
		Be aware that respiratory depression is possible with narcotic medications.
		Provide diversional activities.

Evaluation Each goal must be evaluated to determine how it has been met by the client.

NEOPLASMS OF THE RESPIRATORY TRACT

Neoplasms discussed following include benign neoplasms, lung cancer, and cancer of the larynx.

BENIGN NEOPLASMS

A benign tumor or cyst in the lung has sharply defined edges, as revealed on an x-ray. Peripheral tumors usually have no symptoms. Bronchial tumors may cause obstruction, infection, or atelectasis.

LUNG CANCER

Malignant tumors (carcinomas) of the lung may originate within the lung itself or may result from metastasis from other tumor sites (e.g., breast, colon, or kidney). Men, especially those over 40 years of age, are more likely to suffer from lung cancer than are women. However, the incidence of lung cancer is rising among women and declining among men (American Cancer Society [ACS], 1998). Tobacco smoking is one of the most common causal factors of lung cancer. Air pollution and exposure to carcinogens such as asbestos are also risk factors for developing lung cancer. Prognosis depends on the size of the tumor when diagnosed and the specific cell type (see Figure 18-15).

Most lung cancers are relatively silent, meaning that symptoms develop late in the course of the disease. Peripheral lesions generally have few symptoms. Initially, the client may complain of a chronic cough or wheezing. Central lesions cause obstruction and erosion of the bronchi. As the tumor grows and occludes the air passages, the client may experience shortness of breath, dyspnea, and blood-tinged sputum. Pain occurs relatively late in the course of the disease and indicates that the tumor has grown to a significant size to put pressure on adjacent nerves and other structures. Although some tumors can be seen on chest x-ray, many cannot. Computerized axial tomography (CAT) and MRI scans are more reliable studies when assessing soft-tissue structures. To confirm diagnosis, the physician orders cytology studies on specimens collected via bronchoscopy, needle biopsy, or mediastinoscopy. Lung scans are occasionally useful for diagnosis. Prior to initiating treatment, the client is evaluated for metastatic disease using bone and total body scans.

Family members and significant others often need assistance in coping with their feelings related to the person with lung cancer.

Medical–Surgical Management

Medical

Treatment of lung cancer depends on the type and stage of the cancer.

Surgical

Surgical intervention involves the removal of the tumor and adjacent lung tissue. Pneumonectomy is the removal of an entire lung. Lobectomy is the removal of a lobe of a lung. Segmental resection is the removal of

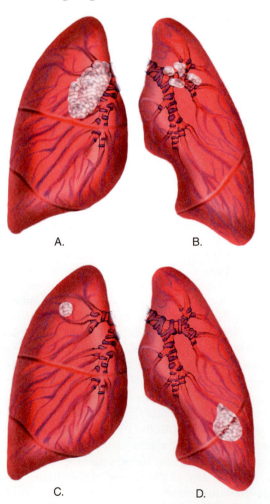

Figure 18-15 Lung Cancers: A. Small-cell carcinoma; B. Epidermoid (squamous-cell) carcinoma; C. Adenocarcinoma; D. Large cell (undifferentiated) carcinoma

CLIENT TEACHING

Tips for Preventing Lung Cancer
- Do not smoke
- Avoid secondhand smoke
- Avoid exposure to air with high concentrations of pollutants
- Support efforts to decrease air pollution
- Protect self from carcinogens in the workplace, such as asbestos

a segment of a lung. The client will have a thoracotomy tube on the operative side. Radiation and chemotherapy are often used in conjunction with surgery. The incidence of lung tumor recurrence following surgery is high. Surgery is often indicated for early non–small-cell carcinomas.

Pharmacological

The specific type of chemotherapy used depends on the cell type and the extent of tumor growth.

Health Promotion

The foremost method of preventing lung cancer is to avoid smoking or to cease smoking. The second-hand smoke of others should also be avoided.

▶ NURSING PROCESS

▶ Assessment

▶ Subjective Data

The client's history is reviewed for history of smoking, exposure to carcinogens, and other causative factors. Information should be gathered regarding the onset, duration, and severity of symptoms. The client may report hoarseness, chronic cough, pain, and shortness of breath. Pain is assessed as to its location, character, duration, and severity.

▶ Objective Data

The color, amount, consistency, and odor of sputum are noted. Prior to surgery, the nurse may hear wheezing or decreased breath sounds on the affected side. Following surgery, breath sounds are diminished or absent on the affected side. The amount and color of drainage from the thoracotomy tube are monitored. The wound is assessed for hemorrhage and infection. Respiratory rate and effort may be increased. Pulse rate may be elevated due to a variety of factors including decreased oxygenation, hemorrhage, and infection. Hypotension occurs with significant blood loss. High blood pressure may indicate pain, anxiety, or other underlying pathology such as essential hypertension.

Nursing diagnoses for a client with lung cancer may include the following:

Nursing Diagnoses	Planning/Goals	Nursing Interventions
▶ *Ineffective Breathing Pattern related to disease process*	The client's respiratory rate and color will be within normal limits.	Frequently monitor the client's level of consciousness, vital signs, color, and respiratory effort.
		Auscultate breath sounds.
		Stagger activities with periods of rest to prevent overtaxing the client's reserves.
		Assist the client in assuming the position that maximizes respiratory effort by positioning the client in semi-Fowler's position or lying on the affected side.
		Assess oxygenation and provide supplemental oxygen as indicated.
		Monitor lab reports for blood gas levels.
▶ *Chronic Pain related to lung cancer*	The client will state pain is decreased on a scale of 1 to 10.	Administer pain medication as ordered.
		Monitor for respiratory depression.
		Provide diversional activities.
		Assist the client in assuming a position of comfort.
▶ *Anticipatory Grieving related to prognosis and perceived separation from significant others*	The client will be able to express to significant others and/or staff feelings related to diagnosis and prognosis.	Aid the client in expressing feelings of grief related to the diagnosis.
		Hope should not be eliminated, but false hope should not be encouraged.
		Allow the client and family time to express their feelings.

Evaluation Each goal must be evaluated to determine how it has been met by the client.

LARYNGEAL CANCER

Cancer of the larynx is more common among men than women. Risk factors for cancer of the larynx include smoking, chronic alcohol abuse, chronic laryngitis, and overuse of the voice. Laryngeal cancer is relatively asymptomatic. The client may experience hoarseness or difficulty speaking above a whisper. If either persists for more than 2 weeks, medical care should be sought. Difficulty swallowing is sometimes present. Laryngeal pain radiating to the ear or a lump in the throat are often signs of metastasis.

Medical–Surgical Management

Treatment is determined by the extent of tumor growth.

CLIENT TEACHING

Daily Stoma Care

After the stoma has healed:
- Use warm water to clean around the stoma;
- Do not use tissues, linty cotton, or soap for cleansing; and
- Wear a bib or dressing over the stoma to filter and warm incoming air.

Surgical

Surgical removal of the larynx, a laryngectomy, is used to treat laryngeal cancer. If the cancer has spread to surrounding tissues, a simple or radical neck dissection may be required. Radiation may be used as an adjunct to surgery or as primary treatment if the tumor is detected in the early stages. Following surgery, a permanent tracheostomy is necessary to allow air to enter the respiratory tract. A small incision is made into the

COMMUNITY/HOME HEALTH CARE

Client with Laryngeal Stoma
- The client's home should be humidified, especially in winter.
- The client and family must know how to suction the respiratory tract, care for the stoma, and care for the respiratory equipment.
- The client should not swim or splash water in the stoma when showering or bathing.
- The client should notify the physician if any signs of respiratory infection develop, such as fever, cough, yellow or green mucus, or redness around the stoma.
- The client must keep follow-up appointments with the physician.

trachea and below the Adam's apple, and a plastic tracheostomy tube is inserted.

▶ NURSING PROCESS

▶ Assessment

▶ Subjective Data

Assessment of the client with laryngeal cancer includes taking a history as to the onset, duration, and severity of symptoms, such as hoarseness or laryngitis and alcohol and tobacco use. The client may describe ear pain and difficulty breathing and swallowing.

▶ Objective Data

The client's respiratory status is evaluated for other respiratory problems that may accompany laryngeal cancer, such as COPD. Sputum is examined for the presence of blood.

Nursing diagnoses for a client with laryngeal cancer may include the following:

Nursing Diagnoses	Planning/Goals	Nursing Interventions
▶ *Impaired Verbal Communication related to removal of the larynx*	The client will be able to communicate needs.	Before surgery, establish a means of communication to be used afterwards. If available, a manual or computer word/picture board works well.
		Keep call light by client's bed.
		Avoid mouthing communications, as this is frustrating to the client and is time consuming.
		As possible, ask questions that require only a "yes" or "no" answer.
		Refer the client to the local support group (Lost Chord Club) or the American Cancer Society.
▶ *Ineffective Airway Clearance related to tracheostomy tube*	The client's respiratory rate and color will be within normal limits, and the client will have clear breath sounds to auscultation.	Suction frequently following surgery to remove static secretions.
		Provide routine tracheostomy care.
		Provide small, frequent feedings of liquid or pureed food to prevent choking.
		Assist client to turn, cough, and deep breathe two to four times an hour.
		Teach client stoma protection.
		Auscultate lung sounds.
		Assess respirations two to four times an hour, if secretions are copious.
		Keep head of bed elevated.
		Provide extra humidity.
▶ *Deficient Knowledge related to tracheostomy care*	The client will verbalize precautions and safety measures for a tracheostomy; how to use equipment; how to suction the respiratory tract; how to change a tracheostomy tube; and actions to take in an emergency.	Teach the client and family how to suction the respiratory tract, care for the tracheostomy, and use respiratory equipment.
		Instruct the client and family in what to do in case of an emergency, such as clogging of the tracheostomy tube with secretions.
		Advise client not to swim and to avoid aspirating water when showering or bathing.
		Suggest that the client avoid extremely cold temperatures. If the tracheostomy site is covered for warming or cosmetic purposes, the covering must be of a porous material without frayed or loose threads.

Evaluation Each goal must be evaluated to determine how it has been met by the client.

DISORDERS OF THE NOSE

The most common disorder of the nose is epistaxis, or nose bleed.

EPISTAXIS

Epistaxis is hemorrhage of the nares or nostrils. It may be either unilateral, which is most common, or bilateral. Epistaxis may be primary in nature, stemming from drying of the nasal mucosa, local irritation, or trauma, or may occur secondary to uncontrolled hypertension or coagulopathies (e.g., thrombocytopenia, anticoagulant therapy). The diffuse vascularity and proximity of blood vessels to the surface of the nasal mucosa make the nares a susceptible avenue for hemorrhage. Blood loss can be minimal to severe. With significant blood loss, hypovolemic shock occurs.

Medical–Surgical Management

Medical

The client with epistaxis usually arrives at an urgent care facility or emergency room following unsuccessful attempts to stop the bleeding. Signs of airway obstruction or aspiration require immediate attention. The goals of treatment are to maintain airway, stop bleeding, identify the cause, and prevent recurrence. Nosebleeds are usually responsive to compression of the nares. Firm pressure should be maintained for 5 minutes. If bleeding persists, the client is instructed to blow the nose and clear the nasal passages. Pressure is then resumed for a full 10 minutes. Epistaxis that continues following these measures requires more aggressive treatment. Bleeding sites that cannot be visualized require packing. Sterile nasal packing is inserted following application of a local anesthetic. In severe cases, a nasostat is inserted. This device resembles a Foley catheter and provides direct compression to the site of bleeding via a balloon. Clients with severe nosebleeds may require fluid and blood replacement to prevent hypovolemic shock. Persistent or recurrent epistaxis may require surgical ligation of the artery supplying the area.

Infection Control: Epistaxis

Wear gloves, goggles or a face mask, and a gown when caring for a client with epistaxis. A cough or sneeze can splatter blood.

Pharmacological

Sites of bleeding that can be visualized are cauterized by the physician. Silver nitrate sticks are used for this purpose. Hemostasis may also be accomplished by packing the affected nostril with epinephrine 1:1000 on cotton packing.

▶ NURSING PROCESS

▶ Assessment

▶ Subjective Data

The client should be questioned about the onset, precipitating events, duration, and frequency of epistaxis, as well as associated symptoms such as nausea, vomiting, headache, and lightheadedness. The client with an occult, or hidden, bleed may complain of needing to swallow frequently.

▶ Objective Data

Blood flow is evaluated for amount, consistency, color, and rate (or severity). Overt bleeding from the nose may be present. This bleeding can vary in flow, from a continuous drip to a pulsating stream of blood. The client who has an occult epistaxis should have the posterior oropharynx visually examined by the nurse or physician to assess blood flow. Vomiting may be present. Lowered blood pressure and rapid heart rate are signs of hypovolemic shock. Conversely, the client with uncontrolled hypertension has an abnormally high systolic blood pressure. Prothrombin time (PT), APTT, INR, and other clotting studies will be abnormal with underlying coagulopathies. Decreased red blood cell count, hemoglobin, and hematocrit are evidence of significant bleeding.

Nursing diagnoses for a client with epistaxis may include the following:

Nursing Diagnoses	Planning/Goals	Nursing Interventions
▶ Impaired Gas Exchange related to airway obstruction	The client's respiratory rate, color, and blood gases will be within normal limits.	Place the client in a high Fowler's position, with the head bent slightly forward.
		Instruct the client to breathe through the mouth and allow the blood to escape freely from the nose and into a container. This aids in preventing obstruction of the airway and swallowing of blood.
		Monitor the client for signs and symptoms of airway obstruction.
		Assess the client's color and respiratory rate and effort.
		Auscultate breath sounds.
		Administer supplemental oxygen as indicated by pulse oximetry or ABG values.
		Monitor pulse oximetry and lab reports of ABGs.

continues

Nursing Diagnoses	Planning/Goals	Nursing Interventions
▶ *Risk for Aspiration related to epistaxis*	The client will develop no complications related to aspiration.	Place the client in the position previously described to aid in preventing aspiration of blood.
		Assess the client for signs of aspiration, such as choking, coarse crackles on auscultation, or elevated temperature.
		Suction the respiratory tract through the mouth to remove secretions and blood.
▶ *Deficient Fluid Volume related to blood loss.*	The client will maintain adequate fluid volume.	With a gloved hand, compress the nares for 5 minutes. If bleeding persists, have client blow nose to clear passages, then compress nares for 10 minutes.
		If bleeding continues following compression attempts, prepare to assist the physician with procedures such as cautery or insertion of nasal packing.
		Administer medications to control blood pressure, as ordered.
		After hemostasis has been established, the clots formed should not be removed or dislodged, as this will lead to recurrence of bleeding.
		Every 30 minutes, evaluate the blood pressure and pulse of the client who shows signs of volume depletion.
		Assess for orthostatic hypotension as a means of measuring volume depletion. A decrease in systolic blood pressure of greater than 10 mm Hg when the position is changed from lying to sitting or standing indicates hypovolemia.
		Administer intravenous fluids, as ordered.

Evaluation Each goal must be evaluated to determine how it has been met by the client.

CASE STUDY

Mrs. White is a 77-year-old female with a history of smoking two to three packs of cigarettes a day for the past 60 years. Mrs. White has been diagnosed with COPD for the past 4 years. She has required supplemental oxygen at 2 L/min for the last 18 months. Three days ago, Mrs. White was admitted with chief complaints of increasing dyspnea on exertion and a productive cough yielding thick, green-yellow sputum. She states that she does "not know why she is coughing up this awful stuff."

Physical examination of Mrs. White this morning revealed vital signs of T = 101.5°F, P = 124, R = 38, BP = 168/74; and sonorous and sibilant wheezes on expiration and in the posterior lung fields, with superimposed coarse crackles heard in the right posterior lower lung field. She is unable to ambulate to the bathroom or complete other ADL due to the dyspnea. Chest x-ray showed a large area of consolidation in the right lower lobe. Sputum culture is still pending.

The following questions will guide your development of a nursing care plan for the case study.

1. List the clinical manifestations that indicate Mrs. White is experiencing an infection concomitant with her COPD.

2. Explain why COPD predisposes a client to respiratory infection.

3. Explain why the physician will increase Mrs. White's oxygen flow to 3 to 4 L/min.

4. List the subjective and objective data the nurse should obtain during the nursing assessment.

5. Identify three nursing diagnoses and client goals that would be pertinent to Mrs. White's care.

6. List the above diagnoses in order of priority, with number one being the highest.

7. Describe client outcomes indicating that Mrs. White's treatment and nursing care regimen have been successful.

SUMMARY

- The primary function of the respiratory system is delivery of oxygen to the lungs and removal of carbon dioxide from the lungs.
- Pneumonia is a lung infection wherein infectious secretions accumulate in the air passages and interfere with gas exchange. Clients with chronic pulmonary disorders or problems of immobility are at increased risk of developing pneumonia.
- Pulmonary TB is an infection of the lung tissue caused by the *Mycobacterium tuberculosis*. Treatment of TB requires the long-term administration of pharmacological agents.
- A common respiratory tract disorder associated with immobility and the administration of anesthetic agents is atelectasis. Clients at risk are encouraged to cough and breathe deeply to aid in preventing atelectasis.
- Obstruction of a pulmonary artery by a bloodborne substance is known as pulmonary embolism. Deep vein thrombosis is a common cause of pulmonary emboli.
- Chronic pulmonary obstructive disease is a collective term used to refer to chronic lung disorders wherein air flow into or out of the lungs is limited. Disorders associated with COPD are asthma, chronic bronchitis, emphysema, and bronchiectasis.
- Traumatic disorders of the respiratory tract include pneumothorax and hemothorax, wherein the underlying lung tissue is compressed and eventually collapses.
- Cigarette smoking is indicated as a major causative factor in the development of respiratory disorders, such as lung cancer, cancer of the larynx, emphysema, and chronic bronchitis.

Review Questions

1. The physician orders 2 to 3 L of oxygen to be delivered to the client with COPD because:

   a. no client ever requires more than 2 to 3 L of oxygen.
   b. the client requests it.
   c. a higher flow rate may suppress the client's drive to breathe.
   d. 2 to 3 L is the maximum flow that a nasal cannula can effectively deliver.

2. A particulate respirator mask is used by the nurse caring for a client with TB because:

   a. regular masks allow the tubercle bacilli to pass through.
   b. this mask is more comfortable for long-term use.
   c. this type of masks allows the nurse to be in close contact with the client for prolonged periods of time.
   d. there is no need for this type of mask when caring for clients with TB.

3. Bronchodilators are used to treat bronchiectasis in order to:

   a. dilate airways that are in bronchospasm due to an antigen–antibody reaction.
   b. dilate airways that have lost their elasticity.
   c. dilate airways that are clogged with secretions.
   d. dilate airways that are chronically narrowed.

4. Incentive spirometry is used to measure the amount of air that:

   a. is exhaled in 1 minute.
   b. is inspired in 1 minute.
   c. is inspired with one inhalation.
   d. is exhaled with one exhalation.

5. Asthma is characterized by:

   a. chronic narrowing of the airways.
   b. intermittent airflow obstruction.
   c. chronic dilation of the airways.
   d. fibrosis of the alveoli.

6. The client with a pneumothorax experiences hypoxia due to:

   a. the entry of air into the thoracic cavity.
   b. compression of the lung tissue underlying the pneumothorax.
   c. impairment of gas exchange.
   d. a lack of surfactant.

Critical Thinking Questions

1. List reasons TB is becoming more prevalent.

2. Compare and contrast the differences and similarities of the disorders classified as COPD.

3. What is the rationale for each nursing intervention given for the possible nursing diagnoses in this chapter?

WEB FLASH!

- Search *tuberculosis* on the Internet. What type of information is available? How can this information be used by clients and families?
- At the end of this book, Internet Web sites are listed in the chapter resources. What information do they provide?

NURSING CARE OF THE CLIENT: CARDIOVASCULAR SYSTEM

CHAPTER 19

MAKING THE CONNECTION

Refer to the following chapters to increase your understanding of the cardiovascular system:

- **Chapter 7, Wellness Concepts**
- **Chapter 10, Fluid, Electrolyte, and Acid-Base Balance**
- **Chapter 12, Health Assessment**
- **Chapter 13, Diagnostic Tests**
- **Chapter 14, Pain Management**

- **Chapter 18, Nursing Care of the Client: Respiratory System**
- **Chapter 20, Nursing Care of the Client: Hematologic and Lymphatic Systems**
- **Chapter 27, Nursing Care of the Client: Endocrine System**

LEARNING OBJECTIVES

Upon completion of this chapter, you should be able to:
- *Define key terms.*
- *Describe the anatomy and physiology of the cardiovascular system.*
- *Relate laboratory results to each disorder.*
- *Describe basic heart dysrhythmias.*
- *Explain the pathophysiology of each disorder.*
- *Describe nursing interventions in caring for clients with cardiovascular conditions.*

KEY TERMS

aneurysm	depolarization
angina pectoris	dyspnea
annulus	dysrhythmia
arteriosclerosis	embolus
ascites	heart sound
atherosclerosis	hemolysis
automatic implant-	Homans' sign
able cardioverter-	hypertrophy
defibrillator (AICD)	myocardial
baseline level	infarction
bradycardia	myocarditis
cardiac cycle	necrosis
cardiac output	orthopnea
cardiac tamponade	palpitation

paroxysmal nocturnal dyspnea	stent
	stroke volume
percutaneous balloon valvuloplasty	tachycardia
	thrombectomy
pericardial friction rub	thrombophlebitis
pericardiocentesis	thrombosis
pericarditis	thrombus
peripheral resistance	transesophageal echocardiography (TEE)
phlebitis	varicosities
phlebothrombosis	vasoconstrict
primary hypertension	vasodilate
repolarization	vein ligation
sclerotherapy	vein stripping
secondary hypertension	Virchow's triad
stasis dermatitis	

INTRODUCTION

Since 1900, heart disease has been the leading cause of death in the United States every year except in 1918 (American Heart Association, 1999a). Approximately 1.1 million Americans experience a myocardial infarction each year with 367,000 of the occurrences ending in death (American Heart Association, 1999b). Congestive heart failure is a contributing factor in approximately 250,000 deaths each year (American Heart Association, 1999a).

Even though these facts are astounding, the death rate for cardiovascular disease has been declining in the last fifteen years. This is due to public education in modifying and decreasing risk factors such as smoking, high-fat diets, and minimal exercise.

This chapter reviews the anatomy and physiology of the cardiovascular system. Pathophysiology, medical management, and nursing interventions related to cardiovascular conditions are discussed with an emphasis on decreasing risk factors and improving lifestyles.

ANATOMY AND PHYSIOLOGY REVIEW

The cardiovascular system consists of the heart and its vasculature and the peripheral vascular system. The heart is located in the lower anterior area of the mediastinum with the apex near the diaphragm. In an average lifetime, the heart will pump 80 million gallons of blood.

The peripheral vascular system consists of arteries, arterioles, capillaries, venules, and veins. The arteries carry oxygenated blood away from the left side of the heart to the body tissues and the veins carry deoxygenated blood back to the right side of the heart. The capillaries connect the arterioles to the venules. In the capillaries, oxygen, nutrients, minerals, and hormones move from the blood to the body cells, and carbon dioxide and waste products move from the body cells into the blood. The venules and veins contain 60% to 70% of the body's total blood volume.

The function of the cardiovascular system is to provide oxygen, nutrients, and hormones to the cells of the body and remove carbon dioxide and waste products of cellular metabolism from body cells. Body temperature is maintained by the distribution of heat throughout the body that has been produced by the metabolic activity of muscles and other body organs.

Structure of the Heart

The heart consists of three layers; endocardium, myocardium, and epicardium. The endocardium is the inner endothelial lining of heart chambers and valves. The myocardium is the thickest part of the heart and consists of cardiac muscle. The epicardium consists of a visceral layer and a parietal layer. The visceral epicardium attaches to the myocardium and is the outer layer of the heart. The parietal epicardium forms the inner layer of a double walled sac called the pericardium that surrounds the heart.

The heart is a hollow muscular organ containing four chambers that fill and empty of blood with each contraction (**depolarization**) and recovery phase (**repolarization**) of the cardiac muscle. The upper chambers are the atria and the lower chambers are the

ventricles (Figure 19-1). When the atria contract, blood is forced into the ventricles. Contraction of the right ventricle pumps blood into the pulmonary arteries and on to the lungs (pulmonary circulatory system). Contraction of the left ventricle pumps blood into the aorta and out to the entire body (systemic circulatory system). The myocardium of the left ventricle is thicker than the right ventricle as more force is needed to pump blood throughout the body.

There are four valves in the heart; tricuspid, bicuspid (mitral), pulmonic, and aortic. One end of fibrous cords called *chordae tendineae* is attached to the cusps of the tricuspid and mitral valves and the other end is attached to papillary muscles on the walls of the ventricles. The chordae tendineae keep the valves from inverting when the ventricles contract, thus preventing blood from flowing back into the atrium. The pulmonic and aortic valves prevent blood from flowing back into the ventricles from the pulmonary artery and aorta during repolarization.

Circulation of Blood

Blood enters the heart through veins and leaves the heart through arteries. With the contraction of the right ventricle, blood is forced through the pulmonic valve into the pulmonary artery. Blood circulates through the pulmonary circulatory system where carbon dioxide is exchanged for oxygen in the lungs. The blood then returns to the left atrium through the pulmonary veins providing oxygenated blood for systemic circulation. When the left ventricle contracts, blood is forced through the aortic valve into the aorta beginning systemic circulation. Blood is then distributed throughout the body and returns to the right atrium of the heart through the inferior and superior vena cava.

Figure 19-1 Internal View of the Heart with Aorta, Vena Cava, and Pulmonary Arteries and Veins

Each time the heart beats, the ventricle pumps 60 to 80 cc of blood. The volume of blood pumped by the ventricle with each contraction is called **stroke volume**. The volume of blood pumped by the left ventricle per minute is known as **cardiac output** and averages 5 liters for an adult at rest. Stroke volume multiplied by the pulse rate yields the cardiac output. If the heart has a strong ventricular contraction, more blood will be pumped by the heart into the systemic circulatory system. Therefore, cardiac output has a direct effect upon the volume of arterial blood being circulated.

Coronary Arteries

Coronary arteries supply nutrients and oxygen to the muscle tissue of the heart. The two coronary arteries are the right coronary artery and the left coronary artery, which branch off the aorta (Figure 19-2). The right coronary artery divides into the posterior descending artery (interventricular artery) and the marginal artery and supplies blood to the anterior area of the right and left ventricles, the posterior area of the right ventricle, the AV node, and the posterior section of the interventricular septum. The left coronary artery divides into the anterior descending artery and the circumflex artery. The left anterior descending (LAD) artery supplies blood to the anterior section of the interventricular septum, anterior area of the left ventricle, and the lateral aspect of the left ventricle. The circumflex artery nourishes the left atrium and ventricle.

Conduction System

The specialized cardiac muscle cells are capable of conducting electrical impulses from one part of the

Figure 19-2 Coronary Arteries that Supply Blood to the Heart Tissue

heart to another. For the heart to beat regularly in a rhythmic sequence, electrical impulses follow a set pattern through the conduction system of the heart. The conduction system consisting of the sinoatrial node (SA node), atrioventricular node (AV node), bundle of His, bundle branches, and Purkinje fibers controls the heartbeat (Figure 19-3).

The SA node initiates electrical impulses that cause the heart to beat, so it is called the pacemaker of the heart. The SA node is located in the superior aspect of

Figure 19-3 A. Conduction System of the Heart; B. Relationship of the Conduction System to an EKG Strip; C. Relationship of S_1 and S_2 Heart Sounds to an EKG Strip

the right atrium. Electrical impulses from the SA node pass through the muscle fibers of the right and left atria causing the atria to contract almost simultaneously. Atrial impulses are transmitted to the AV node located in the lower part of the right atrium. There is a short delay in the impulse at the AV node that allows the atria to complete their contraction and empty the blood into the ventricles. The electrical impulse is transmitted from the AV node into a group of specialized conduction fibers. The group of fibers is called the atrioventricular (AV) bundle or the bundle of His. Once the impulse leaves the AV node, it travels down the fibers of the bundle of His into the interventricular septum. The fibers separate into right and left bundle branches dividing into smaller and smaller branches, called Purkinje fibers. These terminate in the ventricular muscle causing the ventricles to contract. When an impulse has completely gone through the conduction system of the heart and the ventricles have contracted, a **cardiac cycle** has been completed.

Heart Sounds

There are two normal **heart sounds** called S_1 and S_2, heard on auscultation. They yield a sound like "lubb-dubb." S_1, or the "lubb," is the sound of the mitral and tricuspid valves closing simultaneously. It is heard on the left fifth intercostal space. S_2, or the "dubb," is the simultaneous closing of the pulmonic and aortic valves. S_2 is heard on the right second intercostal space. There is a slight pause after the "lubb-dubb" is heard. Clients with congestive heart failure may have a third sound known as S_3. This low-pitched sound occurs after the S_2 sound, or the "dubb," making the heart sound like the word Kentucky ("lubb-dubb-by"). The S_3 sound has also been described as a gallop.

Arterioles and Arteries

The arteries are thick-walled tubes consisting of three layers or tunics as illustrated in Figure 19-4. The inner layer is called the *tunica intima* and consists of a single layer of smooth endothelial cells. The middle layer is the *tunica media* and is composed of smooth muscle cells. The smooth muscle layer of the artery receives nerve stimulation from the sympathetic nervous system. The suppleness of the smooth muscle allows the vessel to **vasoconstrict** (decrease in diameter) and **vasodilate** (increase in diameter). The outer layer, the *tunica adventitia* or *tunica externa,* consists of a connective tissue sheath with some of its collagen fibers fusing with those of the surrounding tissue to hold the vessels in place. The elastic connective tissue allows the artery to expand and recoil with each contraction of the ventricle as an increased volume of blood is pumped through the vessel. The arteries have thick walls so they can withstand the increased pressure from the left ventricle pumping blood through the body.

The arteries divide and branch into smaller vessels called *arterioles,* which are smaller arteries. The same three layers are present in the walls, but as the arterioles approach the capillaries their walls become thinner. The outer layer is reduced to a very thin layer of connective tissue.

Capillaries

Capillaries are very tiny thin vessels that connect the smallest arterioles with the smallest venules. They have only one layer of endothelial cells whose cell membranes are the semipermeable membrane that allows oxygen, nutrients, carbon dioxide, and waste products to be exchanged between the tissues of the body and the blood.

Venules and Veins

Venules are small vessels that emerge from the capillaries and gradually increase in size. As the venules increase in size, they eventually form veins.

Veins have three layers or tunics like the arteries, but the middle layer of a vein is thinner, having less smooth muscle and elastic tissue. This allows the walls of the veins to dilate more easily. Endothelial flaps, called *valves,* are on the inside lining of veins. The valves open and close with each contraction of the surrounding muscles. The purpose of the valves is to assist the blood in returning to the heart. Blood is held by the valves at a certain level until the skeletal muscle contractions cause the blood to move higher in the vein (Figure 19-5).

HEALTH HISTORY

The nurse has three goals when obtaining a health history from a client. The goals are to identify present and potential health problems, identify possible familial and lifestyle risk factors, and involve the client in planning long-term health care.

Figure 19-4 Tunic Layers of Each Type of Vessel

Figure 19-5 Valves in the veins hold the blood at a certain level in the vein. A. Contracted skeletal muscles apply pressure to veins and assist with the circulation of blood. B. Valves prevent the backflow of blood. C. Incompetent valves allow a backflow of blood.

The nurse should ascertain the onset of the symptoms, the predisposing factors that cause the symptoms, and the client's treatment of the symptoms. The nurse should ask if the client has noticed any other bodily changes that occur or have occurred at the same time as the main symptoms. Special attention should be given to the client's activity level or limitations in activity. When asking about dietary habits, the nurse should determine if there has been an increase or decrease in appetite. Asking about sleeping habits will help evaluate the client's ability to sleep, the need for the trunk of the body to be supported with pillows when sleeping, or the need to sleep in a chair.

Major risk factors associated with cardiovascular diseases are age, gender, heredity (including race), smoking, dyslipidemia (presence of increased total serum cholesterol and low-density lipoprotein [LDL]), high blood pressure, physical inactivity, obesity and overweight, and diabetes mellitus. An individual's response to stress may be a contributing factor. Additional contributing factors for women may include menopause, use of birth control pills, and high triglyceride level (American Heart Association, 1999f and 1999g; Mosca, Manson, Sutherland, Langer, Manolio, & Barrett-Connor, 1997).

Advancing age, male gender, diabetes, heredity, and familial history of chest pain or myocardial infarctions are risk factors that cannot be altered. Alterable risk factors are physical inactivity, smoking, contraceptive method, dyslipidemia, obesity and overweight, and triglyceride level. A change in diet may alter the last three factors.

The nurse has a two-fold objective in directing the client toward a healthier lifestyle. The first objective is to educate the client about the risk factors. The second objective is to determine what risk factors the client would like to modify. Once this has been determined, the nurse can assist the client in establishing goals and determining actions to achieve the goals.

ASSESSMENT

Assessment includes clients' self-report of symptoms as well as physical findings and confirming lab data.

Subjective Data

The typical concerns expressed by a client with a cardiac disorder are chest pain, **dyspnea** (difficulty breathing), edema, fainting, palpitations, diaphoresis, and fatigue. When a client talks about having chest pain, it is important to ascertain the onset of the pain, situation occurring at the onset of pain, location and radiation of pain, severity of chest pain, duration, past episodes of chest pain, and methods used to alleviate pain. Women are more likely to express having abdominal pain, dyspnea, nausea, and fatigue (Mosca et al., 1997).

There are several types of dyspnea the client may be experiencing. Exertional dyspnea occurs when a person participates in moderate activity and becomes short of breath. This occurs in the early stages of heart failure and indicates that the heart is not able to meet the demands of the body during moderate activity. **Orthopnea** is when a client has difficulty breathing while lying down and must sit upright or stand to relieve the dyspnea. This occurs in a more advanced stage of heart failure. **Paroxysmal nocturnal dyspnea** is when a person suddenly awakens, is sweating, and is having difficulty breathing. This usually occurs 2 to 5 hours after the person has fallen asleep.

A client may have fainting spells for various physical and psychological reasons. In cardiac clients, fainting occurs because of decreased cardiac output that causes a decreased blood flow to the brain.

A client may describe a "fluttering" or "pounding" sensation in the chest. This is known as **palpitations**. If these sensations occur during exercise, it is a sign that the heart is having to work harder to meet the demands of the body. Palpitations may also be caused by anxiety, ingestion of a large meal, lack of adequate rest, or a large intake of caffeine.

A cardiac client usually will experience fatigue because the heart is not able to keep up with the daily demands of the body. Often the fatigue will increase throughout the day. Frequent rest periods will help alleviate some of the fatigue.

The typical concerns expressed by the client with a peripheral vascular disorder are pain, paresthesia, and/or paralysis in the hands, thigh, calf, ankles, foot, abdomen, or lower back. The quality of the pain (aching, cramping, sharp, or throbbing) and any numbness or tingling should be noted.

Objective Data

In a head-to-toe assessment on a cardiac client, the skin, neck veins, respirations, heart sounds, abdomen, and extremities are carefully assessed. The skin should be observed for cyanosis in the earlobes, lips, fingers, and feet. Assessment of skin turgor could give an indication of fluid volume. If the skin is dry and has poor turgor, the client may be dehydrated from diuretics. If a client has distended neck veins when the head of the bed is at a 45° angle or higher, he or she may be experiencing right-sided heart failure. The nurse should assess the quality of respirations for rate and ease of breathing and also observe for dyspnea and coughing. Heart sounds are assessed for the normal S_1 and S_2 sounds. If the typical lubb-dubb is heard, the valves are closing properly. A pericardial friction rub may be heard if the client has pericarditis. This is an extra sound heard as the heart rubs against the pericardial sac. The sound will be a short, high-pitched squeak.

While listening to the heart, the radial pulse should be palpated to account for every heartbeat. If a heartbeat is heard through the stethoscope but not felt in the radial pulse, the heart has decreased cardiac output to the extremities. If the abdomen is distended, the client may have **ascites**, which is excess fluid in the abdomen. After the heart and lung sounds have been assessed, check the peripheral pulses. Pulses on both sides of the body should be checked at the same time to determine adequate bilateral perfusion. It is important to check pedal pulses in both feet to determine blood flow to each foot. Pulse amplitude can be rated on a scale of 0 to 4: 0 (absent), 1+ (diminished but palpable), 2+ (normal), 3+ (full, increased), and 4+ (bounding).

If the hands and feet are cold or have mottling, this could indicate decreased cardiac output. Capillary refill should be assessed in the fingers and toes.

It should be noted if the feet, ankles, or legs are edematous (Figure 19-6). A client may gain 10 pounds before edema can be detected. It is important that fluid volume be assessed daily on cardiac clients with edema by having the client weighed daily. The weight must be taken on the same scale, at the same time of day, with the client wearing the same amount of clothing.

Assessment of the peripheral vascular system includes assessment of rate, rhythm, and quality of peripheral pulses to give an indication as to the perfusion of the extremities. It is important to compare the two extremities to determine that the pulses are the same in both extremities.

Decreased circulation to an area can result in coolness in the ischemic area, pallor, paresthesia, and paralysis. Paresthesia (decreased sensation in an area) and paralysis result from a lack of oxygenated blood and nourishment to the nerves. Symptoms of paresthesia are numbness and tingling.

If an artery in the leg is occluded, the foot and/or leg becomes reddish in color when the leg is in a dependent position, and pale when elevated. As the ischemia progresses, the leg and/or foot becomes mottled. The skin is smooth and shiny. If the veins are occluded, the

1+ = barely visible   2+ = obviously present

3+ = able to indent, but rebounds when finger removed   4+ = indentation remains when finger removed

Figure 19-6 Edema Rating Scale

foot and/or leg becomes cyanotic when in a dependent position, and has a normal coloration when elevated. Often the anterior area of the lower leg and ankle have a brown pigmentation with venous involvement.

Clients with decreased circulation to the extremities have hardened and brittle nails. The leg will be cool if there is an arterial circulatory problem but warm if there is a venous circulatory problem. Skin ulcerations around the ankles and toes should be assessed.

The client's ankles should be observed for **stasis dermatitis**, an inflammation of the skin due to decreased circulation. Waste products that normally are carried away in the circulatory system remain in the tissues, causing pruritus and irritation of the skin. At first, the ankle area is reddened and edematous, then vesicles form and start oozing. The skin becomes crusted, thickened, and brown in color.

A positive Homans' sign is present in some cases of deep vein thrombosis (DVT). To test for the **Homans' sign**, the nurse dorsiflexes the client's foot. If there is pain in the calf of the leg or behind the knee, the Homans' sign is positive and may indicate the presence of a venous clot.

Table 19–1 COMMON DIAGNOSTIC TESTS FOR CARDIOVASCULAR SYSTEM DISORDERS

Laboratory Tests
Arterial blood gasses (ABGs)
Complete blood count (CBC)
Platelet count
Hemoglobin (Hgb)
Hematocrit (Hct)
Electrolytes
Cardiac enzymes
    Serum aspartate aminotransferase (AST)
    Creatine kinase CPK (CK)
    Lactic dehydrogenase (LDH)
Erythrocyte sedimentation rate (ESR)
Glucose
Prothrombin time (PT)
Partial thromboplastin time (PTT)
International Normalized Ratio (INR)
Serum lipids (lipid profile)
    Cholesterol
    High-density lipoprotein (HDL)
    Low-density lipoprotein (LDL)
    Very low-density lipoprotein (VLDL)
    Triglycerides

Radiologic Tests
Chest x-ray
Cardiac positron emission tomography scan
Radionuclide angiography (multiplegated radioisotope scan, multi-gated aquisition scanning, MUGA)
Technetium pyrophosphate scanning
Thalium scan

Other Diagnostic Tests
Cardiac biopsy
Cardiac catheterization
Echocardiogram
Electrocardiogram (EKG or ECG)
Holter monitor
Magnetic resonance imaging (MRI)
Pericardiocentesis
Pulse oximetry
Stress test
Arterial plethysmography (pulse volume recorder)
Venous plethysmography (cuff pressure test)

COMMON DIAGNOSTIC TESTS

Commonly used diagnostic tests for clients with symptoms of cardiovascular system disorders are listed in Table 19–1. See Chapter 13, Diagnostic Tests, for explanation/normal values and nursing responsibilities.

CARDIAC RHYTHM/DYSRHYTHMIA

As a basis for understanding cardiac dysrhythmias, the normal sinus rhythm must first be understood.

NORMAL SINUS RHYTHM

The electrical conduction of the heart begins with the sinoatrial (SA) (refer back to Figure 19-3) node located in the superior section of the right atrium. From the SA node, the electrical impulse spreads in wave fashion through the atria similar to the ripples from a pebble dropped in water. The firing of the SA node and the electrical impulse spreading across both atria yields a P wave on the EKG. Thus the P wave represents the electrical activity causing the contraction of both atria.

After the atria contract, the electrical impulse then reaches the atrioventricular (AV) node where it pauses for approximately one-tenth second allowing blood to enter both ventricles. The electrical impulse then starts down the AV bundle, also called the *bundle of His,* which divides into right and left bundle branches in the interventricular septum. The electrical impulse continues from the right and the left bundle branches to the Purkinje fibers. The Purkinje fibers transmit the electrical impulse to the myocardial cells causing contractions of the ventricles. On an EKG the QRS complex represents the electrical impulse as it travels through the AV node, bundle of His, bundle branches, Purkinje fibers, and myocardial cells terminating with the ventricles contracting (refer back to Figure 19-3). The Q wave is not always present on the EKG strip.

There is a pause after the QRS complex. The pause is called the ST segment. The ST segment represents the period between the contraction and the beginning of the recovery or repolarization of the ventricular muscles. The T wave represents the repolarization of the ventricles.

After the repolarization of the ventricles, the entire cycle begins all over again at the SA node. In this way the P wave, QRS complex, and T waves are repeated with each heartbeat. Figure 19-7 shows an EKG strip of normal sinus rhythm.

Figure 19-7 An EKG Strip Showing a Normal Sinus Rhythm with the P Wave, QRS Complex, and T Wave Identified

DYSRHYTHMIAS

A **dysrhythmia** is an irregularity in the rate, rhythm, or conduction of the electrical system of the heart. The dysrhythmia can occur in the atria, ventricles, or any part of the conduction system. Specialized cells in the heart muscle have the ability to generate an electrical impulse. Under certain conditions these cells start sending impulses to other cells in the heart causing irregular beats called *ectopic beats*. The most common causes of dysrhythmias are coronary artery disease (CAD), congestive heart failure (CHF), and myocardial infarction (MI). Other causes of dysrhythmias are electrolyte imbalances and drug toxicity.

Symptoms of a client experiencing a dysrhythmia can vary from asymptomatic to cardiac arrest. The client may experience fainting, seizures, fatigue, decreased energy level, exertional dyspnea, chest pain, and palpitations.

BRADYCARDIA

Sinus **bradycardia** is a heart rate of 60 beats/minute or less (Figure 19-8). Causes of sinus bradycardia are myocardial ischemia, electrolyte imbalances, vagal stimulation, heart block, drug toxicity, intracranial tumors, sleep, and vomiting. The treatment for bradycardia is the administration of atropine. Some clients with bradycardia may require a permanent pacemaker.

TACHYCARDIA

Tachycardia is a sinus rhythm with a heart rate ranging from 100 to 150 beats/minute (Figure 19-9). Causes of tachycardia are exercise, emotional stress, fever, medications, pain, anemia, thyrotoxicosis, pericarditis, heart failure, excessive caffeine intake, and tobacco use. When the heart is beating at this rate, there is limited time for the ventricles to fill with blood. This causes a decreased amount of blood to be pumped to the coronary arteries and throughout the body. The client may experience anginal pain. The treatment for sinus tachycardia depends on the cause. If the cause is stress or anxiety, the client is treated for anxiety. Sometimes the heart rate will slow spontaneously. At other times, medications such as beta blockers, calcium channel blockers, and digitalis are needed to treat the underlying cause.

ATRIAL DYSRHYTHMIAS

Atrial dysrhythmias occur from disturbances in the electrical conduction in the atria resulting in premature beats or abnormal atrial rhythms. Common causes for atrial dysrhythmias are myocardial infarction, congestive heart failure, electrolyte imbalances, emotional stress, and drugs.

Premature Atrial Contractions

A premature atrial contraction (PAC) is an ectopic impulse not originating in the sinoatrial node, but rather in the atrial tissue. This causes an atrial depolarization to occur earlier in the cycle than expected, thus the term *premature atrial contraction*.

PACs often do not cause the client to experience physical symptoms depending on how often they occur. Generally they are benign and occur several times a day in healthy individuals. If their occurrence causes an increase or decrease in the pulse rate, they should be evaluated. PACs can be a symptom of myocardial ischemia, developing congestive heart failure, digitalis toxicity, hypokalemia, or an inflammatory condition. Stress, caffeine, and smoking can also cause PACs. PACs can be the first indication that more serious atrial dysrhythmias could occur if not treated properly.

If PACs are occurring because of serious underlying problems, they should be medically managed with antidysrhythmic drugs such as quinidine and procainamide hydrochloride (Procan SR). If stress is the cause of PACs, the nurse can assist with stress reduction techniques. The client may desire counseling to assist with stress reduction. The client is encouraged to decrease or eliminate caffeine intake and to stop smoking.

Atrial Tachycardia

Atrial tachycardia is an ectopic impulse that causes the atria to contract at the rate of 140 to 250 beats/minute. This is sometimes referred to as a *supraventricular dysrhythmia,* meaning the impulse causing the dysrhythmia is occurring above the ventricles. This dysrhythmia can occur as a continuous rhythm or as short, sudden eruptions that start and end spontaneously.

Figure 19-8 Sinus Bradycardia

Figure 19-9 Sinus Tachycardia

Atrial tachycardia occurs with hypokalemia, digitalis toxicity, and ischemia. Potassium supplements are given if the cause of the dysrhythmia is hypokalemia. If an increased level of serum digitalis is the cause, digitalis is withheld until the level returns to normal. An artificial pacemaker may be surgically inserted to regulate the atrial tachycardia dysrhythmia.

Paroxysmal Supraventricular Tachycardia

Paroxysmal supraventricular tachycardia (PSVT) was previously called paroxysmal atrial tachycardia (PAT). PSVT is a rapid atrial beat accompanied by an abnormal conduction in the AV node. The dysrhythmia occurs suddenly (paroxysmally) and is usually initiated by a premature beat. PSVT can stop as abruptly as it begins. It can be caused by myocarditis, caffeine, alcohol ingestion, smoking, and stress. PSVT may also be present in clients with coronary artery disease, mitral valve prolapse, and acute pericarditis.

The client needs to be taught vagal stimulation procedures such as the Valsalva maneuver and carotid sinus pressure or massage, which usually stops the dysrhythmia. If these measures do not work, digoxin (Lanoxin) and propranolol hydrochloride (Inderal) are the drugs of choice. Occasionally, cardioversion is needed to stop PSVT.

Atrial Flutter

Atrial flutter, a rapid contraction of the atria, yields a heart rate of 250 to 350 beats/minute (Figure 19-10). The EKG displays a sawtooth wave pattern. The AV node attempts to block some of the atrial impulses, but usually the ventricles are also contracting at a rate of 300 beats/minute. This causes a decreased blood supply to the body because the atria and ventricles are unable to fill with blood when they are contracting at such a fast rate. This dysrhythmia requires immediate intervention.

Underlying causes of atrial flutter are coronary artery disease, pulmonary embolism, mitral valve disease, acute myocardial infarction, and cardiomyopathy. The client may experience palpitations or go into cardiac shock depending on the underlying cause. If atrial flutter occurs during an MI or with congestive heart failure, it is a sign of poor prognosis.

GERONTOLOGICAL CONSIDERATIONS

Antidysrhythmic Medications
Doses may need to be reduced with the elderly who may have hepatic or renal impairment.

Medications of choice for atrial flutter are digoxin (Lanoxin), which slows the rate, and antiarrhythmic agents such as quinidine or procainamide (Procan SR). Calcium channel blockers such as verapamil hydrochloride (Calan) and nifedipine (Procardia) may be given to block the impulses at the AV node. If the atrial flutter is not controlled with medications, cardioversion can be done.

Atrial Fibrillation

Atrial fibrillation is an erratic electrical activity of the atria, resulting in a rate of 350 to 600 beats/minute (Figure 19-11). Atrial depolarization is so uncoordinated during the dysrhythmia that the atria quiver rather than contract. The AV node is bombarded with impulses and randomly transmits the impulses to the ventricles causing varied irregular contractions of the ventricles with a ventricular rate of 100 to 180 beats/minute. The underlying cause of the dysrhythmia is of an organic nature such as mitral valve disease or dysfunction, CAD, acute MI, hypertensive heart disease, heart failure, cardiomyopathy, and hyperthyroidism. Since the atria are not contracting properly, blood pools in the atria predisposing the person to thrombi forming on the walls of the atria. The clots can dislodge and travel to the brain, lungs, and other parts of the body. Most clients take an aspirin daily to prevent clot formation.

Once the underlying condition is treated, atrial fibrillation may stop. However, it is usually treated with quinidine gluconate (Quinidine Gluconate), procainamide hydrochloride (Procan SR), amiodurone HCL (Cordarone), and digoxin (Lanoxin). A calcium channel blocker, verapamil (Calan) or nifedipine (Procardia), or a beta blocker, atenolol (Tenormin) or timolol maleate (Blocadren), is used for a short time to slow the heart rate. If the dysrhythmia cannot be controlled with medication, cardioversion may be necessary.

Figure 19-10 Atrial Flutter

Figure 19-11 Atrial Fibrillation

Cardioversion should be done with caution if the client has been digitalized. Digitalization causes the heart to be sensitive to cardioversion and the heart may fibrillate from the cardioversion. Anticoagulants should be used before the client undergoes cardioversion so a thrombus is not released into the system.

VENTRICULAR DYSRHYTHMIAS

Ventricular dysrhythmias originate in the ventricles. They are more life threatening than atrial dysrhythmias because the ventricles supply blood to the lungs and the body. These dysrhythmias must be treated promptly.

Premature Ventricular Contractions

Premature ventricular contractions (PVCs) arise from ectopic beats in the ventricles and are the most common ectopic beats (Figure 19-12). PVCs can easily be identified on the EKG because of the wide, bizarre QRS complexes. There are no P waves preceding the QRS complex.

Coronary artery disease is the most common cause of PVCs. Other causes of PVCs are myocardial ischemia, CHF, electrolyte imbalances, digitalis toxicity, anxiety, exercise, hypoxia, caffeine, and excessive alcohol consumption.

The most common pharmacological treatment for PVCs is lidocaine hydrochloride (Xylocaine HCl). Initially lidocaine is given as an IV bolus and then titrated according to the client's response.

Other medications used to treat PVCs are procainamide hydrochloride (Procan SR), quinidine, disopyramide phosphate (Norpace), bretylium tosylate (Bretylol), and magnesium sulfate.

Administering oxygen may increase the oxygen perfusion to the myocardial tissue and decrease the frequency of premature beats.

Ventricular Tachycardia

Ventricular tachycardia (VT) is the occurrence of 3 or more consecutive PVCs. The ventricular rate is 100 beats/minute and may go as high as 140 to 240 beats/minute. The EKG reveals a wide, abnormally shaped QRS complex. Underlying conditions in which VT oc-

curs are cardiomyopathy, hypoxemia, digitalis toxicity, and electrolyte imbalance.

During VT, the client will have a low blood pressure, weak or absent peripheral pulses, body weakness, and may become unconscious. The ventricle is beating so rapidly that it is unable to fill with blood or eject blood properly. This causes blood to back up in the pulmonary circulation leading to pulmonary congestion.

It is important that VT be treated promptly because a ventricular tachycardia rhythm may lead into ventricular fibrillation, a life-threatening dysrhythmia. The client is given oxygen and an intravenous line is inserted if one is not already in place. The drug of choice is procainamide hydrochloride (Procan SR) given intravenously because it slows the electrical conduction in the ventricle. Lidocaine hydrochloride (Xylocaine HCl) is given if PVCs occur with myocardial ischemia or ifarct. If the VT is not controlled with medications, the client may be cardioverted if peripheral pulses are present, or defibrillated if peripheral pulses are absent.

Cardioversion

Cardioversion is the delivery of a synchronized electrical shock to change a dysrhythmia to a rhythm that will circulate more blood to the body tissues and improve oxygenation of the tissues. The electrical shock is set to be delivered on the R wave, as a shock during ventricular depolarization may cause ventricular fibrillation. Cardioversion is done as an elective or emergency treatment. Electrodes are placed to the right of the sternum below the clavicle and at the apex of the heart. The electrodes are lubricated with a special gel or placed on normal saline pads. The electrical current delivered through the electrodes depolarizes the myocardium and allows the heart's pacemaker to reestablish a sinus rhythm.

The client is NPO for 8 hours prior to an elective cardioversion. Diuretics and digitalis preparations are withheld 24 to 72 hours before the cardioversion since the myocardium cells are less responsive to convert to a normal rhythm or may develop a serious dysrhythmia after the cardioversion. Anticoagulants and oral antiarrhythmics are still given before cardioversion. Anticoagulants are given so a thrombus is not released into the system. The client is given a sedative such as diazepam (Valium) or midazolam hydrochloride (Versed) intravenously before the procedure. The client's vital signs and EKG strip are monitored closely for the first hour after the cardioversion and then as ordered by the physician.

Defibrillation

Defibrillation is the delivery of an unsynchronized, high-energy electrical shock during an emergency situation such as a cardiac arrest or pulseless VT to convert the life-threatening dysrhythmia or arrhythmia to a sinus rhythm. Defibrillation is done by a physician or a

Figure 19-12 Premature Ventricular Contraction

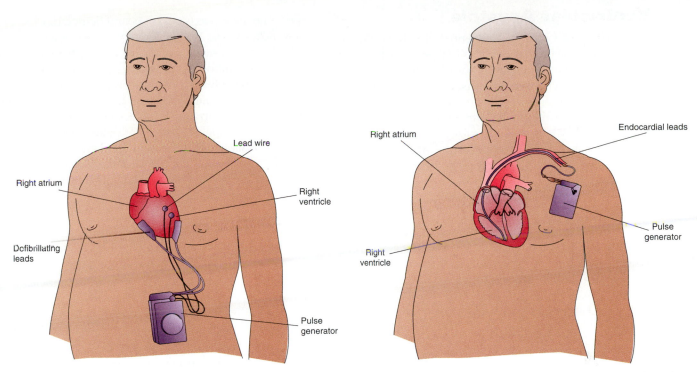

Figure 19-13 Two Different Types of Automatic Implantable Cardioverter-Defibrillators (AICD): A. Pulse generator implanted in the subcutaneous tissue of the abdomen with lead wires and defibrillating leads going to the heart; B. Pulse generator implanted below the collar bone with endocardial leads positioned in the heart through a vein.

nurse who has had special education to handle emergency situations. Paddles are lubricated with a special gel or normal saline pads are applied to the skin where the paddles will be placed. The paddles are placed to the right of the sternum below the clavicle and at the apex of the heart. When the electrical shock is delivered to the client, everyone stands clear of the bed to prevent them from also receiving the electrical shock. More than one electrical shock may be delivered in an attempt to convert the rhythm.

If conservative measures do not control the VT and the client has periodic episodes of VT, an **automatic implantable cardioverter-defibrillator (AICD)** is implanted in the client (Figure 19-13). This device senses the dysrhythmia and automatically sends an electrical shock directly to the heart to defibrillate it.

One type of AICD has leads that are attached to the heart muscle. The pulse generator that initiates the shock is placed in a pocket of subcutaneous tissue in the abdominal wall. The pulse generator is powered by lithium batteries. Another type of AICD has an endocardial lead that is guided through a vein into the right side of the heart. The pulse generator may be placed under the skin below the collarbone or in the abdomen.

The AICD detects VT and ventricular fibrillation (VF) through the leads attached to the heart muscle. Once VT or VF are detected, an electrical shock is sent from the pulse generator. The AICD is capable of delivering three more shocks to the heart muscle if the heart does not return to normal sinus rhythm (NSR). Usually clients are converted to NSR with the first shock. Complications following the insertion of a AICD are atelectasis, pneumonia, pneumothorax, thrombus, and a seroma at the generator site.

Ventricular Fibrillation

The most common cause for VF is CAD. VF is a disorganized, chaotic quivering of the ventricles. The ventricles are unable to contract and no blood is ejected into the circulatory system. The EKG reading is a series of jagged, unidentifiable waves (Figure 19-14). The client will not have a pulse, blood pressure, or respirations. This dysrhythmia is serious. Aggressive measures must be taken to initiate CPR and defibrillate the client immediately.

Figure 19-14 Ventricular Fibrillation

Ventricular Asystole

Ventricular asystole is represented only by a P wave or by a straight line on the EKG (Figure 19-15). The ventricles are not contracting and the client is in cardiac arrest. The client loses consciousness and has no pulse or respirations. Aggressive treatment should be initiated within 1 minute to prevent chemical changes within the body that jeopardize recovery. CPR is started and the client is defibrillated. Atropine sulfate and epinephrine are given intravenously.

ATRIOVENTRICULAR BLOCKS

In atrioventricular blocks the electrical conduction is interrupted to some degree between the atria and ventricles at the AV node. The extent of interruption is classified as first degree, second degree, or third degree.

First Degree AV Block

In first degree block the impulse is delayed in traveling through the AV node (Figure 19-16). The impulse eventually reaches the ventricles, but is delayed. There are no physical symptoms or treatment for first degree block.

Second Degree AV Block

In second degree block some of the impulses pass through the AV node to the ventricles and others are blocked (Figure 19-17). Symptoms include irregular pulse, vertigo, and weakness. A temporary pacemaker may be inserted until the conduction pattern is stabilized. If the dysrhythmia persists, a permanent pacemaker may be implanted.

When the impulse is blocked, the EKG reveals an extended PR interval that is not followed by a QRS complex. There are two types of second degree blocks, type I (Wenckebach or Mobitz I) and type II (Mobitz II). Type I AV block is usually caused by a drug toxicity and is treated by withholding the drug. Type I may also occur with an acute inferior wall myocardial infarction. Type II is more serious than type I and indicates a blockage in the conduction in the bundle of His or the bundle branches (compare Figure 19-16 and Figure 19-17). Type II block occurs most often in clients with an acute anterior septal wall myocardial infarction or fibrosis of the electrical conduction system and may be followed by third degree AV block.

Third Degree AV Block

Third degree heart block is when no impulses are able to pass from the atria through the AV node to the ventricles (Figure 19-18). The atria and ventricles beat independently of each other. The causes of third degree block are myocardial ischemia, drug toxicity, and electrolyte imbalances. Atropine sulfate may be given to improve conduction through the AV node. A permanent pacemaker is usually required to control the dysrhythmia.

 Safety: Pacemaker
The client should wear a medical identification tag indicating the presence of a pacemaker.

Medical–Surgical Management

Pharmacological

Dysrhythmias originating in the atria are treated with a digitalis preparation while dysrhythmias originating in the ventricles are treated with lidocaine hydrochloride (Xylocaine HCl) or other antiarrhythmic agents.

Figure 19-15 Asystole

Figure 19-17 Second Degree AV block: Mobitz's Type II

Figure 19-16 First Degree AV Block

Figure 19-18 Third Degree AV Block

CLIENT TEACHING

Pacemaker

- High-tension wires, high-voltage electrical generators, or MRIs may cause pacemaker malfunction.
- Contact sports should be avoided.
- Pacemakers may activate airport security alarms.

Diet

The client is usually placed on a low-fat, low-cholesterol diet. Caffeine consumption is restricted.

▶ NURSING PROCESS

▶ Assessment

▶ Subjective Data

The nurse should inquire if the client has experienced palpitations, lightheadness, nausea, dyspnea, anxiety, fatigue, or chest discomfort.

▶ Objective Data

If a client is experiencing dysrhythmias, the heart rate, blood pressure, and respirations should be checked. While listening to the apical pulse and respirations, abnormal heart sounds should be noted and breath sounds monitored for crackles. The presence of crackles indicates the lungs are filling with fluid. Observe the skin for pallor and cyanosis. Urine output may decrease.

Nursing diagnoses for a client with dysrhythmias may include the following:

Nursing Diagnoses	Planning/Goals	Nursing Interventions
▶ *Decreased Cardiac Output related to inadequate electrical conduction*	The client will have increased cardiac output.	Apply electrodes for telemetry monitoring. Balance activity with rest periods. Monitor the vital signs during activity and at rest. Listen to the apical pulse, especially noting rate and rhythm. Elevate the extremities so they are not in a dependent position. Perform cardiac resuscitation as needed.
▶ *Anxiety related to fear of potential diagnosis, treatment regimen, and death*	The client will relate fears of potential cardiac problems.	Care for the client in a calm, confident, and efficient manner. Remain with the client and explain procedures and treatments. Encourage client input regarding the care. Encourage the client to verbalize concerns about the dysrhythmia and potential future complications. Teach the client relaxation activities.
▶ *Deficient Knowledge related to electrical conduction of the heart and treatment methods*	The client will describe electrical disorder and treatment methods.	Explain medication administration times, action, side effects, and symptoms that need reporting. Provide written instructions to the client and family. Explain symptoms of dysrhythmias such as fatigue, edema, palpitations, lightheadness, nausea, dyspnea, and anxiety. If a pacemaker is needed, explain the purpose, insertion procedures, and home care. Include the family in all the teaching sessions.

Evaluation Each goal must be evaluated to determine how it has been met by the client.

INFLAMMATORY DISORDERS

Inflammatory disorders include rheumatic heart disease, infective endocarditis, myocarditis, pericarditis, and valvular heart disease.

RHEUMATIC HEART DISEASE

Rheumatic heart disease is a complication of rheumatic fever and is also linked to group A streptococcus following an upper respiratory infection. Rheumatic fever and rheumatic heart disease affect about 1.8 million persons in the United States (American Heart Association, 1999e). Rheumatic fever is a systemic inflammatory disease that occurs 2 to 3 weeks after an inadequately treated pharyngitis caused by the group A *beta-hemolytic streptococcus*. Symptoms of rheumatic fever are a mild fever, polyarthritis, carditis, chorea, and a rash. The endocardium, myocardium, and epicardium can become inflamed with the most damage occurring to the mitral valve. The mitral valve becomes incompetent because of thickening and stenosis of the valve leaflets. Mitral prolapse (valve leaflets fall into the left atrium during systole) may result.

Once afflicted with rheumatic fever, a person is more prone to having it again. It is treated with intravenous antibiotics, anti-inflammatory agents, corticosteroids, and strict bed rest. The main goal is to treat the inflammation, prevent cardiac complications, and prevent the recurrence of the disease. These clients are placed on prophylactic antibiotic therapy prior to dental procedures or invasive surgery. Antibiotic therapy has reduced the mortality from 15,000 in 1950 to 5,000 in 1996 (American Heart Association, 1999e).

INFECTIVE ENDOCARDITIS

Infective endocarditis is an inflammation or infection of the inside lining of the heart, particularly the heart valves. The etiology of inflammatory endocarditis is a collagen-vascular disease or rheumatic fever. Infective endocarditis is caused by bacteria, fungi, or virus. As the microorganisms invade the valves, they form fibrinous substances called *vegetations*. Vegetations cause scar tissue on the valves so they become hard and brittle and do not close properly. When the valve is incapable of holding the blood in the appropriate chamber, blood seeps into the next chamber. The valve is said to be insufficient. Sometimes the vegetations cause the valve flaps to grow together resulting in a narrowing of the opening. This is called a *valvular stenosis*. The mitral valve is more frequently affected than the other valves. When the mitral valve is affected, it is termed *mitral insufficiency* or *mitral stenosis*.

Historically, rheumatic fever was the common cause of endocarditis. More recently, endocarditis is a risk factor for IV drug users, immunosuppressed clients, and clients with valvular heart disease.

The client with endocarditis will have a fever, heart murmur, splenomegaly, and petechiae on the conjunctiva, palate, buccal mucosa, and distal extremities. There are two forms of endocarditis: acute and subacute. Symptoms of acute endocarditis are elevated temperature, tachycardia, pallor, diaphoresis, and symptoms of a systemic infection, such as temperature of 103°F and shaking chills. Clients with subacute endocarditis have low-grade fever, malaise, weight loss, and anemia. Clients with both types of endocarditis may have murmurs and symptoms of congestive heart failure, such as dyspnea, peripheral edema, and pulmonary congestion.

Endocarditis is diagnosed by the client's history and symptoms. A **transesophageal echocardiography (TEE)** can confirm the diagnosis of endocarditis by allowing ultrasonic imaging of the cardiac structures through the esophagus. The erythrocyte sedimentation rate (ESR) and WBC are elevated. A blood culture and sensitivity is done to determine the causative organism and to determine the most effective antibiotic.

Medical–Surgical Management

Surgical

Surgical repair or replacement of a valve is done in severe cases.

Pharmacological

Clients are treated with antimicrobial drugs (endocarditis) and intravenous antibiotics. The antibiotics are usually continued for 2 to 6 weeks. The most commonly used antibiotics are penicillin V potassium (V-Cillin K), vancomycin hydrochloride (Vancocin), and gentamicin sulfate (Garamycin).

Diet

The client is provided a well-balanced nutritious diet with between-meal snacks.

Activity

The client is placed on bed rest to decrease the workload of the heart. A calm, quiet environment should be provided.

Health Promotion

Clients who have previously had endocarditis or have a mitral valve prolapse are more prone to develop endocarditis. They should take antibiotics prophylactically before having dental work and genitourinary or gastrointestinal invasive procedures. Clients prone to developing endocarditis should take amoxicillin trihydrate (Amoxil) 1 hour before the procedure and again after the procedure.

Nursing Management

Oxygen is administered as needed, and blood pressure and pulse measured before and after activity to monitor toleration. Apical pulse rate and rhythm should be noted, and breath sounds assessed for adventitious sounds. Activity should be balanced with rest periods. If a client is on vancomycin hydrochloride (Vancocin) or gentamicin sulfate (Garamycin), BUN and creatinine levels must be monitored as both of these drugs are nephrotoxic.

MYOCARDITIS

Myocarditis is an inflammation of the myocardium of the heart. Lymphocytes and leukocytes invade the muscle fibers of the heart causing the chambers to enlarge and the muscle to weaken. This can lead to congestive heart failure. Myocarditis is caused by bacteria, viruses, fungi, or parasites. It can also be an autoimmune reaction such as in the conditions of rheumatic fever or lupus erythematosus. Usually the cause is a virus. Recently myocarditis has been more prevalent in clients with AIDS.

Acute myocarditis presents itself with flulike symptoms of fever, pharyngitis, myalgias, and gastrointestinal complications. The client will also have chest pain and should be monitored for signs of congestive heart failure. A **pericardial friction rub** is often heard if the pericardium becomes involved. The friction rub is a "squeaky" sound heard through the stethoscope when the two inflamed pericardial surfaces rub together with the contraction of the heart.

Myocarditis diagnostic symptoms are nonspecific. They include elevated ESR and elevated LDH, CK, and SGOT levels. The diagnosis of myocarditis can be confirmed with an endomyocardial biopsy.

Medical–Surgical Management

Pharmacological

Digitalis preparations are given to try to prevent congestive heart failure. Broad spectrum antibiotics are also given to treat the infection. Anti-inflammatory agents may be given to reduce the inflammation. Oxygen is administered as needed.

Activity

The client is placed on bed rest. This decreases the workload of the heart.

Nursing Management

The client should be monitored for symptoms of congestive heart failure or pericarditis. The client is placed in a semi-Fowler's position. A quiet environment and frequent rest periods are important for the client. A pulse oximeter is applied to monitor oxygen saturation.

PERICARDITIS

When the membranous sac surrounding the heart becomes inflamed, the condition is called **pericarditis**. Causative organisms are viral, bacterial, fungal, or parasitic. Inflammation can also occur from rheumatic or collagen-vascular conditions like systemic lupus erythematosus. The most common cause of pericarditis is idiopathic, meaning no known cause. Symptoms of pericarditis are severe precordial pain (pain on the anterior surface of the chest over the heart) and a pericardial friction rub. The pain may radiate to the neck, back, or abdomen and become worse when the client coughs or lies on his left side. If the client sits erect and leans forward, the pain is relieved. Pericardial effusion (excess fluid in pericardial space) may develop. **Cardiac tamponade** will result if the fluid rapidly increases and hinders the functioning of the ventricle. The S_1 and S_2 sounds are often muffled and hard to hear because of fluid accumulation.

With inflammation, scar tissue develops in the pericardial sac. Heart movement is limited by the scar tissue and cardiac failure results.

Medical–Surgical Management

Medical

A **pericardiocentesis** is done to aspirate the excess fluid from the pericardial sac. A needle is inserted through the chest wall into the pericardial space.

Surgical

If fibrotic scar tissue in the pericardium hinders heart performance, a pericardiectomy or pericardial window may be done. Pericardiectomy is removal of the pericardium. When a pericardial window is done, a section of the parietal pericardium is cut and tacked back onto itself allowing fluid to escape from the pericardial sac.

Pharmacological

Clients are given antipyretics, analgesics, and anti-inflammatory agents. The infection is combated with antibiotics. Clients may also be given a digitalis preparation and diuretics to improve the pumping action of the heart and decrease fluid retention.

Nursing Management

The client's apical pulse and blood pressure should be assessed, and the EKG monitored for dysrhythmias. Assessment for signs of cardiac tamponade such as decreased pulse and blood pressure, muffled heart sounds, increased respirations, restlessness, and oliguria is critical. Oxygen can be administered as needed, and the client assisted to a position of comfort. Analgesics, antibiotics, and anti-inflammatory agents should be administered as ordered and the client's responses monitored. The nurse should encourage the client to verbalize concerns and fears.

VALVULAR HEART DISEASES

Valvular heart disease occurs when the valves do not open and close properly. A thickening of the valve tissue, causing the valve opening to be narrow, is called *valvular stenosis*. Valvular insufficiency is the inability of the valve to close completely. When the valve does not close completely, blood leaks back into the chamber from which it was just pumped. This is called regurgitation (Figure 19-19). The client with valvular heart disease often has a history of rheumatic fever.

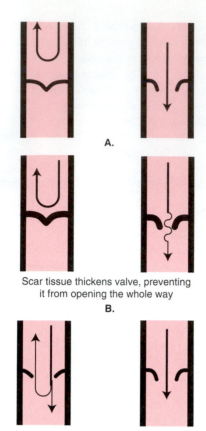

Scar tissue thickens valve, preventing
it from opening the whole way
B.

Scar tissue causes the valve to harden and pull
apart, preventing it from closing completely
and allowing blood to leak backwards
C.

Figure 19-19 A. Normal Valve; B. Stenosed Valve;
C. Insufficient Valve

STENOSIS AND INSUFFICIENCY

The definitions, symptoms, diagnostic findings, medical–surgical management, and nursing interventions for mitral and aortic valve conditions are covered in Table 19–2.

MITRAL VALVE PROLAPSE

Mitral insufficiency can lead to mitral valve prolapse in which the valve leaflets, chordae tendineae, and papillary muscle become damaged. The valve leaflets flip back into the left atrium when the left ventricle contracts. This condition affects more women then men. Often the client remains asymptomatic. The symptoms that a client may experience depend on how seriously the mitral valve is affected. Sometimes

clients experience palpitations and fatigue due to a decreased cardiac output. They also may experience angina, dizziness, and syncope. Some clients have panic attacks. Often a click or murmur can be heard.

Medical–Surgical Management

Medical

Clients with valvular heart disease are to take antibiotics prophylactically before any dental procedures and genitourinary or gastrointestinal invasive procedures.

Surgical

When the activities of a client with valvular heart disease become curtailed because of decreased cardiac output and the symptoms can no longer be controlled by medical means, surgery may be done. The type of surgery performed will depend on the client's overall condition and on the involved valve.

For the mitral valve, surgery alleviates the symptoms, but it does not cure the condition. Surgeries frequently have to be repeated. A commissurotomy is done for mitral stenosis. In this surgery the valve leaflets are surgically separated. For mitral regurgitation or insufficiency, a valvuloplasty is becoming the treatment of choice. A percutaneous mitral valvuloplasty is a repair of perforated cusps or torn chordae tendineae. The risk of a thrombus is less with valvuloplasty than with grafts or prosthetic valves. An annuloplasty, a repair of an **annulus** or valvular ring, can also be done. The annulus is tightened with a pursestring suture or an annular ring. The mitral valve is replaced when other repair measures are not feasible.

The aortic valve is not repaired, only replaced, if the symptoms cannot be controlled by medical means. The preferred treatment for a client with an aortic stenosis is percutaneous aortic valvuloplasty. This treatment is often used in elderly or high-risk surgical clients. A **percutaneous balloon valvuloplasty** can be done in the cardiac catheterization laboratory and no anesthesia is required. A catheter is advanced to the affected valve and a balloon is inflated in the stenosed valve. The narrowed valvular space is expanded by the balloon leaving a wider opening. Later, larger balloons may be used to expand the opening as needed.

There are two types of replacement valves: mechanical and biological. The mechanical valves are the caged-ball valve or the tilting-disk valve (Figure 19-20). There is a higher risk of a thromboembolism with a caged-ball valve. Clients remain on anticoagulant therapy with both types of valves. The biological valves come from calves, pigs, or humans. The disadvantage of the biological valves is tissue degeneration and calcification of the valve.

Table 19-2 MITRAL AND AORTIC VALVE STENOSIS AND INSUFFICIENCY

VALVE CONDITION	DEFINITION	SYMPTOMS	DIAGNOSTIC FINDINGS	MEDICAL–SURGICAL MANAGEMENT	NURSING INTERVENTIONS
Mitral stenosis	The diseased valve becomes narrowed and the leaflets thickened, preventing blood from freely flowing from the left atrium into the right ventricle.	Gradual onset of symptoms: exertional dyspnea, fatigue, orthopnea, paroxysmal nocturnal dyspnea, murmur. **Later symptoms:** peripheral edema, atrial fibrillation, jugular venous distention, hepatomegaly, abdominal distention, hypotension, thrombus from blood pooling in the left atrium.	**Chest x-ray:** hypertrophy and enlargement of left atrium and right ventricle. **EKG:** atrial fibrillation. **Echocardiogram:** fusion of valve leaflets, enlarged left atrium, decreased blood flow through valve.	**Medical management:** diuretics, digitalis, anticoagulants, antidysrhythmics, prophylactic antibiotics for invasive procedures, low-sodium diet, semi-Fowler's position, activity restrictions as needed. **Surgical management:** commissurotomy, percutaneous balloon mitral valvuloplasty, mitral valve replacement.	Encourage rest periods, administer oxygen, elevate head of bed, reposition frequently to decrease pressure points, elevate legs, low-sodium diet, monitor for signs of right and left-sided heart failure, teach stress reduction techniques, daily weight.
Mitral Insufficiency	The valve leaflets become hard and do not close completely. Blood backs up in both the left atria and ventricle, causing both chambers to hypertrophy.	Gradual onset of symptoms: exertional dyspnea, palpitations, fatigue, atrial fibrillation, loud murmur and gallop.	**Chest x-ray:** hypertrophy and enlargement of left atrium and left ventricle. **EKG:** atrial fibrillation.	**Medical management:** same as mitral stenosis. **Surgical management:** valvuloplasty, mitral valve replacement.	Same as mitral stenosis, teach exercise modification.
Aortic Stenosis	The valve cusps become hard and calcify due to rheumatic fever, syphilis, a congenital anomaly, or the aging process.	Syncope, exertional dyspnea, arrhythmias, angina, murmur, and gallop; sudden death may occur. **Later symptoms as the disease progresses:** paroxysmal atrial tachycardia, orthopnea.	**Chest x-ray:** enlargement of left ventricle, calcification of aortic valve. **EKG:** hypertrophy of left ventricle inverted T wave echocardiogram fusion of valve leaflets, regurgitation.	**Medical management:** same as mitral stenosis. **Surgical management:** percutaneous balloon aortic valvuloplasty, aortic valve replacement.	Same as mitral stenosis.
Aortic Insufficiency	The valve cusps become so hardened they do not close completely. The blood no longer flows through the aorta but backs up into the left ventricle.	Palpitations, chest pain, exertional dyspnea, nocturnal angina, dizziness, fatigue, decreased activity, intolerance, paroxysmal nocturnal dyspnea, visible pulsation of the neck veins, murmur, lung congestion.	**Chest x-ray:** hypertrophy and enlargement of left ventricle.	**Medical management:** same as mitral stenosis. **Surgical management:** aortic valve replacement.	Same as mitral stenosis, teach exercise modification.

Figure 19-20 Type of Artificial Valve: St. Jude Medical® Mechanical Heart Valve (St. Jude Medical® is a registered trademark of St. Jude Medical, Inc.) *(Courtesy of St. Jude Medical, Inc. All rights reserved)*

▶ NURSING PROCESS

▶ Assessment

▶ Subjective Data

The nurse must review past medical history for conditions such as rheumatic fever or streptococcal infections. If the client has experienced any dyspnea, palpitations, fatigue, cough, lightheadness, or numbness and tingling in the extremities, this must be documented.

▶ Objective Data

The nurse needs to take the vitals signs and listen to the apical pulse for rate, rhythm, murmurs, and S_3 sound. Breath sound should be auscultated for adventitious sounds. Edema, jugular distention, cyanosis, and equality of peripheral pulses must be noted. Homan's sign should be tested, as dysrhythmias may produce clots.

Nursing diagnoses for a client with cardiac valvular disorders may include the following:

Nursing Diagnoses	Planning/Goals	Nursing Interventions
▶ *Decreased Cardiac Output related to structural changes in valves*	The client will have increased cardiac output.	Administer oxygen as needed.
		Help the client balance activities with rest periods. The pulse should return to the baseline within 10 minutes of activity; if not, activity has been excessive.
		Discourage smoking and refer clients to support groups to assist them to stop smoking. Encourage clients to use Nicoderm or Nicorette gum while attempting to stop smoking if ordered by the physician.
▶ *Excess Fluid Volume related to decreased cardiac output*	The client will have a decrease in edema.	Administer diuretics as needed.
		Support the extremities and do not let them be in a dependent position.
		Encourage the client to maintain a low-sodium diet.
▶ *Anxiety related to threat to or change in health status*	The client will list ways to cope with stressors.	Calmly explain the procedures before doing them.
		Encourage the client's input to decisions regarding care.
		Assist the client and the client's family in identifying ways to cope with stressors.
		Teach relaxation techniques.
▶ *Deficient Knowledge related to disease process and treatment*	The client will relate the disease process and needed self-care management.	Explain the valvular disease process, medication actions, dosage times, and medication side effects to report.
		Refer the client and family members to the dietitian for low-sodium diet instructions.
		Encourage the client to begin an appropriate exercise program.

Evaluation Each goal must be evaluated to determine how it has been met by the client.

OCCLUSIVE DISORDERS

Occlusive disorders include arteriosclerosis, angina pectoris, and myocardial infarction.

ARTERIOSCLEROSIS

Arteriosclerosis is a narrowing and hardening of arteries. A buildup of lipids, collagen, and smooth muscle cells narrows the inner lining of the vessel. Blood flow through the vessel is decreased causing decreased perfusion to body cells beyond the narrowed or hardened area.

There are three types of arteriosclerosis: atherosclerosis, calcific sclerosis, and arteriolar sclerosis. **Atherosclerosis** is fatty deposits on the inner lining, the tunica intima, of vessel walls. The fat deposit is called *plaque*. In calcific sclerosis, calcium deposits are on the middle layer of the wall of the arteries, the tunica media. Hypertension causes a thickening of the arterioles and is called *arteriolar sclerosis*. With these conditions, vessels lose their elasticity resulting in various conditions, such as arteriosclerotic heart disease, angina, myocardial infarction, stroke, and peripheral vascular disease.

ANGINA PECTORIS

When coronary arteries lose elasticity or become narrow due to plaque collection, the heart muscle receives less blood and oxygen. Physical exertion, emotional stress, smoking, exposure to extreme cold, heavy meals, or an arterial spasm may cause a temporary inadequate blood and oxygen supply to the heart. Myocardial ischemia and angina pectoris result. Myocardial ischemia is a temporary inadequate blood and oxygen supply to the myocardial tissues. When this temporary condition occurs, the person experiences chest pain or **angina pectoris**.

At first, the person may experience a squeezing pain under the sternum, which radiates to the left shoulder. For some, the pain may radiate to the right shoulder, jaw, or ear. The discomfort may vary from a mild discomfort to an immobilizing pain. Anginal attacks usually increase in frequency and severity over time. The severity of the condition depends on the amount of collateral circulation that has developed.

Collateral circulation develops as larger vessels gradually narrow or harden. Blood that normally passes through the larger vessels is shunted into surrounding smaller vessels. These vessels enlarge in an attempt to supply blood to the affected area. Collateral circulation increases the blood supply to tissues that suffer from an inadequate blood supply. There is a high incidence of angina pectoris in clients with hypertension and diabetes mellitus.

Many people experiencing ischemic attacks do not experience angina. These people may be having a silent myocardial infarct or ischemia. Symptoms indicative of silent ischemia are chest pressure or heaviness, restlessness, shortness of breath with increased respiratory rate, a sensation of epigastric fullness with noisy belching, numbness or tingling in both arms or shoulders, physical or mental fatigue, and dizziness. The person may also experience a change in sleep patterns and mental alertness. The person may state that he or she "feels funny."

Two other types of angina are unstable angina and Prinzmetal's angina. Unstable angina occurs at rest or with minimal exertion and is not relieved with nitroglycerin. This client is more susceptible to myocardial infarction and sudden death. Prinzmetal's angina is caused by a coronary artery spasm and occurs at rest.

The diagnosis of angina is made after reviewing the client's history, lifestyle, laboratory tests, and stress tests. Cholesterol, low-density lipoprotein (LDL), and high-density lipoprotein (HDL) levels are evaluated. Angina pectoris can be diagnosed by a stress test, thallium scan, or a coronary arteriogram. During a stress test, the heart is placed under stress through increasing physical activity on a treadmill or exercise bicycle. The increased oxygen demand of the body puts an extra load on the heart causing electrocardiogram changes and sometimes pain. Thallium and multigated acquisition (MUGA) scans evaluate the blood supply to the myocardial tissue and determine how well the left ventricle is functioning. A coronary arteriogram shows a narrowing or occlusion of the vessels of the heart.

Medical–Surgical Management

Medical

Treatment for angina includes measures to increase the blood supply to the affected area. This can be accomplished by rest and vasodilation medications.

Silent ischemia is treated in the same way symptomatic ischemia is treated. The client needs to be educated about cardiac risk factors, the importance of following the prescribed medical regimen, and maintaining regular physical checkups.

Surgical

A percutaneous transluminal coronary angioplasty (PTCA) may be done if only one coronary artery is involved and if the atherosclerotic material is small and has not hardened. When a PTCA is done, atherosclerotic matter is pressed against the walls of the coronary vessels to improve circulation to myocardial tissue supplied by that coronary artery (Figure 19-21). A guide

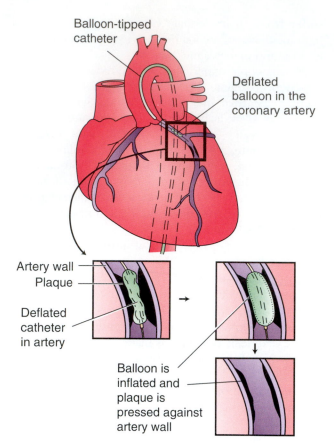

Figure 19-21 Demonstration of the Function of a Balloon-Tipped Catheter During a PTCA Procedure

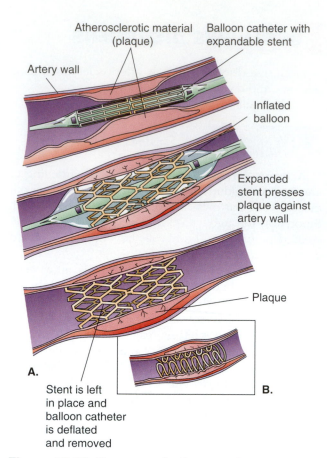

Figure 19-22 Placement of a Stent in a Coronary Artery. A. Palmaz-Schatz Stent; B. Gianturco-Roubin Ex-Stent

wire is inserted to the stenosed area and a special balloon-tipped catheter is placed in the narrowed sclerotic area. When the balloon is inflated, the atherosclerotic material is pressed against the wall of the vessel. The vessel, now open, allows more blood to flow to the myocardial tissue. During this procedure, a piece of the atherosclerotic material may break off and occlude the vessel. If this occurs, the client would have to undergo immediate coronary artery bypass graft (CABG) surgery. Other complications of the procedure are occlusion of the vessel because of a vascular spasm or vessel rupture.

An intracoronary **stent** may be implanted into a stenosed vessel to prevent the vessel from collapsing and to keep the atherosclerotic plaque pressed against the vessel wall. A stent is a tiny metal tube with holes in it (Figure 19-22). The procedure is sometimes done when a vessel collapses after a PTCA or in place of a PTCA. The stent is tightly wrapped around a balloon catheter. When the balloon catheter has been threaded through a vessel to the stenosed area, the balloon is inflated and the stent expands and presses the plaque against the vessel wall. The stent remains in the vessel and the catheter is withdrawn.

Sometimes a transcatheter ablation is done to break up the atherosclerotic areas with a laser. The sclerotic

material is broken into pieces smaller than blood cells and excreted through the kidneys.

With a coronary atherectomy, an atherectomy catheter is inserted into the affected coronary vessel to the atheroma (fatty deposit in the vessel wall). The cutter on the catheter shaves the plaque from the wall of the vessel (Figure 19-23). Depending on the type of catheter, the shavings may be saved in the end of the catheter, suctioned out, or shaved so small they pass through the capillary circulation without damage to the body.

If a CABG is performed, the internal mammary artery, the saphenous vein, or an accordion type of synthetic graft material is used. The vein or synthetic material is grafted to the aorta and passed beyond the obstruction in the coronary vessel (Figure 19-24). The graft provides an increased blood supply to the affected myocardium. The client then experiences reduced angina and has an increased tolerance for activities.

Pharmacological

Vasodilators, such as nitroglycerin tablets, cause the blood vessels to dilate, thus providing an increased blood supply to body tissues. The client may not need as much analgesic medication if beta blockers are given. Beta-adrenergic blockers and calcium channel blockers slow the heart rate and decrease the oxygen

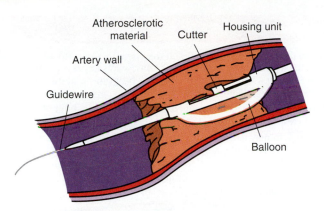

Figure 19-23 A Simpson Coronary AtheroCath cuts the atherosclerotic material (plaque) away from the artery wall.

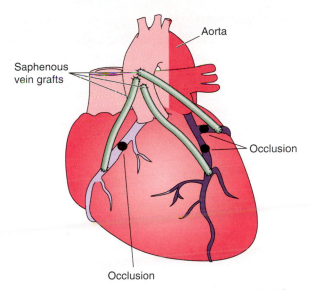

Figure 19-24 Coronary Artery Bypass Graft (CABG) with the Saphenous Vein

demand of the heart. Calcium channel blockers also dilate vessels and decrease spasms of the coronary vessels. All these measures provide an increased blood supply to the myocardium.

Diet

The client is placed on a low-fat, low-cholesterol, salt-restricted diet. Sodium restriction may vary from no salt to 4 grams daily depending on the ability of the client's kidneys to excrete excess sodium.

Activity

Activity should be slower and for shorter periods of time with more rest periods.

Health Promotion

To prevent coronary artery disease from resulting in angina, it is recommended that a person limit fat intake to 30 grams or less per day and exercise 3 to 5 times a week for at least 20 minutes. Simple activities such as parking a car further from an entrance to increase walking distance and taking stairs instead of an elevator improve circulation and help decrease cholesterol

levels. Activities such as gardening or housework are also good.

▶ NURSING PROCESS

▶ Assessment

▶ Subjective Data

The client should be asked to describe the pain as to type, radiation, onset, duration, and precipitating factors.

▶ Objective Data

The client's actions during the anginal attack should be observed and documented. Vital signs should be measured, and the client attached to an EKG monitor and observed for any dysrhythmias.

Nursing diagnoses for a client with angina may include the following:

Nursing Diagnoses	Planning/Goals	Nursing Interventions
▶ *Acute Pain related to decreased oxygen supply to the myocardium*	The client will experience decreased episodes of angina.	Administer nitroglycerin tablets sublingually. The pain should be relieved within 1 to 2 minutes. If the pain has not stopped after 3 doses 5 minutes apart, notify the emergency personnel.
		Once the acute situation is over, administer nitroglycerin as ordered. It is supplied in ointment, transdermal patch, extended-release capsules, and sprays.
		Administer other medication such as beta blockers or calcium channel blockers as ordered and monitor client's response.
▶ *Anxiety related to perceived threat of death or change in lifestyle*	The client will relate concerns and practice stress reduction techniques.	Assist the client in learning to decrease personal expectations and to live within personal activity limitations.
		Emphasize the importance of getting adequate rest and stopping before becoming too exhausted.

continues

Nursing Diagnoses	Planning/Goals	Nursing Interventions
▶ *Deficient Knowledge related to disease process, medications, and treatment regimen*	The client will explain the disease process, medication actions, dosage times and side effects, and self-care practices.	Explain the cause of angina. Teach the client to avoid stressful situations that may produce angina. Other ways to prevent angina are to sleep in a warm room, eat smaller proportions at mealtimes, and not exercise outside in cold weather.
		Inform the client to carry nitroglycerin at all times in a tightly closed container.
		Nitroglycerin may cause orthostatic hypotension, so inform the client to sit after taking it and to change position slowly after taking the medication.
		Encourage the client to start and maintain a regular exercise program as recommended by the physician.

Evaluation Each goal must be evaluated to determine how it has been met by the client.

MYOCARDIAL INFARCTION

A myocardial infarction (MI) is the leading cause of sudden death in men and women, and in 57% of the men and 64% of the women there were no previous symptoms. Of the 367,000 persons who died in 1996 from an MI, 250,000 died within 1 hour of symptom onset and before reaching the hospital (American Heart Association, 1999c). In the United States, 24% of men and 42% of women die within 1 year after having an MI. The most common cause for myocardial infarction is atherosclerosis.

A **myocardial infarction** is caused by an obstruction in a coronary artery resulting in necrosis (death) to the tissues supplied by the artery. The obstruction is usually due to atherosclerotic plaque, a thrombus, or an embolism. The area most commonly affected is the left ventricle.

Obstruction of a large coronary artery damages the myocardial tissue and affects the pumping efficiency of the heart. A client's prognosis is better if a small coronary artery or arteriole is obstructed and there is good collateral circulation to the heart. If a large vessel is obstructed and the client does not have sufficient collateral circulation, the client may die immediately.

The typical symptoms of an MI in men are feelings of chest heaviness or tightness that progresses to a severe gripping pain in the lower sternal area. The pain is not relieved by rest or nitroglycerin. The client may become short of breath (dyspneic), diaphoretic, and anxious. Women are more likely to have upper abdominal pain, dyspnea, nausea, and fatigue as well as chest pain (Kudenchuk, Maynard, Martin, Wirkus, & Weaver, 1996). The client frequently becomes nauseated and vomits. The pulse may be irregular, rapid, and weak and the blood pressure will be low. The skin will be pale and then turn cyanotic. Even though a person may not experience the typical MI symptoms, the condition can still be serious or fatal. Complications such as heart failure and stroke may also occur.

A myocardial infarction can be diagnosed by client symptoms, electrocardiogram tracings, cardiac enzyme values, and a radioactive isotope scan. However, in women the electrocardiographic stress test has less diagnostic value than in men because women are less likely to achieve an adequate heart rate response and more likely to have repolarization abnormalities (Roger, Pellikka, Bell, Chow, Bailey, & Seward, 1997). When an MI is evolving, the EKG has an elevated ST segment, which eventually changes into an inverted T wave. The pattern of the rising and falling values of CK, LDH, and AST are significant in diagnosing a myocardial infarction. The CK level rises within 3 to 6 hours of the infarct, peaks within 12 to 18 hours, and returns to normal in 3 days. The higher the CK level rises the greater the damage to the heart, and the longer the level peaks the more serious the prognosis. AST value increases in 6 hours, peaks in 12 to 14 hours, and returns to normal in 3 to 4 days. LDH level peaks in 72 hours and slowly returns to normal in 11 to 14 days.

The CK and LDH enzymes can be broken down into isoenzyme (a fragment of an enzyme) fractions of the total values of CK and LDH. A CK-MB fraction, which measures an isoenzyme specific to the cardiac muscle, rises in 3 to 6 hours of the onset of a myocardial infarct, peaks in 18 to 24 hours, and returns to normal in 72 hours. CK studies are done as soon as the client is admitted and then every 8 hours until 4 samples have been obtained. A CK-MB fraction above 5% indicated myocardial damage. LCH isoenzymes, LDH_1 and LDH_2 are also specific to heart muscle. An LDH_2 is normally higher than an LDH_1 but after an MI, the LDH_1 is higher than the LDH_2 (referred to as "flipped LDH"). An LDH_1 of more than 40% is indicative of myocardial damage. LDH studies are done upon admission and then every 8 to 12 hours for 24 hours.

Two other important lab values for diagnosing an MI are cardiac tropinin I and myoglobin. Cardiac tropinin I is a protein found in cardiac cells. When cardiac cells are damaged, this protein is released resulting in elevated levels (<0.6 mg) for 7 days. Within an hour of an MI, the myoglobin blood levels elevate, peak in 4 to 12 hours, and return to normal in 18 hours. If an MI is suspected, this lab value must be obtained quickly.

During the first 3 days after the infarction, the client may have a low-grade fever and an increased white cell count. The infarcted heart tissue is soft and necrotic and incapable of responding to electrical stimuli. Life-threatening dysrhythmias are most likely to occur at this time. Four to 7 days after the infarction, the infarcted tissue is the softest and weakest. An aneurysm, or ballooning effect, can occur in the infarcted area with the potential of rupturing. There is a possibility of the ventricle rupturing from the time of the infarct to 2 weeks after the infarct. Collateral circulation begins forming around the edges of the infarct, but it will be 2 to 3 weeks before the collateral circulation will function effectively. Two to 3 months will pass before the heart muscle will regain maximum strength.

Medical–Surgical Management

Medical

Medical–surgical management focuses on reducing oxygen demands, increasing oxygen supply to the myocardium, relieving pain, improving tissue perfusion, and preventing complications and further tissue damage. Immediately after an MI, a client is admitted into a coronary care unit. The client's heart is constantly monitored for dysrhythmias and vital signs are monitored for any changes. Blood pressure is monitored by an arterial line or a noninvasive blood pressure monitoring system.

Three dysrhythmias that may occur following an MI are ventricular fibrillation, bradycardias, and tachycardias. Ventricular fibrillation is treated by defibrillation. Atropine and, if needed, a temporary pacer may be inserted for bradycardias. Two tachycardias that may occur are atrial fibrillation and ventricular tachycardia. Atrial fibrillation is treated with digoxin (Lanoxin) or amiodarone hydrochloride (Cordarone). Ventricular tachycardia is treated with lidocaine or cardioversion. If dysrhythmias continue, magnesium may be given.

Medical complications that can occur following an MI are acute left ventricular failure, cardiogenic shock, pericarditis, embolism and/or thrombosis, and cardiac rupture. The health care team must closely monitor the client for signs of these complications. Women have a worse prognosis and die more often than men after a heart attack or bypass surgery (Mosca et al., 1997).

Surgical

Primary treatment may be PTCA instead of thrombolytic therapy. Along with balloon compression, a stent(s) may be inserted. Clients with multiple vessels occluded, or for whom thrombolytic therapy and PTCA have not been effective, may have the CABG procedure performed.

Pharmacological

Oxygen will be given by a Venturi mask or nasal cannula. Morphine sulfate is given intravenously to control the pain. Nitrates are also given intravenously or sublingually to relieve pain and dilate coronary arteries. Sedatives may be given to help calm and relax the client. A stool softener is given to prevent rectal straining.

Thrombolytic therapy is sometimes used within 3 to 6 hours of the myocardial infarction to dissolve a clot blocking an artery and reperfuse the area. Medications such as streptokinase (Streptase), anistreplase (Eminase), and alteplase recombinant (Activase) are used. A possible complication from thrombolytic therapy is bleeding. Bleeding problems are rare but the nurse should be alert for symptoms of hemorrhaging in the gastrointestinal tract (hematemesis and tarry stools), retroperitoneum (low back pain and numbness in lower extremities), or cerebrum (headache, vomiting, and confusion). Heparin therapy inhibits further clotting. Aspirin or ticlopidine (Ticlid) is given to prevent vasoconstriction and platelet aggregation.

Diet

Until the client is stabilized, a diet is withheld in case a PTCA or CABG procedure is required. Fluids may be offered during the acute stage. A liquid diet is progressed to a regular low-fat, low-cholesterol, low-salt diet. The client may tolerate small frequent feedings better than three large meals. Caffeine and extreme hot and cold foods are avoided.

Activity

It is vital the client receive physical, mental, and emotional rest. The less stimuli the client receives, the less demand is placed upon the heart. Procedures must be explained in simple terms so the client will understand the care being provided.

The client is usually limited to bed rest during the first 24 hours and progressed to sitting in a chair by the second day. If pain returns or other complications occur, the client should be confined to bed rest. Early ambulation is encouraged to prevent thrombosis. During and after each activity, the client's tolerance is assessed by monitoring the heart rate for an increase of 20 beats/minute, checking for a decrease in systolic blood pressure, and observing for dyspnea and dysrhythmias. Verbal and nonverbal statements of fatigue and chest pain are assessed.

Before the client is dismissed, low-intensity exercise tests may be done to determine types of activities in which the client may engage at home. When the client is able to climb two flights of stairs, sexual activity may be resumed.

Health Promotion

A diet of less than 30 grams of fat a day helps reduce the progression of atherosclerosis, but there is no documented evidence that diet will prevent the disease in clients with hereditary hyperlipidemia. Regular exercise, 30 minutes at least 5 days a week, and smoking cessation help prevent an MI.

Participation in a cardiac rehabilitation program provides the client with monitored exercise sessions as well as education and counseling about reducing the risk of future heart problems and coping with a new lifestyle. Because women have a worse prognosis than men, it is critical for women to participate in a cardiac rehabilitation program.

▶ NURSING PROCESS

▶ Assessment

▶ Subjective Data

The nurse should note the medications the client has taken including over-the-counter medications, anticoagulants, and thrombolytic medications. The client's pain should be assessed as to onset, duration, intensity, location, radiation, and precipitating factors; the client can be asked to describe the symptoms. Not all persons having angina or an MI will experience or state having pain. Some may describe feelings of chest heaviness, indigestion, or "something not right." These statements should be explored with the client so the client can explain them in more detail. Dizziness, weakness, and shortness of breath may be expressed. The nurse should ask about how the client tried to relieve pain.

▶ Objective Data

The nurse's assessment will include vital signs, skin changes, breath sounds, and EKG rhythm strips. Vital signs are monitored for an irregular or increased pulse, hypotension, or slight temperature elevation. The client may have pallor, cyanosis, diaphoresis, vomiting, cool clammy skin, or confusion. Breath sounds should be assessed for lung congestion, and the EKG monitored for dysrhythmias. Any client clenching of hands or clutching at the chest should be noted.

Nursing diagnoses for a client with myocardial infarction may include the following:

Nursing Diagnoses	Planning/Goals	Nursing Interventions
▶ *Decreased Cardiac Output related to damaged heart tissue*	The client will have increased cardiac output.	Maintain bed rest with head of bed elevated 30° until the condition is stabilized.
		Auscultate breath sounds every 4 hours.
		Administer oxygen per mask or nasal cannula at 2 to 4 liters per minute.
		Palpate pedal pulses every 4 hours.
		Start an IV so medications such as morphine and antidysrhythmics can be administered.
		If beta-blockers are administered, monitor closely for a drop in heart rate and blood pressure.
		Constantly monitor the client for dysrhythmias. Place a rhythm strip on the chart at least once a shift.
		Monitor I&O.
		Administer medications as prescribed by the physician.
▶ *Acute Pain related to decreased oxygenation of myocardial tissue*	The client will verbalize decrease in frequency and intensity of chest pain.	Maintain client on bed rest.
		Observe for verbal and nonverbal signs of pain such as grimacing, diaphoresis, or increased heart rate.
		Ask the client to rate the pain on a scale of 0 to 10, 0 being no pain and 10 extreme pain.
		Administer analgesic, usually morphine, as ordered.
		Administer oxygen as ordered.
▶ *Risk for Activity Intolerance related to decreased circulation to body tissues*	The client will increase activities with decreased symptoms of angina, dyspnea, cyanosis, and dysrhythmia.	Place objects within reach of the client.
		Balance activity with rest periods.
		Assist the client and partner to discuss their fears and feelings candidly about resuming sexual activity.

continues

Nursing Diagnoses	Planning/Goals	Nursing Interventions
▶ *Death Anxiety related to change in health status and threat of death*	The client will verbalize situations that are causing stress.	Encourage the family and client to verbalize their feelings.
		Provide a quiet, calm environment to relax the client and family.
		Provide the client with periods of uninterrupted rest.
		Administer sedatives to help the client relax.
		Since the myocardial client may be in denial, be aware of denial symptoms such as attempting to conduct business over the phone while hospitalized or statements that the pain is really nothing.

Evaluation Each goal must be evaluated to determine how it has been met by the client.

CONGESTIVE HEART FAILURE

Congestive heart failure (CHF) is often the final stage of many other heart conditions. A weakened muscle wall from a myocardial infarction or a heart that has been stressed over a period of time to meet metabolic needs of the body can cause congestive heart failure. Congestive heart failure develops when the heart is no longer capable of meeting the oxygen needs of the body. The heart is literally failing. The muscle of the left ventricle **hypertrophies** (increases in muscle mass) and often the ventricular chamber enlarges in an attempt to meet the oxygen needs of the body.

Both the right and left ventricles act as pumps for the heart. Each of these pumps can fail separately resulting in two types of heart failure: right-sided heart failure and left-sided heart failure. Heart failure usually begins on the left side. Some of the causes of right-sided failure are untreated left ventricular failure, right ventricular myocardial infarction, chronic obstructive coronary disease, cor pulmonale, and pulmonic valve stenosis. Left-sided failure is caused by left ventricular myocardial infarction, aortic valve stenosis, prolapsed valve complications, and hypertension. Notice that right- and left-sided failure are caused by a defect of the ventricle or an increased resistance in the path of the blood pumped by the ventricles. This causes an increased workload for the involved ventricle.

When left-sided heart failure occurs, the left ventricle is not able to completely empty of blood or effectively pump blood out through the aorta to the body systems. Usually the right ventricle continues to pump adequate quantities of blood. This causes blood to back up in the left ventricle, left atrium, and pulmonary veins. The lungs become congested with fluid as fluid leaks through the capillaries and fills air spaces in the lungs. The client becomes cyanotic, dyspneic, restless, and coughs up blood-tinged sputum. The breath sounds have moist crackles. Often the client has tachycardia with low blood pressure because the heart is not able to pump sufficient blood to meet the body's demands. The client may have decreased urinary output because enough blood is not being pumped through the kidneys. As the blood oxygen level decreases, the client becomes confused.

As the right side of the heart fails, blood becomes congested in the inferior vena cava causing edema first in the extremities and then in the trunk of the body. As the condition progresses, the client experiences edema of the ankles, lower legs, thighs, and finally in the abdomen. The excess abdominal fluid causes the client to be anorectic. Hepatomegaly (enlargement of the liver) and splenomegaly (enlargement of the spleen) develop. The jugular veins in the neck become distended when the client is sitting or standing and pitting edema occurs in the lower extremities. Refer back to Figure 19-6. Oliguria occurs as decreased amounts of blood are pumped through the kidneys.

In the early stages of congestive heart failure, the client experiences fatigue, dyspnea with slight exertion, pedal edema, and a slight cough with a small amount of expectoration. The client may also have paroxysmal nocturnal dyspnea.

Medical–Surgical Management

Medical

Goals for treating congestive heart failure are to improve circulation to the coronary arteries and decrease the workload of the left ventricle. To meet these goals, cardiac efficiency is increased with medication; oxygen

PROFESSIONAL TIP

Heart Failure
- The effects of heart failure can best be understood if blood flow is traced backward from the ventricles.
- Along the path backward from each ventricle is where congestion develops giving rise to the signs and symptoms of right- or left-sided heart failure.

requirements of the body are decreased through bed rest with head elevated 45°; edema and pulmonary congestion are treated with medications, diet, and restricted fluid intake; and fluid retention is monitored by weighing the client daily. A chest x-ray is done to directly visualize the ventricles and check for evidence of lung congestion. An EKG is done and arterial blood gases are evaluated. The client's oxygen saturation level is also monitored by pulse oximetry. Depending on the seriousness of the client's condition, a pulmonary artery catheter may be inserted to determine left ventricular function.

In right-sided failure, the symptoms of edema, hepatomegaly, and neck vein distention are significant diagnostic evidence.

Surgical

Two mechanical devices are available: an intra-aortic balloon pump and a ventricular assist device (VAD). An intra-aortic balloon is threaded through the femoral artery to the descending aorta (Figure 19-25). The pump is synchronized with the contractions of the left ventricle so the balloon inflates during diastole and deflates during systole. Inflation of the balloon increases the blood flow to the coronary arteries, thus increasing oxygenation of the myocardium. Deflation of the balloon allows the left ventricle to pump blood to the body tissues with less peripheral resistance.

The left ventricular assist device has a cannula that takes blood from the left atrium to the aorta bypassing the ineffective left ventricle (Figure 19-26). This gives the left ventricle time to rest and heal. The same process can be done for the right ventricle or both ventricles.

A cardiomyoplasty may be performed to assist the heart's functioning and improve circulation (Figure 19-27). The latissimus dorsi muscle is wrapped around the heart and a cardiomyostimulator and leads are implanted to stimulate contractions of the muscle. The stimulator is programmed to begin functioning 2 weeks after the surgery. After 4 months, the muscle stimulation is at either a 1 : 1 or 1 : 2 heartbeat ratio.

Pharmacological

The client with CHF will receive diuretics such as chlorothiazide (Diuril), furosemide (Lasix), or spironolactone (Aldactone) to decrease fluid retention and a digitalis preparation to increase the strength and contractility of the heart muscle. Vasodilators such as nitroglycerin (Cardabid) are given to dilate the veins so the blood will stay in the peripheral vessels and decrease blood return to the right side of the heart, thereby decreasing the workload on the heart. To reduce blood pressure and peripheral arterial resistance and improve cardiac output, ACE (angiotensin-converting enzyme) inhibitors such as captopril (Capoten) or enalopril (Vasotec) may be given. Morphine sulfate is given in the acute phase to control pain and decrease anxiety.

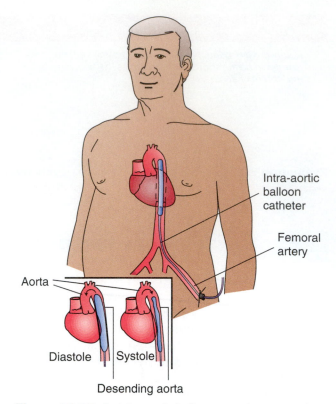

Figure 19-25 An intra-aortic balloon pump increases circulation to the coronary arteries and decreases the workload of the left ventricle.

Figure 19-26 The cannula of the ventricular assist device (VAD) takes blood from the left atrium to the aorta, bypassing the ineffective left ventricle.

Figure 19-27 Cardiomyoplasty: The latissimus dorsi muscle is wrapped around the heart and stimulated by electrical impulses.

Diet

A daily weight and strict intake and output are necessary to assess fluid retention. Sometimes fluid intake is limited. The client is generally on a low-sodium diet.

Activity

Activity orders will depend on the client's activity tolerance. The client's activity may vary from strict bed rest to ambulation depending on the severity of the condition. When in bed, the head of the bed should be elevated 45°. Visitation privileges may be monitored to provide rest periods.

Health Promotion

The most common cause of CHF is left ventricular failure after a myocardial infarction. To prevent CHF following coronary artery disease, a diet low in fat, high in fiber, and balanced in caloric intake to maintain optimum weight is recommended. Stress reduction and a regular exercise program will also decrease the risk of developing CHF. Clients developing CHF from congenital heart defects may not be able to prevent the progression of CHF, but following the prescribed medical regimen may prevent the early development of CHF.

▶ NURSING PROCESS

▶ Assessment

▶ Subjective Data

The nurse should inquire if the client has recently experienced more dyspnea, orthopnea, fatigue, anxiety, weight gain, edema, or pain. Any difficulty in performing activities of daily living should be noted.

▶ Objective Data

The client's level of consciousness should be assessed to determine circulation of blood to the brain and skin color checked for cyanosis or pallor. Assessment of skin turgor will help determine the level of hydration. Jugular distention will give an indication of the functioning level of the right ventricle. Breath sounds should be assessed for adventitious sounds, and heart sounds for gallop or murmurs. Bowel sounds may be hypoactive depending on the amount of fluid retention in the abdomen. Quality of peripheral pulses and capillary refill must be checked to assess the level of circulation to the extremities. Edema in the extremities and abdomen should be documented according to the edema rating scale. The client's daily weight is monitored for possible increase from fluid retention. The physician should be notified if there is a gain of more than 2 pounds in one day. I & O must be monitored and assessment made for oliguria.

Nursing diagnoses for a client with congestive heart failure may include the following:

Nursing Diagnoses	Planning/Goals	Nursing Interventions
▶ *Decreased Cardiac Output related to mechanical failure of heart muscle*	The client's vital signs will remain stable. The client will have decreased adventitious breath sounds.	Take an apical pulse on all cardiac clients, especially checking the rate and rhythm. Monitor the client's heart rate and rhythm by telemetry. Auscultate breath sounds every 4 hours. Administer diuretics, digitalis, and vasodilators as prescribed. Closely monitor the electrolytes, especially the potassium level, as diuretics can deplete the potassium level. Administer potassium supplements as ordered to keep the potassium serum level within the normal level. Take the apical pulse before giving a digitalis preparation. If the heart rate is below 60, withhold the medication and notify the physician. In some institutions the heart rate can drop to 50 before the physician is notified if the client is taking a calcium channel blocker or beta-blocker along with digitalis.

continues

Nursing Diagnoses	Planning/Goals	Nursing Interventions
▶ *Impaired Gas Exchange related to decreased cardiac output and pulmonary edema*	The client will have increased gas exchange.	Provide oxygen by mask or nasal cannula at 2 to 6 liters/minute to assist in the oxygen needs of the body.
		Elevate the head of the bed to a semi-Fowler's or Fowler's position to relieve pressure on the diaphragm.
		Apply a pulse oximeter and monitor the oxygenation status. If the pulse oximeter is ≤90%, notify the physician.
▶ *Excess Fluid Volume related to decreased cardiac output and decreased renal output*	The client will have less edema of the extremities.	Encourage elevation of the client's legs, not letting them hang in a dependent position.
		Monitor daily fluids by obtaining an accurate intake and output.
		Take a daily weight at the same time each day, on the same scales, and with the client wearing the same type of clothing.
		If the client is on a fluid-restricted diet, offer hard candies to quench the thirst.
▶ *Risk for Activity Intolerance related to edema, dyspnea, and fatigue*	The client will have an increased tolerance for activity.	Schedule nursing care so the client is given frequent rest periods with minimal interruptions at night.
		Teach the client to take frequent rest periods and to stop activities before becoming tired.
		Monitor the client's vital signs for an increase or decrease in heart rate or blood pressure, especially after periods of activity.
		Have an occupational therapist assist the client in energy saving methods.
		Instruct the client to call the physician if there is more dyspneic, fatigue, less activity tolerance, or weight gain or loss when at home.
▶ *Anxiety related to change in health status, lifestyle changes, or fear of death*	The client will be able to verbalize anxieties.	Explain procedures to the client and family members.
		Assist the family in identifying stress factors.
		Refer the client to a local support group such as American Heart Association or Mended Hearts, Inc.
▶ *Deficient Knowledge related to disease process, medications, diet, and plan for recovery*	The client will state knowledge of disease process, medications, diet, and plans for recovery.	Make arrangements for a dietitian to explain the sodium and/or fat restricted diet to the client and significant family members.
		Explain that small, frequent feedings, rather than three large meals a day, help prevent feeling distended and dyspneic.
		Suggest adding seasonings and spices to foods to make them more palatable when salt is restricted.
		Teach the client to read the labels on the seasonings for sodium content.
		If taking digitalis, teach the client how to accurately take a pulse before taking the daily dose.
		Teach the route, dosage, administration times, and side effects of each of the medications when the client is given the prescriptions.

Evaluation Each goal must be evaluated to determine how it has been met by the client.

COR PULMONALE

With this condition, the heart is affected because of a lung condition that interferes with the exchange of carbon dioxide and oxygen in the alveoli. The carbon dioxide level increases in the blood. For some unknown reason, the pulmonary arteries vasoconstrict causing pulmonary hypertension. The right ventricle is forced to pump against increased pulmonary pressure. The right ventricle enlarges and finally weakens in the attempt to pump blood into the lungs. The symptoms the client experiences and medical and nursing care are the same as for right-sided heart failure.

CARDIAC TRANSPLANTATION

Cardiac transplantations are done for cardiomyopathy, end-stage coronary artery disease, and valvular disease. Recipients are evaluated for emotional stability, minimal disease involvement, and a good support system. The heart donor and the recipient's tissues are matched.

The transplant is performed by removing the recipient's heart except for posterior sections of the atria. The posterior sections of the atria are removed from the donor's heart and then the heart is sutured to the recipient's posterior atria.

The recipient must remain on an immunosuppressant medication for the remainder of life so the donor heart will not be rejected. Some immunosuppressant medications are azathioprine (Imuran), cyclosporine (Sandimmune), antithymocytic globulin, ATG (Atgam), antilymphocytic globulin (ALG), rapamycin, and FK 506 (Prograf).

PERIPHERAL VASCULAR DISORDERS

Disorders in this category include: venous thrombosis/thrombophlebitis; varicose veins; Buerger's disease; Raynaud's disease; aneurysm; and hypertension.

VENOUS THROMBOSIS/ THROMBOPHLEBITIS

The terms *phlebitis, thrombosis, phlebothrombosis* and *thrombophlebitis* are often used interchangeably even though each word has a separate meaning and etiology. **Phlebitis** is an inflammation in the wall of a vein without clot formation. The formation of a clot in a vessel is a **thrombosis** and a formed clot that remains at the site where it formed is a **thrombus**. If the thrombus moves, it would become an **embolus**, a mass such as a blood clot or an air bubble, that circulates in the bloodstream. **Phlebothrombosis** is the formation of a clot because of blood pooling in the vessel, trauma to the vessel's endothelial lining, or a coagulation problem. With phlebothrombosis, there is little or no inflammation in the vessel. **Thrombophlebitis** is the formation of a clot due to an inflammation in the wall of the vessel.

In 1846, Virchow listed three factors leading to the formation of a clot. These are known as **Virchow's triad**. The three factors are pooling of blood, vessel trauma, and a coagulation problem. Risk factors for thrombi formation are prolonged bed rest, leg trauma, oral contraceptives, obesity, varicose veins, hip fractures, and total hip and knee replacement.

There are two types of thrombi, a superficial thrombus and a deep vein thrombus (DVT). A superficial vein thrombus is a clot in a superficial vein such as the saphenous vein in the leg. A DVT can form in the deep veins of the arms, pelvic area, or legs, but the legs are the most common site. Leg veins in which clots form are the femoral, popliteal, iliac, and deep veins of the calf.

Phlebitis can either form spontaneously or as a result of trauma. IV catheters or cannulas, IV medications such as potassium or antibiotics, or direct trauma to a vein can cause phlebitis. A clot may then form as red blood cells pass over the damaged area, rupture, and start the clotting process.

A phlebitis may manifest as a reddened streak over a vein. If a clot is in a superficial vein, the site becomes reddened, warm, tender, and swollen. The nurse may be able to palpate a hardening in a section of the vein. There may be no symptoms with a deep vein thrombus, or there may be warmth and tenderness at the site, unilateral edema of the affected extremity, positive Homans' sign, dilation of superficial veins, and cyanosis of the foot. The client may say the leg feels "tight" or "heavy." If the clot is in the calf of the leg, the calf may feel tender. If the swelling restricts the arterial blood flow, the leg may be cool and pale. If there are obvious clinical signs of a thrombosis, Homans' sign should not be assessed as the clot may be dislodged and become an embolus.

A complication of a DVT is a pulmonary embolus that results in approximately 50,000 to 60,000 deaths each year in the United States (Beare & Myers, 1998). Symptoms of a pulmonary embolus are sudden and severe chest pain, dyspnea, and tachypnea. Emboli may travel and block other vessels in the heart, brain, or peripheral vessels.

Medical–Surgical Management

Medical

A superficial phlebitis or thrombus should be assessed and may need no further treatment. Warm soaks may be applied to the affected area. Acetaminophen or a nonsteroidal anti-inflammatory drug is given for pain. Elevating the extremity decreases swelling and improves venous return. Some doctors recommend the application of an elastic support hose. If a DVT has been diagnosed, the client is placed on bed rest. Once the client improves and becomes ambulatory, below-the-knee compression stockings are recommended.

Surgical

If a clot has formed in a large vein and all conservative methods have failed, the clot may be removed surgically. This procedure is called a **thrombectomy** and is performed only if the tissue in the area becomes ischemic or gangrenous or if the client has a history of thromboemboli.

Another surgical procedure is a vena cava interruption surgery (venacaval plication) in which a Greenfield vena cava filter or umbrella filter is placed in the inferior vena cava to prevent thromboemboli from traveling from the lower extremities to the lungs, heart, or brain. Figure 19-28 shows these filters and their placement in the vena cava. The procedure is done on clients with a history of pulmonary emboli.

Pharmacological

If a client is at risk for a thrombus or phlebitis, antcoagulant therapy can be initiated. A prophylactic

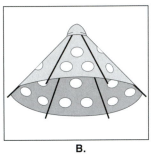

Figure 19-28 A filter in the vena cava prevents an embolus from traveling to the heart, lungs, or brain: A. Greenfield Filter in Place; B. Umbrella Filter

heparin dose is given. Enoxaparin injection (Lovenox), a low-molecular-weight heparin, is used prophylactically after hip replacement surgery. Lovenox is started within 24 hours after surgery and is given subcutaneously twice daily for 7 to 10 days. Lovenox should be used cautiously with clients on oral anticoagulants.

If a clot forms, the client is immediately started on heparin as an IV bolus and then followed with a continuous IV drip of heparin. Before heparin is started, a partial thromboplastin time (PTT) or activated partial thromboplastin time (APTT) and a platelet count are drawn by the laboratory to establish a baseline level. The heparin dose is regulated by the PTT or the APTT. For effective heparin therapy, the client's PTT or APTT level should be two and one-half times the baseline. A **baseline level** is a value at a particular time that will serve as a reference point for future value levels.

Clients are generally given heparin subcutaneously or intravenously in an acute setting. Since warfarin sodium (Coumadin) is taken orally, a client may be discharged on Coumadin. Because of rapid hospital discharges, clients are often started on Coumadin the next day after heparin has been initiated. Once the Coumadin dose is regulated, heparin is stopped.

After the initial Coumadin dose, the daily Coumadin dose is regulated by the prothrombin time (PT) or the International Normalized Ratio (INR). A PT level of 1.3

CLIENT TEACHING

Use of Warfarin Sodium (Coumadin)

- Eat a consistent amount of foods high in vitamin K each day to maintain a consistent therapeutic effect of Coumadin.
- Avoid eating kale or parsley.
- Maintain the same amounts of spinach, turnip, or other greens, broccoli, or Brussels sprouts in the daily diet.
- Avoid drinking alcohol.
- Take the medication at the same time each day.
- Maintain appointments to have the PT or INR level checked.
- Watch for signs of bleeding and avoid aspirin or drugs containing aspirin because it increases the clotting time.
- Notify physician if abdominal pain occurs as this could indicate internal bleeding.

to 1.6 times the hospital laboratory control value indicates effective Coumadin therapy. For a client on Coumadin, an INR of 2 to 3 indicates a therapeutic level. The client generally remains on Coumadin for 3 to 6 months.

Thrombolytic drugs, urokinase (Abbokinase), streptokinase (Streptase) and tissue plasminogen activator, t-PA (Alteplase), are used locally and systemically if there is a massive DVT. Streptokinase should only be used on the same client once every 6 months. If the client has had a recent streptococcal infection, urokinase is given rather than streptokinase because antibodies are present in the blood that will make the streptokinase ineffective (Beare & Myers, 1998). The main complication in a client receiving thrombolytic drugs is bleeding. Heparin and Coumadin are given after the thrombolytic drugs to prevent thrombi formation.

CLIENT TEACHING

Thrombophlebitis

- Drink 2 to 3 quarts of water per day.
- Do not to sit with legs crossed.
- Elevate both legs when sitting.
- Avoid sitting or standing for extended periods.
- Wear support hose.
- When standing, shift weight frequently and occasionally stand on tiptoes to stimulate the calf muscle to pump blood.
- Notify the physician immediately if leg pain, tenderness or swelling, difficulty breathing, or chest pain is experienced.

Diet

Adequate hydration is important for clients at risk for thrombi. This can be accomplished orally or intravenously.

Activity

During the acute stage, the client is placed on bed rest to prevent the clot from dislodging and embolizing. Later the leg is elevated periodically to improve venous return and decrease swelling. The client's leg should never be massaged as a clot could be dislodged and become an embolus.

Health Promotion

Prevention is the best way to treat a DVT. Early ambulation, adequate hydration, alternating pneumatic compression devices, prophylactic anticoagulants, elevation of legs, leg exercises, and deep breathing exercises all contribute to the prevention of thrombi. Figure 19-29 shows an alternating pneumatic compression device used to improve circulation and prevent blood stasis.

▶ NURSING PROCESS

▶ Assessment

▶ Subjective Data

The nurse should ask the client if there has been any recent injury to the extremity, if the affected area is tender to the touch, or if there have been clots previously. It is important to note any chest pain, dyspnea, tachycardia, or hemoptysis.

Figure 19-29 Alternating pneumatic compression device helps prevent thrombi formation. *(Courtesy of Beiersdorf-Jobst, Inc. Charlotte, North Carolina.)*

▶ Objective Data

IV sites are checked at least once a shift to see if a phlebitis or reddened area is developing at the insertion site. If a positive Homan's sign is detected during an assessment, the nurse should notify the physician and not perform another Homan's sign until a clot has been ruled out. The skin should be assessed for redness, tenderness, hardness, or warmth, and both legs are measured to determine baseline measurements. The circumference of the affected leg is measured every shift to determine an increase or decrease in swelling. Peripheral pulses are obtained as baseline data and charted according to the acceptable institutional scale. Peripheral pulses should be checked every 4 hours and more frequently if the client experiences increased pain in the leg, cyanosis of the foot or extremity, or increased swelling. These are signs of an occlusion.

Nursing diagnoses for a client with a venous thrombosis may include the following:

Nursing Diagnoses	Planning/Goals	Nursing Interventions
▶ *Ineffective Tissue Perfusion (Peripheral) related to decreased venous blood flow and/or clot formation*	The client will have adequate tissue perfusion.	Elevate the client's entire affected leg when on bed rest to improve venous return. When elevated, the leg should be slightly flexed at the knee with a pillow under the thigh and calf.
		Apply elastic support or intermittent pneumatic compression stockings on the client.
		If the client has received thrombolytic or anticoagulant drugs, assess for signs of bleeding which include hematuria, bruising, bleeding from the gums, and blood in the stool.
		Monitor pedal pulses and capillary refill.
		Measure thigh or calf circumference daily.
▶ *Acute Pain related to inflammatory process*	The client will state absence of pain.	If the client has a phlebitis, apply warm moist soaks to the affected area.
		Administer acetaminophen or a nonsteroidal anti-inflammatory as ordered for discomfort.
▶ *Anxiety related to possibility of the clot becoming an embolus*	The client will express anxiety about possible embolus.	Encourage client to discuss the possibility of embolus formation.

Evaluation Each goal must be evaluated to determine how it has been met by the client.

VARICOSE VEINS

Varicose veins, also called **varicosities**, are visibly prominent, dilated, and twisted veins. Veins in the lower extremities are more frequently involved, but the veins in the esophagus (esophageal varices) and anus (hemorrhoids) can also be affected. Usually it is the saphenous vein that is affected in the leg. Women are more prone to varicose veins than men (Beare & Myers, 1998). Risk factors for developing varicose veins are a familial tendency, congenital abnormalities, pregnancy, obesity, constrictive clothing, and occupations that require periods of prolonged standing. Pregnancy and obesity cause more pressure in the veins of the legs.

The causes of varicose veins are incompetent valves and veins that have lost their elasticity. The wall of the vessel is weakened from a lack of elastin or collagen and is unable to support the normal pressure of the blood in the vessel. The vein dilates as the blood in it flows backward. As the walls of the vein dilate, the valves become incapable of holding the blood and allow blood to leak backward through the space between the valves. Refer to Figure 19-5C.

Medical–Surgical Management

Medical

Varicose veins are usually treated with conservative measures such as elastic support hose, elevation of the legs when sitting, not crossing legs, and ankle and leg exercises.

Sclerotherapy involves injecting a chemical into the vein, causing the vein to become sclerosed (hardened) so blood no longer flows through it. A compression bandage or elastic stocking is applied to the extremity for 4 to 5 days. The client wears support hose for 5 more weeks. Complications of the procedure are **necrosis** (tissue death) at the injection site, vasospasm, allergic responses, and **hemolysis** (destruction of red blood cells).

Surgical

In more severe cases, varicose veins can be ligated (tied off) or stripped. **Vein stripping** involves introducing a wire into a vein. The wire has collapsible claws on the end. As the wire is withdrawn, the claws expand and strip the walls of the vein. This measure is used when there is a threat of thrombus or leg ulcers. **Vein ligation** is tying off an involved section of a vein with suture.

Pharmacological

Analgesics are given for leg discomfort. Anticoagulants may be given to prevent clot formation.

Activity

The client is encouraged to exercise regularly. Walking is a very good exercise to improve circulation because the blood circulates faster in response to an increased heartbeat. Muscles in the legs also apply pressure to the veins forcing the blood upward toward the heart. Ankle exercises such as rotating the ankle in circular motions also improves circulation.

Health Promotion

Clients with a familial tendency for varicose veins are encouraged to elevate their legs 6 to 10 inches on a small stool when sitting in a chair. Frequent position changes and not standing in one spot for extended times also improve circulation.

Nursing Management

The nurse should assist the client in elevating the legs above the heart when in bed or elevating the feet 6 to 10 inches on a pillow or stool when sitting in a chair.

After a vein stripping, the client is on bed rest for the first 24 hours. Elastic hose are worn continuously for 5 days to compress the blood into the deeper veins. The client continues to wear compression or support hose for 5 weeks after the surgery. Pain medication should be administered 30 minutes before the client ambulates until walking is tolerated without discomfort. Walking and leg exercises are encouraged after the vein stripping.

After sclerotherapy the affected area may be tender and discolored. Most discoloration will disappear in a few weeks, but a darkened pigmentation may last for 6 to 8 months. Repeated sclerotherapy may be needed. The client should be encouraged to maintain a walking exercise program to improve circulation to the legs.

 CLIENT TEACHING

Varicose Veins

Apply support hose after the legs have been elevated for an extended time, 10 to 15 minutes, so the venous blood drains from the legs. Application before getting out of bed in the morning is ideal. Do not fold or roll hose down from the top as this would act like a tourniquet causing pooling of blood. Smooth the hose on the legs as wrinkles or creases may cause extra pressure leading to stasis or pooling of blood or pressure ulcers. Remove hose daily so the leg can be washed and dried before reapplication.

BUERGER'S DISEASE (THROMBOANGIITIS OBLITERANS)

Buerger's disease is an inflammatory disease of small and medium arteries and veins that leads to vascular obstruction. Inflammation occurs in the adventitia and media layers of the vessels and may affect only a portion of the vessel or the entire vessel. Hands and feet are mainly involved, but the wrists and lower extremities may also be affected. The distal tips of the hands and feet are pale, but as the disease progresses, the hands and feet become reddened when held in a dependent position. At first, pain in the palm of the hand and arch of the foot is the main symptom. Pain becomes more severe with disease progression, and as ischemia affects the nerves, the client may experience numbness, burning, pain when at rest, and decreased sensation in the hands and lower extremities. The dorsalis pedis, posterior tibia, and ulnar and radial pulses are weak or absent. Skin color changes, cold sensitivity, ulcers, and gangrene may occur in the later stages.

Buerger's disease occurs primarily in men between the ages of 20 and 40 of Israeli, Indian, and Oriental descent. There is a correlation between smoking and Buerger's disease.

Medical–Surgical Management

Medical

The client is encouraged to stop smoking and may be referred to a smoking clinic or seminar. Buerger-Allen exercises are recommended and explained. Buerger-Allen exercises consist of elevating the legs until they blanch and supporting them at that angle for 2 to 3 minutes. The legs are then lowered to a dependent position until they become red and supported at that level for 5 to 10 minutes. The legs are then placed flat on the bed with the client in a supine position for 10 minutes. The exercises are repeated as tolerated by the client.

Surgical

A sympathectomy may be done to relieve pain and prevent vasospasm in the affected area. Digits and toes may have to be amputated in the later stages of the disease if gangrene occurs.

Pharmacological

Analgesics are given to control pain. Vasodilators are given to increase circulation to the affected area.

Nursing Management

Nursing diagnoses and interventions are the same as for other obstructive vascular conditions and are described under Raynaud's disease.

RAYNAUD'S DISEASE/PHENOMENON

Raynaud's disease or primary Raynaud's disease is an intermittent spasm of the digital arteries and arterioles resulting in decreased circulation to the fingers and toes. Sometimes the tip of the nose and ears can also be affected. The cause of the condition is unknown but seems to be related to vasospastic disorders, a disturbance with the innervation of the sympathetic nervous system, and angiography complications. During a spasm that lasts approximately 15 minutes, the fingers become pale, and then cyanotic. As the circulation returns to the fingers, the fingertips become reddened and the person experiences a tingling or throbbing pain in the fingers. Some people experience only pallor and cyanosis. The episode may last 1 to 2 hours. Symptoms usually occur when the person is exposed to cold or experiences emotional stress. Gangrene is not common but can occur in the fingertips if the disease has been longstanding. Ulcerations can also occur and are difficult to heal because of decreased circulation in the fingers.

The condition is called Raynaud's phenomenon or secondary Raynaud's phenomenon when it is associated with a connective tissue or collagen vascular disease, medications, or occupational trauma. Raynaud symptoms may occur 10 years before the related disease is diagnosed. A 2-year history of signs and symptoms with no evidence of underlying disease, especially an autoimmune disease, is necessary for a diagnosis of Raynaud's disease.

Raynaud's is more prevalent in cool, damp climates. It occurs more frequently in women between the ages of 16 and 40 (Linton et al., 2000). Persons who use vibrating hand tools such as air hammers or grinding wheels or whose hands perform repetitive movements such as typing or playing the piano are also affected.

Diagnostic examinations include a complete blood count, digital blood pressure measurement, digital plethysmography waveforms, and a cold-challenge test. A digital blood pressure of 30 mm Hg below the brachial pressure is indicative of a digital artery obstruction. A sedimentation rate, antinuclear antibody, and rheumatoid factor are done to determine the presence of autoimmune diseases. During a cold challenge test, thermistors are placed on the fingers and a baseline temperature is taken. The hands are submerged into ice water for 20 seconds, then removed. The temperature of the hands is then taken every 5 minutes until it returns to the baseline level. Hand x-rays determine the presence of subcutaneous calcium deposits and narrowing of bone in the digits. The diagnostic tests distinguish between Raynaud's phenomenon and Raynaud's disease. If a client has unilateral or single digit Raynaud's, an obstruction or emboli is suspected.

Medical–Surgical Management

Medical

Raynaud's phenomenon is treated conservatively. The client is assessed regularly for symptoms of autoimmune diseases. If the symptoms of Raynaud's are due to a vasospastic disease, relief is best achieved with medications. Alternative therapies such as relaxation techniques and biofeedback may be beneficial.

Surgical

A sympathectomy (excision of a nerve, plexus, or ganglion of the sympathetic portion of the autonomic nervous system) is sometimes done to alleviate the client's symptoms. However, it usually provides temporary relief and is not a routine treatment.

Pharmacological

Clients may be given nifedipine (Adalat, Procardia) at night for severe cases of Raynaud's phenomenon. Clients may also take the medication 1 to 2 hours before engaging in an outdoor activity during cold weather. They may not need to take the medication during warmer months. Other medications used to improve symptoms in severe Raynaud's phenomenon are diltiazem hydrochloride (Cardizem), verapamil (Calan), nicardipine hydrochloride (Cardene), and captopril (Capoten). Other medications used to improve symptoms in severe Raynaud's phenomenon are calcium channel blockers, vascular smooth muscle relaxants, vasodilators, angiotensin-converting enzyme inhibitors, and alpha-adrenergic blockers. Iloprost and cicaprost, synthetic prostacyclin analogues, are used experimentally as potent vasodilators and antiplatelet agents (McGrath, 1997). Trental is used investigationally to decrease the viscosity of blood and improve the blood flow to peripheral arteries (Spratto & Woods, 1998). Some clients have benefited from topical nitroglycerin and prostaglandin E_2 (Linton et al, 2000). The adrenergic blocker, reserpine (Serpasil) may improve circulation (McGrath, 1997).

Beta blockers, birth control pills, cold medications, and diet pills cause some clients to have Raynaud's phenomenon. These medications should be substituted or discontinued if they are the source of the symptoms. Chemotherapy drugs such as bleomycin sulfate (Blenoxane) and cisplatin, CDDP (Platinol), also cause secondary Raynaud's.

Health Promotion

The client is encouraged to avoid decongestants, caffeine, exposure to cold, repetitive hand movements, and stressful situations. The client is encouraged to quit smoking and avoid secondary smoke as nicotine is a potent vasoconstrictor. Stress management techniques, e.g., biofeedback, may assist in alleviating some distress from the condition. Wearing mittens in cold weather or when handling cold foods keeps fingers warmer than wearing gloves.

▶ NURSING PROCESS

▶ Assessment

▶ Subjective Data

A history must be obtained from the client as to how frequently the vasospastic episodes occur, what symptoms the client experiences, what triggers the episodes, which digits are affected during an episode, and how long the incident lasts. The nurse should inquire about daily activities that the client finds difficult such as tying shoes, washing dishes, or handling frozen foods and should obtain a history of occupational activities.

▶ Objective Data

Pallor, blanching, cyanosis, rubor, coldness, texture, and appearance of the digits should be assessed. If the disease is longstanding, the digits may be tapered and the skin shiny in appearance. There may be ulcerated or gangrenous areas on the fingertips.

Nursing diagnoses for a client with Raynaud's disease may include the following:

Nursing Diagnoses	Planning/Goals	Nursing Interventions
▶ *Ineffective Tissue Perfusion (Peripheral) related to vasospasm of peripheral arteries*	The client will have fewer vasospastic episodes and increased circulation in digits.	Encourage the client to use caution when engaging in activities that may cause a cut or scratch as healing may be impaired because of decreased circulation.
		If a client has ulcers, wash the areas with soap and water and administer prescribed medications such as ciprofloxacin (Cipro) and intravenous iloprost.
▶ *Acute Pain related to decreased circulation in digits*	The client will experience decreased pain as vasospasms are controlled.	Teach client to keep the indoor temperature at a comfortable level to avoid ischemic attacks.

continues

Nursing Diagnoses	Planning/Goals	Nursing Interventions
		Encourage client to avoid dramatic changes in environmental temperatures, e.g., entering a cold air-conditioned room during hot summer months. Encourage the client to wear woolen or wind-proof gloves or mittens and layered clothes when exposed to colder temperatures. Mittens may be better than gloves so the fingers can obtain warmth from each other. Chemical warming devices may be used inside gloves and shoes.
		Encourage the client to stop smoking and make a referral to a smoking cessation clinic.
		Teach the client relaxation exercises that may decrease the number of ischemic attacks.
▶ *Low Self-esteem related to inability of hands to perform activities of daily living*	The client will learn ways to handle activities of daily living.	Encourage client to use mitts or pot holders when removing items from the freezer or handling cold food to decrease the risk of a Raynaud's episode. Clients can wear mittens or socks to bed. Use of insulated mugs, foam rubber holders, or stemware glasses may reduce ischemic attacks.
		Instruct client to wash vegetables under tepid water instead of cold, to bathe in lukewarm water, and to apply lotion regularly to prevent dry and chapped skin.
		Encourage client to use gloves when pushing shopping carts or operating some vibrating machines as this may decrease the cold sensation and soften the vibration.

Evaluation Each goal must be evaluated to determine how it has been met by the client.

ANEURYSM

An **aneurysm** is a localized dilation occurring in a weakened section of an artery's medial layer. The main cause for aneurysms has previously been attributed to atherosclerosis. Recent research indicates a hereditary lack of elastin in the arterial wall as the most common cause of an aneurysm (Beare & Myers, 1998). Another factor indicating a hereditary component is if a person has an abdominal aortic aneurysm (AAA), the risk ratio is 6:1 that a first-degree relative may also develop an aneurysm compared to the general population (Beare & Myers, 1998). Some aneurysms occur because of congenital conditions such as Marfan's syndrome. Others are acquired because of trauma to the vessel wall, infection and/or inflammation, syphilis, or arteritis. Two other possible causes of an aneurysm are an increased turbulence in a section of the vessel and a slower production of smooth muscle cells. Clients have a higher tendency to develop an aneurysm if they smoke cigarettes and have hypertension.

Aneurysms can occur in any artery or peripheral vessel, but occur most often in the abdominal aorta. Abdominal aneurysms occur more frequently in men between the ages of 60 and 70 than in women (Beare & Myers, 1998). Other involved vessels are the ascending, transverse, and descending aorta, thoracic aorta, popliteal arteries, and femoral arteries.

Deposits of atherosclerotic plaque on the tunica intima cause a hardening of the vessel, and the media layer of the vessel loses elasticity. Atherosclerosis and a lack of elastin in the vessel wall predisposes the vessel to a weakened area which develops into an aneurysm.

Symptoms of an aneurysm depend upon the location of the aneurysm in the body. Aneurysms are often asymptomatic until they start leaking or pressing on other structures. A thoracic aneurysm may press on surrounding structures causing dull upper back pain or deep, scattered chest pain. Pressure on the trachea and bronchus may cause dyspnea, coughing, wheezing, and hoarseness. The client experiences dysphagia from pressure on the esophagus.

The most common location of an abdominal aortic aneurysm is between the renal and iliac arteries. There may be no symptoms from an abdominal aortic aneurysm, but as it enlarges and presses on other vessels, organs, and nerves the client may experience abdominal, back, or flank pain. The client may feel a pulse in the abdomen when in a supine position. A tender pulsating mass may be palpated slightly left of the umbilicus. Popliteal and femoral aneurysms may cause decreased pedal pulses. Rupture of an aneurysm is an emergency situation. Signs of rupture may include hypotension, tachycardia, pallor, cool and clammy skin, and intense abdominal, back, or groin pain. An aneurysm is usually diagnosed when a client has an x-ray or ultrasound done for other conditions/symptoms.

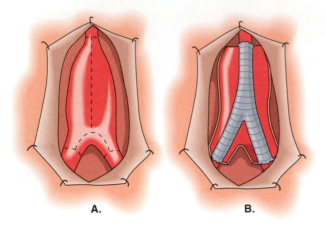

Figure 19-30 A. Aortoiliac Aneurysm; B. Bifurcated Synthetic Graft

Medical–Surgical Management

Medical

If the client has hypertension, control of the hypertension is the focus of care. Aneurysms are monitored for enlargement. Thrombi formation and ischemia may also result.

Surgical

Before elective surgery, the status of the client's carotid arteries and peripheral vessels are checked with a Doppler flow analysis (Doppler ultrasound). The client's cardiac status is usually evaluated by a stress test or cardiac catheterization before surgery is scheduled. The surgeon often orders an angiogram, ultrasound, or CT scan of the affected vessel prior to surgery in order to assess the blood supply to the area surrounding the aneurysm. Prior to surgery, it is common to place 4 to 8 units of blood on hold since hemorrhage is a possibility. The surgeon clamps the aorta, removes the section of the vessel involving the aneurysm, and replaces it with a section of the client's saphenous vein or a synthetic graft (Figure 19-30). Complications that can occur from clamping the aorta are myocardial infarctions, strokes, and renal damage. Vessels below the repaired aneurysm may become occluded because of decreased blood flow during surgery or from plaque that has broken off from the wall of the vessel. A nasogastric tube may be inserted to decrease pressure on the aneurysm repair site and incision. After surgery, the client may be in ICU with mechanical ventilator assistance in breathing.

Pharmacological

Clients with aortic aneurysms may be given propranolol hydrochloride (Inderal) to decrease the pressure of the blood coming from the heart to the affected vessel. Clients with hypertension will be placed on antihypertensive medications and diuretics. Analgesics are given to control pain.

Activity

Any activity that increases blood pressure, especially exercise and lifting, can increase pressure in the arteries and should be avoided.

Health Promotion

Clients are encouraged not to smoke. Education for the hypertensive client includes the importance of closely monitoring the blood pressure and taking antihypertensive medication as prescribed.

▶ NURSING PROCESS

▶ Assessment

▶ Subjective Data

Preoperatively, the client may be concerned about an abdominal pulsation when reclining. The client may also have chest, back, abdominal, or flank pain depending on the location of the aneurysm. Postoperatively the nurse listens for statements of pain and assesses the level of pain according to a scale of 1 to 10, or the appropriate scale used in the facility.

▶ Objective Data

If the client has an AAA, the abdomen should be palpated for a pulsating mass, and vital signs checked. Immediate intervention is needed if symptoms of bleeding or a rupturing aneurysm occur. The peripheral pulses should be checked prior to surgery and the level documented. Pulses can then be compared preoperatively and postoperatively. Postoperatively, the extremities are assessed for color, warmth, peripheral pulses, and sensation.

CLIENT TEACHING

Aneurysms
- Teach the client and significant others the symptoms of a rupturing aneurysm: sudden pain, the sensation of a tearing or ripping, pallor, diaphoresis, and loss of consciousness. If these symptoms occur, the client will need immediate medical attention.
- Aneurysms are a familial disease, so first-degree relatives of a person with an aneurysm are encouraged to share this information with their physician. An ultrasound can rule out an aneurysm.
- Teach clients the name of antihypertensive drugs and possible side effects.

Nursing diagnoses for a client with an aneurysm may include the following:

Nursing Diagnoses	Planning/Goals	Nursing Interventions
▶ *Ineffective Tissue Perfusion (Peripheral) related to decreased arterial blood flow*	The client will have well-oxygenated tissues as manifested by strong pulses and the skin remaining baseline color and warm.	Monitor for symptoms of an occluded vessel (pain, paleness, cyanosis, and coldness). Monitor the temperature, color, and fullness of the peripheral pulses in both extremities and compare them to the preoperative pulses. Assess capillary refill. Assess client's feet for mottling and darkened areas on the toes and soles of the feet. Notify physician immediately if any of these symptoms occur.
▶ *Risk for Deficient Fluid Volume related to hemorrhage*	The client will have adequate fluid volume.	Monitor vital signs closely for signs of hemorrhage. Check the operative site frequently to make sure the dressing is dry. Turn the client to make sure blood is not pooling under the client's body. Monitor for other signs of hemorrhaging. Measure the abdomen for increasing abdominal girth indicating internal bleeding. If the client has low back pain, there may be hemorrhaging in the retroperitoneal space. Other symptoms of hemorrhage are lightheadedness, dizziness, and tachycardia. Check for adequate functioning and drainage of the NG tube to decrease pressure on the aneurysm repair site and incision.
▶ *Ineffective Tissue Perfusion (Renal) related to interruption of blood flow during surgery*	The client will have a urine output above 25 cc/hour.	Measure hourly output to make sure the client has at least 25 to 30 cc of urine per hour. Provide fluids as ordered. Assess for edema which could indicate fluid overload or a vessel occlusion.

Evaluation Each goal must be evaluated to determine how it has been met by the client.

HYPERTENSION

Hypertension (HTN), also known as high blood pressure, is defined as an elevated arterial blood pressure. A systolic blood pressure above 140 or a diastolic blood pressure above 90 is indicative of hypertension. As many as 50 million (1 in 5) people in the United States age 6 and older have hypertension. Of those who have hypertension, 14.8% are not on medication, 26.2% are on medication but blood pressure is not controlled, 27.4% are controlled with medication, and 31.6% are unaware that they have hypertension (American Heart Association, 1999d). In 1996, hypertension was the primary cause of death of 41,634 persons and contributed to the deaths of 202,000 persons in the U.S. (American Heart Association, 1999d)

Prior to age 55, more men than women have hypertension, but after age 55 more women have hypertension (American Heart Association, 1999d). Risk factors include family history of hypertension, smoking, dyslipidemia, obesity, lack of exercise, diabetes mellitus, poor education, and low socioeconomic status (Woods, 1999) (Figure 19-31).

When the cause of hypertension is unknown, it is called **primary hypertension** or "essential hypertension." Ninety-five percent of the clients with hypertension have primary hypertension (Woods, 1999); this is known as **secondary hypertension**. In 5 percent of the cases, the cause of hypertension is due to another condition within the body such as renovascular disease,

Figure 19-31 Risk Factors for Hypertension (*Adapted from Beare and Myers*, Factors Contributing to Hypertension.)

CULTURAL CONSIDERATIONS

Hypertension

African Americans develop hypertension earlier in life, and it is more severe at any decade of life. The estimated prevalence of individuals with hypertension in the population at large is as follows:

POPULATION	MALES	FEMALES
American Indians	26.8%	27.5%
African Americans	35.0%	34.2%
Anglo-Americans	24.4%	19.3%
Asian/Pacific Islanders	9.7%	8.4%
Cuban Americans	22.8%	15.5%
Mexican Americans	25.2%	22.0%
Puerto Ricans	15.6%	11.5%

(American Heart Association, 1999d)

Figure 19-32 Pathophysiology of Renal Diseases and Hypertension

polycystic kidney disease, coarctation of the aorta, Cushing's syndrome, or pheochromocytoma (Woods, 1999); this is known as **secondary hypertension**. Arteriosclerosis, atherosclerosis, hypernatremia (increased sodium in the blood) or prolonged stress may also cause hypertension.

Renal diseases may interfere with the flow of blood to the kidneys causing them to release an enzyme called *renin*. When renin is released, it interacts with plasma proteins forming a vasopressor called *angiotensin*. Vasoconstriction caused by angiotensin increases the blood pressure because more force is required to get the blood through the vessel. Vasodilation decreases vascular or **peripheral resistance** (pressure within a vessel that resists the flow of blood such as plaque buildup or vasoconstriction. Figure 19-32 depicts how renal disease causes hypertension.

Arteriosclerosis causes the vessel walls to have less elasticity, decreasing their ability to expand and recoil.

Since the vessel is not able to expand, more pressure is needed to force the blood through the vessel. Atherosclerosis narrows the vessel lumen, or opening, because of plaque buildup along the wall of the vessel. The plaque buildup causes resistance to the flow of blood through the vessel and more pressure is needed to get the blood through the vessel. Hypernatremia (increased blood sodium) causes vasocongestion. With vasocongestion, the heart must pump with more force, increasing the pressure in the arteries, thus causing HTN.

Stress stimulates the sympathetic nervous system which supplies nerves to the smooth muscles of the arteries, arterioles, veins, and venules. Stimulation of smooth muscles by the sympathetic nervous system causes the vessel to vasoconstrict leading to elevated blood pressure.

Some complications of HTN are cerebral vascular accident (stroke), myocardial infarction, congestive heart failure, and renal failure. Table 19-3 lists the recognized classification of blood pressure and the recommended time frame for follow-up care.

Table 19–3 CLASSIFICATION OF BLOOD PRESSURE AND RECOMMENDED FOLLOW-UP

CATEGORY	SYSTOLIC (MM HG)		DIASTOLIC (MM HG)	RECOMMENDED FOLLOW-UP
Optimal	< 120	and	<80	Recheck 2 years
Normal	< 130	and	< 85	Recheck 2 years
High normal	130–139	or	85–89	Recheck 1 year
Hypertension				
Stage 1 (mild)	140–159	or	90–99	Recheck within 2 months
Stage 2 (moderate)	160–179	or	100–109	Recheck within 1 month
Stage 3 (severe)	> 180	or	> 110	Immediate care

From The Sixth Report of the Joint National Committee on Prevention, Detection, Evaluation, and Treatment of High Blood Pressure, *1997, Bethesda, MD: National Institutes of Health.)*

PROFESSIONAL TIP

Hypertension

Often the hypertensive client may not be experiencing any symptoms and does not see the importance of caring effectively for this condition.

Medical–Surgical Management

Medical

The physician's main goal in caring for a client with HTN is keeping the blood pressure within normal limits. The regimen is referred to as a stepped-care approach. The first step is to encourage the client to try some diet and lifestyle changes. These include losing weight if the client is more than 15% over the optimum weight; limiting sodium, saturated fat, cholesterol, and alcohol intake; exercising on a regular basis; stopping the use of nicotine; and maintaining an adequate intake of calcium, magnesium, and potassium. This step is tried for 3 to 6 months, and if the BP then is less than 140/90, these steps would be continued. If the BP still remains high, the second step would be implemented which would be adding a diuretic or a beta blocker to the client's care regimen. The client would again be evaluated for a period of time, usually 2 months. If the BP still does not return to less than 140/90 within that time frame, the third step of increasing the drug dosage, trying another drug, or adding a second antihypertensive drug from another class of drugs would be implemented. If the BP is maintained at less than 140/90, the regimen would be continued. If the BP is still high, the last step would be implemented by adding a second or third antihypertensive drug.

Pharmacological

Diuretics are usually the first pharmacological step in treating HTN. Diuretics increase the renal excretion of sodium and water from the body decreasing the total fluid volume. When less fluid is in the body, less pressure or force is needed to pump the blood through the body.

Beta-adrenergic blocking agents are given to block the epinephrine and norepinephrine receptor sites. With these receptor sites blocked, the vessels will not constrict and the blood will have less resistance flowing through the vessel. Diuretics and antihypertensive medications may cause impotence.

Other medications used to lower blood pressure are alpha$_1$-receptor blockers, angiotensin-converting enzyme (ACE) inhibitors, calcium channel blockers, centrally acting alpha$_2$-agonists, peripherally acting adrenergic antagonists, and direct vasodilators. Refer to Table 19–4 for a list of antihypertensive medications.

Table 19–4 ANTIHYPERTENSIVE MEDICATIONS
Alpha-adrenergic Blockers   clonidine hydrochloride (Catapres)   doxazosin mesylate (Cardura)   methyldopa (Aldomet)   phentolamine mesylate (Regitine)   prazosin hydrochloride (Minipress)   terazosin hydrochloride (Vasocard, Hytrin)
Angiotensin-converting Enzyme (ACE) Inhibitors   captopril (Capoten)   enalapril maleate (Vasotec)
Beta-andrenergic Blockers   propranolol hydrochloride (Inderal)   timolol maleate (Blocardren)   atenolol (Tenormin)
Calcium Channel Blockers   diltiazem hydrochloride (Cardizem)   nifedipine (Procardia)   verapamil (Calan, Isoptin)
Ganglionic Blockers   trimethaphan camsylate (Arfonad)
Loop Diuretics   bumetanide (Bumex)   furosemide (Lasix)
Potassium-sparing Diuretics   amiloride hydrochloride (Midamor)   spironolactone (Aldactone)   spironolactone with HCTZ (Aldactazide)   triamterene (Dyrenium)
Thiazide Diuretics   chlorothiazide (Diuril)   hydrochlorothiazide (Esidrex, HydroDIURIL)   methyclothiazide (Enduron)   metolazone (Zaroxolyn)   hydrochlorothiazide with triamterene (Dyazide)
Thiazide-like Diuretics   chlorthalidone (Hygroton)   indapamide (Lozol)
Peripherally Acting Adrenergic Antagonists   reserpine (Serpasil)
Direct Vasodilators   diazoxide (Hyperstat)   hydrolazine hydrochloride (Apresoline)   nitroprusside sodium (Nipride)

Diet

The hypertensive client is encouraged to have a low-fat, low-cholesterol, and low-sodium diet. Restricting sodium intake to 2.3 grams of sodium or 6 grams of sodium chloride a day assists in decreasing blood pressure. Slight lifestyle changes such as avoiding processed foods, carbonated drinks, and most cereals help decrease sodium intake. The client should have an adequate intake of potassium, magnesium, and calcium. These minerals can be obtained by eating fresh oranges, bananas, broccoli, and collards. Fresh foods are better sources for minerals than frozen foods. Yogurt is a good calcium supplement. The National Committee on Prevention, Detection, Evaluation, and Treatment of High Blood Pressure recommends that clients with hypertension not consume more than 2 ounces of alcohol at a time and no more than twice a week.

Activity

A regular aerobic exercise regimen assists in lowering blood pressure. The client is to gradually increase the exercise period to 30 to 45 minutes 3 to 5 times per week with a pulse rate at 75% of the target heart rate (target heart rate = $220 - age \times 0.75$). Walking, swimming, and jogging are excellent aerobic exercises.

Health Promotion

Measures to prevent hypertension are exercising regularly; reducing sodium in the diet; maintaining an optimum weight; reducing and managing stress; maintaining intake of potassium, calcium, and magne-sium; decreasing alcohol consumption; and ceasing smoking.

▶ NURSING PROCESS

▶ Assessment

▶ Subjective Data

The hypertensive client should be asked about general lifestyle habits such as smoking, alcohol consumption, exercise routine, dietary intake, and family history of hypertension. Any dizziness, blurred vision, and headache in the occipital region upon rising in the morning is noted.

▶ Objective Data

The basic assessment for HTN is taking the blood pressure. An accurate blood pressure is obtained if the bladder of the blood pressure cuff surrounds two-thirds of the client's arm, the arm is supported at heart level, and the blood pressure is taken in both arms in supine and sitting positions. Before taking the blood pressure, the client should rest quietly for 5 minutes. If the client has an elevated BP, a repeat blood pressure should be taken 15 minutes later and compared to previous readings. Client height and weight is recorded, and heart sounds and peripheral pulses measured.

Nursing diagnoses for a client with hypertension may include the following:

Nursing Diagnoses	Planning/Goals	Nursing Interventions
▶ *Ineffective Health Maintenance related to lack of knowledge about lifestyle habits contributing to hypertension*	The client will relate needed changes in lifestyle habits to decrease blood pressure.	Make referrals to the appropriate personnel to teach the client lifestyle changes. These may include a dietitian, smoking cessation clinic, fitness center, or stress management seminars. Explain the pathophysiology, risk factors, lifestyle changes, medication actions and side effects, and complications of hypertension.
▶ *Noncompliance related to individual's value system (lack of physical symptoms and expense of medication)*	The client will keep appointments for regular check-ups and take medications as prescribed.	Regularly inquire about the client's satisfaction in regard to the prescribed regimen of diet, exercise, and prescribed medication(s). If the client cannot afford needed medications, refer the client to financial assistance programs. Encourage the client to become an active participant in the treatment as this will give the client a sense of control over the condition. Encourage the client to record BP readings, weekly weight, exercise activities, and dietary intake as a way of giving a sense of control and encouraging compliance.
▶ *Imbalanced Nutrition: more than body requirements, related to excess caloric intake and excess sodium intake*	The client will maintain weight at no more than 15 percent over optimum weight and have no more than 2.3 grams of sodium per day.	Give basic dietary instructions as stated under medical management or make a referral to a dietitian. Weigh the client at scheduled appointments.
▶ *Sexual Dysfunction related to altered body structure or function and side effects of antihypertensive medications*	The client will state satisfaction with sexual function while taking antihypertensive medications.	Since diuretics and antihypertensive medications may cause impotence, discuss this effect in an open and candid manner, so the client and spouse will be more open to discuss difficulties in this area.

Evaluation Each goal must be evaluated to determine how it has been met by the client.

SAMPLE NURSING CARE PLAN

THE CLIENT WITH HYPERTENSION

Thomas Liggins, a 28-year-old African American, is in his last year of law school and is clerking for a prestigious law firm. He and his fiancé are planning to be married as soon as he graduates. During the last week he has had 4 dizzy spells and has had a headache at the base of his skull upon awakening for the last 2 days. His father has a history of hypertension, so Thomas is aware that his symptoms may be indicative of high blood pressure. Thomas stops by the clinic on his way home from work and asks to have his blood pressure checked. The nursing assessment has the following data.

Subjective data: States he has had 4 dizzy spells and has awakened with a headache in the occipital lobe the last 2 mornings. Thomas has been having 1 glass of wine at lunch and 2–3 beers in the evening to relax from the tension of school and work. Most of his meals have been at fast-food establishments and have a high fat content. Thomas does not smoke. He used to jog 4 mornings a week but quit when he starting clerking. He has been getting up twice in the night to urinate for the last 3 weeks. He is not taking any medication. Thomas states he is concerned about having hypertension because he does not want to take medication.

Objective data: T 98.6 P 78 R 16 BP 142/92 Wt 190 (optimum weight 160). No edema noted in hands, feet, or legs.

Nursing Diagnosis 1 *Ineffective Health Maintenance related to ineffective individual coping as evidenced by high-fat diet, lack of exercise, stressful job, and alcohol intake*

PLANNING/GOALS	NURSING INTERVENTIONS	RATIONALE	EVALUATION
Thomas will change lifestyle habits by engaging in aerobic exercises at least 3 times a week for 30 to 45 minutes, stating three ways to reduce stress, and limiting alcohol consumption to 2 ounces twice a week.	Refer Thomas to a dietitian to learn ways to cut fat and sodium in his diet.	Knowledge of a low-sodium, low-fat diet will encourage compliance.	Thomas starts exercising with his fiancé 3 times a week. Thomas uses breathing techniques and a hot shower to reduce daily stress. Thomas limits alcohol consumption to 1 beer a day.
	Discuss ways Thomas can exercise and still meet responsibilities of work, school, and personal and social life.	Thomas will be more willing to exercise if he sees ways that he can still meet responsibilities of life.	
	Explain that alcohol consumption should be limited to 2 ounces of alcohol twice a week.	Knowledge of alcohol content in alcoholic beverages will encourage compliance.	

Nursing Diagnosis 2 *Imbalanced Nutrition: more than body requirements, related to excessive caloric intake as evidenced by 30 pounds overweight and high-fat diet*

PLANNING/GOALS	NURSING INTERVENTIONS	RATIONALE	EVALUATION
Thomas will lose 30 pounds and maintain a low-fat, low-sodium diet.	Refer Thomas to a weight support group.	It will be easier for Thomas to change life habits if others are encouraging him.	Thomas and his fiancé are maintaining a diet low in sodium and no

continues

Encourage Thomas to maintain a weekly weight record and to monitor daily intake of fat grams.	Monitoring personal diet and recording weight weekly promotes self-care and personal involvement in health maintenance.	more than 30 grams of fat per day. Thomas keeps a weekly record of his weight.

Nursing Diagnosis 3 *Anxiety related to threat to or change in health status and stress as evidenced by alcohol consumption to relax and statement of not wanting to take medications*

PLANNING/GOALS	NURSING INTERVENTIONS	RATIONALE	EVALUATION
Thomas will state preventive measures to reduce blood pressure.	Have Thomas identify stress factors in life.	Thomas may not be aware of some stressors in his life. Action to cope with stressors can be taken only if stressors are identified.	Thomas states 4 ways to reduce blood pressure.
	Discuss stress reduction techniques with Thomas.	Knowledge of ways to reduce stress will promote compliance.	
	Discuss risk factors of hypertension and ways to reduce blood pressure.	Knowledge of risk factors will promote identification of risk factors in personal life.	
	Explain to Thomas and his fiancé that hypertension is a chronic condition, possibly without symptoms, and with some potentially serious complications.	Knowledge of disease process promotes compliance. It is important for client and client's support system to understand disease process so lifestyle changes can be made more easily.	

CASE STUDY

Mr. Lance Jeffers, a 55-year-old truck driver, is admitted to the emergency room with a feeling of heavy squeezing pressure in his sternal area. The pain is radiating to his left shoulder. He is diaphoretic, short of breath, and nauseated. He states the sternal pain came on suddenly while watching a football game. He had been mowing his yard and decided to rest. The emergency physician gives Mr. Jeffers a nitroglycerin tablet and connects him to an EKG monitor. Cardiac enzymes with isoenzyme fractions and a chest x-ray are requested STAT. Morphine sulfate 2 mg is given intravenously. Oxygen is given by mask at 4 liters/minute. Mr. Jeffers's apical pulse is 102 and his blood pressure is 130/88. A cardiac catheterization with fluoroscopy is ordered to determine the patency of the coronary blood vessels and functioning of the heart muscle. Three hours after admission, crackles are heard in the lungs.

The following questions will guide your development of a nursing care plan for the case study.

1. List symptoms/clinical manifestations, other than Mr. Jeffers's, a client may experience when having a myocardial infarction.
2. List two reasons morphine sulfate was given to Mr. Jeffers.
3. List two other diagnostic tests that may have been ordered for Mr. Jeffers.
4. List subjective and objective data a nurse would want to obtain about Mr. Jeffers.
5. Write three individualized nursing diagnoses and goals for Mr. Jeffers.
6. Mr. Jeffers is moved from the critical care unit. List pertinent nursing actions a nurse would do in caring for Mr. Jeffers related to:

    oxygenation

    cardiac output

    comfort/rest

    activity

    medications

    teaching
7. List teachings that Mr. Jeffers will need before his discharge.
8. List at least three successful client outcomes for Mr. Jeffers.

SUMMARY

- The function of the heart is to pump blood through the vascular system. Blood is the medium by which oxygen and nutrients are provided to the body cells and carbon dioxide and waste products are removed from the body cells.
- The volume of blood pumped into the circulatory system depends on the cardiac output.
- The coronary arteries supply blood to the heart. If the blood flow through these vessels becomes diminished or occluded, ischemia to the heart tissue occurs resulting in angina or a myocardial infarction.
- Typical symptoms experienced by a person with cardiac problems include chest pain, dyspnea, edema, fainting, palpitations, diaphoresis, and fatigue.
- A lipid profile and cardiac enzymes, including the CK and LDH isoenzymes, provide diagnostic infor-

mation as to the risk of heart disease and the occurrence of a myocardial infarction.
- A dysrhythmia is an irregularity in the rate, rhythm, or conduction of the electrical system of the heart.
- Inflammatory or infectious conditions of the heart include endocarditis, myocarditis, and pericarditis. Endocarditis may cause valvular heart disease with the possibility of the valve needing to be surgically repaired (valvuloplasty) or replaced with a mechanical (caged-ball valve or tilting-disk valve) or biological valve from a calf, pig, or human.
- Arteriosclerosis and atherosclerosis cause a narrowing and occluding of vessels and are the primary causes of angina and myocardial infarction.
- Surgical treatment for angina includes a PTCA, intracoronary stent, transcatheter ablation, or a coronary artery bypass graft.

- Nursing interventions for CHF are monitoring vital signs with each client activity; administering digitalis, diuretics, and vasodilators as ordered; administering and observing the effects of oxygen; weighing the client daily; obtaining accurate I & O; and teaching healthy lifestyle changes.
- Congestive heart failure is often the final stage of many other heart conditions in which the heart is no longer able to fulfill the demands of the body and is literally failing.
- To assess the peripheral vascular system, the nurse assesses pain, pulse, pallor, paresthesia, and paralysis.
- Three factors leading to the formation of a clot—pooling of blood, vessel trauma, and a coagulation problem—are called Virchow's triad.
- A client with a DVT may be asymptomatic or may have warmth and tenderness at the site, edema of the extremity, a positive Homans' sign, cyanosis of the foot, and a sensation of heaviness or tightness in the extremity.
- Treatment for a thrombus includes bed rest, warm soaks, elevation of the extremity, and application of elastic stockings or intermittent pneumatic compression. It is important for the nurse to measure the leg circumference every shift and check peripheral pulses.
- The cause of varicose veins is incompetent valves and veins that have lost their elasticity.
- Primary Raynaud's disease is an intermittent spasm of the digital arteries and arterioles resulting in decreased circulation to the digits.
- An aneurysm is a localized dilation of a weakened section of the medial layer of an artery.
- Symptoms of an aneurysm depend upon the location of the aneurysm in the body and are often asymptomatic until they start leaking or pressing on other structures.
- Hypertension is an elevated arterial blood pressure of 140/90.

Review Questions

1. The nurse may assist in relieving the chest pain of a client with pericarditis by having the client:
   a. lie flat and turn on the right side.
   b. lie flat and turn on the left side.
   c. sit in a semi-Fowler's position.
   d. sit erect and lean forward.

2. To assess a client with right-sided heart failure, the nurse would:
   a. listen for a pericardial friction rub.
   b. listen for a muffled S_1 and S_2 heart sound.
   c. check for distended neck veins with the bed at a 45° angle.
   d. assess for radiation of the squeezing sensation under the sternum.

3. A diagnostic test for a myocardial infarction is:
   a. cardiac enzymes.
   b. arterial blood gases.
   c. cardiac biopsy.
   d. pulse oximetry.

4. It would be important to teach a client with angina to:
   a. take antibiotics before having dental work.
   b. carry nitroglycerin tablets at all times.
   c. perform the Valsalva maneuver daily.
   d. massage the carotid sinuses in the neck.

5. A client with the diagnosis of a myocardial infarction has just been admitted to the ER. To relieve chest pain, the physician orders:
   a. amoxicillin (Amoxil).
   b. ibuprofen (Motrin).
   c. digoxin (Lanoxin).
   d. morphine sulfate.

6. A cardiac dysrhythmia that has an erratic electrical activity of the atria resulting in a rate of 350 beats/minute to 600 beats/minute is:
   a. atrial fibrillation.
   b. bradycardia.
   c. ventricular asystole.
   d. third degree AV block.

7. A nursing intervention to improve cardiac output is:
   a. encouraging the client to verbalize fears.
   b. teaching the side effects of new medications.
   c. a referral to a dietitian for low-sodium diet instructions.
   d. administer oxygen per physician orders.

8. The most appropriate nursing diagnosis for a client with coronary artery disease is:
   a. decreased cardiac output.
   b. social isolation.
   c. fatigue.
   d. altered nutrition.

9. Instructions to a client on anticoagulant therapy include:
   a. taking Coumadin twice a day.
   b. watching for symptoms of bleeding.
   c. taking over-the-counter medications as needed.
   d. no dietary or activity limitations.

10. When assessing a client with a possible DVT, the nurse:
    a. routinely does a Homans' sign.
    b. massages the calf of the leg.
    c. gently touches the affected area and checks for warmth.
    d. calls the physician immediately.

11. A nurse is assigned to care for a client who has just had a hysterectomy. To prevent the formation of a thrombus, the nurse:

    a. encourages the client to lie in bed with the knee gatch activated.

    b. encourages the client to ambulate with assistance according to the physician's orders.

    c. assesses Homans' sign as part of the routine postop assessment.

    d. checks peripheral pulses every 4 hours.

12. A client, admitted with the diagnosis of AAA, states he can feel a pulsation when he lies flat in bed. To assess the pulsation, the nurse would palpate:

    a. the epigastric area.

    b. the right lower quadrant.

    c. one inch above the symphysis pubis.

    d. left of umbilicus.

13. The symptoms a client with an aneurysm pressing on the inferior vena cava would most likely experience are:

    a. low dull back pain and a pulsating mass in the abdomen.

    b. dyspnea, wheezing, and hoarseness.

    c. bloating, nausea, and vomiting.

    d. edema in the extremities and possible cyanosis.

14. The first step of the stepped-care approach in treating hypertension is:

    a. changes in lifestyle.

    b. diuretics.

    c. beta-blockers.

    d. adding a second or third antihypertensive.

Critical Thinking Questions

1. What lifestyle changes could a person take to decrease the risk factors for a myocardial infarction?

2. Prepare a teaching strategy to teach the hypertensive client ways to modify the present lifestyle.

3. What is the rationale for each nursing intervention given for the nursing diagnoses in this chapter?

WEB FLASH!

- Search the Internet for information about the disorders covered in this chapter. What information is available? For whom is the information suitable?
- What Internet information do the chapter resources at the end of the book provide?

NURSING CARE OF THE CLIENT: HEMATOLOGIC AND LYMPHATIC SYSTEMS

CHAPTER 20

MAKING THE CONNECTION

Refer to the following chapters to increase your understanding of the hematologic and lymphatic systems:

- **Chapter 10, Fluid, Electrolyte, and Acid-Base Balance**
- **Chapter 12, Health Assessment**
- **Chapter 14, Pain Management**
- **Chapter 17, Nursing Care of the Oncology Client**
- **Chapter 18, Nursing Care of the Client: Respiratory System**
- **Chapter 19, Nursing Care of the Client: Cardiovascular System**
- **Chapter 22, Nursing Care of the Client: Immune System**
- **Chapter 27, Nursing Care of the Client: Endocrine System**

LEARNING OBJECTIVES

Upon completion of this chapter, you should be able to:
- *Define key terms.*
- *Relate anatomy and physiology of the blood and lymph systems to disease processes.*
- *Relate diagnostic test results to the blood and lymph disorders.*
- *Describe nursing interventions in caring for clients with blood and lymph disorders.*
- *Assist in developing a nursing care plan for clients with blood and lymph disorders.*

KEY TERMS

agranulocytosis	idiopathic
apheresis	induction dose
bands	leukocytosis
blastic phase	leukopenia
combination	lymphoma
chemotherapy	maintenance therapy
erythrocytapheresis	median survival time
fibrinolysis	microthrombi
hemarthrosis	phlebotomy
hematocrit	purpura
hematopoiesis	reticulocyte
hemolysis	sickled
hyperuricemia	thrombocytopenia

INTRODUCTION

The hematological system of the body is comprised of blood and blood-forming organs. Blood consists of formed elements (red blood cells, white blood cells, and platelets) and plasma. As blood is pumped through the body, it carries essential substances to the tissues and removes waste products from the tissues. Disorders of the hematological system usually result from abnormal production or functioning of the cells. Some of these disorders are the result of genetics, environment, or pathogenic organisms.

The lymph system consists of lymph vessels, nodes, and organs. Lymph vessels collect and return lymph fluid to the blood vessels through the right and left lymphatic ducts at the right and left subclavian veins. The functions of the lymph system are to assist with immunity, control edema, and absorb digested fats.

Medical management and nursing diagnoses, goals, and interventions are given for each blood and lymph disorder. It is important for the nurse to have a complete understanding of the blood and lymph disorders when providing nursing care to clients.

ANATOMY AND PHYSIOLOGY REVIEW

The blood and lymphatic systems are discussed following.

Blood

The heart pumps 5–6 liters of blood per minute through the circulatory system of an adult. Blood is an aqueous mixture consisting of plasma and cells (Figure 20-1).

Plasma

Plasma is a straw-colored liquid consisting of approximately 90% water and 10% proteins. The water component assists in transporting body nutrients, hormones, antibodies, electrolytes, and waste; regulating blood volume; and controlling body temperature. The proteins are albumin, globulins, and fibrinogen. Albumin controls the volume of the blood and blood pressure by osmotic pressure that pulls tissue fluid into the capillary system. There are three types of globulins: alpha, beta and gamma. Alpha and beta globulins are secreted by the liver and are carrier molecules for substances. Gamma globulins are antibodies important in the immune response of the body. Fibrinogen changes into fibrin, a solid, that controls bleeding in the blood clotting mechanism of the body. The formed elements in plasma are red blood cells (RBCs), white blood cells (WBCs), and platelets.

Red Blood Cells

Red blood cells, also called erythrocytes, are the most numerous blood cells in the body, generally 4.5 to 6.1 million/mm^3 in an adult. RBCs are biconcave disks that do not have a nucleus. They are about the size of the smallest capillary but are flexible and capable of changing shape so they can squeeze through the capillaries.

RBCs in conjunction with the respiratory and circulatory systems oxygenate body tissues. In the capillary bed of the alveoli, blood receives oxygen (O_2), and carbon dioxide (CO_2) is eliminated. The O_2-enriched RBCs (oxyhemoglobin) carry O_2 to systemic capillaries, where O_2 is exchanged for CO_2. The carbon dioxide–laden blood then returns the CO_2 to the alveoli in the lungs, where it is again exchanged for oxygen. The CO_2 is exhaled from the body with each breath. Hemoglobin is a protein in the RBC that carries O_2 and is responsible for the exchange of O_2 and CO_2.

The average life span for an RBC is 120 days. Blood cells originate from a single stem cell that proliferates and differentiates into lymphoid stem cells or blood stem cells (Figure 20-2). The lymphoid stem cells further divide and differentiate into T cells and B cells. The blood stem cells divide and differentiate into RBCs, WBCs, and platelets. The process of blood cell production and development is called **hematopoiesis**. RBCs are produced daily by the bone marrow according to the demand of the body. When the partial pressure of O_2 drops, a renal hormone, erythropoietin, stimulates the bone marrow to produce more immature RBCs (**reticulocytes**), which are released into the bloodstream. These reticulocytes develop into mature red blood cells. The number of circulating reticulocytes can be used as a diagnostic tool for RBC disorders.

As RBCs age, their outer membrane deteriorates and they are destroyed by large macrophages in the liver and are filtered out of the body by the spleen. The iron from heme in the old RBCs is used in the production of new RBCs.

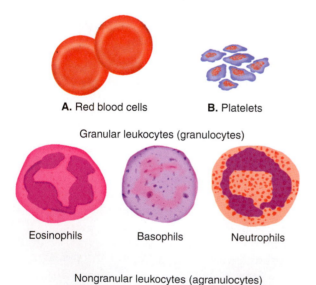

A. Red blood cells   **B.** Platelets

Granular leukocytes (granulocytes)

Eosinophils   Basophils   Neutrophils

Nongranular leukocytes (agranulocytes)

Lymphocytes   Monocytes

C. Granular and nongranular white blood cells

Figure 20-1 The Cells in Blood: A. Red blood cells (erythrocytes); B. Platelets (thrombocytes); C. White blood cells (leukocytes).

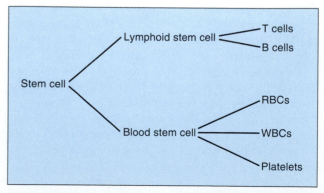

Figure 20-2 Origin of T cells, B cells, RBCs, WBCs, and Platelets

Hematocrit is the percentage of blood cells in a volume of blood. A normal hematocrit is 42% to 45% of blood volume; that is, 42% to 45% of a certain amount of blood consists of cells.

White Blood Cells

White blood cells, also called leukocytes, fight infection and assist with immunity. The life span of a WBC varies from hours to years, depending on the type of WBC. Neutrophils, basophils, and eosinophils live from a few hours to days, whereas lymphocytes and monocytes live from days to years. The normal WBC count is 5,000 to 10,000/mm³ of blood (Pagana & Pagana, 1999). An increased number of WBCs (**leukocytosis**) may signify the presence of an infection, inflammation, tissue necrosis, or leukemia. A decreased number of WBCs (**leukopenia**) may indicate bone marrow failure, a massive infection, dietary deficiencies, a drug toxicity, or an autoimmune disease.

WBCs are classified as granulocytes or polymorphonuclear leukocytes (PMNs, or polys), and agranulocytes. The granulocytes have granules (grainy substances) in their cytoplasm, and the agranulocytes do not have granules. Granulocytes are divided into three types: the neutrophils, eosinophils, and basophils. Agranulocytes are classified into two groups, monocytes and lymphocytes. Neutrophils are the most numerous WBCs, making up approximately 60% of the total number of WBCs. The main function of neutrophils is to digest and kill microorganisms. If a client has an acute infection, the bone marrow is stimulated to produce more neutrophils, resulting in an increased circulation of immature neutrophils called **bands**. An increased production of neutrophils indicates the presence of an acute infection. An increased number of basophils and especially of eosinophils indicates an allergic response.

Monocytes become macrophages, cells that destroy dead and injured cells and bacteria. There are two types of lymphocytes, T cells and B cells, which are involved in the body's immune response.

Platelets

Platelets (thrombocytes) are not typical cells but nonnucleated, granular ovoid, or spindle-shaped cell fragments. The normal life span of a platelet is approximately 10 days. Platelets are active in the clotting mechanism of the body. When platelets flow over a rough or damaged area in a vessel, they adhere to the area and release thromboplastin and clotting factors that start the blood-clotting process. They also secrete prostaglandins and serotonin, which cause the vessel to constrict, thereby decreasing the blood flow through the area. Prothrombin, thromboplastin, and calcium ions form thrombin which joins with fibrinogen to form fibrin. The fibrin strands seal the opening or area and a clot is formed (Figure 20-3).

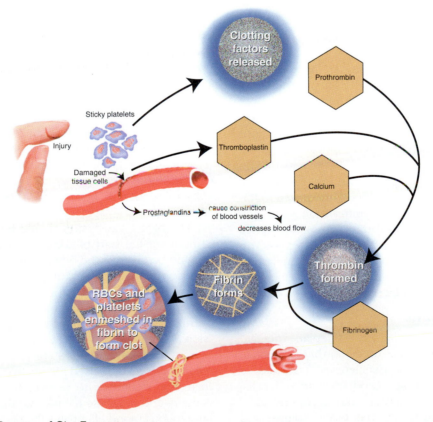

Figure 20-3 The Process of Clot Formation

Blood Types

On the surface of RBC membranes are genetically determined antigens called agglutinogens. The A and B antigens constitute the ABO blood group. If the A antigen is on the RBC membrane, the client has type A blood. If the B antigen is on the RBC membrane, the client has type B blood. If both an A and a B antigen are present, the client has type AB blood, and if no antigen is present, the client has type O blood.

Anti-A or anti-B antibodies are present in the serum of every person with type A and type B blood. Type A blood has anti-B antibodies in the serum, and type B blood has anti-A antibodies. If a person with type A blood receives type B blood during a transfusion, the anti-B antibodies will attack the infused RBCs and hemolyze (destroy) them. The hemoglobin released when these cells are hemolyzed can lead to kidney damage.

A person with AB blood does not have anti-A or anti-B antibodies. People with AB blood are theoretically universal recipients because they can receive blood from all blood types. Type O blood does not have any antigens that the antibodies can attack. Persons with type O blood can theoretically give blood to persons having any type of blood. Persons with type O blood are called universal donors. The terms *universal recipient* and *universal donor* are only theoretical because during blood transfusions, blood incompatibilities can occur because of other types of antigens.

There are fourteen different blood groups and over 100 different antigens. The different blood groups vary in number with different ethnic groups.

Rh Factor

Another factor to consider during blood transfusions is the Rh factor. Persons who have Rh antigens (the D antigen) are Rh positive. Those who do not have Rh antigens on their RBC membranes are Rh negative. Approximately 85% of Caucasian people have Rh-positive blood and 15% have Rh-negative blood. The African-American population has 90% and 10% respectively (Lewis, Heitkemper, & Dirksen, 2000).

If a person with Rh-negative blood is exposed to Rh-positive blood during a blood transfusion or during childbirth, anti-Rh antibodies form in the blood serum. When a person with Rh-negative blood is exposed a second time to Rh-positive blood, the anti-Rh antibodies will react with the Rh-positive blood and cause hemolysis of the infused blood and a severe blood reaction.

Blood Transfusions

Blood transfusions are given to replace needed blood components because of hemorrhage, anemia, clotting disorders, or blood deficiencies. Transfusable blood products are whole blood, packed red cells, platelets, fresh frozen plasma, and cryoprecipitate. Whole blood is given to increase blood volume and the various blood components. Packed red cells are given for anemia. Platelets assist in controlling bleeding. Fresh frozen plasma is administered for clotting disorders. Cryoprecipitate corrects fibrinogen deficiencies.

Before blood products are given, the lab does a type and crossmatch to check compatibility between the donor blood type and Rh factor and the client's blood type and Rh factor. The lab also checks all blood products for HIV and hepatitis B and C viruses. Blood must be handled gently so as not to damage the cells. Administration of the blood should begin within 30 minutes of obtaining it from the laboratory refrigerator.

The nurse takes baseline vital signs—temperature, pulse, and blood pressure—before administering the blood product. Once the transfusion is started, temperature and pulse are measured after 15 minutes, 30 minutes, and then hourly; blood pressure is measured hourly during the transfusion. Blood is generally administered through a peripheral vein using an 18- or 19-gauge cannula. A large cannula is used so the blood cells do not break when passing through the cannula.

Before the transfusion, two nurses check the compatibility of the blood product and the client's blood. The first 50 cc is given within 5 to 10 minutes. The client is observed closely for a hemolytic blood reaction during this time.

There are three types of blood reactions: hemolytic, febrile, and allergic. Symptoms of a hemolytic reaction include chest pain, dyspnea, flushing, oliguria, hypotension, and shock. It is usually a severe reaction occuring within 15 minutes. The transfusion should be stopped immediately and the physician notified. A client with a febrile reaction has a temperature above 101.4°F, often with severe shaking, sweating, and tachycardia. This is usually a mild reaction occuring within 30–90 minutes but may occur up to several hours after the transfusion. An allergic reaction includes symptoms of pruritus, urticaria, and possibly anaphylactic shock. This reaction may be mild or severe and usually occurs within 30 minutes, but it may occur up to several hours after the transfusion.

If a client experiences any symptoms of a reaction, the infusion must be stopped immediately and the physician notified. Institutional protocol should be followed.

The blood transfusion should be completed within 4 hours of the start of administration. No medications should be given at the blood administration site during infusion. The only solution given during a blood transfusion is 0.9% sodium chloride.

Autotransfusion If time and the client's condition permit, autotransfusion or autologous blood transfusion ("from self") blood as opposed to homologous ("from a donor") blood is collected and saved for the client. This may be used for elective surgeries. An alternative procedure is to recover the blood lost during surgery and transfuse it back into the client. The use of autologous blood eliminates the possibility of a transfusion reaction and prevents the transmission of disease.

CULTURAL CONSIDERATIONS

Jehovah's Witnesses and Blood

- Many Jehovah's Witnesses will agree to autologous blood transfusions.
- Some Jehovah's Witnesses will allow the use of certain blood volume expanders and will carry a card identifying the expanders to be used.

Lymphatic System

The lymphatic, or lymph, system is a separate vessel system. The two main functions of the lymph system are to transport excess fluid from the interstitial spaces to the circulatory system and to protect the body against infectious organisms.

Lymph Fluid and Vessels

Lymph fluid is a pale yellow fluid. Fluid and substances move from the plasma through the capillary walls and become interstitial fluid. As fluid accumulates in the interstitial space, pressure within the interstitial space increases. The interstitial fluid then diffuses through the lymphatic vessel wall into the lymph vessel. The flow of fluid is illustrated in Figure 20-4.

Semilunar valves in the lymphatic vessels assist the lymph system in returning the interstitial fluid, which is now called lymph, to the venous system. When the valves do not work properly or the vessels become ob-

structed, edema occurs. The pumping action or contractions of the skeletal muscles and the rhythmic action of the respiratory muscles assist in the movement of the lymph toward the subclavian veins. The right lymphatic duct drains lymph from the right side of the head, neck, thorax, and arm into the right subclavian vein. The lymph from the rest of the body drains into the left subclavian vein through the thoracic duct.

Lymph Nodes

Lymph nodes are scattered throughout the body along the lymph vessels (Figure 20-5) and contain dense patches of lymphocytes and macrophages. Lymphocytes act against such foreign particles as viruses and bacteria. Macrophages ingest and destroy foreign substances, damaged cells, and cellular debris. Lymph nodes can be superficial or deep. Those located superficially such as in the neck, axilla, and groin can be palpated, especially if they become infected and swollen. The tonsils in the pharynx and Peyer's patch in the mucosal lining of the ileum are located deeper within the body and cannot be palpated.

As lymph is collected from body tissues, cancer cells may enter the lymphatic system and escape into the circulation or to other body tissues, such as the lungs. Wherever the cancer cells collect, more cancer cells may be produced. In this way cancer can spread to other body parts. Lymph nodes are biopsied to check for the spread of cancer.

Lymph Organs

The spleen and thymus are lymph organs. The spleen removes old RBCs, platelets, and microorganisms from the blood. Approximately 350 mL of blood are stored in the spleen and approximately 200 mL can be pumped out within a minute into the body as needed (Thibodeau & Patton, 1999). During an infection, the spleen enlarges to produce and release monocytes and lymphocytes. Lymphocytes in the lymph tissue differentiate into T lymphocytes (T cells) and B lymphocytes (B cells).

In infancy and childhood, the thymus gland is large but decreases in size with age. In advanced age, it is replaced with fat and connective tissue. The thymus performs an important role in the special processing and proper functioning of the thymus-derived T lymphocytes (T cells). The T cells are actively involved in immunity.

ASSESSMENT

Information is based on client report, physical examination, and diagnostic tests.

Subjective Data

Biological and demographic data including age, sex, ethnic background, and race are important for

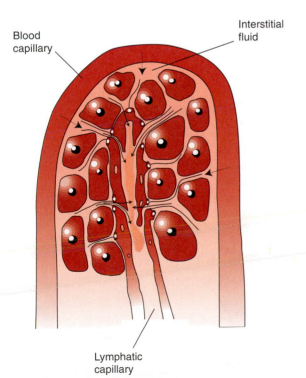

Blood capillary

Interstitial fluid

Lymphatic capillary

Figure 20-4 Flow of Fluid from the Blood into the Lymphatic System

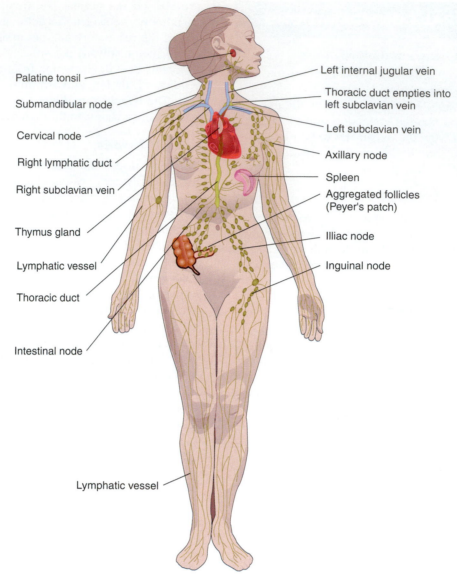

Palatine tonsil

Submandibular node

Cervical node

Right lymphatic duct

Right subclavian vein

Thymus gland

Lymphatic vessel

Thoracic duct

Intestinal node

Left internal jugular vein

Thoracic duct empties into left subclavian vein

Left subclavian vein

Axillary node

Spleen

Aggregated follicles (Peyer's patch)

Illiac node

Inguinal node

Lymphatic vessel

Figure 20-5 The Lymphatic System

many hematological problems. The nurse should inquire about the client's occupation and hobbies as there may be exposure to radiation or chemicals. Past military experience is also important, as some military personnel have been exposed to toxic chemicals. A medication history should be obtained from the client, including prescription and over-the-counter medications. Recent or recurring infections, night sweats, palpitations, bleeding problems, previous blood transfusions and any complications should be noted.

Neurological functioning is assessed by asking if the client has experienced any cognitive or mental difficulties or numbness and tingling of the extremities. A headache may be indicative of a low erythrocyte count or intracranial bleeding. Hearing or vision difficulties must also be noted.

The nurse should ask the client about past surgeries and any complications from surgeries; if the client has

had a duodenal, gastric, or ileal resection, the absorption of iron and vitamin B_{12} may be affected. Alcohol use may be important because alcohol may affect vitamin intake and is caustic to the GI tract. The client should be asked about the presence of blood in the stool or urine and any anorexia, nausea, vomiting, oral discomfort, or problems with taste perception. A history of dietary intake is helpful when reviewing the erythrocyte level. The nurse needs to inquire if the client has difficulty accomplishing ADLs because of decreased energy.

Objective Data

The assessment begins by obtaining the client's height, weight, and vital signs. An elevated temperature may indicate an infection. Recent weight gains or losses should be noted.

Laboratory tests are very important when assessing

the hematological and lymphatic systems. It is important to compare past laboratory tests and present laboratory results.

The lymph nodes in the neck, axillae, and groin are palpated; normal findings include small (0.5–1.0 cm) nodes that are freely movable, firm, and nontender. Tender nodes are indicative of inflammation. Hard, fixed nodes may be malignant.

Next, the skin and extremities are inspected for petechiae, bruises, lesions, and brittle nails. Urine and stool should be checked for blood. Dyspnea, an enlarged abdomen, or swollen joints should be documented.

COMMON DIAGNOSTIC TESTS

Commonly used diagnostic tests for clients with symptoms of blood and lymph system disorders are listed in Table 20–1. See Chapter 13, Diagnostic Tests, for explanations, normal values, and nursing responsibilities.

RED BLOOD CELL DISORDERS: ANEMIAS AND POLYCYTHEMIA

Red blood cell disorders discussed in this section are the anemias and polycythemia vera. The nursing process for anemias is presented after the discussion of sickle-cell anemia because the nursing diagnoses, goals, and interventions are similar for all anemias.

Anemia is a common hematopoietic disorder in which the client has a decreased number of RBCs and a low hemoglobin level. The causes for anemia are a decreased production of RBCs, an increased destruction of RBCs, or a loss of blood. The types of anemia discussed in this section are iron deficiency anemia, hypoplastic (aplastic) anemia, pernicious anemia, acquired hemolytic anemia, and sickle-cell anemia.

IRON DEFICIENCY ANEMIA

Iron deficiency anemia is the most common type of anemia and occurs when the body does not have enough iron to synthesize functional Hgb. The decrease in iron may be due to a decreased dietary intake, a decreased iron absorption from the gastrointestinal tract, chronic intestinal or uterine blood loss, or an increased bodily need for iron such as during growth periods or pregnancy. Iron deficiency anemia is more frequently found in premature or low-birthweight infants, adolescent girls, alcoholics, and the elderly. The symptoms are fatigue, loss of appetite, decreased ability to concentrate, and pallor. Clients with chronic anemia may have tachycardia, exertional dyspnea, hypotension,

Table 20–1 COMMON DIAGNOSTIC TESTS FOR BLOOD AND LYMPHATIC SYSTEM DISORDERS

Partial thromboplastin time (PTT)
Activated partial thromboplastin time (APTT)
Bleeding time
Blood culture and sensitivity
Coombs' test (direct antiglobulin test)
D dimer test
(Fragment D-dimer, Fibrin degradation fragment)
Erythrocyte sedimentation rate (sed rate, ESR)
Folic acid (Folate level)
Hematocrit (Hct)
Hemoglobin (Hgb)
Hemoglobin electrophoresis
Platelet count
Prothrombin time (PT, Protime)
Red blood cells (RBCs)
Schilling test
Sickledex (Sickle cell test)
Total iron binding capacity (TIBC)
White blood cells (WBCs)
Differential count (WBCs)
Granulocytes
   Basophils
   Eosinophils
   Neutrophils
   Bands
Agranulocytes
   Lymphocytes
   Monocytes
Bone marrow aspiration
Gastric analysis, tube and tubeless test
Radiologic lymphangiogram

dysphagia, stomatitis, glossitis, and brittle nails. Diagnostic tests of a client with iron deficiency anemia would reveal decreased RBCs, a low Hgb level, a low Hct, a low serum iron, and a high total iron binding capacity (TIBC).

Medical–Surgical Management

Pharmacological

Oral iron preparations are ferrous gluconate (Fergon), ferrous fumarate (Feostat), and ferrous sulfate (Feosol). These preparations are not given with milk because milk interferes with iron absorption. The administration of iron with meals, with orange juice, or vitamin C–rich drinks increases iron absorption. Iron dextran (Infed), an intramuscular iron preparation, is given by Z-track technique.

Diet

The treatment for iron deficiency anemia is iron supplements and a diet high in iron. Foods rich in iron are red meats, fish, raisins, apricots, dried fruits, dark green vegetables, dried beans, eggs, and iron-enriched whole grain breads. An increase of vitamin C in the diet assists in the absorption of iron. If the client has a loss of appetite, small frequent snacks may be tolerated better than three large meals.

Activity

Daily activities should be spaced to provide rest periods between times of exercise.

HYPOPLASTIC [APLASTIC] ANEMIA

The bone marrow decreases or stops functioning in a client with aplastic anemia. The client with aplastic anemia has pancytopenia, a drop in the number of red blood cells, white blood cells, and platelets. It develops without a known cause and is thought to be congenital. Secondary aplastic anemia is caused by exposure to viruses, chemicals (benzene or airplane glue), radiation, or medications. Some medications that cause aplastic anemia are chloramphenicol (Chloromycetin), mephenytoin (Mesantoin), trimethadione (Tridione), mechlorethamine or nitrogen mustard (Mustargen), methotrexate (Folex PFS), 6-mercaptopurine or 6-MP (Purinethol), and phenylbutazone (Butazolidin). Symptoms include fatigue, weakness, tachycardia, dyspnea, susceptibility to infection, petechiae, gingival bleeding, and epistaxis. Clients with aplastic anemia are extremely ill. Diagnosis is confirmed by a bone marrow aspiration.

Medical–Surgical Management

Medical

The cause of aplastic anemia is removed if possible. Another treatment is antithymocyte globulin or ATG (Atgam) immunosuppressive therapy, which is given to suppress the reaction causing the aplastic anemia and to allow the client's bone marrow to recover. ATG is given daily through a central venous catheter for 7 to 10 days. A client who has a good response to ATG will improve in 3 to 6 months. The sooner the diagnosis is made and ATG started, the better the prognosis. Transfusions of packed red cells and platelets may be given.

Surgical

Bone marrow transplants are done if the client's bone marrow fails to start functioning. Cyclosporine (Sandimmune), an immunosuppressant, is given for a bone marrow transplant to decrease the graft rejection. The best response occurs in a young client who has

PROFESSIONAL TIP

Bone Marrow–Depressing Medication
When a client is taking medications that cause bone marrow depression. Monitor the blood cell count closely.

not previously had a transfusion because transfusions increase bone marrow graft rejection. Bone marrow transplants from a human leukocyte antigen- (HLA-) matched sibling donor is the treatment of choice for clients less than 45 years of age. The treatment of choice for an older adult or a client who does not have a HLA-matched sibling donor is immunosuppression with ATG or cyclosporine. (Bone marrow transplants are discussed in the section on acute myelocytic leukemia.)

Pharmacological

Infections are treated with antibiotics. Steroids and androgens are also sometimes used to stimulate the bone marrow.

PERNICIOUS ANEMIA

The parietal cells of the gastric mucosa secrete a protein intrinsic factor that is essential for the proper absorption of vitamin B_{12}. Pernicious anemia is an autoimmune disease in which the parietal cells are destroyed and the gastric mucosa atrophies. Without the secretion of the intrinsic factor, vitamin B_{12} cannot be absorbed in the distal portion of the ileum.

The onset of the disease occurs between 50 and 60 years of age. Pernicious anemia occurs most frequently in those of Northern European and African American descent. African American women are especially affected with the disease and often severely. Pernicious anemia can occur in clients who have had a gastrectomy with the section of the stomach removed that secretes the intrinsic factor. A gastric analysis and Schilling test are confirming diagnostic tests.

Pernicious anemia has an insidious onset, and it may take several months for the symptoms to be fully manifested. Symptoms include extreme weakness, a sore tongue, numbness and tingling of the extremities, edema of the legs, ataxia, dizziness, dyspnea, headache, fever, blurred vision, tinnitus, jaundice with pallor, poor memory, irritability, and loss of bladder and bowel control. The client may have decreased sensitivity to heat and pain because of neurological involvement. Clients with pernicious anemia are highly susceptible to gastric carcinoma and should be monitored closely for symptoms.

PROFESSIONAL TIP

Vitamin B$_{12}$ Deficiency

Strict vegetarians are at risk for vitamin B$_{12}$ deficiency. A dietary supplement of Vitaming B$_{12}$ is the treatment.

Medical–Surgical Management

Pharmacological

Topical anesthetics are given to relieve oral discomfort during the acute phase of the disease. Vitamin B$_{12}$, cyanocobalamin, (Rubramin PC) or hydroxocabalamin crystalline (Hydro Cysti$_{12}$) is given IM daily for 2 weeks and then weekly until the Hct returns to a normal level. Then cyanocobalamin is usually administered monthly for the rest of the client's life. The frequency of administration will depend on the client's symptoms and response to the medication. Oral administration of vitamin B$_{12}$ is not effective because vitamin B$_{12}$ cannot be absorbed without the intrinsic factor. Folic acid or folate (Folvite) is prescribed. The client is encouraged to increase folic acid in the diet by eating green leafy vegetables, meat, fish, legumes, and whole grains. Iron is usually not prescribed because once the condition is corrected with regular administration of cyanocobalamin, erythrocytes are produced and the Hgb and Hct return to normal.

ACQUIRED HEMOLYTIC ANEMIA

In hemolytic anemias, **hemolysis**, or destruction of RBCs, occurs and iron and hemoglobin are released. Several causes for acquired hemolytic anemia are an autoimmune reaction, radiation, blood transfusion, chemicals, arsenic, lead, or medications. Sulfisoxazole (Gantrisin), penicillin, and methyldopa (Aldomet) are medications that can cause hemolysis. A substance produced by the bacterium *Clostridium perfringens* can also cause hemolysis. Symptoms may go unnoticed, or there may be a severe reaction. Symptoms are mild fatigue and pallor. More severe symptoms include jaundice, palpitations, hypotension, dyspnea, and back and joint pain. Diagnostic tests would reveal a low Hgb and Hct and an elevated LDH. LDH is an enzyme in the heart, liver, kidneys, skeletal muscle, brain, red blood cells, and lungs. As these tissues are damaged, LDH is released into the bloodstream, causing an elevated LDH.

Medical–Surgical Management

Medical

Treatment is aimed at removing the cause of the hemolytic anemia, if possible. The client may be given blood transfusions or **erythrocytapheresis** (a procedure that removes abnormal RBCs and replaces them with healthy RBCs).

Surgical

The function of the spleen is to destroy RBCs. In severe cases of hemolytic anemia, a splenectomy may be done in an attempt to stop the destruction of RBCs.

Pharmacological

Corticosteroids are administered to decrease the autoimmune response. Folic acid may also be given to increase the production of RBCs.

SICKLE CELL ANEMIA (INHERITED HEMOLYTIC ANEMIA)

Sickle cell anemia is also known as inherited hemolytic anemia or sickle cell disease. This genetic disorder has abnormal hemoglobin S rather than hemoglobin A in the RBCs. Sickle cell anemia is caused by a recessive gene or genes that are passed through the generations (Figure 20-6). The client with one s gene has sickle cell trait (Hb sA) and is asymptomatic but is a carrier of the disease. The client with sickle cell anemia has two s genes (Hb ss) and manifests symptoms.

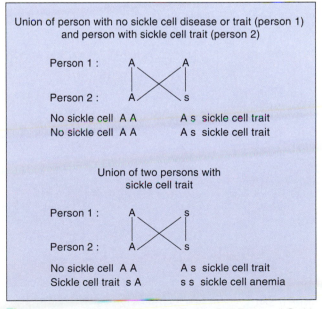

Figure 20-6 Inheritance of the Sickle Cell Trait and Sickle Cell Anemia

The condition occurs most frequently in African Americans, with an estimated 1 of 12 persons being sickle cell carriers (Phipps, Cassmeyer, Sands, and Lehman, 1999). It also occurs in persons from Asia Minor, India, and the Mediterranean and Caribbean areas.

Sickle cell tests are done on infants to diagnose sickle cell trait or disease. A screening test to detect the presence of Hb S is Sickledex or sickle cell test. If Hb S is present, a hemoglobin electrophoresis is done to distinguish between sickle cell trait and sickle cell disease. If the hemoglobin electrophoresis test is negative, the client has the sickle cell trait and not sickle cell disease.

Situations that precipitate sickle cell crisis are dehydration, fatigue, infection, emotional stress, exposure to cold, anesthesia, blood loss, and alcohol consumption. In these situations that compromise oxygenation, the more fragile RBCs with Hb S become **sickled** (crescent-shaped and elongated) and obstruct capillaries and larger vessels (Figure 20-7). Sickled cells cause circulatory problems by obstructing vessels and rupturing. The area normally supplied by these obstructed blood vessels becomes infarcted and ischemic. The rupturing of sickled RBCs causes chronic anemia, causing the heart to enlarge in an attempt to circulate more blood for adequate oxygenation of body tissues. Other symptoms include fatigue, jaundice, chronic leg ulcers, tachypnea, dyspnea, and arrhythmias. Periodically, the client experiences a sickle cell crisis with symptoms of fever, severe pain, and loss of blood supply to various organs because of obstructed vessels. Areas most frequently affected are the joints, bone, brain, lungs, liver, kidneys, and penis. Joints become

CLIENT TEACHING

Sickle Cell Anemia
- Encourage client to avoid high altitudes and nonpressurized airplanes.
- It is important for the client to have adequate fluid intake as dehydration causes a sickle cell crisis.
- All infections should be promptly treated.
- Client should avoid tight-fitting, restrictive clothing, and strenuous exercise, smoking, and cold temperatures.
- Encourage client to receive yearly flu vaccine and pneumococcal vaccine.

painful, swollen, and immobile. The client may experience cerebrovascular accidents, renal failure, pulmonary infarction, shock, and priapism (a continuous, painful erection).

It is important for the nurse to assess extremity circulation frequently by doing capillary refill, peripheral pulses, and temperature. Application of warm compresses to painful areas relieves pain. Encourage the client to avoid restrictive clothing and anything that may restrict circulation. It is important for the clients to avoid high altitudes and have adequate fluid intake.

Medical–Surgical Management

Medical

Medical management of sickle cell disease is still evolving in administration of medications and treatments. Infections are treated promptly with antibiotics. Large amounts of oral and intravenous fluids (3–5 L/day) are given to remove the by-products of broken RBCs. Skin grafting may be necessary for chronic leg ulcers.

Genetic counseling is recommended for clients with sickle cell trait and sickle cell anemia. There may be more openness to counseling if the counselor is from the same community as the client.

Pharmacological

Folic acid or folate (Folvite) is administered daily to assist in the production of RBCs. Cetiedil citrate has an antisickling effect by changing the RBC membrane. Pentoxifylline (Trental) reduces blood viscosity, increases RBC flexibility, and lengthens the time between sickle cell crises. Blood transfusions may be given during a crisis.

Patient-controlled analgesia (PCA) with morphine is effective during a crisis. The client is progressed from narcotics to nonnarcotic analgesics as indicated.

Normal red blood cell   Sickle-shaped red blood cell

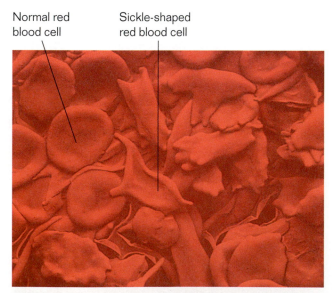

Figure 20-7 Blood cells magnified through a scanning electron microscope show normal and sickle-shaped red blood cells. *(Courtesy of Philips Electronic Instruments Company.)*

▶ NURSING PROCESS

▶ Assessment

▶ Subjective Data

A history of the client's medical problems is obtained, including a history of familial hematopoietic illnesses. Some anemias may be caused by drugs and environmental conditions, so gathering information about medications taken and about environmental situations at work and in recreational settings is important. The client should be asked about fatigue, dyspnea with exertion, palpitations, dizziness, pain, petechiae, tingling and numbness in the extremities, blurred vision, and oral discomfort.

▶ Objective Data

The client's weight and vital signs; apical pulse and peripheral pulses; breath sounds; sensation and movement in the extremities; abdominal tenderness; and edema, pallor, and signs of bruising or jaundice must all be assessed. A thorough assessment of the cardiac system is completed because severe anemia can cause cardiac enlargement and arrhythmias.

Nursing diagnoses for a client with decreased erythrocytes and hemoglobin may include the following:

Nursing Diagnoses	Planning/Goals	Nursing Interventions
▶ *Deficient Knowledge related to prescribed treatment regimen*	The client will relate the prescribed treatment regimen.	Teach the cause of the particular type of anemia and, if possible, ways to avoid the occurrence of that anemia in the future.
		For iron deficiency anemia, teach the importance of taking iron and increasing iron in the diet.
		Instruct clients with pernicious anemia to obtain a vitamin B_{12} injection at regularly scheduled times.
		Teach clients with hemolytic anemias the significance of following the prescribed regimens.
▶ *Activity intolerance related to imbalance between oxygen supply and demand.*	The client will increasingly tolerate activity.	Assist the client as needed with activities of daily living.
		Teach the client the importance of alternating periods of rest with activity.
▶ *Ineffective Tissue Perfusion (Peripheral) related to a decreased hemoglobin concentration in the blood.*	The client will have increased tissue perfusion.	Administer oxygen as needed to relieve symptoms of dyspnea.
		Monitor Hgb, Hct, RBCs, ABGs, and electrolytes.
		Monitor vital signs and mental alertness.
		Monitor for symptoms of obstructed vessels such as pain, leg ulcerations, abdominal tenderness, dyspnea, confusion, and blurred vision.
		Administer blood products as ordered.
		Monitor the client closely after blood transfusions for possible reactions such as chills, fever, dyspnea, pruritus, wheezing, and pain in the lumbar region.

Evaluation Each goal must be evaluated to determine how it has been met by the client.

SAMPLE NURSING CARE PLAN

THE CLIENT WITH SICKLE CELL ANEMIA

Reggie Thompson, a 19-year-old African American, was diagnosed with sickle cell anemia 5 years ago. Reggie works for a computer company and has been working 12-hour days to get a system installed. He has felt fatigued lately and decided to relax by playing golf on a warm Saturday morning. After the seventh hole, Reggie experienced dyspnea and tingling and numbness in his legs. After the next hole, he experienced severe pain in his ankles and knees. He was taken to the local medical center, where he was admitted. The physician ordered oxygen by nasal cannula, IV fluids, and a PCA pump with morphine sulfate.

continues

Nursing Diagnosis 1 *Acute Pain related to occlusion of small vessels by sickled cells as evidenced by severe pain in the knees and ankles*

PLANNING/GOALS	NURSING INTERVENTIONS	RATIONALE	EVALUATION
Reggie will state pain has been relieved as the analgesic becomes effective.	Assess pain type, location, and intensity.	Other vessels to the brain, heart, lungs, spleen, gallbladder, kidney, and penis may become occluded, causing pain.	The morphine in the PCA pump relieved Reggie's pain, and oral analgesics were ordered.
	Monitor analgesic administration by PCA pump.	Analgesic administration is monitored to assess relief from pain.	
	Support joints and lower extremities with pillows.	Support of joints and lower extremities relieves joint pain.	
	Keep bed linens off knees and ankles with a bed cradle.	Use of a bed cradle keeps linen from putting pressure on painful areas.	

Nursing Diagnosis 2 *Ineffective Tissue Perfusion (Cardiopulmonary and Peripheral) related to a decreased number of RBCs and decreased oxygenation as evidenced by dyspnea and tingling and numbness in his ankles and knees*

PLANNING/GOALS	NURSING INTERVENTIONS	RATIONALE	EVALUATION
Reggie will experience improved circulation in his extremities as RBCs increase in number.	Elevate the head of the bed and administer oxygen as needed to relieve symptoms of dyspnea.	Lungs can expand more fully if the head of the bed is elevated, and oxygen administration increases blood oxygen level.	Circulation in lower extremities has improved as manifested by prompt capillary refill and strong pedal and popliteal pulses. Extremities are warm to touch.
	Administer IV fluids as ordered.	Adequate hydration decreases the possibility of RBCs' sickling.	
	Encourage Reggie to drink eight to ten glasses of water daily.	Dehydration causes RBCs to sickle.	
	Monitor for symptoms of obstructed vessels such as pain, leg ulcerations, abdominal tenderness, dyspnea, confusion, and blurred vision.	Since RBCs are sickling, vessels supplying blood to other vital organs can become obstructed.	

continues

| | Administer blood products as ordered. | Administration of blood products increases the number of normal RBCs, which improves the blood oxygen concentration. | |
| | Closely monitor for possible blood transfusion reactions such as chills, fever, dyspnea, pruritus, wheezing, and pain in the lumbar region. | Administration of blood products may cause adverse reactions. | |

Nursing Diagnosis 3 *Activity intolerance related to imbalance between oxygen supply and demand, as evidenced by weakness, fatigue, dyspnea, tingling, and numbness*

PLANNING/GOALS	NURSING INTERVENTIONS	RATIONALE	EVALUATION
Reggie will tolerate some activity.	Assist Reggie as needed with activities of daily living.	Assistance with daily activities would conserve energy resources.	Reggie takes periods of rest after each period of activity. He acknowledges that he had been working too hard and not getting enough rest before hospitalization.
	Teach Reggie the importance of alternating periods of rest with activity.	Conservation of energy is important. Impaired circulation to the brain may cause dizziness when ambulating.	

Nursing Diagnosis 4 *Deficient Knowledge related to prescribed treatment regimen as evidenced by a lack of rest and working long hours*

PLANNING/GOALS	NURSING INTERVENTIONS	RATIONALE	EVALUATION
Reggie will relate the prescribed treatment regimen before discharge.	Teach Reggie the pathophysiology related to sickle cell disease.	An understanding of the disease process improves compliance with the medical regimen.	Reggie states his RBCs have Hgb S rather than Hgb A, and a lack of oxygen causes his RBCs to sickle. Situations that may cause sickling are fatigue, lack of oral fluids, emotional and physical stress, infection, exposure to cold and anesthesia. He knows the purpose and side effects of each of his medications and the times he is to take them. Reggie states he is to avoid high altitudes.
	Encourage Reggie to take medications as ordered.	Medications will improve circulation and postpone sickle cell crisis situations.	
	Explain the importance of avoiding stressful situations and the symptoms of infection.	Clients with sickle cell disease should avoid situations that increase oxygen demands. Lack of oxygen can precipitate a sickle cell crisis.	
	Explain the importance of adequate rest on a routine basis.	Allows adequate oxygenation and reduces stress.	Reggie states that he will try to routinely have enough rest.

POLYCYTHEMIA

Polycythemia is a disease in which there is an increased production of red blood cells. Usually the numbers of white blood cells and platelets are also increased. The increased production of cells increases the blood volume and viscosity and decreases the ability of the blood to circulate freely. There are two types of polycythemia: polycythemia vera (primary polycythemia) and secondary polycythemia. Polycythemia vera occurs most frequently in the middle-aged and in Jewish men. The etiology of the disease is unknown. Secondary polycythemia results from long-term hypoxia, as from chronic obstructive pulmonary disease, chronic heart failure, smoking, or living in a high altitude. It is a compensatory mechanism as the body makes more red blood cells as a response to the low oxygenation caused by the previously mentioned situations.

Symptoms of the two types are the same. As the blood viscosity and volume increase the client experiences headaches, epistaxis, dizziness, tinnitus, blurred vision, fatigue, weakness, pruritus, exertional dyspnea, angina, and increased blood pressure and pulse. The client's complexion becomes ruddy (reddish), and the lips become reddish purple. The client may have petechiae and bruise easily because of a platelet dysfunction. The client is susceptible to thrombi formation because of the increased viscosity of the blood. The increased destruction of RBCs causes **hyperuricemia** (increased uric acid blood level). The RBC cell count is over 6 million, Hgb is over 18 mg/dL, and the Hct is over 55% (Williams & Hopper, 1999).

Medical–Surgical Management

Medical

The treatment for polycythemia is **phlebotomy**, which is the removal of blood from a vein. Generally 350 mL to 500 mL of blood is withdrawn every other day until the Hct level is 40% to 50%. Radioactive phosphorus (^{32}P) and radiation therapy may be used to decrease the production of blood cells in the bone marrow.

Complications that can occur from the disease process are cerebral vascular accident, thrombosis, myocardial infarction, and hemorrhage.

Pharmacological

Antineoplastic drugs such as busulfan (Myleran), chlorambucil (Leukeran), cyclophosphamide (Cytoxan), and mechlorethamine or nitrogen mustard (Mustargen) are also used to decrease bone marrow production. Allopurinol (Zyloprim) is given to decrease the

CLIENT TEACHING

Polycythemia
- Drink at least 3 L of water daily.
- Elevate feet when resting.
- Avoid tight or restrictive clothing.
- Wear support hose.
- Take medications as ordered.
- Report chest pain, joint pain, fever, or activity intolerance to physician.
- Keep appointments for laboratory testing and physician checks.

production of uric acid. Pruritus can be relieved with the administration of antihistamines.

Diet

The client is placed on a diet that has increased calories and protein. A diet low in sodium decreases fluid volume. Iron-containing foods should be avoided.

Activity

Activities of daily living may need to be adjusted so the client can have regular periods of rest to relieve fatigue.

▶ NURSING PROCESS

▶ Assessment

▶ Subjective Data

The client should be asked about the history of symptoms, especially difficulty breathing, chest pain, dizziness, headache, pruritus, tinnitis, blurred vision, and sensitivity to hot and cold. Nutritional status of the client must be assessed as there may be an inadequate dietary intake due to GI symptoms of fullness and dyspepsia.

▶ Objective Data

The nurse observes the skin for bruises and changes in skin color. The cardiovascular system can be assessed by checking for distention of neck vessels, listening to the apical pulse, taking radial and pedal pulses, and checking for Homans' sign and edema. The respiratory system can be assessed by observing for epistaxis and dyspnea and listening to the breath sounds. The central nervous system is checked through pupil response and presence of numbness or tingling.

Nursing diagnoses for a client with polycythemia may include the following:

Nursing Diagnoses	Planning/Goals	Nursing Interventions
▶ *Deficient Knowledge related to disease process and treatment*	The client will relate disease process and treatment.	Explain the cause of the disease, possible symptoms, side effects of medications, and possible future complications to report. Teach client to report headache, chest pain, dyspnea, or redness, swelling, or tenderness in the arms or legs to the physician or nurse practitioner immediately.
▶ *Ineffective Tissue Perfusion (Peripheral) related to decreased blood circulation*	The client will have increased circulation.	Administer oxygen as needed for dyspnea. Check vital signs frequently. Assess Homans' sign and signs of thrombi formation. Explain process of phlebotomy.
▶ *Risk for Injury related to dizziness*	The client will relate measures to avoid injury.	Encourage the client to change positions slowly to prevent dizziness. Encourage activities of daily living when the client is feeling well. Teach client to avoid activities in which bruising or trauma may occur.

Evaluation Each goal must be evaluated to determine how it has been met by the client.

WHITE BLOOD CELL DISORDERS

White blood cell disorders include leukemia and agranulocytosis.

LEUKEMIA

Leukemia is a malignancy of blood-forming tissues in which the bone marrow produces increased numbers of immature white blood cells that are incapable of protecting the body from infections. The increased number of WBCs crowds out the other cells in the bone marrow, causing a decreased production of RBCs and platelets. Anemia and bleeding result from the decreased number of RBCs and platelets,

Leukemia has two classifications: acute and chronic. The acute leukemias are subclassified into acute myelocytic leukemia (AML) and acute lymphocytic leukemia (ALL). Chronic leukemias are subclassified into chronic myelocytic leukemia (CML) and chronic lymphocytic leukemia (CLL).

Because of the increased production of immature WBCs, clients with acute leukemia generally are fighting persistent infections and have a fever and chills. The decreased number of RBCs causes symptoms of anemia such as fatigue, pallor, malaise, tachycardia, and tachypnea. The decreased platelet production causes bleeding tendencies, and the client will experience petechiae, bruising, epistaxis, melena, gingival bleeding, and increased menstrual bleeding. The client

may also experience weight loss, night sweats, and swollen lymph nodes. As the malignant cells invade the central nervous system, the client will experience headaches and visual disturbances. Some clients experience bone pain because the rapid production of WBCs causes cells to become crowded in the bone marrow. Refer to Table 20–2 to see the relationship of leukemia symptoms to laboratory results.

Table 20–2 RELATIONSHIP OF LABORATORY TESTS TO LEUKEMIA SYMPTOMS

LAB RESULT	OVERALL SYMPTOM	SYMPTOM MANIFESTATION
Immature WBCs	Persistent infections	Fever Chills
Decreased RBCs	Anemia	Fatigue Pallor Malaise Tachycardia Tachypnea
Decreased platelets	Bleeding	Petechiae Bruising Epistaxis Melena Gingival bleeding Increased menstrual bleeding

ACUTE LEUKEMIA

Acute leukemias have a rapid onset and must be treated quickly for a good prognosis. ALL usually occurs in children between the ages of 2 and 6 and has a more rapid onset than AML. Left untreated, clients with ALL have a **median survival time** (average length of life) of 4 to 6 months. Approximately 90% of clients have complete remissions with present chemotherapy (Phipps et al., 1999).

AML occurs most frequently in adolescence and after 55 years of age (Phipps et al., 1999). The median survival time for clients with untreated AML is approximately 2 to 3 months (Phipps et al., 1995). With chemotherapy, complete remission occurs in approximately 50% to 75% of AML clients, with a median survival time of 2 to 3 years (Phipps et al., 1999).

Medical–Surgical Management

Medical

Diagnosis of acute leukemia is confirmed with a CBC and a bone marrow biopsy. A lumbar puncture determines the presence of malignant cells in the central nervous system. An x-ray, MRI, or CT scan of the chest and skeleton determine the presence of infection and bone marrow tissue involvement.

Surgical

Bone marrow transplants are used with relapsed ALL clients and AML clients. High doses of chemotherapy and radiation therapy are given to the client to destroy the bone marrow. Leukemic white blood cells and healthy bone marrow cells are both destroyed, placing the client at a high risk for infection and death. Identical human leukocyte antigen (HLA) bone marrow from a sibling, the client, or an antigen-matched donor is given intravenously in a manner similar to a blood transfusion. The transfused bone marrow finds its way to the client's bone marrow and starts producing WBCs, RBCs, and platelets. The bone marrow is matched in a process very similar to the process of crossmatching blood. If the client's own bone marrow is used, it is removed from the client, treated with chemotherapy, and then reinfused into the client.

Pharmacological

Initial doses of chemotherapy are called **induction doses**. Small doses of chemotherapy given every 3 to 4 weeks to maintain remission are called **maintenance therapy**. Induction doses of chemotherapy for ALL consists of vincristine (Oncovin) and prednisone (Deltasone). Maintenance therapy consists of giving 6-mercaptopurine or 6-MP (Purinethol) and methotrexate or amethopterin (Methotrexate). Usually vincristine (Oncovin) and prednisone (Deltasone) are given periodically with the maintenance therapy.

Leukemic cells can lie dormant in the brain and

Table 20–3 CHEMOTHERAPEUTIC AGENTS TO TREAT LEUKEMIA

LEUKEMIA	CHEMOTHERAPEUTIC AGENTS
Acute lymphocytic leukemia (ALL)	vincristine (Oncovin)
	prednisone (Deltasone)
	6-mercaptopurine or 6-MP (Purinethol)
	methotrexate (Methotrexate)
Acute myelocytic leukemia (AML)	daunorubicin HCl (Cerubidine)
	cytarabine or ara-C (Cytosar-U)
	6-thioguanine (Thioguanine)
	doxorubicin HCl (Adriamycin)
Chronic myelocytic leukemia (CLL)	chlorambucil (Leukeran)
	COP (Cytoxan, Oncovin, and prednisone)
Chronic lymphocytic leukemia (CML)	busulfan (Myleran)
	hydroxyurea (Hydrea)
	DAT (daunorubicin, ara-C, thioguanine)

spinal area because the chemotherapeutic drugs are unable to pass through the blood-brain barrier. Intrathecal (within the spinal canal) administration of methotrexate has decreased recurrences of ALL. Methotrexate is given by a lumbar puncture into the cerebrospinal fluid or through a subcutaneous cerebrospinal reservoir. Sometimes radiation therapy is also used on the brain and spinal area.

AML is treated with chemotherapeutic agents, blood products, and antibiotics. Refer to Table 20–3 for a review of chemotherapeutic agents used in treating acute leukemia.

Diet

Extremely hot or cold foods and drinks should be avoided. A bland, high-protein, high-carbohydrate diet is usually ordered. Drinking alcohol should be avoided.

Activity

Clients should alternate periods of rest with activity. They should keep frequently used items nearby to conserve energy.

CHRONIC LEUKEMIA

Chronic leukemia generally occurs in adults with a gradual increase in the white cell count over months or years. The prognosis depends on the severity of the disease at the time of diagnosis. Clients with CLL have a median survival time of 4½ to 5½ years (Phipps et al., 1999).

CLL clients have increased abnormal B lymphocytes, with a WBC count between 20,000 and 100,000

(Phipps et al., 1999). CLL develops with advanced age and has a higher incident rate in men than in women (Phipps et al., 1999).

CML is characterized by the Philadelphia chromosome, indicating a possible genetic link. Clients with CML have a poor prognosis with a median survival rate of 5 years (Phipps et al., 1999). The WBC count ranges from 15,000 to 500,000 (Phipps et al., 1999). Most clients feel good and maintain a relatively normal life until later in the disease process when the chronic recessed phase changes into an intensified stage that resembles an acute phase of leukemia. This acute phase is called a **blastic phase** in which there is an increased production of WBCs. Approximately 50% to 60% of CML cases develop a later blastic phase (Phipps et al., 1999). When this occurs, the general condition spirals downhill and the client soon dies. The most common cause of death in the leukemic client is viral and fungal pneumonia.

Medical–Surgical Management

Medical

Diagnosis of chronic leukemia is confirmed with a CBC and a bone marrow biopsy.

Surgical

In the CML chronic phase, the HLA-identical allogenic bone marrow is given, and the client's own treated bone marrow is given in the blastic phase.

Pharmacological

Refer to Table 20–3 for a review of chemotherapeutic agents used in treating CLL and CML. Chemotherapy does not extend the length of life but seems to give a better quality of life by prolonging the chronic phase. In a recent clinical trial, interferon increased the survival time to 61 months as opposed to 41 months (Campbell, 1995).

Diet

The client is on a diet high in protein, carbohydrates, and vitamins. A bland, nonirritating diet prevents oral mucosal irritation. Alcohol should be avoided.

Activity

The decreased RBC level causes the client to have symptoms of anemia that include weakness and increased respirations. It is important for the client to learn methods to conserve energy, such as placing frequently used items nearby.

▶ NURSING PROCESS

▶ Assessment

▶ Subjective Data

A thorough history of the symptoms the client has experienced is needed. The nurse should ask the client or family about chromosomal abnormalities, exposure to chemicals, viral infections, and previous chemotherapy or radiation therapy. The client should describe the location, type, and duration of pain, especially in bones or joints. Symptoms of infection such as the presence of a cough or pain or burning on urination should be noted. A history of bleeding such as epistaxis, gingival bleeding, melena, or hematuria should be documented. Fatigue, malaise, and irritability are often described.

▶ Objective Data

Signs of infection, bleeding, and chemotherapy complications must be noted. Common sites for infection include the mouth, pharynx, lungs, skin, bladder, and perianal area. During chemotherapy the reduced white cell count may stop the formation of pus, so infection may manifest as redness, swelling, and pain.

Assessment for bleeding includes monitoring the platelet count as bleeding occurs easily if the platelet count falls below 50,000. Clients can bleed from any orifice, so it is important for the nurse to inspect any discharge from the body. Occult blood may be present in the urine and stool.

Chemotherapy complications are nausea, vomiting, and stomatitis. Alopecia occurs 1 to 2 weeks after treatments are initiated.

Nursing diagnoses for a client with leukemia may include the following:

Nursing Diagnoses	Planning/Goals	Nursing Interventions
▶ *Deficient Knowledge related to disease process and treatment.*	The client will relate treatment methods and possible complications of chemotherapy.	Teach the client to observe for signs of infection and bleeding. Review side effects of chemotherapy and radiation with the client, family members, and significant others. Explain bone marrow transplant methods.

continues

Nursing Diagnoses	Planning/Goals	Nursing Interventions
▶ *Risk for Infection related to increased production of immature white blood cells*	The client will describe ways to prevent infection.	Follow good handwashing techniques.
		Teach proper handwashing to the family and friends who come into contact with the leukemic client.
		Use antimicrobial soaps for the client's daily bath.
		Provide frequent oral care with a soft toothbrush and nonirritating mouthwash to prevent open sores and stomatitis.
		Wash the perianal area after each bowel movement to decrease bacterial contamination and prevent rectal fissures.
		Avoid taking a rectal temperature and giving suppositories.
		Monitor the temperature every 4 hours for signs of infection.
		Report any temperature over 100°F to the physician.
		Administer antibiotics and antifungals as ordered.
		Closely monitor respiration rate and breath sounds as the client is prone to respiratory infections.
▶ *Risk for Injury related to decreased production of platelets*	The client will identify ways to avoid injury and prevent bleeding.	Frequently observe the client for signs of bleeding such as epistaxis, gingival bleeding, petechiae, ecchymoses, hematemesis, enlarged abdomen, hematuria, melena, and confusion, which can occur from intracranial hemorrhage.
		Administer stool softeners frequently to prevent anal irritation from hard stools.
		Use cotton swabs instead of a toothbrush for oral care.
		Encourage the client to use an electric razor.
		Avoid giving injections as much as possible.
		If a catheter is needed, lubricate it well to avoid trauma to the mucosal lining of the urethra.
▶ *Imbalanced Nutrition: Less than body requirements related to effects of disease process and chemotherapy on gastrointestinal tract*	The client will choose nonirritating, high-protein, high-carbohydrate meals and snacks.	Administer antiemetics as ordered to relieve nausea and vomiting.
		Suggest that the client may tolerate small frequent feedings better than three large meals.
		Provide the client with a high-protein, high-carbohydrate diet to prevent infection and provide needed energy.
		Administer vitamin supplements as ordered.
		Teach the client to avoid raw fruits and vegetables as these foods may contain more bacteria than cooked foods.
▶ *Ineffective Coping related to uncertainty about treatment of disease and prognosis*	The client will identify ways to cope with concerns about disease process.	Inform the client of the possibility of alopecia from therapy treatments.
		Encourage the client to voice concerns and fears related to having leukemia.
		Teach the client, family members, and significant others to monitor and report signs of infection and bleeding.
		Refer to support groups, social workers, and clergy as needed.

Evaluation Each goal must be evaluated to determine how it has been met by the client.

AGRANULOCYTOSIS

A severely reduced number of granulocytes (basophils, eosinophils, and neutrophils) is called **agranulocytosis**. The primary cause is an adverse reaction to medication or medication toxicity, especially with administration of phenylbutazone (Butazolidin), chloramphenical (Chloromycetin), penicillin derivatives, cephalosporins, phenytoin (Dilantin), antihistamines, vincristine (Oncovin), propythiouracil, diuretics, chlorpromazine hydrochloride (Thorazine), fluphenazene (Prolixin), promazene hydrochloride (Sparine), and sulfonamides and its derivatives. Other causes of agranulocytosis are neoplastic disease, chemotherapy, radiation therapy, and bacterial and viral infection. The causative agent suppresses the bone marrow, reducing the production of leukocytes.

The client exhibits the symptoms of infection: headache, fever, chills, and fatigue as well as mucous membrane ulcerations of the nose, mouth, pharynx, vagina, and rectum. The white blood count and neutrophils will be low.

Medical–Surgical Management

Medical

The main goals of treatment are to remove the cause of the bone marrow suppression and either prevent or treat any infection. When the client's temperature is elevated, blood cultures may be performed; if mucosal ulcerations occur, they may be cultured. Blood transfusions are given to provide mature leukocytes. Filgrastim (Neupogen), a human granulocyte colony stimulating factor, may be given. Protective isolation may be instituted.

Pharmacological

Antibiotics specific for cultured microorganisms are given.

Diet

A soft, bland diet that is high in calories, protein, and vitamins is ordered.

Activity

Periods of activity must be balanced with periods of rest to prevent weakness and fatigue.

Infection Control: The Client with Agranulocytosis

- Caregivers must thoroughly wash their hands and follow aseptic technique when caring for the client.
- The client's environment must be kept very clean.
- The client should avoid crowds.
- Visitors are screened so no one with a cold or any type of infection is allowed to see the client.
- Teach client to avoid hot or cold environments.
- Ensure that the client reports any signs or symptoms of infection.

▶ NURSING PROCESS

▶ Assessment

▶ Subjective Data

The client may describe having extreme fatigue, weakness, headache, chills, and fever. Inquire about all medications taken, including over-the-counter and prescription drugs.

▶ Objective Data

Assess vital signs especially for a temperature over 100.6°F. Mucosal ulcerations may be reddened. Auscultate the lungs for crackles and wheezes.

Nursing diagnoses for a client with agranulocytosis may include the following:

Nursing Diagnoses	Planning/Goals	Nursing Interventions
▶ *Risk for Infection related to decreased leukocyte production*	The client will not have signs and symptoms of infection.	Thoroughly wash hands before caring for the client.
		Screen all persons for signs of infection before allowing them near the client.
		Monitor vital signs for signs of infection.
		Use strict asepsis for all procedures.
		Encourage the client to drink an adequate amount of fluids.
		Monitor WBC count.
		Provide personal hygiene to prevent infection.
		Provide client with periods of rest between activities.

Evaluation Each goal must be evaluated to determine how it has been met by the client.

COAGULATION DISORDERS

Coagulation disorders include disseminated intravascular coagulation, hemophilia, and thrombocytoperia.

DISSEMINATED INTRA-VASCULAR COAGULATION

Disseminated intravascular coagulation (DIC) is not a disease in itself but a syndrome that occurs because of a primary disease process or condition. A few of the conditions in which DIC may occur are burns, acute leukemia, metastatic cancer, polycythemia vera, pheochromocytoma, shock, acute infections, septic abortion, abruptio placenta, blood transfusion reactions, and trauma.

DIC is a condition of alternating clotting and hemorrhaging. The primary disease stimulates the clotting mechanism, causing many **microthrombi** (very small clots) to form and block the circulation in the arterioles and capillaries. With the formation of the numerous small clots, the body's fibrinolytic process responds in an attempt to stop the clot formation, thus causing hemorrhaging (Figure 20-8). This can be a very serious and potentially fatal condition.

The occlusion of blood vessels with the clots causes infarcts and necrosis of organs and tissues. The kidneys are the most commonly affected organ.

If a client with a predisposing condition develops **purpura** (reddish purple patches on the skin indicative of hemorrhage), bleeding tendencies, or renal impairment, the nurse should assess for DIC. Symptoms of DIC may present as oozing from a venipuncture, mucus membrane, or surgical wound. The oozing may progress rapidly into a hemorrhage within a few hours to a day. The client may have decreased urine output from decreased blood flow or renal infarction.

Figure 20-8 Pathophysiology of DIC

Medical–Surgical Management
Medical

DIC is diagnosed by the client's symptoms and laboratory tests. With DIC there is an increased prothrombin time, partial thromboplastin time, thrombin time, and a decreased fibrinogen and platelet count. A laboratory test that confirms the diagnosis is the D dimer, which measures a fibrin split product that is released when a clot breaks.

The primary disease or condition must be treated. For example, if the primary disease is an infection, an antibiotic is given. If cancer is the primary disease, chemotherapy is given.

DIC is treated by administering whole blood or blood products to normalize the clotting factor levels. Platelets and packed red cells are given to replace those lost during hemorrhage. Cryoprecipitate or fresh-frozen plasma is given to normalize clotting factor levels.

Pharmacological

Heparin has no effect on the thrombi that are already formed but may be given to prevent the formation of more microthrombi. The administration of heparin is controversial because of the risk of hemorrhage. After thrombi formation has been controlled with heparin, aminocaproic acid (Amicar) can be given to stop the bleeding because it stops the fibrinolytic process. **Fibrinolysis** is the process of breaking fibrin apart.

▶ NURSING PROCESS

▶ Assessment

▶ Subjective Data

The client should be asked about previous conditions such as infectious processes, trauma, or cancer. Client statements of joint pain may indicate bleeding into the joint. Recent visual changes should also be documented.

▶ Objective Data

The nurse observes and records the amount of bleeding from any wound or body orifice. I&O is monitored closely. Purpura on the chest and abdomen is a common first sign. Abdominal tenderness is often present. Presence of pulmonary edema, hypotension, tachycardia, absence of peripheral pulses, confusion, restlessness, convulsions, and coma are noted.

Nursing diagnosis for a client with DIC may include the following:

Nursing Diagnoses	Planning/Goals	Nursing Interventions
▶ *Risk for Injury related to altered clotting factors*	The client will experience a minimal amount of injury.	Monitor vitals signs, peripheral pulses, neurological checks, and urine output.
		Check urine and stool for the presence of blood. Assess for abdominal bleeding by checking for abdominal firmness or rigidity.
		If abdominal bleeding is suspected, measure the abdominal girth every 4 hours.
		Assess surgical wounds and all body orifices for bleeding.
		Assess color, warmth, sensation, and movement of extremities.
		Observe for changes in mental status.
		Apply pressure to any oozing site.
		Avoid giving injections and venipunctures as much as possible.
		Observe for signs of orthostatic hypotension.

Evaluation Each goal must be evaluated to determine how it has been met by the client.

HEMOPHILIA

Hemophilia is an inherited bleeding disorder in which there is a lack of clotting factors. Approximately 20,000 persons in the United States have hemophilia (Beare & Myers, 1998). There are two types of hemophilia: hemophilia A is lacking clotting factor VIII, and hemophilia B (Christmas disease) is lacking clotting factor IX. The hemophilia trait is carried on the recessive X chromosome, so a mother is asymptomatic but can pass the trait to the son, who then manifests the symptoms of hemophilia (Figure 20-9). In the male population, hemophilia A occurs at the rate of 1 : 10,000 and hemophilia B occurs at the rate of 1 : 100,000 (Phipps et al., 1999). Genetic counseling is often advantageous for clients who are carriers or who have hemophilia.

There are three classifications of hemophilia: severe (factor level less than 1% of normal), moderate (factor level 1% to 5% normal), and mild (factor level 40% of normal). The main symptom of hemophilia is bleeding. The client with severe hemophilia bleeds when there is minor trauma to an area but can also bleed spontaneously. **Hemarthrosis** (bleeding into the joints) occurs most frequently, causing pain, swelling, redness, and fever. The client can have spontaneous ecchymoses and bleed from the mouth and gastrointestinal and urinary tracts. The most common cause of death is intracranial hemorrhage. Clients with mild hemophilia will not have spontaneous muscle and joint bleeding but will bleed after minor or major surgery. This condition could prove fatal if the diagnosis is not determined promptly.

Medical–Surgical Management

Medical

Hemophilia is diagnosed by a deficient or absent blood level of factors VIII or IX. The prothrombin time (PT), thrombin time, platelet count, and bleeding time are normal, but the partial thromboplastin time (PTT) is usually prolonged.

The treatment for hemophilia is the administration of clotting factors VIII and IX. Clients with hemophilia A are given fresh frozen plasma and cryoprecipitate that has factor VIII. Clients with hemophilia B are given fresh frozen plasma that contains factor IX. Hemophiliacs who received blood products before 1984 often tested seropositive for HIV later in life (Beare & Myers, 1998). This risk has been greatly reduced by heat-treating human-derived factor VIII. The heat treatment inactivates viruses. Factor IX can also be treated in a similar manner. A genetically engineered product called *recombinant factor VIII* is viral safe and relatively economical.

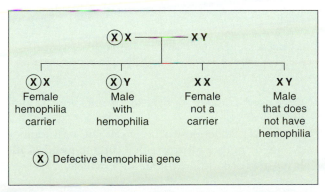

Figure 20-9 Hemophilia Inheritance Pattern between a Female Hemophilia Carrier and a Male without Hemophilia

COMMUNITY/HOME HEALTH CARE

Hemophilia

It is important for the client and family to understand the disease process, learn how to recognize signs and symptoms of bleeding, and be able to administer treatments at home. Inform the client to:
- Obtain medical care for trauma, cuts, edema, or pain in muscles and joints.
- Wear a Medic-Alert tag.
- Not take aspirin.
- Use soft-bristled toothbrush and carefully perform oral hygiene.
- Prevent injuries: wear gloves and long-sleeved clothing when doing household chores, participate in noncontact sports and activities.

Pharmacological

Desmopressin acetate (DDAVP) and aminocaproic acid (Amicar) can be given to mild hemophiliacs to decrease the fibrinolytic process.

▶ NURSING PROCESS

▶ Assessment

▶ Subjective Data

The client should be assessed for pain and asked what measures had been used in the past to relieve pain and bleeding.

▶ Objective Data

The nurse assesses the client for bleeding by checking for petechiae, ecchymoses, hematuria, hematemesis, melena, epistaxis, hemarthrosis, abdominal firmness and rigidity, and frank bleeding. Edematous or immobile joints should be noted.

Nursing diagnoses for a client with hemophilia may include the following:

Nursing Diagnoses	Planning/Goals	Nursing Interventions
▶ *Deficient Knowledge related to disease process*	The client will relate symptoms to report and treatment methods if bleeding occurs.	Discuss ways to improve the safety of the client's home environment. Advise client not to take aspirin. Encourage the client to use an electric razor and soft-bristled toothbrush. Teach family members or significant others administration of clotting factors for prophylactic purposes and if injury occurs. Encourage client to wear Medic-Alert bracelet. Refer for genetic counseling.
▶ *Acute Pain related to bleeding into tissues and joints*	The client will have minimal pain.	Assess the client for bruising, swelling, and joint discomfort. Apply ice and pressure to bleeding sites. When a joint is hurting, immobilize it in a flexed position with a supportive device. Give analgesics as needed. Aspirin is not given because of the anticoagulant effect.
▶ *Risk for Injury related to altered clotting factors*	The client will take precautions to avoid injury.	Transfuse clotting factors as ordered. Encourage the client to avoid activities that may cause trauma. Post emergency medical numbers in convenient places in case of future need.

Evaluation Each goal must be evaluated to determine how it has been met by the client.

THROMBOCYTOPENIA

Thrombocytopenia is a decrease in the number of platelets in the blood. The decrease may be related to:

- Decreased platelet production as in aplastic anemia, tumors, leukemia, and chemotherapy
- Decreased platelet survival as in infection or viral illnesses
- Increased platelet destruction as in DIC or thrombocytopenic purpura that is either drug induced or **idiopathic** (occurring without a known cause)

Withdrawal of the causative drug will usually allow the platelet count to return to normal in 1 to 2 weeks.

The acute form of idiopathic thrombocytopenic purpura (ITP) is an autoimmune process caused by an autoantibody destroying platelet antigen.

Petechiae, ecchymoses, and bleeding from mucous membranes are observed. Bleeding may occur in internal organs. The platelet count is very low; the bleeding time is prolonged; Hgb and Hct may be low; and bone marrow aspiration shows mostly immature platelets.

Medical/Surgical Management

Medical

Transfusions of platelet concentrates may be given, or **apheresis** (removal of unwanted components) may be performed on the client's blood to remove the autoantibodies.

Surgical

A splenectomy may be performed because the spleen is the primary site of platelet destruction. This treatment is usually reserved until all other treatments have been unsuccessful.

Pharmacological

Corticosteroids are given to prolong platelet life and strengthen the capillaries. Immunosuppressive drugs, gamma globulin, and vitamin K may be given.

Diet

A high-fiber diet is used to prevent constipation and the need to strain when having a bowel movement.

CLIENT TEACHING

Thrombocytopenic Purpura
- Use electric razor for shaving.
- Use soft toothbrush.
- Wear shoes or slippers at all times.
- Do not take aspirin.
- Eat high-fiber diet.
- Blow nose gently, if at all.

Activity

Activity should be undertaken thoughtfully and carefully to prevent any trauma.

▶ NURSING PROCESS

▶ Assessment

▶ Subjective Data

The client should be asked about medications being taken and any recent infection.

▶ Objective Data

Observe for petechiae, ecchymoses, and any signs of blood or internal bleeding.

Nursing diagnoses for a client with thrombocytopenia may include the following:

Nursing Diagnoses	Planning/Goals	Nursing Interventions
▶ *Acute Pain related to hemorrhage*	The client will verbalize having less pain.	Assess client's pain on 0 (least) to 10 (most) pain scale.
		Assess client's ability to cope with pain.
		Administer analgesic as ordered.
		Note client's response to analgesic.
▶ *Risk for Injury related to thrombocytopenia*	The client will have minimal injury.	Monitor client's vital signs and neurological and mental status.
		Assess client's skin and excretions for signs of bleeding.
		Handle client very carefully when turning, assisting out of bed, and in all other care situations.

Evaluation Each goal must be evaluated to determine how it has been met by the client.

LYMPH DISORDERS

A **lymphoma** is a tumor of the lymphatic system. Two malignant lymphomas discussed in this chapter are Hodgkin's disease (HD) and non-Hodgkin's lymphoma (NHL). The overview and medical management of each disease will be presented separately. The nursing process for both diseases will be presented together since the nursing diagnoses, goals, and interventions are the same for HD and NHL.

HODGKIN'S DISEASE

Hodgkin's disease is a rare lymphoma that usually arises as a painless swelling in a lymph node. The diagnosis is confirmed when Reed-Sternberg cells are biopsied from the swollen lymph node. The incidence is highest in adolescents and young adults (Leukemia Society of America, 1998a). The 5-year survival rate has doubled from 40% in 1960 to 81% in 1998 (Leukemia Society of America, 1998b). In children, the 5-year survival rate is 94% (Leukemia Society of America, 1998b).

The cause of Hodgkin's disease is unknown. Researchers are investigating genetic factors. Some researchers suspect an infectious origin especially in connection with infectious mononucleosis. Other researchers suspect a viral origin associated with the oncovirus and Epstein-Barr virus (Beare & Myers, 1998).

Clients with Hodgkin's disease most commonly have painless enlarged lymph nodes in the neck, in the area above the clavicles, and in the groin. Lymph nodes in the mediastinum may also be enlarged but are not usually diagnosed until the nodes enlarge and press on the mediastinal structures causing dyspnea and a cough. A chest x-ray or a computed tomography (CT) scan confirms the involvement of the mediastinal lymph nodes. Other symptoms are weight loss, anorexia, fatigue, pruritis, fever, chills, night sweats, anemia, thrombocytopenia, and lowered resistance to infections.

If a client has painless, enlarged lymph nodes and the symptoms of an elevated temperature, night sweats, pruritus, and weight loss of more than 10% of the body weight in a 6-month period, the prognosis is worse than if only enlarged lymph nodes are present. Hodgkin's disease spreads throughout the body in a predictable pattern. From the site of the original swollen gland, the disease spreads to nearby lymph nodes then to other lymphatic tissue in the body such as the liver, spleen, and bone marrow.

The invasion of other nodes and lymphatic tissue determines the prognosis of the disease. As more tissue is invaded, the disease process moves through different phases which is known as staging. The Ann Arbor Staging Classification is used to classify the progression of HD and NHL within the body (Figure 20-10). A classification of A or B is added to each stage depending on whether the client has symptoms other than swollen lymph nodes. A client who has lymph node enlargement only is asymptomatic (A). A client

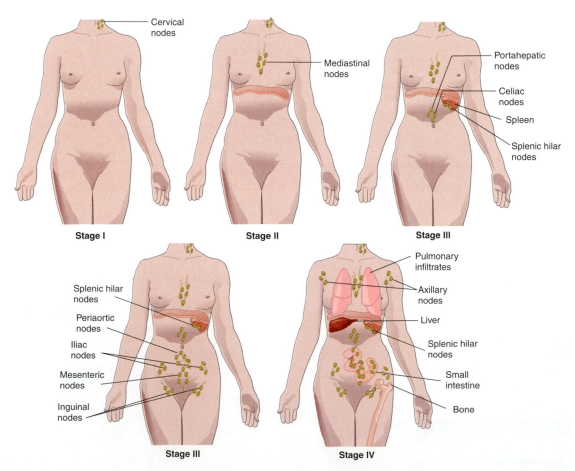

Figure 20-10 Staging of Hodgkin's Disease and Non-Hodgkin's Lymphoma (*From* Medical-Surgical Nursing: Assessment and Management of Clinical Problems (*5th ed.), by S. Lewis, M. Heitkemper, & S. Dirksen, 2000, St. Louis: Mosby, Inc. Reprinted with permission.)

who has symptoms other than lymph node enlargement is symptomatic (B).

Medical–Surgical Management

Medical

Based on the history and physical examination, diagnostic tests to determine the staging of the disease include CBC, platelet count, bone marrow aspiration, chest x-ray, abdominal CT scan, lymphangiogram, and lymph node biopsy.

Localized Hodgkin's disease stages I and II are treated with radiation therapy over a 4-week period. Clients with massive mediastinal involvement and those who have relapsed after radiation therapy alone are treated with radiation therapy and chemotherapy.

During radiation therapy the client may experience symptoms of toxicity, which are weight loss, nausea and vomiting, skin reactions, esophagitis, fatigue, and bone marrow suppression. The client's blood count is monitored closely during the therapy treatments to check for infections and bleeding tendencies. If the WBC level drops too low, the client will be more susceptible to infections. A decrease in RBCs and platelets causes a bleeding tendency. Long-term complications from radiation therapy include hypothyroidism, radiation pneumonitis, immune system impairment, herpes zoster, and the development of a second cancer.

Generalized Hodgkin's disease, stages III_1, III_2, and IV, are treated with **combination chemotherapy**, which is administering a series of combined drugs over a set period of time. Serious late complications of chemotherapy are infertility and a secondary malignancy or cancer.

Surgical

Sometimes a laparotomy is done to see if the liver and spleen are involved. The rationale of performing the procedure is being questioned since the overall treatment plan is not altered.

Pharmacological

During radiation therapy antiemetics, such as ondansetron HCl (Zofran), are given for nausea and vomiting. Analgesics can be given for esophagitis discomfort.

Chemotherapy drugs are often given in combinations such as MOPP and ABVD. MOPP combines mechlorethamine or nitrogen mustard (Mustargen), vincristine sulfate (Oncovin), procarbazine HCl (Matulane), and prednisone (Deltasone). ABVD combines doxorubicin HCl (Adriamycin PFS), bleomycin sulfate (Blenoxane), vinblastine sulfate (Velban), and dacarbazine (DTIC-Dome). These drugs are usually administered through an implanted venous port. Allopurinol (Zyloprim) is given to prevent uric acid renal stones caused by the rapid destruction of cells during therapy.

Diet

During therapy the client is on a high-calorie, high-protein diet. An intake of 2,500 mL of fluid per day is encouraged to prevent the formation of renal stones.

Activity

Extra rest periods may be necessary to cope with fatigue that occurs with Hodgkin's disease.

NON-HODGKIN'S LYMPHOMA

Non-Hodgkin's lymphoma (NHL) is more common than Hodgkin's disease and is the seventh most common cause of cancer-related deaths in the United States. Approximately 55,700 new cases occurred in 1998 (Leukemia Society of America, 1998a). The 5-year survival rate has increased from 31% in 1960 to 51% in 1998; in children, the 5-year survival rate has increased from 18% in 1960 to 73% in 1998 (Leukemia Society of America, 1998c).

NHL originates from the B lymphocytes and the T lymphocytes. NHL arising from the B lymphocyte occurs in the older adult population; NHL arising from the T lymphocytes manifests in malignant skin diseases such as mycosis fungoides or Sezary syndrome. More men are affected than women. NHL does not have the Reed-Sternberg cell present. The incidence for non-Hodgkin's lymphoma has nearly doubled since 1970 probably because of exposure to certain infectious agents and chemicals.

Symptoms of NHL are enlarged tonsils and adenoids and diffuse enlarged painless, rubbery lymph nodes in the cervical, axillary, and inguinal areas. Symptoms include fever, night sweats, weight loss, excessive tiredness, indigestion, abdominal pain, loss of appetite, and bone pain.

Medical–Surgical Management

Medical

The diagnosis of NHL is confirmed by a lymph node biopsy. Physicians use a staging system to define the progression of the disease within the body and to determine the appropriate treatment and prognosis of the disease. (Refer to Figure 20-10.)

Pharmacological

There are three different chemotherapy regimens, CHOP, CVP, and COPP: CHOP combines cyclophosphamide (Cytoxan), doxorubicin HCl (Adriamycin), vincristine sulfate (Oncovin), and prednisone (Deltasone); CVP combines cyclophosphamide (Cytoxan), vincristine sulfate (Oncovin), and prednisone (Deltasone); COPP combines cyclophosphamide (Cytoxan), vincristine sulfate (Oncovin), procarbazine HCl (Matulane), and prednisone (Deltasone).

▶ NURSING PROCESS

▶ Assessment

▶ Subjective Data

Ask if the client is experiencing pruritus, night sweats, weight loss, decreased appetite, fever, fatigue, weakness, or chest pain.

▶ Objective Data

The nursing physical assessment consists of weighing the client, taking the vital signs, and assessing for skin infections; dyspnea; cough; voice changes; enlarged lymph nodes in the neck, axilla, and groin; and edema in the extremities. Bone scan shows fractures and tumor infiltration. Review blood tests. Blood tests show hypercalcemia if bone lesions are present, and a CBC often indicates anemia. When the client is having radiation or chemotherapy treatments, the assessment includes observing for dysphagia, nausea and vomiting, skin rashes, and alopecia.

Nursing diagnoses for a client with Hodgkin's disease or non-Hodgkin's disease may include the following:

Nursing Diagnoses	Planning/Goals	Nursing Interventions
▶ *Ineffective Breathing Pattern related to tracheobronchial obstruction from enlarged mediastinal nodes*	The client will complete activities of daily living without dyspnea.	Elevate the head of the bed to assist the client's breathing.
		Encourage the client to take frequent deep breaths to expand the lungs and prevent infection.
		Assess the client's breathing pattern every shift and as needed for dyspnea.
▶ *Risk for Infection related to radiation/chemotherapy treatments, decreased WBCs and pruritus*	The client will remain free of infection.	Monitor the lab results for lowered WBCs.
		Teach the client the importance of avoiding situations where there is exposure to infections.
		Provide cool sponge baths or oral medication to relieve pruritus.
		Assess the radiated skin areas for redness or breaks in the skin.
		Encourage the client to report symptoms of dyspnea, sore throat, and burning or frequency of urination.
▶ *Imbalanced Nutrition: Less than body requirements related to decreased appetite*	The client will consume an adequate amount of a nutritional diet.	Serve attractive high-calorie, high-protein meals in a pleasant environment.
		Offer six to eight smaller meals throughout the day to decrease a feeling of fullness.
		Offer a soft, bland diet, which may be more palatable during radiation or chemotherapy treatments.
		Avoid hot, spicy foods as they are caustic to mucous membranes and may lead to infection.
		Encourage an adequate intake of fluids to prevent constipation and renal stones.
		Weigh the client biweekly or more frequently if needed.
▶ *Anxiety related to disease and therapy treatments*	The client will cope effectively with disease process and therapy treatments.	Listen to the concerns of the client regarding the effect of the disease on life-style, family, and finances.
		Encourage the family to express their concerns and discuss effective ways to deal with the diagnosis and treatment.
		Refer the client and family to clergy and social agencies when appropriate.

Evaluation Each goal must be evaluated to determine how it has been met by the client.

PLASMA CELL DISORDER

The main plasma cell disorder is multiple myeloma.

MULTIPLE MYELOMA

There were an estimated 13,800 new cases of multiple myeloma diagnosed in 1998, and an estimated 11,300 persons died from it (Leukemia Society of America, 1998d). Most cases occur in men over age 60.

The plasma cells, mainly in bone marrow, become malignant, crowd out normal cell production, destroy normal bone tissue, and thereby cause pain. The normal production of antibodies is changed, making the client susceptible to infections. The first sign of multiple myeloma is often bone pain, especially in the ribs, spine, and pelvis. The long bones ache; joints are swollen and tender; and a low-grade fever and general malaise are present. The client tires easily and has weakness from anemia. The weakened bones fracture easily. The cause of multiple myeloma is not known.

Diagnosis is made with bone marrow biopsy showing large numbers of immature plasma cells and x-rays showing demineralization and osteoporosis. Bence Jones protein is found in the urine of many clients with multiple myeloma. The client will also have hypercalcemia, hyperuricemia, anemia, and hypercalciuria.

Medical–Surgical Management

Medical

Multiple myeloma is not curable, so treatment is symptomatic. Both radiation and chemotherapy are used to reduce tumor size and slow tumor growth.

Surgical

A laminectomy may be required if any vertebrae collapse. If the client gets kidney stones from the large amount of calcium in the blood and urine, surgery may be required.

Pharmacological

Steroids such as prednisone (Metcorten) along with antineoplastic drugs such as cyclophosphamide (Cytoxan), chlorambucil (Leukeran), or melphalan (Alkeran) are given. An analgesic is given for pain relief.

It is important for the nurse and client to monitor the level of blood calcium. Hypercalcemia can cause confusion, weakness, fatigue, diarrhea, polyuria, and renal stones. If the serum calcium level rises above 10 mg/dl, the physician may order an IV of normal saline infused at a high rate followed by diuretics.

CLIENT TEACHING

Multiple Myeloma
- Drink 3 to 4 L of fluids per day.
- Exercise to decrease bone demineralization.
- Monitor for symptoms of hypercalcemia and notify physician if symptoms occur.

Diet

Six small meals a day are often tolerated better than the usual three meals a day; nutritious meals based on the client's food preferences are recommended. A fluid intake of 3 to 4 L/day is essential to minimize the complications of excessive calcium in the blood and urine.

Activity

It is important to keep the client mobile as much as possible. Walking stimulates calcium resorption and decreases demineralization. When the client is in bed, it is important to reposition the client frequently using a lift sheet to decrease the risk of pathological fractures.

▸ NURSING PROCESS

▸ Assessment

▸ Subjective

The client describes constant pain that increases with movement. The pain is usually in the back, ribs, or pelvis. Achiness in the long bones and joints and general malaise may also be described.

▸ Objective

Pain should be assessed using a 0 (none) to 10 (most) pain scale. Temperature may be elevated. The client's ability to perform activities of daily living should be evaluated and the level of blood calcium should be monitored.

Nursing diagnoses for a client with multiple myeloma may include the following:

Nursing Diagnoses	Planning/Goals	Nursing Interventions
▸ *Chronic Pain related to disease process*	The client will express a decrease in pain level.	Administer analgesic as ordered. Monitor the client's response to the analgesic. Assess the client's pain level with pain scale.
▸ *Risk for Injury related to bone demineralization*	The client will have minimal injuries.	Handle client gently. Reposition the client using a lift sheet. Keep the client's personal items within easy reach.

continues

Nursing Diagnoses	Planning/Goals	Nursing Interventions
▶ *Risk for Infection related to disease process and pharmaceutical agents*	The client will have few infections.	Thoroughly wash hands before caring for the client.
		Teach the client and family proper handwashing.
		Assist the client with personal hygiene as needed.
		Screen visitors for signs of infections before allowing them to visit the client.

Evaluation Each goal must be evaluated to determine how it has been met by the client.

CASE STUDY

James Johns, 46, owns a hobby shop. He has had a cold for 3 weeks that has recently settled in his chest. He has been tired lately and takes naps each evening before the evening meal. His wife noticed several bruises on his arms and legs, but James could not recall any particular injury. James has gradually lost 10 pounds over the last 3 months but has not been concerned about it. When James went to the clinic for some antibiotics for his cold, the nurse practitioner completed a physical assessment, and ordered a chest x-ray and CBC. The nurse practitioner noticed the WBCs were 250,000/mm^3; RBCs, 4.2 million/mm^3 and platelets, 100,000/mm^3. After several other tests were performed over the next few days, a diagnosis of chronic myelocytic leukemia (CML) was confirmed.

The following questions will guide your development of a nursing care plan for the case study.

1. List the symptoms occurring in James Johns that are typical of CML.
2. List five other typical symptoms of CML that were not stated in the case study.
3. List other diagnostic tests that could be done to confirm the diagnosis of CML.
4. List subjective and objective data the nurse would obtain about James Johns.
5. Write three individualized nursing diagnoses and goals for James Johns.
6. List nursing interventions for James Johns.
7. List community resources specific to locale that could assist James and his family during his illness with CML.
8. List discharge teaching the nurse would give to James and his family.
9. List successful client outcomes for James Johns.
10. List chemotherapeutic agents and side effects of the agents that may be prescribed for James.
11. List other medical treatments that may be ordered for James.
12. What measures could the nurse take to meet the emotional needs of James and his family?

SUMMARY

- The main formed components of the blood are red blood cells, white blood cells, and platelets.
- The lymphatic system is composed of lymph vessels that drain lymph into the venous system and lymph nodes that filter microorganisms in the body.
- Sickledex and hemoglobin electrophoresis are diagnostic tests for sickle cell anemia.
- A client with anemia has a decreased number of RBCs and low hemoglobin and hematocrit levels.

- Some of the symptoms of anemia are fatigue, pallor, exertional dyspnea, and tachycardia.
- Symptoms of polycythemia vera are headache, epistaxis, dizziness, tinnitus, blurred vision, fatigue, weakness, pruritus, exertional dyspnea, angina, and increased blood pressure and pulse.
- Polycythemia vera is treated with chemotherapeutic agents.
- DIC is not a disease but a syndrome that occurs because of a client's having a primary disease or condition. The primary disease causes the client to

alternate between forming many small clots and hemorrhaging.

- Hemophilia is a recessive X chromosome inherited bleeding disorder in which the client is lacking clotting factors. The main symptom is spontaneous bleeding or bleeding due to trauma.
- The two types of malignant lymphomas are Hodgkin's disease and non-Hodgkin's lymphoma. Clients with both types of lymphoma have enlarged lymph nodes.
- Hodgkin's disease is diagnosed by the presence of the Reed Sternberg cell in the swollen lymph nodes. Non-Hodgkin's lymphoma arises from the B lymphocytes and T lymphocytes and does not have the Reed Sternberg cell in the lymph system.

Review Questions

1. The diagnostic test for sickle cell anemia is the:
   a. D dimer.
   b. sickledex.
   c. hemoglobin electrophoresis.
   d. Schilling test.

2. For improved iron absorption, a client with iron deficiency anemia takes Feosol with:
   a. milk.
   b. an orange.
   c. water.
   d. processed cheese.

3. A thorough assessment of the cardiac system on a client with sickle cell anemia is important because:
   a. the heart enlarges in an attempt to provide the oxygen needs to the body tissues.
   b. cells sickle more easily in the heart chambers.
   c. more cardiac force is needed to pump RBCs with Hbg S.
   d. people with sickle cell anemia are prone to bradycardia.

4. Clients with leukemia are prone to infections because:
   a. there are too many WBCs.
   b. the bone marrow is not producing WBCs.
   c. the bone marrow is producing too many cells.
   d. the WBCs are incapable of fighting infections.

5. A nursing action for a client with pernicious anemia is to:
   a. inquire about exposure to radiation and chemicals.
   b. administer cyanocobalamin (vitamin B_{12}) as ordered.
   c. teach the importance of increasing iron in the diet.
   d. administer oral vitamin B_{12} as ordered.

6. Nursing care for a client with polycythemia vera includes:
   a. doing a Homans' sign to check for blood clots.
   b. administering folic acid as ordered.
   c. observing for blood in the stool and urine.
   d. observing for petechiae and ecchymotic spots.

7. Symptoms that alert a nurse that a client may have DIC are:
   a. tinnitus and numbness and tingling in the extremities.
   b. jaundice, palpitations, and dyspnea.
   c. purpura, bruising, and decreased urine output.
   d. ruddy complexion, epistaxis, and tinnitus.

8. A client with hemophilia is taught to:
   a. adminster clotting factors as needed.
   b. administer cyanocobalamin (vitamin B_{12}) as needed.
   c. maintain a high-calorie, high-protein diet.
   d. report night sweats.

9. Encourage a client with non-Hodgkin's lymphoma to:
   a. use an electric razor.
   b. take folic acid as prescribed.
   c. apply ice and pressure to bleeding sites.
   d. avoid exposure to infections.

Critical Thinking Questions

1. Explain how the symptoms of iron deficiency anemia are related to a decreased red blood cell count and a decreased hemoglobin.

2. Compare the etiologies and symptoms of iron deficiency anemia, hypoplastic (aplastic) anemia, pernicious anemia, acquired hemolytic anemia, and sickle cell anemia.

3. Compare the diagnostic tests, symptoms, and treatments stated in the text to an assigned client in the clinical setting.

⚡ **WEB FLASH!**

- Search the Internet for the various disorders discussed in this chapter. What new or experimental treatments are discussed?
- What Internet information do the resources at the end of the book provide for this chapter? For whom is this material intended?

UNIT
5
Body Defenses

NURSING CARE OF THE CLIENT: INTEGUMENTARY SYSTEM

MAKING THE CONNECTION

Refer to the following chapters to increase your understanding of the integumentary system:

- **Chapter 10, Fluid, Electrolyte, and Acid-Base Balance**
- **Chapter 12, Health Assessment**
- **Chapter 13, Diagnostic Tests**
- **Chapter 17, Nursing Care of the Oncology Client**

- **Chapter 22, Nursing Care of the Client: Immune System**
- **Chapter 35, Nursing Care of the Older Client**

LEARNING OBJECTIVES

Upon completion of this chapter, you should be able to:
- *Define key terms.*
- *Describe common disorders of the integumentary system.*
- *Relate the pathophysiology of each skin disorder.*
- *Discuss the common diagnostic tests used to differentiate skin disorders.*
- *State the usual treatment for each skin disorder.*
- *Assess the nursing care needs of a client with a disorder of the integument.*
- *Plan and implement effective nursing care.*

KEY TERMS

alopecia	keloid
angiogenesis	keratin
angioma	lipoma
blanching	melanin
cyanosis	nevi
debride	pallor
ecchymosis	petechiae
erythema	purulent exudate
eschar	sebaceous cyst
friction	sebum
granulation tissue	serosanguineous
hemorrhagic exudate	exudate
hemostasis	serous exudate
hyperthermia	shearing
hypothermia	telangiectasia
inflammation	vitiligo
ischemia	wound
jaundice	

INTRODUCTION

As an old adage asserts, the health of the skin mirrors the health of the body. Many systemic diseases have skin manifestations. Psychological stress can affect the condition of the skin, and skin rashes can be a complication of drug therapy. As the largest and the most visible system in the body, the integumentary system (skin, hair, scalp, nails, and mucous membranes) is vulnerable to injury and is susceptible to a number of primary diseases. It is estimated that skin-related problems account for 5% to 10% of all ambulatory client visits in the United States (Deters, 1996).

While the outward appearance of the skin is important for psychological well-being, the healthy, intact status of the skin also is essential for physiologic well-being. Maintaining this status of the integumentary system is, therefore, an important independent nursing function. The focus of this chapter will be to describe common skin disorders, identify the usual treatment modalities for these disorders, and discuss measures that nurses can implement to provide effective nursing care for clients with disorders of the integument.

ANATOMY AND PHYSIOLOGY REVIEW

As the external covering of the body, the skin performs the vital function of protecting internal body structures from harmful microorganisms and substances. The skin is continuous with mucous membranes at external body openings of the respiratory tract, the digestive system, and the urogenital tract. As appendages of the skin, the hair and nails also have protective functions. In addition to its vital protective role, the skin also plays other roles in the normal functioning of the human organism. These roles include participating in the regulation of body temperature, functioning as a sensory organ, helping to maintain fluid and electrolyte balance, producing vitamin D, and excreting certain waste products from the body.

Structure of the Skin

The skin is composed of three layers: the epidermis, the dermis, and the subcutaneous fatty tissue (Figure 21-1).

Epidermis

The epidermis is a layer of squamous epithelial cells. Most of the cells are keratinocytes that produce a tough, fibrous protein called **keratin**. As new cells are produced in the deep layers of the epidermis, old cells are pushed to the surface of the skin. As these cells move from the deeper epidermal layers to the surface, they undergo a process of keratinization in which they become filled with keratin, thus hardening the outer layer of epidermal cells. The keratin creates a barrier that repels bacteria and foreign matter and is impermeable to most substances. The epidermal cells on the palms of the hands and soles of the feet, areas of the body subjected to increased friction and pressure, contain larger amounts of keratin, resulting in thickened skin and callouses.

The epidermis also contains specialized cells called melanocytes. These cells produce **melanin**, the pigment that gives the skin its color. The more melanin present, the darker the skin color. Moles and birthmarks (**nevi**), pigmented areas in the skin, are aggregations of melanocytes. In **vitiligo**, melanocytes are destroyed, causing milk-white patches of depigmented skin surrounded by normal skin. Exposure to ultraviolet light (sun) causes an increase in the production of melanin, which darkens (tans) the skin and provides some protection against the harmful effects of suntanning.

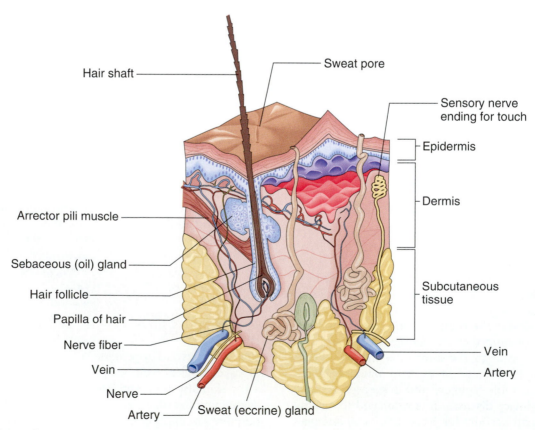

Figure 21-1 Cross Section of the Skin

Dermis

The dermis is dense, irregular connective tissue composed of collagen and elastic fibers, blood and lymph vessels, nerves, sweat and sebaceous glands, and hair roots. The sebaceous glands secrete an oily substance called **sebum** that lubricates the skin, helping to keep it soft and pliable. Sweat (eccrine) glands are found in the skin over most of the body surface. Another type of sweat gland, apocrine glands, is concentrated in the axillae, anal region, scrotum, and labia majora. These glands secrete an organic substance that is odorless at first but is quickly metabolized by skin bacteria causing the characteristic odor commonly referred to as body odor (Seeley, Stephens, & Tate, 1995). Intradermal injections, such as the TB skin test, are given in the dermis.

Subcutaneous Tissue

The subcutaneous tissue is primarily connective and adipose (fatty) tissue. Here the skin is anchored to muscles and bones. An individual's nutritional status and genetic makeup dictate the amount of subcutaneous tissue present. Emaciated persons have very little subcutaneous tissue while obese persons may have several inches of subcutaneous tissue. The amount of subcutaneous tissue is an important factor in body temperature regulation.

Functions of the Skin

Understanding the functions of the skin and contiguous mucous membranes guides the nurse in planning and implementing appropriate nursing care. Because intact, healthy skin and mucous membranes serve as the first line of defense against harmful agents, maintaining skin integrity is one of the most important independent functions of the nurse. Nursing interventions such as providing daily hygiene care and regularly turning and repositioning dependent clients are aimed at preventing skin breakdown.

Protection

The first and most important function of the skin is protection. As long as the skin is intact and healthy, it is a barrier against microorganisms and numerous substances that could be harmful to the individual. Not only is the skin a barrier to keep harmful substances out, it is also a barrier to keep essential substances such as water and electrolytes inside the body.

Temperature Regulation

The body produces heat as a result of metabolism of food. Exercise, fever, or a hot environment can raise body temperature. Through several mechanisms, the skin can either release or conserve body heat to maintain normal body temperature. Radiation is the primary means of heat loss. As body heat increases, arterioles in the dermis dilate, bringing body heat to the skin surface. By the process of radiation, waves of heat from uncovered body surfaces are released to the environment. Layering clothes in winter, for example, helps to prevent excess loss of body heat by radiation. Heat is also lost by conduction. In conduction, heat is transferred from warmer surfaces to cooler ones. Placing a cool washcloth on a client's forehead is an example of using the principle of conduction. The washcloth becomes warmer, the forehead cooler. Evaporation is another way in which excess body heat is lost. As moisture on the skin, either from perspiration or from a tepid sponge bath, dries the body is cooled. To conserve (prevent excess loss) body heat, arterioles in the dermis contract to decrease the flow of blood to the skin surface, thus decreasing heat lost by radiation. The phenomenon of "goose flesh" is another method of conserving body heat. Tiny hairs standing on end create a layer of air insulation decreasing loss of body heat to the environment.

Sensory Perception

The skin contains receptors for pain, touch, pressure, and temperature. The sensory receptors help protect the body from environmental dangers as well as provide sensations of comfort and pleasure.

Fluid and Electrolyte Balance

The skin helps to maintain the stability of the internal environment by preventing loss of body fluids and electrolytes and by preventing subcutaneous tissues from drying out. Skin damage, such as that occurring with severe burns, results in rapid loss of large quantities of fluid and electrolytes. This can lead to shock, circulatory collapse, and death.

Structure of Hair

Hair is composed of dead epidermal cells that begin to grow and divide in the base of the hair follicle. As the cells are pushed toward the skin surface, they become keratinized and die. Hair color is genetically determined.

Hair Growth and Replacement

Scalp hair grows for 2 to 5 years, then the follicle becomes inactive. When the growth cycle begins again, a new hair is produced and the old hair is pushed out. Approximately 50 hairs are lost each day. Sustained hair loss of more than 100 hairs each day usually indicates that something is wrong (Martini, 2000).

Function of Hair

There are 5 million hairs covering the entire human body except for the lips, palmar and plantar surfaces, nipples, and the glans penis. The amount and texture of hair vary with age, gender, race, and body part.

- Vellus hair: Fine "peach fuzz" hair that covers most of the body
- Terminal hair: Coarser, darker, sometimes curly hair on the head, eyebrows, and eyelashes; axillary and pubic hair become terminal with the onset of puberty
- Intermediate hair: Have intermediate characteristics such as the hairs on the arms and legs

Hair on the head protects the scalp from the ultraviolet rays from the sun and cushions blows to the head. Eyelashes help prevent foreign particles from entering the eyes just as the hairs in the nostrils and external ear canals help keep particles from entering the nose and ears.

Structure and Function of Nails

Nail production occurs in the nail root, an epithelial fold that cannot be seen from the surface (Figure 21-2). The nail plate covers the nail bed. The blood vessels under the nail bed give the nails their pink color.

The nails protect the ends of the fingers and toes.

Structure and Function of Mucous Membranes

Mucous membranes have epithelium overlying a layer of loose connective tissue. Specialized cells within the mucous membrane secrete mucus.

The cavities and tubes that open to the outside of the body are lined with mucous membranes. These include the oral and nasal cavities and the tubes of the respiratory, gastrointestinal, urinary, and reproductive systems. Mucous membranes perform absorptive or secretory functions depending on their placement.

Effects of Aging

With advancing years, the blood flow to the skin is reduced. The skin becomes thinner and is more easily injured. Older skin breaks down easily from prolonged pressure. The long accepted rule of thumb is to turn clients every 2 hours, but for the ill elderly client, every

GERONTOLOGICAL CONSIDERATIONS

Effects of Aging on the Skin

- Skin vascularity and the number of sweat and sebaceous glands decrease, affecting thermoregulation.
- Inflammatory response and pain perception diminish, increasing the risk of adverse effects from noxious stimuli.
- A thinning epidermis and prolonged wound healing make the elderly more prone to injury and skin infections.
- Skin cancer is more common among the elderly.
- Use of skin lotions containing alcohol can cause drying of the skin, increasing the risk of injury. Moisture-enhancing products should be used instead.

2 hours may not be often enough. Significant skin damage can occur in just 1 hour of unrelieved pressure. Preventing skin breakdown in the elderly client depends on an accurate assessment of both the client's skin condition and mobility status.

Loss of subcutaneous tissue causes skin sagging and wrinkling. The activity of sebaceous and sweat glands diminishes, resulting in dry skin and a decreased ability to adapt to changes in environmental temperature. Extremes in temperature pose hazards for older adults. In very hot weather they are susceptible to **hyperthermia**, a condition in which the core body temperature reaches 106°F. In hyperthermia, the hypothalamus no longer functions appropriately. Sweating stops, the skin becomes dry and flushed, and the person becomes confused and eventually comatose. Each summer many elderly persons die from the effects of hyperthermia. Winter puts older adults at risk for **hypothermia**, a condition in which the core body temperature drops below 95°F. The hypothermic client may become confused and disoriented. As the core body temperature continues to drop, the person becomes comatose. Each winter some older adults die from severe hypothermia (Seeley et al., 1995).

On the hands and face, melanocytes increase in number, causing the age spots commonly seen in older adults. Gray hair occurs from a lack of melanin production. Skin exposed to sunlight ages faster.

ASSESSMENT

Assessing clients with disorders of the integument includes obtaining a health history and performing a physical assessment of the skin, hair, nails, and mucous membranes. The nurse's assessment skills along with an understanding of the anatomy and physiology

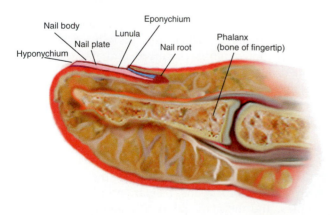

Figure 21-2 Structure of the Fingernail

Table 21–1 OBTAINING A CLIENT HISTORY OF SKIN PROBLEMS

- When did you first notice this problem?
- Where did the first symptom appear?
- What did the rash/lesion look like when it first appeared?
- Describe what happened in the days/weeks after the first symptom appeared.
- Are the symptoms worse at any particular time? Season?
- Have you experienced any itching or burning sensations?
- Are the lesions painful?
- What do you think might have caused this problem?
- Have you ever had a skin problem like this before?
- Has anyone in your family ever had a problem like this?
- What have you been doing to treat this problem?
- What kind of skin care products do you normally use?
- Have you changed any of your usual products/habits/routines?
- Is there anything else you would like to tell me about this problem?

of the integumentary system ensure a complete, factual database from which to plan and implement appropriate nursing care. Table 21–1 contains a list of questions to use in obtaining a health history.

Assessment of Skin

There are seven parameters that should be examined when performing a physical assessment of the skin. They are integrity, color, temperature and moisture, texture, turgor and mobility, sensation, and vascularity. Inspection and palpation are the two assessment techniques used when examining the skin. Good lighting is essential for accurate assessment. Table 21–2 outlines these parameters with the normal and abnormal findings.

Any skin lesions should be identified according to type and described as to color, size, and location. The nurse should describe the amount, color, odor, and appearance of any drainage that might be present. Assessment findings must be documented clearly, concisely, and completely. The intent of nursing care is to maintain the integrity of intact skin and to restore damaged skin or mucous membranes to an intact state. Aging changes skin texture, moisture, and mobility requiring increased nursing vigilance to maintain skin integrity. Daily hygiene products should be selected to meet the client's individual skin care needs.

Table 21–2 SKIN ASSESSMENT PARAMETERS

PARAMETER	NORMAL	ABNORMAL
Integrity	Skin intact; no diseased or injured tissue.	Broken skin; open areas such as fissures, ulcers, excoriations. Rash or lesions such as papules, nodules, vesicles, pustules, wheals, scales (Figures 21-3 and 21-4).
Color	Varies with skin type and race: pink, tanned, olive, brown.	**Pallor**—pale skin, especially in face, conjunctiva, nail beds, and oral mucous membranes. **Cyanosis**—bluish discoloration noticed in lips, earlobes, and nail beds. **Jaundice**—a yellowing of the skin, mucous membranes, and sclera. **Erythema**—reddish hue to the skin as in sunburn and inflammation.
Temperature and moisture	Usually warm and dry, depending on environmental temperature.	Cool, cold, moist, clammy, or warmer than normal.
Texture	Smooth, soft. Thickness varies in different areas.	Loose, wrinkled, rough, thickened, thin, oily, flaking, scaling.
Turgor and mobility	An assessment of skin hydration. Normally skin moves freely. A pinched fold of skin returns immediately to normal position (Figure 21-5).	Taut with edema; slack with dehydration. Rigid in some diseases such as scleroderma.
Sensation	Distinguishes hot and cold, sharp and dull.	Numbness, tingling, insensitive to pressure and sharp objects.
Vascularity	Clear; no discoloration.	**Telangiectasia** (permanent dilation of groups of superficial capillaries and venules); **Petechiae** (pinpoint hemorrhagic spots); **Ecchymosis** (large, irregular, hemorrhagic areas) (Figure 21-6).

NONPALPABLE

(A)

Macule:
Localized changes in skin color of less than 1 cm in diameter
Example:
Freckle

(B)

Patch:
Localized changes in skin color of greater than 1 cm in diameter
Example:
Vitiligo, stage 1 of pressure ulcer

PALPABLE

(C)

Papule:
Solid, elevated lesion less than 0.5 cm in diameter
Example:
Warts, elevated nevi

(D)

Plaque:
Solid, elevated lesion greater than 0.5 cm in diameter
Example:
Psoriasis

(E)

Nodules:
Solid and elevated; however, they extend deeper than papules into the dermis or subcutaneous tissues, 0.5–2 cm
Example:
Lipoma, erythema nodosum, cyst

(F)

Tumor:
The same as a nodule only greater than 2 cm
Example:
Carcinoma (such as advanced breast carcinoma); not basal cell or squamous cell of the skin

(G)

Wheal:
Localized edema in the epidermis causing irregular elevation that may be red or pale
Example:
Insect bite or a hive

FLUID-FILLED CAVITIES WITHIN THE SKIN

(H)

Vesicle:
Accumulation of fluid between the upper layers of the skin; elevated mass containing serous fluid; less than 0.5 cm
Example:
Herpes simplex, herpes zoster, chickenpox

(I)

Bullae:
Same as a vesicle only greater than 0.5 cm
Example:
Contact dermatitis, large second-degree burns, bullous impetigo, pemphigus

(J)

Pustule:
Vesicles or bullae that become filled with pus, usually described as less than 0.5 cm in diameter
Example:
Acne, impetigo, furuncles, carbuncles, folliculitis

(K)

Cyst:
Encapsulated fluid-filled or a semi-solid mass in the subcutaneous tissue or dermis
Example:
Sebaceous cyst, epidermoid cyst

Figure 21-3 Types of Primary Skin Lesions (*From* Health Assessment & Physical Examination, *2nd edition, by M. E. Z. Estes, 2002, Albany, NY: Delmar. Copyright 2002 by Delmar. Reprinted with permission.*)

ABOVE THE SKIN SURFACE

(A)

Scales:
Flaking of the skin's surface
Example:
Dandruff or psoriasis, xerosis

(B)

Lichenification:
Layers of skin become thickened and rough as a result of rubbing over a prolonged period of time
Example:
Chronic contact dermatitis

(C)

Crust:
Dried serum, blood, or pus on the surface of the skin
Example:
Impetigo

(D)

Atrophy:
Thinning of the skin surface and loss of markings
Example:
Striae, aged skin

BELOW THE SKIN SURFACE

(E)

Erosion:
Loss of epidermis
Example:
Ruptured chickenpox vesicle

(F)

Fissure:
Linear crack in the epidermis that can extend into the dermis
Example:
Chapped hands or lips, athlete's foot

(G)

Ulcer:
A depressed lesion of the epidermis and upper papillary layer of the dermis
Example:
Stage 2 pressure ulcer

(H)

Scar:
Fibrous tissue that replaces dermal tissue after injury
Example:
Surgical incision

(I)

Keloid:
Enlarging of a scar past wound edges due to excess collagen formation (more prevalent in dark skinned persons)
Example:
Burn scar

(J)
Excoriation:
Loss of epidermal layers exposing the dermis
Example:
Abrasion

Figure 21-4 Types of Secondary Skin Lesions (*From* Health Assessment & Physical Examination, *2nd edition, by M. E. Z. Estes, 2002, Albany, NY: Delmar. Copyright 2002 by Delmar. Reprinted with permission.*)

Assessment of Hair, Nails, and Mucous Membranes

Hair should be smooth, shiny, and resilient. Excess hair loss can result from drugs, radiation, dietary or hormonal factors, stress, and high fever.

Nails should be pink, smooth, and shiny and feel firm yet flexible when palpated. An angle of approximately 160° should be present between the nail body and the eponychium (Figure 21-7).

Mucous membranes normally appear pink and moist.

Figure 21-5 Assessment of Skin Turgor

A.

B.

C.

Figure 21-6 A. Telangiectasia (Spider Veins); B. Petechiae (*Courtesy of Dr. Mark Dougherty, Lexington, KY*); C. Ecchymosis (bruise)

Normal nail angle

Normal nail: Has an angle of approximately 160° between the fingernail and nail base; nail feels firm when palpated.

Clubbing: Hypoxia causes an angle greater than 180° between the fingernail and nail base; nail feels springy when palpated.

Koilonychia (spoon nail): Characterized by concave curves; associated with iron deficiency anemia.

Beau's line: Characterized by transverse depression in the nails; associated with injury and severe systemic infections.

Paronychia: Characterized by an inflammation at the nail base (may be swollen, red, or tender); associated with trauma and local infection.

Figure 21-7 Nail Variations (*Photos of clubbing and Beau's line courtesy of Robert A. Silverman, MD, Clinical Associate Professor, Department of Pediatrics, Georgetown University*)

PROFESSIONAL TIP

Possible Signs of Physical Abuse

Areas of ecchymosis are one sign of trauma that could be the result of physical abuse. Injuries noted at the base of the skull or on the face, buttocks, breasts, abdomen, or any area such as the top of the back that the client could not reach, are suspicious for abuse. Unusual marks on the skin such as cigarette burns and belt buckle or bite marks may also be signs of abuse. Injuries that are inconsistent with the client's story may also be the result of abuse.

Institutional policies generally relate to reporting and to whom to report when the situation of possible physical abuse is encountered. This is usually based on state laws about reporting physical abuse. Nurses must know the reporting laws of the state in which they are employed.

COMMON DIAGNOSTIC TESTS

Commonly used diagnostic tests for clients with integumentary disorders are listed in Table 21–3. Refer to Chapter 13, Diagnostic Tests, for explanation/normal values and nursing responsibilities.

WOUNDS

A disruption in the integrity of body tissue is called a **wound**.

Physiology of Wound Healing

When an injury is sustained, a complex set of responses is set into motion, and the body begins a three-phase process of wound healing. Understanding these physiological responses will assist the nurse in caring for clients with impaired skin integrity and promoting optimal wound healing.

Defensive (Inflammatory) Phase

The defensive phase occurs immediately after injury and lasts about 3 to 4 days. The major events that

Table 21–3 COMMON DIAGNOSTIC TESTS FOR INTEGUMENTARY DISORDERS

Biopsy
Patch testing
Tzanck smear
Immunofluorescence (IF testing)
Wood's light examination
Skin scrapings
Culture and sensitivity

occur in this phase are hemostasis and inflammation. **Hemostasis**, or cessation of bleeding, occurs by vasoconstriction of large blood vessels in the affected area. Platelets, activated by the injury, aggregate to form a platelet plug and stop the bleeding. Activation of the clotting cascade results in the eventual formation of fibrin and a fibrinous meshwork, which further entraps platelets and other cells. The result is fibrin clot formation, which provides initial wound closure, prevents excessive loss of blood and body fluids, and inhibits contamination of the wound by microorganisms.

Inflammation is the body's defensive adaptation to tissue injury and involves both vascular and cellular responses. During the vascular response, tissue injury and activation of plasma protein systems stimulate the release of various chemical mediators, such as histamine (from mast cells), serotonin (from platelets), complement, and kinins. These vasoactive substances cause blood vessels to dilate and become more permeable, resulting in increased blood flow and leakage of serous fluid into the surrounding tissues. The increased blood supply carries nutrients and oxygen, which are essential for wound healing, and transports leukocytes to the area to participate in phagocytosis, or the envelopment and disposal of microorganisms. The increased blood supply also removes the "debris of battle," which includes dead cells, bacteria, and exudate, or material and cells discharged from blood vessels. The area is red, edematous, and warm to touch, and it has varying amounts of exudate.

During the cellular response, leukocytes move out of the blood vessel into the interstitial space. Neutrophils are the first cells to arrive at the injured site and begin phagocytosis. They subsequently die and are replaced by macrophages, which arise from blood monocytes. Macrophages perform the same function as neutrophils but remain for a longer time. In addition to being the primary phagocyte of debridement, macrophages are important cells in wound healing because they secrete several factors, including fibroblast activating factor (FAF) and angiogenesis factor (AGF). FAF attracts fibroblasts, which form collagen or collagen precursors. AGF stimulates the formation of new blood vessels. The development of this new microcirculation supports and sustains the wound and the healing process.

Reconstructive (Proliferative) Phase

The reconstructive phase begins on the third or fourth day after injury and lasts for 2 to 3 weeks. This phase contains the process of collagen deposition, angiogenesis, granulation tissue development, and wound contraction.

Fibroblasts, normally found in connective tissue, migrate into the wound because of various cellular mediators. They are the most important cells in this phase because they synthesize and secrete collagen. Collagen is the most abundant protein in the body and is the material of tissue repair. Initially, collagen is gel-like, but within several months it cross-links to form collagen fibrils and adds tensile strength to the wound. As the wound gains strength, the risk of wound separation or rupture is less likely. The wound can resist normal stress such as tension or twisting after 15 to 20 days. During this time, a raised "healing ridge" may be visible under the injury or suture line.

Angiogenesis (formation of new blood vessels) begins within hours after the injury. The endothelial cells in preexisting vessels begin to produce enzymes that break down the basement membrane. The membrane opens, and new endothelial cells build a new vessel. These capillaries grow across the wound, increasing blood flow, which increases the supply of nutrients and oxygen needed for wound healing.

Repair begins as granulation tissue, or new tissue, grows inward from surrounding healthy connective tissue. Granulation tissue is filled with new capillaries that are fragile and bleed easily, thus giving the healing area a red, translucent, granular appearance. As granulation tissue is formed, epithelialization, or growth of epithelial tissue, begins. Epithelial cells migrate into the wound from the wound margins. Eventually, the migrating cells contact similar cells that have migrated from the outer edges. Contact stops migration. The cells then begin to differentiate into the various cells that comprise the different layers of epidermis.

Wound contraction is the final step of the reconstructive phase of wound healing. Contraction is noticeable 6 to 12 days after injury and is necessary for closure of all wounds. The edges of the wound are drawn together by the action of myofibroblasts, specialized cells that contain bundles of parallel fibers in their cytoplasm. These myofibroblasts bridge across a wound and then contract to pull the wound closed.

Maturation Phase

Maturation, the final stage of healing, begins about the 21st day and may continue for up to 2 years or more, depending on the depth and extent of the wound. During this phase, the scar tissue is remodeled (reshaped or reconstructed by collagen deposition and lysis and debridement of wound edges). Although the scar tissue continues to gain strength, it remains weaker than the tissue it replaces. Capillaries eventually disappear, leaving an avascular scar (a scar that is white because it lacks a blood supply).

Types of Healing

Tissue may heal by one of three methods, which are characterized by the degree of tissue loss. Primary intention healing occurs in wounds that have minimal tissue loss and edges that are well-approximated (closed). If there are no complications, such as infection, necrosis, or abnormal scar formation, wound healing occurs with minimal granulation tissue and scarring.

Secondary intention healing is seen in wounds with extensive tissue loss and wounds in which the edges cannot be approximated. The wound is left open, and granulation tissue gradually fills in the deficit. Repair time is longer, tissue replacement and scarring are greater, and the susceptibility to infection is increased because of the lack of an epidermal barrier to microorganisms.

Tertiary intention healing, also known as delayed or secondary closure, is indicated when primary closure of a wound is undesirable. Conditions in which healing by tertiary intention may occur include poor circulation or infection. Suturing of the wound is delayed until the problems resolve and more favorable conditions exist for wound healing.

Kinds of Wound Drainage

Chemical mediators released during the inflammatory response cause vascular changes and exudation of fluid and cells from blood vessels into tissues. Exudates may vary in composition, but all have similar functions. These functions include the following:

- Dilution of toxins produced by bacteria and dying cells
- Transport of leukocytes and plasma proteins, including antibodies, to the site
- Transport of bacterial toxins, dead cells, debris, and other products of inflammation away from the site

The nature and amount of exudate vary depending on the tissue involved, the intensity and duration of the inflammation, and the presence of microorganisms.

Serous exudate is composed primarily of serum (the clear portion of blood), is watery in appearance, and has a low protein level. This type of exudate is seen with mild inflammation resulting in minimal capillary permeability changes and minimal protein molecule escape (e.g., seen in blister formation after a burn).

Purulent exudate is also called pus. It generally occurs with severe inflammation accompanied by infection. Purulent exudate is thicker than serous exudate because of the presence of leukocytes (particularly neutrophils), liquefied dead tissue debris, and dead and living bacteria. The process of pus formation is called suppuration, and bacteria that produce pus are referred to as pyogenic bacteria. Purulent exudates may vary in color (e.g., yellow, green, brown) depending on the causative organism.

Hemorrhagic exudate has a large component of red blood cells (RBCs) due to capillary damage, which allows RBCs to escape. This type of exudate is usually present with severe inflammation. The color of the exudate (bright red versus dark red) reflects whether the bleeding is fresh or old.

Mixed types of exudates may also be seen, depending on the type of wound. For example, a **serosanguineous exudate** is clear with some blood tinge and is seen with surgical incisions.

Factors Affecting Wound Healing

Wound healing is dependent on multiple influences, both intrinsic and extrinsic. Wounds may fail to heal or may require a longer healing period when unfavorable conditions exist. Factors that may negatively influence healing include age, oxygenation, smoking, drug therapy, and diseases such as diabetes. Such factors reduce local blood supply and, therefore, impair wound healing. Nutrition and diet can also affect the healing process.

Hemorrhage

Some bleeding from a wound is normal during and immediately after initial trauma and surgery, but hemostasis usually occurs within a few minutes. Hemorrhage (persistent bleeding) is abnormal and may indicate a slipped surgical suture, a dislodged clot, or erosion of a blood vessel. Swelling in the area around the wound or affected body part and the presence of sanguineous drainage from the surgical drain may indicate internal bleeding. Other evidence of bleeding may include the signs and symptoms seen in hypovolemic shock (decreased blood pressure, rapid thready pulse, increased respiratory rate, diaphoresis, restlessness, and cool clammy skin). A hematoma (localized collection of blood underneath the tissues) may also be seen and appears as a reddish-blue swelling or mass. External hemorrhaging is detected when the surgical dressing becomes saturated with sanguineous drainage. It is also important to assess the linen under the client's wound site because it is possible for the blood to seep out from under the sides of the dressing and pool under the client. The risk for hemorrhage is greatest during the first 24 to 48 hours after surgery.

Infection

Bacterial wound contamination is one of the most common causes of altered wound healing. A wound can become infected with microorganisms preoperatively, intraoperatively, or postoperatively. During the preoperative period, the wound may become exposed to pathogens because of the manner in which the wound was inflicted, such as in traumatic injuries. Nicks or abrasions created during preoperative shaving may also be a source of pathogens. The risk for intraoperative exposure to pathogens increases when the respiratory, gastrointestinal, genitourinary, and oropharyngeal tracts are opened.

If the amount of bacteria in the wound is sufficient or the client's immune defenses are compromised, clinical infection may result and become apparent 2 to 11 days postoperatively. Infection slows healing by prolonging the inflammatory phase of healing, competing for nutrients, and producing chemicals and enzymes that are damaging to the tissues.

Wound Classification

Many different classification systems are used to describe wounds. These systems describe either how the wound was acquired, how clean it is, or which tissue layers are involved. A classification system will assist the nurse in planning wound care management. The following are commonly used classification systems.

Cause of Wound

Intentional wounds occur during treatment or therapy. These wounds are usually made under aseptic conditions. Examples include surgical incisions and venipunctures.

Unintentional wounds are unanticipated and are often the result of trauma or an accident. These wounds are created in an unsterile environment and therefore pose a greater risk of infection.

Cleanliness of Wound

This classification system ranks the wound according to its contamination by bacteria and risk for infection (Schwartz, Shires, & Spencer, 1994).

- *Clean wounds* are intentional wounds that were created under conditions in which no inflammation was encountered and the respiratory, alimentary, genitourinary, and oropharyngeal tracts were not entered.
- *Clean-contaminated wounds* are intentional wounds that were created by entry into the alimentary, respiratory, genitourinary, or oropharyngeal tract under controlled conditions.
- *Contaminated wounds* are open, traumatic wounds or intentional wounds in which there was a major break in aseptic technique, spillage from the gastrointestinal tract, or incision into infected urinary or biliary tracts. These wounds have acute nonpurulent inflammation present.
- *Dirty and infected wounds* are traumatic wounds with retained dead tissue or foreign material or intentional wounds created in situations where purulent drainage was present.

Depth of Wound

The third classification system is based on the depth of the wound, taking into account the skin layers involved.

- *Superficial wounds* are confined to the epidermis layer, which comprises the four outermost layers of skin.
- *Partial-thickness wounds* involve the epidermis and part of the dermis, which is the layer of skin beneath the epidermis.
- *Full-thickness wounds* involve the entire epidermis and dermis. Deeper structures such as fascia, muscle, and bone may be involved.

Assessment

Nurses are confronted with wounds that are extremely diverse. The wound may have occurred traumatically just before the client presents to the emergency room, or the wound may be a slow-healing chronic ulcer. Despite all this diversity, the nurse should approach assessment of the wound in a systematic manner, evaluating the wound's stage in the healing process. The nurse also needs to show sensitivity to the client's pain and tolerance levels during assessment and must always follow Standard Precautions to prevent transfer of pathogens. Following are some basic criteria for wound assessment.

Location

Assessment begins with a description of the anatomical location of the wound, for example, "5-inch suture line on the right lower quadrant of the abdomen." This task often becomes difficult if the client has multiple wounds close to each other, as is common in burn or multiple trauma victims. Use of a skin documentation form that incorporates drawings of the body (Figure 21-8) allows the nurse to draw circles and write numbers to depict the location of the various wounds.

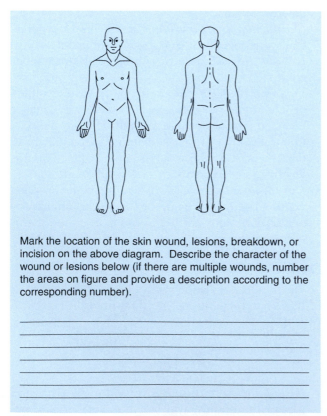

Mark the location of the skin wound, lesions, breakdown, or incision on the above diagram. Describe the character of the wound or lesions below (if there are multiple wounds, number the areas on figure and provide a description according to the corresponding number).

_____
_____
_____
_____
_____
_____
_____

Figure 21-8 Documenting Location and Character of Wounds *(From* Fundamentals of Nursing: Standards & Practice, *by S. DeLaune and P. Ladner, 1998, Albany, NY: Delmar. Copyright 1998 by Delmar. Reprinted with permission.)*

Size

The length (head to toe), width (side to side), and depth of a wound are measured in centimeters. Single-use measurement guides (tape measures) often come with dressing supplies. To determine the depth of a wound, a sterile cotton swab is inserted into the deepest point of the wound and marked at the skin surface level. Then the swab can be measured and the wound depth in centimeters documented. Tunneling, also called undermining, can be measured by using a cotton swab to gently probe the wound margins. If tunneling is noted, the location and depth are documented. For clarity in describing the location of the tunneling, the hands of the clock can be used as a guide, with 12 o'clock pointing at the client's head. Example: "Tunneling occurs at 1 o'clock and its depth is 2 cm."

For extremely irregularly shaped wounds, the wound edges can be traced on a plastic surface. A plastic bag or piece of plastic sheeting folded in half is placed on the wound, and the wound margins are traced. The side of the plastic that has been placed against the skin is cut off and discarded. The rest of the plastic can be placed in the chart.

General Appearance and Drainage

A general description of the color of the wound and surrounding area helps to determine the wound's present phase of healing. The edges of the wound should be gently palpated for swelling, and the amount, color, location, odor, and consistency of any drainage documented.

Pain

The nurse should document and notify the physician of any pain or tenderness at the wound site. Pain may indicate infection or bleeding. It is normal to experience pain at the incision site of a surgical wound for approximately 3 days. If there is any sudden increase in pain accompanied by changes in the appearance of the wound, the physician must be notified immediately.

Laboratory Data

Cultures of the wound drainage are used to determine the presence of infection and the identity of the causative organism. The sensitivity results list the antibiotics that will effectively treat the infection. An elevated WBC count is indicative of an infectious process. A decreased leukocyte count may indicate that the client is at increased risk for developing an infection related to decreased defense mechanisms. Albumin is a measure of the client's protein reserves; if the albumin is decreased, the client will have decreased resources of protein for wound healing.

Nursing Diagnoses

Nursing diagnoses for clients with wounds focus on prevention of complications and promotion of the healing process through proper wound care and client teaching. Following are NANDA-approved nursing diagnoses with a partial list of related factors:

- *Impaired Tissue Integrity related to surgical incision, pressure, shearing forces, decreased blood flow, immobility, mechanical irritants*
- *Risk for Infection related to malnutrition, decreased defense mechanisms*
- *Acute Pain related to inflammation, infection*
- *Disturbed Body Image related to changes in body appearance secondary to scars, drains, removal of body parts*
- *Deficient Knowledge (wound care) related to lack of exposure to information, misinterpretation, lack of interest in learning*

Planning/Outcome Identification

After identifying the nursing diagnoses, the nurse establishes targeted outcomes for wound healing based on the client's identified needs and individualized to the client's condition. Changes in the health care delivery system have brought about early discharge from the hospital, so clients are often sent home with wounds that need continued care; the goals for clients with wounds generally focus on promoting wound healing, preventing infection, and educating the client.

Implementation

Nursing interventions to promote wound healing and prevent infection include emergency measures to maintain homeostasis (state of internal constancy of the body), and cleansing and dressing of the wound.

Emergency Measures

The nurse assesses the type and extent of injury that the client has sustained. If hemorrhage is detected, sterile dressings and pressure should be applied to stop the bleeding, and the physician notified immediately. Standard Precautions are always implemented. The client's vital signs should be monitored frequently.

When dehiscence or evisceration occurs, the client should be instructed to remain quiet and to avoid coughing or straining. The client should be positioned to prevent further stress on the wound. Sterile dressings, such as ABD pads soaked with sterile normal saline, should be used to cover the wound and internal contents. This will reduce the risk of bacterial contamination and drying of the viscera. The surgeon should be notified immediately and the client prepared for surgical repair of the area.

Cleansing the Wound

The goal of cleansing the wound is to remove debris and bacteria from the wound bed with as little trauma to the healthy granulation tissue as possible.

PROFESSIONAL TIP

Wound Cleansing

Following are the major principles to keep in mind when cleansing a wound:

- Use Standard Precautions at all times.
- When using a swab or gauze to cleanse a wound, work from the clean area out toward the dirtier area. For example, when cleaning a surgical incision, start over the incision line, and swab downward from top to bottom. Change the swab and proceed again on either side of the incision, using a new swab each time.
- When irrigating a wound, warm the solution to room temperature, preferably to body temperature, to prevent lowering of the tissue temperature. Be sure to allow the irrigant to flow from the cleanest area to the contaminated area to avoid spreading pathogens.

Choice of cleansing agent depends on the physician's prescription as well as agency protocol. It is recommended that isotonic solutions such as normal saline or lactated Ringer's be used to preserve healthy tissue.

Dressing the Wound

Following are the three purposes of a wound dressing:

1. To keep the wound moist and therefore enhance epithelialization
2. To clean the wound or keep it clean
3. To protect the wound from physical trauma or bacterial invasion

Keeping these three purposes in mind, an appropriate dressing for the client's wound is determined. There are thousands of different wound care products on the market. The physician may prescribe a specific dressing, or agency policy is followed. It is important to remember that the dressing plans must be modified as the wound changes.

Monitoring Drainage of Wounds

During the inflammatory response, exudates develop within a wound. When excessive drainage accumulates in the wound bed, tissue healing is delayed. If the outer surface is allowed to heal while the drainage remains entrapped within the wound, infection and abscess formation may occur. To facilitate drainage of any excess fluid, the physician may insert a tube or drain.

Evaluation

The nurse needs to evaluate the client's achievement of the goals established during the planning phase to achieve or maintain skin integrity. Goals for clients with wounds generally focus on wound healing, prevention of infection, and client education. If the goals are not achieved, the nurse will need to examine the nursing interventions and strategies that were employed and revise the nursing care plan accordingly. Reviewing techniques and procedures, especially those performed by the client or other caregivers in the client's support system, is especially important.

BURNS

Burns are among the most devastating injuries that an individual can suffer. Burns can be painful and disfiguring, requiring long hospitalizations. Many are fatal. Most accidental burns occur in the home and are preventable. Frequently, the burn injury is the result of the individual's own action. Feelings of anger and guilt can complicate recovery. Often the individual suffers self-image disturbances, and family relationships can be strained.

Major Causes

There are many different causes for burns to the skin. A major source of burn injury for all ages is overexposure to the sun. The greatest number of burn injuries to adults are associated with cigarette smoking and cooking. The elderly are more likely to suffer burns by spilling hot liquid on themselves or by catching their clothes on fire as they cook or smoke. Young children are especially prone to burn injuries from spilling scalding liquids on themselves and playing with matches or cigarette lighters. Industrial accidents account for a significant number of burn injuries in young adults.

Severity

Burns are classified according to the depth of the burn and the extent of skin surface involved. First- and second-degree burns are partial-thickness (within the epidermis/dermis) burns. First-degree burns involve only the epidermis. The skin is hot, red, and painful. A sunburn is an example of a first-degree burn. First-degree burns heal in about a week without scarring. Second-degree burns damage the dermis and the epidermis. The skin is red, hot, and painful; blisters form and tissue around the burn is edematous, or swollen, with an excessive amount of fluid. An example of a second-degree burn is spilling boiling water on the skin. Usually, second-degree burns heal in about 2 weeks without scarring. However, if deep layers of the dermis are involved, healing might take months and scarring can occur. Second-degree burns involving deep layers of the dermis may appear white, tan, or red in color.

When the dermis and epidermis are completely destroyed and deeper tissues are involved, burns are classified as full-thickness burns. Third-degree and fourth-degree burns are full-thickness burns. In third-degree burns all dermal structures are destroyed and cannot be regenerated. Subcutaneous tissue is also damaged. Full-thickness burns can be white, tan, brown, black, charred, or bright red in color. Fourth-degree burns, which extend to the underlying muscles and bones, appear white to black or charred with dark networks of thrombosed capillaries visible inside the wound. Fourth-degree burns result from fires, explosions, and nuclear radiation. Figure 21-9 depicts the various layers of skin involved in burn injuries.

Severely burned individuals generally have both partial-thickness and full-thickness burns. While first- and second-degree burns are painful, third- and fourth-degree burns themselves are not painful because of the destruction of sensory nerve endings. The client, however, will still be in severe pain. Body movement causes pain in areas of first- and second-degree burns that often surround the full-thickness burns. Skin can regenerate only from the edges of full-thickness burns. Scarring is inevitable. Skin grafting is necessary to promote healing because the section of skin destroyed by the burn cannot regenerate itself.

Prognosis in burn cases depends upon the severity of the burn, the surface area of the body burned, and the preinjury health status of the individual. If the client's health status before the burn was good, a burn covering 40% of the body will require a minimum of 40 days to heal (Fritsch & Yurko, 1995). Elderly burn victims whose physiologic reserves are already reduced as an effect of aging will have an extended recovery period and a greater risk of complications.

Documenting the extent of the burn injury can be done by using a burn assessment chart such as the Rule-of-Nines method (Ogden, 1998). The Rule-of-Nines method of estimating the body surface area burned is used for adults. The body is divided into areas that are about 9% (or multiples of 9%). The head comprises 9% (4.5% anterior and 4.5% posterior). Each arm is 9% (4.5% anterior and 4.5% posterior). The anterior trunk and posterior trunk are each 18%. Each leg is 18% (9% anterior and 9% posterior). The genitalia comprise the remaining 1% (Figure 21-10).

Complications

Destruction of the skin renders it unable to fulfill its functions. Vast amounts of internal fluids and electrolytes are lost. The ability to maintain body temperature is altered, and the individual is susceptible to serious infections. Initially the complications that are the most life threatening are respiratory failure and massive loss of body fluids.

Figure 21-9 Skin Layers Involved in Burn Injuries: A. First-degree burn; B. Second-degree burn; C. Third-degree burn; D. Fourth-degree burn *(Photos courtesy of the Phoenix Society for Burn Survivors, Inc.)*

Smoke Inhalation and Carbon Monoxide Poisoning

Heat and smoke can cause serious damage to the respiratory tract. Facial burns, singed nasal hairs, and carbon-tinged sputum are signs that the client may have suffered respiratory tract damage (Ogden, 1998).

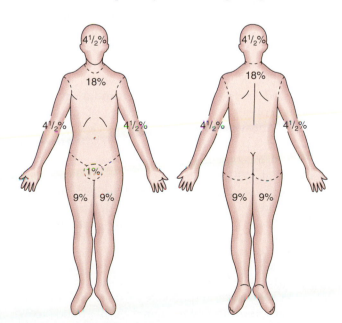

Figure 21-10 Rule-of-Nines

Inhaling heat and smoke in a closed-space fire causes airway inflammation and edema of the respiratory mucosa. The carbon monoxide that is inhaled along with the heat and smoke attaches to hemoglobin, forming the compound, carboxyhemoglobin. A high level of carboxyhemoglobin in the blood means that oxygen is not being delivered to vital body tissues. The client may be stuporous because of cerebral anoxia. Keeping an open airway and administering 100% humidified oxygen are essential for treating these two conditions. Intubation is often necessary.

Shock

Severely burned clients may suffer both hypovolemic shock (a life-threatening condition caused by massive loss of blood and circulating fluids) and neurogenic shock (a form of shock that occurs when peripheral vascular dilation occurs causing hypotension). Fluids and electrolytes must be replaced as fast as they are being lost. Tremendous amounts of fluids are lost through the burn wounds themselves as well as into surrounding tissues in the form of edema. The fluid loss shock that results can lead to circulatory collapse and renal shutdown. Using the Rule-of-Nines to assess the extent of the burn can be helpful in guiding fluid replacement. Expect at least two large-bore venous catheters to give large volumes of fluid rapidly.

Infection

Once the client has been stabilized, infection poses a serious risk. *Staphylococcus aureus,* an ever-present organism in the environment, is a common cause of infections. Of grave concern is an infection caused by methicillin-resistant *Staphylococcus aureus* (MRSA) because this strain of staphylococcus is resistant to all antibiotics except vancomycin hydrochloride (Vancocin). This antibiotic has serious side effects, especially to the otic nerve and to the liver, and is used only when other antibiotics fail.

All persons coming into contact with the burn client must wear gowns, gloves, masks, and caps to help prevent the introduction of organisms such as *Staphylococcus aureus, Pseudomonas aeruginosa,* or coliform bacilli into burn wounds. Sterile technique is used for wound care and dressing changes. Care of severely burned clients in special burn units reduces the chance of infection because of stringent infection control precautions and a carefully controlled environment.

Medical–Surgical Management

Medical

Immediate Care Initially, medical management of the client involves keeping an open airway, maintaining an adequate level of oxygenation, replacing body fluids and electrolytes, monitoring kidney function, controlling pain, and protecting the burns with sterile dressings to minimize the loss of body temperature and the risk of infection. In cases of severe burns, the client usually requires endotracheal intubation and administration of 100% humidified oxygen. A multiport central venous catheter or two large-bore peripheral venous catheters are needed for fluid and electrolyte replacement. A Foley catheter is used and urine output measured hourly to help monitor kidney function.

Pain can be controlled with small intravenous doses of narcotics. Emotional and psychological trauma can intensify pain perception. The client will be anxious, not only for his survival but also about his physical appearance and the effect this injury will have on his family. Prophylactically the client receives tetanus toxoid.

Stabilized Care Once the client's condition has been stabilized, care focuses on promoting healing, preventing complications, controlling pain, and restoring function. During the recovery phase, preventing infection is an important priority. Burn wounds may require daily cleansing and dressing changes. Because of the nature of the injury, burn wounds contain a large amount of dead tissue along with fluids and proteins, making them highly susceptible to infection even with the best of care. Antibiotics and strict aseptic technique are essential. The dead tissue of full-thickness burns forms a dry, dark leathery **eschar** (a scab of denatured protein) within 48 to 72 hours. Infection can

often begin under the eschar, causing tissue sloughing. Loose eschar must be **debrided** before skin grafting can occur. Debriding, removing dead and damaged tissue or foreign material within the burn wound, can sometimes be done mechanically by hydrotherapy, either by submersion in a whirlpool bath or by placing the client on a spray table and directly spraying the wound with a hose system that controls both the force and the temperature of the solution (Fritsch & Yurko, 1995). Burn wounds may require surgical debridement. The base of the wound must be free of infection and necrotic tissue before it can be covered with skin grafts.

Infection Control: Debridement
Strict aseptic techniques must be followed during burn debridement procedures.

Use of specialty beds such as fluidized or alternating air-filled mattresses minimizes pressure on skin surfaces, thus promoting comfort. Limiting movement and maintaining normal body alignment with the use of splints can also help alleviate client discomfort.

Surgical

Skin grafts cover the burn wound to promote healing. Four types of skin grafts might be used:

1. Autograft—the client's own skin that is removed from an unburned area and applied to the wound
2. Homograft—skin obtained from a cadaver within 6 to 24 hours after death
3. Heterograft—skin obtained from an animal, such as a pig
4. Synthetic skin substitute—a man-made product that has properties similar to skin (Fritsch & Yurko, 1995)

Homografts, heterografts, and synthetic skin substitutes are temporary grafts that facilitate healing. These grafts prevent water, electrolyte, and protein loss. They decrease pain and allow more freedom of movement for the client. When the client's condition is stable and the wound beds have healthy **granulation tissue** (delicate connective tissue consisting of fibroblasts, collagen, and capillaries), permanent closure of the burn wounds is done with autographs. Granulation tissue is red in color and provides a base for healing (Seeley et al., 1995).

Autografts are taken from areas of healthy skin. They may be either split-thickness grafts or full-thickness grafts. Split-thickness grafts include the epidermis and part of the dermis. They are not so deep as to prevent regeneration of skin at the donor site.

Infection Control: Skin Grafts
Follow strict aseptic care of both the donor sites and the newly grafted burn wounds to prevent infection.

The application of pressure dressings during the rehabilitative phase reduces the development of hypertrophic scarring, a condition in which the scar becomes elevated and has a "Swiss cheese" appearance (Beare & Myers, 1998). Pressure dressings, which may be elastic wraps, stockinettes, or custom-made pressure garments, must be worn constantly and are to be removed only for daily hygiene care. Full maturation of the burn scar may take 1 to 2 years. As the physical wounds heal, so do the emotional and psychological wounds. The client's ability to cope with daily stresses and resume social and work activities typically coincides with the physical healing process.

Pharmacological

Dressing changes, wound debridement, as well as any movement or manipulation are extremely painful for clients. Many clients become extremely anxious, fearing pain as well as permanent disfiguration and loss of function. Intravenous narcotics, usually morphine, may be administered 10 to 15 minutes prior to procedures. By decreasing anxiety and fear, daily doses of psychotropic drugs can enhance the effectiveness of pain medications and help the client cope with the prospect of long-term rehabilitation.

Treatment of the burn wound with topical agents can decrease infection and promote healing. Common topical agents used are mafenide acetate (Sulfamylon); silver sulfadiazine (Silvadene); povidone-iodine (Betadine); nitrofurazone (Furacin); and antibiotic agents such as neomycin sulfate (Myciguent), bacitracin (Baciguent), and gentamicin sulfate (Garamycin). Mafenide acetate (Sulfamylon) can penetrate thick eschar and is effective against gram-negative and gram-positive organisms, including *Pseudomonas aeruginosa*. Silver sulfadiazine (Silvadene) is effective against many gram-positive and gram-negative organisms as well as *Candida* organisms. It is painless and somewhat soothing but may cause a skin rash. Povidone-iodine (Betadine) has broad-spectrum microbial action against a wide variety of bacteria, fungi, yeasts, viruses, and protozoa. Application of povidone-iodine to large open areas could lead to elevated serum iodine levels. Nitrofurazone (Furacin) has broad-spectrum activity and is effective against *Staphylococcus aureus*. It is not absorbed systemically and has a low incidence of sensitivity.

Antibiotic ointments are used to decrease infection. Neomycin sulfate (Myciguent) and gentamicin sulfate (Garamycin) can be absorbed systemically and have serious side effects of ototoxicity and nephrotoxicity. Bacitracin (Baciguent) has minimal antimicrobial activity, but it is especially useful to prevent drying of the wound. Topical agents must be applied in a thin layer with a sterile glove. The wound may be left open to air or covered with a gauze dressing, depending on the properties of the medication and the physician's orders. Application of these medications can be painful

PROFESSIONAL TIP

Silver Nitrate Therapy

Silver nitrate therapy, commonly used in the past, is prescribed less often now. Silver nitrate has bacteriostatic effects, lessens pain, and reduces odor, but the dressings must be kept constantly wet. The procedure for dressing changes is involved and painful. Silver nitrate also stains dark purple everything it touches (Fritsch & Yurko, 1995).

because of manipulation of the burned tissue. Administration of pain medication may be necessary before providing wound care. The surrounding skin should be assessed for any allergic rashes.

Diet

Following a moderate to severe burn, the need for calories and protein increases. Actual protein loss occurs with the burn injury itself. Additionally, some protein is metabolized to meet the increased energy requirements brought on by stress. For tissue repair and healing to occur, daily protein needs may increase by 2 to 4 times the normal daily protein requirement (Fritsch & Yurko, 1995). Twice the normal caloric requirement may be needed to meet the body's energy needs. Supplemental vitamins and minerals are also given.

Initially, the client's daily nutritional needs may be met with total parenteral nutrition (TPN) because of a paralytic ileus and gastric dilation. Following a severe burn, decreased enteric circulation leads to slowed or stopped peristalsis. Food and fluids cannot be given orally or by tube feeding until peristalsis is restored. Hearing active bowel sounds is one indication of peristaltic activity in the bowel. Immobility, stress, and the negative nitrogen balance brought on by protein catabolism depress appetite. Meeting the client's nutritional needs can be a challenge. Six to 8 small feedings daily and high-protein milk shakes or protein supplements can help meet daily nutritional needs. Involving the family in bringing in favorite foods can also stimulate the client's appetite.

PROFESSIONAL TIP

Serving Meals

Serve foods attractively and put an occasional small "surprise" on the tray (e.g., a flower, a small, brightly colored seasonal decoration, a funny card) so that the client will look forward to meals.

Activity

Contractures are among the most serious complications of severe burns. They can be prevented with a program of positioning, splinting, exercising, and ambulating. When repositioning, the client's body must be kept in correct alignment. Pillows can be used to keep limbs in alignment. Splints can be used on limbs to prevent contractures or to immobilize joints following skin grafting. Range-of-motion exercises maintain joint mobility. Whenever possible, active rather than passive range-of-motion exercises should be encouraged. Active exercise increases circulation, maintains joint flexibility, and improves muscle tone. As the client recovers, activities of daily living can be increased and ambulation can be initiated.

▶ NURSING PROCESS

▶ Assessment

▶ Subjective Data

Emotional status needs to be assessed. Clients with burns are likely to be frightened and anxious. Feelings of guilt, anger, and depression are also common following burns. Nonverbal behavior such as grimacing should be noted. The client should be asked to describe the pain according to location, intensity, and duration, and also to rate the pain on a scale of 0 to 10. Hypoxia or fluid and electrolyte imbalances can cause confusion, disorientation, and decreased level of consciousness. The client may be nauseated.

▶ Objective Data

Vital signs, level of consciousness, and breath sounds should be assessed. If the client has a productive cough, the amount and color of sputum should be noted. Black/gray sputum indicates smoke inhalation. Clients suffering from smoke inhalation may also have crackles, wheezing, or diminished breath sounds. Burn wounds should be observed for signs of infection such as redness, swelling, purulent drainage, and a foul odor. Urine output must be measured hourly. Intake and output and daily weight must be monitored. Bowel sounds and vomiting should be checked. As rehabilitation progresses, the nurse must continue to assess wounds for signs of healing such as a moist, clean, red wound base and decrease in the size of the wound. The client's mobility status and degree of involvement in care should be noted. Daily dietary intake should be assessed. Laboratory test results need to be monitored:

GERONTOLOGICAL CONSIDERATIONS

Burn Injuries in the Elderly

- Normal physiologic changes that occur with aging delay recovery and put the older adult at greater risk for complications following a burn injury.
- As a person ages, the physiologic reserves of organ systems decrease.
- While the older person may have adequate pulmonary and cardiac functions at rest, the stress of a severe burn can leave the body unable to cope with demands for increased oxygen and increased cardiac output.
- Renal changes that occur with aging, such as decreased renal blood flow, fewer nephrons, and a decreased glomerular filtration rate, put the older adult at higher risk for kidney failure following a severe burn.
- With loss of subcutaneous tissue and decreased secretion of sebum, the older person's skin is normally more fragile.
- Circulation, especially in the lower extremities, may already be compromised, so healing will be delayed.
- Skin grafting procedures may not be successful because of impaired circulation and impaired tissue nutrition.

- Red blood cell count and hemoglobin level give information about the body's ability to meet oxygen demands of body tissues and organs.
- Creatinine and blood urea nitrogen as well as the specific gravity of the urine give information about kidney function.
- Total protein and albumin levels yield information about the ability to maintain the volume of circulating fluid as well as information about nutritional status.
- White blood cell count indicates the presence of infection and the body's ability to fight it.
- Wound culture and sensitivity data indicate the specific organisms causing infection and the specific antibiotics that are effective against these organisms.
- Electrolytes yield information about the homeostasis of body fluids. Alterations in pH and electrolyte levels affect cell function in every body tissue, particularly vital body organs such as the heart and cerebrum.

Nursing diagnoses for a client with a burn injury may include the following. Initially, the greatest dangers to the client will be:

Nursing Diagnoses	Planning/Goals	Nursing Interventions
▶ *Impaired Gas Exchange related to edema and inflammation of the respiratory tract*	The client will achieve a regular respiratory pattern and oxygen saturation level >90%.	Monitor the client's vital signs every 4 hours if stable; otherwise, every 1 to 2 hours.
		Listen to breath sounds, especially noting respiratory pattern and effort.
		If the client is on continuous oximetry, note the oxygen saturation reading each time vital signs are assessed.
		Assess the client's color and level of consciousness.
		Document assessments and keep the physician informed about the client's condition.
		Elevate the head of the bed 30° to facilitate full chest expansion with each breath.
▶ *Deficient Fluid Volume related to increased capillary permeability with loss of large amounts of fluid through open burn wounds*	The client will maintain electrolytes within normal limits and an hourly urine output >30 mL per hour.	Administer intravenous fluids at the ordered rate.
		Monitor for signs and symptoms of fluid overload such as shortness of breath, crackles auscultated in lung bases, changes in heart rate and/or heart sounds, changes in blood pressure, increased anxiety, or changes in mental status.
		Measure urine output hourly, report outputs below 30 mL to the physician.
		Record intake and output. Involve the client and family in keeping a bedside record of fluid intake.
		Weigh client daily, preferably before breakfast, and in the same type of clothing each day.
		When the client can tolerate oral fluids, set a fluid intake goal for each shift (e.g., 1,200 mL during the day; 800 mL during the evening; 500 mL during the night).
		Explain to the client and family the reasons for a high fluid intake.
		Involve family members in helping the client achieve the fluid maintenance goal.
		Keep fluids available at the bedside, including within dietary restrictions, the client's favorite fluids.
		Monitor for signs and symptoms of electrolyte imbalances such as increased muscle weakness, muscle cramps, cardiac arrhythmias, fatigue, nausea, dizziness.
		Monitor the client's laboratory results.

During the stabilization and recovery period following a burn, the nursing diagnoses may include the following:

Nursing Diagnoses	Planning/Goals	Nursing Interventions
▶ *Risk for Infection related to risk factors of tissue destruction and inadequate primary defenses*	The client's burn wounds will exhibit signs of healing without serious or life-threatening infections.	Wear clean gloves when giving client care.
		Wash hands with an antibacterial skin cleanser before and after gloving.
		Wear an isolation gown over your uniform when giving client care.
		Whenever the client's wounds are exposed, wear gown, cap, mask, and sterile gloves.
		Use sterile technique for wound care and dressing changes.
		Monitor wound daily for signs of infection: redness, swelling, purulent drainage, pain.
		Assess for signs of systemic infections.
		Observe for increased pulse and respirations, decreased blood pressure, and fever.
		Observe for any changes in mentation such as disorientation and delirium.
		Note urinary output.
		Assess for hypoactive bowel sounds.

continues

Nursing Diagnoses	Planning/Goals	Nursing Interventions
		Monitor the client's white blood cell count.
		Assist client with personal hygiene, and keep noninjured areas of the body clean.

Other nursing diagnoses common to most clients with burns include the following:

Nursing Diagnoses	Planning/Goals	Nursing Interventions
▶ *Acute Pain related to physical injury*	The client will verbalize that pain is controlled at a tolerable level.	Assess for pain every 2 to 4 hours by asking client to rate pain level on a scale of 0 to 10.
		Observe for nonverbal signs of pain such as grimacing or crying.
		Administer pain medications as ordered, especially prior to wound care or exercise and mobilization activities.
		Monitor and document response to medications.
		Implement comfort and diversional measures:
		a. Reposition client; use pillows or foam supports to keep all body parts in good alignment.
		b. Teach client to use progressive relaxation exercises or to use guided imagery.
		c. Encourage the client to use diversionary activities of his choice such as television or music, or place him so that he can see into the hallway.
▶ *Imbalanced Nutrition: Less than body requirements, related to increased caloric requirements and difficulty ingesting sufficient quantities of food*	The client will ingest sufficient calories daily to meet increased metabolic needs.	If the client is currently on TPN or enteral tube feedings, administer the ordered nutrients at the correct rate and closely monitor the client's reaction.
		When oral intake is tolerated, encourage the client to eat 90% to 100% of daily diet.
		Provide oral hygiene before meals to stimulate salivation and eliminate any bad taste in the client's mouth.
		Give 6 to 8 small feedings daily of the client's favorite foods within dietary restrictions and encourage family members to bring in home-prepared foods and eat with the client.
		When permitted, encourage the client to sit up in a chair for each meal.
		Plan care so that painful procedures are not done immediately before meals. A rest period of 20 to 30 minutes before meals helps the client feel more like eating.
		Determine the time of day when the client feels most like eating and does indeed eat most of the meal, and serve the highest calorie/protein nutrients at that time.
▶ *Impaired Physical Mobility related to pain and decreased muscle strength*	The client will participate in daily activity to maintain joint mobility and prevent contractures.	Perform passive ROM exercises 4 times a day by supporting the limb above and below the joint and performing exercises slowly and smoothly.
		As the client is able, instruct him to perform active ROM exercises every 3 to 4 hours.
		Use small pillows and foam supports to keep the client's body in good alignment.
		Turn and reposition the client every 2 hours.
		Use splints as ordered by the physician to keep hands, wrists, feet, and ankles in natural alignment and explain the reason for these activities to the client.
		As healing and rehabilitation progress, encourage progressive ambulation and self-care activities.
		Gradually guide and assist the client to resume activities of daily living (ADL).
		Encourage family members to participate in ADLs and provide positive reinforcement as the client becomes involved in his care.

continues

Nursing Diagnoses	Planning/Goals	Nursing Interventions
▶ *Disturbed Body Image related to change in physical appearance with loss of body tissues or body parts*	The client will state realistic expectations for recovery and participate in rehabilitation.	Provide time for the client to express feelings (fear, anger, frustration, regret, and depression are commonly expressed by clients with burns) and practice active listening.
		Explain the healing process to the client.
		Give the client daily updates on the degree of wound healing and on his progress in rehabilitation.
		Encourage the client to look at the wounds, to show evidence of healing. Stress that wound healing following serious burn injuries proceeds slowly and that complete healing with improved skin appearance may take a year or more.
▶ *Interrupted Family Processes related to the shift in health status of a family member*	The client and family members will verbalize feelings to nurses and each other and will participate in client care.	Involve family members in the client's care and encourage daily visits.
		Encourage family members to express their fears and concerns, especially any feelings of anger, blame, or guilt.
		Guide family members in recognizing and reflecting to the client small, step-by-step progress that is made.
		Maintain an honest, open approach with the client and family but do not give false reassurance.
		Collaborate with counselor, social worker, and chaplain to help the client and family cope with the condition.
		Assist the family to appraise the situation and plan for discharge. What is at stake? What is realistic for the future? What can they expect during the rehabilitation phase? What are their choices? Where can they get help?

Evaluation Each goal must be evaluated to determine how it has been met by the client.

NEOPLASMS: MALIGNANT

Skin cancer is one of the most common malignant neoplasms in the United States and is the most preventable cancer. Basal cell carcinoma, squamous cell carcinoma, and malignant melanoma are the three most common skin cancers; mycosis fungoides is another type of malignancy. Exposure to the sun is the leading cause of skin cancer. Skin damage from sun exposure is cumulative. The ability of skin to tan is not fully developed until the teenage years, meaning that most of the long-term skin damage from sun exposure occurs during childhood. By age 20, most adults have already experienced significant skin damage; however, it takes 10 to 20 years before unprotected sunbathing results in skin cancer.

BASAL CELL CARCINOMA

Basal cell carcinoma, the most frequent type of skin cancer, arises from the epidermis. Prolonged sun exposure, poor tanning ability, and previous therapy with x-rays for facial acne are associated with basal cell carcinoma (Figure 21-11).

As the disease develops, it extends into the dermis and may form an open ulcer. Surgical removal cures this type of cancer.

SQUAMOUS CELL CARCINOMA

Squamous cell carcinoma appears as a nodular lesion in the epidermis. It is much less common than basal cell carcinoma. Risk factors include prolonged sun exposure and exposure to gamma radiation and x-rays. The sun-exposed lower lip is a common site for squamous cell carcinoma. Without treatment it can extend into the dermis and ultimately metastasize to other body tissues, causing death (Figure 21-12). The

Figure 21-11 Basal Cell Carcinoma *(Courtesy of Robert A. Silverman, MD, Clinical Associate Professor, Department of Pediatrics, Georgetown University)*

Figure 21-12 Squamous Cell Carcinoma *(Courtesy of Robert A. Silverman, MD, Clinical Associate Professor, Department of Pediatrics, Georgetown University)*

lesion may be excised surgically or it may be treated with chemosurgery, which involves application of a dressing with a fixative paste such as zinc chloride. When the dressing is removed, tumor cells trapped in the dressing are removed also. Dressings are reapplied and removed in this fashion until all malignant tissue has been removed (Weaver, 1995).

MALIGNANT MELANOMA

In malignant melanoma, atypical melanocytes are present in both the dermis and epidermis. Malignant melanoma is the most serious of the three types of skin cancers and may begin in a preexisting mole (nevus). These moles have an irregular shape. Contrasted to normal moles, they are larger than 6 mm in diameter and do not have a uniform color. Malignant melanoma can metastasize to every organ in the body through the bloodstream and lymphatic system.

The incidence of malignant melanoma is increasing in the United States as a result of increased sun exposure. Deters (1996) succinctly summarizes the incidence of malignant melanoma: "The incidence is doubling every 10 years. . . . The peak incidence is between 21 and 45 years of age. . . . At present there is no cure." Clearly the best hope of preventing skin cancer lies in education. Limiting sun exposure and using sunscreen products on exposed skin markedly reduce damage from ultraviolet rays and ultimately decrease the risk of skin cancer. Figure 21-13 shows lentigo malignant melanoma.

MYCOSIS FUNGOIDES

Mycosis fungoides, also known as cutaneous T-cell lymphoma, is a malignant disease involving T-helper cells that have both skin manifestations and multiple organ system manifestations. In the early stages it re-

Figure 21-13 Lentigo Malignant Melanoma *(Courtesy of Robert A. Silverman, MD, Clinical Associate Professor, Department of Pediatrics, Georgetown University)*

sembles psoriasis or seborrheic dermatitis. Later, fissures and skin ulcers develop. Pruritus can be severe. Even if the skin condition can be improved with topical steroids and chemotherapeutic agents, the disease is ultimately fatal because of the involvement of vital organ systems (Nicol, 1997). Clients with AIDS can develop mycosis fungoides.

Medical–Surgical Management

Surgical

Electrosurgery, cryosurgery, and surgical excision are the primary methods of treatment for malignant neoplasms. Electrosurgery uses electric current to destroy and remove malignant tissue. It is best used for small lesions 1 to 2 cm in diameter. Cryosurgery destroys tumor tissue by freezing it. A special type of needle apparatus directs liquid nitrogen through the tumor until a temperature of –40° to –60°C is reached at the base of the tumor (Deters, 1996). In addition, regional perfusion chemotherapy can be used to treat malignant melanomas of the extremities. The circulation of the involved extremity is isolated and a high dose of a cytotoxic drug is perfused directly into the tumor area (Deters, 1996). This method of treating just the area of the malignancy minimizes systemic effects of cytotoxic drugs. Because most skin cancers are treated by excision, client teaching and follow-up care focus on proper wound care to promote healing and prevent infection.

Nursing Management

Careful assessment of the client's skin condition can reveal suspicious skin lesions. Clients who have had one skin cancer are likely to have more. Early referral and prompt care can ensure a good prognosis. Clients who have just had skin cancers removed need to be taught good wound care to prevent infection and facilitate healing. Many clients will experience body image disturbance; the nurse will need to help the client cope with this. All other nursing care should be focused on prevention.

NEOPLASMS: NONMALIGNANT

Benign tumors of the skin include a variety of lesions such as skin tags, lipomas, keloids, sebaceous cysts, nevi (moles), and angiomas. In general, they do not require medical or nursing intervention except for cosmetic reasons or unless they are subject to continual irritation that might predispose to a break in skin integrity and infection. **Lipomas** (benign, fatty tumors) or **sebaceous cysts** (distended sebaceous glands filled with sebum) might cause pressure on surrounding nerves or interfere with normal body function. In these instances they would be surgically removed. A **keloid** is abnormal growth of scar tissue that is elevated, rounded, and firm with irregular, clawlike margins. Surgical removal is not always successful; healing following surgery can again result in a keloid. Steroids or radiation have been helpful in some conditions. **Angiomas**, commonly known as birthmarks, are vascular tumors involving skin and subcutaneous tissue. They can be raised, bright red nodular lesions (strawberry birthmarks) or dark red/purple patches (port-wine angiomas). Cosmetics can be used to camouflage them. According to Deters (1996), the argon laser is being used on some angiomas with some success.

INFECTIOUS DISORDERS OF THE SKIN

Given an accessible portal of entry and decreased host resistance, virulent organisms can invade the skin, causing inflammation, infection, itching, and pain. Bacteria, viruses, fungi, or parasites can cause infectious disorders of the skin (Figure 21-14). Treating the client's disease is only one aspect of the treatment plan; preventing the spread of infection is the other. Table 21–4 outlines several disease conditions and identifies the organism responsible, clinical manifestations, and the medical management for each disorder.

▶ NURSING PROCESS

▶ Assessment

▶ Subjective Data

The client should be asked how long the problem has existed, if there is any itching or pain, and what

Figure 21-14 Infectious Disorders of the Skin: A. Impetigo contagiosa; B. Herpes zoster (shingles); C. Herpes simplex type 1; D. Tinea (ringworm); E. Scabies; F. Pediculosis (lice) (A, C, and E courtesy of Robert A. Silverman, MD, Clinical Associate Professor, Department of Pediatrics, Georgetown University; B and D courtesy of the Centers for Disease Control and Prevention, Atlanta, GA; F courtesy of Reed and Carnrick Pharmaceuticals)

Table 21-4 INFECTIOUS DISORDERS OF THE SKIN

DISEASE	ORGANISM	CLINICAL MANIFESTATIONS	MEDICAL MANAGEMENT
Bacterial Infections			
Impetigo contagiosa	*Staphylococcus aureus*	Begins as a small vesicle; becomes a weeping lesion; forms a light brown crust. Usually on the face and upper trunk (Figure 21-14A). More common in children. More common in spring and fall. Poor hygiene coupled with warm weather facilitates the spread of the disease.	Cleanse the affected area at least 3 times a day. Apply an antibiotic ointment. Occasionally, systemic antibiotics are needed.
Carbuncle	*Staphylococcus aureus*	Begins as infected hair follicles in the dermis. Symptoms are redness, swelling, pain. Yellow cores of pus develop. Carbuncles usually occur on the nape of the neck and upper back. Obese or malnourished persons with poor hygiene as well as diabetics are most susceptible to carbuncles.	Warm, moist soaks may help "bring the boil to a head." Once the carbuncle ruptures or is incised and drained, pain subsides. Carbuncles tend to recur. The staphylococcus organism may be resistant to topical antibiotics. Systemic antibiotics may be needed.
Viral Infections			
Herpes zoster (shingles)	V-Z (varicella-zoster)	Clusters of small vesicles over the course of a peripheral sensory nerve. Two-thirds of clients have lesions just in the thoracic region. Lesions can occur over the trigeminal nerve, affecting the face, scalp, and eyes (Figure 21-14B). Crusts develop in several days. Symptoms are mild to severe pain, itching, fever, malaise. In older adults, pain can last for months or years. Persons who have not had chickenpox risk contracting the disease if they care for herpes zoster clients with open lesions. Persons who previously had chickenpox, but developed only partial immunity to it, may still be susceptible to herpes zoster.	Acyclovir (Zovirax) is given to clients in severe pain or to immunosuppressed clients. Analgesics help control the pain. Narcotic analgesics are prescribed for severe pain. Antipruritic topical medications decrease the itching.
Herpes simplex, type 1 and 2 (fever blisters, cold sores) Type 2 (genital)	*Herpes simplex virus*	Type 1—a cluster of vesicles on an erythematous base occurring most commonly at the corners of the mouth (Figure 21-14C) or at the edge of the nostrils. Type 2—lesions in the vagina or cervix of a woman or on the penis of a man. The lesions itch, burn, and frequently break open, forming a crust. Healing occurs in about 10 days.	Topical use of antiviral agents such as acyclovir decreases discomfort. Even with treatment cold sores and fever blisters tend to recur, especially with fever, upper respiratory infections, and stress. Oral administration of acyclovir helps to prevent recurrence of genital herpes.
Warts	Human papillomavirus	Seen as small, painless round papules on hands, face, and neck. On the bottom of the feet, warts grow inward from the pressure and are painful (plantar warts). Warts in the anogenital region itch. Genital warts increase the risk of cervical cancer.	No treatment is indicated for painless warts; they tend to disappear eventually. Plantar warts may be removed by cryosurgery or with locally applied chemicals such as nitric acid. Warts are not highly contagious from person to person but may be spread on the person's own body by rubbing or scratching. Genital warts are spread by sexual intercourse.
Fungal Infections			
Tinea (ringworm) Tinea capitis (ringworm of the scalp) Tinea corporis (ringworm of the body) Tinea cruris ("jock itch") Tinea pedis (athlete's foot)	*microscorim audouini*	Tinea is a superficial infection of the skin, called ringworm because of its circumscribed appearance, typically round, and reddened with slight scaling (Figure 21-14D). Lesions of tinea corporis have a pale center. Itching is common with tinea cruris. Itching and burning occur with tinea pedis. Tinea is spread easily. Jock itch and athlete's foot are more common among men than women.	Treat mild infections with a topical antifungal drug such as miconazole nitrate (Micatin) or tolnaftate (Aftate). Severe infections are treated with oral administration of griseofulvin microsize (Grisactin).

continues

Table 21–4 INFECTIOUS DISORDERS OF THE SKIN (*continued*)

DISEASE	ORGANISM	CLINICAL MANIFESTATIONS	MEDICAL MANAGEMENT
Parasitic Infections			
Scabies	*Sarcoptes scabiei* (female itch mite)	The itch mite burrows under the skin, lays eggs, and deposits fecal material. Short, dark-red wavy lines may be seen on hands, wrists, elbows, axillary folds, nipples, waistline, and gluteal folds (Figure 21-14E). Pruritis is severe and can persist for up to 3 months after treatment. Scratching leads to secondary infection. Scabies is spread by prolonged contact and is frequently seen in several members of a family.	Apply the scabicide, lindane (Kwell), topically to the entire body at bedtime so that the medication remains on the skin 8 to 12 hours. Treat all family members even if they do not have symptoms. Wash all underclothing and bed and bath linens in hot water. Change linens daily.
Pediculosis (lice)	*Pediculus capitis* (head lice) *Pediculus corporis* (body lice) *Phthirus Pubis* (pubic lice)	Eggs, or nits, of pediculosis capitis attach themselves firmly to a hair shaft on the head or in a beard (Figure 21-14F). Nits have a gray, pearly appearance. The pubic louse resembles a tiny crab that attaches itself to pubic hair. Body lice live in the seams of clothing. The bite of the louse causes severe pruritis. Scratching leads to secondary infection.	Lindane (Kwell) is applied topically to the hair as a shampoo or to the body as a cream or lotion. Repeat the treatment again in 8 to 10 days. Wash or dry-clean clothing and linens. Disinfect combs and brushes. Vacuum carpets and furniture; then spray with a pediculicide.

treatment has been used. Clients with infectious disorders of the skin may feel shame or embarrassment because of stigmas attached to some of these conditions, so the client's mood should also be noted.

▶ Objective Data

A complete skin assessment is in order, describing the size, appearance, and distribution of any lesions, as well as any drainage present.

CLIENT TEACHING

Herpes Zoster
- Take full course of prescribed medications.
- Use topical measures along with NSAIDs for pain management.
- Avoid persons who have not had chickenpox, especially pregnant women, so they do not get chickenpox.
- When dark crusts form over pustules, the client is no longer contagious.
- In older adults, pain may last for months or years.

Nursing diagnoses for a client with an infectious disorder of the skin may include the following:

Nursing Diagnoses	Planning/Goals	Nursing Interventions
▶ *Impaired Skin Integrity related to invasion of skin structures by pathogenic organisms*	The client will regain skin integrity.	Wear gloves when caring for the client with skin lesions.
		Cleanse the skin thoroughly, but gently. In the case of bacterial infections or lesions with secondary infections, use an antibacterial soap.
		Gently remove crusts, scales, and traces of old medication before applying fresh creams or lotions.
		Administer prescribed medications; apply creams and lotions; then monitor their effectiveness.
		Explain what you are doing and why.
▶ *Acute Pain, related to itching, burning, and infection*	The client will report less pain.	Instruct the client to keep the environmental temperature cool because warmth increases itching.
		Cleanse skin lesions with tepid water, not hot.
		Stress the importance of not scratching the lesions.

continues

Nursing Diagnoses	Planning/Goals	Nursing Interventions
▶ *Disturbed Body Image related to unsightly skin lesions and embarrassment*	The client will verbalize a positive body image.	Encourage the client to ask questions and to talk about feelings.
		Provide positive reinforcement as the client learns to care for the skin lesions.
		When possible, suggest ways to camouflage the lesions or minimize their appearance.
		When there is no danger of spreading the infection, encourage the client to participate in social and work activities.

Evaluation Each goal must be evaluated to determine how it has been met by the client.

SAMPLE NURSING CARE PLAN

THE CLIENT WITH SCABIES

Emma Evans, 68, has had a skin rash for the past 2 weeks. The dark red lesions occur mainly on her hands, wrists, and elbows, around her nipples, at her waistline, and in her gluteal folds. The itching has become increasingly intense. She states that she has been scratching the lesions, sometimes until they are open and bleeding. Upon examination, some of the lesions are open with small amounts of serosanguineous drainage. Other lesions are scabbed. She lives with her daughter and 2 teenaged granddaughters. Because the lesions were getting steadily worse, her daughter finally convinced her to seek medical attention. She was horrified when the doctor told her that she had scabies. She had always associated "the itch" with "dirty people who didn't take care of themselves."

Nursing Diagnosis 1 *Impaired Skin Integrity related to scratching scabies lesions as evidenced by open lesions draining serosanguineous fluid, scabbed lesions, and client statements of scratching the lesions until they bleed*

PLANNING/GOALS	NURSING INTERVENTIONS	RATIONALE	EVALUATION
Mrs. Evans will follow the prescribed treatment protocol to promote healing of skin lesions and regain skin integrity.	Instruct Mrs. Evans to cleanse lesions carefully using an antibacterial soap and tepid water. Depending upon the condition of the lesions and the severity of the itching, the lesions will need to be cleaned 1 to 3 times daily.	Maintaining cleanliness of the skin reduces the number of microorganisms present and decreases the risk of infection. Tepid water does not intensify itching as hot water does.	Mrs. Evans's lesions are still red, but none are open and draining. Some lesions are still scabbed. No new open lesions have developed. Mrs. Evans states that the recommended measures "help," but that the itching is still "pretty bad." Goal of promoting healing of skin lesions is being met. Encourage Mrs. Evans to continue outlined protocols. Reassure her that itching will gradually subside as healing progresses.
	Teach Mrs. Evans to apply antipruritic lotions as prescribed by the doctor after cleansing the skin.	Cleansing removes dirt, oils, and microorganisms. Lotion applied to clean skin is more effective. Lotions applied just after bathing help to retain skin moisture.	
	Instruct Mrs. Evans to keep fingernails short with smooth edges.	Short fingernails with smooth edges are less likely to break the skin if	

continues

the client does scratch the scabies lesions.

Teach Mrs. Evans to press itching lesions, and not to scratch them.

Pressing the skin stimulates nerve endings and can reduce the sensation of itching. Pressing itching skin areas rather than scratching them prevents breaks in the skin, which would be portals of entry for microorganisms.

Explain that itching can persist up to 3 months following treatment with the scabicide and that persistent itching does not mean that treatment to kill the itch mite was ineffective.

Skin reaction to the toxins and secretions of the itch mite can persist for up to 3 months after the itch mites are killed by the scabicide.

Keep room temperature between 68° and 72°F and humidity constant at 30% to 35%.

Itching is intensified in hot, humid environments. Maintaining room humidity at a constant level decreases drying of the skin and increases comfort.

Nursing Diagnosis 2 *Deficient Knowledge (infection control measures), related to lack of familiarity with treatment and prevention protocols as evidenced by client's inability to recognize the skin lesions as infectious and by statements about scabies happening only to people with poor hygiene*

PLANNING/GOALS	NURSING INTERVENTIONS	RATIONALE	EVALUATION
Mrs. Evans will apply the scabicide correctly and state ways to avoid spreading infection to others.	Assess Mrs. Evans' knowledge of scabies, its treatment regimen and infection control measures. Ask specific questions.	Building on knowledge that Mrs. Evans already has provides a frame of reference for the client, which helps her relate new information and integrate it into her behavior.	Mrs. Evans and her family did apply the scabicide as prescribed. The client can describe how scabies are transmitted, but continues to express fear that she will give "this awful thing to somebody." Goal of correctly applying scabicide met. Although Mrs. Evans can state how scabies are transmitted, she still has doubts; hence, the goal of stating ways to avoid spreading the infection to others
	Explain that scabies is transmitted by skin-to-skin contact or by contact with articles freshly contaminated by infected persons and in the United States, infection with scabies affects persons of all social, economic, and age levels.	Teaching that does not "talk down" to the client communicates respect.	
	Stress the importance of following treatment protocol exactly. Review salient	Failure to apply the scabicide as directed and/or failure to leave the lotion	

continues

points such as (1) Shower before applying the scabicide; (2) apply the scabicide to the entire body surface, including skin without scabies lesions; and (3) apply the scabicide at bedtime so that the medication remains on the skin 8 to 12 hours.

Give Mrs. Evans step-by-step written instructions.

Instruct Mrs. Evans to wash hands under warm running water with plenty of soap (preferably an antibacterial soap) for at least 10 seconds after touching lesions and clean carefully under fingernails while washing hands.

Advise to not share washcloths, towels, clothing, pillows, or bed linens with other family members.

Instruct to wash underclothing and bed and bath linens in detergent and hot water and dry outside in sunlight or in a dryer on the hot setting.

Advise to shower daily, use an antibacterial soap, rinse thoroughly, and dry carefully, especially in skin folds and between toes, using a towel and washcloth only once before laundering it.

on the skin for the prescribed length of time will not kill the itch mite.

Giving the client written step-by-step instructions enhances compliance with the treatment regimen.

Thorough handwashing is the single most effective means of preventing the spread of infection. Large numbers of bacteria reside under the fingernails.

Disease-causing microorganisms can be spread to well individuals indirectly when their skin comes into contact with contaminated items.

Soap reduces surface tension. When fat or protein substances that shield organisms are broken down, the organisms are exposed to the killing effects of heat. Prolonged exposure to heat or ultraviolet rays from direct sunlight kills microorganisms.

Regular cleansing reduces the number of microorganisms on the skin. Antibacterial soap further decreases the number of microorganisms on the skin. Moisture in skin folds and between toes encourages the growth of microorganisms. Laundering the towel and washcloth after only one use prevents the indirect transfer of the itch mite.

has only been partially met. Reinforce that even though red skin lesions are still visible, the itch mites were killed by treatment and cannot be transmitted to others even if the client does shake hands, hug, or touch someone else.

continues

Assess lesions daily for signs of healing. Report any signs and symptoms of infection in secondary lesions such as redness, swelling, pain, drainage (describe characteristics of the drainage) to the physician or clinic.

Early recognition of signs of infection increases the probability of effective treatment with fewer complications.

Teach Mrs. Evans and family members the early signs and symptoms of scabies infection, such as any reddened papules with wavy, threadlike lines visible on the skin around the papules and severe itching, especially at night.

Early recognition and treatment of scabies can minimize the severity of the infection.

Instruct them to assess their skin daily.

A daily examination allows treatment to begin as soon as the problem is identified.

Nursing Diagnosis 3 *Disturbed Body Image related to unsightly lesions and embarrassment as evidenced by distribution of lesions on exposed skin areas and client statements of being horrified about the diagnosis and associating scabies with "dirty people"*

PLANNING/GOALS	NURSING INTERVENTIONS	RATIONALE	EVALUATION
Mrs. Evans will assume self-care of lesions and maintain relationships with family and friends.	Encourage Mrs. Evans to express her feelings about herself and her opinions about scabies.	Allowing the client to express feelings and opinions brings them out into the open where they can be dealt with appropriately.	The client has assumed self-care responsibilities. She does interact with her family but emphasizes that she "doesn't want to get too close to them until these things are completely gone." She has refused to go to church, social gatherings, or activities outside of the house.
	Provide information to correct any misconceptions she might have.	If the client has any misconceptions, accurate information can dispel them and lead to an improved self-image.	
	Encourage Mrs. Evans to verbalize the perceptions she has about her family's and friends' feelings about persons with scabies.	If the client perceives that her friends have derogatory opinions of her, she is likely to socially isolate herself from them.	Goal has been partially met in that the client does follow proper procedures when caring for her skin lesions, but goal has not been met in so far as maintaining relationships is concerned. Encourage the
	Be alert to verbal and nonverbal messages.	Nonverbal behavior gives insight into the client's real feelings. Identifying and discussing feelings can lead to behavioral changes.	
	Reassure her that she will not infect friends and fam-	The client will be unlikely to avoid friends or make	

continues

ily members by going places with them, sitting beside them, or being in the same room with them for prolonged periods.

Share with Mrs. Evans that wearing long-sleeved cotton blouses or dresses will hide most of the visible lesions.

Explain that by using the scabicide, lindane (Kwell), as directed and by following measures to prevent secondary infection of the scabies lesions, she can expect complete healing of the lesions without any visible scars within a few weeks.

disparaging remarks about herself when she realizes that she is not a danger to them.

Covering unsightly skin lesions makes the client less self-conscious and embarrassed. Cotton fabric allows good air circulation. When the skin feels cooler, itching is less intense.

Reassurance that scabies can be cured enhances the client's self-image.

client to talk about her feelings, particularly feelings of embarrassment. Point out to her the evidence that her lesions are healing. Emphasize that symptoms of intense itching, worsening of present skin lesions, and signs of more skin lesions would be present if the itch mites were alive and still spreading. Encourage her to go on at least 1 outing with her family during the coming week. Reevaluate in 1 week.

INFLAMMATORY DISORDERS OF THE SKIN

Included in this category are dermatitis and psoriasis.

DERMATITIS

By definition, dermatitis is an inflammatory condition of the skin. In current usage, eczema has almost become synonymous with dermatitis, although eczema tends to be used most often to refer to chronic forms of dermatitis. Other types of this inflammatory disorder include contact dermatitis and exfoliative dermatitis.

ECZEMA

Eczema is an atopic dermatitis often associated with allergic rhinitis and asthma. It is a chronic superficial

GERONTOLOGICAL CONSIDERATIONS

Skin Integrity in the Elderly
With thinning and drying of the skin secondary to aging, elderly clients are more susceptible to irritants that cause dermatitis. Restoring skin integrity in elderly clients takes longer and requires persistent nursing effort.

inflammation that evolves into pruritic, red, weeping, crusted lesions (Estes, 1998). See Figure 21-15.

CONTACT DERMATITIS

In contact dermatitis the skin reacts to external irritants such as (1) allergens like poison ivy or cosmetics, (2) harsh chemical substances like detergents or insec-

Figure 21-15 Eczema *(Courtesy of the Centers for Disease Control and Prevention, Atlanta, GA)*

GERONTOLOGICAL CONSIDERATIONS

Exfoliative Dermatitis

Elderly clients have a greater risk of fatal complications from exfoliative dermatitis. As body systems age, they are less able to respond quickly and effectively to the stress of illness.

Figure 21-16 Allergic Contact Dermatitis from Poison Oak: Note Linear Pattern to Lesions (*Courtesy of the Centers for Disease Control and Prevention, Atlanta, GA*)

ticides, (3) metals such as nickel, (4) mechanical irritation from wool or glass fibers, and (5) body substances like urine or feces. Symptoms include pruritus, burning, and erythema. Often a maculopapular rash or a combination of papules and vesicles develops. Scratching the lesions may spread the dermatitis as well as lead to secondary infections of the skin (Figure 21-16).

EXFOLIATIVE DERMATITIS

In exfoliative dermatitis, inflammation of the skin gradually worsens. Localized symptoms include erythema, severe pruritus, extensive scaling, and loss of skin surface. Exfoliative dermatitis affects the entire body, not just the skin. Systemic symptoms include chills, fever, and malaise. With the loss of large areas of skin surface, the individual has difficulty maintaining body temperature, loses body fluids and electrolytes, and is susceptible to infection.

In most cases, the cause of exfoliative dermatitis is unknown. Severe reactions to drugs such as penicillin may sometimes cause exfoliative dermatitis. It may also be associated with other types of dermatitis or lymphoma. Exfoliative dermatitis can be fatal, primarily because of overwhelming systemic infections and/or massive loss of body fluids and electrolytes.

Medical–Surgical Management

Medical

Clients with contact dermatitis can be treated as outpatients. Patch testing may identify a specific allergen that is causing the dermatitis. Taking precautions to avoid the allergenic substance may prevent future cases of contact dermatitis. In some cases, application of topical corticosteroids may be all that is needed. When weeping lesions are present, treatment with Burow's solution (1:40 dilution of aluminum acetate) for 20 minutes 4 times a day relieves symptoms and promotes healing (Weaver, 1995).

When clients are hospitalized with exfoliative dermatitis, medical management is directed toward maintaining fluid balance, preventing infection, decreasing inflammation, and promoting comfort. The client requires intravenous fluids to maintain the volume of circulating fluid, corticosteroids to decrease inflamma-

tion, and antibiotics to treat infection. Medicated baths, topical steroids, and mild analgesics may be prescribed to ease the pruritus.

Nursing Management

As with other skin disorders, nursing management is directed toward promoting healing, providing comfort, preventing infection, and fostering a positive attitude to help the client cope with an altered body image. Nursing diagnoses may include *Skin Integrity, Impaired; Infection, Risk for; Pain;* and *Body Image Disturbance.* These clients will need to know how to care for the lesions, how to prevent infection, how to cope with conditions that alter their physical appearance and psychological well-being, and how to keep their physical discomfort at a tolerable level. Client teaching focuses on identifying and avoiding substances that cause dermatitis.

PSORIASIS

Psoriasis, a chronic, inflammatory, noninfectious disease of the skin, affects a fairly large segment of the population, especially young adults. The parts of the body most commonly affected are the scalp, hands, arms, knees, lower back, and genitalia (Weaver, 1995) (Figure 21-17). The exact cause of psoriasis is unknown, although a genetic component may be involved. Emotional stress, infections, trauma, and seasonal and hormonal changes trigger exacerbations of psoriasis. It may improve for a while only to recur. This process of subsiding and recurring continues to occur throughout the client's life. Psoriasis is not curable. In psoriasis the process of keratinization has gone awry. Instead of producing cells that provide a natural barrier against harmful substances and microorganisms, abnormal keratinization causes large, red patches covered with thick silvery scales in the outermost layer of the epidermis (Seeley et al., 1995). If these scales are scraped away, bleeding occurs. When fingernails are affected, pitting and yellow discoloration will be seen.

Figure 21-17 Psoriasis *(Courtesy of Robert A. Silverman, MD, Clinical Associate Professor, Department of Pediatrics, Georgetown University)*

Medical–Surgical Management

Medical

Treatment is directed toward slowing down the rate of cell formation in the epidermis or toward altering the abnormal process of keratinization. Treatment regimens can be effective in reducing the scaling and itching; however, the client must recognize that psoriasis can only be controlled, not cured. Further, the client must be committed to lifetime therapy.

Pharmacological

Keratolytic agents such as salicylic acid preparations and coal tar preparations are applied topically to the lesions. Corticosteroids may also be used to reduce inflammation. Ultraviolet light and methotrexate (Mexate) inhibit DNA synthesis in the epidermal cells, thus slowing down the rate of cell division and the process of abnormal keratinization. Because of its toxicity to the liver, methotrexate is used only in severe cases of psoriasis that do not respond to any other form of

treatment. The Goeckerman regimen, which combines the use of coal tar and ultraviolet light, is one of the oldest treatments available but is effective and is still widely used (Weaver, 1995).

Photochemotherapy is used for severe psoriasis. Photochemotherapy (psorafen ultraviolet A-range, or PUVA) combines the use of methoxsalen (Oxsoralen) with ultraviolet A light waves. The dose of Oxsoralen is based on body weight and must be taken 2 hours before exposure to ultraviolet A light waves. Oxsoralen is a photosensitizing agent that reacts with ultraviolet A light waves to markedly reduce DNA synthesis, thereby slowing cell division in psoriasis lesions and relieving symptoms. While the treatment is generally effective, the results are not seen immediately (Hill, 1998).

Etretinate (Tegison), a compound related to retinoic acid vitamin A, is used in severe psoriasis not amenable to other therapies. It may be used alone or in combination with ultraviolet A light waves. Etretinate has numerous adverse effects, including liver damage and severe birth defects. The client must be monitored closely. Women of childbearing age must use effective contraception during treatment and for at least 1 month after treatment.

▶ NURSING PROCESS

▶ Assessment

▶ Subjective Data

Psoriasis lesions are generally very visible and likely to make the client feel quite self-conscious as well as very uncomfortable. These clients also tend to suffer self-esteem and body image disturbances, and sometimes depression, because psoriasis requires lifelong treatment. The treatment can be time-consuming, bothersome and, from the client's point of view, not completely effective. The client should be encouraged to verbalize feelings. Itching, burning, and discomfort, as well as the client's mood, should all be assessed.

▶ Objective Data

A careful skin assessment, noting the distribution, size, and appearance of lesions, should be performed. Signs of infection such as redness, swelling, pain, or drainage must be noted.

Nursing diagnoses for a client with psoriasis may include the following:

Nursing Diagnoses	Planning/Goals	Nursing Interventions
▶ *Deficient Knowledge related to psoriasis and its treatment*	The client will discuss condition and adhere to treatment.	Help the client gain an understanding of psoriasis and comply with the treatment regimen.
		Support and encourage the client.
		Explain the purpose of each medication.

continues

Nursing Diagnoses	Planning/Goals	Nursing Interventions
▶ *Risk for Infection related to open lesions*	The client will not get an infection.	Teach the client how to prevent infections by proper handwashing and not scratching the lesions.
▶ *Disturbed Body Image related to scaly lesions*	The client will identify positive attributes about self.	Listen actively and encourage the client to express feelings and frustrations. Reinforce positive behavior.
▶ *Situational Low Self-Esteem related to appearance*	The client will demonstrate behaviors that promote self-esteem.	Guide the client in identifying effective coping techniques. Help the client focus on personal attributes that contribute to effective functioning and a positive self-image. Encourage work and social interactions.

Evaluation Each goal must be evaluated to determine how it has been met by the client.

ULCERS

The two most common types of ulcers of the skin are stasis ulcers and pressure ulcers.

STASIS ULCERS

Poor venous circulation, especially in lower extremities, can lead to a condition known as stasis dermatitis (Figure 21-18). The skin changes in texture, turgor, and

Figure 21-18 Venous Stasis Ulcer *(Courtesy of Carrington Laboratories, Inc., Irving, TX)*

color. The skin develops a brownish discoloration and a brawny induration, that is, skin in the affected area becomes dry and looks rough; subcutaneous tissue atrophies; and the texture loses its usual resiliency and feels hard to the touch. Body hair is lost in this area of the skin. Pruritus is common. Scratching or small injuries can lead to ulcer formation because of the poor circulation.

Venous stasis ulcers begin as small, tender, inflamed areas above the ankle. Any slight trauma to the area causes an open area that develops into an ulcer. Some edema surrounds the ulcer, which can easily become infected, most often with staphylococcus or streptococcus. Healing is very slow. In an effort to decrease venous congestion and improve circulation, varicose veins, if present, may be removed. Ulcers that do not heal may require surgery. If diagnostic testing reveals adequate circulation, skin grafting will result in the healing of large venous stasis ulcers. In severe cases that do not respond to treatment, the affected leg has to be amputated.

Medical–Surgical Management

Medical

Vacuum-assisted closure (VAC) therapy may be used for chronic open wounds such as stasis ulcers. Applying negative pressure to the wound is painless for the client. The negative pressure stretches or distorts the cells, causing the epithelial cells to multiply rapidly and form granulation tissue. As the vacuum pulls fluid from the surrounding tissues, reducing edema that compressed blood vessels, blood flow to the wound is improved.

A sterile foam sponge is fitted into the wound, the vented end of pliable vacuum tubing is placed on the sponge, and an occlusive adhesive dressing applied over all. The occlusive adhesive dressing keeps the wound moist, prevents bacteria from entering, and maintains the vacuum pressure. The amount of internal negative pressure and suction (continuous or intermittent) is set on the pump. Dressings are usually changed 3 times a week.

Enzyme preparations such as fibrinolysin and dexsoxyribonucleas (ELASE) or wet-to-dry dressings may be used to debride the ulcer. Normal saline is the solution most often used in wet-to-dry dressings because it is not irritating to healthy tissue.

Pharmacological

For healing to occur, the ulcer must have adequate circulation and be free of infection and necrotic tissue. Usually antibiotics are prescribed. For small ulcers, especially in ambulatory clients, an Unna's boot may be ordered. The "boot" is a special type of gauze impregnated with gelatin, glycerin, and zinc oxide paste that is applied in a spiral fashion around the leg. It hardens around the client's leg, providing even, constant support during ambulation. Unna's boot can achieve a 70% healing rate (Dennison & Black, 1997).

Diet

A diet high in protein and vitamin C is needed for tissue regeneration. If the client is anemic, lean meats, whole grains, and green, leafy vegetables should be encouraged.

▶ NURSING PROCESS

▶ Assessment

▶ Subjective Data

The client should be asked to describe any pain and rate its severity on a scale of 1 to 10. It should be noted whether the pain is worse with the leg in a dependent position or when the client is standing. Measures used to relieve the pain should be documented. If the skin around the ulcer itches, this must be noted. The length of time the client had the ulcer prior to seeking care, and any palliative measures tried, should also be noted.

▶ Objective Data

The size and location of the ulcer must be described, as well as the appearance of the ulcer and surrounding skin. The nurse should observe for necrotic tissue inside the ulcer. It may be yellow and look like thin strands of fibers. The base of the ulcer may have a dark red, "beefy" appearance. The color and appearance of the extremity in both a dependent and an elevated position should be assessed. Any drainage needs to be noted, including its odor and characteristics. Edema may be present, and the lower extremity may appear swollen. Hardened and indurated tissue surrounds the ulcer. Tissue farther away from the ulcer may "pit" with firm pressure. Peripheral pulses must be assessed.

Nursing diagnoses for a client with a stasis ulcer may include the following:

Nursing Diagnoses	Planning/Goals	Nursing Interventions
▶ *Ineffective Tissue Perfusion (Peripheral) related to edema and pooling of venous blood*	Client will follow prescribed measures to improve peripheral circulation.	Encourage the client to elevate legs while sitting or when in bed.
		Advise the client to avoid standing for more than a few minutes at a time.
		Advise client to wear elastic stockings when walking and that new stockings should be purchased every few months because continual wear and laundering tend to decrease the elasticity of the stockings. Instruct not to wear garters, tight girdles, or sit with legs crossed.
		Note the client's hemoglobin level since anemic clients will have difficulty meeting tissue demands for oxygen.
▶ *Chronic Pain related to exposed sensory nerve endings and edema*	Client will report decreased pain after implementing recommended measures.	Encourage client to elevate legs.
		Cleanse ulcer with prescribed solutions.
		Keep ulcer covered with prescribed medications and dressings.
▶ *Risk for Infection related to poorly nourished tissue in and around the ulcer and to nonintact skin*	Client will describe and implement measures to minimize the risk of infection.	Assess the ulcer daily for signs of healing.
		Assess the client's ability to care for the ulcer physically and financially.
		Review diet with the client and instruct in food choices as needed. Encourage foods high in iron such as fortified cereal, lean meats, whole grains, and leafy green vegetables.

Evaluation Each goal must be evaluated to determine how it has been met by the client.

PRESSURE ULCERS

Pressure ulcers, also known as bedsores or decubitus ulcers, are localized areas of tissue necrosis that tend to develop when soft tissue is compressed between a bony prominence and an external surface such as a mattress or chair seat for a prolonged period of time. Pressure ulcers are due to **ischemia**, local and temporary decrease in blood supply, and commonly occur in areas subject to high pressure from body weight on bony prominences.

Physiology of Pressure Ulcers

A pressure ulcer occurs when pressure on the skin is sufficient to cause collapse of blood vessels in the area. Ischemia and redness can occur at the site within 1 hour; when pressure continues for more than 2 hours, necrosis (tissue death) may occur in the involved area. Bony prominences such as the occipital skull, pinna of ears, sacrum, ischial tuberosities, trochanter area of hips, ankles, and heels are the areas most likely to develop a pressure ulcer. By far the most common location is the sacrum (Barczak, Barnett, Childs, & Bosley, 1997).

Other forces acting in conjunction with pressure contribute to pressure ulcer formation. **Shearing** is the force exerted against the skin by movement or repositioning. The skin and subcutaneous tissue tend to adhere to the bed surface and remain stationary while deeper underlying tissues pull away and slide in the direction of movement. This action results in stretching and tearing of blood vessels, reduced blood flow, and necrosis.

Friction is the force of two surfaces moving across one another. When a client moves or is pulled up in bed, rubbing of the skin against the sheets creates friction. Friction can remove the superficial layers of the skin, making it more prone to breakdown.

The reduction of blood flow causes **blanching** (white color) of the skin when pressure is applied. When pressure is relieved, the skin takes on a brighter color (reactive hyperemia) due to vasodilation, the body's normal compensatory response to the absence of blood flow. If this area blanches with fingertip pressure or if the redness disappears within an hour, no tissue damage is anticipated. If, however, the redness persists and no blanching occurs, then tissue damage is present.

Pressure ulcers are staged to classify the degree of tissue damage (Figure 21-19). The National Pressure Ulcer Advisory Panel (NPUAP) (United States Department of Health and Human Services [USDHHS], 1992) recommends the following staging system:

- Stage I: Nonblanchable erythema of intact skin; the heralding lesion of skin ulceration.

- Stage II: Partial-thickness skin loss involving epidermis, dermis, or both. The ulcer is superficial and presents clinically as an abrasion, blister, or shallow crater.
- Stage III: Full-thickness skin loss involving damage or necrosis of subcutaneous tissue that may extend down to, but not through, underlying fascia. The ulcer presents clinically as a deep crater with or without undermining of adjacent tissue.
- Stage IV: Full-thickness skin loss with extensive destruction, tissue necrosis, or damage to muscle, bone, or supporting structures. Undermining and sinus tracts may also be associated with stage IV pressure ulcers.

The National Pressure Ulcer Advisory Panel (1999) has developed an assessment tool, Pressure Ulcer Scale for Healing (PUSH Tool). It uses three parameters: the surface area of the wound, amount of exudate, and type of tissue present in the wound. The scores for each are added together and plotted to show wound healing or worsening. This PUSH Tool is available on the Internet.

Risk Factors for Pressure Ulcers

Pressure ulcers can be prevented if at-risk individuals are identified and the specific factors placing them at risk are reduced or eliminated. More than 1 million clients each year have pressure ulcers, and most of these clients are in their 70s and 80s (National Decubitus Foundation, 1998). Both intrinsic and extrinsic factors may influence tissue response to pressure. Intrinsic factors include impaired immobility, incontinence, nutritional status, and altered level of consciousness. Extrinsic factors include pressure, shearing, friction, and moisture. Any condition that decreases tissue perfusion,

A. Stage 1   **B.** Stage 2

C. Stage 3   **D.** Stage 4

Figure 21-19 Pressure Ulcers *(Courtesy of Emory University Hospital, Atlanta, GA)*

such as edema, anemia, or atherosclerosis, also increases the risk. Other factors are decreased mental status, diminished sensation, and age-related changes.

Individuals should be assessed for pressure ulcer risk on admission to acute care hospitals, nursing homes, and other health care facilities and at least weekly thereafter.

Medical–Surgical Management

Medical

Sterile technique is followed in the care of all pressure ulcers to prevent secondary infection. The wound should be cleansed with normal saline or a noncytotoxic wound cleaner at each dressing change. Such agents as povodine-iodine, iodophor, sodium hypochlorite, hydrogen peroxide, or acetic acid should not be used because they can damage the cells. A 35 mL syringe with a 19 gauge needle or angiocatheter provides enough pressure to cleanse the wound and enhance wound healing without causing trauma to the tissue.

Debridement must be done as needed. Topical enzyme agents may be applied or a mechanical method of wet-to-dry dressings, or hydrotherapy may be used. Refer to the discussion of VAC therapy in the section on stasis ulcers; this therapy can also be used for pressure ulcers.

There are many commercial products available for treatment and dressing of pressure ulcers. Whichever products the physician prescribes, everyone should be taught how to use them and have a commitment to use them properly.

Support Surfaces and Beds A variety of support surfaces and beds is available to support the entire body and evenly distribute pressure. These devices are used to help reduce pressure and prevent ulcers, but they are no substitute for frequent positioning. There is no evidence that any one support surface works consistently better than any other (USDHHS, 1992).

In addition to pressure reduction or relief, many support surfaces reduce shear and friction and control moisture. Pressure-reducing support surfaces include overlays filled with foam, gel, or water.

- *Eggcrate mattress:* The eggcrate mattress is composed of thick foam with a unique, eggcrate design (Figure 21-20). The purposes of the eggcrate mattress include minimizing pressure and shearing force. The open design of the mattress surface allows air to circulate to dissipate heat and moisture. Eggcrate foam is also used as wheelchair cushions, heel-ankle protectors, wrist restraint cushioning pads, and ulnar protectors. They are used in acute care hospital settings and for long-term use.
- *Air-filled mattresses:* The air-filled mattress is placed over the mattress of the hospital bed. The purpose

Figure 21-20 Eggcrate Pressure Relief Aids: A. Mattress; B. Wheelchair cushion (*Courtesy of Graham-Field, Inc., Hauppauge, NY*)

of the air-filled mattress is weight redistribution. Varieties of air-filled mattresses include some with a pump and alternating bands of inflation and deflation and some that are inflated continuously with air. Mattresses are covered with a sheet for client comfort. These types of mattresses are frequently used in long-term care situations.
- *Clinitron® bed:* A Clinitron® bed is a specialized bed that has a mattress filled with small glass sand particles. Moisture from urine, stool, or drainage flows through the mattress, preventing moisture exposure to the skin. Because warm air is circulating through the mattress, the accumulation of moisture next to the skin is inhibited. The mattress aids in positioning the client because it is constructed to mold against the client's body. Figure 21-21 shows a Clinitron® bed.
- *Kin Air bed:* A Kin Air bed, another type of specialized bed, has a mattress of air-inflated pillows divided in sections for the head, back, seat, legs, and feet. The pressure can be adjusted in each of the sections for the client's specific needs. Air flows from the mattress to eliminate moisture. The bed frame can be adjusted for various positions such as Fowler's, Trendelenburg, prone, or supine. A trapeze can be connected to the bed frame (Figure 21-22).

Figure 21-22 Kin Air Bed

Figure 21-21 Clinitron® Air Fluidized Therapy Unit Model CII *(Courtesy of Hill-Rom, Batesville, IN)*

Figure 21-23 Avoiding Pressure Points with the 30° Lateral Position

- *Roto Kinetic bed:* A Roto Kinetic bed is a specialized bed that rocks slowly from side to side, thus relieving pressure areas and countering the effects of immobility. The client is placed on the mattress, with dividers between the legs and dividers between the trunk and arms. Clients can be maintained in traction while on this bed.

Regardless of the type of surface or bed on which the client is lying, the 30° side-lying position prevents pressure on the sacrum and trochanters. This position is illustrated in Figure 21-23.

Surgical

Occasionally, surgical debridement may be necessary.

Pharmacological

Vitamin and mineral supplements may be ordered. Antibiotics may also be ordered.

Diet

Eating a well-balanced diet should be encouraged, including 2 half-cup servings of orange juice or other juice high in vitamin C and 6 ounces of a high-protein drink.

Activity

Active ROM exercises should be performed, if possible. If not, passive ROM exercises should be performed with the client several times a day.

PROFESSIONAL TIP

Preventing Pressure Ulcers

- Establish written repositioning/turning schedule for clients, including those on pressure-reducing support surfaces.
- Use 30° position when side-lying position is used.
- Prevent direct contact between bony prominences by using pillows and foam wedges.
- Use a lifting sheet.
- Encourage clients in wheelchairs to shift their weight every 15 minutes.
- Raise heels off the bed with pillow lengthwise to support legs.
- Use knee gatch when head of bed is elevated.
- Keep head of bed elevated to less than 30° except at mealtimes.
- Limit sitting time to 1 hour at a time whether in bed, chair, or wheelchair.
- Use proper positioning, transferring, and turning techniques.
- Inspect skin at least once a day.
- Use mild cleansing agent, but avoid hot water for bathing.
- Avoid massage over bony prominences.
- Use moisturizer on skin.
- Use protective barrier on skin if client is incontinent.
- Cleanse skin at time of soiling and at routine intervals.

▶ NURSING PROCESS

▶ Assessment

▶ Subjective Data

Statements such as, "I'm tired of lying on my side"; "I wish I could move more"; or "my hips (back, heels, and so on) are sore" may be expressed.

▶ Objective Data

Symptoms may include any of the risk factors already mentioned; shiny, erythematous area; small blisters or erosions or ulcerations. The nurse should check for reddened areas and blanching of those areas.

Nursing diagnoses for a client at risk for pressure ulcers or who has a pressure ulcer may include the following:

Nursing Diagnoses	Planning/Goals	Nursing Interventions
▶ *Risk for Impaired Skin Integrity related to immobility*	The client will maintain skin integrity.	Assess skin 3 times a day for pressure areas.
		Provide daily bath and skin care as needed for incontinence of urine or stool.
		Use mild cleansing agents with warm water.
		Use moisturizing lotion and minimize exposure to cold and low humidity.
		Avoid massage over bony prominences.
		Keep bed linen clean, dry, and free from wrinkles.
		Encourage adequate fluid intake and a well-balanced diet, including 2 half-cup servings of orange juice or other juice high in vitamin C and 6 ounces of a high-protein drink.
		Encourage active ROM exercises or provide passive ROM exercises.
		Turn and reposition client at least every 2 hours. If reddened area does not blanch when you press it, turn the client more often.
		Use the 30° lateral position to avoid pressure on the sacrum and trochanters.
		Use pressure-reducing surfaces. Do not use donut-shaped cushions because they just put pressure around the pressure ulcer.
▶ *Impaired Skin Integrity related to pressure ulcer formation*	The client will show healing of pressure ulcer.	Assess skin daily, identifying the stage of pressure ulcer development (size, color, odor, and exudate).
		Continue all preventive nursing interventions.
		Position client on unaffected areas.
		Protect skin surface and affected area as per facility protocol or as ordered.
		Monitor temperature.
		Administer antibiotics as ordered.
▶ *Disturbed Body Image related to trauma or injury (pressure ulcer)*	The client will make a positive statement about body image.	Encourage client to discuss meaning of pressure ulcer to the client.
		Provide information as requested by client.
▶ *Anxiety related to threat to or change in health status (pressure ulcer)*	The client will discuss concerns about pressure ulcer with caregivers.	Schedule time to be with client, other than care times.
		Provide information as requested by client.
		Encourage client to discuss fears and concerns.

Evaluation Each goal must be evaluated to determine how it has been met by the client.

ALOPECIA

Alopecia, which is partial or complete baldness or loss of hair, can be caused by illness, malnutrition, effects of certain drugs such as those used in cancer therapy, hormonal imbalances, or diseases that affect the scalp.

There are many types of alopecia, ranging from head or beard hair loss to loss of all hair over the entire body. Treatment depends on the cause. Hair transplants may be performed on the head, but this is very expensive. In some clients, minoxidil (Rogaine) can promote hair growth, but hair growth stops when the drug is stopped. This also is very expensive.

CASE STUDY

Maude Murphy, age 68, noticed that the skin on the outside of her left lower leg just above the ankle was changing in color and texture. The skin felt rigid and did not move as easily as skin on the upper part of her leg did. Itching was becoming a problem. Inadvertently she would scratch the area, sometimes causing small excoriations. One day she bumped her leg against the rough edge of the outside steps as she was going into the house. The cut was only an inch long and was not very deep. Over the next few weeks, she noticed that instead of healing, it was getting bigger and was becoming quite painful. The skin around the wound was red and swollen. The yellow drainage coming from the wound had a bad smell. She had never had this kind of problem before. She did have varicose veins in that leg, and while she knew that she was uncomfortable if she was standing for long periods, she did not think the problem was serious. When she went to the doctor, he diagnosed a venous stasis ulcer and cultured the drainage. He ordered the following treatment:

1. *Cefaclor (Ceclor) 500 mg p.o. every 8 hours for 2 weeks (culture of the wound identified Staphylococcus aureus).*
2. *Wet-to-dry dressings with normal saline solution. Change every 8 hours.*
3. *Bed rest with left leg elevated. May have bathroom privileges and be up for meals.*

The doctor explained that he would be ordering an Unna's boot after the wound was debrided and the infection controlled so that she could be ambulatory, but that even after the Unna's boot was applied, he would want her to have rest periods during the day with her leg elevated. Mrs. Murphy thought she could learn to change the dressings, but she expressed doubt that she could stay in bed most of the time. She was used to being up and active and getting her work done each day.

The following questions will guide your development of a nursing care plan for the case study.

1. List the clinical manifestations of a venous stasis ulcer.
2. What is the usual medical treatment?
3. List the subjective and objective assessment data that the nurse should obtain from Maude Murphy.
4. Write 2 to 4 individualized nursing diagnoses to address these problems.
5. What will be the goals (expected outcomes) of nursing treatment?
6. List appropriate nursing actions for each diagnosis. Include basic nursing care measures. Be specific about client education needs. Address nutrition and pharmacologic implications. Give a rationale for each action.
7. Describe how to evaluate goal achievement for Maude Murphy.

SUMMARY

- Maintaining intact skin and mucous membranes to protect internal body structures from harmful substances and from invasion by microorganisms is an important independent nursing responsibility.
- Burns are devastating, traumatic injuries that can often be prevented.
- In general, skin cancers can be prevented by avoiding excessive sun exposure.
- Treatment of benign skin tumors such as nevi, lipomas, keloids, sebaceous cysts, and angiomas depends on the kind of tumor and its location.
- Psoriasis is a chronic skin condition that can be treated, but not cured.

- Skin infections caused by bacteria, viruses, fungi, or parasites can be effectively treated with medications and supportive nursing care.
- Dermatitis, an inflammation of the skin, can be a contact dermatitis or an exfoliative dermatitis.
- Eczema is a term that is often used for chronic forms of dermatitis.
- Venous stasis ulcers are more common in older persons, heal slowly, and often recur following a slight injury.
- Alopecia, or baldness, can be caused by illness, drugs, hormonal imbalances, or heredity.

Review Questions

1. The skin has a vital role in the normal functioning of the human organism. That role is:

   a. production of antibodies.
   b. protection from invasion by microorganisms.
   c. support for internal organs.
   d. regulation of cellular oxygenation.

2. The nurse charted that the client's skin was loose, wrinkled, and thin with mild scaling. The nurse was describing:

   a. integrity.
   b. texture.
   c. turgor and mobility.
   d. vascularity.

3. An effective nursing intervention related to the care of open burn wounds that require daily dressing changes would be:

   a. keep the head of the bed elevated 30° with all four side rails up.
   b. set a fluid intake goal of 2,500 mL/24 hours (1,200 mL during the day; 950 mL during the evening; 350 mL during the night).
   c. wear a cap, gown, mask, and sterile gloves when providing wound care.
   d. weigh daily, preferably before breakfast, and in the same type of clothing each day.

4. The client has lesions on his scalp and on his arms near his elbows. The lesions appear as red patches covered with thick silvery scales. The most likely cause of these lesions is:

   a. herpes zoster (shingles).
   b. pemphigus vulgaris.
   c. psoriasis.
   d. tinea (ringworm).

5. A nursing care plan for a client with an infectious disorder of the skin would include interventions to teach the client:

   a. how to avoid spreading the infection to others.
   b. how to do range-of-motion exercises to maintain joint flexibility.
   c. ways to conserve energy.
   d. which foods are most likely to cause allergic reactions.

6. Which of the following is a malignant tumor?

   a. Angioma
   b. Lipoma
   c. Melanoma
   d. Sebaceous cyst

Critical Thinking Questions

1. How might a person's self-image be affected when the person has a skin disorder on the face or hands?

2. Prepare a teaching plan related to preventing the spread of skin infections.

3. Identify the rationale for each nursing intervention given for the possible nursing diagnoses in this chapter.

 WEB FLASH!

- Search the Internet for information on new medications or treatments for the disorders in this chapter. Share the information with classmates.
- What type of information do the resources for this chapter have on the Internet? How can the information benefit a student nurse, client, family, or professional caregiver?

NURSING CARE OF THE CLIENT: IMMUNE SYSTEM

CHAPTER 22

MAKING THE CONNECTION

Refer to the following chapters to increase your understanding of the immune system:

- **Chapter 3, Legal Responsibilities**
- **Chapter 5, Communication**
- **Chapter 7, Wellness Concepts**
- **Chapter 10, Fluid, Electrolyte, and Acid-Base Balance**
- **Chapter 12, Health Assessment**
- **Chapter 14, Pain Management**
- **Chapter 17, Nursing Care of the Oncology Client**
- **Chapter 18, Nursing Care of the Client: Respiratory System**
- **Chapter 19, Nursing Care of the Client: Cardiovascular System**
- **Chapter 20, Nursing Care of the Client: Hemotalogic and Lymphatic Systems**

- **Chapter 21, Nursing Care of the Client: Integumentary System**
- **Chapter 23, Nursing Care of the Client: HIV and AIDS**
- **Chapter 24, Nursing Care of the Client: Musculoskeletal System**
- **Chapter 25, Nursing Care of the Client: Neurological System**
- **Chapter 28, Nursing Care of the Client: Gastrointestinal System**
- **Chapter 32, Nursing Care of the Client: Sexually Transmitted Diseases**
- **Chapter 34, Nursing Care of the Client: Substance Abuse**

LEARNING OBJECTIVES

Upon completion of this chapter, you should be able to:

- *Define key terms.*
- *Identify three allergic reactions with a systemic response.*
- *Describe symptoms of anaphylaxis and appropriate first aid.*
- *Recall common diagnostic tests used to evaluate immunological functioning.*
- *Discuss the medical/surgical management of clients with immunological disorders.*
- *Relate signs and symptoms of complications clients with immunological disorders could experience.*
- *Use the nursing process to plan the care of clients with immune system disorders.*

KEY TERMS

allergen
anaphylaxis
angioedema
antibodies
antigen
autoimmune disorder
autologous
cellular immunity
diplopia
exacerbation
histamine
homologous
human leukocyte
   antigen

humoral immunity
hypersensitivity
immune response
immunity
immunotherapy
myasthenia gravis
ptosis
remission
rheumatoid arthritis
systemic lupus
   erythematosus
urticaria

INTRODUCTION

Immunity is the body's ability to protect itself from foreign agents or organisms. This occurs through the complex interaction of the tissues within the immune system. Constant surveillance of cells within the body occurs to differentiate self from nonself. Those identified as nonself are then neutralized or destroyed. Dead or damaged cells are eliminated and homeostasis is maintained. When alterations in the system develop, immunological conditions develop. They may be hypersensitivity responses such as allergies; immunological deficiencies, such as those associated with corticosteroid medications; or **autoimmune disorders**, where the body identifies its own cells as foreign and activates mechanisms to destroy them. Rheumatoid arthritis, systemic lupus erythematosus, and myasthenia gravis are examples of autoimmune disorders. Immunosuppressive disorders suppress the body's natural immune response to an antigen. Kaposi's sarcoma and non-Hodgkin's lymphoma are examples of immunosuppressive disorders. HIV and AIDS are discussed in detail in Chapter 23.

ANATOMY AND PHYSIOLOGY REVIEW

The human body has a variety of natural physical and chemical mechanisms that enhance immunological functioning. The skin, eyelashes, cilia in the nose and respiratory system, gastric acidity, intestinal mucosa, and pH of vaginal mucosa all act to protect against invading organisms. In addition, all body tissues are linked together via lymphatic ducts and blood vessels to the organs and cells of the immune system.

Organs of the Immune System

The organs of the immune system are classified as primary or peripheral lymphoid organs. Primary lymphoid organs are bone marrow and the thymus gland. Within bone marrow, stem cells, the parent cells for all blood cells, are produced. Peripheral lymphoid organs are lymph nodes, spleen, tonsils, appendix, Peyer's patches of the small intestines, and the liver. Lymph nodes, located throughout the body, connected by an elaborate ductal system, filter lymphatic fluid, removing destroyed matter. Enlargement of lymphoid organs indicates an infectious or malignant process is occurring. The spleen serves as a reservoir for macrophages, lymphocytes, and plasma cells. The tonsils, appendix, and Peyer's patches also contain plasma cells and lymphocytes. The Kupffer cells of the liver house monocytes that ingest and destroy foreign organisms in hepatic circulation.

Cells of the Immune System

Leukocytes, white blood cells (WBCs), are vital components of the immune system. They are formed mostly in the bone marrow and partially in the lymph tissue. After formation, they are transported to different parts of the body where they fight infectious organisms. There are 6 types of WBCs normally found in the blood. They are neutrophils, eosinophils, basophils, monocytes, lymphocytes, and plasma cells (Guyton & Hall, 1996). Adults have about 7,000 WBCs/mm³ of blood. Each type is a percentage of the total number of WBCs (Table 22–1).

Those cells with granules in the cytoplasm are called *granulocytes,* while those lacking them are called *agranulocytes* (Figure 22-1). Eosinophils, neutrophils, and basophils are granular leukocytes. Monocytes and lymphocytes are agranular leukocytes. Each has its own unique function. Eosinophils come into play during allergic reactions or parasitic invasions. Neutrophils are useful in ingesting bacteria. Basophils secrete **histamine**, a substance released during allergic reactions, and heparin. Monocytes travel to the sites of invading organisms and transform into macrophages, capable of ingesting large quantities of microorganisms and damaged cells, a process known as *phagocytosis.* They also secrete Interleuken-1, which stimulates the activation of specific lymphocytes. Granulocytes, also called *polymorphonuclear leukocytes,* make up the greatest number of WBCs.

B-lymphocytes, or B-cells, and T-lymphocytes, or T-cells, play a vital role in the immune response. B-cells are responsible for **humoral immunity**, or immunity dominated by antibodies (Table 22–2). They stimulate plasma cells to secrete **antibodies** (proteins that react with antigens to neutralize or destroy them) in response to **antigens** (any substance identified by the body as nonself). Antibodies are also called *immunoglobulins.* IgA, IgD, IgE, IgG, and IgM are common antibodies found in plasma. When an antibody-antigen reaction occurs, the complement system, a complex sequential immunological process, is activated. This system is composed of plasma proteins made in the

Table 22–1 PERCENTAGES OF DIFFERENT WBC TYPES	
Neutrophils	55%–70%
Eosinophils	1%–4%
Basophils	0.5%–1.0%
Monocytes	2%–8%
Lymphocytes	20%–40%

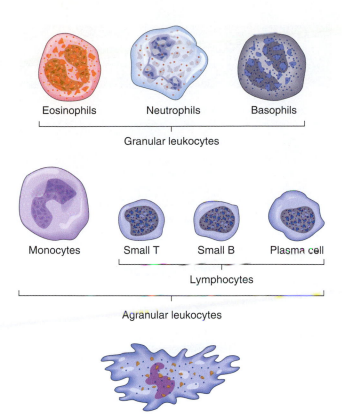

Figure 22-1 Cells of the Immune System

Table 22–2 HUMORAL AND CELLULAR RESPONSES	
HUMORAL RESPONSE (B-CELL RESPONSE)	**CELLULAR RESPONSE (T-CELL RESPONSE)**
• B-lymphocytes stimulate plasma cells, which manufacture antibodies in response to an antigen and release them into the bloodstream. • Predominant role in response to: Bacteria and some viral infections Allergic reactions Autoimmune diseases	• Plasma cells are transformed into special T-lymphocyte cells, which detect, attack, and destroy invading antigens. • Predominant role in response to: Viral and some bacteria infections Delayed hypersensitivity (TB testing) Transplant rejection Graft-versus-host disease Fungal and parasitic infections Detection and destruction of tumor cells

liver. They alter cell membranes in the antibody-antigen reaction, facilitating the cellular breakdown of the invading antigen, and attract macrophages and granulocytes to the antibody-antigen reaction site. When a B-cell identifies an antigen, it places the characteristics of that antigen in a memory bank. B-cells also produce "memory cells" capable of identifying the antigen, if and when it is introduced to the body again.

T-cells are responsible for **cellular immunity**, a type of acquired immunity involving T-cell lymphocytes. (again, see Table 22–2). With T-cell mediated immunity, there is a formation of large numbers of activated lymphocytes that are specifically designed to destroy the foreign agent. T-cells include helper cells (CD4), suppressor cells (CD8), and killer (cytotoxic) cells. CD4 and CD8 are molecules on the T-helper and T-suppressor cells and are important in understanding how HIV attacks the immune system.

Types of Immunity

There are 2 types of immunity: natural (innate) and acquired (adaptive) (Table 22–3). One is born with natural immunity. It is species specific. For example, humans have an innate resistance to distemper while dogs never develop measles or syphilis. Acquired immunity develops after birth and may be active or passive. Active acquired immunity is the result of exposure to the disease itself or its vaccine. As a result, the body develops antibodies and memory cells for the causative microorganism. A repeated exposure results in rapid activation of these components of the immune system and annihilation of the invading agent. Passive acquired immunity utilizes antibodies produced by another human being or an animal. Injection of these immunoglobulins temporarily prevents development of

Table 22–3 COMPARISON OF NATURAL AND ACQUIRED IMMUNITY		
	ACQUIRED IMMUNITY	
NATURAL IMMUNITY	**ACTIVE ACQUIRED IMMUNITY**	**PASSIVE ACQUIRED IMMUNITY**
• Innate immunity • Present at birth • Includes physical and chemical barriers to invading antigens	• Long-term immunity • Antibodies develop as a result of exposure to a disease or vaccine • Antibodies neutralize future invasions of the same antigen	• Temporary immunity • Antibodies obtained from an animal or another human who has been exposed to an antigen • Examples are gamma-globulin or antiserum

the disease once exposed. Transmission of antibodies through fetal circulation is an example of passive acquired immunity.

Factors Influencing Immunity

Although the exact physiological mechanisms involved are unknown, it has been well documented that a number of factors influence the **immune response** (body's reaction to substances identified as nonself, neutralization of antigen). These include age, sex, nutritional status, stress, and treatment modalities. As one ages, the immune system becomes less effective. Sex hormones affect immunity; estrogen enhances immunological functioning, while androgen suppresses it. Therefore, women are especially prone to autoimmune diseases, while men are more prone to immunosuppressive disorders. Poor nutritional status and emotional stress lead to increased susceptibility to infections. Radiation therapy and a variety of medications, such as corticosteroids and chemotherapeutic agents, suppress the immune system.

ASSESSMENT

Physical assessment of the immune system involves the entire body. The skin and mucous membranes are evaluated for urticaria, inflammation, or bleeding. Superficial head, neck, supraclavicular, axilla, and inguinal lymph nodes are inspected and palpated for redness, tenderness, or swelling. Elevated temperature may indicate infection. Joints must be evaluated for possible tenderness, swelling, or limited range of motion. Changes in the rate and rhythm of respirations, presence of a cough, or abnormal lung sounds may indicate immunological conditions. Cardiovascular status, including rate, rhythm, arrhythmias, and peripheral vascular circulation, must be assessed. Enlarged liver or spleen and gastrointestinal conditions, such as nausea, vomiting, or diarrhea, may have an immunological basis. Alterations in vision, hearing, urinary habits, and neurological function may occur.

COMMON DIAGNOSTIC TESTS

Commonly used diagnostic tests for clients with symptoms of immune system disorders are listed in Table 22–4. See Chapter 13, Diagnostic Tests, for explanation/normal values and nursing responsibilities.

HYPERSENSITIVE IMMUNE RESPONSE

Hypersensitive immune responses include allergies, anaphylaxis, transfusion reactions, transplant rejection, and latex allergy.

Table 22–4 COMMON DIAGNOSTIC TESTS FOR IMMUNE SYSTEM DISORDERS

- Antinuclear antibodies (ANA)
- Complement assay (Total complement, C3 and C4)
- C-reactive protein test (CRP)
- CD4 T-cells
- Enzyme-linked immunosorbent assay (ELISA)
- Erythrocyte sedimentation rate (ESR or Sed Rate Test)
- Human leukocyte antigen DW4 (HLA-DW4)
- Lupus erythematosus test (LE Prep)
- Polymerase chain reaction (PCR)
- Red blood cell count (RBC count)
- Rheumatoid factor (RF)
- Total white blood cell count
  Differential count
  Neutrophils
  - Segs (mature neutrophils)
  - Bands (immature neutrophils)
  Eosinophils
  Basophils
  Lymphocytes
  Monocytes
- Western blot

ALLERGIES

Allergic disorders are the result of a **hypersensitivity** (excessive reaction to a stimulus) of the immune system to **allergens** (a type of antigen commonly found in the environment). Allergens may be inhaled, injected, ingested, or contacted. There are four types of hypersensitivity reactions based on how tissue is injured.

Type I reactions occur immediately upon exposure to a specific antigen. Upon first exposure to an allergen, IgE antibodies are produced. They adhere to mast cells. When a subsequent exposure occurs, these cells attach to the antigen and activate the release of chemical mediators, such as histamine, bradykinin, and serotonin. These chemicals cause vasodilation, enhanced capillary permeability, and bronchoconstriction (Figure 22-2).

The most common Type I reactions include allergic rhinitis, urticaria, and angioedema. Anaphylaxis is the most severe and is covered separately. Drug and food allergies are also Type I hypersensitivity.

Allergic rhinitis, also known as *hay fever* or *pollinosis,* is a common allergy in our society caused by airborne allergens such as pollen, mold, animal dander, dust, and ragweed. Symptoms include nasal congestion, thin, clear, watery discharge, sneezing, itching, swelling, and redness of the eyes. Headaches and ear infections may also develop. An estimated 10% or 26 million persons in the United States are affected by al-

Allergic response

First exposure

Second or subsequent exposure

Figure 22-2 Allergic Response

lergic rhinitis (National Institute of Allergy and Infectious Diseases [NIAID], July 1999a).

Urticaria (hives) are raised pruritic, red, nontender wheals on the skin. They are usually on the trunk and on the areas of the extremities closest to the trunk.

Angioedema, edema of subcutaneous layers and mucous membranes, is painless and only slightly pruritic. Urticaria and angioedema together affect approximately 15% of the United States population each year (NIAID, July 1999a).

Any drug potentially may cause a drug reaction, but common ones include penicillin, cephalosporins, insulin, vaccines, and local anesthetics. Reactions vary from mild to severe. Usually symptoms do not occur until the client has taken several doses of the medication, although they can occur at first exposure. The most common reaction is the sudden development of a bright red, itchy rash, often appearing initially on the trunk or arms. Occasionally, a client may develop an anaphylactic reaction. Approximately 2% to 3% of hospitalized clients have an allergic reaction to drugs, especially penicillin and cephalosporins (NIAID, July 1999a).

Although individuals may be allergic to any edible substance, certain foods, such as milk, fish, chocolate, and nuts, are common allergens that cause diarrhea as a result of immunological reaction in the intestinal mucosa. Headache, nausea, vomiting, rash, itching, and wheezing may also develop.

Type II reactions are the destruction of cells or substances with antigens attached that either immunoglobulin G (IgG) or immunoglobulin M (IgM) senses as being foreign. Antibodies cause either lysis of the cells or accelerated phagocytosis. Hemolytic transfu-

sion reactions are this type of reaction. Transfusion reactions are discussed in further detail later.

Type III reaction involves IgG immune antigen-antibody complexes. It is a local reaction evident after several hours that may change from red skin to hemorrhage and tissue necrosis. Occasionally this is noted after penicillin or sulfonamide use.

Type IV is a delayed reaction involving sensitized T-lymphocytes coming in contact with the allergen. Contact dermatitis and transplant rejection are examples of this type of reaction. Poison ivy and poison oak are the most common causes of contact dermatitis. Latex rubber is a more recently discovered cause of contact dermatitis or occasionally a Type 1 (anaphylactic) reaction. Transplant rejection and latex allergy are covered separately.

Medical–Surgical Management

Medical

Medical management of clients experiencing an allergic response (reaction to allergen) includes drug therapy to treat symptoms and identification of precipitating agents. Once the allergen(s) have been identified, **immunotherapy** (treatment to suppress or enhance immunological functioning) is begun. This involves repeated injections of the diluted allergen. Subsequently, decreased levels of histamine are released upon exposure to the allergen.

Pharmacological

A number of medications are employed to treat the symptoms of an allergic response. Antihistamines counteract the effects of histamine. They may be taken orally, topically, or intravenously, depending upon the type of allergic response and urgency for treatment. Nasal decongestants help relieve respiratory symptoms. Topical corticosteroids effectively relieve inflammation associated with contact dermatitis and dermatitis medicamentosa. Oral or injectable forms of corticosteroids may be used either alone or in combination with antihistamines and nasal decongestants.

Skin testing by a physician can determine the specific causative allergen.

Diet

Individuals allergic to certain foods should be taught to check food labels carefully, be aware of how food is prepared, and not eat any product that could lead to a reaction. This includes restaurant foods and foods prepared in another person's home.

Activity

Avoidance of the causative allergen prevents allergic reactions. Activities should be centered around doing this, if at all possible. For instance, individuals who are allergic to pollen may need to stay in air-conditioned environments on those days when the pollen count is extremely high.

▶ NURSING PROCESS

▶ Assessment

▶ Subjective Data

A detailed, comprehensive client history should include information about previous allergic reactions, foods eaten or medications taken recently, and contact with environmental pollutants or anything not normally encountered.

▶ Objective Data

Physical assessment includes gastrointestinal and respiratory functioning, and cardiovascular and neurological status. It is also important to assess for the presence of urticaria and angioedema.

Nursing diagnoses for clients with allergies may include the following:

Nursing Diagnoses	Planning/Goals	Nursing Interventions
▶ *Risk for Injury related to an allergic reaction*	The client will identify factors that increase the potential of a reaction.	Assist client in identifying those factors that increase the potential for a reaction.
▶ *Health-Seeking Behaviors related to causative allergen, therapeutic modalities, and/or preventive measures*	The client will relate methods to avoid exposure to allergens.	Assist client in planning lifestyle changes that will help in avoiding exposure to allergens.
▶ *Deficient Knowledge related to lack of information about allergens, treatment, or preventive measures*	The client will demonstrate an understanding of and compliance with therapeutic modalities if a reaction occurs. The client will demonstrate an understanding of and compliance with preventive measures to avoid subsequent allergic reactions.	Teach client about allergy treatments and what to do if a reaction occurs.

Evaluation Each goal must be evaluated to determine how it has been met by the client.

ANAPHYLACTIC REACTION

Anaphylaxis is a type I systemic reaction to allergens and is the most serious type of allergic reaction. It occurs in individuals who are extremely sensitive to an allergen. Symptoms develop suddenly and can progress to severe levels within minutes. Foods, drugs, hormones, insect bites, blood, and vaccines all are associated with anaphylactic reactions. Shellfish, eggs, nuts, berries, and chocolates are the most common foods involved. Any medication has the potential of causing a reaction, but antibiotics (especially penicillin), insulin, muscle relaxants, and x-ray dyes are the most frequent precipitating agents. Bee, wasp, hornet, and snake bites may also cause anaphylactic reactions. At least 40 deaths in the United States each year are the result of insect sting anaphylaxis (NIAID, July 1999a).

Anaphylactic reactions may be life-threatening. Symptoms involve the skin, GI tract, and cardiovascular and respiratory systems. Clients experience peripheral tingling, flushing, fullness in the mouth, throat/nasal congestion, tearing and swelling around the eyes, itching, cough, laryngeal edema, bronchospasms, severe dyspnea, vasodilation, and cyanosis. If untreated, these catastrophic effects lead to respiratory failure, severe hypotension, anaphylactic shock, and death. Therefore, it is crucial that symptoms be identified early and treatment initiated immediately, as death can occur in minutes.

Medical–Surgical Management

Medical

Medical management centers around establishing an intravenous line, administering fluids and emergency drugs, and maintaining an airway. Oxygen is provided via nasal cannula or face mask. In severe cases, endotracheal intubation or a tracheotomy may be required.

CLIENT TEACHING

Severe Allergies

- Advise clients with severe allergies wear a Medic Alert tag.
- Encourage clients allergic to insect stings to carry an emergency anaphylactic kit containing epinephrine at all times.

Pharmacological

Epinephrine is administered subcutaneously as soon as symptoms develop to dilate bronchioles, increase heart contractions, and constrict blood vessels. Antihistamines, such as diphenhydramine hydrochloride (Benadryl), block the effects of histamine in bronchioles, blood vessels, and the GI tract. Corticosteroids are given for their anti-inflammatory effect. Vasopressors, such as norepinephrine bitartrate (Levophed) or dopamine hydrochloride (Intropin) may be needed to increase blood pressure. If bronchoconstriction and spasms are severe, albuterol (Proventil), metaproterenol sulfate (Alupent), and/or aminophylline (Aminophyllin) may be administered.

Diet

Clients will be NPO until normal respiratory and circulatory function have been restored.

Activity

Clients will remain on bedrest until vital signs are stable and normal breathing patterns have been restored. Those experiencing severe anaphylactic responses are generally transferred to intensive care units for continued treatment and observation.

▶ NURSING PROCESS

▶ Assessment

▶ Subjective Data

Client history may reveal a previous anaphylaxis reaction. The client may describe feelings of uneasiness, anxiety, weakness, itching, dizziness, nausea, peripheral tingling, and a generalized warm sensation throughout the body.

▶ Objective Data

Since anaphylaxis is a sudden, unexpected event, nurses must be aware that variations in a client's cardiovascular and respiratory status may be signs of an impending anaphylactic reaction. The first symptoms are sweating, sneezing, tachycardia, hypotension, dysrhythmias, cyanosis, edema of tongue and larynx, wheezing, bronchospasms, vascular collapse, and cardiac arrest. Regularly assessing client's vital signs and cardiovascular, respiratory, and neurological status will detect changes before the severe signs of respiratory distress and impending shock develop.

Nursing diagnoses for clients with anaphylaxis may include the following:

Nursing Diagnoses	Planning/Goals	Nursing Interventions
▶ Ineffective Tissue Perfusion (Peripheral) related to increased capillary permeability and vasodilation	The client will have adequate tissue perfusion.	Monitor vital signs frequently. Monitor I & O. Place client in Trendelenburg position for hypotension. Administer IV fluids and medications as ordered.
▶ Ineffective Breathing Patterns related to bronchoconstriction, laryngeal edema, and increased secretions	The client will have effective breathing patterns.	Monitor vital signs. Suction secretions as needed. Maintain patent airway. Administer oxygen and medications as ordered.
▶ Deficient Knowledge related to causative allergen, therapeutic modalities, and/or preventive measures	The client will relate causative allergen, therapeutic modalities, and preventive measures.	Teach client importance of avoiding allergen. Advise client to provide the name of the causative agent and a description of reaction experienced when asked about allergies. Document allergy on all medical records. Teach client and family symptoms of anaphylactic reactions.

Evaluation Each goal must be evaluated to determine how it has been met by the client.

TRANSFUSION REACTIONS

Blood components, such as whole blood, packed or frozen RBCs, leukocytes, platelets, and plasma, may be administered to clients when their own bodies are incapable of manufacturing them at a rate required to maintain vascular homeostasis. Any client receiving blood products that are **homologous** or from a donor of the same species may develop a transfusion reaction. For this reason, some clients are arranging to have their own blood collected, saved, and available for infusion, if needed, during or following elective surgeries. This is known as an **autologous** blood transfusion. Immunological reactions do not develop with this type of blood transfusion.

There are 5 types of transfusion reactions: febrile nonhemolytic, allergic urticarial, delayed hemolytic, acute hemolytic, and anaphylactic. Febrile nonhemolytic reactions are the most common and occur in clients who have had previous blood transfusions. It is the result of an antibody-antigen reaction to WBCs. Symptoms may develop soon after the infusion has started or up to 5 to 6 hours after completion. Fever is the classic symptom and may be accompanied by chills, nausea, headache, hypotension, and respiratory problems. Clients who have allergic urticarial reactions develop a skin rash during or within 1 hour following the transfusion. A delayed hemolytic reaction may occur days to weeks following the transfusion. The client's hemoglobin level falls due to incompatibility of RBC antigens. This type of reaction is often misdiagnosed and thought to be related to the condition that created the need for blood replacement rather than a transfusion reaction. An acute hemolytic reaction is potentially a life-threatening situation. Symptoms, resulting from the incompatibility of ABO groups usually occur during the first 15 minutes of administration, but can develop anytime during the transfusion. Clients complain of chills, nausea, and back pain. Fever, drop in blood pressure (hypotension), vomiting, hematuria, or oliguria may be observed. As the condition progresses, chest pain, dyspnea, anuria, and shock develop. Anaphylactic reactions, although rare, are also life-threatening. Symptoms of acute gastrointestinal malfunctioning and cardiovascular and respiratory collapse develop moments after the transfusion has started.

Medical–Surgical Management

Medical

Medical management of clients experiencing a blood transfusion reaction depends on the type of reaction. Treatment of a febrile nonhemolytic reaction includes stopping the blood, infusing normal saline, and treating the symptoms. For clients experiencing an allergic urticarial reaction, the transfusion should be slowed and an antihistamine administered. Delayed hemolytic reactions often go undetected and untreated. Both an acute hemolytic reaction and anaphylactic reactions are medical emergencies. The transfusion must be stopped immediately. Normal saline and emergency drugs are given intravenously.

Pharmacological

If a febrile nonhemolytic or allergic urticarial reaction occurs, diphenhydramine (Benadryl) and a corticosteroid (hydrocortisone or prednisone) are administered to counteract the immunological response. Antipyretics are ordered to control fever. For life-threatening conditions, emergency medications are employed. (Refer back to Anaphylactic Reaction.)

Diet

Clients should not be fed if a reaction is occurring, especially if respiratory symptoms have developed, as aspiration could occur.

Activity

Clients should remain in bed until symptoms of the reaction have subsided.

▶ NURSING PROCESS

▶ Assessment

▶ Subjective Data

Occasionally, clients verbalize the feeling of something "not being right" or "something strange is going on in my body" before actual symptoms become apparent. They may have itching, headache, or low back pain.

▶ Objective Data

Clients receiving blood components need to be carefully assessed for any signs of a transfusion reaction, such as fever, chills, or respiratory problems.

A nursing diagnosis for clients with transfusion reactions may be:

Nursing Diagnoses	Planning/Goals	Nursing Interventions
▶ *Risk for Injury related to infusion of homologous blood components*	The client will not have injury from infusion of homologous blood products.	Follow protocol for blood products and administration.
		Check client's identification and blood product with another nurse.
		If a reaction occurs, stop transfusion immediately, then call the physician.
		Administer medications as ordered.
		Send blood tubing and a urine specimen to the lab for analysis.
		Monitor and document client's condition.
		Teach client who has a blood transfusion reaction to inform health care providers whenever questioned about allergies.

Evaluation Each goal must be evaluated to determine how it has been met by the client.

TRANSPLANT REJECTION

In 1995, more than 20,000 organ transplants were performed in the United States (NIAID, July 1999b). The success of these procedures is directly related to matching antibodies and antigens of the donor and recipient and to the effectiveness of immunosuppressive medications in preventing rejection. Even with the use of immunosuppressive drugs, 10% to 15% of transplanted organs fail (NIAID, July 1999b). Immunosuppressive medications make the client prone to the development of infections and cancers. Clients must have a regular medical check-up, including cancer screening tests.

Medical–Surgical Management

Medical

Although blood components are the most common type of tissue transplants, today it is possible to transplant bone marrow, corneal tissue, skin, kidneys, pancreas, hearts, livers, and lungs. Bone marrow and blood components often employ autologous donations. Homologous donations may be from living related donors or living nonrelated donors. Cadaveric donations are harvested from individuals after they are pronounced clinically dead. It is important to match ABO blood groups and **human leukocyte antigen** (antigens present in human blood), to prevent rejection when homologous and cadaveric donors are used.

Pharmacological

A combination of immunosuppressive medications is used to hinder rejection. Steroids such as prednisone (Deltasone) and methylprednisolone sodium succinate (Solu-Medrol) decrease the inflammatory response. Cyclosporine (Sandimmune), antithymocyte globulin (equine), ATG (Atgam), and tacrolimus (Prograf) inhibit T-cells. Azathioprine (Imuran) inhibits purine synthesis. Muromonab-CD3 (Orthoclone, OKT 3) prevents acute rejection in kidney transplant clients. Clients taking immunosuppressive medications are especially prone to developing infections. Antibiotics may be prescribed prophylactically.

Steroids cause fluid and sodium retention, low potassium level, elevated blood pressure, moon face, muscle wasting, elevated glucose level, impaired wound healing, mood swings, and masculinization in women. Cyclosporine may be toxic to the kidneys and liver. Imuran may cause hair loss and lower platelet level. OKT 3 also causes fluid retention.

Activity

Activity is dependent upon the type of transplant. Clients who receive a major organ, such as a heart, lung, pancreas, or liver, are placed in reverse isolation in the hospital setting for at least 2 weeks. They are carefully observed for signs of rejection. Exposure to others is limited. Prior to discharge, they are taught to avoid contact with any one who may have an infection and to wear a mask whenever out in public.

▶ NURSING PROCESS

▶ Assessment

▶ Subjective Data

Client history may reveal fear of possible transplant rejection. The client generally describes tenderness at the transplant site.

▶ Objective Data

Following transplantation, clients' vital signs, nutritional status, fluid balance, urinary output, mental status, and respiratory and cardiovascular functioning need to be carefully monitored. Daily weight should be taken. Wound sites should be checked frequently. Signs of rejection include fever, weight gain, and swelling or tenderness at the transplant site.

Nursing diagnoses for clients with organ transplants may include the following:

Nursing Diagnoses	Planning/Goals	Nursing Interventions
❯ *Fear related to possible transplant rejection.*	The client will relate less fear regarding rejection.	Allow client to verbalize concerns and develop realistic expectations. Set aside time to sit down and talk to client.
❯ *Deficient Knowledge related to home care following transplantation*	The client will discuss signs and symptoms of rejection. The client will demonstrate an understanding of the side effects of immunosuppressive drugs and lifestyle changes to adapt to their effects.	Teach client and family about signs of rejection and infection. Teach client and family ramifications of taking immunosuppressive medications. Teach client to watch for side effects and report them to physician.
❯ *Risk for Infection related to immunosuppressive medications*	The client will demonstrate appropriate wound care. The client will be free of infection.	Teach client and family appropriate wound care and proper handwashing. Teach client importance of taking antibiotics as ordered. Teach the client to wear a mask whenever out in public. Teach client importance of regular checkups, including cancer screening tests.

Evaluation Each goal must be evaluated to determine how it has been met by the client

LATEX ALLERGY

Since 1987, when universal precautions (now called Standard Precautions) were mandated, exposure to latex by health care workers has dramatically increased. Between 1988 and 1992, more than 1,000 systemic allergic reactions to natural rubber latex were reported (NIAID, July 1999a). By June 1996, 28 latex-related deaths had been reported to the Food and Drug Administration (FDA) (Burt, 1998).

The latex proteins can enter the body through the skin and mucous membranes, intravascularly, and by inhalation. The cornstarch powder on gloves absorbs the latex proteins and becomes airborne when the gloves are put on or taken off. From the air, the latex proteins may be inhaled or may be in contact with the skin and mucous membranes. Anyone, client or health care worker, who after exposure to latex develops red, watery, itchy eyes; sinus or nasal irritation; hives; shortness of breath; dry cough; wheezing; chest tightness; or flushing, tachycardia, and hypotension should be suspected of latex allergy.

There are more than 20,000 medical products containing latex (Burt, 1998). Synthetic versions of products are often available. An individual product may be "latex free," but an environment is "latex safe" only when all items of latex that might come in contact with the allergic individual are removed.

Safety: Latex Allergy
A MedicAlert tag stating "latex allergy" should be worn by any individual with a latex allergy.

AUTOIMMUNE DISEASES

Disorders in this category include rheumatoid arthritis, systemic lupus erythematosus, and myasthenia gravis.

RHEUMATOID ARTHRITIS

Rheumatoid arthritis (RA) is a chronic, systemic autoimmune disease characterized by joint stiffness. It affects 2.1 million people in the United States, including 1.5 million women and 600,000 men (Arthritis Foundation, 1999a). It affects people of all races, usually beginning between the ages of 25 and 50, but RA is reported in persons of all ages (Arthritis Foundation, 1999b).

The cause of RA is unknown, but there seems to be a genetic predisposition (susceptibility) in many, but not all, persons affected. It is believed that something must trigger the disease process such as a virus, bacterium, hormonal factors, or stress. The person's immune system attacks the cells inside the joint(s), producing substances that act as antigens. Immune complexes are formed within the joint, causing inflammation, swelling, and increased synovial fluid. As this chronic, systemic condition progresses, surrounding cartilage, tendons, and ligaments become involved. Thickening of synovial tissue eventually leads to calcification of the joint, joint pain, limited mobility, and deformity.

It is believed that the damage to the bones begins within the first two years of the onset of RA. Early diagnosis and aggressive treatment are important to control the disease. Usually, the joints of the hand and wrist are affected initially. As the disease progresses, shoulder, elbow, hip, knee, ankle, and cervical spine joints become affected. The pattern of joint involvement is symmetrical, that is, if a joint is affected on the right side of the body, the same joint will also be affected on the left side (Arthritis Foundation, 1999c). Other areas of the body where connective tissue is present may also be involved, such as blood vessels, lining of the lungs, and pericordial sac.

Clients experience periods of **remission**, a decrease or absence of symptoms, and **exacerbations**, an increase in symptoms. Both physical and emotional stressors lead to increased symptomatology. This means that simple tasks such as answering the telephone or buttoning clothes may become very challenging.

Medical–Surgical Management

Medical

Medical management centers around reducing inflammation, relieving pain, maintaining normal joint function, and promoting general health. Therapeutic regimen includes medications, exercise, rest, hot and cold applications, and stress management.

Surgical

Hip, knee, and finger joints may be surgically replaced. Refer to Chapter 24, Nursing Care of the Client: Musculoskeletal System, for a discussion of joint replacement.

Pharmacological

Nonsteroidal anti-inflammatory drugs (NSAIDs) and salicylates have the potential to relieve symptoms such as joint pain, stiffness, and swelling but do not control the disease. Disease-modifying anti-rheumatic drugs (DMARDs) have the potential for modifying the disease and should be given early in the disease to control progression. The commonly used DMARDs include prednisone (Deltasone), gold salts, and sulfasalazine (Azulfidine EN-Tabs) (Table 22–5). Because of the large doses required to control inflammation and the long-term use due to the chronicity of this condition, side effects often develop. In severe cases, azathioprine (Imuran), hydroxychloroquine sulfate (Plaquenil Sulfate), D-penicillamine (Depen), or methotrexate sodium (Rheumatrex) may be used. These medications also have serious side effects.

Table 22–5 MEDICATIONS USED TO TREAT RHEUMATOID ARTHRITIS

DRUG	USE/ACTIONS	SIDE EFFECTS	NURSING CONSIDERATIONS
Salicylates • aspirin	Inhibit prostaglandin synthesis resulting in decreased pain. (Analgesia) antipyretic and anti-inflammatory effects.	GI upset, tinnitus, easy bruising, nausea, prolonged bleeding time.	Instruct client to take with food or take enteric coated aspirin and to report ringing in ears. Do not give to clients on oral anticoagulants. Assess for bleeding/bruising.
Nonsteroidal Anti-inflammatory Drugs (NSAIDs) • ibuprofen (Motrin, Rufen) • naproxen (Naprosyn) • phenylbutazone (Butazolidin) • nambumetone (Relafen)	Inhibit prostaglandin synthesis. Reduce joint swelling stiffness. Analgesic and antipyretic properties.	GI irritation, nausea, vomiting, heartburn. GI bleeding and ulceration, dizziness, headache, liver toxicity.	Administer with food. May prolong bleeding time, may require frequent blood count.
Indole Analogues • indomethacin (Indocin) • sulindac (Clinoril)	Analgesic anti-inflammatory effect.	Gastric bleeding, headaches, dizziness, psychiatric disturbances.	Administer with food. Instruct client to report any bleeding (tarry stools, hematemesis). Avoid giving aspirin.
Corticosteroids • prednisone (Deltasone)	Decreases inflammation.	GI irritation, muscle weakness, fluid retention, moon face, muscle wasting, impaired wound healing.	Administer with food. Weigh daily. Monitor BP, sleep pattern, and serum potassium.
Antimalarials • hydroxychloroquine sulfate (Plaquenil Sulfate)	Not a drug of choice.	Visual disturbances, nightmares, skin lesions, nausea, diarrhea, low blood count.	Monitor CBC and liver function tests. Discontinue after 6 months if no beneficial effects noted.

continues

Table 22–5 MEDICATIONS USED TO TREAT RHEUMATOID ARTHRITIS *continued*

DRUG	USE/ACTIONS	SIDE EFFECTS	NURSING CONSIDERATIONS
Gold Salts			
• auranofin (Ridaura)	Anti-inflammatory effect.	Diarrhea, nausea, vomiting, jaundice.	Remind client to keep all physician appointments. Beneficial effects may take 3 months to appear.
Chelating Agent			
• penicillamine (Depen)	Palliative when other medications have failed.	Bone marrow depression, fever, rashes, blood dyscrasias, liver toxicity.	Give on empty stomach. Have epinephrine 1:1,000 handy for anaphylaxis. Fluids to 3,000 mL/day to prevent renal failure.
Sulfonamide			
• sulfasalazine (Azulfidine EN-TABS)	For clients who do not respond well to NSAIDs.	Anorexia, headache, nausea, vomiting, gastric distress, reversible oligospermia.	Give with food. May discolor urine or skin yellow-orange. Take at least 2–3 L/day of water. May increase sensitivity to sun.

Diet

Clients need to be taught to eat a nutritious, well-balanced diet. Poorly nourished individuals are prone to infections. For clients with RA, an infection results in exacerbation of symptoms. Foods high in iron are encouraged when RBCs are low.

Activity

Since joint mobility is a major problem, occupational and physical therapists are part of the therapeutic team. Range of motion exercises, resting splints, and assistive devices such as canes and hand rails are often employed to promote mobility.

▶ NURSING PROCESS

▶ Assessment

▶ Subjective Data

Client history frequently reveals a gradual development of symptoms, beginning initially with early morning stiffness and pain in finger joints. Eventually, other joints become involved. Fatigue, weight loss, temperature elevation, and anemia develop. Subjective data often include malaise, loss of appetite, fatigue, and muscle weakness. Information about periods of remissions and exacerbations should be obtained, as well as the clients' understanding of and compliance with the treatment regimen.

▶ Objective Data

Assessment of the hands may reveal the classic deformities associated with RA: boutonniere deformity (fixed flexion of the proximal interphalangeal joint and hyperextension of the distal interphalangeal joint), ulnar drift (deviation of the fingers to the ulnar side of the hand), and swan-neck deformity (fixed flexion of the distal interphalangeal joint and hyperextension of the proximal interphalangeal joint). Figure 22-3 illustrates these changes in the hands.

Skin may show the presence of ulcers, due to vasculitis, and moveable, subcutaneous skin nodes, known as *rheumatoid nodules*. Eye tissue may be inflamed. Reduction in tear and saliva production can occur, causing dryness of the eyes, mouth, and mucous membranes. This is known as Sjogren's syndrome. The client may have weight loss and an elevated temperature.

X-rays demonstrate the amount and degree of deformity. There is no specific laboratory test that confirms a diagnosis of RA, though alterations in the following may occur: RBCs decrease (anemia) as the disease progresses, elevation of WBCs, erythrocyte sedimentation rate (ESR), antinuclear antibodies (ANAs), C-reactive proteins, and platelet count. The rheumatoid factor (RF) is present in about 80% of adult clients with RA (Arthritis Foundation, 1999d).

Figure 22-3 Arthritic Hands (*Courtesy of the Arthritis Foundation*)

Nursing diagnoses for clients with rheumatoid arthritis may include the following:

Nursing Diagnoses	Planning/Goals	Nursing Interventions
▶ *Chronic Pain related to swollen, inflamed joints*	The client will relate appropriate use of anti-inflammatory medications. The client will relate methods to decrease pain.	Teach client about prescribed analgesics and anti-inflammatory medications. Encourage client to practice relaxation techniques and take warm shower to relieve early morning joint stiffness and pain. Use hot and cold packs to decrease muscle spasms. Teach client proper body alignment and to avoid using pillows under the knees, which leads to pooling of blood in the feet.
▶ *Impaired Physical Mobility related to edema, and joint immobility*	The client will demonstrate measures to maintain joint mobility. The client will demonstrate use of adaptive devices.	Teach hospitalized clients to use the overhead trapeze when moving in bed and to change position frequently. Assist with ROM exercises. Maintain planned rest periods. Teach client use of assistive devices, such as handrests, tools to pick up objects, or three-legged canes, as needed. Check with occupational and physical therapists for available equipment. Assist client to use handrails in tub, shower, and toilet; raised toilet seat; and rubber-tipped walker or cane.
▶ *Bathing/Hygiene and Dressing/Grooming Self-care Deficit related to joint inflammation or deformity*	The client will bathe, dress, and groom to abilities.	Recommend shoes with Velcro® closures. Encourage client to stop and rest when getting tired. Teach self-care using assistive devices, as required. Assist with routine plan for ADLs.
▶ *Fatigue related to chronic inflammatory process*	The client will state less fatigue. The client will establish priorities for daily activities. The client will balance daily activities with periods of rest.	Explain that fatigue is a common symptom of autoimmune disorders. Allow the client to express feelings about altered lifestyle. Inform client of community services such as Meals on Wheels. Plan rest periods between activities. Help identify activities client should perform and what can be delegated. Instruct client to record level of fatigue and activities performed on an hourly basis for 24 hours. One method uses 0 to 10 scale (0 = not tired, peppy; 10 = totally exhausted). Help plan important tasks during high-energy periods and distribute difficult ones throughout the week.

Evaluation Each goal must be evaluated to determine how it has been met by the client.

SYSTEMIC LUPUS ERYTHEMATOSUS

Systemic lupus erythematous (SLE) is a chronic, progressive, incurable autoimmune disease affecting multiple body organs. It is characterized by periods of exacerbation and remission. SLE occurs most commonly in women during their childbearing years and develops 3 times more frequently in African Americans and is more common in Hispanic, Asian, and Native Americans than in the white population (National Institute of Arthritis, Musculoskeletal, and Skin Diseases [NIAMS], 1999). More people have lupus than AIDS, cerebral palsy, multiple sclerosis, sickle-cell anemia, and cystic fibrosis combined (Lupus Foundation of America, 1995). In clients with SLE, abnormal B-lymphocyte cells produce autoantibodies that destroy body cells. Immune complexes are formed and circulate in serum, causing inflammation and tissue damage in the skin, brain, kidney, lung, heart, or joints. Production of these autoantibodies is influenced by genetic predisposition, medications, infections, stress, and sunlight (ultraviolet light rays).

No single test is conclusive for a diagnosis. The American Rheumatism Association has established criteria for SLE. If 4 or more of these criteria are present, a diagnosis of SLE is confirmed (Table 22–6).

Medical–Surgical Management

Medical

Medical treatment is aimed at decreasing tissue inflammation and destruction. A knowledgeable client

Table 22–6   THE ELEVEN CRITERIA USED FOR THE DIAGNOSIS OF LUPUS ERYTHEMATOSUS

CRITERION	DEFINITION
Malar Rash	Rash over the cheeks
Discoid Rash	Red raised patches
Photosensitivity	Reaction to sunlight, resulting in the development of or increase in skin rash
Oral Ulcers	Ulcers in the nose or mouth, usually painless
Arthritis	Nonerosive arthritis involving 2 or more peripheral joints (arthritis in which the bones around the joints do not become destroyed)
Serositis	Pleuritis or pericarditis (inflammation of the lining of the lung or heart)
Renal Disorder	Excessive protein in the urine (greater than 0.5 gm/day or 3+ on test sticks) and/or cellular casts (abnormal elements in the urine, derived from red and/or white cells and/or kidney tubule cells)
Neurologic Disorder	Seizures (convulsions) and/or psychosis in the absence of drugs or metabolic disturbances which are known to cause such effects
Hematologic Disorder	Hemolytic anemia or leukopenia (white blood count below 4,000 cells per cubic millimeter) or lymphopenia (less than 1,500 lymphocytes per cubic millimeter) or thrombocytopenia (less than 100,000 platelets per cubic millimeter). The leukopenia and lymphopenia must be detected on two or more occasions. The thrombocytopenia must be detected in the absence of drugs known to induce it.
Antinuclear Antibody	Positive test for antinuclear antibodies (ANA) in the absence of drugs known to induce it.
Immunologic Disorder	Positive anti-double stranded anti-DNA test, positive anti-Sm test, positive antiphospholipid antibody such as anticardiolipin, or false-positive syphilis test (VDRL).

To assist the physician in the diagnosis of lupus, the American College of Rheumatology (ACR) in 1982 issued a list of 11 symptoms, or signs, that help distinguish lupus from other diseases. This was revised in 1998.

Adapted from "The 1982 revised criteria for the classification of SLE," by E. M. Tan et al., 1982, Arth. Rheum., *25, pp. 1271–1277. Used with permission.*

can assist in controlling the disease process through stress management, rest, exercise, taking medications as prescribed, and immediately reporting symptoms to the health care provider. During acute exacerbations, plasmapheresis may be used. This treatment modality involves removal of the client's plasma, processing it through a special machine to eliminate various cellular elements, and reinfusing the cleansed plasma. In SLE, autoantibodies are removed.

CLIENT TEACHING

Systemic Lupus Erythematosus
- Get adequate rest.
- Use stress-reduction techniques such as visualization, guided imagery, meditation, or yoga.
- Avoid exposure to sunlight; use sunscreen.
- Involve family and friends in care.
- Report fever, chills, anorexia, or symptom worsening to health care provider immediately.
- Never just stop taking medications.
- Contact the Lupus Foundation of America, Inc., for information and support (see Resources at the end of the book).

Since clients with SLE are prone to a variety of complications, they are carefully monitored for renal, cardiac, pulmonary, hematological, and neurological damage. A large percentage of SLE clients eventually develop renal failure, requiring dialysis to maintain life.

Pharmacological

NSAIDs are used for muscle and joint pain. The lowest possible dose of corticosteroid is used to suppress immune system activity. During periods of exacerbations, higher doses may be required. Prolonged use of these medications leads to multiple side effects. Hydroxychloroquine sulfate (Plaquenil sulfate), an antimalarial agent, is used. Although the exact mechanism involved is unknown, it does work effectively in decreasing joint and skin problems. It can lead to the development of retinal toxicity; therefore, clients should have yearly eye exams. Cyclophosphamide (Cytoxan) or azathioprine (Imuran) may be used for severe SLE or for those clients who are steroid-resistant (Johnson, 1999).

Diet

Clients on corticosteroids are prone to developing hypernatremia, hyperglycemia, hypokalemia, and fluid retention. Diet should be low in sodium and glucose and high in potassium. Excessive fluid intake should be discouraged.

PROFESSIONAL TIP

RA and SLE

Clients with RA and SLE have common nursing diagnoses of fatigue and impaired mobility. Clients with SLE have an additional risk for infection if WBC count is low.

Activity

Clients should be encouraged to sleep at least 8 hours a night and rest periodically during the day. Regular exercise helps prevent muscle weakness and fatigue.

▶ NURSING PROCESS

▶ Assessment

▶ Subjective Data

The client should be asked when the disease began, what symptoms have developed, and how they have been treated. Information about medications the client is taking and side effects should be elicited, and activity level and degree of fatigue noted. The nurse should determine client's understanding of the disease process, how lifestyle has changed, and how effectively client is coping. The client may describe having malaise, photosensitivity, pain in joints, irregular menses, irritability, confusion, or hallucinations.

▶ Objective Data

A complete head-to-toe assessment is needed. Most common findings include joint swelling and pain, fever, swollen glands, nausea, vomiting, anorexia, hypertension, respiratory and cardiac infections, renal involvement, enlarged liver and spleen, and skin lesions, especially the classic "butterfly" rash. Figure 22-4 shows an individual with a "butterfly rash." If exposed to the cold, Raynaud's phenomenon, intermittent attacks of diminished blood supply to fingers, toes, ears, and nose, may develop.

Laboratory tests frequently reveal serum antinuclear antibodies (ANA) and anti-DNA antibodies. Lupus erythematosus cells (LE cells) are present in most clients. Anemia, leukopenia, and thrombocytopenia are evident.

Figure 22-4 Butterfly Rash (*Courtesy of the American Academy of Dermatology*)

Nursing diagnoses for a client with SLE may include the following:

Nursing Diagnoses	Planning/Goals	Nursing Interventions
▶ *Impaired Skin Integrity related to presence of butterfly rash, skin lesions, Raynaud's phenomenon, and/or oral ulcers*	The client will participate in a plan to promote wound healing.	Teach client to clean and dry area prior to application of topical corticosteroids. Warn client that sunlight and ultraviolet rays increase symptoms and tanning sessions are contraindicated. Encourage client to wear protective clothing, sunscreen of at least SPF 15, and sunglasses. In cold weather, client should wear a hat and gloves. Encourage client in regular oral care to promote healing of mouth sores.
▶ *Deficient Knowledge related to adapting lifestyle with treatment and prevention of complications*	The client will describe disease process, factors contributing to symptoms, and regimen for control.	Teach client effects of disease and methods to control complications. Teach stress management techniques. Allow client to vent feelings. Help client plan methods to adapt lifestyle. Encourage client to visit the physician on a regular basis to monitor for early symptoms of major organ involvement. Advise client to have regular eye exam if taking Plaquenil Sulfate. Inform client of community support groups available through the Lupus Foundation of America, Inc. (see Resources).

Evaluation Each goal must be evaluated to determine how it has been met by the client.

MYASTHENIA GRAVIS

Myasthenia gravis (MG) is an autoimmune disease characterized by extreme muscle weakness and fatigue due to the body's inability to transmit nerve impulses to voluntary muscles. It is thought that clients with MG develop antibodies that act to decrease the number and effectiveness of acetylcholine receptor sites at neuromuscular junctions. Voluntary muscles are most commonly involved, especially those innervated by cranial nerves. Muscle weakness increases during periods of activity and improves after a period of rest.

Severity of symptoms varies. In mild conditions known as Group I ocular myasthenia, only the eye muscles are involved. As severity increases, symptoms of Group II generalized myasthenia develop. Facial, neck, skeletal, and respiratory muscles become affected. The thymus gland is enlarged in most clients. It is in this organ that anti-ACh receptor antibodies are produced. MG affects men more frequently than women with the onset of symptoms after age 50. Periods of remission and exacerbation occur, usually during the first few years.

There are 3 possible complications: respiratory distress, myasthenic crisis, and cholinergic crisis. Clients need to be carefully monitored for early signs of respiratory distress, such as dyspnea, tachypnea, tachycardia, and diaphoresis.

Myasthenia crisis is an acute emergency characterized by increased muscle weakness; difficulty swallowing, chewing, or talking; and respiratory distress. It occurs in newly diagnosed clients who are not responding to anticholinesterase medications following infections, surgery, or delivery of a child.

Cholinergic crisis is the result of an overdose of anticholinesterase medications. Physical symptoms of both myasthenia crisis and cholinergic crisis are the same. An edrophonium chloride (Tensilon) test is used to differentiate between the two. Tensilon is administered intravenously; symptoms of clients experiencing a myasthenia crisis will be relieved within seconds, while clients in cholinergic crisis will show no response. Atropine is administered to counteract the effects of excessive amounts of anticholinesterase drugs. The treatment goal for both is restoration of normal respiratory functioning and alleviation of symptoms.

Medical–Surgical Management

Medical

Medical management involves the use of anticholinesterase medications and plasmapheresis. Plasmapheresis removes anti-ACh receptor antibodies. Since it affords only temporary relief of symptoms, it is used primarily for clients in acute crisis who are not responding to drug therapy or prior to a thymectomy. A client's relief of symptoms is a good indicator of how successful surgery might be.

Surgical

Surgical removal of the thymus gland has shown the best results in young people early in the course of the disease. Clients with disease onset after the age of 60 seldom show substantial improvement after thymectomy (Howard, 1997).

Pharmacological

Anticholinesterase medications, such as pyridostigmine bromide (Mestinon), neostigmine bromide (Prostigmin), and ambenonium chloride (Mytelase), are prescribed early in the course of the disease and act to increase acetylcholine at the neuromuscular junction. Dosages need to be individually determined. Early side effects of overdosage include nausea, abdominal cramping, vomiting, diarrhea, increased saliva, diaphoresis, and low pulse rate. Variation may occur in muscle group responses for the same client. Steroids are also prescribed to slow down the immunological response.

Diet

Clients need to be encouraged to eat a snack prior to taking anticholinesterase medications to avoid GI irritation. If the client's ability to chew and swallow is affected, the diet may need adjustment.

Activity

Symptoms of MG increase with exercise. Clients should avoid excessive muscular activity and should rest periodically throughout the day. ROM exercises, braces, splints, and walkers assist in keeping the client independent.

▶ NURSING PROCESS

▶ Assessment

▶ Subjective Data

Client describes muscle weakness, fatigue, and possibly difficulty chewing or swallowing.

PROFESSIONAL TIP

Myasthenia Gravis

Clients with myasthenia gravis experience problems similar to those with RA and SLE, i.e., fatigue and impaired physical mobility. Although the cause, in this case, is due to weakness of voluntary muscles, client goals and nursing interventions are the same.

▶ Objective Data

The nurse must assess level of muscle groups affecting the eyes, face, neck, and chest, looking for **diplopia** (double vision), **ptosis** (drooping upper eyelids) and facial symmetry. Chewing or swallowing problems should be noted. Vocal tones and breath sounds should be assessed. Level of weakness in arm and legs muscles as well as muscles used for breathing should all be noted.

ACh receptor antibody and LE cell tests are often positive. X-rays and CT scans of the thymus gland are used to detect enlargement. Electromyogram (EMG) determines the extent of muscle damage.

Nursing diagnoses for a client with MG may include the following:

Nursing Diagnoses	Planning/Goals	Nursing Interventions
▶ *Ineffective Breathing Pattern related to muscle weakness*	The client will have normal respiratory rate and rhythm and normal breath sounds bilaterally.	Monitor client's respiratory rate and rhythm and breath sounds frequently. Administer oxygen as ordered. Elevate head of client's bed. Notify physician immediately if respiratory problem develops.
▶ *Risk for Aspiration related to impaired swallowing*	The client will not experience aspiration.	Have client eat in a sitting position or with head of the bed elevated. Teach client to chew food well and swallow only small bites. Request a special diet of thickened, soft foods. Suction oral secretions as required. Teach client to suction secretions as needed.
▶ *Deficient Knowledge related to disease process and understanding of methods to control disease and prevent complications*	The client will describe disease process, factors contributing to symptoms, and regimen for control. The client will practice health behaviors needed to manage the effects of MG and methods to prevent complications.	Teach client stress management techniques and methods to avoid infections. Teach clients to take medications at regularly scheduled times to maintain appropriate level. Encourage client to wear a MedicAlert bracelet indicating the name and dosage of medications being taken. Refer to the Myasthenia Gravis Foundation for information and support groups (see Resources).

Evaluation Each goal must be evaluated to determine how it has been met by the client.

SAMPLE NURSING CARE PLAN

THE CLIENT WITH MYASTHENIA GRAVIS

Mrs. Henry, a 29-year-old mother of two preschool children, was diagnosed with myasthenia gravis 2 years ago. Initially, she had double vision and drooping eyelids, but after beginning a course of pyridostigmine bromide (Mestinon), she went into remission. Recently, she has been experiencing facial, neck, and chest muscle weakness and is now admitted to the hospital for evaluation. Occasionally, she has difficulty swallowing and breathing. Her thymus gland is enlarged. She has asked the nurse to teach her some strategies for managing this chronic illness.

Nursing Diagnosis 1 *Ineffective Breathing Pattern related to respiratory muscle fatigue as evidenced by facial, neck, and chest weakness*

PLANNING/GOALS	NURSING INTERVENTIONS	RATIONALE	EVALUATION
Mrs. Henry's respiratory rate and rhythm and	Assess Mrs. Henry's breathing patterns q2h.	Frequent client assessment detects early signs of respiratory distress.	Mrs. Henry's respiratory rate and rhythm have

continues

breath sounds will remain within normal limits.	Inform Mrs. Henry to notify the nurse immediately if she begins to develop any breathing difficulties.	Some clients are reluctant to call the nurse and need to be encouraged to do so.	remained within normal limits.
	Notify physician immediately if respiratory problems develop.	When respiratory problems develop, the physician needs to determine the exact cause and if a tracheostomy is needed.	

Nursing Diagnosis 2 *Risk for Aspiration related to impaired swallowing as evidenced by difficulty swallowing*

PLANNING/GOALS	NURSING INTERVENTIONS	RATIONALE	EVALUATION
Mrs. Henry will not experience aspiration.	Position Mrs. Henry to eat in a sitting position.	Eating in a sitting position promotes the passage of food into the stomach.	Mrs. Henry has not aspirated. She makes a point of always sitting up when eating.
	Teach Mrs. Henry the importance of thoroughly chewing food, and swallowing only small bites.	Swallowing big bites of food can cause aspiration.	
	Have oral suctioning available at the bedside.	If food or secretions become caught in the mouth or throat, suctioning may be required.	

Nursing Diagnosis 3 *Deficient Knowledge related to disease process and understanding of methods to control effects of myasthenia gravis and prevent complications as evidenced by verbalization of need for future teaching*

PLANNING/GOALS	NURSING INTERVENTIONS	RATIONALE	EVALUATION
Mrs. Henry will practice health behaviors needed to manage the effects of MG and prevent complications.	Assess Mrs. Henry's prior knowledge of MG and methods of controlling the effects of prescribed medications and preventing complications.	Assessing a client's prior knowledge provides a basis for planning teaching.	Mrs. Henry and her husband related information about MG, action and side effects of Mestinon, signs and symptoms to watch for, and when to notify the physician. She has obtained a MedicAlert bracelet and has con-
	Include Mrs. Henry's family members in teaching sessions.	Including family members in the teaching session fosters imple-	

continues

Teach Mrs. Henry and family members basic information about MG, the actions of anticholinesterase medication, the need to take it on a regular basis with a snack, side effects of overdose, and the importance of notifying the physician of any signs of respiratory problems or infection.

Information about one's disease, medications, and when to notify the physician is essential knowledge the client and family members need in order to effectively manage this chronic illness.

mentation of the teaching in the home setting.

tacted the MG Foundation. She plans to attend the next local chapter meeting.

Encourage Mrs. Henry to wear a MedicAlert bracelet, which lists her name, diagnoses, and dosage of prescribed medications.

A MedicAlert bracelet provides accurate information to medical personnel in case of an emergency.

Provide Mrs. Henry with the address and telephone number of the Myasthenia Gravis Foundation and encourage her to contact them for additional information and support.

Providing a resource for additional information facilitates future attainment of knowledge and possible involvement with a support group.

CASE STUDY

Sharon is a thirty-four-year-old divorced African American woman. Five years ago she was diagnosed with SLE. Recently, she developed a urinary tract infection that has not responded to medication. Yesterday, when she visited her physician, she complained that the pain in her hands and wrists is getting worse. She was admitted to the hospital for evaluation and rehabilitation.

Sharon has three children, ages 16, 12, and 8. Her husband divorced her several years ago. She tells you "He just couldn't take it anymore. He was working full time. When he came home he would have to do all the housework and care for the children." She now lives with her mother. Sharon used to work as an aide in a nursing home, but due to constant fatigue she had to quit.

Upon admission Sharon's vital signs were as follows: temperature 100.6, blood pressure 170/94, pulse 84, respirations 20. Physical exam revealed the presence of a butterfly rash. This is the first symptom she developed. She had hoped it would go away after she started taking prednisone (Meticorten), but it has remained. She relates that she does not go out in public anymore because everyone stares at her. The assessment revealed that the joints in her hands are stiff; she stated that she has difficulty using her fork.

continues

CASE STUDY *continued*

Initial lab results are:
Urinalysis - Bacteria count greater than 100,000/milliliter
ESR - 24 mm/hr
RBCs - 3.2
WBCs - 15,035
LE Cell Test - Positive
Hemoglovin - 9.2
ANA - Positive

The following questions will guide your development of a nursing care plan for the case study.

1. List signs and symptoms, other than those identified, that clients with SLE might experience.
2. Since Sharon has a history of long-term use of corticosteroids, what side effects might she experience?
3. What diagnostic tests might be ordered to evaluate her arthritic condition?
4. Write three nursing diagnoses and goals for Sharon.
5. Identify nursing interventions to help Sharon deal with the nursing diagnoses identified in number 4.
6. What teaching would be done for Sharon's home care?
7. Identify resources available to help Sharon cope with this chronic condition.

SUMMARY

- The immune system identifies substances as self or nonself and protects the body by neutralizing or destroying foreign organisms.
- Immunity to a disease is either natural or acquired.
- Age, sex, nutritional status, medications, and stress influence the immune response.
- Clients receiving blood transfusions must be carefully monitored, especially during the first half hour, for signs of a reaction.
- Anaphylactic reactions, which may occur as a result of exposure to foods, medications, blood, or insect bites, can potentially be life-threatening.
- Organ transplant clients must understand the implications of taking immunosuppressive medications.
- Clients with rheumatoid arthritis must be taught methods of adapting to the effects of synovial joint inflammation, immobility, and deformity.
- Systemic lupus erythematosus affects multiple body systems.
- Clients with myasthenia gravis experience extreme muscle weakness and fatigue and must be carefully monitored for signs of respiratory distress, and myasthenic or cholinergic crisis.

Review Questions

1. Ms. Caldwell has just been diagnosed with syphilis and has an order for 1,000,000 units of penicillin I.M. She has no history of allergies to medications. She has never had penicillin. When giving her the injection in the right upper outer quadrant of her buttocks, you note a tattoo. Several minutes after receiving the injection, she tells you she feels anxious and weak. You note she is diaphoretic, scratching her forearm, and is breathing faster than normal. Based upon this assessment data, you would conclude:

   a. she is embarrassed because you saw her tattoo.
   b. she is probably anxious since you know she has a sexually transmitted disease.
   c. her syphilis is getting worse.
   d. these are early signs of an anaphylactic reaction.

2. Which of the following is a potentially life-threatening transfusion reaction?

   a. Acute hemolytic reaction
   b. Allergic urticarial reaction
   c. Delayed hemolytic reaction
   d. Febrile nonhemolytic reaction

3. Sensitivity to sunlight, a butterfly rash, and renal failure are symptoms of which of the following conditions?

   a. Anaphylaxis
   b. Myasthenia gravis
   c. Rheumatoid arthritis
   d. Systemic lupus erythematosus

4. Rheumatoid arthritis is:

   a. an autoimmune disease characterized by abnormal IgG antibodies.
   b. associated with abnormal B-cell lymphocytes.
   c. curable if the client takes large doses of Plaquenil Sulfate.
   d. the results of a hypersensitivity reaction.

5. Increased muscle weakness, difficulty chewing or swallowing, and shortness of breath in clients with myasthenia gravis are signs of:

   a. cholinergic crisis.
   b. myasthenia crisis.
   c. both cholinergic crisis and myasthenic crisis.
   d. reaction to plasmapheresis.

Critical Thinking Questions

1. What are the lifestyle implications of being diagnosed with a chronic disease such as rheumatoid arthritis or systemic lupus erythematosus?

2. List the pros and cons of receiving a blood transfusion from a donor.

WEB FLASH!

- Search the Internet for the disorders discussed in this chapter. Can information be found for all of them? What type of research is being performed for these disorders? What type of drugs are available? Diagnostic tests? Other treatments?
- Search the Web for the resources listed for this chapter at the end of this text. How many of them have a Web page? What other information is provided?

CHAPTER 23

NURSING CARE OF THE CLIENT: HIV AND AIDS

MAKING THE CONNECTION

Refer to the following chapters to increase your understanding of HIV and AIDS:

- **Chapter 3, Legal Responsibilities**
- **Chapter 5, Communication**
- **Chapter 7, Wellness Concepts**
- **Chapter 10, Fluid, Electrolyte, and Acid-Base Balance**
- **Chapter 12, Health Assessment**
- **Chapter 14, Pain Management**
- **Chapter 17, Nursing Care of the Oncology Client**
- **Chapter 18, Nursing Care of the Client: Respiratory System**
- **Chapter 19, Nursing Care of the Client: Cardiovascular System**

- **Chapter 20, Nursing Care of the Client: Hemotalogic and Lymphatic Systems**
- **Chapter 21, Nursing Care of the Client: Integumentary System**
- **Chapter 24, Nursing Care of the Client: Musculoskeletal System**
- **Chapter 25, Nursing Care of the Client: Neurological System**
- **Chapter 28, Nursing Care of the Client: Gastrointestinal System**
- **Chapter 32, Nursing Care of the Client: Sexually Transmitted Diseases**
- **Chapter 34, Nursing Care of the Client: Substance Abuse**

LEARNING OBJECTIVES

Upon completion of this chapter, you should be able to:

- *Define key terms.*
- *Describe symptoms of HIV and AIDS.*
- *Recall common diagnostic tests used to evaluate HIV and AIDS.*
- *Discuss the medical/surgical management of clients with HIV and AIDS.*
- *Relate signs and symptoms of complications clients with HIV and AIDS could experience.*
- *Explain the modes of transmission of HIV.*
- *Identify methods of risk reduction of HIV for health care workers.*
- *Use the nursing process to plan the care of clients with HIV and AIDS.*

KEY TERMS

acquired immuno-deficiency syndrome
cytomegalovirus
enzyme-linked immuno-sorbent assay
HIV-wasting syndrome
human immunodeficiency virus
Kaposi's sarcoma
Mycobacterium avium complex
opportunistic infection
Pneumocystis carinii pneumonia
seroconversion
viral load test
Western blot test

INTRODUCTION

While allergies are hypersensitive immune responses, and autoimmune diseases literally have the body attacking itself, acquired immunodeficiency syndrome (AIDS) is a disease that causes an inadequate immunological response by the body. The human immunodeficiency virus (HIV) may be acquired anytime after conception.

The **human immunodeficiency virus** (HIV), a retrovirus that causes **acquired immunodeficiency syndrome** (AIDS), was first reported in the United States in 1981. AIDS is a progressively fatal disease that destroys the immune system and the body's ability to fight infection. By the end of 1998, it was estimated that 33.4 million people in the world were living with HIV/AIDS (National Institute of Allergy and Infectious Diseases [NIAID] and National Institutes of Health [NIH], May 1999). In the United States, 688,200 cases of AIDS had been reported by the end of 1998, and as many as 900,000 may be infected with HIV (NIAID and NIH, March 1999).

Following exposure to HIV and an incubation period of 2 to 4 weeks, some individuals, but not all, will experience flulike symptoms such as fever, sweats, headache, myalgia, neuralgia, sore throat, GI distress, and photophobia (Figure 23-1). Many persons, if tested at this time, will test negative because antibodies may not yet be present in the blood. In 2 or 3 weeks, these symptoms disappear. Infected individuals are very infectious during this period with large quantities of HIV present in genital secretions.

Most individuals will remain symptom free for years (10 or more), but some may begin to have symptoms in a few months. During this "asymptomatic" period, HIV is multiplying, infecting, and killing the CD4 T-cells of the immune system.

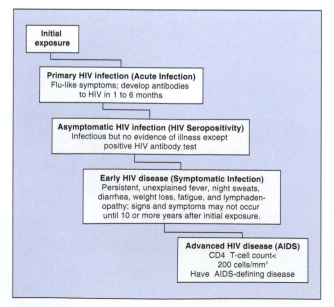

Figure 23-1 Continuum of HIV Disease

PROFESSIONAL TIP

Retroviruses

HIV is a retrovirus. Retroviruses use RNA to make DNA copies that then become part of the genetic material of the human cell. It is because this is a reversal of the usual DNA-to-RNA transcription of genetic information that these viruses are called retroviruses.

HIV infection affects the immune system and the brain. In the immune system, the main characteristic of HIV infection is progressive depletion of the CD4 T-helper cells. The normal ratio of T-helper cells to T-suppressor cells (CD4:CD8 ratio) is 2:1. As immunodeficiency worsens, it is not uncommon for the CD4:CD8 ratio to fall to as low as 0:1. The altered T-helper cells cause malfunction of the B-cells and macrophages, which leads to collapse of the immune system. HIV also affects the CD4 molecule present on microglial cells in the brain, causing memory loss and other brain dysfunctions.

A variety of symptoms become evident as the CD4 T-cells disappear. Lymph nodes enlarged for more than 3 months are one of the first symptoms. Others may include weight loss, lack of energy, fevers and sweats, persistent skin rashes or flaky skin, persistent or frequent oral or vaginal yeast infections, PID that does not respond to treatment, and short-term memory loss. Oral, genital, or anal herpes infection or shingles may also develop.

When the CD4 T-cell count is less than 200 cells/mm^3 (healthy persons have 1,000 or more CD4 cells/mm^3) and the individual has 1 or more of the 26 clinical conditions that affect persons with advanced HIV disease, the individual is considered to have AIDS. Most of the AIDS-defining conditions are **opportunistic infections** (infections in persons with a defective immune system that rarely cause harm in healthy individuals). *Pneumoncystis carinii* pneumonia is the most frequent AIDS-defining diagnosis in the United States and Europe (Lisanti & Zwolski, 1997).

The **enzyme-linked immunosorbent assay** (ELISA) is the basic screening test to detect antibodies to HIV. A positive test result is always retested to rule out false-positive results and/or technician error. A confirmatory test, the **Western blot** test, is always employed when the ELISA test is positive. Results of both the ELISA and Western blot taken together have an extremely high accuracy rate.

Obtaining a signed informed consent for testing is often a nursing responsibility. Most states mandate a consent form solely for HIV testing. Some states allow verbal consent and a statement of the client's consent signed by the health care provider (Figure 23-2).

**PATIENT CONSENT TO RECEIVE
COMMUNICABLE DISEASE BLOOD TEST**

I, _____ , am a patient of Dr. _____ ("Physician"). My physician/infection control officer has informed me that he/she recommends that I receive a blood test for the virus which is the probable cause of Acquired Immune Deficiency Syndrome ("AIDS").

I understand that the blood tests for the virus which is the probable cause of Acquired Immune Deficiency Syndrome ("AIDS") are not 100% accurate, and that these blood tests sometimes produce false positive or false negative test results. I further understand that the presence of antibodies means that a person probably has been infected with the AIDS virus, but does not necessarily mean that a person will develop AIDS.

I acknowledge the following:
1. That the general nature of my condition has been explained to me.
2. That the above stated test and information regarding the test have been explained to me.
3. I understand that when the blood sample is taken, I may have some slight discomfort at the site of entry of the needle and a small bruise may develop; otherwise there is litttle risk of physical injury.
4. I understand that a positive test does not mean that I have AIDS.
5. I understand that there is a slight chance that I may have the AIDS virus even if my test is negative.
6. I understand that a positive test result could cause psychological stress for me and that a positive test could be used to discriminate against me should it not be kept confidential.
7. That reasonable alternatives to the above stated test have been explained to me.
8. That my consent to the above stated test is voluntary.

I understand that the Physician will notify me of the results of the blood tests and the results will be explained to me. (Place your initials below where applicable)

_____ I authorize the Hospital to furnish my insurance companies and other third party payers with any and all information it has or may hereafter have, either written or oral, pertaining to or in any manner connected with the tests authorized herein, that may aid in payment of any account presented to me or us, jointly or severally, and I further agree that no person, firm or corporation shall be held liable in any manner for furnishing or having furnished such information.
_____ I do not consent to the release of the nature of the test(s) to my insurance company or medical assistance program.

Subject to the foregoing, the Hospital, to the best of its ability, will not disclose the results of this test to others except to the extent required by law or except to the extent such disclosure is required in order to safeguard the well-being of patients and employees at the Hospital or other persons at risk.

On this basis, I authorize the Hospital, Physician and anyone authorized by them to perform the blood test as described, and I understand that my signature below acknowledges:
1. My understanding of the plan described herein;
2. My understanding of the information about AIDS and the blood test that has been given to me;
3. I have been given full opportunity to ask questions to obtain further information;
4. All of my questions have been answered to my satisfaction;
5. My refusal or consent to the testing described is shown by my signature below;
6. That the test results may be disclosed as provided herein.

I consent to the test described herein.

_____   _____
(Patient signature)   (Date)

_____   _____   _____
(Physician/infection control officer signature)   (Date)   (Witness over eighteen years of age)

I refuse the test described herein.

_____   _____
(Patient signature)   (Date)

_____   _____   _____

Figure 23-2 Informed Consent—Communicable Disease Blood Test

DEMOGRAPHICS OF AIDS IN THE UNITED STATES

Demographics are viewed in terms of clients' age, gender, and race.

Age

AIDS mainly affects people during the most productive years of their life. As of December 1998, AIDS is now the fifth leading cause of death among persons ages 25 to 44 (NIAID and NIH, May 1999). Children under the age of 13 made up 1% (8,461) of cases reported to the CDC by the end of 1998 (NIAID and NIH, May 1999).

Gender

Trends in HIV-related mortality reflect changes in the demographic patterns of the HIV epidemic. Although more men than women are infected with HIV, the number of AIDS cases in women in the United States has increased from 7% in 1985 to 16% in 1998. Of 688,200 cases of AIDS that had been reported to the CDC by the end of 1998, 570,425 (83%) were males 13 years old and older, and 109,311 (16%) were females 13 years old and older (NIAID and NIH, May 1999).

PROFESSIONAL TIP

HIV Testing

Although physicians are responsible for client counseling, the nurse must know the information to be able to answer questions and clarify the client's knowledge. Pretest counseling should include the following:

- Ask why the client believes the test should be done.
- Explain the meaning of a positive or negative test result and the possibility of a false-negative result.
- Discuss risk reduction and ways to modify behavior.
- Share state reporting requirements.
- Ensure confidentiality of test results.
- Explain that there is often stress related to test results and possible reactions to learning the results, such as depression or anxiety.
- Discuss the potential negative social consequences of positive results.
- Assist the client in making a decision about testing.
- Arrange a return appointment for the client to receive test results.

Posttest counseling should include the following:

- Review the test results with the client.
- Assess the client's understanding of the test results.
- Allow the client to express feelings about the test results.
- Review routes of HIV transmission.
- Assess the client's psychological condition including the risk for suicide.
- Assess the client's risk behavior and strategies for reducing risk.
- Provide information about support groups and national/local resources.

Race

Of the new AIDS cases reported in the United States in 1998:
- African Americans accounted for 66.4/100,000 population.
- Hispanic Americans accounted for 28.1/100,000 population.
- Whites accounted for 8.2/100,000 population.
- American Indian/Alaska Natives accounted for 7.4/100,000 population.
- Asian American/Pacific Islanders accounted for 3.8/100,000 population (NIAID and NIH, May, 1999)

The HIV/AIDS epidemic is growing most rapidly among some minority populations and is a leading cause of death of African American males. The CDC reports that the prevalence for AIDS is 6 times higher in African Americans and 3 times higher in Hispanic Americans than among whites (NIAID and NIH, March 1999).

MODES OF TRANSMISSION

There are many ways to become infected with HIV. The virus may be found in blood, semen, vaginal secretions, and breast milk of infected individuals. There is no evidence that HIV is spread through sweat, tears, urine, or feces. The saliva of infected individuals has the virus, but there is no evidence that it is spread to others through kissing. The risk of infection from "deep kissing" and oral sex is unknown. Tissue transplantation (including artificial insemination), blood transfusion, and needle sticks are high-risk situations but are relatively rare methods of transmission in the United States today. Having another sexually transmitted disease such as chlamydia, genital herpes, syphilis, or gonorrhea seems to make an individual more susceptible to becoming infected with HIV during sexual intercourse with an infected partner. Theoretically, HIV is present in sufficient quantities in amniotic fluid, cerebrospinal fluid, pleural fluid, peritoneal fluid, and pericardial fluid whereby infection could occur with exchange of these body fluids, particularly in health care settings where contact with these fluids may occur. Behaviors associated with increased risk of sexual transmission of HIV by infected persons include unprotected sexual intercourse, multiple sex partners, failure to disclose HIV status, and trading sex for money or drugs (CDC, 1996b). Transmission of HIV can also take place by having contact with infected blood or sharing needles or syringes; it may also transmit from mother to fetus during pregnancy or birth.

Sexual intercourse (anal, oral, vaginal) without using a condom is the most frequently reported risk behavior for infection with HIV. Among individuals reported with AIDS in the United States in 1998, 45% of the men and 38% of the women had unprotected sex (NIAID and NIH, May 1999). Injection-drug use is the second most frequently reported risk behavior for infection with HIV. Among individuals reported with AIDS in the United States in 1998, 21% of the men and 29% of the women reported injection-drug use. When HIV seropositive women take zidovudine (AZT) during pregnancy and labor and zidovudine is given to the newborn, perinatal transmission is significantly reduced.

Medical–Surgical Management

Medical

The goal of care is to keep the disease from progressing for as long as possible. The client's chance of disease progression can now be monitored by a **viral load test** that measures copies of HIV RNA. The approved viral load test is the Amplicor HIV-1 Monitor test, better known as the *polymerease chain reaction (PCR) test* (AIDS Treatment Data Network, May 1999). It can be used to see if individuals with HIV are at risk for getting sick, for checking the effects of drugs taken by individuals with HIV to see if they are working against the virus, and to distinguish the difference between actual HIV infection in a newborn and maternally acquired antibodies. The "ultra-sensitive" PCR test can measure as few as 50 copies/mL of HIV RNA.

Pharmacological

The goal of anti-HIV treatment is to keep the viral load as low as possible for as long as possible, ideally below what the viral load test can detect (AIDS Treatment Data Network, May 1999). Currently available antiretroviral drugs do not cure HIV/AIDS. Treatment is usually begun at the time of **seroconversion** (evidence of antibody formation in response to disease or vaccine). In high-risk occupational exposures, treatment may be started immediately.

One group of drugs, called *nucleoside analog reverse transcriptase inhibitors (NRTIs)*, interrupt HIV's life cycle at an early stage. The spread of HIV in the body may be slowed and the onset of opportunistic infections may be delayed by NRTIs, but these drugs *do not* prevent HIV transmission to other individuals. This group includes zidovudine (Retrovir), formerly known as AZT, zalcitabine (Hivid), didanosine (Videx), stavudine (Zerit), lamivudine (Epivir), and abacavir (Ziagen). A combination of zidovudine and lamivudine (Combivir) is now available. Zidovudine (Retrovir) may cause depletion of red or white blood cells. If this depletion is severe, the drug must be discontinued. Painful nerve damage and pancreatitis may be caused by didanosine (Videx).

Non-nucleoside reverse transcriptase inhibitors (NNRTIs) are available to be used only in combination with other antiretroviral drugs. These include delavirdine (Rescriptor), nevirapine (Viramune), and efavirenz (Sustiva).

The protease inhibitors interrupt HIV's life cycle at a later step. These include ritonavir (Norvir), saquinavir mesylate (Fortovase, Invirase), indinavir sulfate (Crixivan), and nelfinavir mesylate (Viracept). Nausea, diarrhea, and other GI symptoms are common side effects of protease inhibitors. Some individuals have an abnormal redistribution of body fat (NIAID and NIH, March 1999).

HIV can become resistant to each type of drug, so combination treatments are necessary to effectively suppress the virus. Current guidelines recommend drug therapy for any client with symptomatic HIV disease (evidence of opportunistic infections or tumors).

For asymptomatic HIV-positive clients, drug therapy is recommended if:

- Viral load test results are greater than 500 copies/mL, or
- The client's CD4 T-cell count is under 500 cells/mm³ (Kirsten & Whipple, 1998).

Health Promotion

The CDC and the Occupational Safety and Health Administration (OSHA) have developed recommendations to reduce the risk of health care personnel exposure to blood and body fluids. These recommendations are called Standard Precautions. Personal protective equipment should be worn while caring for all clients when there is a reasonable likelihood of contact with any blood or body fluids.

COMMON DIAGNOSTIC TESTS

Commonly used diagnostic tests for clients with symptoms of HIV and AIDS are listed in Table 23–1. See Chapter 13, Diagnostic Tests, for explanation/normal values and nursing responsibilities.

PULMONARY OPPORTUNISTIC INFECTIONS

Conditions discussed following include *pneumocystis carinii* pneumonia, histoplasmosis, and tuberculosis.

PNEUMOCYSTIS CARINII PNEUMONIA

***Pneumocystis carinii* pneumonia** (PCP) is the most common opportunistic infection associated with advanced HIV disease (CDC, 1995b). A marked decrease in the number of AIDS clients diagnosed with PCP is due to initiation of prophylactic treatment when the CD4 T-cell count is 200 or less/mm³. Although *Pneumocystis carinii* is found primarily in the lungs, it has also been reported in the adrenal glands, bone marrow, skin, thyroid, kidneys, and spleen of persons with AIDS.

Table 23–1 COMMON DIAGNOSTIC TESTS FOR HIV AND AIDS
- CD4 T-cells
- Enzyme-linked immunosorbent assay (ELISA)
- Polymerase chain reaction (PCR)
- Western blot

Clinical signs and symptoms include fever, shortness of breath, nonproductive cough, and crackles. Initial diagnosis is made by chest x-ray, which shows diffuse infiltrates. Fiberoptic bronchoscopy is the procedure of choice to obtain a definitive diagnosis. During the bronchoscopy, sputum is obtained to demonstrate the presence of the organism.

Current standard treatment for PCP includes either intravenous pentamidine isethionate (Pneumopent, Pentam 300) or sulfamethoxazole-trimethoprim (Bactrim, Septra), given orally or intravenously. Oral sulfamethoxazole-trimethoprim is the treatment of choice; however, approximately one-third of people with AIDS eventually develop hypersensitivity reactions and must switch to pentamidine for primary therapy. Prophylaxis against PCP is a therapeutic necessity for all persons infected with HIV when the CD4 T-cell count is 200 or less. Primary prophylaxis refers to therapy for those considered at risk for PCP based on the CD4 count to prevent infection with PCP. Secondary prophylaxis refers to therapy to prevent recurrences in clients who have already had PCP. Current guidelines recommend either oral sulfamethoxazole-trimethoprim or aerosolized pentamidine for prophylaxis. For those allergic to sulfamethoxazole-trimethoprim, pentamidine diluted in sterile water administered by a Respigard II nebulizer can be used.

HISTOPLASMOSIS

Histoplasmosis is an infection caused by the fungus *Histoplasma capsulatum*. The fungus has been isolated in bird droppings, dirt from chicken coops, and caves. The spores from the fungus are introduced into the body by inhalation. Histoplasmosis is not specific to the lung. In most clients with HIV disease, histoplasmosis is disseminated (spread out). Histoplasmosis should be suspected if the person presents with fever of uncertain origin, cough, and malaise.

The diagnosis is confirmed by culture or biopsy of the bone marrow, blood, lymph nodes, lungs, or skin. Initial treatment of histoplasmosis consists of IV amphotericin B (Amphotericin B) (Muma, Lyons, Borucki, & Pollard, 1997). Oral ketoconazole (Nizoral) can be used for maintenance therapy. The CDC has recommended prophylaxis against reoccurrence of histoplasmosis with itraconazole (Sporanox) (CDC, 1995b).

TUBERCULOSIS

Mycobacterium tuberculosis, an acid-fast aerobic bacterium, is the cause of tuberculosis (TB). It is spread through airborne particles and enters the body by inhalation. The particles usually lodge in the apex of the lungs; however, one-half to two-thirds of cases of HIV-associated or AIDS-associated TB involve organs outside the lungs as well. Tuberculosis is more prevalent in medically underserved populations, foreign-born persons from areas of the world with a high prevalence, homeless persons, correctional-facility inmates, alcoholics, injection-drug users, the elderly, and people with compromised immune systems.

Clinical manifestations include fever, night sweats, cough, and weight loss. People with AIDS will commonly present with a productive cough and pleuritic pain. Diagnosis is made by a combination of tests: skin testing with purified protein derivative (PPD); examination and culture of sputum, urine, and other fluids; x-rays; and other tests such as IVP.

The most common test for exposure to TB is the Mantoux skin test, which consists of injecting 0.1 ml of (PPD) intradermally. A negative reaction does not rule out infection. HIV-positive clients with a CD4 count lower than 200/mm^3 may no longer have an immune response to the PPD. The chest x-ray may reveal middle and lower lobe infiltrates. A sputum specimen is smeared and stained with an acid-fast stain, then examined under the microscope for acid-fast bacillus (AFB). Other body fluids such as urine, blood, and stool may also be tested for AFB.

The risk of transmission of TB to health care workers is highest during and immediately after procedures that induce coughing. In the home and health care setting, cough-inducing procedures should be performed only in well-ventilated areas.

Infection Control: TB

A densely woven, snug-fitting mask (particulate respirator) should be worn by all persons in contact with the person who has TB until the person has received treatment for 2 to 3 weeks. Persons with TB should also be taught to cover their mouths while coughing and should wear a particulate respirator when they are out of their room for tests.

Due to the upsurge of multidrug-resistant TB (MDR-TB), the CDC recommends treating with multiple medications (CDC, 1994). Treatment is provided in two phases. In the initial treatment phase, the client receives isoniazid (Laniazid), rifampin (Rifadin), pyrazinamide, and ethambutol HCl (Myambutol) or streptomycin sulfate for 2 to 6 months, depending on whether *Mycobacterium tuberculosis* is identified outside the lungs. In the continuation phase, treatment with 2 to 4 of the medications used in the initial phase is indicated for 4 to 6 months longer.

▶ NURSING PROCESS
▶ Assessment
▶ Subjective Data

The nurse must assess the client's ability to dress, bathe, ambulate, and so on. The client's perception of breathlessness should be noted.

▶ Objective Data

The client's respiratory rate, depth, and breath sounds should be assessed. Cough (productive or nonproductive), cyanosis, dyspnea, use of accessory muscles, and fever must be noted. Arterial blood gas (ABG) results are monitored for decreased PaO_2, increased $PaCO_2$, and decreased pH.

Nursing diagnoses for the HIV-positive client with pulmonary disorders may include the following:

Nursing Diagnoses	Planning/Goals	Nursing Interventions
▶ *Ineffective Airway Clearance related to chronic, unrelieved cough, pain, or viscous secretions*	The client will mobilize secretions effectively.	Administer 2.5–3 L of fluid per day (oral or IV) to decrease thick secretions. Administer medications as ordered to suppress cough and decrease pain. Reposition client every 2 hours and PRN.
▶ *Impaired Gas Exchange related to inadequate ventilation/oxygenation*	The client will maintain an $SaO_2 > 90\%$.	Administer oxygen as ordered. Encourage use of incentive spirometer, if not contraindicated.
▶ *Ineffective Breathing Pattern related to fatigue*	The client will pace activities to minimize fatigue.	Plan care to allow rest periods.

Evaluation Each goal must be evaluated to determine how it has been met by the client.

GASTROINTESTINAL OPPORTUNISTIC INFECTIONS

Disorders discussed following include: *Mycobacterium avium* complex, cytomegalovirus, cryptosporidiosis, hepatitis, and HIV-wasting syndrome.

MYCOBACTERIUM AVIUM COMPLEX

Mycobacterium avium and *Mycobacterium intracellulare* are two closely related mycobacteria that are grouped together and called **Mycobacterium avium complex** (MAC). For humans, the source of exposure to MAC is contaminated water although it has been isolated from soil, dust, sediments, and aerosols. In persons with AIDS, MAC involvement of the bowel is usually extensive, suggesting that the gastrointestinal tract may be the site of initial infection, with spread to other organs after that. The microorganism can fill the bone marrow and lymph nodes.

The most common symptoms of MAC include chronic fever, malaise, anemia, weight loss, diarrhea, and abdominal pain. Often the client will appear cachectic due to malabsorption. Because the symptoms are nonspecific, MAC is often difficult to distinguish from other AIDS-related infections. MAC is usually disseminated at the time of diagnosis. Diagnosis is made by tissue biopsy and cultures of the lung, bone marrow, lymph nodes, liver, or blood.

Treatment for MAC infection may include one or more of the following medications: clarithromycin (Biaxin Filmtabs) to treat disseminated MAC; and a combination of amikacin sulfate (Amikin), azithromycin (Zithromax), ciprofloxacin hydrochloride (Cipro), cycloserine (Seromycin), and ethionamide (Trecator-SC). For persons with AIDS who have a CD4 count of less than $75/mm^3$, rifabutin (Mycobutin) is recommended for prevention of disseminated MAC (CDC, 1995b).

CYTOMEGALOVIRUS

Cytomegalovirus (CMV) belongs to the herpes virus group. Thus, it shares the same phenomena of latency and reactivation. The virus lies dormant in tissues waiting to be reactivated in the immunocompromised client. The potential for infection with CMV is increased during two periods: the perinatal period through the preschool years, and later during the sexually active years.

CMV causes disease by destroying the brain, lung, retina, and liver. CMV infection has been identified in all parts of the gastrointestinal tract from the oral cavity to the perianal area. CMV can be life-threatening for persons with suppressed immune systems. Persons with HIV infection or AIDS may develop severe infections including CMV retinitis that can lead to blindness.

Signs and symptoms of CMV include weight loss, fever, diarrhea, and malaise. The diagnosis of CMV is based on microscopic identification of CMV from specific organs such as the brain, lung, liver, or adrenal gland. Ganciclovir sodium (Cytovene) is the drug of choice for treating individuals infected with CMV. Maintenance therapy is required to prevent relapse.

Intravenous foscarnet sodium (Foscavir) has been approved as an alternative therapy.

CRYPTOSPORIDIOSIS

Cryptosporidium, a protozoan causing cryptosporidiosis, usually infects the epithelial cells that line the digestive tract. Transmission is often by the fecal-oral route, but can be spread from animal to person as well as person to person. *Cryptosporidium* can also be spread by ingesting contaminated food and water.

Clinical signs and symptoms include profuse watery diarrhea, up to 20 liters per day (Lisant & Zwolski, 1997). Abdominal pain, serious weight loss, abdominal cramping, anorexia, low-grade fever, dehydration, electrolyte imbalance, and malaise may also be present. Diagnosis is made by identifying the organism in fresh stool specimens.

There is no effective treatment for cryptosporidiosis. Antidiarrheals such as diphenoxylate hydrochloride with atropine sulfate (Lomotil), loperamide hydrochloride (Imodium), and opium tincture (Paregoric) should be given on a programmed schedule rather than PRN. Treatment is palliative and focused toward the symptoms. This includes fluid and electrolyte replacement (orally if possible), analgesics, and occasionally the use of total parenteral nutrition. Anticryptosporidial agents are under investigation. Protecting the integrity of the client's perianal skin is extremely important. A low-residue, high-protein, high-calorie diet helps maintain nutritional status.

HEPATITIS

Only 3 of the 5 hepatitis viruses are commonly seen with HIV infection (Paar, 1997). They are hepatitis B virus (HBV), hepatitis C virus (HCV), and hepatitis D virus (HDV). All 3 viruses have been associated with chronic infection and have similar transmission and risk factors. Risk factors include exposure to blood or blood products, exposure to contaminated needles and syringes, and multiple sexual contacts.

Signs and symptoms include malaise, weakness, anorexia, nausea, vomiting, and right upper quadrant pain. Abnormalities in bilirubin and hepatic enzymes may also occur. Diagnosis is made by serologic assays identifying antigens and antibodies.

Interferon has been approved for treatment of chronic HBV and HCV and is being investigated for the treatment of HDV. Response to therapy varies but is decreased with HIV infection. Clients with a CD4 count greater than 400 mm^3 respond best to this therapy (Parr, 1997).

HIV-WASTING SYNDROME

HIV-wasting syndrome is defined as unexplained weight loss of more than 10% of body weight accompanied by weakness, chronic diarrhea, and fever in those infected with HIV (NIAID and NIH, May 1997). Weight loss and malnutrition are related to reduced food intake, malabsorption of nutrients, and altered metabolism of nutrients. Some of the factors related to reduced intake include anorexia, oral or esophageal lesions, nausea, neurologic or psychiatric conditions, fatigue, inadequate finances, and side effects of medications. Nutritional malabsorption is related to injury of the small intestine caused by opportunistic infections or by HIV infection of the cells in the gastrointestinal tract. Opportunistic infections produce fever that depletes the body's energy stores and causes weight loss.

Signs and symptoms of HIV-wasting syndrome are anorexia, diarrhea, nausea, vomiting, changes in taste and smell, aphthous ulcers of mouth and esophagus, and abdominal pain.

Symptom control is the major focus for HIV-wasting syndrome. Medications to control nausea and vomiting should be given routinely and not PRN. Treatment of anorexia includes megestrol acetate (Megace) or dronabinol (Marinol). Antimotility drugs such as loperamide hydrochloride (Imodium), luminal acting agents such as kaolin and pectin mixture (Kaopectate), and hormonal agents such as octreotide acetate (Sandostatin) are used to treat diarrhea. The aphthous ulcers are safely and effectively healed with the drug thalidomide (NIAID and NIH, May 1997). This makes eating much easier. Oral nutritional supplements are most frequently used for weight loss. Total parenteral nutrition (TPN) is usually considered a final option except in cases of severe malnutrition, because of the risk and expense involved.

▶ NURSING PROCESS

▶ Assessment

▶ Subjective Data

The client should be asked about bowel habits, and what causes and relieves diarrhea. The nurse should inquire about alcohol consumption since excessive alcohol intake depletes B vitamins and provides no nutrition. Activities that cause fatigue are noted. Food likes/dislikes, food intolerances, and food intake for the previous 3 days should be discussed.

▶ Objective Data

The nurse should assess the client's skin integrity including temperature, moisture, color, vascularity, texture, lesions, areas of excoriation, and poor wound healing. Fever, weight, and daily nutritional intake must be noted. Laboratory values of nutritional status including serum albumin, total protein, hemoglobin, and hematocrit, as well as stool specimens for ova and parasites, should all be assessed.

Nursing diagnoses for the HIV-positive client with gastrointestinal disorders may include the following:

Nursing Diagnoses	Planning/Goals	Nursing Interventions
❯ *Deficient Fluid Volume related to nausea, vomiting, diarrhea, or inadequate oral intake*	The client will have normal skin turgor and decreased frequency and amount of stools.	Suggest client use hard candy or chewing gum to stimulate saliva production if mouth is dry.
		Encourage client to drink liquids between (not with) meals.
		Monitor and record intake and output.
		Monitor client for evidence of electrolyte imbalance (hypokalemia, hypochloremia, confusion, muscle weakness).
❯ *Imbalanced Nutrition: Less than body requirements related to anorexia, dysphagia, malabsorption, or side effects of medications*	The client will eat 75% of prescribed diet and maintain current weight.	Provide the prescribed diet (usually low-residue, high-caloric, high-protein) in small frequent meals at room temperature.
		Offer commercially prepared nutritional supplements between meals.
		Administer supplemental vitamins and minerals as prescribed.
		Provide oral hygiene before and after meals to enhance taste sensation.
		Administer antiemetics and antidiarrheals as ordered.
		Weigh client daily.
		Advise client to keep a food diary and a log of exacerbation and remission of signs and symptoms.
❯ *Risk for Impaired Skin Integrity related to diarrhea, malnutrition, decreased mobility*	The client will maintain skin integrity.	Monitor stool for presence of blood, fat, undigested food.
		Monitor stool cultures for evidence of new infections.
		Protect the perirectal area by keeping it clean and using compounds such as Aloe Vesta cream.
		Avoid prolonged pressure on bony prominences by a scheduled turning plan.
		If nonambulatory, provide client with a pressure relief mattress.
		Teach client to use nondrying soaps and to pat skin dry.
		Use soft sheets on the bed and avoid wrinkles.

Evaluation Each goal must be evaluated to determine how it has been met by the client.

ORAL OPPORTUNISTIC INFECTIONS

Candidiasis and leukoplakia are discussed following.

ORAL AND ESOPHAGEAL CANDIDIASIS

Oral candidiasis (thrush) is a fungal infection caused by *Candida albicans* (Figure 23-3), which occurs in more than 90% of AIDS clients (Lisanti & Zwolski, 1997). Many clients complain of an unpleasant taste or mouth dryness. Other clinical signs and symptoms include creamy, white oral plaques and mucosal tenderness. When the white oral plaques are wiped off, they leave an erythematous or even bleeding mucosal lesion (Lisanti & Zwolski, 1997). Esophageal candidiasis, an AIDS-defining disease, causes dysphagia and painful swallowing.

Figure 23-3 Oral Candidiasis (Thrush)

These symptoms may interfere with the client's eating, nutrition, and weight. Diagnosis is established by the presence of the characteristic lesions in the oral cavity. Microscopic examination of oral or esophageal lesions reveals budding yeast cells.

Treatment for esophageal candidiasis is oral fluconazole (Diflucan). Oral candidiasis is treated with nystatin suspension (Mycostatin) and clotrimazole (Mycelex Troches). Another medication used to treat candidiasis is ketoconazole (Nizoral). Amphotericin B (Amphotericin B) is used to treat disseminated candida infection. The antiulcer drug sucralfate (Carafate) may be used in a slurry form to relieve mouth pain prior to eating.

Figure 23-4 Oral Hairy Leukoplakia (*Courtesy of Dr. Joseph Konzelman, School of Dentistry, Medical College of Georgia.*)

ORAL HAIRY LEUKOPLAKIA

Oral hairy leukoplakia (OHL) usually appears as a white patch on the lateral borders of the tongue as shown in Figure 23-4. It is caused by the Epstein-Barr virus. The lesions are rarely in other areas of the mouth and are different in appearance from candidiasis. The irregular surface of the lesion appears as projections that resemble hairs and cannot be scraped off. Diagnosis is made by visual inspection of the lesion. OHL is not usually bothersome to the client and may regress spontaneously. No treatment is necessary for most cases of OHL; however, oral acyclovir (Zovirax) may be given to selected clients. More than 50% of clients with OHL develop AIDS within 30 months (Lisanti & Zwolski, 1997).

▶ NURSING PROCESS

▶ Assessment

▶ Subjective Data

The client's history of symptoms and oral hygiene habits should be assessed, and the client asked about recent nutritional intake, use of alcohol and tobacco, and current medications.

▶ Objective Data

The client's lips, tongue, and buccal mucosal surfaces are assessed for lesions, white cheesey patches, and bleeding. Any difficulty swallowing should be noted.

A nursing diagnosis for an HIV-positive client with oral manifestations may be:

Nursing Diagnosis	Planning/Goals	Nursing Interventions
▶ *Impaired Oral Mucous Membrane related to oral lesions*	The client will be free from oral lesions.	Administer prescribed medications.
		Frequently assess the oral cavity.
		Instruct client to avoid commercial mouthwashes containing alcohol or glycerine.
		Provide oral hygiene with a small soft toothbrush before and after meals.

Evaluation Each goal must be evaluated to determine how it has been met by the client.

GYNECOLOGICAL OPPORTUNISTIC INFECTIONS

Gynecological infections discussed include vaginal candidiasis and cervical intraepithelial neoplasia.

VAGINAL CANDIDIASIS

Vaginal candidiasis is a fungal infection caused by *Candida albicans*. It is the most common initial infection occurring in HIV-infected women. Clinical manifestations include a white, clumped-appearing vaginal discharge, vaginal wall inflammation, and vaginal itching. Diagnosis is made by microscopic identification of yeast.

Most cases of vaginal candidiasis are treated with topical antifungal agents such as clotrimazole (Gyne-Lotrimin). For clients who do not respond to treatment with clotrimazole, ketoconazole (Nizoral) or fluconazole (Diflucan) is recommended.

CERVICAL INTRAEPITHELIAL NEOPLASIA

Women infected with HIV have a much higher incidence of cervical intraepithelial neoplasia (CIN) than women who are not infected. CIN and cancer of the cervix are considered to be on a continuum of abnormal cervical cells, ranging from mild abnormality (Grade I) to severe abnormality and cancer (Grade III). CIN in HIV-infected women progresses more rapidly and is less responsive to standard treatments than in noninfected women. Factors related to increased risk of CIN in HIV-positive women include a decreased number of CD4 T-cells and infection with human papilloma virus (HPV). It is thought that HIV activates HPV, causing cellular abnormalities.

The early stages of CIN have no symptoms. Clinical manifestations of cervical cancer include painless postcoital bleeding and blood-tinged vaginal discharge. As CIN progresses, back pain, abdominal or pelvic pain, weight loss, anorexia, and leg edema caused by obstruction of lymph nodes may occur. Initial diagnosis is made by Pap smear to determine the presence of abnormal cells. Clients with abnormal Pap smears are referred for cervical biopsy and colposcopy.

Treatment for CIN includes laser therapy, conization, and hysterectomy. Treatment for invasive cervical cancer depends on the stage of the disease and may include chemotherapy, surgery, and radiation.

▶ NURSING PROCESS

▶ Assessment

▶ Subjective Data

Assess the client's history of symptoms, and ask the client about bleeding after intercourse, abdominal and pelvic pain, and vaginal itching or discharge.

▶ Objective Data

Vaginal discharge is assessed for white or blood-tinged secretions. Weight loss and edema are noted.

Nursing diagnoses for a female HIV-positive client with gynecological manifestations may include the following:

Nursing Diagnoses	Planning/Goals	Nursing Interventions
▶ *Impaired Tissue Integrity related to vaginal mucosal lesions*	The client will be free of vaginal infections.	Teach the client to have Pap smears every 6 months.
		Assess the frequency and consistency of vaginal discharge.
		Teach client to keep the vaginal area clean and dry and to wear loose fitting cotton underwear to prevent irritation.
▶ *Disturbed Body Image related to chronic vaginal infections or surgery, radiation, or removal of cervix*	The client will verbalize feelings and concerns about body image.	Encourage client to verbalize feelings and concerns about body image.
		Refer client to a support group for women with HIV.

Evaluation Each goal must be evaluated to determine how it has been met by the client.

CENTRAL NERVOUS SYSTEM OPPORTUNISTIC INFECTIONS

Disorders covered include AIDS dementia complex, toxoplasmosis, and cryptococcosis.

AIDS DEMENTIA COMPLEX

The most common central nervous system complication in persons with AIDS is AIDS dementia complex (ADC). Without early treatment with zidovudine (Retrovir), the chance of developing ADC is approximately 33% (Lisanti & Zwolski, 1997). This disorder is chronic and progressive with cognitive, motor, and behavioral dysfunction. ADC is caused by infection of glial cells in the brain with HIV. Signs and symptoms are sometimes vague during the initial stages of ADC. Early signs include poor concentration, forgetfulness, loss of balance, leg weakness, apathy, and social withdrawal. Clients with advanced ADC may exhibit psychotic behaviors and delirium and progress to a catatonic-like state with minimal responsiveness to the environment.

Diagnosis is made by neurological testing of cognitive, motor, and behavioral functioning. Other diagnostic tests include brain imaging to look for cerebral atrophy. Cerebrospinal fluid analysis can show elevated proteins and will exclude other pathogens. Clients treated with zidovudine (Retrovir) have shown improvement in cognitive and motor skills, but the effect only lasts about 12 months (Lisanti & Zwolski, 1997).

TOXOPLASMOSIS

Toxoplasmosis is caused by the protozoan *Toxoplasma gondii*. Cats and other animals serve as a reservoir for this organism. It is spread to humans by ingestion of oocytes found in contaminated water, soil, or food, especially raw or undercooked meat. After entering the body, *Toxoplasma gondii* reproduces and spreads via the blood or lymph system. A person with an intact immune system may have no symptoms or mild symptoms, and the organism may remain dormant for years. In the immunocompromised person, the infection may be reactivated (secondary) or occur with the ingestion of oocytes from contaminated sources. Clinical signs and symptoms may be vague and nonspecific, or range from a mild headache, fever, and lethargy to poor coordination, seizures, and coma. Diagnosis is made by identification of a lesion through brain imaging (computerized tomography or magnetic resonance imaging), presence of serum antibodies to *Toxoplasma gondii,* and recent onset of a neurologic abnormality.

The treatment of choice is oral pyrimethamine (Daraprim) and sulfadiazine (Microsulfon). Lifelong suppressive therapy of pyrimethamine plus sulfadiazine and leukovorin calcium (Wellcovorin) is required (CDC, 1995b).

CRYPTOCOCCOSIS

Cryptococcosis is a fungal infection caused by *Cryptococcus neoformans*. Cryptococcosis is the most life-threatening fungal infection associated with AIDS (Lisanti & Zwolski, 1997). The organism is acquired in the environment, usually from bird droppings. In the noncompromised host, the fungus is inhaled and con-tained in the lungs. In the immunocompromised host with AIDS, *Cryptococcus neoformans* can be disseminated, remain in the lungs, or infect the brain and meninges. Clinical manifestations include fever, headache, nausea and vomiting, dizziness, photophobia, mental status changes, seizures, and a stiff neck. Detection of cryptococcal antigen in cerebrospinal fluid, urine, or blood can be used for diagnosis. If untreated, this is a fatal condition.

Treatment for acute cryptococcal infections includes intravenous amphotericin B (Fungizone Intravenous) to be given for at least 2 weeks, followed by fluconazole (Diflucan) for 10 to 12 weeks. Once treatment for acute infection is complete, lifelong suppressive therapy with oral fluconazole daily is recommended (Lisanti & Zwolski, 1997).

▶ NURSING PROCESS

▶ Assessment

▶ Subjective Data

Ask the client about forgetfulness, missing appointments, ability to complete activities of daily living, and if there have been any recent falls or accidents. Ask the client's family and significant others about behavior changes such as social withdrawal or unusual behavior.

▶ Objective Data

Assess the client for subtle mental status changes such as poor concentration and inability to remember instructions or previous conversations. Assess the client for motor impairment such as dropping things, poor coordination, or changes in writing ability. Assess the client's ability to remember usual medication schedule. Observe the environment for safety.

Nursing diagnoses for an HIV-positive client with central nervous system manifestations include the following:

Nursing Diagnoses	Planning/Goals	Nursing Interventions
▶ *Disturbed Thought Processes related to mental status changes*	The client will maintain cognitive functioning.	Assess mental and neurologic status. Evaluate client's emotional, cognitive, and motor skills. Provide cues for reorientation (clock, calendar). Monitor client for adherence to medical regimen.
▶ *Social Isolation related to alteration in mental status*	The client will have contact and interact with significant others.	Encourage family and significant others to visit client. Provide structured activities and environment for social interaction. Encourage client to verbalize feelings and concerns.

Evaluation Each goal must be evaluated to determine how it has been met by the client.

OPPORTUNISTIC MALIGNANCIES

Kaposi's sarcoma and non-Hodgkin's lymphoma are discussed.

KAPOSI'S SARCOMA

Kaposi's sarcoma (KS) is a vascular malignancy that can occur any place in the body, including internal organs. The first lesions often appear subtly on the face or in the oral cavity. The more immunosuppressed the person is, the more aggressive the spread of KS. Clinical manifestations of KS are red to purple lesions, which are painless, nonblanching, and palpable (Figure 23-5). These lesions are sometimes mistaken for bruises. Edema in the face, penis, scrotum, and legs can occur as a result of blockages in the lymphatic system. KS can also be found in the GI tract and lungs. Diagnosis is made by tissue biopsy.

Treatment involves a variety of options depending on whether the lesions are local or systemic. Radiation therapy, intralesional therapy with interferon alpha 2a or 2b (Roferon A, Intron A) or vinblastine sulfate (Velban), laser therapy, and cryotherapy are used on single

Figure 23-5 Kaposi's Sarcoma *(Courtesy of Daniel J. Barbaro, MD, Fort Worth, Texas.)*

or isolated KS lesions. For clients with advanced widespread symptomatic disease, single or combination chemotherapeutic regimens include vinblastine sulfate (Velban), vincristine sulfate (Oncovin), etoposide (VePesid), bleomycin sulfate (Blenoxane), doxorubicin HCl (Rubex), and mitoxantrone HCl (Novantrone).

SAMPLE NURSING CARE PLAN

THE CLIENT WITH KAPOSI'S SARCOMA

Mr. Williams, a twenty-three-year-old singer, is HIV positive. Until recently, Mr. Williams was very active and enjoyed socializing with family and friends. He was diagnosed with Kaposi's sarcoma and has prominent lesions on his forehead and nose. He is unable to make decisions, has called in "sick" to work several times per week, and has not returned telephone calls to family and friends. At his clinic appointment he states how "ugly" his face looks.

Nursing Diagnosis 1 *Disturbed Body Image related to facial lesions as evidenced by the statement "My face looks ugly."*

PLANNING/GOALS	NURSING INTERVENTIONS	RATIONALE	EVALUATION
Mr. Williams will express positive feelings about himself.	Provide Mr. Williams opportunities to discuss his feelings.	As Mr. Williams explores his feelings (positive and negative), he may need reassurance that the nurse is willing to listen to all of his concerns.	Mr. Williams was able to discuss his feelings with the nurse and contacted a local AIDS service organization for peer counseling.
	Provide Mr. Williams with information about intralesional treatment.	Providing Mr. Williams with information empowers him to see	

continues

		alternatives to his current situation.	
	Encourage Mr. Williams to contact his local AIDS Service Organization for peer support/counseling.	Interacting with someone who has been through the experience is helpful in adjustment.	
	Assist Mr. Williams in identifying positive aspects of himself.	Identifying positive aspects of himself will enhance Mr. Williams' well-being.	
	Explore possibility of covering lesions with theatrical makeup.	Learning to cover lesions contributes to self-esteem.	

Nursing Diagnosis 2 *Ineffective Coping related to situational crisis of changed physical appearance as evidenced by impaired decision-making ability*

PLANNING/GOALS	NURSING INTERVENTIONS	RATIONALE	EVALUATION
Mr. Williams will verbalize awareness of own coping abilities.	Assist Mr. Williams to identify previous ways of dealing with life problems.	Enables Mr. Williams to identify patterns of successful coping.	Mr. Williams was able to discuss his diagnosis with his pastor.
	Encourage Mr. Williams to evaluate perceptions of his current coping abilities.	Self-awareness leads to new insight and possible solutions.	
	Assist Mr. Williams in identifying sources of strength.	By identifying sources of strength such as religious beliefs or positive personal attributes, Mr. Williams is able to acknowledge current resources.	
	Develop a therapeutic relationship using active listening.	Provides a safe environment for problem-solving.	

Nursing Diagnosis 3 *Social Isolation related to altered physical appearance as evidenced by decreased interpersonal interactions and absence from work*

PLANNING/GOALS	NURSING INTERVENTIONS	RATIONALE	EVALUATION
Mr. Williams will verbalize willingness to be involved with others.	Develop a written plan of action with Mr. Williams that includes daily contact with others.	Provides Mr. Williams with a reference for action.	Mr. Williams agreed to have face-to-face contact with at least one other person on a daily basis.
	Facilitate Mr. Williams' interactions with others diagnosed with KS.	Provides Mr. Williams with an opportunity to discuss shared	

continues

		problems with others and decreases feelings of aloneness.
	Involve family members and friends in treatment plan.	Assists Mr. Williams in identifying a network of support and acceptance.
	Encourage Mr. Williams to explore temporary work arrangements with employer.	Initiating discussions about work-related absences enables Mr. Williams to begin to deal with consequences of social isolation.

NON-HODGKIN'S LYMPHOMA

Lymphomas are malignant tumors of the immune system. B-cells are the origin of malignancy for the majority of clients with AIDS-related non-Hodgkin's lymphoma (NHL). Clinical manifestations are nonspecific and may include fever, night sweats, and weight loss. Confusion, lethargy, and memory loss may be present in persons with CNS involvement.

Diagnosis of NHL is complicated because of the nonspecific symptoms. Examination of tissue is the recommended diagnostic procedure. There is no standard treatment of NHL. Individualized treatment may include a combination of chemotherapy, antiretroviral agents, prophylaxis against opportunistic infections, and colony-stimulating factors to enhance bone marrow production of blood cells. However, in many clients with advanced HIV disease, treatment of NHL is withheld because it is not tolerated well and may even lead to earlier death.

▶ NURSING PROCESS

▶ Assessment

▶ Subjective Data

The client must be asked about frequency, onset, and persistence of current symptoms. The effect of current symptoms on ability to perform activities of daily living and relationships with others should be noted, as well as the effect of treatment plan on quality of life.

▶ Objective Data

Skin lesions should be assessed. Increased frequency, intensity, or recurrence of nonspecific symptoms including fever, night sweats, and weight loss should be documented.

Nursing diagnoses for an HIV-positive client with a malignancy may include the following:

Nursing Diagnoses	Planning/Goals	Nursing Interventions
▶ *Risk for Impaired Skin Integrity related to lesions or treatment*	The client will maintain skin integrity.	Teach client to avoid scratching skin lesions, to avoid drying soaps, and to make sure clothing and linen have been thoroughly rinsed of detergent.
▶ *Social Isolation related to change in appearance*	The client will maintain usual social interactions and identify factors that enhance quality of life.	Facilitate the client's interaction with others. Keep client and significant others aware of treatment plan. Encourage significant others to participate in the care of client. Encourage physical closeness between the client and significant others. Provide client with access to clergy, social worker, or HIV counselor. Encourage the client to join a support group or obtain peer support. Assist client in identifying positive coping strategies.

Evaluation Each goal must be evaluated to determine how it has been met by the client.

CASE STUDY

Jim Hayes, a 37-year-old male, suspects that he is HIV positive. He enters the medical unit with chronic symptoms such as fever, night sweats, diarrhea, weight loss, shortness of breath, and a nonproductive cough. On the initial assessment, he is alert and oriented, color is pale, temperature 100.6°F, pulse 92, respirations 36, and blood pressure 140/70. He has generalized lymphadenopathy. His height is 5'11", and his weight is 125 pounds. Jim states that he is not currently taking any medications although he is "familiar" with the drug zidovudine (Retrovir).

The following questions will guide your development of a nursing care plan for the case study.

1. List symptoms/clinical manifestations, other than Mr. Hayes's, that a client may experience when HIV positive.
2. List 2 reasons zidovudine (Retrovir) may be initiated for Mr. Hayes.
3. List 2 diagnostic tests that will confirm the diagnosis of HIV.
4. List subjective and objective data the nurse would want to obtain about Mr. Hayes.
5. Write 3 individual nursing diagnoses and goals for Mr. Hayes.
6. List pertinent nursing actions the nurse would perform in caring for Mr. Hayes related to:

   hydration

   fatigue

   nutrition

   oxygenation

   medications
7. List resources that could assist Mr. Hayes with his diagnosis.
8. List teaching Mr. Hayes will need before leaving the medical unit.

SUMMARY

- Diagnosis of HIV/AIDS is made by the ELISA and Western blot test. These tests determine the presence of antibodies to HIV, not the virus itself.
- *Pneumocystis carinii* pneumonia is the most common opportunistic infection associated with HIV.
- Oral candidiasis can be painful and interfere with the client's nutritional status.
- AIDS dementia complex is a progressive disorder with cognitive, motor, and behavioral dysfunction.

Review Questions

1. Which of the following statements shows that the client understands a diagnosis of HIV positive?

   a. "Being HIV positive means that I have AIDS."
   b. "Since I am only HIV positive I cannot infect others."
   c. "Because I am HIV positive I have the virus that causes AIDS."
   d. "I became infected by donating blood."

2. The drug of choice for treating *Pneumocystis carinii* pneumonia (PCP) is:

   a. co-trimoxazole (Septra).
   b. ganciclovir (Cytovene).
   c. megestrol acetate (Megace).
   d. fluconazole (Diflucan).

3. The nurse is caring for an HIV client who is experiencing diarrhea and weight loss. Which of the following nursing interventions is appropriate for him?

   a. Encourage fluids with meals
   b. Substitute a milk shake for lunch
   c. Offer small, frequent meals
   d. Suggest he eat more sweets

4. The nurse is caring for a client who asks when zidovudine (Retrovir) is normally started. Which of the following would be the nurse's correct response?

   a. When the client becomes symptomatic
   b. When CD4 level reaches 500/mm^3

c. After the client's first opportunistic infection

d. As soon as the client is diagnosed as HIV positive

5. The nurse is discussing transmission of HIV with a client. Which of the following statements indicates that the client needs more education?

a. "I should not share needles with anyone."
b. "I can spread the virus through sexual contact."
c. "I can no longer donate blood."
d. "I should not hug or kiss anyone."

6. The only opportunistic infection that is found when the CD4 cell count is normal is:

a. AIDS dementia complex.
b. Kaposi's sarcoma.
c. *Pneumocystis carinii* pneumonia.
d. oral candidiasis.

Critical Thinking Questions

1. How would you tell your family and friends if you were diagnosed HIV positive?

2. How might a person's lifestyle change after receiving a diagnosis of HIV positive?

WEB FLASH!

- Search the Internet for HIV and AIDS.
- What new research information is available for clients with HIV and AIDS? What type of drugs are available? Diagnostic tests? Other treatments?
- Search the Web for the resources listed for this chapter at the end of this text. What other information is provided?

NURSING CARE OF THE CLIENT: MUSCULOSKELETAL SYSTEM

MAKING THE CONNECTION

Refer to the following chapters to increase your understanding of the musculoskeletal system:

- **Chapter 7, Wellness Concepts**
- **Chapter 12, Health Assessment**
- **Chapter 14, Pain Management**
- **Chapter 17, Nursing Care of the Oncology Client**
- **Chapter 19, Nursing Care of the Client: Cardiovascular System**
- **Chapter 22, Nursing Care of the Client: Immune System**
- **Chapter 35, Nursing Care of the Older Client**

LEARNING OBJECTIVES

Upon completion of this chapter, you should be able to:
- *Define key terms.*
- *List the diagnostic tests used in the evaluation of orthopedic disorders and diseases.*
- *Describe preventive nursing care of the orthopedic client, i.e., positioning, mobility, and so on.*
- *Identify the various types of casts used in the treatment of orthopedic disorders.*
- *Describe nursing care of clients with orthopedic devices.*
- *List four types of fractures and their related treatment.*
- *Discuss the nursing care of the client undergoing a total hip replacement.*
- *Utilize the nursing process to plan nursing care including physical and emotional needs of the orthopedic client.*

KEY TERMS

amphiarthrosis	lordosis
amputation	open reduction
arthroplasty	orthopedics
bruxism	osteoporosis
closed reduction	paresthesia
contracture	phantom limb pain
crepitus	scoliosis
diarthrosis	sprain
dislocation	strain
fracture	subluxation
Heberden's nodes	synarthrosis
kyphosis	tophi
locomotor	windowing

INTRODUCTION

Orthopedics, also spelled orthopaedics, is the branch of medicine that deals with the prevention or correction of the disorders and diseases of the musculoskeletal system. It involves the muscles, skeleton, joints, and supporting structures such as ligaments and tendons.

The prime concern of the nurse caring for a client with **locomotor** (pertaining to movement or the ability to move) disorders is the prevention of **contractures** (permanent shortening of a muscle) or deformities. The objective of all caregivers is to maintain good body position, preserve muscle tone, and continue joint motion for the client with acute or long-term therapeutic or rehabilitative needs. Caring for orthopedic clients also requires an understanding of basic principles that apply to all of these clients whether they are in traction, casts, or recovering from surgery.

ANATOMY AND PHYSIOLOGY REVIEW

The musculoskeletal system consists of bones, muscles, tendons, ligaments, cartilage, and joints. When it is functioning properly, the musculoskeletal system allows an individual to stand erect and ambulate. Figure 24-1 identifies the bones of the skeleton.

The skeletal system consists of bones attached to each other by cartilage and strong ligaments. The functions of the skeleton are to:

- provide the body with structural framework.
- act as a protective casing for internal organs such as the brain, heart, and lungs.
- allow movement by muscles attached to the skeleton.
- store calcium, phosphorus and magnesium and release these minerals when the body requires them.
- manufacture blood cells in the red bone marrow.

Bones in the skeletal system are classified as long, short, flat, or irregular. Examples include the humerus, a long bone; the phalanges of the finger, short bone; occiput, flat bone; and the vertebrae, irregular bone. Figure 24-2 illustrates these bones.

There are two types of bone. One type of bone is cancellous, which resembles a sponge with spaces and is found in the epiphysis or end of the long bones as well as in all other bones. The other type is cortical bone, which is compact bone and is found in the diaphysis or shaft of the long bones. Short bones consist of cancellous bone covered by a layer of compact bone. Flat bones are made of cancellous bone layered between compact bone. Generally, the makeup of irregular bones is similar to that of flat bones.

The muscular system is composed of muscle fibers and tendons innervated by nerves (Figure 24-3). The muscle fibers vary in size and shape and are arranged according to a muscle's function. The muscles act as motors controlled by nerve impulses from the cerebral cortex. The muscles and the skeleton work together to permit body movement. Muscles are attached to bones by tendons.

Figure 24-1 Anterior and Posterior Views of the Adult Human Skeleton

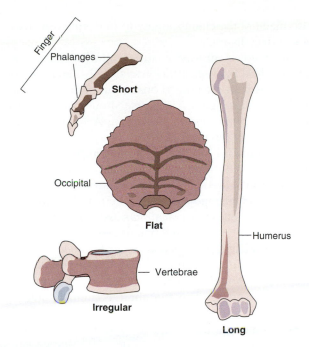

Figure 24-2 Bone Shapes

The action of muscles is to contract or shorten. Muscles are arranged within the body as opposing pairs to act as antagonists to each other. For example, the biceps flex the forearm and the triceps extend it.

Muscles are surrounded and divided by fibrous envelopes called *fascia*. In the extremities, the muscles surround and give support to main blood vessels and nerves. Muscles also give support to and keep the body erect as well as give shape to the body.

Movement of the muscles may be either voluntary or involuntary. Muscles attached to bone can function at the will of the person (voluntary). Involuntary muscles are found within body organs and the actions are not under the person's control. They regulate the physical activity of the organs so the organs can perform their functions. Involuntary muscles are located in the intestinal tract, the pupil of the eye, and in the heart and blood vessels.

A joint is a junction of two or more bones. There are three types of joints: diarthrosis, synarthrosis, and amphiarthrosis. **Diarthrosis** joints are freely movable joints such as the hinge (elbow, knee), ball and socket (hip and shoulder), pivot (skull and first vertebrae), gliding (wrist), and saddle (thumb). **Synarthrosis** joints are immovable, such as the suture line between the temporal and occipital bones of the skull. **Amphiarthrosis** joints are slightly movable, such as the vertebrae and pelvic bones separated by fibrous cartilage. Figure 24-4 illustrates types of joints.

The ends of articulating joints are covered with a smooth articular cartilage. The joint capsule is composed of an outer fibrous layer and an inner synovial

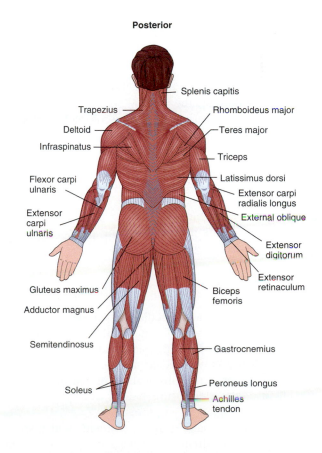

Figure 24-3 Muscular System: Anterior and Posterior Views

Figure 24-4 Joints Classified by the Degree of Movement Permitted

layer that secretes synovial fluid. This clear fluid acts as a lubricating fluid for the joints.

Other structures related to the musculoskeletal system include bursa, fascia, tendons, and ligaments. Bursae are sacs filled with fluid that facilitate joint movement by making it possible for muscles and tendons to move or glide over ligaments or bones. Fascia is connective tissue that covers a muscle. Tendons are strong fibrous tissue attaching muscle to bones, providing mobility. Ligaments grow out of the periosteum and lash bones together more firmly.

ASSESSMENT

Assessment of the musculoskeletal system ranges from a basic assessment of functional abilities done by the nurse to a complete physical exam by the physician for diagnosis of specific muscle and joint disorders. The extent of the physical exam will depend on the client's complaints, the health history, and any other physical signs or symptoms.

The nurse, in making an assessment, will inspect and palpate to evaluate bone integrity, posture, joint function, muscle strength, and gait. An assessment is also made of the client's ability to perform basic activities of daily living.

The medical history includes information on any past medical or surgical disorders. It also includes any symptoms with relation to onset, duration, or location of discomfort or pain. The nurse should ask if activity makes symptoms better or worse. A family medical history should also be obtained.

Assessment of the bony skeleton includes notation of any deformities, body alignment, abnormal growths due to bone tumors, shortened extremities, amputations, abnormal angulation other than at the joints, and **crepitus,** a grating or crackling sensation or sound.

Assessment of the spine will necessitate exposure of the client's back, buttocks, and legs for adequate visualization. Differences in the height of the shoulders or iliac crests should be noted. Gluteal folds should appear symmetrical. The vertebral column should be straight and perpendicular to the floor with the spine convex through the thoracic portion and concave through the cervical/lumbar portion.

Three common spinal curvatures are: scoliosis, kyphosis, and lordosis. A lateral curving deviation is known as **scoliosis**. Scoliosis (crooked back) is seen most frequently in schoolage children and adolescents. **Kyphosis** (hump back) is seen as an increased roundness of the thoracic spinal curve. This condition is frequently seen in the older person with osteoporosis. **Lordosis** (sway back) is an exaggeration of the lumbar spine curvature as seen in pregnancy as a woman's body adjusts to the center of gravity. These three curvatures are illustrated in Figure 24-5.

Figure 24-5 Curvatures of the Spine

Assessment of the articular system includes: range of motion (limited, active, and passive), stability of joints, deformities and any nodular formation, and pulses in the extremities.

Range of motion (ROM) includes assessment of the client's ability to change position, muscle strength and coordination, and the size of individual muscles. When assessing passive range of motion, the nurse should remember to keep the motion steady and avoid causing any pain.

Joints are examined for excessive fluid. The knee is the most common site for fluid accumulation. Edema and an elevated temperature may be signs of active inflammation in the joint. Normal joint movement is stable and smooth. If there is a snap or crack sound when a joint is passively moved, it may be indicative of a ligament slipping over a bony prominence.

Deformities may be due to several factors including contractures, dislocations, and **subluxation** (a partial separation of an articular surface). Nodular formations are produced by musculoskeletal diseases such as gout, rheumatoid arthritis, and osteoarthritis.

Pulse points in the extremities are palpated to assess for weak or absent pulses. The strength of the pulse in affected extremities is compared with that of nonaffected extremities. Skin color and temperature are noted, and capillary refill is checked by pressing down on the client's fingernail or toenail for a few seconds, then releasing and noting the time it takes for the client's nail to return to normal color. The color should return immediately (less than 2 seconds); if a client has an arterial disorder, the color will take longer than 2 seconds to return to normal.

COMMON DIAGNOSTIC TESTS

Commonly used diagnostic tests for clients with symptoms of musculoskeletal system disorders are listed in Table 24–1. See Chapter 13, Diagnostic Tests, for explanation/normal values and nursing responsibilities.

MUSCULOSKELETAL TRAUMA

Trauma to the musculoskeletal system may cause a variety of injuries to clients of all ages. Such injuries include strains, sprains, dislocations, fractures, and compartment syndrome.

STRAIN

A **strain** is an injury to a muscle or tendon due to overuse or overstretching. A strain may be either acute or chronic. An acute strain may be caused when an individual performs unaccustomed exercises vigorously.

Table 24–1 COMMON DIAGNOSTIC TESTS FOR CLIENTS WITH MUSCULOSKELETAL DISORDERS
Laboratory Tests
Antinuclear antibodies (ANA)
Complete blood count (CBC)
• WBC
• Hg
C-reactive protein (CRP)
Erythrocyte sedimentation rate (ESR)
Rheumatoid factor (RF)
Serum calcium
Uric acid
• serum
• urine
Radiologic Studies
Arthrogram/graphy
Computed tomography (CT scan)
Electromyography (EMG)
Magnetic resonance imaging (MRI)
Radiograph (x-ray)
Other Tests
Arthrocentesis
Arthroscopy

A chronic strain may develop after repeated overuse of certain muscles. Individuals suffering acute strains experience sudden severe pain while the onset is gradual in chronic strains, with the affected part feeling only stiff and sore.

Chronic strains require no specific treatment, but acute strains will require rest and possibly immobilization. Immediately following injury cold packs may be applied for 20- to 30-minute periods, then removed for 1 hour during a 24-hour period to reduce any edema. Heat may then be applied for the client's comfort. In the case of a severe strain when the muscle may be completely ruptured, surgical repair may be necessary.

SPRAIN

A **sprain** is an injury to ligaments surrounding a joint caused by a sudden twist, wrench, or fall. Symptoms include pain, edema, loss of motion, and ecchymosis. X-ray will reveal soft tissue edema but no evidence of joint or bone injury. Immediate treatment is RICE (rest, ice, compression, and elevation). The client rests and ice is applied to the injured area. The part may then be immobilized with an elastic compression bandage or a brace, and elevated. After the edema has decreased significantly, a cast may be applied.

DISLOCATION

Dislocation occurs when articular surfaces of a joint are no longer in contact. The bones are literally "out of joint." The displaced bone may hinder the blood supply, damage nerves, tear ligaments, or rupture muscle attachments. Traumatic dislocations are considered orthopedic emergencies. Congenital dislocations are present at birth, while spontaneous or pathologic dislocations are caused by diseases affecting joints.

Symptoms of a dislocation include localized joint pain, loss of function of the joint, and a change in the length of the extremity and contour of the joint. Diagnosis is based on the symptoms, physical exam, and x-rays. X-rays reveal either a complete or partial separation of the articulating surfaces.

FRACTURE

A **fracture** is a break in the continuity of a bone. Fractures occur when the forces from outside the body become greater than the strength of the bone, causing the bone to break. Fractures usually involve soft tissue (edema and bleeding), damaged nerves, and tendons. Most fractures are caused by accidents. These may be the result of direct force, torsion or twisting, or violent contractions of highly developed muscles. Other fractures may be the result of a disease process that weakens the bone. This type of fracture is known as pathologic or spontaneous. Individuals considered at high risk for fractures include those who have predisposing bone conditions such as metastatic or primary bone tumors or osteoporosis, poor coordination, diminished vision, dizzy spells, or general weakness.

There are more than 90 different classifications of fractures. Some of the more common types include:

greenstick or incomplete, simple or closed, compound or open, impacted or telescoped, spiral, and comminuted.

In a greenstick fracture, the continuity of the bone is not completely disrupted but has splintering on one side and bending on the other. This fracture is seen most frequently in children. An uncomplicated (clean) fracture in which the skin remains intact is called a closed or simple fracture; the fractured surfaces are not contaminated by outside air. In a compound or open fracture, the bone is broken and the skin is also broken, allowing the bone to protrude and be susceptible to a greater chance for infection. An impacted fracture is also called a telescoped fracture; one portion of a bone fragment is forcibly driven into another. A spiral fracture twists around the shaft of the bone. This type of fracture may occur from a twisting force. In a comminuted fracture, the bone is splintered into many unaligned fragments. Various types of fractures are shown in Figure 24-6.

Healing time for fractures is affected by the age of the client and the type of injury or any underlying disease process, and may take weeks, months, or even years before the healing is complete. The sequence of healing takes place beginning with the formation of a hematoma, then granulation tissue formation, callus formation, callus ossification, and ultimately remodeling.

Hematoma formation begins with the formation of a clot that serves as a fibrin network. Bleeding comes from ruptured vessels within the bone as well as from tears in the periosteum and adjacent tissues. The hematoma is not absorbed but develops into granulation tissue. Granulation tissue forms a soft tissue callus that surrounds the fracture site and serves as a temporary splint. Callus ossification is the result of deposits of calcium salts in the callus forming rigid bone in excess as a protective measure. The formation of bone binds the bone ends together. Remodeling is completed by osteoclastic activity, whereby excess bone is

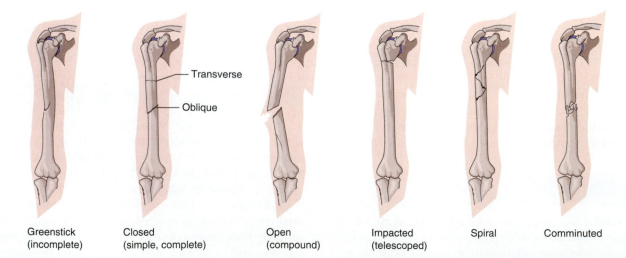

Greenstick (incomplete) Closed (simple, complete) Open (compound) Impacted (telescoped) Spiral Comminuted

Figure 24-6 Types of Bone Fractures

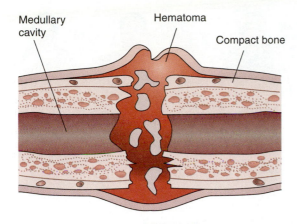

A. A hematoma forms from blood from ruptured vessels.

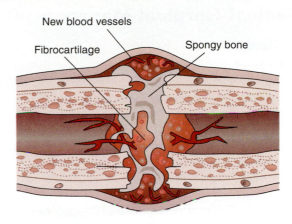

B. Spongy bone forms close to developing blood vessels; fibrocartilage forms away from new blood vessels.

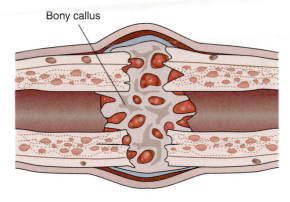

C. Bony callus replaces fibrocartilage.

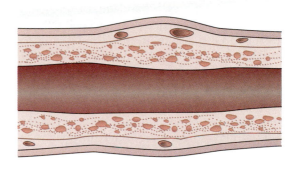

D. Excess bony tissue is removed by osteoclasts.

Figure 24-7 Steps of Bone Repair

gradually reduced and removed by absorption until the original shape and outline of the fractured bone is reestablished. Figure 24-7 outlines the healing sequence.

Complications of a fracture include infection, fat embolism, and compartment syndrome. Complications may delay healing or be life threatening.

Infections may result from an open fracture in which the bone extends through the skin, allowing contamination from the outside. They may also occur following surgical repair of a fracture using an internal fixation device. Any infection may lead to a delayed union of the bone.

A fat embolism occurs when a particle of fat from the marrow of a broken bone travels in the bloodstream toward the heart and lungs. It is usually associated with fractures of the long bones, multiple fractures, or crushing injuries. An embolus usually occurs within 24 to 72 hours following a fracture but may occur up to a week after injury. When a small area of the lungs is involved, the symptoms are pain, tachycardia, and dyspnea. Larger areas of lung involvement produce more pronounced symptoms, including severe pain, dyspnea, cyanosis, restlessness, and shock. Petechiae may appear over the neck, upper arms,

chest, or abdomen. Treatment consists of bed rest, gentle handling, oxygen, and IV fluids.

COMPARTMENT SYNDROME

Compartment syndrome is a form of neurovascular impairment that may lead to permanent injury of an affected limb caused by the progressive constriction of blood vessels and nerves. It can occur with any orthopedic injury as a result of bleeding into the tissue, tissue edema, or pressure from a cast or tight dressing. If untreated, in 4 to 6 hours it may lead to irreversible damage to nerves and muscles and within 24 to 48 hours permanent loss of normal limb function. A neurovascular assessment that reveals pain which is not relieved by narcotic analgesics, diminished capillary refill, weak or unequal pulses, **paresthesia** (numbness or tingling), and paralysis is indicative of this orthopedic emergency. Treatment consists of relieving pressure by removing the cast or dressing or by performing a fasciotomy. A surgical fasciotomy is an incision into the fascia to relieve pressure on the nerves and blood vessels.

Medical–Surgical Management

Medical

The treatment of a fracture requires immediate attention. The most important objectives are to: (1) realign the fracture, (2) maintain the alignment, and (3) regain the function of the injured part. The method of treatment will depend on the first aid given; the site, severity, and type of the fracture; and the age and condition of the client.

Closed Reduction Repair of a fracture accomplished without surgical intervention is called **closed reduction**. External manipulation is used to correct bone position. This manipulation requires three maneuvers: traction and countertraction, angulation, and rotation. Following the reduction, x-rays are taken to visualize the fracture alignment. The part is then immobilized by using a cast, bandage, or traction. Local or general anesthesia may be used to make the reduction easier and less painful to the client.

Casts A well-made and applied cast is as perfect a fixation apparatus as can be devised for the human body. Casts are made either from plaster bandages or synthetic materials such as fiberglass. Synthetic casts are used for non-weight bearing parts of the body. The cast should include the joint above and below the affected part. The major purposes of casts are: immobilization, support and protection of the affected part, prevention of deformities that may be the result of conditions such as arthritis, and the correction of deformities like scoliosis.

A dry cast should be odorless, shiny in appearance, resonant when percussed, and have a temperature similar to the room air. Moisture occurring from any underlying drainage will give the cast a musty smell, dullness on percussion, a lusterless color, and cool temperature.

Numerous types of casts exist. Long and short arm casts allow the fingers to be visible; long and short leg

Figure 24-8 Casts Used to Correct Musculoskeletal Disorders

casts allow the toes to be visible. A spica cast is used for hip, shoulder, and thumb dislocations or injuries. The hip spica has an abduction bar that keeps the cast in the correct position. A walking cast with a cast shoe facilitates client ambulation. Body casts are used to immobilize the spine following surgical spinal fusions, unstable spinal injuries, or for degenerative disorders. Figure 24-8 shows different types of casts.

After the application and drying of a cast, it may be necessary for the doctor to order a cast cut to allow visualization of a body area or to relieve pressure. This procedure is known as **windowing**. An arm cast may be cut in order to take a radial pulse or to dress a wound. Abdominal distention may be a reason to window a hip spica.

When a cast is removed, the client may become conscious of aches and discomforts caused by the constricted joint structures and immobilized muscles. The client's discomfort may be minimized by supporting the joint and maintaining the part in the same position as it was in the cast. The skin will be cool and pale with mottling and edema present. A yellow exudate, which is part dead skin and part secretions from oil sacs, will be on the skin. This exudate should not be rubbed or forced off.

Traction The principle of traction is to have two forces pulling in opposite directions. Traction consists of weights and counterweights. Countertraction forces can be provided by the weight of the client's body or other weight such as elevating the foot of the bed. Traction may be used to reduce a fracture, immobilize an extremity, lessen muscle spasms, or correct or prevent a deformity.

Types of traction are skeletal, skin, and manual. Skeletal traction requires the surgical insertion of pins (Steinmann) or wires (Kirschner) through the bones.

CLIENT TEACHING

Casts

Since plaster casts dry from the inside out, they should not be covered or dried with a hairdryer or heat lamp. Moisture and heat from the drying cast should be allowed to evaporate naturally. Clients should be informed that the heat they feel during the application, drying, and setting process is normal and should subside after 10 to 15 minutes. To avoid indentation, a drying cast should be placed on pillows and not on a hard surface. For the same reason, when handling the cast, only the palms of the hands should be used. Synthetic casts dry in minutes.

Figure 24-9 Types of Traction Devices: A. Skeletal traction; B. Head tongs

Skeletal traction is continuous and is used most frequently for fractures of the femur, tibia, and cervical spine. Head tongs (e.g., Gardner-Wells tongs) are fixed in the skull to apply traction that immobilizes cervical fractures. Figure 24-9 shows examples of traction devices.

Skin traction is a nonsurgical method of providing necessary pull for shorter periods of time, such as Buck's traction (Figure 24-10). Materials used include tapes, traction strips, cervical halters, and pelvic belts. Skin traction is frequently used to temporarily immobilize a part or stabilize a fracture. The disadvantage of skin traction for adult use is that it does not adequately control rotation and cannot be maintained for the length of time necessary for adult healing. Tapes and bandages should be applied smoothly to prevent any pressure areas.

A nurse caring for a client in traction should know the purpose of the traction, how it accomplishes its purpose, and any complications associated with the use of the traction. It is also important to know the extent of the injury and the movements and positions allowed. Care of the client should include maintenance of the injured part, general body alignment, the alignment of the traction apparatus, and range of motion in as many joints as possible.

Rehabilitation The physician will determine when the bone has healed sufficiently for rehabilitation. Healing is monitored by periodic x-rays and physical examinations. The major objective of rehabilitation is to assist the client to return to the former level of functioning. Rehabilitation programs vary depending on the injury and the client.

Physical therapy may be started with the use of parallel bars or other exercise equipment before the client is allowed to exercise independently. The nurse has a major role in client education reinforcing the directions of both the physician and the physical therapist. Patience and encouragement are extremely important in assisting the client to feel comfortable in learning self-care techniques. The client should be taught to report any unusual signs or symptoms to the physician.

The client will also need to learn the proper use of equipment such as crutches, canes, or walkers. Crutches allow ambulation with limited or no weight bearing on the affected extremity. Walkers allow limited weight bearing and provide stability while the client ambulates. Canes allow the client to walk with balance and support.

The tripod position is the basic stance for crutch walking. Tips of the crutches are placed approximately 8 to 10 inches in front of and beside the client's feet. The client must place his weight on the handpiece of the crutches and not on the axilla. Crutch gaits depend on the client's disability and are prescribed by the physician. See Figure 24-11 for basic crutch walking gaits.

Canes are held in the hand opposite the affected extremity. In normal walking, the opposite arm and leg move together. This same action should be done when walking with a cane. Walkers provide more support than canes or crutches. They are especially useful for clients who have poor balance. The client should

Figure 24-10 Buck's Traction, a Type of Skin Traction

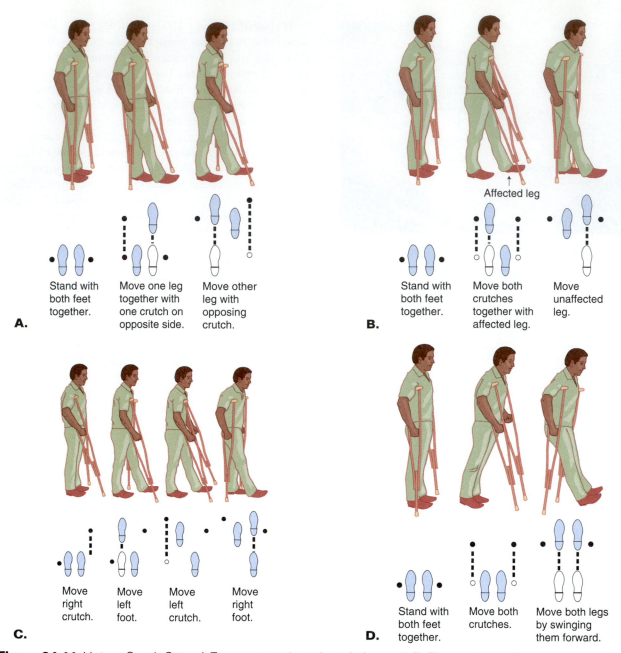

Figure 24-11 Various Crutch Gaits: A Two-point gait (partial weight bearing); B. Three-point gait (partial or non-weight bearing); C. Four-point alternate crutch gait (partial or full weight bearing); D. Swing through gait (non-weight bearing)

place the walker 12 to 18 inches in front and walk toward the walker holding onto the hand grips.

Surgical

Open reduction is a surgical procedure that enables the surgeon to reduce (repair) the fracture under direct visualization. When an open reduction/internal fixation (ORIF) is done, orthopedic devices are used to maintain the reduction. Some of the devices used include pins, screws, nails, plates, wires, and rods. These internal fixation devices may be inserted through bone fragments or fixed to the sides of the bones.

The major disadvantage of the open reduction is the possibility of introducing infection into the bone.

Other disadvantages include impaired circulation and accidental injury to major nerves, blood vessels, and bone caused by the fixation devices. X-rays may be taken during and after the open reduction to evaluate the alignment of the fracture.

Pharmacological

Analgesics may be given to relieve pain. Muscle relaxants, such as cyclobenzaprine hydrochloride (Flexeril), may also be prescribed for muscle spasms. Severe or continued pain may indicate complications and should be given immediate attention. Stool softeners, such as docusate sodium (Colace), may be given to prevent constipation in the immobilized client.

Diet

The client should be encouraged to eat regular meals. The meals should include foods that provide fiber, protein, calcium, phosphorus, and fluids. For the client whose dietary intake is inadequate, vitamin and mineral supplements, especially calcium and phosphorus, may be included. Consultation with a dietitian regarding food preferences of the client may be necessary.

Activity

Client activity and exercise are important in maintaining muscle strength and tone, and minimizing cardiovascular problems. Joints that are not immobilized should be exercised either actively or passively to maintain function. Isometric (maintaining constant resistive force) exercises help to maintain muscle strength of immobilized muscles.

▶ NURSING PROCESS

▶ Assessment

▶ Subjective Data

The neurovascular assessment of a client with a fracture may reveal subjective data of pain, especially on movement; muscle spasms; and paresthesia.

▶ Objective Data

Edema, shortening and deformity of the affected limb, and pallor may be found. Pulses in the affected and unaffected extremity must be checked and compared. The client's vital signs should be taken routinely, and the general physical and mental condition of the client should be noted. The skin, especially over

PROFESSIONAL TIP

Neurovascular Assessment

- Circulation, movement, and sensation (CMS) assessments are performed on clients following musculoskeletal trauma; after surgery, if nerve or blood vessel damage is possible; and following casting, splinting, and bandaging.
- The CMS assessment is performed every 15 to 30 minutes for several hours, and then every 3 to 4 hours.
- All findings must be documented.
- Tingling and numbness may be relieved by flexing fingers or toes or repositioning extremity.
- The nurse should remember 5 Ps when performing a CMS assessment:
  1. Pain
  2. Pallor (slow capillary return)
  3. Paresthesia (unrelieved tingling or numbness)
  4. Puffiness (edema)
  5. Pulselessness

bony prominences, should be checked for color and temperature.

The client who has a cast applied must have all cast edges checked for smoothness. The cast should also be checked for spots indicating wound drainage including the color and amount. Extremities including fingers, toes, hands, and feet should be assessed for changes in skin color, pulse, or temperature. All traction wires, pulleys, and weights should be checked. Weights should hang free.

Nursing diagnoses for a client with musculoskeletal trauma may include the following:

Nursing Diagnoses	Planning/Goals	Nursing Interventions
▶ Acute Pain related to fracture	The client will have relief of pain with medication.	Provide comfort measures.
		Administer medications for pain as ordered.
▶ Risk for Impaired Skin Integrity related to immobility	The client will experience no skin breakdown.	Change client position, if allowed, maintaining correct body alignment.
		Check bony prominences and keep the client's skin clean and dry.
		For the client in a cast, check the edges of the cast for roughness, keep the exposed skin next to the cast clean and dry.
		Inspect all body pressure points including the head, ears, and heels; turn the client as orders direct; and check for friction rubs.
		Instruct clients not to poke anything under the cast or use objects to scratch, causing skin breakdown or infections.
		Avoid getting the cast wet.

continues

Nursing Diagnoses	Planning/Goals	Nursing Interventions
▶ *Impaired Physical Mobility related to loss of integrity of bone structures*	The client will perform range of motion exercises in unaffected joints. The client will demonstrate use of adaptive devices to improve mobility.	If the client in a cast is allowed to turn, use an overhead trapeze. Assist client in performing ROM exercises. Assist client in use of adaptive devices.

Evaluation Each goal must be evaluated to determine how it has been met by the client.

INFLAMMATORY DISORDERS

Inflammatory disorders involve inflammation of the joints and include conditions such as rheumatoid arthritis, bursitis, polymyositis, and osteomyelitis.

RHEUMATOID ARTHRITIS

Rheumatoid arthritis is a chronic systemic disease of unknown etiology, with recurring inflammation involving the synovium or lining of the joints. It can also affect the lungs, heart, blood vessels, muscles, eyes, and skin. Rheumatoid arthritis is a potentially destructive and disabling disease. The course is variable with either slow or rapid progress and/or periods of remissions. Women are affected more often than men. Rheumatoid arthritis can occur at any age; however, it most commonly affects young adults. In children it occurs in a form known as juvenile rheumatoid arthritis (Still's disease). See Chapter 22 for more information on rheumatoid arthritis.

BURSITIS

Bursitis is inflammation of the bursa, a sac filled with synovial fluid that facilitates joint movement. Major bursae are found in the shoulder, knee, hip, and elbow. The inflammation is usually the result of trauma or repetitive movements. The client experiences painful joint movement. Diagnosis is made from the client's symptoms and x-ray which shows a calcified bursa. Treatment includes rest of the joint and the administration of anti-inflammatory drugs including salicylates and NSAIDs. For some clients, corticosteroids may be injected into the bursa.

POLYMYOSITIS

Polymyositis is an inflammatory disease involving striated muscle. The etiology of this disease is unknown, but probably is an autoimmune mechanism. It is primarily a disease of skeletal muscle; however, the heart, gastrointestinal tract, and lungs are also frequently involved. Symptoms include muscle weakness with activities like climbing the stairs, getting out of a chair, or combing the hair. The muscles of swallowing may also become involved. This weakness is the result of degeneration and necrosis of parts or entire groups of muscle fibers. Some individuals have arthralgia and Raynaud's phenomenon.

Medical–Surgical Management

Pharmacological

Treatment is symptomatic and begins initially with high doses of prednisone (Deltasone). The doses are then modified in response to muscle enzymes. Reduction of the muscle enzymes may take several months, thus requiring long-term maintenance treatment.

Diet

If the neck flexor muscles are involved, the client may need frequent small meals and antacids for reflux esophagitis.

Activity

Physical therapy is begun to preserve muscle strength and prevent contractures. Complete bed rest with the head of the bed elevated is eventually required.

▶ NURSING PROCESS

▶ Assessment

▶ Subjective Data

Questions regarding muscle or joint pain, appetite, dyspnea, and gastrointestinal symptoms are appropriate.

▶ Objective Data

Objective data is gathered from observations of the client's ability to complete activities of daily living and any evidence of respiratory difficulty. Muscles and joints should be palpated for tenderness or pain.

Nursing diagnoses for a client with polymyositis may include the following:

Nursing Diagnoses	Planning/Goals	Nursing Interventions
▶ Impaired Physical Mobility related to muscle weakness	The client will perform physical activity as tolerated.	Assist client and encourage physical mobility, provide rest periods before and after activity.
▶ Bathing/Hygiene, Dressing/Grooming, and Feeding/Toileting Self-Care Deficit related to muscle weakness	The client will perform ADLs as able.	Assist the client in activities whenever necessary. Provide frequent position change and ROM exercises to prevent contractures.
▶ Imbalanced Nutrition: Less than body requirements related to difficulty in swallowing	The client will maintain adequate nutritional status.	Provide small, frequent, high-caloric feedings.

Evaluation Each goal must be evaluated to determine how it has been met by the client.

OSTEOMYELITIS

Osteomyelitis is the inflammation of the bone and bone marrow. The most common cause of osteomyelitis is the introduction of pathogenic bacteria into a penetrating injury such as an open fracture. Bone infections may also result from the spread of infection from another site such as infected teeth, tonsils, or an upper respiratory infection. The most common pathogen causing osteomyelitis is *Staphylococcus aureus*. Other organisms found in osteomyelitis are *Pseudomonas* and *Escherichia coli*. Osteomyelitis may become a chronic disabling problem affecting the quality of life. The affected bone may have spontaneous fractures.

Local symptoms of an acute infection are sudden pain and tenderness of the affected bone, warmth, redness, edema, and pain on movement. General symptoms with acute severe bone infections may include chills, elevated temperature, rapid pulse, and marked leukocytosis.

A bone sheath forms around the sequestrum (dead bone) giving the appearance of healing. However, chronically infected sequestrum has the tendency to produce recurrent abscesses throughout the life of the individual.

Surgical

A sequestrectomy to remove the dead bone tissue may need to be performed. Strict aseptic technique must be maintained when changing any dressings. Because infected bone may be extremely painful, unnecessary movement should be avoided and the affected extremity should be handled very gently.

Pharmacological

Vigorous antibiotic therapy and analgesics are the medications used for the treatment of osteomyelitis. Wound irrigations with antiseptics or antibiotics are often prescribed by the physician. Specific drugs given are determined by the causative organism.

Medical–Surgical Management

Medical

The client is placed on bed rest and the infected bone is kept at rest with the use of sandbags or casts. Antibiotics are given as soon as osteomyelitis is suspected. Unless the infective process is controlled early, a bone abscess forms (Figure 24-12). Cultures of the abscess may indicate a need for change in the antibiotic therapy. The abscess may drain naturally; however, it usually requires an incision allowing it to drain. The abscess cavity of dead bone tissue does not liquefy easily, drain, and heal as in soft tissue abscesses.

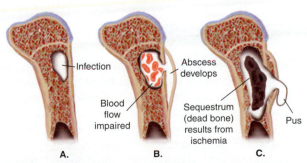

Figure 24-12 A. Osteomyelitis; B. Without early treatment, an abscess forms; C. Bone dies (sequestrum) and pus forms.

Diet

A high-caloric, high-protein diet is generally ordered for the client with osteomyelitis. Dietary supplements of vitamins and calcium are also given. Fluids should be increased as tolerated.

Activity

There should be absolute rest of the affected extremity. Excessive handling of the extremity is very painful and should be avoided. The extremity should be handled in a smooth unhurried manner, supporting the joints above and below the affected area.

▶ NURSING PROCESS

▶ Assessment

▶ Subjective Data

Inquire about pain, muscle spasms, and tenderness in the bone. Ask about any traumas, surgeries, and other diseases.

▶ Objective Data

Observe the client for signs of infection, including chills, elevated temperature, pain, redness, and edema of the affected extremity. The client may also experience headaches, restlessness, and irritability.

Nursing diagnoses for a client with osteomyelitis may include the following:

Nursing Diagnoses	Planning/Goals	Nursing Interventions
▶ *Impaired Physical Mobility related to pain*	The client will maintain movement of unaffected extremities.	Encourage and assist client to maintain active ROM or perform passive ROM to unaffected extremities.
▶ *Risk for Impaired Skin Integrity related to immobility*	The client will maintain skin integrity.	Handle the affected extremity gently, protect it from injury, keep it in good body alignment and level with the body.
		Irrigate wound as ordered.
		Use aseptic technique when irrigating the affected area and when changing the dressing.
		Assess skin and bony prominences for reddened areas.
		Encourage adequate fluid intake.
▶ *Acute Pain related to inflammation*	The client will verbalize reduction of pain.	Protect client from jerky movements and falls.
		Assess wound appearance and new sites of pain.
		Provide diet high in protein and vitamin C.
		Administer pain medications as ordered.

Evaluation Each goal must be evaluated to determine how it has been met by the client.

DEGENERATIVE DISORDERS

Conditions discussed following include osteoporosis, degenerative joint disease, and total joint arthroplasty.

OSTEOPOROSIS

Osteoporosis is an increase in the porosity of bone. It is a common disorder in bone metabolism in which both mineral and protein matrix components are diminished and the bone becomes brittle and fragile. There is an increased susceptibility to fractures of the hip, spine, and wrist.

Ten million individuals in the United States have osteoporosis and another 18 million have low bone mineral density which places them at risk for osteoporosis (Dowd & Cavalieri, 1999; National Osteoporosis Foundation [NOF], 1999b; National Institute of Arthritis and Musculoskeletal and Skin Diseases [NIAMS], October

1998). Of those affected by osteoporosis, 80% are women (NOF, 1999c). More than 1.5 million fractures occur annually related to osteoporosis, including 300,000 hip fractures, 700,000 vertebral fractures, 250,000 wrist fractures, and more than 300,000 fractures of other types (NOF, 1999c).

Osteoporosis has been called the "silent disease" because there are no symptoms of bone loss. Bone loss may be 50% before pain or a fracture occurs (Darovic, 1997). Because the bone tissue loses its density, fractures and kyphosis may occur. Very slight trauma may fracture the brittle bones. With multiple vertebral fractures, the individual may experience a loss of height.

The only way to determine if an individual has osteoporosis is to measure bone mineral density (BMD). There are several methods of measuring BMD; all are painless, noninvasive, and safe. They include:

- DXA or DEXA (dual energy X-ray absorptiometry) measures spine, hip, or total body.

PROFESSIONAL TIP

Osteoporosis

Risk factors for osteoporosis include being female, having thin or small bones, advanced age, family history of osteoporosis, postmenopause without estrogen replacement therapy, amenorrhea, eating disorders, low calcium intake, inactive life style, smoking, excessive alcohol intake, use of corticosteroids or anticonvulsant medications, and low testosterone level in men.

- SXA (single energy X-ray absorptiometry) measures wrist or heel.
- DPA (dual photon absorptiometry) measures spine, hip, or total body.
- Ultrasound measures heel, shin bone, and kneecap (NOF, 1999b).

Medical–Surgical Management

There is no cure for osteoporosis. Prevention through diet, regular exercise, and eliminating tobacco and alcohol use is the best defense against osteoporosis (Dowd and Cavalieri, 1999).

Pharmacological

Four medications are approved for postmenopausal women to prevent and/or treat osteoporosis; no medications are as yet approved for men (NOF, 1999c). Estrogen is used both for prevention and treatment. It is the primary choice for prevention in postmenopausal women. Alendronate sodium (Fosamax) is used for prevention and treatment. Calcitonin (Miacalcin) for treatment of osteoporosis is available as a nasal spray. To obtain its full therapeutic effect, the client should also take calcium and vitamin D supplements. To prevent osteoporosis, raloxifene (Evista) may be used. It prevents bone loss throughout the body, but may cause venous thrombosis.

Testosterone replacement therapy may be used for men with low testosterone levels.

Nonnarcotic analgesics may be prescribed for relief of pain. The client may also be advised to take supplemental calcium.

Diet

The client is encouraged to maintain an adequate balanced diet rich in calcium and vitamin D. A reduction in the consumption of caffeine, alcohol, excess protein, and the use of cigarettes is recommended.

Activity

The client is encouraged to practice good body mechanics and posture. Walking, preferably outdoors for the benefits of sunshine (vitamin D), is also encouraged. This is effective in preventing further bone loss and stimulating new bone formation.

▶ NURSING PROCESS

▶ Assessment

▶ Subjective Data

This includes the client's gender, age, and family health history. Any symptoms the client expresses regarding altered body image or back or neck pain that worsens when coughing, sneezing, straining, or standing should be noted. A nutritional history should be taken. Lifestyle patterns such as smoking, inactivity, or immobilization should be noted. A medical history regarding any medications is also important.

▶ Objective Data

This includes a dowager's hump, gait impairment, and posture.

CULTURAL CONSIDERATIONS

Osteoporosis

- Significant risk has been reported in persons of all ethnic backgrounds.
- White women over age 65 have twice as many fractures as African American women (NOF, 1999c).
- White men are at greater risk for osteoporosis, but osteoporosis is found in men from all ethnic groups (NOF, 1999d).

COMMUNITY/HOME HEALTH CARE

Osteoporosis

- Maintain physical activity—walking, isometric exercises.
- Remove potential hazards—throw rugs.
- Eat a diet high in calcium and vitamin D.
- Be out in the sun 10 to 15 minutes a day.
- Move items down from top shelves of cupboards as it is difficult to see or reach what is up there due to curvature changes in the spine.

Nursing diagnoses for a client with osteoporosis may include the following:

Nursing Diagnoses	Planning/Goals	Nursing Interventions
▶ *Chronic Pain related to disease process*	The client will express minimal discomfort.	Administer analgesics as ordered; teach the client about the medications.
		Handle the client carefully; instruct the client to avoid any twisting movements.
		The bed should have a firm mattress or bed board for support.
▶ *Risk for Injury related to disease process*	The client will practice correct body mechanics.	Teach client correct body mechanics.
▶ *Impaired Physical Mobility related to disease process*	The client will maintain physical activity.	Teach client about types of exercises and physical activities that will help maintain bone mass and isometric exercises to strengthen muscles.
		Encourage ambulation with the client using a walker or cane if necessary.

Evaluation Each goal must be evaluated to determine how it has been met by the client.

DEGENERATIVE JOINT DISEASE (OSTEOARTHRITIS)

Since osteoarthritis is not an inflammatory disorder, as the name implies, the term *degenerative joint disease* (DJD) is often used to better reflect the pathophysiology. Osteoarthritis is considered a "wear and tear" disease and is characterized by the slow and steady progressive destructive changes of the joint. It is a nonsystemic, noninflammatory disorder causing bones and joints to degenerate. It is the most common type of arthritis. The etiology is unknown but predisposing factors include obesity, an injury to a joint, poor posture, or occupations that put strain on joints. Recent studies suggest that there may also be a genetic cause of osteoarthritis (NIAMS, May 1998). The weight bearing joints of the lower extremities as well as the hands and cervical and lumbar vertebrae are the joints most frequently affected. The cartilage covering the bone becomes thin and then wears off. The synovial membrane thickens and fibrous tissue around the joint ossifies. The effects of degenerative changes on the knee joint are shown in Figure 24-13.

The onset of osteoarthritis begins during middle age, and by age 60 most people have some degeneration. Symptoms include early morning stiffness and pain after physical activity. There is joint enlargement and characteristic hypertrophic spurs, called **Heberden's nodes,** in the terminal interphalangeal finger joints. More women are affected with DJD, especially in the hands. The hips are more affected in men.

Diagnosis is made from the client's symptoms and examination of the joints that are enlarged and tender. X-ray shows a narrowing of joint spaces and gross irregularities of joint structure. A CT scan or MRI may be used to show vertebral joint involvement.

Medical–Surgical Management

Medical

No treatment exists to stop the degenerative process; therefore, treatment focuses on the relief of the client's discomfort. Medical management includes local heat and rest for the affected joint, weight reduction for obese clients to relieve strain on affected joints, and orthotic devices (braces, canes, crutches) to support the inflamed joints. Physical therapy can provide exercises to strengthen muscles and teach self-management skills.

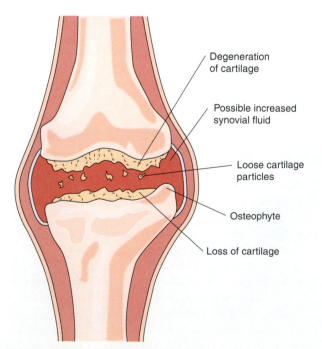

Figure 24-13 Degenerative Changes in the Cartilage of the Knee Due to Osteoarthritis

CLIENT TEACHING

Degenerative Joint Disease

- Set priorities each day, and do the most important activities first.
- Do not plan too many activities for one day.
- Plan rest periods during the day between activities.
- Prevent rushing and stressful situations by planning ahead.
- Lose weight, if necessary.
- When knees or hips are affected, avoid climbing stairs, bending, stooping, or squatting.

Surgical

Surgical procedures such as total hip or knee replacement may be recommended for clients with severe osteoarthritis. Osteotomy may help correct malalignment situations. Refer to the section on total joint arthroplasty in this chapter.

Pharmacological

Pharmacological treatment includes the use of aspirin or NSAIDs. Narcotics should be avoided because of the chronic nature of the disease. Steroids may be used and are sometimes injected into a joint to provide immediate relief of pain and to stop the degenerative process temporarily. If the client has vertebral involvement with muscle spasms, cyclobenzaprine hydrochloride (Flexeril) may be given to relax the muscles.

▶ NURSING PROCESS

▶ Assessment

▶ Subjective Data

The client may describe nonspecific symptoms such as general musculoskeletal pain, joint stiffness especially on rising, and joint pain or tenderness. Weight gain and occupation and any conditions or situations that may exacerbate the client's joint pain should be noted. Some of these situations may include cold weather, overexercising, or extreme fatigue. The client's understanding of the disease and its effect on lifestyle and ability to perform activities of daily and social living should also be assessed.

▶ Objective Data

This includes edema and tenderness around the joints and bony enlargements of distal interphalangeal joints (Heberden's nodes).

Nursing diagnoses for a client with osteoarthritis may include the following:

Nursing Diagnoses	Planning/Goals	Nursing Interventions
▶ *Chronic Pain related to joint tenderness and edema*	The client will express minimal discomfort.	Handle the affected extremity gently and apply heat as ordered. Administer prescribed analgesic and evaluate its effectiveness.
▶ *Impaired Physical Mobility related to joint deterioration*	The client will maintain mobility within the parameters of the disease process.	Coordinate with physical therapy and assist in a planned exercise program as ordered. Advise the client to plan rest periods during the day.

Evaluation Each goal must be evaluated to determine how it has been met by the client.

TOTAL JOINT ARTHROPLASTY

Joint replacement or **arthroplasty** is the replacement of both articular surfaces within a joint capsule. The hip, knee, shoulder, and fingers are the joints most frequently replaced in this procedure. Replacements consist of metal and polyethylene and may be cemented in the prepared bone with methyl methacrylate which has properties similar to bone. See Figure 24-14 for knee and hip replacement components.

Newer techniques use porous-coated cementless artificial joint components. These allow bone to grow into the joint component and securely fix the prosthesis. This reduces the incidence of prosthesis failure.

Joint replacement is usually an elective procedure and clients may wish to have autologous blood transfusions whereby they pre-donate their own blood in case a blood transfusion is needed.

TOTAL HIP REPLACEMENT

Total hip replacement is the replacement of a severely damaged hip with an artificial joint. This procedure is usually reserved for clients over 60 with severe pain or irreversibly damaged hip joints. However, with improved prosthetic materials and operative techniques, younger clients with severely damaged hips are being considered for total hip replacement surgery. Potential problems with the hip replacement include

Figure 24-14 A. Total hip and knee replacement; B. Radiograph of a total knee replacement (anterior-posterior view). Because the patella is plastic, it is not visible here.

dislocation of the prosthesis, excessive wound drainage, and infection.

Following a total hip replacement the client's hip and leg should be kept in a position of abduction and extension. The knees are kept apart by using foam wedges, several pillows, or an abductor pillow. The client may lie on the unaffected side. When the client turns from the back to a side-lying position, the entire leg should be supported with pillows to keep the hip abducted. The client should be instructed to avoid acute flexion of the hip. The legs should not be crossed nor the hips flexed to pull up a blanket or sheet. A fracture bedpan should be used until the client can ambulate to the bathroom. In the bathroom a raised toilet seat should be used. Any specific client turning, movement, and positioning will be ordered by the physician. Vital signs and circulation, movement, and sensation (CMS) checks should be done routinely.

Dressings should be inspected frequently. If the surgical site is drained with a portable suction device, it should be monitored for patency, and the type and amount of drainage. Initially drainage might be 200 to 500 cc. Within 48 hours the drainage should decrease to 30 cc or less and the suction device can be removed.

The goal for clients who have total hip or knee joint replacement is to ambulate independently. Ambulatory activity progresses rapidly for clients with joint replacement. Clients who have total hip replacement are usually out of bed the night of surgery or early the next day. Gait training may begin with the use of a walker and progress to the use of crutches or a cane.

The client should avoid hip flexion of more than 90 degrees. Stair climbing should be avoided for at least 3 months.

TOTAL KNEE REPLACEMENT

Total knee replacement, like the hip replacement, is considered for clients experiencing severe pain and functional disability related to joint destruction. The prosthesis chosen for the replacement provides the client with a painless, stable, and functional joint. Following total knee replacement surgery, clients may use a continuous passive motion (CPM) machine. This machine helps to increase circulation to the operative area and promotes flexibility within the knee joint. The surgeon orders the frequency of use and the amount of tension, flexion, and extension produced by the machine.

Following knee arthroplasty, the client's knee may be immobilized with a firm compression dressing and an adjustable soft knee immobilizer. The client may transfer out of bed to a wheelchair with the immobilizer in place. No weight bearing is allowed on the knee until it is prescribed by the surgeon. If ordered, a sequential compression device (SCD) may be used or antiembolism stockings worn to minimize the development of thrombophlebitis.

Rehabilitation generally starts the second day for clients who have total knee arthroplasty. When the client sits in a chair, the knee should be elevated. Ambulation with assistive aids and weight bearing limits is usually started 1 to 2 days after surgery.

▶ NURSING PROCESS

▶ Assessment

▶ Subjective Data

This involves assessing for irritability, restlessness, orientation, and neurovascular assessment of the affected extremity for pain, numbness, tingling, and paresthesia.

▶ Objective Data

This involves assessing the incision for approximation, redness, and drainage. Assessment of skin over all bony prominences should also be made, as well as assessment for tachypnea, dyspnea, hypoxemia, and crackles and wheezes in the lungs (signs of fat em-bolism). Vital signs, pedal pulses, and I & O are also assessed.

The client with a total hip replacement should be assessed for position of the affected hip. The hip should be maintained in a position of abduction and extension. The most prominent symptom of a dislocation is a clicking, popping sound. Other symptoms are a sudden sharp pain that is unrelieved by narcotic analgesics, loss of leg motion, and edema of the affected hip. The client should not be moved and the physician should be notified immediately.

Assessment of the client with a total knee replacement includes the neurovascular status of the leg, the dressing and drainage device, keeping the knee elevated, and monitoring the CPM machine. Vital signs, intake and output, and the color and temperature of the extremity are also assessed.

Nursing diagnoses for the client undergoing arthroplasty surgery may include the following:

Nursing Diagnoses	Planning/Goals	Nursing Interventions
▶ *Impaired Skin Integrity related to immobility and surgical incision*	The client's skin will remain free from redness or any other signs of breakdown.	Maintain a clean and dry dressing. If a drainage device is used, assess functioning. Keep client's skin and bed clean and dry. Assess bony prominences for redness. Provide high-protein diet with dairy products and vitamin C.
▶ *Impaired Physical Mobility related to surgery*	The client will ambulate following physician's direction.	Keep client in a position of abduction. Use an abductor pillow or wedge to maintain the position when turning the client. Assist the client in accomplishing activities of daily living. Encourage client to use the trapeze to raise hips off the bed to use the bedpan.
▶ *Ineffective Tissue Perfusion (Peripheral) related to surgery and immobility*	The client will have adequate circulation of extremity.	Encourage the client to cough and deep breathe. Monitor vital signs until stable. Assess pedal pulses and capillary refill in both extremities.

Evaluation Each goal must be evaluated to determine how it has been met by the client.

MUSCULOSKELETAL DISORDERS

Musculoskeletal disorders discussed include amputations, temporomandibular joint disease/disorder, and carpal tunnel syndrome.

AMPUTATIONS

An **amputation** is the removal of all or part of an extremity. Amputations are done in response to injuries resulting in extensive laceration of arteries or nerves, or diseases such as malignant tumors, infections, and peripheral vascular disorders. Other disease conditions that may require amputation include extensive osteomyelitis, or congenital disorders. In severe trauma situations, an amputation may be done to save the client's life.

Recent advances in microsurgical techniques have allowed replantation (limb reattachment) in some injuries. These procedures involve the use of microscopes and highly specialized instruments to reconnect severed nerves and blood vessels. Amputations involving the hand or wrist are more likely to be considered for replantation rather than an injury involving a large muscle mass because of extensive tissue, bone, and muscle damage. Any amputation creates a major physical and psychological adjustment for the client.

Medical–Surgical Management

Medical

Rehabilitation for the client with an amputation requires the effort of the entire rehabilitation team. The client's physical and psychological responses to the amputation are monitored by all members of the team. If appropriate, counseling and job training will enable many clients to return to their jobs.

Surgical

Before surgery the surgeon must evaluate the client and make several decisions. These decisions include: necessity of an amputation, type of amputation (open or closed), level of amputation, potential for rehabilitation, and type of prosthesis and rehabilitation program.

The surgeon will try to save as much of the limb as possible. A closed amputation is done by using skin flaps to cover the bone end of the extremity. This type of amputation is done when there is no evidence of infection. Sometimes a Guillotine (open) amputation is necessary. This amputation requires a straight cut and allows for free drainage of infectious material. Tissue, bone, and vessels are severed at the same level without skin flaps. The major indication for doing an open amputation is infection.

The level of an amputation is determined by the vascular supply and is never higher than absolutely necessary. If the blood flow at the site of the incision is normal, the amputation is performed at that level. If the bleeding is scant, a higher level of amputation is performed to ensure adequate postoperative healing.

Pharmacological

Narcotic analgesics may be required immediately following surgery. After several days pain may be controlled with nonnarcotic analgesics. If infection exists, appropriate antibiotic therapy will be ordered.

Diet

A balanced diet with adequate vitamins and protein is essential for adequate wound healing. Many elderly clients are poorly nourished or require special diets. Nutritional care plans should be discussed with the physician and a dietitian.

Activity

Postoperative positioning of the stump will be determined by the surgeon. The stump may be placed in an extended position or elevated on pillows for short periods. The client should also be encouraged to spend some time in the prone position. This position helps to stretch the flexor muscles and to prevent contractions of the hip. One to 2 days following surgery the client may begin bed exercises. These exercises, taught by the physical therapist, are done to prevent contractures and increase muscle strength. Ambulation begins in physical therapy after transfer techniques are learned by the client. Ambulation progresses according to whether the client is to be fitted with a prosthesis immediately or at a later time.

▶ NURSING PROCESS

▶ Assessment

▶ Subjective Data

This should include pain, sensations felt on extremity to be amputated, and the emotional status of the client. If a client has experienced chronic pain prior to the amputation, pain may seem mild following the surgery. Severe pain may indicate a hematoma or excessive pressure from a cast or elastic bandage on a bony prominence. The client may confuse **phantom limb pain** with the incisional pain. Phantom limb pain is the sensation that there is pain, soreness, and stiffness in the amputated limb. Phantom pain will decrease as inflammation subsides at the incisional site.

▶ Objective Data

This includes the color and temperature of the skin, pulse, and responses to limb movement. The unaffected extremity should also be assessed for function and circulation.

Nursing diagnoses for the client who has an amputation may include the following:

Nursing Diagnoses	Planning/Goals	Nursing Interventions
▶ *Impaired Skin Integrity related to amputation*	The client will remain free from infection.	Inspect the incision for any inflammation, excessive drainage, edema, increased pain, and hypersensitivity to touch.
		Use aseptic technique for all dressing changes.
		Monitor vital signs.

continues

Nursing Diagnoses	Planning/Goals	Nursing Interventions
▶ *Disturbed Body Image related to loss of limb*	The client will participate in the care of the residual limb.	Handle the residual limb gently and treat it as though a prosthesis will be worn.
		Encourage client to watch dressing change and eventually assist with and do the dressing changes.
		Encourage the client to express feelings and concerns about the amputation.
▶ *Impaired Physical Mobility related to loss of limb*	The client will demonstrate improved physical mobility.	Encourage the client to participate in physical therapy.
		Assist the client when ambulating with assistive devices.
		Encourage client to perform ROM exercises.

Evaluation Each goal must be evaluated to determine how it has been met by the client.

SAMPLE NURSING CARE PLAN

THE CLIENT WITH A BELOW THE KNEE AMPUTATION

Mrs. Spencer is a 76-year-old resident in a retirement home. She has remained active since her retirement from the secretarial job she held for 20 years. Her health history indicates she has had circulatory problems with inadequate peripheral circulation resulting from atherosclerosis. Her physician has hospitalized her for a planned below the knee amputation on the left leg and has ordered an arteriogram to assist in determining the site for the amputation. The arteriogram will help determine the circulatory status of her leg necessary to promote wound healing.

The nurse's assessment of Mrs. Spencer's vital signs indicated B/P 120/68, pulse 72, and respirations 18. Femoral pulses were present in both extremities; however, the pedal pulse in her left foot was barely palpable, and the skin was cool and pale. She stated that lately her left foot is always cold and is a "bluish-black" color. Mrs. Spencer has expressed concern about her ability to take care of herself after she loses her foot.

Nursing Diagnosis 1 *Disturbed Body Image related to scheduled amputation as evidenced by statement of concern over losing foot*

PLANNING/GOALS	NURSING INTERVENTIONS	RATIONALE	EVALUATION
Mrs. Spencer will communicate her concerns and feelings about the changes in her body image.	Involve Mrs. Spencer in participating in her daily care.	Gives sense of independence.	Mrs. Spencer has demonstrated beginning acceptance of body changes by taking an active interest in her appearance.
	Encourage Mrs. Spencer to voice her concerns.	Helps resolve concerns.	
	Provide positive reinforcement when Mrs. Spencer attempts to adapt to body changes.	Encourages her to continue adapting.	

Nursing Diagnosis 2 *Situational Low Self-Esteem related to loss of body part as evidenced by expression of concern about ability to care for self*

PLANNING/GOALS	NURSING INTERVENTIONS	RATIONALE	EVALUATION
Mrs. Spencer will identify at least two positive qualities about herself.	Encourage Mrs. Spencer to express her feelings about herself.	Listening helps Mrs. Spencer identify positive qualities.	Mrs. Spencer has voiced two positive qualities about herself.

continues

| | Involve Mrs. Spencer in the decision-making process regarding her care. | Helps Mrs. Spencer maintain a sense of control over her life. | |
| | Provide Mrs. Spencer with positive feedback. | Gives Mrs. Spencer a feeling of approval. | |

Nursing Diagnosis 3 *Anticipatory Grieving related to loss associated with amputation as evidenced by her expression of concern*

PLANNING/GOALS	NURSING INTERVENTIONS	RATIONALE	EVALUATION
Mrs. Spencer will express her feelings about the loss of her foot.	Encourage Mrs. Spencer to express her feelings by talking, crying, writing.	Some people are uncomfortable expressing their feelings; gives several options for expression.	Mrs. Spencer expresses feelings about her potential loss.
	Spend a specific amount of nonnursing time each shift with Mrs. Spencer to allow for uninterrupted conversation.	Allows expression of feelings and shows concern and understanding.	
	Inform Mrs. Spencer and her family about support groups and organizations in the community.	May help Mrs. Spencer find new ways of adapting to loss.	

Nursing Diagnosis 4 *Deficient Knowledge related to postoperative care and activity as evidenced by concern about ability to care for self*

PLANNING/GOALS	NURSING INTERVENTIONS	RATIONALE	EVALUATION
Mrs. Spencer will perform stump wrapping correctly.	Encourage Mrs. Spencer to participate in the care of the residual limb.	Encouraging participation helps client adjust to body changes.	Mrs. Spencer demonstrated the ability to care for the residual limb by wrapping the stump correctly.
	Demonstrate how to wrap her stump, then allow her to do it several times.	Discharge instructions help clients to know how to take care of themselves.	

TEMPOROMANDIBULAR JOINT DISEASE/DISORDER

Temporomandibular joint disease/disorder (TMD) is commonly referred to as TMJ by the general public. It is a collection of conditions affecting the temporomandibular joint and/or the muscles of mastication.

Over 10 million people in the United States have TMD. It affects both males and females, but 90% of those seeking treatment are females between puberty and menopause (The TMJ Association, 1998). The majority of clients will get better with or without treatment (The TMJ Association, 1998).

The temporomandibular joint is the articular surface

between the mandible and temporal bone of the skull. It is a combined hinge and gliding joint. Normally, the mandible moves smoothly, appears symmetrical, and is without deformity. Causes for TMD include: trauma, stress, teeth clenching or grinding (**bruxism**), and joint diseases such as rheumatoid arthritis or osteoarthritis. Common symptoms of TMD include limited jaw movement, clicking or crepitus when the jaw moves, popping when chewing or talking, and radiating pain in the face, neck, or shoulders. The clicking is caused by displaced cartilage. The jaw may lock as a result of muscle spasms.

Diagnosis of TMD may include an x-ray to evaluate the bony structure, a CT scan, to evaluate any degenerative changes, an MRI or arthrography, and an evaluation of the teeth and jaw in a bite position. Nursing assessment of the joint includes movement and appearance. If the mandible protrudes, it may indicate a mandibular dislocation.

Medical management consists of moist heat to promote muscle relaxation, cold therapy to reduce muscle spasms, and analgesics or nonsteroidal anti-inflammatory drugs. Clients may be fitted with a dental retainer or bite plate to prevent teeth clenching or grinding, or splints to help realign malocclusions. Procedures such as arthroscopy or surgery to reshape the joint may be done in some cases that do not respond to medical treatment.

A soft diet allows the jaw and muscles to relax. Clients should be advised against chewing gum.

CARPAL TUNNEL SYNDROME

Carpal tunnel syndrome occurs when the median nerve in the wrist is compressed by inflamed, edematous flexor tendons and tenosynovium (Figure 24-15). Symptoms include pain, paresthesia, and weakness of the thumb, index, middle and part of ring fingers but never the little finger. Persons working in occupations requiring repetitious movement of hands and fingers, such as computers, typing, intense quilting, or crocheting, have a higher incidence of this syndrome. Arthritis or fractures may also be a cause. Diagnosis is based on a physical examination and the subjective symptoms of the client and may be confirmed by motor nerve velocity studies.

Medical–Surgical Management

Medical

Treatment consists of rest for the hands. Splints to immobilize the hand and wrist may also be used to help relieve some of the discomfort.

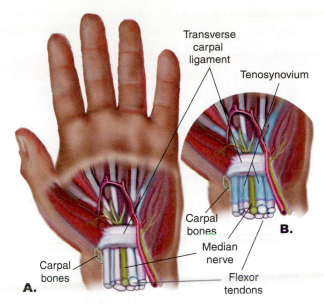

Figure 24-15 Carpal Tunnel Syndrome: A. Cross-section of carpal tunnel showing nerves and tendons; B. Inflamed flexor tendons and tenosynovium put pressure on the median nerve.

Surgical

If conservative treatment does not control the symptoms, surgery may be necessary to relieve the pressure on the median nerve. After surgery, the hand is elevated and may be in a splint for up to 2 weeks. Lifting is restricted for several weeks.

Pharmacological

Anti-inflammatory drugs may decrease inflammation and edema and reduce symptoms. NSAIDs may provide pain relief. If symptoms are not controlled with these measures, cortisone may injected into the carpal tunnel.

▶ NURSING PROCESS

▶ Assessment

▶ Subjective Data

This consists of the client's description of tingling in the hands, and numbness in the thumb, index, middle and part of the ring fingers. The client may also state that there is a feeling of "puffiness" in the affected hand and that the client is unable to grasp or hold small objects. Waking in the middle of the night with pain and a feeling that the entire hand is asleep is very common.

▶ Objective Data

This may include atrophy of the padded area at the base of the thumb.

Nursing diagnoses for a client with carpal tunnel syndrome may include the following:

Nursing Diagnoses	Planning/Goals	Nursing Interventions
▶ *Acute Pain related to inflammation and swelling causing pressure on the median nerve*	The client will have less discomfort.	Administer analgesics as ordered and teach client about use, side effects, and dosage. Encourage client to wear wrist brace. Encourage client to refrain from repetitive hand movements.
▶ *Risk for Disuse Syndrome related to tingling and numbness of hand and wrist*	The client will use fingers and hand.	Teach client to do ROM exercises, and to prevent twisting and turning of wrist.

Evaluation Each goal must be evaluated to determine how it has been met by the client.

SYSTEMIC DISORDERS WITH MUSCULOSKELETAL MANIFESTATIONS

Disorders discussed following include gout and lyme disease.

GOUT

Gout is a metabolic disease of ineffective purine metabolism resulting from deposits of needlelike crystals of uric acid in connective tissue, joint spaces, or both. It affects 2.1 million individuals in the United States (Arthritis Foundation, 1998). Middle-aged men are most commonly affected, but it may occur in women after menopause. Gout may be primary (an inherited problem with purine metabolism), secondary (complication from another disease or from use of certain drugs), or idiopathic (unknown cause). Up to 18% of clients with gout have a family history of the disease (NIAMS, January 1999). The excessive use of alcohol interferes with uric acid removal from the body and may contribute to or exacerbate symptoms.

The attack generally begins abruptly with severe constant pain. The joint becomes swollen, red, and tender. The great toe is the joint most frequently involved; however, any joint may be affected. The course of gout is variable with 1 to 2 attacks being severe. If the disease is untreated, the attacks may occur with increasing frequency. Clients with symptoms of gout may develop **tophi** which are subcutaneous nodular deposits of sodium urate crystals appearing in various parts of the body including the rim of the ears, the knuckles, and great toe. Diagnosis is made from the client's health history and an examination of the affected joint. Aspiration of the joint synovial fluid will show urate crystals. The client should be instructed to avoid foods high in purine. These foods include liver, sardines, sweetbreads, anchovies, gravies, and aspara-

gus. Oral fluid intake should be increased to 3,000 mL/day to reduce the possibility of urate stone formation in the kidneys.

To reduce inflammation, NSAIDs are given, especially indomethacin (Indocin) and naproxen (Anaprox, Naprosyn). Colchicine may be used if NSAIDs are ineffective. When tophi develop, medicine to reduce hyperuricemia may be used, such as allopurinol (Zyloprim) and probenecid (Benemid).

LYME DISEASE

Lyme disease is caused by a spirochete *Borrelia burgdorferi* carried by deer ticks. In the United States it has been reported in nearly all states, but most cases are in the coastal northeast, mid-Altantic states, Minnesota, and northern California (National Institute of Allergies and Infectious Diseases [NIAID], 1999).

These ticks should be removed by using a tweezers. Early manifestations occur from spring through late fall. People living in states with a high incidence of Lyme disease should wear protective clothing and check for ticks frequently. Insect repellent containing DEET should be applied to exposed parts of the body and to clothing. Household pets should wear a flea and tick collar and also be checked frequently for ticks.

For most individuals, the first symptom is a red rash called erythema migrans. It starts as a red spot at the site of the tick bite and expands resembling a bull's eye. Other symptoms are headache, neck stiffness, fever, and pain. For those individuals untreated with antibiotics, arthritis (joint swelling and pain), fatigue, and neurological abnormalities like facial palsy, meningitis, and encephalitis become evident. The antibody test ELISA is used to identify antibodies to *B. burgdorferi* in blood or spinal fluid specimens. Antibiotics such as doxycycline (Vibramycin), cefuroxime exetil (Ceftin), or amoxicillin (Amoxil) speed healing of the rash and prevents arthritis and neurological symptoms.

CASE STUDY

George Ellis, a 40-year-old truck driver, was getting ready to help unload his cargo. He was climbing into the truck when he lost his balance and fell to the ground, twisting his left leg. He stated he was in severe pain and was unable to stand. His coworkers called the emergency ambulance service to transport him to the hospital. Upon arrival in the emergency room, the nurse immediately took Mr. Ellis's vital signs. His vital signs were temperature 98.6°F, pulse 92, respirations 24, and blood pressure 158/90. The nurse also noted that Mr. Ellis's face was flushed and his left leg was shorter than his right.

The following questions will guide your development of a nursing care plan for the case study.

1. List five types of fractures.
2. Based on the action of the fall, what type of fracture do you think Mr. Ellis may have received?
3. What diagnostic measures will determine whether or not Mr. Ellis has a fracture of his left leg?
4. What immediate care should have been given to Mr. Ellis?
5. List four nursing interventions for clients in traction.
6. What options may be considered for treatment of Mr. Ellis's injury?
7. List objective and subjective information the nurse would obtain regarding Mr. Ellis's injury.

SUMMARY

- When assessing the client with a musculoskeletal disorder, the nurse should evaluate any changes in appearance including alignment, loss of motion, and any signs of circulatory impairment.
- Treatment of a fracture may include any one or more of the following methods: closed reduction, open reduction that may include internal fixation, casts, and traction.
- Complications of a fracture include infection, fat embolism, and compartment syndrome.
- Compartment syndrome is a serious form of neurovascular impairment. Symptoms include severe pain that is not relieved with narcotic analgesics, sluggish capillary refill, weak pulses, numbness, and paralysis.
- When a client is in traction it is important to remember to preserve body alignment, maintain continuous pull and countertraction, keep the ropes moving freely through the pulleys, use the prescribed amount of weights, and keep the weights hanging freely.
- Osteoarthritis is characterized by slow progressive degeneration of joint articular cartilage.
- Hips, knees, and fingers are the joints most frequently considered for replacement.
- Following total hip replacement, the hip should be kept in a position of abduction and extension.
- Following total knee replacement surgery, some clients may use a CPM machine that promotes knee joint flexibility and increased circulation to the operative area.
- Individuals at greatest risk for developing osteoporosis are postmenopausal women and older adults who are generally inactive.
- Carpal tunnel syndrome occurs in individuals who perform jobs requiring repetitive wrist and hand movements. The resulting trauma causes inflammation and edema that compresses the median nerve, causing numbness, pain, and impaired mobility to the hand and fingers.

Review Questions

1. A fracture caused by forceful twisting is known as a:
   a. comminuted fracture.
   b. spiral fracture.
   c. transverse fracture.
   d. greenstick fracture.

2. The primary goal in the treatment of a fracture is to:
   a. aid in the formation of osteoclasts.
   b. aid in the formation of granulation tissue.
   c. establish a callus between the broken ends of bone.
   d. prevent further injury to the fractured limb.

3. A closed reduction of a fracture:
   a. always requires surgery.
   b. is completed by manual manipulation.
   c. never requires a cast.
   d. requires the use of immobilizing plates.

4. The nurse knows that proper body positioning and alignment of an immobilized client is always maintained to prevent:
   a. scoliosis.
   b. lordosis.
   c. contractures.
   d. atony.

5. One of the first symptoms a client with arthritis may complain of is:
   a. nausea after each meal.
   b. joint stiffness especially on arising.
   c. an increased appetite.
   d. muscle spasms after exercising.

6. Traction is frequently used to treat clients with a musculoskeletal problem. One of the primary reasons for traction is to:
   a. heal a fracture.
   b. maintain a corrected position.
   c. stop muscle spasms.
   d. prevent infection.

7. Osteomyelitis:
   a. affects mainly the hip bone.
   b. is a bacterial infection of the bone.
   c. occurs most often in adults.
   d. causes a great deal of deformity.

Critical Thinking Questions

1. Prepare a teaching plan for a client to learn how to use crutches.

2. How would you explain "phantom limb pain" to a client?

3. What is the rationale for each nursing intervention for the nursing diagnoses given in this chapter?

WEB FLASH!

- Search the Internet for information about the disorders in this chapter. What new diagnostic tests or treatments are being tested?
- Share the Internet information focused for clients' use with your classmates.

NURSING CARE OF THE CLIENT: NEUROLOGICAL SYSTEM

CHAPTER 25

MAKING THE CONNECTION

Refer to the following chapters to increase your understanding of the neurological system disorders:

- **Chapter 12, Health Assessment**
- **Chapter 17, Nursing Care of the Oncology Client**
- **Chapter 19, Nursing Care of the Client: Cardiovascular System**
- **Chapter 24, Nursing Care of the Client: Musculoskeletal System**

- **Chapter 27, Nursing Care of the Client: Endocrine System**
- **Chapter 35, Nursing Care of the Older Client**
- **Chapter 36, Rehabilitation, Home Health, Long-Term Care, and Hospice**

LEARNING OBJECTIVES

Upon completion of this chapter, you should be able to:
- *Define key terms.*
- *Identify basic functional areas of the human nervous system.*
- *Perform a neurological screening and a basic neurological examination.*
- *Prepare a client for common neurological diagnostic examinations.*
- *Derive a Glasgow Coma Scale score for a client.*
- *Recognize common symptoms of neurological disorders.*
- *Plan interventions for a client with a neurological disorder.*

INTRODUCTION

The human nervous system is highly complex, controlling and integrating all other body systems. The purpose of the nervous system is to control motor, sensory, and autonomic functions of the body. This is accomplished by coordination and initiation of cellular activity through the transmission of electrical impulses and various hormones.

KEY TERMS

affect	homonymous
agnosia	hemianopia
anosognosia	Kernig's sign
aphasia	meningitis
areflexia	mentation
ataxia	neuralgia
aura	neurogenic shock
automatism	neurotransmitter
autonomic nervous system	nuchal rigidity
bradykinesia	nystagmus
central nervous system	orientation
cephalalgia	paraplegia
chorea	peripheral nervous system
dysarthria	quadriplegia
dysphagia	responsiveness
emotional lability	sclerotic
encephalitis	somatic nervous system
fasciculation	spinal shock
Glasgow Coma Scale	status epilepticus
graphesthesia	stereognosis
hemiparesis	unilateral neglect
hemiplegia	vertigo

ANATOMY AND PHYSIOLOGY REVIEW

The nervous system is divided into the **central nervous system**, consisting of the brain and spinal cord; the **peripheral nervous system**, which consists of the cranial nerves and spinal nerves; and the **autonomic** **nervous system**, which is part of the peripheral nervous system and consists of the sympathetic and parasympathetic systems.

Central Nervous System

The central nervous system (CNS) comprises the brain and the spinal cord (Figure 25-1).

Figure 25-1 The central nervous system includes the brain, spinal cord, and meninges. A. Structures of the brain; B. Functional areas of the brain. (*From* Health Assessment & Physical Examination, *2nd edition, by M. E. Z. Estes, 2002, Albany, NY: Delmar. Copyright 2002 by Delmar.*)

The Brain

The brain, composed of gray matter and white matter, controls, initiates, and integrates body functions through the use of electrical impulses and complex molecules. The gray matter, on the outer part of the brain, contains billions of neurons. Neurons, the basic cells of the nervous system, have three major components: the cell body, the axon, and the dendrites (Figure 25-2). The axon carries impulses away from the cell body, and the dendrites carry impulses toward the cell body. The cell body controls the function of the neuron. Functions include the conduction of impulses and the release of neurotransmitters. **Neurotransmitters** are chemical substances that excite, inhibit, or modify the response of another neuron (Hickey, 1997).

The white matter of the inner structures of the brain contains association and projection pathways that transmit nerve impulses to communicate information to the different areas of the brain. These communication pathways are necessary for integration of brain activity (Hickey, 1997).

The brain is contained within the skull, or cranium, which is a bony, rigid box that protects the brain tissue. There are three coverings of the brain, called meninges. They are the dura mater, arachnoid mater, and pia mater. The purpose of these coverings is to provide protection, support, and small amounts of nourishment. The meninges are separated by spaces.

The brain is divided into two hemispheres. The right side of the brain receives information from and controls the left side of the body. The left hemisphere receives information from and controls the right side of the body. Both hemispheres of the brain communicate through nerve fibers in the corpus callosum. A predominate hemisphere exists for special tasks so that confusion does not occur. The right side specializes in the perception of physical environment, art, nonverbal communication, music, and spiritual aspects. The left hemisphere generally specializes in analysis, calculation, problem solving, verbal communication, interpretation, language, reading, and writing.

The Spinal Cord

The spinal cord is a continuation of the brain stem. It exits the skull through the foramen magnum, an opening in the base of the skull. The spinal cord is approximately 45 centimeters, or 18 inches, in length and is the thickness of one finger. The cord is divided into right and left halves and has a shallow groove, called the posterior median sulcus, on the dorsal side and a deep groove, called the anterior median fissure, on the ventral side. The cord tapers to a thin tip, called the conus medullaris, at the first lumbar vertebrae, and terminates as a thin cord of connective tissue, called the filum terminale, which continues as far as the second sacral vertebrae (Figure 25-3). The vertebral column provides vertical support for the cord. The meninges

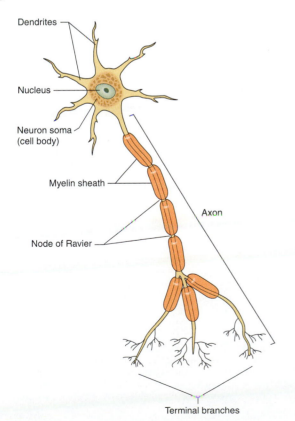

Figure 25-2 Neuron (Nerve Cell) Structure

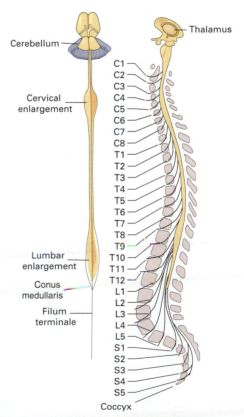

Figure 25-3 The Spinal Cord (Adapted from Health Assessment & Physical Examination, 2nd edition, by M. E. Z. Estes, 2002, Albany, NY: Delmar. Copyright 2002 by Delmar.

cover the spinal cord, providing protection. Reflex activity is initiated within the spinal cord.

There are 31 pairs of spinal nerves originating from the spinal cord. Each pair contains a dorsal, or posterior, nerve root and a ventral, or anterior, nerve root. The dorsal nerve roots carry sensory impulses from the body to the brain; the ventral nerve roots carry motor impulses from the spinal cord to the body. The spinal cord has an **H**-shaped appearance of gray matter within the white matter. The horns forming the **H** shape are referred to as the anterior (ventral) horns, the posterior (dorsal) horns, and the lateral horns. These horns contain the cell bodies of neurons that innervate the skeletal muscles.

Cerebrospinal Fluid

Cerebrospinal fluid (CSF) is produced primarily in the choroid plexus. Five hundred milliliters of CSF are produced daily, with excess being reabsorbed by the arachnoid villi in the subarachnoid space. The circulation of CSF is from the lateral ventricles to the third and fourth ventricles. From there, it enters the subarachnoid space to flow around the spinal cord and the brain.

Cerebrospinal fluid provides for shock absorption and bathes the brain and spinal cord. It contains glucose, protein, urea, and salts. These nutritive substances are delivered to the CNS cells, and the waste and toxic substances are removed.

Peripheral Nervous System

All of the nerve tissue outside of the CNS is part of the peripheral nervous system (PNS). The PNS consists of the cranial nerves and the spinal nerves and has both sensory and motor components. The PNS can be divided into the **somatic nervous system** and the autonomic nervous system. The somatic portion connects the CNS to the skin and skeletal muscles. It is involved in conscious activities such as walking. The autonomic portion connects the CNS to visceral organs such as the heart, stomach, intestines, and various glands. It is involved in unconscious activities, such as breathing.

Cranial Nerves

The twelve pairs of cranial nerves have sensory, motor, or mixed functions. Table 25–1 lists functions and describes assessment of cranial nerves. The cranial nerves originate from the brain or brain stem, with most originating from the brain stem. Although always identified by Roman numerals, the cranial nerves also have names.

Table 25–1 CRANIAL NERVES

CRANIAL NERVE	FUNCTION	ASSESSMENT	EXPECTED FINDINGS
Olfactory (I)	Sensory: smell	Have client identify smells such as coffee or alcohol, with one nostril occluded; repeat for opposite nostril.	Correct identification of smell or ability to choose smell from a list of choices.
Optic (II)	Sensory: vision	Ask client to read printed material, identify number of fingers held in front of client, or read from Snellen eye chart. Test visual fields by having client identify when the examiner's finger enters visual field.	Vision intact or correctable with lenses. Visual field intact.
Oculomotor (III)	Motor: pupil constriction	Cranial nerves III, IV, and VI are tested together. Inspect for ptosis, or drooping of eyelid. Assess extraocular eye muscles by having client follow the examiner's finger to each quadrant of the visual field. Assess for accommodation by asking the client to look at the examiner's finger held 4 to 6 inches from the client's nose, and then to follow the finger to 18 inches from the client's nose. Ask client about double vision.	Pupils are equal and round and react equally to light. No ptosis or double vision. Eyes move smoothly and consensually inward and downward. As the examiner's finger moves away from the client, the pupil will accommodate by dilating; as the finger moves closer; the pupil will normally constrict.
Trochlear (IV)	Motor: upper eyelid elevation, extraocular eye movement	See oculomotor (III).	Eyes should move smoothly and consensually upward and outward without nystagmus or diplopia.
Trigeminal (V)	Sensory: cornea, nose, and oral mucosa Motor: mastication	Test corneal reflex by lightly touching cornea with a small piece of cotton. Check sensation of face by touching lightly with a cotton ball while the client's eyes are closed and asking the client whether sensation is pres-	Corneal reflex as evidenced by rapid blinking when cotton swept across cornea. Feeling cotton ball on face indicates that facial sensation is intact. Jaw movement symmetrical and able to overcome resistance.

continues

Table 25–1 CRANIAL NERVES continued

CRANIAL NERVE	FUNCTION	ASSESSMENT	EXPECTED FINDINGS
		ent. Check motor function by having client clench jaws shut while the examiner palpates the contraction of the temporalis and masseter muscles.	
Abducens (VI)	Motor: extraocular eye movement	See oculomotor (III)	Eyes move outward.
Facial (VII)	Motor: facial muscles; Sensory: taste (anterior two-thirds of tongue)	Ask client to smile, show teeth, wrinkle forehead, or whistle. Have client close eyes lightly and keep them closed against the examiner's trying to open them. Have client identify salt and sugar when dabbed on tongue.	Facial movement symmetrical; sense of taste intact.
Acoustic (VIII)	Sensory: hearing, equilibrium	Assess ability to hear ticking watch or whispered voice. Observe gait for swaying. Perform Romberg test (refer to assessment of motor function).	Sense of hearing intact; no swaying or loss of balance.
Glossopharyngeal (IX)	Sensory: sensation to throat and taste (posterior one-third of tongue) Motor: swallowing	Have client identify taste of salt and sugar on back of tongue. Have client say "ah" and assess for symmetrical position of uvula. Test gag reflex by touching back of pharynx with tongue depressor. Observe swallowing ability and speech patterns.	Taste sensation intact; uvula raises symmetrically; gag reflex intact; swallowing and speech intact.
Vagus (X)	Motor and sensory	Test along with glossopharyngeal nerve.	
Spinal accessory (XI)	Motor: movement of uvula, soft palate, sternocleidomastoid muscle, trapezius muscle	Place examiner's hand on side of client's face and ask client to turn head against resistance; have client shrug shoulders against resistance of the examiner's hand.	Ability to move shoulder and head against resistance.
Hypoglossal (XII)	Motor: tongue movement	Ask client to stick out tongue and observe for symmetry, deviation to side; have client push tongue against tongue depressor and move tongue from side to side.	Tongue should be centrally aligned, able to push against resistance of tongue depressor; no **fasciculations** (involuntary twitching of muscle fibers) should be present.

Spinal Nerves

Thirty-one pairs of spinal nerves exit from the spinal cord through the vertebral column (Table 25–2). The dorsal, or posterior, nerve roots carry sensory impulses to the brain. The ventral, or anterior, nerve roots carry motor impulses from the spinal cord and brain to the muscles. Motor and sensory impulses are transmitted from the body and internal organs.

Reflex activity is a stereotypical response to a stimulus that is initiated by the nervous system (Hickey, 1997). The three classifications of reflexes are: muscle stretch, or deep tendon; superficial, or cutaneous; and pathological (see section on assessment of reflexes). Reflex activity requires the function of five areas in the nervous system: the sensory fibers, the neuron relaying the impulse, the association center in the brain, the neuron relaying the motor impulse from the brain to the body, and the specific organ involved. Disease processes at any of these areas can cause an abnormal reflex response.

Autonomic Nervous System

The main function of the autonomic nervous system (ANS) is to maintain internal homeostasis. There are two subdivisions of the ANS: the sympathetic system

Table 25–2 SPINAL NERVES

NERVES	NUMBER OF PAIRS
Cervical	8
Thoracic	12
Lumbar	5
Sacral	5
Coccyx	1

and the parasympathetic system. The sympathetic system, activated by stress, prepares the body for the "fight or flight" response. The activity of the sympathetic system causes increased heart rate, increased blood pressure, vasoconstriction, decreased peristalsis, dilated pupils, increased secretions of epinephrine and sweat, and decreased secretions of digestive juices and saliva (Table 25–3).

The parasympathetic system conserves, restores, and maintains vital body functions (Hickey, 1997), slowing heart rate, increasing gastrointestinal activity, and activating bowel and bladder evacuation.

The sympathetic and parasympathetic systems work antagonistically to regulate the smooth muscles, the heart, and the glands of the body. When one system increases an action, the other system decreases the action. Thus, when one stimulates, the other inhibits; when one dilates, the other one constricts, and so forth. The purpose is to maintain a stable internal environment (Hickey, 1997). Both systems function simultaneously, but one can dominate the other as needed.

NEUROLOGICAL NURSING ASSESSMENT

A complete health history and a neurological screening assessment allow the nurse to identify areas of dysfunction in order to focus the neurological assessment. Observation (inspection) is necessary for the majority of the assessment; palpation, auscultation, and percussion are also used.

Health History

A baseline assessment is essential to ascertaining changes in neurological functioning. Any change from the baseline assessment must be identified and early intervention initiated. A thorough health history includes asking the client about headaches; clumsiness; loss of or change in function of an extremity; seizure activity; numbness or tingling; change in vision; pain; extreme fatigue; personality changes; and mood swings.

Neurological Assessment

The neurological screening involves assessment of level of consciousness and verbal responses to specific questions; selected cranial nerves for eye movement and visual acuity; muscle strength; movement; gait for motor function; and tactile and pain sensation of extremities for sensory screening.

A complete nursing assessment of neurological function includes assessment of the following areas: cerebral function, cranial nerve function, motor function, sensory function, and reflexes. Neurological nursing assessment is discussed in more detail following.

Cerebral Function

Areas of assessment of cerebral function include level of consciousness, mental status, intellectual function, emotional status, pupil reaction, and communication.

Level of Consciousness Level of consciousness is assessed by determining the client's responsiveness and orientation and is the most important indicator of

Table 25–3 SYMPATHETIC AND PARASYMPATHETIC RESPONSES

SYSTEM	SYMPATHETIC RESPONSE	PARASYMPATHETIC RESPONSE
Neurological	Pupils dilated Heightened awareness	Pupils normal size
Cardiovascular	Increased heart rate Increased myocardial contractility Increased blood pressure	Decreased heart rate Decreased myocardial contractility Vasodilation
Respiratory	Increased respiratory rate Increased respiratory depth Bronchial constriction	Bronchial relaxation
Gastrointestinal	Decreased gastric motility Decreased gastric secretions Increased glycogenolysis Decreased insulin production Sphincter contraction	Increased gastric motility Increased gastric secretions Sphincter dilatation
Genitourinary	Decreased urine output Decreased renal blood flow	Normal urine output

GERONTOLOGICAL CONSIDERATIONS

Neurological Changes with Aging

Remember the following with regard to the elderly client:

- Nerve impulse transmission slows.
- Cardiovascular system changes that lead to a decreased oxygen supply to the brain affect mental acuity, sensory interpretation, and motor ability.
- The amount of neurotransmitters produced diminishes, and the enzyme activity that degrades neurotransmitters increases.
- Changes in neurotransmitters affect sleep, temperature control, and mood.
- The brain tends to atrophy, leaving the cortical bridging veins, which connect the brain to the meninges, vulnerable to trauma and bleeding.

Table 25–4 LEVELS OF CONSCIOUSNESS

Alert	Oriented, opens eyes spontaneously, responds appropriately.
Lethargic	Sleepy; slow to respond, but responds appropriately; oriented; opens eyes in response to verbal stimuli.
Stuporous	Aroused only in response to painful stimuli; never fully awake; conversation, if present, is confused or unclear; opens eyes to painful stimuli.
Semicomatose	May move in response to painful stimuli; does not converse; protective blink, swallowing, and pupil reflexes are present.
Comatose	Unresponsive except to severe pain; protective reflexes are absent; pupils are fixed; no voluntary movement.

change in neurological status. **Responsiveness** is the person's ability to perceive environmental stimuli and body reactions and then respond with thought and action. The client's responsiveness state can be described in terms of consciousness, such as alert, lethargic, stuporous, semicomatose, or comatose (see Table 25–4).

A more objective assessment is made using the **Glasgow Coma Scale**, an objective tool for assessing consciousness in clients, most frequently in clients with head injuries. With the Glasgow Coma Scale, eye opening, verbal response, and motor response are scored using measurable criteria (Table 25–5). The scores are then totalled to indicate severity of coma. A score of 15 indicates a fully oriented person. A score of 3 is the lowest possible score and is indicative of deep coma. A score of 7 or less is considered a state of coma.

Changes in the Glasgow Coma Scale indicate changes in client condition. To prevent further damage to the brain in instances of decreasing scores, the nurse must act quickly. The physician must be notified immediately and measures must be taken to decrease intracranial pressure (see section on increased intracranial pressure).

Orientation is the person's awareness of self in relation to person, place, and time. In some instances, awareness of situation is also a necessary measure. Using open-ended communication techniques, the nurse will instruct the client to "tell me who you are," "tell me what day of the week it is," "tell me where you are," and so on in order to ascertain the client's level of orientation.

Mental Status Assessment of mental status requires observation of the client's appearance, behavior, posture, mood, gestures, movements, and facial expressions. The nurse compares these behaviors to expected behaviors based on the client's age, health status, educational level, and social position. Mood is assessed by observation and asking the client about moods and feelings.

Intellectual Function Intellectual function is the ability of the brain to perform thought processes. Ability

Table 25–5 GLASGOW COMA SCALE

BEHAVIOR	RESPONSE	SCORE
Eye opening response	Spontaneous	4
	To verbal command	3
	To pain	2
	No response	1
Best verbal response	Oriented, conversing	5
	Disoriented, conversing	4
	Use of inappropriate words	3
	Incomprehensible sounds	2
	No response	1
Best motor response	Obeys verbal commands	6
	Moves to localized pain	5
	Flexion withdrawal to pain	4
	Abnormal posturing—decorticate	3
	Abnormal posturing—decerebrate	2
	No response	1
Total		3 to 15

CULTURAL CONSIDERATIONS

Neurological Assessment

- Consider language and cultural norms when performing the mental status assessment.
- An interpreter may be required to ensure that the client understands the questions or directions.

to concentrate, memory function (both long-term and short-term), recall, calculation activities, and abstract reasoning are all aspects of intellectual function.

Nursing assessment of intellectual function involves asking individuals to perform certain tasks, such as the following:

- Repeating a series of numbers, such as 1, 3, 7, 1
- Telling what the individual ate for breakfast
- Adding a couple of numbers, for example, 2 + 6
- Explaining a proverb such as "the early bird gets the worm"

The nurse will determine the client's ability to process thoughts by evaluating the responses to questions such as these. For purposes of comparison, the client's ability to perform these tasks prior to assessment should be ascertained by asking the family. For example, if the client was math illiterate prior to the nursing assessment, the client will still not be able to add or subtract.

Emotional Status Emotional status is assessed by observation of the client's **affect** (emotional response or mood). Is affect appropriate for the situation? Is affect labile (prone to rapid change)? Is affect consistent with verbal communication?

Pupil Reaction Size, equality, and roundness of pupils are assessed (Figure 25-4). Size is measured in millimeters. Pupils are evaluated for symmetry of size and for reaction to light. The nurse should briefly shine a penlight into the client's eye by passing the light from the outer edge of the eye toward the center of the eye (Figure 25-5). Reaction is assessed as being brisk, sluggish, or nonreactive; consensual reaction (the opposite pupil responding at the same time) is also noted. Accommodation is assessed as described in Table 25–1.

The abbreviation PERRLA is used for documenting pupils that are equal, round, and reactive to light and that demonstrate accommodation. This abbreviation can be used only when pupil reaction is normal. If any part of the assessment is abnormal in one or both eyes, the assessment findings must be written out for clarity.

Communication Both written and oral communication are assessed. Various specialized areas of the

Figure 25-4 A. Unequal Pupils; B. Dilated, Fixed Pupils

Figure 25-5 Pupil Assessment: A. Starting position, with penlight to side of pupil; B. Moving penlight directly in front of pupil

PROFESSIONAL TIP

Assessment of Pupils

To ensure accuracy in assessing direct light reflex and consensual light reflex, the beginning examiner should focus the beam of light a total of four times, twice in each eye.

Table 25-6 MUSCLE STRENGTH

SCORE	DEFINITION
5/5	Full power of contraction
4/5	Fair or moderate power of contraction
3/5	Just able to overcome force of gravity
2/5	Can move, but cannot overcome power of gravity
1/5	Minimal contractile power
0/5	No movement

nervous system are involved in communication. The inability to communicate, termed **aphasia**, can be caused by the inability to form words or the inability to understand written or spoken words. To assess communication function, various approaches are necessary. The client is asked to follow a simple command such as "Close your eyes." A written card instructing the client to complete a simple task such as "Touch your nose" should also be used. The ability to form words; appropriate use of words; speech patterns, clarity, rate, and flow; and voice modulation are all noted. The client's ability for verbal and written expression of self is noted during the health history by asking the client about expectations of health care. The ability to write is evaluated by having the client write his name and address on paper.

Cranial Nerve Function

Cranial nerve function essentially reflects brain stem activity. A complete cranial nerve examination, if required, is usually performed by the physician or advanced practice nurse.

Motor Function

The neurological screening includes assessment of muscle strength, arm and leg movement, and gait. A complete motor function assessment is performed if a deficit is identified. A complete motor function assessment includes evaluating muscle size, symmetry, tone, and strength; coordination; balance; and posturing.

Muscle Size and Symmetry Muscle size and symmetry are assessed by palpating major muscle groups of the arms and legs and then comparing them to the muscle groups of the opposite side of the body. Unilateral atrophy may indicate a nervous system problem.

Muscle Tone Muscle tone is assessed during palpation of major muscle groups for size and symmetry, while at rest and during passive movement. Muscle tone is described as normal, flaccid, spastic, or rigid. Flaccid muscles are hypotonic, or soft and flabby. Spastic muscles are at first resistant to passive movement, but then release resistance. Rigid muscles may have tremors but are constantly rigid. Rigidity is a more constant state of spasticity, with fewer periods of release of resistance.

Muscle Strength To assess muscle strength, each extremity is placed through passive movement. The client is then asked to move the extremity, first against gravity, by lifting the extremity off the bed, then against resistance, by lifting against slight resistance exerted by the nurse's hand pushing on the extremity. Strength is graded on a scale of 0 to 5 (Table 25–6).

Coordination Coordination, a function of the cerebellum, is assessed by asking the client to perform repetitious movement. The client should close her eyes and repeatedly, rapidly touch her own nose with alternate index fingers (Figure 25-6). Lower extremity coordination is assessed by asking the client to run the heel of one foot down the opposite shin, and then repeat with the other heel (Figure 25-7). Inability to perform these movements is termed **ataxia**, incoordination of voluntary muscle action.

Figure 25-6 Assessment of Coordination: Fingertip-to-Nose Touch

Figure 25-7 Assessment of Coordination: Heel Slide

Balance Balance is evaluated by using the Romberg test. The client stands with the feet together, arms extended in front, and eyes closed. Balance is observed; a slight swaying is normal.

Safety: Romberg Test
Always stand in front of the client during the Romberg test, anticipating that the client might fall.

Posturing Abnormal posturing occurs with injury to the motor tract. Two types for which to observe are decorticate and decerebrate posturing. Decorticate posturing is characterized by flexion of the arms, adduction of the upper extremities, and extension of the lower extremities. Lesions of the cerebral hemispheres or internal structures of the brain cause decorticate posturing. Decerebrate posturing is caused by brain stem injury and is characterized by an arcing of the back, backward flexion of the head, adduction and hyperpronation of the arms, and extension of the feet (Figure 25-8).

Abnormal posturing may be present either at all times or in response to stimuli such as loud noises, bright lights, or painful stimuli. The nurse must note whether bilateral or unilateral posturing is present, and, if intermittent, the cause of the posturing. The presence of either type of posturing should be reported at once, because either represents an ominous sign of cerebral dysfunction. Decerebrate posturing represents greater dysfunction than does decorticate

Figure 25-8 Abnormal Posturing: A. Decorticate posturing; B. Decerebrate posturing *(Courtesy John White, Corpus Christi, TX)*

PROFESSIONAL TIP

Assessing Coordination
Ensure that clients who wear eyeglasses have their glasses on prior to the assessment being performed.

PROFESSIONAL TIP

Assessing Pain and Temperature Sensory Function
- Test upper and lower extremities
- Begin with the upper arms, moving down to the hands; then work from thighs to feet (proximo–distal)

posturing, and any change from decorticate to decerebrate posturing indicates a worsening of condition.

Sensory Function

A subjective examination of sensory function, performed with the client's eyes closed, is generally done only when a dysfunction is suspected. Different pathways are used to transmit different sensory impulses. To evaluate all pathways, the examiner must test tactile sensation, pain and temperature, vibration, proprioception, stereognosis, graphesthesia, and integration of sensations.

Tactile Sensation Tactile sensation is tested by using a cotton ball to lightly touch the client's arms, hands, upper legs, and feet. Comparison is done side to side. The client, with eyes closed, indicates whether the cotton ball is felt.

Pain and Temperature Sensations of pain and temperature are transmitted along the same pathways and are evaluated using a sharp and dull touch. A paper clip or cotton-tipped applicator is used.

Safety: Assessing Pain Sensation
Do not use a safety pin to test pain because skin integrity may be compromised.

The nurse touches the client with the rounded end of a paper clip or cotton-tipped applicator to test for dull sensation, and the pointed end of paper clip or uncovered end of the applicator to test for sharp sensation. The client's ability to distinguish sharp and dull is noted, again comparing both sides of the body.

Vibration Vibration is tested using a tuning fork. The nurse strikes the tuning fork on the palm, holding only the handle, then places the end of the handle first on the client's wrists and then on the ankles and asks whether the vibrations are felt (Figure 25-9). The client's eyes should be closed during the test.

Proprioception Proprioception is the sense of joint position in space. With the client's eyes remaining closed, the nurse moves a joint of the client's finger or extremity up or down in space and asks the client to distinguish the direction of movement of the digit or extremity as being either up or down.

Stereognosis Stereognosis is the ability to recognize an object by feel. Placing a familiar object such as a coin or key in the client's hand and asking that the

Figure 25-9 Assessment of Vibration

Figure 25-10 Assessment of Stereognosis

Figure 25-11 Assessment of Graphesthesia

object be identified is a test of stereognosis. This sensation is a function of the brain, not of the spinal pathways (Figure 25-10).

Graphesthesia **Graphesthesia** is the ability to identify letters, numbers, or shapes drawn on the skin. The nurse holds the client's hand and, with the stick end of a cotton-tipped applicator or a closed pen, traces an outline on the open palm, ensuring that the letter, number, or shape is right side up for the client (Figure 25-11).

Integration of Sensation Integration of sensation is a higher cortical function. A two-point discrimination test is performed by touching the client simultaneously on opposite sides of the body with a sharp object and asking the client to ascertain the number of objects felt. The normal response is two. If only one is felt, the brain function of integration is abnormal.

Reflexes

Both deep tendon reflexes and superficial reflexes are assessed. Deep tendon reflexes are involuntary contractions of muscles or muscle groups responding to brisk stretching near the insertion site of the muscle (Smeltzer & Bare, 1996). Testing of these reflexes is generally the responsibility of the physician or registered nurse, although the licensed practical/vocational nurse should be familiar with these assessments, as abnormal reflex responses may be an early indicator of motor or sensory dysfunction.

Superficial, or cutaneous, reflexes are elicited by irritating the skin on the area being assessed. They are diminished or absent with dysfunction of the reflex arc.

Examination A reflex hammer held loosely between the thumb and index finger is used to examine deep tendon reflexes. The insertion site of the muscle is directly struck with the hammer or indirectly struck by placing the thumb of the examiner over the insertion site and then striking the thumb. The muscle must be relaxed and the joint in midposition. Deep tendon reflexes commonly tested are the Achilles, patellar, biceps, and triceps (Figure 25-12).

A.

B.

C.

D.

Figure 25-12 Assessment of Deep Tendon Reflexes: A. Achilles; B. Patellar; C. Biceps; D. Triceps

The superficial reflexes generally assessed are the plantar and abdominal. To assess the plantar reflex, the handle of the reflex hammer is used. The outer aspect of the sole of the foot is stroked from the heel and across the ball of the foot to just below the big toe. Plantar flexion, or curling under of the toes, should occur.

To assess the abdominal reflex, the stick end of a cotton-tipped applicator is used to stroke the skin of the abdomen. An upward and outward contraction of the upper abdominal muscles and a contraction of the lower abdomen muscles should occur.

Table 25–7 REFLEX GRADING SCALE

GRADE	DEFINITION
4	Hyperactive with clonus (alternating muscle contractions between antagonistic muscles)
3	Hyperactive
2	Normal
1	Hypoactive
0	Absent

Description or Grading of Response Reflexes are generally described as present, absent, or diminished. If a grading scale is used, it is important to note whether a four-point or five-point scale is used. The description of each number varies between agencies, but a typical scale is presented in Table 25–7.

Abnormal Reflexes The absence of deep tendon reflexes in clients is considered an abnormal finding. A fanning of the toes and dorsiflexion of the big toe in response to the assessment of the plantar reflex is called a positive Babinksi's reflex (Figure 25-13). This abnormal response is indicative of corticospinal disease and is the most important abnormal superficial reflex.

COMMON DIAGNOSTIC TESTS

Commonly used diagnostic tests for clients with symptoms of nervous system disorders are listed in Table 25–8. See Chapter 13, Diagnostic Tests, for explanation/normal values and nursing responsibilities.

HEAD INJURY

Head injuries involve trauma to the scalp, skull, or brain.

Table 25–8 COMMON DIAGNOSTIC TESTS FOR NERVOUS SYSTEM DISORDERS

- Lumbar puncture (LP)
- Electroencephalogram (EEG)
- Electromyogram (EMG)
- Imaging procedures: computerized tomography (CT), positron emission tomography (PET), single photon emission computed tomography (SPECT), magnetic resonance imaging (MRI)
- Cerebral angiography
- Brain scan
- Myelogram

 GERONTOLOGICAL CONSIDERATIONS

Reflexes

The absence of the Achilles reflex in the elderly client is not considered abnormal.

Figure 25-13 Pathologic Reflex: Babinski

SCALP

Scalp injuries bleed profusely because of the abundance of blood vessels in the scalp. As with any break in skin integrity, infection is of major concern. The wound is cleansed and irrigated to remove foreign matter before closing the wound with sutures or butterfly dressings.

SKULL

Skull injuries and fractures of the skull may occur with or without brain injury. A fracture is usually caused by extreme force. Skull fractures are considered closed if the dura mater is intact, and open if the dura mater is torn. The clinical manifestation of skull fracture is localized pain. If the brain is injured, other symptoms may occur.

Types of skull fractures are linear fracture, comminuted fracture, depressed fracture, and basilar fracture. Linear fractures are nondisplaced cracks in the bone. Comminuted fractures occur when the bone is broken into fragments. Depressed fractures have bone fragments pressing into the intracranial cavity. Basilar skull fractures are of the bones in the base of the skull.

Basilar fractures are of particular concern because of the close proximity of the fragile sinus bones and the adhesion of the dura mater to this area. The dura mater can easily tear, and CSF can leak from the ears or nose. The internal carotid artery and cranial nerves can also be damaged easily with a basilar skull fracture.

BRAIN

Brain injuries are caused by primary injuries of acceleration–deceleration force, rotational force, or penetrating missile. Acceleration injuries are caused by moving objects striking the head, such as a baseball bat. Deceleration injuries result when the head is moving and strikes a solid object such as a car dashboard. Rotational injuries are hyperextension, hyperflexion, or lateral flexion of the head, which cause twisting of the cerebrum on the brain stem, such as a whiplash injury. Penetrating missile injuries are a direct penetration of an object, such as a bullet, into brain tissue (Thelan, Davie, & Urden, 1998).

Open Injury

Brain injuries from skull fractures and penetrating injuries are referred to as open head injuries. Hemorrhaging from the nose, pharynx, or ears; ecchymosis over the mastoid area (Battle's sign); or blood in the conjunctiva may occur in conjunction with open head injuries. Cerebrospinal fluid may leak from the ears or nose. A computed tomography (CT) scan or magnetic resonance imaging (MRI) is performed to determine the extent of injury. Neurological deficits depend on the extent and area of injury.

Closed Injury

Closed head injuries are caused by blunt force to the head. Coup injuries are caused by the impact of the head against an object. Contrecoup injuries are caused by the impact of the brain against the opposite side of the skull (Figure 25-14).

Types of closed head injuries are concussion, contusion, and laceration. Concussions are transient neurological deficits caused by the shaking of the brain. Clinical manifestations may include immediate loss of consciousness lasting from minutes to hours, momentary loss of reflexes, respiratory arrest for several seconds, and amnesia for the period immediately prior to and following the event. Headaches, drowsiness, confusion, dizziness, irritability, visual disturbances, and unsteady gait may also occur (Hickey, 1997).

Post-concussion syndrome may develop following the injury, as manifested by headache and dizziness. Nervousness, irritability, emotional lability, fatigue, insomnia, loss of **mentation** (ability to concentrate, remember, or think abstractly), and sometimes other neurological deficits occur. This syndrome may last from several weeks up to a year (Hickey, 1997).

Contusions are surface bruises of the brain. Symptoms depend on the area of injury. Frequently, the

client is unconscious for a longer period of time than with a concussion. The client may become conscious only to drift back into unconsciousness. Pulse, blood pressure, and respirations are below normal. Skin is cool and pale. Cerebral edema may occur in conjunction with widespread injury (see section on cerebral edema).

Return of consciousness may be followed by cerebral irritability to stimuli. Headache and dizziness may be present for an indefinite period. Permanent damage may cause either changes in mental function or seizure disorders. Prognosis ranges from full recovery to death.

Cerebral laceration is the tearing of cortical tissue. Symptoms of brain stem injury include deep coma from time of impact, decerebrate posturing, autonomic dysfunction, nonreactive pupils, and respiratory difficulty. The ability to relay nerve impulses from high levels in the brain is lost. Diffuse axonal injury (DAI) usually occurs in conjunction with brain stem injuries. This widespread damage to nerve cells in the white matter of the brain causes immediate coma, decerebration, and increased intracranial pressure.

Hemorrhage

Intracranial hemorrhage is a common complication of any head injury. Bleeding may occur in the epidural space, subdural space, subarachnoid space, or ventricles or intracerebrally. Neurological change is caused by pressure on the brain resulting from the space-occupying hemorrhage. With epidural hematoma (bleeding in the epidural space), momentary unconsciousness is followed by a conscious state of a few hours to a week, depending on the rapidity of the bleeding. As the bleeding continues, neurological status begins to deteriorate, with decreasing level of consciousness; headache; seizures; hemiparesis; decerebration; and dilated, fixed pupils. Treatment is surgery to evacuate the hematoma, stop the bleeding, and relieve pressure on the brain.

Subdural hematomas (bleeding in the subdural space) cause immediate pressure on the brain. Classification of subdural hematomas is acute (within 48 hours of injury), subacute (from 2 to 14 days following injury), and chronic (from 2 weeks to months following injury). Common symptoms are headache, drowsiness, slow mentation, and confusion. The symptoms slowly progress as the size of the subdural clot increases, causing increased pressure on the brain. Small hematomas are usually reabsorbed. Large hematomas require surgical removal.

Subarachnoid (below the arachnoid) and intraventricular (within the ventricles of the brain) hemorrhages are common in severe head injury. The symptoms include those listed for hematoma, as well as **nuchal rigidity**, stiffness or inability to bend the neck. Blood in the subarachnoid space interferes with the reabsorption of CSF, further increasing intracranial pressure.

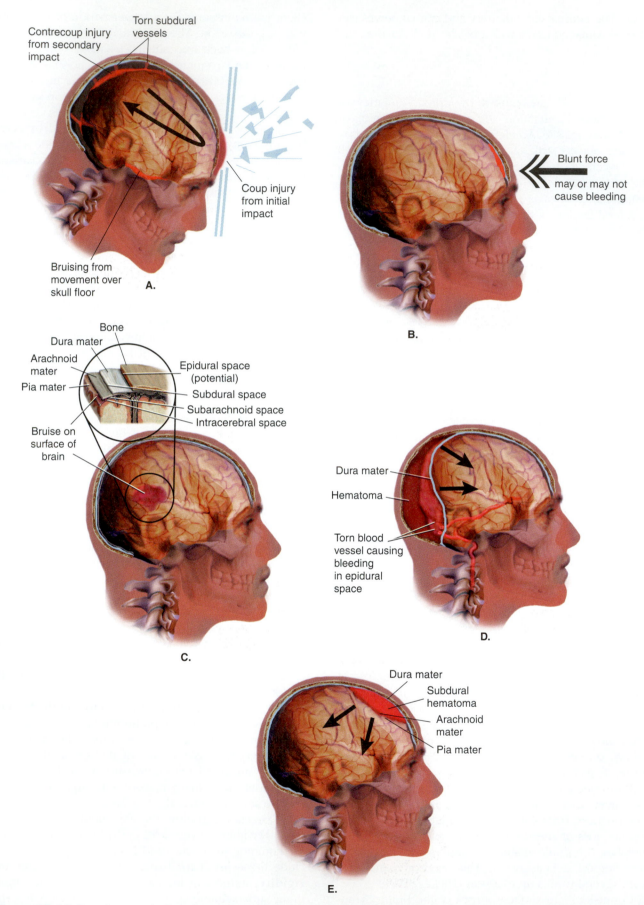

Figure 25-14 Brain Injuries: A. Coup/contrecoup; B. Concussion; C. Contusion; D. Epidural hematoma; E. Subdural hematoma

Intracranial hematomas from contusions usually occur in the temporal or frontal lobes; from shearing forces, they usually occur deep in the brain. The hematoma usually expands rapidly. The injury may cause immediate unconsciousness. Headache, deteriorating level of consciousness, hemiplegia, and dilated pupils are initial signs of an internal hematoma. As intracranial pressure increases, herniation of the brain stem occurs, causing changes in pupils, respirations, and vital signs. Craniotomy along with evacuation and control of bleeding may be performed depending on the condition of the client, extent of cerebral contusion, and accessibility of the bleeding site.

Signs and symptoms of increased intracranial pressure include a deterioration in level of consciousness; confusion; difficulty in rousing; and, initially, restlessness. Other signs and symptoms are changes in pupil size or reaction to light. The pupil gradually dilates and becomes less responsive to light. Muscle weakness progressing to **hemiplegia**, paralysis of one side of the body, or **paraplegia**, paralysis of lower extremities, and abnormal posturing may occur. Headache and vomiting are experienced by some clients. Vital sign changes generally do not occur until the increased intracranial pressure has progressed to the point of involving the brain stem. An increase in systolic blood pressure and a widening pulse pressure accompanied by a slowing pulse are the effects of pressure on the brain stem.

Cerebral Edema and Increased Intracranial Pressure

The brain is contained in a rigid container, the skull. The only normal opening to the adult skull is the foramen magnum at the base of the skull. Intracranial pressure is a result of the pressure exerted by the contents of the skull, which are the brain, blood, and CSF.

Regulatory mechanisms maintain intracranial pressure between 0 and 15 mm Hg. The Monroe-Kellie hypothesis states that when one component of the cranial contents increases in volume, the volumes of the other components decrease in order to compensate and maintain intracranial pressure between 0 and 15 mm Hg. As long as this ability to compensate remains effective, no neurological changes occur.

In decompensation, the volume increase is so excessive that intracranial pressure cannot be maintained below 15 mm Hg by decreasing the volume of the remaining components. Neurological changes are exhibited because of cellular hypoxia and displacement of the brain, which compresses neurons, especially in the brain stem. These changes include deteriorating level of consciousness; decreased motor response to commands; fixed, dilated pupils; and vital sign changes known as Cushing's triad or reflex. Cushing's triad refers to bradycardia, widening pulse pressure along with increasing

systolic pressure, and respiratory irregularities. Respiratory changes include periods of apnea, decreased respiratory rate and depth, and irregular respirations.

Causes of increased intracranial pressure are increased blood volume resulting from vascular vasodilatation; increased volume of brain tissue resulting from edema, infection, tumor, or hemorrhage; or increased volume of CSF resulting from overproduction, decreased reabsorption, or interruption of CSF circulation. If intracranial pressure continues to increase, brain herniation will occur at the tentorial notch or through the foramen magnum, resulting in death.

Medical–Surgical Management

Management of head injury is focused on early recognition and treatment of increasing intracranial pressure and maintenance of normal body functions.

Medical

Suctioning may be necessary but is never done through the nose on a head injury client because of the possibility of CSF leakage. Oxygen is given to maintain cerebral perfusion. Arterial blood gases (ABGs) are checked.

If the client has an endotracheal tube in place, the $PaCO_2$ level can drop below normal. This causes a slightly alkaline pH, which decreases vasodilation and, thus, intracranial pressure.

Surgical

Decompression is performed surgically by removing a bone flap from the skull to allow room for the expansion of the brain. A space-occupying lesion such as a tumor, hematoma, or abscess may be surgically removed. Excess CSF may be drained from the ventricles.

Pharmacological

Corticosteroids such as dexamethasone (Decadron) are given to reduce cerebral edema. Antacids, such as Mylanta or Maalox, or histamine receptor antagonists,

---

 CLIENT TEACHING

Surgery for Head Injury

Inform the client of the following:

- The head will be shaved in the area of the incision.
- Edema of the head and face may be present after surgery but will gradually disappear.
- A mechanical ventilator may be used for a day or two following surgery.

such as cimetidine (Tagamet), are given to decrease both the side effects of corticosteroids and stress-induced gastric acidity. Osmotic diuretics such as mannitol (Osmitrol), are administered to rapidly reduce fluid in the brain tissue; muscle relaxants, sedatives, barbiturates, or muscle paralyzing agents are administered to decrease activity and reduce the oxygen need of the brain.

Antipyretic drugs are used to decrease body temperature and the metabolic needs of the brain, thereby reducing the volume of blood sent to the brain to supply oxygen and glucose. Anticonvulsants are given to prevent or treat seizure activity.

Activity

Activity is limited to keep the metabolic needs of the brain at a minimum. Increased metabolic needs require more oxygen and glucose supplied by increases in blood volume in the cranium, which, in turn, further increases intracranial pressure.

▶ NURSING PROCESS

▶ Assessment

Nursing assessment for any head injury is focused on neurological status.

▶ Subjective Data

Subjective data to be gathered includes a history of what happened, including type of trauma (acceleration, deceleration, or missile), site of blow, and any loss of consciousness, including timing, length, and ability to be roused.

▶ Objective Data

A neurological screening is done to obtain a baseline neurological status; then, a more in-depth neurological exam is performed to identify any early signs of increasing intracranial pressure.

Frequent assessment of neurological status including level of consciousness, motor function, eye movement, pupil size and reaction, protective reflexes, and vital signs allows for early recognition of and intervention for increasing intracranial pressure. Nursing observation also includes assessing for double vision, headache, nausea, and bleeding from any orifice. Ipsilateral pupil reaction (reaction of the pupil on the same side as the injury or lesion), may occur as a result of pressure on the oculomotor nerve caused by increased intracranial pressure or cerebral edema. Recognition of factors that cause increased intracranial pressure is a necessary aspect of assessment.

For the client undergoing intracranial surgery, an assessment of teaching needs of the client and family must be performed. Emotional and psychosocial needs and support systems are also assessed.

Longer-term care involves assessment of bowel elimination status to prevent the need for straining; skin assessment to prevent skin breakdown, and assessment for complications of immobility.

Nursing diagnoses for a client with a head injury may include the following:

Nursing Diagnoses	Planning/Goals	Nursing Interventions
▶ *Ineffective Tissue Perfusion (Cerebral) related to disruption in cerebral blood flow*	The client will demonstrate improvement or maintenance on Glasgow Coma Scale.	Assess neurological status of client every 15 to 60 minutes. Note findings on Glasgow Coma Scale. Compare findings to previous assessments to uncover changes in condition.
		Administer oxygen as ordered to supply a high concentration of oxygen to the brain.
		Position client with head of the bed up 30° to 40° and client's head at midline to promote venous drainage from the head.
		Minimize physical activity to prevent increasing metabolic demands. Maintain blood $PaCO_2$ between 25 and 30 mm Hg to prevent vasodilatation.
▶ *Ineffective Breathing Pattern related to neurological impairment of respiratory status or mechanical ventilation*	The client will have an effective breathing pattern.	Assess respiratory status every 15 to 60 minutes.
		Provide mechanical ventilation if necessary.
		Continually assess ABG levels or pulse oximeter readings to identify need for assisting respirations to prevent vasodilatation in the brain and increasing intracranial pressure.
		Administer oxygen as ordered to maintain blood oxygen concentration.

continues

Nursing Diagnoses	Planning/Goals	Nursing Interventions
▶ *Interrupted Family Processes related to sudden crisis*	The client and/or family will demonstrate effective coping mechanisms.	Assess family's coping mechanisms.
		Provide information about the client in an ongoing fashion. Provide teaching about the injury and pathophysiology involved.
		Prepare family for possible outcomes of the injury, such as paralysis or death.
		Collaborate with clergy, social services, mental health counselors, and support groups.
		Involve the family in client care as appropriate.
		Teach the family to report increased drowsiness, arm/leg weakness, muscle twitching, nausea or vomiting, visual or hearing disturbances, and so on.
		Inform the family that the client may not be aware of the symptoms and that signs and symptoms of the head injury may not be immediately apparent.

Evaluation Each goal must be evaluated to determine how it has been met by the client.

BRAIN TUMOR

Brain tumors are space-occupying intracranial lesions, either benign or malignant. Classification of brain tumors is by location or tissue type. Intracranial lesions may be primary lesions, which develop initially in brain tissue; extensions of tumors of the meninges, cranial nerves, or pituitary gland; or metastatic lesions from tumors originating in other body systems.

Pathophysiology of brain tumors depends on the increase in volume of brain tissue. The etiology is unknown. Clinical manifestations differ according to the area of the lesion and the rate of growth. Intracranial pressure increases as compensatory mechanisms are no longer able to balance tumor growth. Clinical manifestations commonly include alterations in consciousness, decreased mental functioning, headaches, seizures, or vomiting (sometimes sudden and projectile). Other signs and symptoms are relative to the functions of areas involved, such as visual problems resulting from occipital lobe tumors.

Diagnostic evaluation is by CT scan, MRI, or electroencephalogram (EEG). Total body scans, chest x-rays, and needle biopsies of the tumor may be performed to identify the type of tumor and, thus, serve as a basis for medical treatment.

Medical–Surgical Management

Medical

Medical management is based on tissue type, growth rate, and assessment of the client. Radiation therapy may be administered for treatment of specific tumor types or for inoperable tumors. The goal is to destroy the tumor cells, which are more susceptible to radiation than are normal cells. Radiation is also used in conjunction with surgery and chemotherapy.

Surgical

Surgical intervention, conventional or laser, includes resection of tumors (benign or malignant) to decrease the space occupied by the lesion or to obtain tissue for biopsy. Some CSF may be removed to relieve increased pressure.

Pharmacological

Pharmacological interventions are based on presenting symptoms. Dexamethasone (Decadron) is administered to decrease cerebral edema. Phenytoin (Dilantin) is given to prevent seizure activity. Antacids and H_2 blockers such as cimetidine (Tagamet) are given to prevent gastric irritation. Analgesics, NSAIDs, or codeine are used for headaches, and stool softeners are administered to prevent straining. Antineoplastic agents may be administered based on tumor type and whether the client meets the requirements for receiving the drug.

▶ NURSING PROCESS

▶ Assessment

▶ Subjective Data

Subjective assessment involves asking the client about fatigue, pain, headache, weakness, and ability to perform daily activities. Sensory alterations such as hearing, visual, or olfactory changes should be noted.

The nurse must assess the client's pain and evaluate effectiveness of interventions. A thorough psychosocial assessment, including changes in personality or judgment, serves as the basis for providing emotional support.

▶ Objective Data

Included is assessment of functional ability, mobility, and mental status, including motor strength, gait, ability to perform activities of daily living (ADL), and level of consciousness. Signs of neurological changes, deficits, or increased intracranial pressure, such as restlessness, changes in logic, changes in vital signs, pupil responses, speech abnormalities, seizure activity, or changes in respiratory patterns, must all be noted.

Nursing diagnoses for a client with a brain tumor may include the following:

Nursing Diagnoses	Planning/Goals	Nursing Interventions
▶ *Anxiety related to fear of unknown and treatment plans*	The client will demonstrate effective use of coping mechanisms.	Allow client to verbalize feeling of anxiety and discuss coping patterns previously used.
		Observe for verbal and nonverbal cues of anxiety.
		Provide emotional support by listening and guiding client to explore feelings of helplessness, fear of the unknown, and potential impending death.
		Teach client and family about diagnostic tests, treatments, and expected outcomes.
		Collaborate with pastoral care, physician, social services, and family to provide emotional support.
		Maintain a calm demeanor.
		Teach relaxation exercises and techniques such as slow, deep breathing and progressive muscle relaxation.
		Administer tranquilizers and sedatives as ordered.
▶ *Fatigue related to effects of treatment*	The client will verbalize lessened fatigue with frequent rest periods.	Allow client to discuss feelings of fatigue.
		Involve client in planning daily schedule that includes frequent rest periods.
		Assess client's ability to perform ADL, need for assistance to conserve energy.
		Cluster care activities to provide frequent rest periods that coincide with peak effectiveness of analgesics.
▶ *Imbalanced Nutrition: Less than body requirements related to side effects of treatment and disease process*	The client will maintain weight within 5 pounds of initial weight.	Assess client's weight every other day.
		Provide frequent small feedings of high-calorie and high-protein foods.
		Offer foods of client's choice.
		Use nutritional supplements to maintain weight. Offer fluids frequently.

Evaluation Each goal must be evaluated to determine how it has been met by the client.

CEREBROVASCULAR ACCIDENT/TRANSIENT ISCHEMIC ATTACKS

Cerebrovascular accident (CVA), or stroke, is a sudden loss of brain function accompanied by neurological deficit. Stroke is the third highest cause of death in the United States. Death rates from stroke have steadily declined from 120 per 100,000 in 1970 to 26 per 100,000 in 1992 (National Stroke Association, 1998a). The first rise in death rates in 35 years occurred in 1993, with 26.5 per 100,000, and again in 1995, with 26.7 per 100,000. Deaths totaled 157,991 in 1995. The rise in deaths in two groups among this population is noteworthy: rates for African American women ages 45 to 60 increased by 15% and rates for African American men over age 65 increased by 10% (National Stroke Association, 1995). Reasons for this sharp rise have not

CLIENT TEACHING

Stroke-Prevention Guidelines

- Have an annual blood pressure check
- Be aware of cholesterol level
- Consume lesser amounts of sodium (salt) and fat

(National Stroke Association, 1998b)

PROFESSIONAL TIP

Risk Factors for Stroke

- The major risk factor for stroke is hypertension.
- Other risk factors are diabetes mellitus, atherosclerosis, aneurysm, cardiac disease, high blood cholesterol, obesity, sedentary lifestyle, smoking, stress, drug abuse (especially of cocaine), and use of oral contraceptives. Clients with more than one risk factor are at even greater risk.

been determined. A proposed cause is decreased mortality from other diseases such as heart disease.

Strokes are caused by ischemia (oxygen deprivation) resulting from a thrombus, embolus, severe vasospasm, or cerebral hemorrhage. Blood supply to the brain is interrupted, causing neurological deficits of sensation, movement, thought, memory, or speech. The loss of function can be temporary or permanent.

Transient ischemic attacks (TIAs) frequently precede a CVA. A TIA is a temporary or transient episode of neurological dysfunction caused by temporary impairment of blood flow to the brain. The loss of motor or sensory function may last from a few seconds to minutes to 24 hours. A classic symptom is fleeting blindness in one eye. A reversible ischemic neurological deficit (RIND) is a TIA that lasts 24 to 48 hours.

Clinical manifestations of TIA or CVA vary according to the location of interrupted blood supply in the brain. As with head injury, the specific functions of the involved area of the brain are interrupted, causing the symptoms. Common neurological deficits are motor deficits of hemiplegia (paralysis of one side of the body on the side opposite of the brain lesion), **hemiparesis** (weakness of one side of the body), **dysarthria** (impairment of speech due to muscle dysfunction), and dysphagia (impairment of swallowing muscles). **Emotional lability** (loss of emotional control), inability to control behavior, and inability to process multiple pieces of information are also common manifestations of a stroke.

Sensory deficits include visual deficits of double vision, decreased visual acuity, and **homonymous hemianopia**, the loss of vision in half of the visual field on the same side of both eyes. Other possible sensory deficits include decreased sensation to touch, pressure, pain, heat, and cold. The client also may be confused and disoriented.

Intellectual deficits include memory impairment, poor judgment, short attention span, difficulty organizing thoughts, and inability to reason or calculate. Emotional deficits include depression and decreased tolerance to stressors.

Most clients experience initial bowel and bladder dysfunction. With early recognition of the problem and use of bowel and bladder retraining programs, however, most clients regain continence of bowel and bladder.

Differences in the affected side of the brain have been identified. Clients with left-side CVA tend to have communication deficits of aphasia, or inability to communicate. These clients tend to be slow and cautious in behavior and have intellectual impairments such as memory deficits or loss of problem solving skills. Defects in the right visual field occur, and hemiplegia occurs on the right side.

Clients with right-side CVA have left-sided paralysis and defects in the left visual field. Spatial–perceptual defects, called **agnosia**, cause the inability to recognize familiar objects such as a hairbrush. These clients demonstrate poor judgment and impulsive behavior and are unaware of the deficits. This is called **anosognosia**, which is gross or unconscious denial of the stroke or neurological deficit. Furthermore, these clients are easily distracted and usually show **unilateral neglect**, or the failure to recognize or care for the affected side of the body.

Cerebral edema and increased intracranial pressure may further complicate neurological status. Cerebral edema maximizes in 3 to 5 days following CVA. Neurological deficits begin to resolve within 2 days as cerebral edema decreases. Gradual progression in the return of various functions from proximal to distal can occur for 1 to 2 years.

Medical–Surgical Management

Medical

Medical management of the client with CVA is directed toward airway maintenance and supportive therapy during the first 24 to 48 hours. Early diagnosis of the cause and type of stroke is necessary to determine the appropriate treatment. Maintaining adequate cerebral perfusion and preventing cerebral edema reduce neurological deficit. Respiratory failure is treated with mechanical ventilation; temperature is regulated, with the help of a hypothermia blanket if necessary. (See the section on increased intracranial pressure for information on prevention and treatment.)

PROFESSIONAL TIP

Medication and Cerebrovascular Accident
Calcium channel blockers should not be used for the client with CVA, as they dilate blood vessels and increase cerebral perfusion.

To prevent further loss of function, a focus on rehabilitation must begin on admission. Self-care and mobility that remain must be maintained.

Surgical

Surgical removal of the thrombus (thrombolectomy) or embolus (embolectomy) may be necessary to relieve pressure on the brain.

Pharmacological

Antihypertensive agents are used to control blood pressure. To prevent further clot formation in cases of stroke caused by thrombi, anticoagulants, aspirin, heparin, or coumadin are used. To dissolve the clot, thrombolytic agents such as alteplase (Activase), anistreplase (Eminase), streptokinase (Streptase), or urokinase (Abbokinase) may be ordered. A stroke caused by bleeding would not be treated with thrombolytic agents. Dexamethasone (Decadron) may be used to reduce intracranial pressure. Anticonvulsants such as phenytoin (Dilantin) may be used if convulsions are present.

Diet

Fluids may be restricted for a few days following a CVA. The client will, however, be given intravenous fluids or tube feedings. The gag reflex must be assessed to identify choking risk, and food restrictions implemented accordingly.

PROFESSIONAL TIP

Caregivers for Client with CVA
To provide consistency in understanding of the CVA client's needs, assign the same caregiver to the client whenever possible.

Activity

In cases of an embolic or thrombolic stroke, the client's bed is kept flat to increase cerebral perfusion. In the event of a hemorrhagic stroke, the head of the bed is elevated to decrease cerebral perfusion. The type of CVA and the physician's judgment determines the length of time the client stays in bed.

Other Therapies

Both following the initial acute phase and during rehabilitation, physical, occupational, and speech therapy are vital for the client to reach the optimal functional level of recovery.

▶ NURSING PROCESS

▶ Assessment

▶ Subjective Data

Subjective data collected include client statements regarding how the client is feeling, frustration level with limitations, reports of pain, numbness, tingling, and sensory deficits of vision or hearing

▶ Objective Data

Specific attention must be paid to objective findings of assessment of level of consciousness, respiratory status, hemiparesis, hemiplegia, mobility, and cognitive perceptual functioning including the inability to think clearly and the ability to understand the condition.

COMMUNITY/HOME HEALTH CARE

Post-CVA Care
- Consult with the family to evaluate the home for safety and use of wheelchair or walker, if needed
- Evaluate the client's ability to perform self-care so that assistive devices or personal assistance can be obtained
- Determine whether a hospital bed or other medical equipment will need to be rented

Nursing diagnoses for a client with a CVA may include the following:

Nursing Diagnoses	Planning/Goals	Nursing Interventions
▶ *Deficient Knowledge related to home care*	The client and/or family will verbalize or demonstrate home health care management.	Assess client's and family's needs for discharge teaching, knowledge level about necessary home care.
		Develop a multidisciplinary plan for client and family teaching.
		Provide education in verbal, written, and picture forms to accommodate the varying possible impairments from the stroke.

continues

Nursing Diagnoses	Planning/Goals	Nursing Interventions
		Teach small segments of information at a time and reinforce teaching, then, to ascertain effectiveness of teaching, have client and family return demonstrate or verbalize knowledge. Primary areas of teaching are medication administration; dosages, actions, and side effects to report to the physician; mobility needs; self-care needs; safety factors; communication; swallowing; elimination; and skin care.
▶ *Impaired Verbal Communication related to neuromuscular impairment*	The client will communicate needs to the caregiver.	Assess communication deficits and consult a speech therapist to determine a method of communication, if deficits are apparent.
		Allow time for the client to attempt to communicate needs; anticipate needs to prevent client frustration in trying to communicate.
		Use gestures, pictures, and closed questions (those requiring only a "yes" or "no" answer). Provide paper and pencil if dominant side is unaffected.
▶ *Unilateral Neglect related to neuromuscular impairment*	The client will move paralyzed extremities with assistance from functioning extremities.	Adapt environment to prevent injury of the client with unilateral neglect by positioning water and personal items on the unaffected or unneglected side. Approach the client from the unneglected side.
		Gradually cue client to remind to tend to the neglected side.
		Remind client of safety factors such as arm trailing over edge of wheelchair or close proximity of a wall on the neglected side.
		Teach client and family to place small bites of food on unaffected side and to check for food in the cheek on the affected side after meals.
		Instruct client to scan environment for safety factors at all times.
		Teach client how to dress and tend to neglected side.
		Place arm either in a sling, if client is ambulatory, or on a wheelchair tray, if client is in a wheelchair.

Evaluation Each goal must be evaluated to determine how it has been met by the client.

EPILEPSY/SEIZURE DISORDER

Epilepsy is a disorder of cerebral function in which the client experiences sudden attacks of altered consciousness, motor activity, or sensory phenomenon. Convulsive seizures are the most common type of attack. Most recurrent seizure patterns are due to epilepsy. Most clinicians and authors use the term "seizure disorder" for epilepsy or seizures (Hickey, 1997).

A seizure is initiated by an electrical disturbance in the neurons, which, in turn, causes an aberrant discharge of electrical activity from any part of the cerebral cortex and possibly from other areas of the brain (Samuels, 1999). This electrical discharge may cause involuntary episodes of loss of consciousness, excessive muscular movement or loss of muscle tone, and changes in behavior, mood, sensation, and/or perception (Smeltzer & Bare, 2000).

The etiology of the electrical disturbance may be birth trauma, hypoxia, infection, tumor, alcohol toxicity, drugs, drug withdrawal, carbon monoxide or lead poisoning, vascular abnormalities such as CVA, hypoglycemia electrolyte imbalance, or fever. Often, the cause is idiopathic, or unknown.

Seizures are classified as generalized or partial. In generalized seizures, the entire brain is affected simultaneously, causing bilateral, symmetrical reactions. Generalized seizures are classified as tonic and/or clonic (grand mal), absence (petit mal), or myoclonic.

Tonic–clonic seizures involve rigid tonic contractions of muscles and loss of postural control followed by a clonic stage of intermittent contraction and relaxation. Loss of continence of stool or urine is common. Absence seizures involve loss of conscious activity without the muscular involvement of tonic–clonic seizures. Myoclonic seizures may be very mild, sudden, involuntary contractions of a muscle group or may be rapid, forceful movements. They usually occur in the trunk or extremities and involve no loss of consciousness.

Partial seizures initiate in a focal point in the brain and involve the function of those specific neurons. Partial seizures are either simple or complex. In simple partial seizures, the area affected may be a hand, a finger, the ability to talk, or a sense such as smell. Consciousness is not lost.

Complex partial seizures generally involve loss of consciousness and may produce cognitive, affective, psychosensory, or psychomotor symptoms. The client may perform inappropriate purposive behaviors, called **automatisms**, or mechanical, repetitive motor behaviors performed unconsciously, such as lip-smacking.

Auras, peculiar sensations that precede the seizure and may take the form of a taste, smell, sight, or sound; dizziness; or a "funny" feeling. After the seizure, the client typically cannot remember the episode.

Diagnostic testing to determine the type of seizure activity includes the EEG to identify abnormal electrical activity and/or the focal point of the seizure. Sleep and video EEGs are performed to document changes in electrical activity of the brain. Computerized tomography scans are used to identify or rule out lesions, degenerative changes, or vascular abnormalities.

Medical–Surgical Management

Surgical

Surgical intervention may be indicated for a very small percentage of clients. Microsurgery may be utilized to irradiate focal points of abnormal electrical discharge caused by tumor, vascular abnormality, or abscess.

Pharmacological

The primary method of controlling seizure activity is pharmacological. Seizure activity in 75% of clients is controlled with an anticonvulsant agent or a combination of anticonvulsants (Hickey, 1997). Phenytoin (Dilantin), phenobarbital (Phenobarbital), carbamazepine (Tegretol), valproic acid (Depakene), and primidone (Mysoline) are often used. Anticonvulsant agents are started one at a time in gradually increasing doses. The client's blood level is monitored for therapeutic range, and the client is assessed for side effects of the drug and signs of drug toxicity, such as drowsiness, dizziness, gastric distress, rash, blood dyscrasias, and ataxia.

The goal is to obtain seizure control with minimal side effects. Any anticonvulsant should be gradually discontinued. Abrupt withdrawal can cause **status epilepticus,** an acute prolonged episode of seizure activity lasting at least 30 minutes with or without loss of consciousness (Smeltzer & Bare, 2000). Status epilepticus is a medical emergency that can result in respiratory arrest and irreversible brain damage.

Diet

Nutritionally balanced meals are required. The client should never consume alcohol.

PROFESSIONAL TIP

Long-Term Use of Dilantin

The client on Dilantin requires good oral hygiene because of hyperplasia of the gums, which become edematous and enlarged.

Activity

Adequate rest is required. Driving, operating machinery, and swimming are not allowed until seizures are controlled.

Safety: Precautions During a Seizure

If the client is in bed:
- Be sure the side rails are up, and
- Put padding (blankets) on the side rails to prevent injury.

If the client is out of bed:
- Carefully ease the client to the floor,
- Move nearby objects so that the client will not be injured, and
- Place a soft item beneath the client's head.

Whether the client is in or out of bed:
- Never leave the client alone,
- Do not restrain the client,
- Do not attempt to put anything in the client's mouth after the seizure has begun,
- Loosen any restrictive clothing around the client's neck,
- Turn the client's head to the side, and
- Monitor seizure activity carefully, noting the exact time that the seizure began and ended.

After the seizure:
- Call the client by name and ask to perform a simple command,
- Test the client's memory by asking to remember two words,
- Ask the client whether an aura was experienced before the seizure,
- Check the oral cavity—especially the tongue—for injury,
- Offer comfort and reassurance, as the client may be frightened and embarrassed, and
- Document everything observed.

▶ NURSING PROCESS

▶ Assessment

▶ Subjective Data

This includes client statements of experiences prior to the seizure and what activity the client was performing when the seizure occurred. The nurse must determine whether an aura was experienced and the sensations that were manifested, and ascertain if the client has a prior history of seizure disorder.

▶ Objective Data

Assessment of the nature of the seizure and sequencing of events is important in determining cause and management of seizure activity. During the seizure, the nurse assesses the client's respiratory status and observes for muscular stiffness or flaccidity, the position of the eyes and head, the size and equality of the pupils, automatism, any cry or sounds made, and incontinence of urine or stool. The duration of the phases of the seizure, total duration, and whether unconsciousness occurred are noted. If the onset of seizure activity was observed, this should be noted along with what the client was doing when the seizure began.

Following the seizure the client should be observed for postictal signs of paralysis of arms or legs, inability to speak, sleep following seizure, difficulty in awakening from sleep, confusion, or general dazed affect (Smeltzer & Bare, 2000; Hickey, 1997). The postictal phase can last from several minutes to hours. The client should be assessed for signs of injury and vital signs. Clients on anticonvulsant therapy need a thorough nursing assessment because of the wide variety of side effects involving multiple body systems.

Nursing diagnoses for a client with a seizure may include the following:

Nursing Diagnoses	Planning/Goals	Nursing Interventions
▶ Ineffective Airway Clearance related to mucus accumulation during the seizure and uncontrollable tonic–clonic muscle contractions involving the respiratory muscles	The client will maintain an effective airway during seizure activity.	Following tonic–clonic activity, turn client to the side to allow secretions to drain from the airway.
		Prepare to suction oropharynx if necessary to clear airway.
		Assess skin color and respiratory rate and depth during and following seizure.
		Administer oxygen as needed.
		Insert oral airway or epistick if client's jaw is not clenched. Never insert an object if the jaw is already clenched. Do not place fingers between client's teeth. Loosen restrictive clothing.
▶ Risk for Injury related to seizure activity	The client will be free of injury related to seizure activity.	During seizures in bed, use blankets or protective pads to pad side rails.
		If client is standing or sitting, ease client to the floor when seizure activity begins. Place client in a supine position, but do not physically restrain client.
		Remove objects from around client so that he or she will not hit them.
		Following the seizure, turn client to the side to allow secretions to drain from the mouth.
		Maintain a low-stimulus environment to prevent further seizure activity.
		Observe client for injuries, i.e., tongue lacerations; broken bones; body lacerations or bruising.
		Teach client about ways of maintaining a safe environment, including driving restrictions; lying down in a safe area if an aura is experienced; showering instead of tub bathing; either avoiding swimming or swimming with a partner if the physician allows; and wearing a medical identification tag.
▶ Ineffective Coping related to anxiety secondary to seizure disorder and altered self-concept	The client will verbalize fears and concerns about seizure activity; and will use effective coping methods.	Allow client to verbalize fears and concerns.
		Explore coping mechanisms with client.
		Collaborate with mental health counselor or clergy to assist client in development of coping mechanisms.

Evaluation Each goal must be evaluated to determine how it has been met by the client.

HERNIATED INTERVERTEBRAL DISK

Herniated intervertebral disks are a major cause of chronic back pain. Most clients with herniated disks are 30 to 50 years of age. The majority of herniated disks occur in the lumbar or cervical spine because of the flexibility of these regions (Hickey, 1997). This can occur either suddenly from trauma, lifting, or twisting or gradually from aging, osteoporosis, or degenerative changes. Most herniated disks are caused by trauma, such as falls, accidents, or repeated lifting. Degenerative

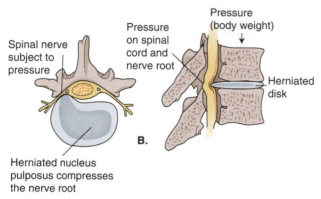

Figure 25-15 A. Normal Intervertebral Disc; B. Herniated Disc

changes related to arthritis, aging, or repeated minor injuries predispose the client to herniated intervertebral disks.

The intervertebral disk is a cartilaginous cushion between vertebral bodies (Figure 25-15). In herniation, or rupture of the disk, the nucleus pulposus protrudes into the fibrous ring, the annulus fibrosus. This protrusion presses on the spinal cord and nerve roots, causing pain, motor changes, sensory changes, and alterations in reflexes.

The nerve root affected and the degree of compression lead to specific symptoms. Ninety percent to 95% of lumbar herniations occur at the L-4 to L-5 and S-1 levels (Hickey, 1997). Low-back pain that radiates across the buttock and down the leg along the path of the sciatic nerve is the most common symptom. The affected leg tingles and is numb. Sneezing, straining, stooping, standing, sitting, blowing the nose, and jarring movements aggravate the pain. Positions of comfort are lying on the back, with knees flexed and a small pillow under the head, or lying on the unaffected side, with the affected knee flexed.

Motor weakness may be experienced. Paresthesia and numbness of the leg and foot occur. Knee and ankle reflexes are diminished or absent. Lasegue's sign, pain experienced upon gentle raising of the fully extended leg of the supine-positioned client to 20° to 60°, stems from stretching of the inflamed sciatic nerve. Inflammation in the nerve roots may also be present as indicated by a positive finding for **Kernig's sign**. To test for Kernig's sign, the client is placed in a dorsal recumbent position and attempts to flex the hip and knee and then extend the knee. Normally, the client should be able to extend the knee to 90°. With a low-back herniated disk, however, the client will be unable to extend the knee because of severe pain radiating down the hip and leg. Symptoms vary with the area and degree of nerve root compression.

Cervical herniation commonly occurs at levels C-5 to C-6 or C-6 to C-7. Symptoms of lateral herniation include pain and paresthesia in the neck, arms, and shoulders. Loss of muscle strength and reflexes may also occur, as may muscle atrophy.

Because of anatomic position, cervical disks may herniate centrally more frequently than do lumbar disks, thereby compressing the spinal cord. Symptoms are weakness of the lower extremities and unsteady gait. Spasticity and hyperactive reflexes may develop in the lower extremities. Difficulty in voiding and sexual dysfunction may occur.

Degenerative spinal cord disease can follow compression from a herniated disk. Spinal cord tumors and herniated lumbar disk are differential diagnoses that are ruled out through the use of MRI or CT scans.

Medical–Surgical Management

Medical

Conservative medical treatment, providing rest, stress reduction and immobility of the spine, and pain relief, is often tried for several weeks.

Surgical

Surgery to remove the herniated disk is done when neurological deficit or pain are not responsive to conservative treatment or when symptoms require immediate surgical intervention.

Pharmacological

Narcotic analgesics, such as hydrocodone bitartrate with acetaminophen (Vicodin), and nonnarcotic analgesics, such as tramadol hydrochloride (Ultram), are ordered for pain control. Antiinflammatory drugs, steroids, or NSAIDs such as ibuprofen (Motrin) or naproxen (Anaprox) are prescribed to reduce the inflammatory response. Muscle relaxants such as methocarbamol (Robaxin) are given to reduce spasms of surrounding muscles, which decreases the pain. Antianxiety medications such as diazepam (Valium) are given to decrease muscle tension and promote rest.

Diet

To decrease the workload on the involved muscles, weight reduction is advocated if the client is overweight. A high-protein diet with calcium, vitamin D, and phosphorus is necessary for bone repair and prevention of osteoporosis. Fiber is necessary for bowel function, because constipation is a common side effect of analgesics.

Activity

Bed rest, a support garment (back brace) or cervical collar, a firm mattress, and traction may be used to decrease stress on the affected vertebrae. Postoperatively, log-roll turning is used to prevent injury to the vertebrae and spine.

The client may not lift or carry more than 5 pounds for at least 8 weeks. Twisting movements are to be avoided. The client cannot drive a car until the surgeon permits. Sitting should be limited during the early postoperative period; the client should either stand or lie down. Physical therapy is focused on muscle strengthening and client comfort. Heat therapy, ultrasound, and exercises are often used to promote comfort and healing.

▶ NURSING PROCESS

▶ Assessment

▶ Subjective Data

Assessment includes eliciting client statements about motor and sensory function, pain, and effectiveness of comfort measures.

▶ Objective Data

Assessment entails a neurological evaluation of motor and sensory function of the extremities innervated below the herniated area. Reflex testing may be a part of the nursing assessment in some facilities. Range of motion (ROM) of the affected extremity is assessed. The nurse assesses the client's knowledge about the disease process, the planned treatment including pain management and surgery, and the postsurgical care. Status of bowel and bladder elimination is assessed for potential nerve involvement or effects of immobility. Gait alteration and limited bending should also be noted.

Nursing diagnoses for a client with a herniated intervertebral disk may include the following:

Nursing Diagnoses	Planning/Goals	Nursing Interventions
▶ *Chronic Pain related to nerve compression or surgical intervention*	The client will experience increased comfort.	Assess pain intensity and location, as well as activities or position when pain began. Have the client rate pain on a scale of 1 to 10.
		Maintain activity level as ordered by physician.
		Place client in position of comfort, usually on back, with knees slightly flexed and a small pillow beneath head, or on unaffected side, with affected extremity flexed and a pillow between the legs.
		Maintain immobility of vertebrae with corset, brace, or traction.
		Apply moist heat as prescribed and administer medications to relieve pain, relax muscles, and relieve inflammation and anxiety, as ordered. Document effectiveness.
		Provide diversional activities.
▶ *Impaired Physical Mobility related to nerve compression or surgical intervention*	The client will have no complications of immobility.	Assess for complications of immobility.
		Turn client every 1 to 2 hours. The client will tend to limit position to one of comfort.
		Assist the client to log roll, that is, move the body as a unit without twisting the back.
		Ambulate as ordered by the physician.

Evaluation Each goal must be evaluated to determine how it has been met by the client.

SPINAL CORD INJURY

Spinal cord injury (SCI) occurs from trauma to the spinal cord or from compression of the spinal cord due to injury to the supporting structures. Each year, almost 10,000 new spinal cord injuries occur. Most of the victims are males between the ages of 16 and 30 years. Leading causes of injury are motor vehicle accidents; acts of violence; falls; and sporting accidents (Beare & Meyers, 1998; Hickey, 1997; National Spinal Cord Injury Statistical Center, 1998).

Numerous classification systems exist for SCIs. Spinal cord injuries may be classified by level of injury, mechanism of injury, or neurological or functional level (Figure 25-16). The injury may be considered complete or incomplete. When injury is complete, no

Figure 25-16 Spinal Cord—Levels of Injury: A. Areas of sensory function; B. Areas of motor function

impulses are carried below the level of injury. There is complete disruption of the spinal cord functions including motor (voluntary) movement, sensation, and reflexes to areas innervated by the spinal nerves at and below the level of the injury. In an incomplete injury, some of the spinal cord tracts are affected while others are able to carry impulses normally.

The mechanism of injury is usually an acceleration–deceleration event that causes hyperflexion, hyperextension, axial loading, or excessive rotation injury (Hickey, 1997). Hyperflexion is the extreme forward movement of the head, which causes compression of the vertebral bodies and damage to the posterior ligaments and intervertebral disks. Hyperextension is the extreme backward movement of the head, causing injury to the posterior vertebral structures and the anterior ligaments. Axial loading or compression occurs when extreme pressure is placed on the spinal column, such as in diving accidents or falls landed on feet or buttocks. Compression of the vertebrae causes shattering of the vertebral body. Compression fractures and posterior ligament injury can also be caused by excessive rotation, or turning the head beyond the normal range.

Classification of injury by cause includes concussion, contusion, laceration, transection, hemorrhage, or damage to blood vessels supplying the spinal cord. Immediately following injury to the spinal cord, an autodestructive process begins, with chemical and vascular changes that lead to ischemia and necrosis of the spinal cord.

Spinal shock (cessation of motor, sensory, autonomic, and reflex impulses) and **areflexia** (the absence of reflexes) occur immediately upon transection of the spinal cord or upon injury to the spinal cord. Flaccid paralysis of all skeletal muscles; loss of spinal reflexes; loss of sensation; and absence of autonomic function below the level of injury also occur. The diaphragm is innervated at levels C3 through C5. Injuries in this area cause partial or complete disruption of respiratory function. The client does not perspire below the level of the injury. Bowel and bladder function may be lost either for a few days to months, or permanently, though this loss generally lasts from 1 to 6 weeks.

As spinal shock resolves, reflex activity returns below the level of injury. The client with a lower motor neuron injury continues to experience flaccid paralysis, areflexia, hypotonic bowel and bladder function, and sexual dysfunction. Lower motor neuron injury causes paraplegia, or paralysis of lower extremities.

Neurogenic shock, a hypotensive situation resulting from the loss of sympathetic control of vital functions from the brain, may occur during spinal shock. This happens in clients with injury above the sixth thoracic vertebra. The client develops orthostatic hypotension, bradycardia, decreased cardiac output, loss of ability to sweat below the level of injury, and subnormal temperature.

Upper motor neuron injury results in spastic paralysis, loss of voluntary skeletal muscle movement, and reflexive bowel, bladder, and sexual responses. Complete upper motor neuron injury results in **quadriplegia**, or dysfunction or paralysis of both arms, both legs, bowel, and bladder. Injuries above C5 affect respiratory function because of innervation of the diaphragm and accessory respiratory muscles. Mechanical ventilation is required to keep the client alive. Fractures below the cervical vertebrae result in diaphragmatic breathing, if the phrenic nerve is functioning.

The client with an injury above the sixth thoracic vertebra is at risk for developing autonomic dysreflexia or autonomic hyperreflexia. Autonomic dysreflexia is an emergency situation resulting in a hypertensive crisis and possibly stroke or seizure activity. The cause is noxious stimuli such as a full bladder, a fecal impaction, a wrinkle in clothing, menstrual cramps, an erection, an ingrown toenail, a bladder infection, or sitting on catheter tubing. Autonomic reflexes below the level of the injury cause vasoconstriction in this area. The controlling impulses from the higher cortical levels do not transmit past the level of injury but cause bradycardia and vasodilatation above the level of injury. Skin above the level of injury is warm and moist, but skin below the level of injury is cold, with goose flesh (Beare & Meyers, 1998; Hickey, 1997).

The noxious stimuli must be removed, if possible, and the client placed in a sitting position immediately. Blood pressure must be assessed immediately and monitored every few minutes until within normal limits (Huston & Boelman, 1995). The drug of choice, nitroprusside sodium (Nipride), may be given if the conservative measure does not work. Autonomic dysreflexia must be prevented when possible, recognized when it develops, and treated immediately. Once autonomic dysreflexia is relieved, the client may develop hypotension from the decreased sympathetic response and the residual effects of medication and positioning changes. A pattern of individual response to stimuli and of sympathetic response is soon identified for the client. However, the client with an upper motor neuron injury above T-6 is always at risk for developing autonomic dysreflexia. Some clients experience the first episode years after the injury.

The extent of permanent injury cannot be determined immediately, because of necrosis, edema, and spinal shock. Functional loss depends on the level, degree, and type of injury.

Medical–Surgical Management

Medical

Medical management of the client with spinal cord injury begins prior to reaching the hospital. Further damage to the spinal cord is prevented by immobilizing the head, neck, and vertebral column with devices such as rigid cervical collars and splinting backboards. All trauma clients are treated as potential spinal cord injuries. When the client reaches the emergency room, x-rays of the spine are taken prior to removing the immobilizing devices.

Respiratory function is continuously assessed, and ventilatory support is provided as necessary. The client may have multiple injuries, necessitating astute diagnostic skills by the emergency room physician. Assessment of the trauma client must involve evaluating for internal hemorrhaging, cardiac contusion, head injury, hemorrhagic shock, and spinal shock resulting from the spinal cord injury. A thorough assessment is done to specifically evaluate the degree of deficit and to establish the level or degree of injury.

Immobilization of the spinal cord continues to be the focus of care during early medical management of the client. Traction may be used to maintain alignment of the spinal column. Cervical tongs and halo devices are used to apply traction and to immobilize the cervical spine. Under local anesthesia, cervical tongs and halo rings are applied with spring-loaded pins that are embedded into the scalp. Antiseptic solution is used to cleanse the scalp, and a local anesthetic is injected into the insertion sites. Traction weights are applied to the cervical tongs or halo rings after the insertion pins are firmly embedded (Figure 25-17). Body casts, jackets, or braces are used to immobilize thoracic and lumbar fractures.

Figure 25-17 Halo Vest *(Courtesy of DePuy AcroMed)*

Surgical

Surgical interventions are performed for decompression, realignment, and stabilization of the vertebral column, depending on the nature of the injury. A laminectomy may be performed to decompress the spinal cord with fusion or placement of Harrington rods to stabilize the vertebral column. Realignment is maintained by surgical manipulation of the vertebral column.

If the client has respiratory involvement, an endotracheal tube is put in place to provide mechanical ventilatory support. Following urgent treatment, a tracheostomy will be performed to continue ventilation.

Pharmacological

Steroid therapy with dexamethasone (Decadron) is administered to prevent and reduce edema in the injured spinal cord. To decrease and prevent edema and to improve blood flow, high loading doses of the steroid methylprednisolone sodium succinate (Solu-Medrol) are given immediately, with tapering dosages being given over the next 1 to 2 weeks. Mannitol, an osmotic diuretic, may be administered to decrease and prevent cord edema. Hydralazine hydrochloride (Apresoline) or nifedipine (Procardia) is frequently or-

dered to reduce blood pressure in cases of autonomic dysreflexia.

Activity

Initially, immobilization of the spinal column is necessary. In the acute phase, ROM for all joints is performed to prevent mobility loss and muscle contracture. As the spine is stabilized, the client's activity progresses to sitting up in a chair, performing strengthening exercises, and increasing endurance. The nurse must observe for the complication of orthostatic hypotension.

Orthostatic hypotension is caused by the venous pooling of blood in the lower body and extremities resulting from impairment of the sympathetic nervous system. The client becomes hypotensive and develops bradycardia and syncope. Asystole may even occur. To maintain mean arterial pressure (MAP) between 80 and 90 mm Hg and to improve spinal cord perfusion during the acute phase, vasopressor agents such as dopamine hydrochloride (Intropin) are given. Prevention of orthostatic hypotension also requires the application of full leg support stockings and pneumatic boots and the gradual lowering of the lower extremities. The client's vital signs are monitored throughout the mobilization process to ascertain tolerance to the procedure.

After spinal shock has subsided, active rehabilitation begins, with the interdisciplinary team optimizing the functional capabilities of the client. The physical therapist plays a major role in the activity level; the occupational therapist, in ADL; and the speech therapist, in swallowing ability and communications.

Other Therapies

An interdisciplinary approach is used for rehabilitation. Rehabilitation begins immediately, with a focus on preventing disabilities and maximizing and strengthening remaining functional ability. Neurological function can be regained for up to 1 year.

▶ NURSING PROCESS

▶ Assessment

▶ Subjective Data

Subjective assessment involves eliciting input from the client regarding sensation, pain, and history of the accident. How the client is coping with the injury, the resulting disability, and the major lifestyle changes that have occurred should all be noted. How the family or support system is coping with the changes is also evaluated.

▶ Objective Data

In the acute phase of care of the client with a spinal cord injury, nursing assessment focuses on the critical factors of airway, breathing, circulation, disability, and exposure.

Assessment of circulatory status involves monitoring vital signs and observing for complications of neurogenic shock; orthostatic hypotension; hypertensive episodes of autonomic dysreflexia; and hemorrhaging.

Disability is assessed by performing a baseline neurological assessment (as described under the Components of Neurological Assessment section in this chapter).

Exposure refers to removing the client's clothing to perform a thorough assessment of the client's body for skin condition and for entrance and exit wounds. Body temperature must be monitored because of the neurological deficit in temperature regulation as caused by dysfunction of the autonomic nervous system.

Subacute assessment is based on the level of injury and neurological functioning of the client. With upper motor neuron injuries, the client is at higher risk of developing autonomic dysreflexia; thus, assessment includes monitoring for these signs.

All clients with spinal cord injury are assessed for skin condition, bowel and bladder function, respiratory status, and signs and symptoms of complications of immobility. Psychosocial assessment is also very important to the well-being of the client.

Nursing diagnoses for the client with a spinal cord injury in the subacute phase of care may include the following:

Nursing Diagnoses	Planning/Goals	Nursing Interventions
▶ *Risk for Injury related to motor and sensory deficits secondary to spinal fractures*	The client will not experience additional injury.	Assess the client's risk factors for additional injury.
		Monitor skin condition for pressure areas or shearing injuries from sliding across sheets or the mats in physical therapy.
		Turn client frequently to prevent pressure areas.
		Use enough personnel to turn client correctly to maintain alignment of client's spinal column.
		Provide call light that client can operate; teach to call nurse for assistance as necessary.
		Reinforce wheelchair safety factors and observe client for use of wheelchair.
		Prevent falls when transferring client to wheelchair.
		Prevent foot drop.
		Provide passive and active ROM exercises.
		Maintain adequate fluid intake and nutrition.
		Provide routine care for halo device by opening vest on one side to cleanse skin under vest at least daily and to assess for skin breakdown. Repeat procedure on the other side.
		Monitor pin sites of halo device every shift for placement.
		Perform pin site care using facility protocol.

continues

Nursing Diagnoses	Planning/Goals	Nursing Interventions
▶ *Powerlessness related to changes in motor and sensory function and in lifestyle*	The client will make decisions regarding care, treatment, and future.	Explain all procedures and care options.
		Establish an open, trusting relationship with client to foster therapeutic communication.
		Allow time for client to express concerns, anger, and fears.
		Foster a positive environment for client to explore feelings and accept disability.
		Allow client to participate in care decisions.
		Assess for signs and symptoms of depression.
		Collaborate with mental health professional to provide assistance in coping with lifestyle changes.
		Collaborate with family and support people to include them in the plan of care.
▶ *Autonomic Dysreflexia related to noxious stimulation secondary to overstimulation of autonomic nervous system*	The client will state factors that cause autonomic dysreflexia, describe treatment, and notify the nurse if experiencing symptoms of dysreflexia.	Teach client causes and symptoms of autonomic dysreflexia: increased blood pressure, sudden throbbing headache, chills, pallor, goose flesh, nausea, and/or metallic taste in mouth.
		Prevent bladder distention and fecal impaction by implementing a bowel and bladder training program.
		Observe for bradycardia, vasodilatation, flushing, and diaphoresis above the level of spinal cord injury. If these symptoms occur, immediately notify the physician and administer medications as ordered to decrease blood pressure. Raise head of bed and lower legs to reduce blood pressure. Then, remove the noxious stimuli, which may include constrictive clothing, shoes, splints, or linens.
		Assess client for a distended bladder and empty the bladder if distended.
		Observe urine for signs of infection and obtain a urine specimen for culture, if needed to identify the cause of the reaction.
		Check for fecal impaction using xylocaine viscous per physician's order to decrease stimulation.
		Monitor blood pressure every few minutes.

Evaluation Each goal must be evaluated to determine how it has been met by the client.

PARKINSON'S DISEASE

Parkinson's disease is a chronic, progressive, degenerative disease affecting the area of the brain controlling movement. The cause is unknown in most cases, but toxicity, hypoxia, or encephalitis may precede the onset of Parkinson's disease. Vascular and genetic factors have been implicated. Drugs such as cocaine, reserpine (Serpasil), haloperidol (Haldol), and chlorpromazine (Thorazine) may cause a parkinsonian syndrome. The theory is that these drugs interfere with the synthesis or storage of dopamine.

Typical signs and symptoms of Parkinson's Disease are muscular rigidity, **bradykinesia** (slowness of voluntary movement and speech), resting tremors, muscular weakness, and loss of postural reflexes. Muscular rigidity along with bradykinesia impairs the person's ability to perform daily activities and speech.

Rigidity is noted along with increased muscle tone when the client is at rest. Stiffness of the trunk, head, and shoulders is present. The rigidity causes loss of

arm swing when walking. A cogwheel phenomenon results from the muscle contractions breaking through the muscular rigidity. The alternating rigidity and rhythmic contractions causes a jerking-like movement. Motor impairment progressively affects facial expressions, eye blink, and voice, causing a typical presentation of a mask-like face and a monotone voice.

Resting tremors, usually in the upper extremities, are present when the hand is motionless. The hand moves in a "pill-rolling" motion. When the client is moving or sleeping, the tremors are usually absent. Tremors also occur in other areas including the feet, lip, tongue, or jaw. The tremors usually begin unilaterally in one area and progress to other areas and then to the opposite side of the body. Anxiety and concentration tend to increase the degree of tremors.

The posture and gait of people with Parkinson's disease is characterized by bowed head, forward-bent trunk, drooped shoulders, and flexed arms. The gait is characterized by shuffling movement and small steps. Balance is affected, resulting in a tendency to fall forward. Figure 25-18 shows the classic posture of a client with Parkinson's disease.

Autonomic dysfunction includes drooling, **dysphagia** (difficulty swallowing), excessive sweating, hyperactivity of oil glands, and constipation. Orthostatic hypotension may occur from loss of the peripheral autonomic response. Urinary incontinence and frequency occur.

Mental changes may also occur. Intelligence is not impaired, but problems with judgment and emotional stability may occur. Dementia is present 10% to 15% of the time. Depression frequently accompanies Parkinson's disease. Depression may occur from the chemical changes in dopamine level or in reaction to the disorder. Cognitive, perceptual, or memory deficits may occur. The major cause of death is from the complications of immobility or injury. Fatigue increases all signs and symptoms. Since there is no diagnostic test specific for Parkinson's disease, diagnosis is made from clinical signs and symptoms. In cases of early onset, it is important to differentiate from Wilson's disease, which is an increased absorption of copper, for which testing is available.

Medical–Surgical Management

Medical

The goals of medical management are to control the symptoms, provide supportive therapy and maintenance, maintain function via physiotherapy, and provide psychotherapy as necessary.

Surgical

Stereotactic thalamotomy, a surgical procedure to disrupt the transmission of motor impulses, is occasionally used to treat the tremors and muscular rigidity. This invasive procedure does not treat the disease, but, rather, alleviates the tremors.

Pharmacological

Drug therapy is used to control the symptoms of Parkinson's disease. L-dihydroxyphenylalanine (L-Dopa) is converted into dopamine in the basal ganglia to replace the deficit of dopamine. Dopamine itself is not given orally because it is metabolized before reaching the brain. L-Dopa, a precursor to dopamine, is given orally and reaches the brain to be converted into dopamine.

Dopadecarboxylase inhibitors such as carbidopa-levodopa (Sinemet) prevent the conversion of L-Dopa to dopamine in peripheral tissue. Dopamine in the peripheral tissue can cause numerous side effects as well as decrease the amount of L-dopa available to the brain. Dopadecarboxylase inhibitors that do not cross the blood–brain barrier are used to inhibit the enzyme that changes L-dopa to dopamine so that the conversion in the brain is not inhibited.

Figure 25-18 Progression of Parkinson's Disease: A. Flexion of affected arm; B. Shuffling gait; C. Need for sources of support to prevent falling; D. Progression of weakness to point of needing assistance for ambulation; E. Profound weakness

Anticholinergic drugs such as trihexyphenidyl hydrochloride (Artane), cycrimine hydrochloride (Pagitane hydrochloride), and benztropine mesylate (Cogentin), are administered to control tremors and rigidity. Anticholinergics are used alone for mild symptoms or if L-dopa is contraindicated. In other instances, they may be administered in conjunction with L-dopa.

PROFESSIONAL TIP

Pallidotomy

Pallidotomy, an operation of the 1950s for Parkinson's disease, is being used again. Improved surgical equipment and clients who no longer benefit from medications are causing a resurgence in the use of pallidotomy.

Using MRI and stereotactic equipment, the physician can pinpoint the area of the brain that is causing the unwanted symptoms. A probe is then inserted into the brain through a small hole in the client's head. A small lesion is made deep in the brain to interrupt the electrical pathways that cause the rigidity and tremors. The surgery relieves symptoms but does not cure Parkinson's disease. Furthermore, associated risks such as paralysis and bleeding must be considered (Raine, 1997).

Amantadine hydrochloride (Symmetrel), an antiviral agent, is effective in treating Parkinsonian symptoms. The mechanism by which the drug works is not known, but the theory is that it either releases dopamine storage areas or delays the reuptake of dopamine Ethopropazine hydrochloride (Parsidol), a phenothiazine derivative, is used in combination with other anti-Parkinson drugs to alleviate symptoms. Dopamine agonist-ergot derivatives, such as pergolide mesylate (Permax), directly stimulate the dopamine receptors to improve the use of available dopamine. The monoamine oxidase (MAO) inhibitor selegiline hydrochloride (Eldepryl) inhibits dopamine breakdown. The tricyclic antidepressants amitriptyline hydrochloride (Elavil) and imipramine hydrochloride (Tofranil) alleviate depression as well as other symptoms.

Diet

Pureed foods or tube feedings may be required because of dysphagia. Maintenance of weight may require high- or low-calorie diets. A diet that discourages formation of free radicals is being researched as a deterrent to progression of the disease. Free-radical formation is thought to be discouraged by diets high in complex carbohydrates (such as those found in whole grain breads and lentils), low in fat, and high in vitamins A and E. Large doses of supplemental vitamins A and E are also given. A high-fiber diet will help in preventing constipation.

PROFESSIONAL TIP

Drug Therapy for Parkinson's Disease

- Numerous side effects, such as blurred vision, drowsiness, disorientation, and delirium may be noted.
- Dosage requirements vary greatly among individuals.
- Symptom control varies in the same individual from day to day.
- To maintain a constant therapeutic level for better symptom control, Sinemet solution may be ordered hourly while the client is awake.

 Safety: Mealtime

The client with Parkinson's disease must be monitored for choking while eating because of dysphagia.

Activity

Ambulation with assistance is necessary to maintain joint mobility and to prevent injury. The client should not be hurried, as the bradykinesia becomes worse when the client is attempting to hurry.

Other Therapies

Physical therapy is directed toward the maintenance of joint mobility, posture, and gait. Occupational therapy focuses on maintaining optimal functioning in achieving ADL. Speech therapy is used to promote

COMMUNITY/HOME HEALTH CARE

Adaptations for the Client with Parkinson's Disease

- Arrange for bathroom facilities and bedroom on first floor
- Remove crepe- or rubber-soled shoes from the client, as they may drag on the floor, especially on carpeting
- Remove throw rugs or other obstacles over which the client may trip
- Install handrails at steps and in hallways and the bathrom
- Have no highly waxed floors
- Provide assistance to client as needed

communication and maintain swallowing function. Psychotherapy addresses the implications of living with a chronic disease; depression; and the possible psychiatric side effects of the medication regimen.

▶ NURSING PROCESS

▶ Assessment

▶ Subjective Data

Nursing assessment focuses on functional ability and activities. It includes eliciting client statements about symptom control and emotional status. Bowel and bladder elimination patterns are ascertained.

▶ Objective Data

Objective assessment involves evaluation of tremors, muscular rigidity, movement, posture, and gait for degree of impairment. Assessment of swallowing ability is necessary to maintain adequate nutrition and prevent aspiration. Mental/emotional status is evaluated for signs and symptoms of depression or dementia.

Skin is assessed for diaphoresis, or excessive oil production; skin integrity; and signs of injury from falls. Supine, sitting, and standing blood pressures are obtained to assess for orthostatic hypotension.

CLIENT TEACHING

Parkinson's Disease

Advise caregivers to:

- Encourage the client to be as independent as possible,
- Protect the client from injury, and
- Protect the client from unnecessary stress and fatigue.

Advise the client to:

- Use adaptive devices (cane, walker, feeding utensils),
- Take medications at scheduled times to maintain level in the body,
- Avoid taking multivitamins, foods high in vitamin B_6, and high-protein foods when taking L-dopa,
- Prevent constipation by drinking plenty of water and, possibly, using a stool softener, and
- Have intraocular pressure measured frequently if client has glaucoma.

Nursing diagnoses for a client with Parkinson's disease may include the following:

Nursing Diagnoses	Planning/Goals	Nursing Interventions
▶ *Impaired Physical Mobility related to muscle rigidity, gait disturbance, and bradykinesia*	The client will maintain optimal mobility.	Assess degree of muscle involvement by testing ROM, muscular rigidity, tremors, and gait.
		Administer medications within the time window that provides a constant therapeutic level for symptom control.
		Perform passive and active ROM exercises to maintain function.
		Ambulate, as client is able to tolerate.
		Frequently turn client in bed.
▶ *Bathing/Hygiene and Dressing/Grooming Self-care Deficit related to immobility, tremors, and bradykinesia*	The client will maintain optimal independence in self-care.	Assess client's ability to perform self-care.
		Encourage client to perform as much self-care as possible.
		Consult with occupational therapy for methods to increase the ability to perform self-care.
		Assist with daily care that the client is unable to perform alone.
▶ *Impaired Swallowing related to neuromuscular impairment*	The client will swallow with minimal choking and coughing and no aspiration.	Position client sitting upright when eating.
		Position client's head slightly forward and never extended to facilitate swallowing.
		Encourage client to take small bites.
		Provide small bites of food or pureed foods to prevent client from choking.
		Have suction equipment available during meals.

Evaluation Each goal must be evaluated to determine how it has been met by the client.

MULTIPLE SCLEROSIS

Multiple sclerosis (MS) is a chronic, progressive, degenerative disease wherein scattered nerve cells of the brain and spinal cord are demyelinated. The cause of MS is unclear. Research suggests, however, that it is an immune-mediated process with a viral trigger. The disease is more prevalent in colder climates and in people who lived in colder climates before the age of 15 years. In 75% of the cases, onset of symptoms is in adults between the ages of 20 and 40 (Frozena, 1997). Women are affected slightly more often than are men.

The white matter of the brain and spinal cord consists of axons covered by a white, lipid substance called myelin. This myelin sheath is an insulator that is involved in the conduction of impulses.

Multiple sclerosis is a central nervous system disease characterized by a loss of myelin in the brain, spinal cord, or both and by the occurrence of **sclerotic** (hardened) patches (Figure 25-19). The disease interferes with the conduction of impulses. The neurological deficit that occurs depends on which nerve cells are affected (Frozena, 1997).

As sclerotic tissue replaces the myelin, neurological function returns. Nerve fibers begin to degenerate as periods of exacerbation become more frequent. Degeneration of the nerve fibers leads to permanent neurological deficits.

Signs and symptoms of MS vary according to the areas of demyelination. The client may have one symptom or a combination of symptoms. Periods of exacerbation and remission also make diagnosis difficult. Symptoms may vary from hour-to-hour or day-to-day. Medical diagnosis is generally based on history and on elimination of other possible diagnoses. Magnetic resonance imaging and CT scan can be used to identify lesions of sclerotic tissue as the disease progresses. Cerebrospinal fluid reveals increased white blood cells, protein, and immunoglobulin (IgG), a diagnostic indicator.

Frozena (1997) classifies client symptoms as sensory, motor, or other disturbances. Sensory symptoms

Figure 25-19 A. Normal Nerve Fiber and Myelin Sheath; B. Multiple Sclerosis Destruction of Myelin Sheath

CLIENT TEACHING

Temperature Sensation

Because the client has a decreased sense of temperature, advise to:

- Be careful when cooking or otherwise around the kitchen stove,
- Use a bath thermometer to test bath or shower water so as to prevent burning, and
- Use only the low setting on a heating pad.

may include visual disturbances, numbness, paresthesia (burning, prickling, tingling), pain, and decreased sense of temperature. Motor symptoms may include decreased muscle strength, spasticity, paralysis, or bowel and bladder incontinence or retention.

Ataxia (loss of balance or coordination), **nystagmus** (constant, involuntary eye movements in any direction), speech disturbances, tremors, and **vertigo** (dizziness) may occur. Other possible symptoms are sexual dysfunction and mood changes ranging from depression to euphoria. Profound fatigue is common.

Exacerbations are frequently precipitated by periods of emotional or physical stress, such as infections, pregnancy, trauma, or fatigue. Hot baths or strenuous exercise may aggravate motor symptoms. Periods of exacerbation may last hours to months. Commonly, the periods of exacerbation become more frequent as the disease progresses. Complications such as urinary tract infection, pneumonia, pressure ulcers, contractures, and depression frequently occur. As the disease progresses and permanent neurological deficits occur, the client may become bedridden, have difficulty speaking and handling oral secretions, and/or develop emotional and intellectual disturbances.

Medical–Surgical Management

There is no cure or specific treatment for MS. Treatment goals are to limit exacerbations, prevent complications, and maintain functional level.

Pharmacological

According to Rudick (1997), the treatment of choice for relapsing–remitting MS is interferon beta (Avonex, Betaseron). For 2 or 3 months, clients usually experience flu-like symptoms after each injection. For clients who cannot take either of these two drugs, glatiramer acetate (Copaxone) is an option. The steroids adrenocorticotropic hormone (ACTH) or prednisone (Delasone) are used to decrease periods of exacerbation. Muscle relaxants such as dantrolene sodium (Dantrium) or baclofen (Lioresal) are used for muscle spasticity.

The immunosuppressive agents azathioprine (Imuran), cyclophosphamide (Cytoxan), or cyclosporine (Sandimmune) are administered to decrease immune response. Propantheline bromide (ProBanthine) is often used for urinary frequency and urgency. Bethanechol chloride (Urecholine) may be helpful for the client with a neurogenic bladder. Trimethoprim sulfamethoxazole (Bactrim or Septra) or nitrofurantoin macrocrystals (Macrodantin) is given prophylactically when urinary tract infections are a problem.

Diet

A well-balanced diet complete with roughage is necessary to promote bowel elimination. Plenty of fluids are also necessary. If the client is obese, a dietitian should be consulted for meal planning to help the client lose weight while maintaining adequate nutrition.

Activity

The goal of maintaining the highest possible functional level must be individualized to each client. Daily exercise is necessary for clients with limited motor involvement. Physical therapy may be necessary to prevent contractures, maintain muscle strength, or prevent loss of function from spasticity, or for gait training. Passive/active ROM exercises should be done several times per day. Occupational therapy may be used to maintain or attain self-care. Daily skills of cooking, doing laundry, or maintaining a job may also be encouraged.

▶ NURSING PROCESS

▶ Assessment

▶ Subjective Data

Subjective assessment includes eliciting client statements of symptoms and an historical accounting of exacerbations and remissions. Subjective data should

COMMUNITY/HOME HEALTH CARE

Adaptive Devices

To assist the client in self-care:

- Purchase a raised toilet seat,
- Use a long-handled comb and shoe horn, and
- Modify clothing so that the client can dress self.

CLIENT TEACHING

Risk of Falling

Advise the client to:

- Use assistive devices such as a walker or cane,
- Wear high-topped (above the ankles) shoes, with laces, and
- Watch feet when walking so as to know where they are.

include incidence of visual disturbances, hazy vision, loss of central vision, or diplopia (double vision). Symptoms of weakness, numbness, fatigue, bowel or bladder problems, sexual dysfunction, emotional instability, vertigo, changes in gait, urinary incontinence or retention, constipation, or difficulty swallowing must all be noted. Pain is not common.

▶ Objective Data

Objective assessment includes observation of gait for spastic or ataxic gait and a complete neurological examination.

Nursing diagnoses for a client with MS may include the following:

Nursing Diagnoses	Planning/Goals	Nursing Interventions
▶ *Impaired Physical Mobility related to muscle weakness, ataxia, spasticity, or perceptual impairment*	The client will maintain optimal mobility within physical limitations.	Assess motor status every 4 to 24 hours.
		Provide active and passive ROM every 8 hours.
		Turn bedridden clients every 2 hours.
		Use pillows, splints, high-topped (above the ankles) shoes with laces to maintain proper body alignment.
		Encourage client to perform daily activities as able given the limitations of the disease.
		Ambulate client four times daily with use of assistive devices as necessary.
▶ *Impaired Urinary Elimination related to changes in innervation of the bladder*	The client will have adequate bladder elimination with minimal post-void residual, urinary tract infections, and episodes of incontinence.	Assess for bladder retention or incontinence.
		Maintain fluid intake of 1,000 cc/day.
		Catheterize as necessary for retention or post-void residual.

continues

Nursing Diagnoses	Planning/Goals	Nursing Interventions
		Develop bladder program to meet individual needs of client. Toilet client at scheduled times even if no urge to go.
		Assess for signs and symptoms of urinary tract infection, such as elevated temperature and burning on urination.
▶ *Situational Low Self-esteem related to neuro-muscular and perceptual impairment*	The client will verbalize positive statements of self-esteem.	Assess client's concept of self in relation to changes brought about by the disease process.
		Allow client to verbalize feelings.
		Assist client in methods of adapting to change.
		Collaborate with other health care providers, such as mental health counselors and physicians.
		Teach client about the disease process.
		Refer client to local support groups (see Resources).
▶ *Sexual Dysfunction related to changes in sensation, genitalia, and musculature, and psychological response to diagnosis*	The client will seek counseling concerning sexual dysfunction.	Allow client to verbalize concerns.
		Suggest adaptations (planning time for sexual contact so as to conserve energy, alternatives to sexual intercourse, such as touching or holding).
		Refer client to appropriate health care providers.

Evaluation Each goal must be evaluated to determine how it has been met by the client.

SAMPLE NURSING CARE PLAN

THE CLIENT WITH MULTIPLE SCLEROSIS

Mrs. Donna Britton, a 37-year-old wife and the mother of two children, ages 3 years and 5 years, was diagnosed with MS two days ago. She presents with decreased sensation (paresthesia) in the lower extremities and muscle weakness of the right lower extremity. She has also experienced episodes of loss of central vision. Fatigue has affected her ability to care for her children and perform household tasks. She states, "I do not know what is going to happen to me." She is crying and states, "I do not know about multiple sclerosis or how I am going to take care of my children," and "I cannot get my housework done, and my children need more from me than I can give right now."

Her employer is concerned about her ability to perform her teaching responsibilities, but because he values her excellence as a teacher, he is willing to give her a few weeks off. She has bruises on her thigh, face, and arm from a fall that she experienced several days ago. The client presents in an outpatient clinic for follow-up care.

Nursing Diagnosis 1 *Deficient Knowledge related to disease process and lifestyle changes as evidenced by client statements, "I do not know what is going to happen to me, I do not know about multiple sclerosis or how I am going to take care of my children"*

PLANNING/GOALS	NURSING INTERVENTIONS	RATIONALE	EVALUATION
Mrs. Britton will verbalize knowledge of the disease process, pathophysiology, prognosis, and treatment, including the need to reduce stressors in her life, eat	Assess Mrs. Britton's knowledge of diagnosis, treatment regimen, and lifestyle changes. Ask specific questions.	Building on the knowledge base that Mrs. Britton already has provides a frame of reference for Mrs. Britton, helping her to relate new information and	Mrs. Britton verbalizes accurate information regarding the disease process, prognosis, and treatment. She states that by reducing

continues

a balanced diet, drink adequate fluids, and get adequate rest.

Begin teaching information about the pathophysiology and signs and symptoms of MS.

Discuss lifestyle changes that need to be made, such as planning rest periods, avoiding stressors, eating a balanced diet, and drinking plenty of fluids.

Emphasize the importance of keeping a diary of symptoms, activities, and overall feelings in order to identify stressors that exacerbate symptoms.

Provide information about the Multiple Sclerosis Society and offer available pamphlets. Provide the name and telephone number of a contact from the local MS support group or of another client who is willing to share.

integrate it into her behavior.

By keeping a diary of symptoms, activities, and overall feelings, Mrs. Britton can identify activities that exacerbate the symptoms.

Written material and contact with a national organization can provide more resources to strengthen Mrs. Britton's knowledge base.

Having an individual or support group with whom to discuss similar concerns can provide a great deal of emotional support as well as practical solutions to problems.

stressors, maintaining a balanced diet, taking in adequate fluids, and obtaining plenty of rest, she can prevent exacerbations of MS.

Nursing Diagnosis 2 *Impaired Home Maintenance related to fatigue, neuromuscular impairment, and difficulty in performing child care and household tasks as evidenced by client statements, "I cannot keep my housework done, my children need more from me than I can give right now" and by objective data including decreased sensation in lower extremities, muscle weakness, and fatigue*

PLANNING/GOALS	NURSING INTERVENTIONS	RATIONALE	EVALUATION
By the next appointment, Mrs. Britton will identify concerns and solutions to accomplishing home maintenance management.	Allow Mrs. Britton to verbalize concerns about home maintenance management.	By verbalizing fears and concerns, Mrs. Britton can begin to plan to organize tasks and responsibilities within her ability to perform home maintenance management.	Mrs. Britton identifies that she is able to care for her children with the assistance of her husband and her mother, but that she does not have the strength to maintain the housekeeping
	Assist Mrs. Britton in identifying areas of	Mrs. Britton can investigate methods of solving	

continues

concern, items that can be delegated, and possible solutions.

Assess the extended family's ability to assist with home maintenance management.

Ask Mrs. Britton to start identifying ways to decrease workload and to set priorities in expending energy.

Collaborate with social services to identify social agencies that can be of assistance.

Plan activities around rest periods.

Identify peak energy times and plan activities with peak energy in mind.

her home maintenance problems once she identifies concerns and explores possible solutions.

Assisting Mrs. Britton in assessment of extended family's ability to assist with home maintenance management may uncover opportunities that she had not considered.

Setting priorities helps Mrs. Britton focus on needed changes.

Exploration of available resources gives Mrs. Britton other possible solutions to achieving home maintenance management.

Planned rest periods can conserve Mrs. Britton's strength and prevent fatigue.

Mrs. Britton can accomplish more by using peak energy times to perform responsibilities.

responsibilities. Following further discussion of family commitments and availability of social supports, Mrs. Britton agrees to request weekly assistance from the women's group at her church.

Nursing Diagnosis 3 *Risk for Injury related to muscle weakness, decreased sensory perceptual deficits (vision, tactile, kinesthetic), and fatigue as evidenced by recent falls*

PLANNING/GOALS	NURSING INTERVENTIONS	RATIONALE	EVALUATION
Mrs. Britton will remain free of injury.	Teach Mrs. Britton to identify risk factors in the environment.	Mrs. Britton can avoid injury by recognizing and preventing environmental risk factors.	Injuries have been prevented by increasing Mrs. Britton's awareness of the risks involved with the disease process.
	Teach Mrs. Britton to identify risk factors of the disease process.	Mrs. Britton can reduce her risk of injury by identifying risk factors associated with the disease process, such as decreased sensation, weakness in the legs, and visual deficits.	

continues

Teach Mrs. Britton to avoid hot baths, hot tubs, saunas, and so on, because muscle weakness and paraesthesia can be exacerbated by the heat.	By avoiding hot baths, hot tubs, saunas, and so on, Mrs. Britton can prevent exacerbation of weakness and decreased sensation, thereby reducing her risk of injury.
Teach safety factors of wearing well-fitting, oxford-style shoes.	Wearing well-fitting tie shoes decreases the risk of falling by providing support for feet.

AMYOTROPHIC LATERAL SCLEROSIS (LOU GEHRIG'S DISEASE)

Amyotrophic lateral sclerosis (ALS) is a progressive, fatal disease characterized by the degeneration of motor neurons in the cortex, medulla, and spinal cord. The cause of the disease is not known, but a viral–immune response is suggested by current research. A genetic defect is also being researched. Age at onset is 40 to 70 years; men are affected two to three times more often than are women. Average time from onset to death is 3 years, but some have remained active 10 to 20 years after diagnosis.

The upper and lower motor neurons degenerate and deteriorate, causing atrophy of the muscles innervated by those neurons. The involved motor neurons are in the anterior horns of the spinal cord and lower brain stem. The muscles of the hands, forearms, and legs usually atrophy first. As the disease progresses most body muscles are affected. Muscle spasticity and reduced muscle strength result when upper motor neurons are involved. Lower motor neuron involvement causes muscle flaccidity, paralysis, and muscle atrophy. Sensory and intellectual function are not af-

fected. Respiratory function, ability to communicate, and emotional lability are affected as the disease progresses. Drooling, inability to handle oral secretions, and impaired swallowing occur.

Medical–Surgical Management

There is no known cure for ALS. The focus of medical management is to treat the symptoms and to promote independence for as long as possible.

Pharmacological

Muscle relaxants including diazepam (Valium), baclofen (Lioresal), and dantrolene sodium (Dantrium) are used to reduce spasticity. Quinidine is prescribed for muscle cramping. Increased salivation is treated with trihexyphenidyl hydrochloride (Artane), clonidine hydrochloride (Catapres), or amitriptyline hydrochloride (Elavil).

Diet

A regular diet adapted to provide soft, easily chewed food is maintained as long as the client can swallow. Tube feeding may be required to prevent aspiration as chewing and swallowing difficulties arise.

Activity

Ambulation and other activities are encouraged as long as possible.

Other Therapies

Physical and occupational therapy are used to maintain ROM and independence as much as possible. Speech therapy promotes maintenance of communication skills. Mental health counseling assists individual and family coping with the fatal disease.

PROFESSIONAL TIP

Advance Directives

Before the client with ALS becomes unable to communicate, suggest some advantages of drawing up a living will or giving someone power of attorney for health care.

▶ NURSING PROCESS

▶ Assessment

▶ Subjective Data

Subjective data gathered include the client's and family's emotional status and knowledge status. The client may also indicate chewing or swallowing difficulties as well as dyspnea and fatigue.

▶ Objective Data

Objective assessment includes evaluation of muscle weakness, muscle atrophy, spasticity of upper extremities, flaccid paralysis, difficulty chewing and swallowing, and respiratory status.

Nursing diagnoses for a client with ALS may include the following:

Nursing Diagnoses	Planning/Goals	Nursing Interventions
▶ *Impaired Physical Mobility related to muscle atrophy, weakness, and spasticity*	The client will maintain the highest possible functional ability within limitations of the disease.	Provide active and passive ROM at least twice daily. Use assistive devices to prevent contractures, for ambulation, and for muscle strengthening. Assess breath sounds for presence of congestion; skin for pressure areas; and legs for thrombophlebitis. Turn every 2 hours.
▶ *Impaired Verbal Communication related to weakness of muscles used for speech*	The client will communicate verbally or through an alternate communication method as speech muscles deteriorate.	Prolong verbal communication with speech therapy interventions consisting of voice projection and speech devices. Develop alternate methods of communicating prior to the loss of verbal skills. Eye-blinking for "yes" and "no"; communication boards, if any arm movement remains; and computer programs can be used.
▶ *Ineffective Breathing Pattern related to weakness of respiratory muscles and to fatigue*	The client will maintain an adequate PaO$_2$ level.	Assess breathing patterns frequently and observe for aspiration and the loss of the swallow reflex. Assess breath sounds every 4 to 8 hours, depending on the progress of the disease. Provide good pulmonary hygiene to prevent aspiration and pneumonia by liquifying secretions and suctioning. Turn from side to side to allow oral secretions to drain from mouth; suction oral pharynx, as necessary. Provide ventilation support, as ordered.
▶ *Powerlessness related to loss of control over life; physical dependence; and presence of a fatal disease*	The client will inform significant others of wishes while still able to communicate, so as to maintain some control over decisions.	Explore client and family emotional status and coping abilities. Allow client to verbalize feelings while still able to communicate and make decisions in daily care. Promote discussion of client's wishes with family, health care team, and legal representative while client is still able to speak. Provide client education about the disease process, support groups, and counseling to provide support.

Evaluation Each goal must be evaluated to determine how it has been met by the client.

ALZHEIMER'S DISEASE

Alzheimer's disease (AD) is a progressive, degenerative neurological disease wherein brain cells are destroyed. The cerebral cortex atrophies, and neuron loss and changes within the brain cells occur. Identified risk factors are advanced age, female gender, head injury, a history of thyroid disorders, and chromosomal abnormalities.

The cause of AD is unknown. Some hypothesized causes are genetic, viral, toxic, immunologic, traumatic, biochemical, or nutritional. The neurons of the frontal and medial temporal lobes are affected, with resultant biochemical and structural changes. Characteristic physiologic changes are neurofibrillary tangles and neuritic plaques (deposits of protein), which interfere with the cells' ability to transmit impulses (Figure 25-20). These changes are found in the association areas and scattered throughout the cortex. The hippocampus, that part of the limbic system responsible for learning, memory, and emotions, is affected. Those cells most affected are neurons that use acetylcholine as the

Figure 25-20 At autopsy, the cerebral cortex displays changes (white spots) caused by Alzheimer's disease. *(Photo courtesy of the Alzheimer's Association)*

neurotransmitter. The size of the brain and the amount of acetylcholine both decrease. An increased amount of aluminum is found in the brain tissue on autopsy (Hickey, 1997; Smeltzer & Bare, 2000).

Diagnosis is difficult because of the variety in clinical manifestations and the lack of a test specific to AD. Diagnosis is thus based on the clinical picture and the exclusion of other conditions that can cause similar clinical patterns, such as overmedication, metabolic disorders, depression, thyroid imbalance, or brain tumors. Computerized tomography or MRI is used to both measure brain atrophy and rule out other conditions.

The stages of AD are scaled from early to late. Different authors identify from three to six stages of the disease. The time frame for each stage varies from person to person. Table 25–9 lists clinical manifestations of early, middle, and late stages of AD.

COMMUNITY/HOME HEALTH CARE

Safe Environment for the Client with Alzheimer's Disease

- Keep furniture in the same place
- Orient client to surroundings and reorient as necessary
- Keep floors free of clutter
- Provide adequate lighting
- Monitor temperature of hot water and food
- Maintain monitoring system to prevent outside wandering
- Prevent access to sharp items such as knives and razors; hot items such as coffee pot and heaters; poisonous solutions such as cleaning supplies, paints, medications, and insecticides; and hazardous items such as power tools, guns, and electric fans

Table 25–9 STAGES OF ALZHEIMER'S DISEASE

STAGE	CLINICAL MANIFESTATIONS
Stage 1: Early	Forgetfulness, often subtle and masked by client
	Indecisiveness
	Increasing self-centeredness; decreasing interest in others, environment, social activities
	Difficulty in learning new information
	Slowed reaction time
	Beginnings of compromised performance at home and at work
Stage 2: Middle	Progressing forgetfulness, inability to remember names of family members or close friends
	Tendency to lose things
	Confusion
	Fearfulness
	Easily induced frustration and irritability; sometimes, angry outbursts
	Repetitive storytelling
	Beginnings of communication problems (inability to remember words, apparent aphasia)
	Inability to follow simple directions
	Difficulty in calculating numbers
	Beginnings of getting lost in familiar places
	Evasive or anxious interactions with others
	Physical activity (pacing, wandering)
	Changes in sleep–rest cycle (with frequent activity at night)
	Changes in eating patterns (possible constant hunger or none at all)
	Neglect of ADL and personal hygiene; changes in bowel and bladder continence; and dressing difficulties
	Inability to maintain safety without supervision
	Losses of social behaviors
	Paranoia
Stage 3: Late	Inability to communicate
	Inability to eat
	Incontinence (urine and feces)
	Inability to recognize family or friends
	Confinement to bed
	Total dependence relative to care

In late stages of the disease, EEG may indicate general slowing of brain waves. Definitive diagnosis is determined on autopsy with a brain biopsy. Though generally a disease of older people, AD does occur in people ages 40 to 50.

The family caring for a member who has Alzheimer's becomes more tied down as the disease progresses. Many clients with advanced Alzheimer's cannot be left alone. Respite care is important for the physical and mental health of the caregiver. With respite care, someone else (e.g., another family member, a friend, or a hired professional licensed practical/vocational nurse or registered nurse) comes in to care for the client with Alzheimer's while the primary caregiver gets away for a time. Respite care should be carried out on a routine basis, such as every 2 or 3 weeks or as often as is feasible.

Medical–Surgical Management

There is no curative treatment for AD. Management of the client is geared toward controlling undesirable symptoms. Other conditions such as drug reaction, depression, brain tumor, pernicious anemia, or hormonal imbalances must be ruled out.

Pharmacological

Antipsychotics, sedatives, antianxiety agents and antidepressants may be used to treat behavioral symptoms, though medications often make symptoms worse. Several medications that affect transmission of chemicals across synapses are under study. Tacrine hydrochloride (Cognex), an anticholinesterase, has demonstrated effectiveness in increasing cognitive function of clients with Alzheimer's, though there is a high incidence of liver toxicity, nausea, and vomiting with the use of this drug.

Diet

A high-fiber diet is used to prevent constipation. A high-calorie diet is needed for hyperactive clients. Fre-quent feedings of high nutritive value are preferable to three meals a day.

▶ NURSING PROCESS

▶ Assessment

▶ Subjective Data

Data about sleeping and eating habits must be collected. Each client must be assessed for individual signs and symptoms. The client is an expert at hiding these deficits in the early stages of the disease. A family interview may be helpful in ascertaining health and personal history.

▶ Objective Data

An objective neurological examination with particular attention to memory loss and gradual loss of thought processes and impaired judgment is important. Eating patterns, bowel and bladder control, aggressiveness, depression, ambulation, agitation, restlessness, sleep patterns, vision, and hearing should all be assessed. The client's ability to provide self-care, manage finances, drive, prepare meals, use the telephone, perform housekeeping, communicate needs, and perceive the environment also must be assessed. Attention must be directed to assessing the support system, the family caregiver, support groups, and availability of respite care for the caregiver. The care of the caregiver is often the focus of nursing care of the client with AD.

Nursing diagnoses for the client with Alzheimer's may include the following:

Nursing Diagnoses	Planning/Goals	Nursing Interventions
▶ *Risk for Injury related to inability to perceive danger in the environment, confusion, impaired judgment, and weakness*	The client will not experience injury.	Assess client's ability to perceive environmental hazards.
		Maintain a safe environment: eliminate clutter, position furniture/equipment in same place, monitor temperature of hot water and food, maintain monitoring system to prevent wandering into adverse climate or into traffic, provide adequate lighting, orient client and family to surroundings and reorient as necessary.
		Teach family to provide a safe home environment.
		Ensure that the client wears well-fitting tie shoes to reduce risk of falls.
▶ *Disturbed Thought Processes related to neuron degeneration, sleep deprivation*	The client will maintain optimal cognitive ability.	Assess for cognitive, memory, and communication deficits.
		Develop memory aids and cues to help client remember.
		Maintain a consistent environment and daily schedule.
		Approach client in a quiet, nonthreatening manner.
		Do not confront client with reality if it will only upset and agitate him. For example, do not tell a 90-year-old client who wants his mother that she is dead.
		Attend to nonverbal cues for unmet needs (e.g., pacing, grimacing, crying, agitation). The client may be hungry, have a full bladder, or be unable to ask to be repositioned.

continues

Nursing Diagnoses	Planning/Goals	Nursing Interventions
		Obtain a photo of client that can be recognized by the client. A current photo of client may appear as a stranger to the client, but a photo of the client at age 20 or 30 may be remembered.
		Give simple, single instructions.
▶ *Disturbed Sleep Pattern related to disorientation or irritability*	The client will sleep 4 to 5 hours each night.	Advise the client to avoid caffeine.
		Maintain a quiet environment.
		Provide a night light.
		Increase daytime activities to tolerance and use exercise to tire client.
		Provide comfort measures.

Evaluation Each goal must be evaluated to determine how it has been met by the client.

GUILLAIN-BARRÉ SYNDROME (POLYRADICULONEUROPATHY)

Guillain-Barré syndrome is an acute inflammatory process primarily involving the motor neurons of the peripheral nervous system. The cause of Guillain-Barré syndrome is not known, but most cases are preceded by a nonspecific infection. There may be an autoimmune or viral basis for this syndrome. Both spinal and cranial motor nerves can be involved. Sensory neurons may also be affected. The demyelination process begins in distal nerves and ascends symmetrically. Remyelination occurs from proximal to distal (Hickey, 1997).

Clinical manifestations occur in differing patterns, but include motor weakness and areflexia, or absence of reflexes. Characteristically, motor weakness begins in the legs and progresses up the body. Respiratory failure results from loss of respiratory muscle function. Cranial nerve involvement results in facial muscle deficits, difficulty in swallowing, and autonomic dysfunctions. Autonomic functions possibly affected are cardiac rhythm, blood pressure regulation, gastrointestinal mobility, and urine elimination.

Sensory involvement causes paresthesia and pain in the hands and feet. The pain progresses up the body and can interfere with sleep.

The three stages of Guillain-Barré syndrome are acute onset, lasting 1 to 3 weeks, the plateau period, lasting several days to 2 weeks, and the recovery phase, which involves remyelination and may last up to 2 years.

Diagnosis is based on the clinical picture of a recent viral infection and motor and possibly sensory deficits, along with characteristic diagnostic results. These results include both an elevated protein level in CSF without elevation of red blood cells or white blood cells and electromyelogram (EMG) showing slowed nerve conduction velocity of paralyzed muscles.

Medical–Surgical Management

Medical

The goal of medical management is prevention and treatment of complications such as immobility, infection, and respiratory failure.

Plasma exchanges have been found to decrease the severity and duration of symptoms. Plasmapheresis is performed in severe cases, this complete plasma exchange removes the antibodies affecting the myelin sheath. Three to four exchanges 1 to 2 days apart are initiated within the first 2 weeks of diagnosis of Guillain-Barré. Plasmapheresis may also be used late in the disease process for continued demyelination or lack of progress in remyelination. Mechanical ventilatory support will be initiated for decreased or lost respiratory function. Blood gas monitoring is used to assess respiratory function.

Surgical

Those who develop respiratory failure may require a tracheostomy along with mechanical ventilation.

Pharmacological

Steroids, such as adrenocorticotropic hormone (ACTH) and prednisone (Detasone) and immunosuppressive agents such as azathioprine (Imuran) or cyclophosphamide (Cytoxan), are prescribed to slow the demyelination process. Low doses of anticoagulants such as heparin are ordered to prevent thrombophlebitis.

Diet

A balanced diet is necessary to prevent tissue and muscle breakdown and to promote healing. If severe paralysis is present, a gastrostomy tube may be used to provide adequate nutrition.

Activity

Range of motion and muscle strength are maintained through physical therapy. Occupational therapy activities teach the client to maintain optional self-care within the limitation of the disease process. Pool therapy, or exercising in a swimming pool, is often used to maintain and strengthen muscles.

▶ NURSING PROCESS

▶ Assessment

▶ Subjective Data

Subjective data collected include client statements about return of sensation; pain; respiratory function; and knowledge.

▶ Objective Data

Assessment includes the status of motor and sensory functions which are monitored continuously in the acute phase of the illness. Progression of loss of function from distal to proximal is monitored, with particular emphasis on respiratory status. Decreased depth and quality of respirations and diminished breath sounds may be found. Status of autonomic functions is monitored by assessment of blood pressure, cardiac rhythm, urinary elimination, and bowel sounds. Assessment for complications of immobility includes breath sounds; signs of thrombophlebitis; loss of ROM; skin condition; and temperature.

Nursing diagnoses for a client with Guillain-Barré syndrome may include the following:

Nursing Diagnoses	Planning/Goals	Nursing Interventions
▶ *Ineffective Breathing Pattern related to loss of respiratory muscle function*	The client will be adequately ventilated.	Monitor respiratory status of client by assessing breath sounds, respiratory rate, and respiratory quality.
		Position client to facilitate maximal expansion of the chest wall for optimal breathing.
		Monitor oxygenation by assessing skin color, mental status, pulse oximeter readings, and blood gas values.
		Administer oxygen as ordered. Report failing respiratory status to the physician.
		Provide mechanical ventilation for respiratory failure.
▶ *Impaired Physical Mobility related to progressive loss of motor function*	The client will avoid complications of immobility (pneumonia, thrombophlebitis, pressure areas, and loss of ROM).	Monitor status of motor and sensory functions in an ongoing fashion.
		Have client turn, deep breathe, and cough every 2 hours.
		Suction client as necessary.
		Perform respiratory assessment for diminished breath sounds or congestion.
		Monitor vital signs (blood pressure, pulse, respiration, and temperature) every 4 to 8 hours.
		Assess for calf tenderness, redness, or increased warmth.
		Monitor for positive Homan's sign, indicative of deep vein thrombosis.
		Perform ROM to lower extremities every 2 to 4 hours.
		Use plexipulse boots, which are intermittent-pumping boots that promote return blood flow from the lower extremities.
		Administer low doses of heparin or other anticoagulants as prescribed.
		Apply antiembolism stockings.
		Assess condition of skin for pressure areas.
		Use specialty mattress.
		Massage client's back and pressure points with lotion three times a day.
		Assist client to sitting positions in wheelchair two to three times daily.
		Progress to ambulation as motor function returns.
		Apply high-topped shoes to keep feet in correct alignment.

continues

Nursing Diagnoses	Planning/Goals	Nursing Interventions
▶ *Dressing/Grooming Self-care Deficit related to decreased motor function*	The client will have self-care needs met.	Encourage self-care within the limitations of the neurological deficits.
		Maintain muscle strength and ROM with physical therapy.
		Provide ROM to all extremities three to four times daily.
		Provide daily care needs that client is unable to perform.
		Initiate rehabilitation following acute phase of illness with strengthening exercises, occupational therapy, and getting client out of bed several times per day to build strength and endurance.

Evaluation Each goal must be evaluated to determine how it has been met by the client.

HEADACHE

Headache, or **cephalalgia**, the condition of pain in the head, is caused by stimulation of pain-sensitive structures in the cranium, head, or neck. Headaches are classified as symptoms rather than a disease.

The pain-sensitive areas of the intracranial structure include the peripheral nerves, cerebral vasculature, and parts of the dura mater. The external supporting structures of the skin, muscles, and nasal passages are also sensitive to pain. The skull, brain tissue, and most of the meninges are insensitive to pain.

More than 45 million people in the United States each year suffer from headaches that require treatment by a physician (American Academy of Neurology [AAN], 1997a). Headaches are generally classified as either primary or secondary.

PRIMARY HEADACHES

Primary headaches are not caused by an underlying medical condition. They include tension-type, migraine, and cluster headaches (AAN, 1997a) (Table 25–10).

Tension-Type Headache

The most common type of headache is the tension type, affecting 75% of the population each year. The ache is steady rather than throbbing, affects both sides of the head, and occurs frequently, sometimes daily.

Migraine Headaches

Up to 18% of women experience migraine headaches each year, compared to 6% of men. Migraine headaches are vascular and recurrent. The initial vasoconstriction can cause neurological symptoms or an aura prior to the vasodilatation that causes the headache. The aura is a visual disturbance typically consisting of brightly colored or blinking lights or a pattern moving across the field of vision. When only the aura occurs, and there is no pain in the head, the migraine

is termed "silent." Serotonin levels increase in the initial phase prior to the onset of the headache, indicating involvement of neurotransmitters in the pathophysiology. Recent studies demonstrate that migraine pain results from inflammatory changes in blood vessels induced by activation of certain nerves (AAN, 1997a). Some migraine headaches may be triggered by certain foods or chemicals.

Cluster Headaches

A cluster headache develops around or behind one eye and is very severe. Generally, it awakens the person from sleep. The affected eye may tear and the nose become congested on the same side. These headaches occur in clusters daily for weeks or months, then disappear for a year or more. Most cluster headaches occur in men.

SECONDARY HEADACHES

Secondary headaches are the result of pathological conditions such as aneurysm, brain tumor, or inflamed cranial nerves. The headache is caused by compression, inflammation, or hypoxia of pain-sensitive structures.

Medical–Surgical Management

Medical

Medical management is based on the underlying cause of the headache. A thorough history of headache pattern, dietary pattern, and coping pattern is essential. Underlying pathology of brain tumor, aneurysm, and infection must be ruled out. If pathology is identified, secondary headache is diagnosed and therefore treatment will be based on findings. If no cause is found, management of primary headache will be based on symptoms.

Surgical

Surgical management may include clipping of an aneurysm or resection of a brain tumor.

Table 25–10 PRIMARY HEADACHE PATTERNS

TYPE	AURA	PAIN	TYPICAL PATTERN	DURATION
Tension	None	Steady ache	Usually begins gradually in frontal or temporal areas; affects both sides of the head; occur frequently, maybe daily	Hours
Classic Migraine	Duration of 15 to 30 minutes; sensory, usually visual (bright spots, zig-zag lines), unilateral or bilateral numbness or tingling in lips, face, or hand; difficulty thinking; confusion or drowsiness; sometimes preceded by premonition 24 hours before	Throbbing, intense; unilateral; tenderness in scalp; muscle contractions in neck and scalp followed by feelings of exhaustion	Periodic, recurrent; usually begins on awakening; begins in childhood or early adolescence; tends to be familial; nausea and vomiting typical; sensitivity to light and sound	Hours to days
Cluster	None	Intense throbbing; unilateral pain in orbitotemporal area	Causes awakening two to three times during the night; accompanied by watering eyes, nasal congestion, runny nose, facial flushing over the throbbing area; after cluster headaches for days, weeks, or months may be free of symptoms for a year or more; same side of head usually involved; usually in men	30 minutes to 2 hours

Pharmacological

Management is either abortive, to stop the headache, or prophylactic, to prevent reccurrence or to decrease frequency of headaches. Abortive therapy for vascular headaches includes ergotamine tartrate (Ergostat), administered orally, sublingually, rectally, intramuscularly, or subcutaneously at the beginning of a migraine headache. Cafergot, containing ergotamine and caffeine, is also used for abortive therapy. These agents cause vasoconstriction and block serotonin uptake. Promethazine hydrochloride (Phenergan) is often used to control nausea and vomiting. Narcotic or nonnarcotic analgesics are administered for pain relief.

Prophylactic treatment includes the beta blockers propranolol hydrochloride (Inderal) and methysergide maleate (Sansert), which prevent dilation of the blood vessels and interrupt the serotonin mechanism. Clonidine hydrochloride (Catapres) directly affects the ability of the blood vessels to constrict or dilate. Tricyclic antidepressants such as amitriptyline hydrochloride (Elavil), block the uptake of serotonin.

Diet

A strict food diary should be kept to identify precipitating foods. After all suspect foods have been eliminated from the diet, skin testing for allergies may be performed. Introduction of suspect foods may be done one at a time to identify triggering foods. Alcohol; cured meats containing nitrates; aged cheeses; monosodium glutamate (MSG); citrus fruits; chocolate; and red wines are common precipitating foods.

Activity

Activities that precipitate headaches must be identified and eliminated if possible. Stressful situations are frequently precipitating agents. Biofeedback, relaxation techniques, stress reduction, and development of coping mechanisms are useful in reducing the occurrence of headaches caused by stress and tension.

CLIENT TEACHING

Headaches

Advise the client to:

- Keep a diary of headache history to ascertain pattern,
- Avoid foods that trigger headache,
- Reduce salt intake, and
- Practice relaxation techniques.

Nursing Management

Nursing interventions focus on relieving pain and assisting the client in managing the pain. Identifying methods of decreasing pain, such as effective use of medications and managing the environment to minimize stimulation from light, noise, activity, are also nursing priorities.

The client should be assisted in developing a plan for accomplishing daily activities when incapacitated by a headache. Teaching the client to keep a diary of headache history to determine patterns in headache development is essential. The nurse must assist the client in changing lifestyle to decrease the incidence of headaches in ways such as minimizing stress, avoiding certain foods, reducing salt intake during premenstrual time frame, and using relaxation techniques.

TRIGEMINAL NEURALGIA (TIC DOULOUREUX)

Trigeminal neuralgia is a condition of cranial nerve V and is characterized by abrupt paroxysms of pain and facial muscle contractions. **Neuralgia** is nerve pain. The pain follows one of the three branches of the trigeminal nerve: the ophthalmic, maxillary, or mandibular. The last two branches are most commonly affected (Figure 25-21).

The etiology of trigeminal neuralgia is not known, but injury, dental caries, dental work, and anatomic

position of the nerves have been identified as possible causes. Pain is precipitated when trigger points are stimulated, causing periods of intense pain and facial twitching lasting from seconds to minutes. These periods may last several weeks to months. Periods of remission interspersed with exacerbations occur with increasing frequency with advancing age (Hickey, 1997).

Medical–Surgical Management

Drug therapy, nerve blocks, and surgery are treatment modalities for trigeminal neuralgia.

Surgical

Surgical approaches to relieve pain include percutaneous electrocoagulation with radio frequency. This procedure affects the pain-sensory fibers but causes little damage to the touch, proprioception, and motor fibers. Longer-term relief or permanent relief may be obtained.

Pharmacological

Phenytoin (Dilantin) and carbamazepine (Tegretol) are used to shorten the length of the paroxysmal pain. Nerve blocks using alcohol and phenol injections into the nerve provide temporary relief for 8 to 16 months.

Nursing Management

Goals of nursing interventions are relief of pain, prevention of injury, prevention of self-care deficits, and promotion of social interaction. The client with trigeminal neuralgia frequently experiences such severe pain that grooming, talking, and eating are avoided. It is especially important to provide good oral hygiene if the client is on phenytoin (Dilantin), because the medication causes hyperplasia of the gums. The client should be taught to identify both the trigger points that stimulate the pain and ways to avoid those areas without neglecting daily needs.

The client who has had surgery may have lost the mechanisms that protect the eye from injury, and will

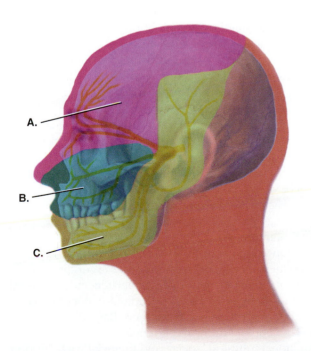

Figure 25-21 Areas of Face Innervated by the Trigeminal Nerve (CN-I): A. Ophthalmic; B. Maxillary; C. Mandibular

CLIENT TEACHING

Dental Work in the Client with Trigeminal Neuralgia

The client with trigeminal neuralgia should:

- Plan to have dental work done during a period of remission,
- Inform the dentist of the condition, and
- Maintain good dental hygiene, especially during remission.

need to be taught not to touch his eye and to observe for redness of the eye and conjunctiva. Following surgery, the client may not feel pain caused by dental caries, so it is important to encourage routine visits to the dentist for oral examination.

ENCEPHALITIS, MENINGITIS

Encephalitis is inflammation of the brain. **Meningitis** is inflammation of the meninges. The most common cause of encephalitis or meningitis is a virus. Bacteria, fungi, or parasites can also be causative factors. The virus or other causative agent enters the brain either through the bloodstream as a direct extension of trauma or by nerve pathways.

The inflammatory process causes demyelination of white matter and degeneration of neurons. Cerebral edema, hemorrhage, and necrosis of brain tissue can also occur. Clinical manifestations vary depending on the causative agent, area of involvement, and degree of damage to nerve tissue. Fever, headache, nuchal rigidity, photophobia, irritability, lethargy, nausea, and vomiting are typical signs and symptoms. As the disease progresses, level of consciousness may decrease and other neurological dysfunctions occur, including motor weakness, aphasia, seizures, behavioral changes, or even death. A lumbar puncture is performed to test CSF for the causative agent, presence of white blood cells or red blood cells, and elevated protein level. A complete blood count is done to identify the presence of viral or bacterial infection.

Medical–Surgical Management

Medical

Treatment is supportive and based on presenting symptoms. The aim of treatment is to prevent or decrease intracranial pressure and to minimize neurological deficits. Intravenous fluids are given to rehydrate the client.

Pharmacological

Antibiotics or antiinfectives are administered in massive doses as appropriate for the causative agent. They may be given intravenously or intrathecally into the spinal canal. Most viral agents do not respond to antibiotics or antiinfectives. Glucocorticosteroids are administered to prevent cerebral edema. Osmotic diuretics may be used to reduce cerebral edema. To prevent seizures, anticonvulsants are often ordered. Antipyretics are often given to reduce fever.

Diet

Optimal nutritional status must be maintained to promote response to the infection.

Activity

A quiet environment with minimal stimulation from noise, light, or client activity is maintained. Routine turning, ROM exercises, pulmonary hygiene, and skin care are required to prevent the complications of immobility.

Nursing Management

In the acute stage, the client must be monitored for changes in neurological status, especially for changes in level of consciousness and for signs of increasing intracranial pressure. A quiet environment will decrease external stimulation. The client must be observed for seizure activity and protected from injury. Comfort measures such as oral hygiene, tepid baths, and administration of analgesics for relief of headaches should be offered.

HUNTINGTON'S DISEASE OR CHOREA

Huntington's disease is a chronic, progressive hereditary disease of the nervous system. It is characterized by a progressive involuntary choreiform movement and progressive dementia.

The cells of the basal ganglia, which control movement, die prematurely. Cells in the cerebral cortex also die, interfering with thought processes, memory, perception, and judgment. Age of onset is usually 35 to 45 years, with death occurring 10 to 15 years following onset of symptoms (Smeltzer & Bare, 2000). The theorized cause is lack of γ-aminobutyric acid (GABA), a neurotransmitter. Each child of a person with Huntington's disease has a 50% chance of developing the disease. A genetic marker has been discovered that indicates whether the person will develop the disease. However, there is no cure for this devastating progressive disease.

Clinical manifestations are **chorea**, abnormal involuntary, purposeless movements of all musculature of the body. Facial tic, grimacing, difficulty in chewing and swallowing, speech impairment, disorganized gait, and bowel and bladder incontinence also occur. Mental or intellectual impairment progresses to dementia. The client may experience paranoia, hallucinations, or delusions. Emotions are labile, from outbursts of anger to profound depression, apathy, or euphoria. A ravenous appetite is usually present, but because of the constant movement, the client is often emaciated and exhausted. Death usually results from heart failure, pneumonia, infection, or an accident (Smeltzer & Bare, 2000).

The entire family experiences this disease in an emotional, physical, social, and financial way. Supportive care is required as the family progresses through life with a loved one with Huntington's disease. Because of the hereditary factor, genetic counseling is necessary.

Medical–Surgical Management

Pharmacological

Medications used to decrease choreiform movement are dopamine receptor blockers, chlorpromazine (Thorazine), haloperidol (Haldol), thiothixene (Navane), and reserpine (Serpasil), which depletes presynaptic dopamine. Antidepressants, such as desipramine hydrochloride (Norpramin) and fluoxetine hydrochloride (Prozac), and antipsycotics, such as fluphenazine hydrochloride (Prolixin), are used for emotional disturbances.

Diet

The diet must be high in calories to provide for the high energy needs caused by the continuous movement. Chewing and swallowing difficulties necessitate foods that are easy to chew or foods cut into small pieces to prevent choking.

Activity

Ambulation is maintained as long as possible. A safe environment must be maintained to prevent injury from falls or from sharp objects. Driving is usually restricted when choreiform movement or impaired judgment interferes with the ability to drive safely.

Nursing Management

Nursing interventions include a holistic approach to the client's care. Collaboration with the social worker, the chaplain, the physician, and the mental health worker is necessary.

Teach the client and family about the disease process, the progress of the disease, and the genetic factors involved. Safety factors must be considered. Fall prevention measures, such as removing throw rugs and small objects from the floor, and injury prevention measures, such as removing sharp or dangerous objects such as guns and knives from the home, are implemented. The hazard of choking also must be addressed, by teaching the family to cut the client's food into small pieces and to serve soft foods and by teaching the Heimlich maneuver.

GILLES DE LA TOURETTE'S SYNDROME

Gilles de la Tourette's syndrome is a neurological movement disorder that also has prominent behavioral manifestations. Clinical manifestations include motor tics, and involuntary repetitive movements of the mouth, face, head, or neck muscles. The trunk and extremities may also be involved. Motor tics may take the form of forceful eye blinking or toe touching. Vocal tics or repetitive involuntary vocalizations, may take the form of sniffing, grunting, throat clearing, or coprolalia (involuntary and inappropriate swearing). Other complex motor and vocal tics that may also be present include copropraxia, involuntary and effectively appropriate use of obscene gestures; echolalia, involuntary repetition of the speech of others; and palilia, involuntary repetition of the person's own speech (Hyde & Weinberger, 1995). The obsessive–compulsive symptoms of repetitive handwashing or checking rituals may also be exhibited.

Structural abnormalities in the basal ganglia and prefrontal cortex have been identified in research as the possible cause of Tourette's syndrome (Hyde & Weinberger, 1995). Attention deficit hyperactivity disorder and obsessive–compulsive disorders may also coexist with Tourette's syndrome.

Onset is prior to age 18 years, with males being more commonly affected than females. Estimates of prevalence range from 2.9 to 49.5 per 100,000 children. Tourette's is a genetic disorder, with the affected individual having a 50% chance of passing the gene on to children (AAN, 1997b).

Medical–Surgical Management

Pharmacological

Tics may be controlled with clonadine (Catapres), haloperidol (Haldol), or primozide (Orap). Coexisting attention deficit hyperactivity disorder may be controlled with clonidine (Catapres), methylphenidate (Ritalin), or pemoline (Cylert). Clomypramine (Anafranil) or fluoxetine (Prozac) can be used to keep obsessive–compulsive behaviors under control (Kurlan, 1998). Acetaminophen (Tylenol) may help the discomfort of muscle spasms.

Other Therapies

As they age, clients may learn to suppress tics in social situations. Psychotherapy and family counseling are beneficial in coping with social stigma and adjustment problems.

Nursing Management

The client and the family with Tourette's syndrome need a great deal of emotional support and will benefit from knowing about the availability of support groups for clients with Tourette's syndrome. The nurse should teach about the disease process and expectations for the client. Behavioral modification techniques are generally effective; the nurse must know which modification techniques are being used and must follow through with consistent responses.

CASE STUDY

Mr. Domingo Ochoa, a 76-year-old retired farmer, was admitted to the emergency room with left-sided hemiplegia, difficulty swallowing, and inability to speak. He was awake and watching the staff upon admission. He moved his right arm to indicate that Mrs. Ochoa was his wife, but was unable to speak or form sounds. Mrs. Ochoa stated that her husband was working in the garden, picking tomatoes and cucumbers, when he fell to the ground 30 minutes before admission. The emergency room nurse administered oxygen through nasal cannula at 2 liters per minute and obtained vital signs. His blood pressure was 182/98, pulse was 88, respirations were 20, and temperature was 100.5°F. The emergency room physician ordered an MRI scan of the head, a complete blood count, and prothrombin time (PT). The MRI indicated that Mr. Ochoa experienced a CVA caused by a bleeding into the brain.

The following questions will guide your development of a nursing care plan for the case study.

1. List clinical manifestations other than the ones Mr. Ochoa experienced that can occur with a CVA.

2. List subjective and objective data that a nurse would obtain.

3. Identify three individualized nursing diagnoses and goals for Mr. Ochoa.

4. Mr. Ochoa is transferred to a general medical unit for 3 days, then is transferred to a rehabilitation center for intensive therapy. What pertinent nursing actions should a nurse perform in caring for Mr. Ochoa in the acute setting and the rehabilitation setting related to:

     Mobility
     Safety
     Elimination
     Skin integrity
     Comfort and rest

5. What teaching will Mr. Ochoa need before discharge from the rehabilitation facility?

6. List at least three client outcomes for Mr. Ochoa.

SUMMARY

- The nervous system controls all bodily functions, from movement, to thinking, to processing information, to autonomic responses.

- The frontal lobe of the cerebrum specializes in emotional attitudes and responses, formation of thought processes, motor function, judgment, personality, and inhibitions.

- The parietal lobe of the cerebrum is a purely sensory region for interpretation of all senses except smell; the purpose is to analyze sensations, including pain, touch, and temperature, from receptors in the skin.

- The temporal lobe of the cerebrum houses Wernicke's area, the primary auditory association area, where words that are heard are interpreted. Memory is also a function of the temporal lobe, especially memories that are highly detailed or involve multiple sensations.

- A special interpretive area located at the junction of the temporal, parietal, and occipital lobes integrates somatic, auditory, and visual sensory interpretations.

- The occipital lobe of the cerebrum is responsible for visual interpretation and visual association.

- Disorders of the nervous system cause complex dysfunctions; the nurse must use assessment skills and quickly recognize changes in condition.

- Teaching about injury prevention and the effects and prognosis of the disorder are required to meet the physical and psychosocial needs of the client and family.

- Many neurological disorders potentiate injury. Nursing care must include providing the client and family with necessary safety information.

- In order to maintain and restore functional ability, rehabilitation is initiated from the first contact with the client.

Review Questions

1. The most important indicator of change in neurological status is:

   a. level of consciousness.
   b. pupil reaction.
   c. vital signs.
   d. motor function.

2. Cranial nerves III, IV, and VI all have functions affecting:

   a. special senses.
   b. facial movement.
   c. eye movement.
   d. gag reflex.

3. Assessment of intellectual function requires that the nurse:

   a. have knowledge of the client's prior ability to function.
   b. administer a written test to determine the client's IQ level.
   c. utilize auscultation, percussion, and palpation skills.
   d. observe the client's behavior, posture, and facial expression.

4. Contusion of the brain is a (an):

   a. shaking of the brain.
   b. bleeding into the brain tissue.
   c. open head injury.
   d. bruising of the brain.

5. Benign brain tumors can be:

   a. more anxiety producing than are malignant tumors.
   b. more life threatening than are malignant tumors.
   c. treated with radiation therapy.
   d. the cause of increased intracranial pressure.

6. Miss Webster, a 24-year-old client with Guillain-Barré Syndrome, can be told which of the following?

   a. The nerve degeneration slowing continues to progress in this chronic degenerative nerve disease.
   b. The disease is an acute inflammatory process with most clients regaining complete function.
   c. Respiratory failure requiring chronic ventilatory support may occur.
   d. Motor function deficit will occur, but sensation will remain.

Critical Thinking Questions

1. What are the similarities between Parkinson's disease and Alzheimer's disease?

2. What are the most important things to teach a client with multiple sclerosis?

3. Identify the rationale for each nursing intervention given for the possible nursing diagnoses in this chapter.

WEB FLASH!

- Try to locate each of the disorders in this chapter on the Internet. Share information on new medications, diagnostic tests, treatments, or nursing care found on the web sites.
- What sites could you recommend to families and individuals coping with any of these disorders?
- List books, videos, or other media on these disorders found on the Internet.

NURSING CARE OF THE CLIENT: SENSORY SYSTEM

CHAPTER 26

MAKING THE CONNECTION

Refer to the following chapters to increase your understanding of the sensory system:

- **Chapter 5, Communication**
- **Chapter 7, Wellness Concepts**
- **Chapter 9, Loss, Grief, and Death**
- **Chapter 12, Health Assessment**
- **Chapter 14, Pain Management**

- **Chapter 16, Nursing Care of the Surgical Client**
- **Chapter 25, Nursing Care of the Client: Neurological System**
- **Chapter 35, Nursing Care of the Older Client**

LEARNING OBJECTIVES

Upon completion of this chapter, you should be able to:
- *Define key terms.*
- *Compare and differentiate common disorders of the special senses.*
- *Identify the structure and function of the major parts of the eye and ear.*
- *Explain the purpose of the common diagnostic tests for sensory problems.*
- *List the nursing assessments and common nursing diagnoses related to sensory impairment.*
- *Assist in planning nursing care for clients with sensory disorders.*
- *List some of the common sensory aids for the visual and hearing impaired.*

INTRODUCTION

From the moment we wake in the morning until we fall asleep at night, we are inundated with information from the outside world through our senses. Although most of us do not consider our senses as organs of protection, we depend on visual and auditory alarms to keep us from harm. This chapter reviews the structure and function, identifies appropriate nursing diagnoses, and presents the medical and nursing management of the five senses: hearing, vision, taste, smell, and touch.

KEY TERMS

acoustic neuroma
affect
afferent nerve
  pathways
arousal
astigmatism
awareness
cataract
cerumen
chalazion
cognition
conductive hearing
  loss
conjunctivitis
consciousness
disorientation
efferent nerve
  pathways
glaucoma
hallucination
hyperopia
illusion
judgment
keratitis

macular
  degeneration
Ménière's disease
myopia
nystagmus
orientation
otitis externa
otitis media
otosclerosis
perception
presbycusis
presbyopia
sensation
sensorineural hearing
  loss
sensory deficit
sensory deprivation
sensory overload
sensory perception
strabismus
stye
tinnitus
vertigo

SENSATION, PERCEPTION, AND COGNITION

Sensation is the ability to receive and process stimuli through the sensory organs. There are two types of stimuli; external and internal. External stimuli are received and processed through the senses of sight (visual), hearing (auditory), smell (olfactory), taste (gustatory), and touch (tactile). Internal stimuli are received and processed through kinesthetic (an awareness of the position of the body) and visceral (feelings originating from large organs within the body) modes.

Perception is the ability to experience, recognize, organize, and interpret sensory stimuli. **Sensory perception** is the ability to receive sensory impressions and, through cortical association, relate the stimuli to past experiences and form an impression of the nature of the stimulus.

Perception is closely associated with **cognition**, the intellectual ability to think. The processes of organizing and interpreting stimuli are dependent on a person's level of intellectual functioning. Cognition includes the elements of memory, judgment, and orientation. The well-being of an individual is dependent on the functions of sensation, perception, and cognition because it is through these mechanisms that the person fully experiences and interacts with the environment.

Sensory, perceptual, and cognitive alterations can be either temporary or progressive in their manifestations and can result from disease or trauma. Whatever the status or cause of the alterations, these conditions usually lead to social isolation and increased dependence on others. In addition, impairment in sensory, perceptual, and cognitive functions can place the individual at risk for injury to self or to others.

ANATOMY AND PHYSIOLOGY REVIEW

Sensation, perception, and cognition are neurological functions. The nervous system is composed of two major subsystems: the central nervous system (CNS) and the peripheral nervous system (PNS), which consists of the somatic and autonomic nervous systems (Figure 26-1). The CNS and PNS act in unison to accomplish three purposes: collection of stimuli from the receptors at the end of the peripheral nerves; transport of the stimuli to the brain for integration and cognition processing; and conduction of responses to the stimuli from the brain to responsive motor centers in the body. Refer to Chapter 25 for the anatomy of the neurological system.

Sensory perception involves the function of both the cranial and peripheral nerves. The cranial nerves arise from the brain and govern the movement and function of various muscles and nerves throughout the body. The peripheral nerves connect the CNS to other parts of the body (Figure 26-2).

Figure 26-1 The Nervous System (*From* Fundamentals of Nursing Standards & Practice, *by S. DeLaune and P. Ladner, 1998, Albany, NY: Delmar. Reprinted with permission.*)

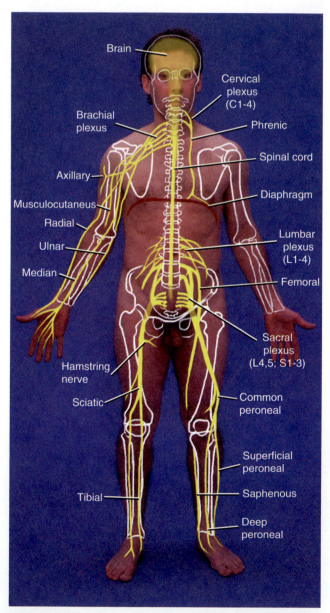

Figure 26-2 The Peripheral Nerves (*From* Fundamentals of Nursing Standards & Practice, *by S. DeLaune and P. Ladner, 1998, Albany, NY: Delmar. Reprinted with permission.*)

Components of Sensation and Perception

The sensory system is a complex network that consists of **afferent nerve pathways** (ascending pathways that transmit sensory impulses to the brain), **efferent nerve pathways** (descending pathways that send sensory impulses from the brain), the spinal cord, the brainstem, and the cerebrum.

Components of Cognition

Cognition includes the cerebral functions of memory, affect, judgment, perception, and language. In order for these higher functions to occur, consciousness must be present.

Consciousness

Consciousness is a state of awareness of self, others, and the surrounding environment. It affects both cognitive (intellectual) and affective (emotional) functions. An alert individual (one who is aware of self and stimuli) is able to perceive reality accurately and to base behavior on those perceptions. The components of consciousness provide a foundation for behavior and emotional expression, thereby contributing to the uniqueness of each individual's personality. Consciousness may be altered by various metabolic, traumatic, or other factors such as the pharmacological actions of drugs that affect mental status. The primary components of consciousness are arousal and awareness, both of which must be present before higher cognitive functioning occurs.

Arousal The degree of **arousal** (state of wakefulness and alertness) is indicated by a person's general response and reaction to the environment. People exhibit arousal by behaving in an alert and aware manner and by experiencing periods of wakefulness. The degree of an individual's arousal is indicated by the general response and reaction to the environment. Impaired arousal can exist when a sleep pattern deficit is experienced. There may be an inability to take advantage of opportunities for activity because of inadequate periods of rest.

Awareness Awareness is the capacity to perceive sensory impressions and react appropriately through thoughts and actions. An essential element in

PROFESSIONAL TIP

CNS Deficits and Illness

Specific conditions, such as diabetes mellitus and atherosclerosis, can impair neurosensory pathways and result in deficits in sensation, perception, and cognition. Diseases of the CNS can result in loss of sensory function and paralysis.

PROFESSIONAL TIP

Effects of Medications on Sensation
Certain medications have the potential to alter or depress the neurosensory system. For example, sedatives and narcotics can alter the perception of sensory stimuli. Medications such as analgesics can alter the level of consciousness.

awareness is **orientation** (perception of self in relation to the surrounding environment). When awareness is impaired, orientation to time is frequently the first area affected. The degree of disorientation is worse when the individual loses awareness of place and self (person).

Memory

There are three types of memory: immediate, recent, and remote. Immediate memory is the retention of information for a specified and usually short period of time. The recall of a telephone number long enough to dial it is an example of immediate memory. Recent memory is the ability to recall events that have occurred over the past 24 hours, such as remembering the foods eaten for dinner the previous night. Remote memory is the retention of experiences that occurred during earlier periods of life, such as an adult's memories of childhood or school days. The ability to learn is dependent on remote memory.

Affect

Affect (expression of mood or feeling) is an important component of cognition in that variations of mood can affect one's thinking ability. For example, a client with a flat affect due to depression may have difficulty sustaining concentration or attention.

Judgment

Judgment, the ability to compare or evaluate alternatives in order to arrive at an appropriate course of action, is closely related to reality testing and depends on effective cognitive functioning. Behaviors indicative of impaired judgment include impulsiveness, unrealistic decision making, and inadequate problem-solving ability.

Perception

Perceptions are considered in the context of the individual's awareness of reality. Misperceptions of reality can occur in the form of an **illusion** (an inaccurate perception or misinterpretation of sensory stimuli) or a **hallucination** (a sensory perception that occurs in the absence of external stimuli and is not based on reality).

Clients who are anxious and fearful or who are on therapeutic regimens involving the use of certain

PROFESSIONAL TIP

Remote Memory

Remote memory should be assessed only when client responses about past events can be validated, either by others or by written account.

medications may experience misperceptions of environmental stimuli. For example, a postoperative client, after receiving analgesic medication for pain, may see the belt from his bathrobe lying on the floor and become terrified because he thinks there is a snake in the room. Once the nurse determines that the client is experiencing an illusion, appropriate reassurance and reality orientation can be implemented to reduce the client's anxiety.

Language

Language is one of the most complex of cognitive functions, involving not only the spoken word but also reading, writing, and comprehension. Characteristics of speech are fluency (ability to talk in a steady manner), prosody (melody of speech that conveys meaning through changes in the tempo, rhythm, and intonation), and content.

ASSESSMENT

When caring for clients with sensory, perceptual, and cognitive alterations, the nurse must obtain a health history and perform a physical examination to identify existing or potential problems in this area of functioning. The physical examination focuses specifically on the client's ability to hear, see, taste, smell, and touch. Refer to Chapter 25 for assessment of cranial nerves. Table 26–1 provides some guidelines helpful in assessing sensory perceptual status.

When assessing clients for sensory, perceptual, and cognitive alterations, the level of consciousness (LOC) must also be evaluated. Refer to Chapter 25 for the Glasgow Coma Scale, developed to assess LOC objectively.

Safety: Sensory Impairments
Vision—Risk of tripping, falling
Hearing—Lack of awareness of warning sounds such as automobile horns, sirens, smoke alarms
Olfactory—Inability to perceive warning odors such as burning food, escaping gas
Gustatory—Inability to recognize spoiled or contaminated food or beverages
Tactile—Lack of awareness of excessive pressure on a body part; at risk for exposure to extreme temperatures (frostbite, burns)

Table 26–1 ASSESSING SENSORY PERCEPTUAL STATUS

SENSATION BEING ASSESSED	ASSESSMENT FOCUS
Visual	• Presence of visual problems, including: —Decreased acuity —Blurred vision —Double vision —Blind spots —Rainbows or halos around objects —Photosensitivity —Loss of peripheral field (narrowing) • Difficulty seeing far or near • Family history of visual problems (such as glaucoma, cataracts) • Use of contact lenses or eyeglasses • Date of last eye examination
Auditory	• Presence of hearing problems • Recent changes in hearing ability • Ability to distinguish sounds (tone and pitch) • Presence of buzzing or ringing noises • Use of a hearing aid
Gustatory	• Changes in ability to taste • Difficulty in differentiating salty, sweet, sour, and bitter tastes • Changes in appetite
Olfactory	• Changes in ability to smell • Ability to distinguish common smells (such as food, perfume, flowers)
Tactile	• Difficulty in feeling temperature changes in extremities • Impairment of pain perception in extremities • Presence of unusual sensations in extremities (such as tingling or numbness)

From Fundamentals of Nursing Standards & Practice, *by S. DeLaune and P. Ladner, 1998, Albany, NY: Delmar. Reprinted with permission.*

The Ear

The human ear can be divided into three main anatomical components: the outer ear, middle ear, and inner ear (Figure 26-3). Each part plays a major role in hearing. Similar to other paired organs in the body, dysfunction of part or all of one ear does not affect the function of the other.

Outer Ear

The outer ear is composed of the auricle (pinna), a cartilaginous flap on the temporal sides of the head,

Sensory Changes in the Elderly
- When the eye lens yellows and becomes cloudy, the ability to discern colors, especially greens and blues, is impaired.
- The elderly need more light to see because the pupils become smaller, letting in less light.
- It takes the elderly longer to accommodate (adjust) to darkness and glare.
- Tear production decreases with age, predisposing to dry eye syndrome and corneal irritation.
- The most common hearing loss is sensorineural, which can be helped by a hearing aid.
- Taste sensation may be dulled with age.

and the external ear canal, or external auditory meatus. The outer ear is responsible for collecting, conducting, and amplifying sound waves. The auricle directs sounds through the external ear canal to the tympanic membrane (eardrum). This canal is lined with ceruminous glands that secrete **cerumen** (ear wax), a yellowish brown protective substance that guards against certain bacteria and small insects, and traps dust and debris that may damage the inner ear. Normally, the cerumen works its way out of the ear as we eat, chew,

or speak. However, cerumen can build up and actually cause significant hearing loss in the affected ear.

The tympanic membrane (TM) serves as a boundary between the outer and middle ear. As sound waves vibrate against the membrane, the motion is transmitted to the bones of the inner ear. In an acute ear infection, fluid fills the middle ear, creating significant pressure on the tympanic membrane.

Middle Ear

The three bones of the middle ear are collectively referred to as the ossicles and include the malleus (hammer), incus (anvil), and stapes (stirrup), so named because they resemble the tools of a blacksmith's trade. The malleus is attached to the upper, inner portion of the tympanic membrane. The head of the malleus connects with the incus which then joins the stapes. The flat oval bone of the stapes, called the footplate, rests on the oval window (part of the inner ear). The vibration created by sound waves passes through the outer ear canal to the tympanic membrane and then to these three bones.

The eustachian tube opens into the pharynx from the middle ear. It is approximately 3 to 4 cm long, and its primary function is to equalize pressure on both sides of the eardrum by providing a path (via the nasal passages) to relieve the pressure. In addition to pressure equalization, the functions of the middle ear include amplification of the sound waves and stimulation of the oval window to move the fluids of the inner ear.

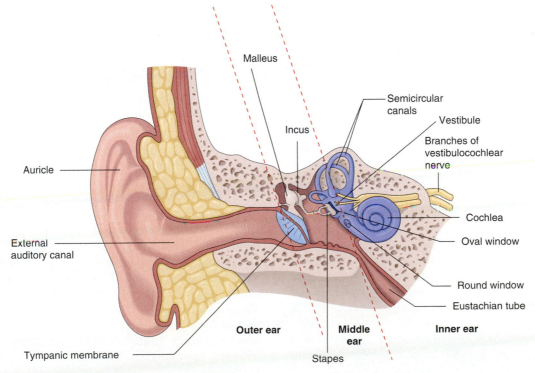

Figure 26-3 Structures of the Ear

PROFESSIONAL TIP

Tympanic Membrane

The tympanic membrane is normally concave on otoscopic exam, so a convex or bulging tympanic membrane is an important sign of an acute infectious process.

Inner Ear

The inner ear has two main functions: hearing and equilibrium. It consists of a complex series of interconnected, fluid-filled chambers and tubes called the labyrinth. It can be divided into three main parts: the semicircular canals, the vestibule, and the cochlea, all located in the temporal bone. The semicircular canals, which function in providing the sense of balance, open into the vestibule. The vestibule is the central chamber of the inner ear. The cochlea is a snail-shaped structure that contains the auditory organ for the sense of hearing.

Vibration of the stapes creates pressure and causes the nerves to respond to different sounds and initiate neural responses that are sent along the auditory nerve (VIII cranial nerve) to the brain. Thus, mechanical information is translated into nerve impulses and sent to the brain, which translates the sound into meaningful impressions and language.

The Eye

The eyes are a pair of spherical organs located in bony orbital cavities in the front of the skull. They are the sensory receptor organs of the visual system that transduce light from the environment into electrical impulses, which the optic nerve then transmits to the brain where they are interpreted as the sensation of vision. The adult eyeball measures about 1 inch in diameter. Of its total surface area, only the anterior one-sixth is exposed. The remainder is recessed and protected by the bony orbit into which it fits. Anatomically, the eye can be divided into three separate coats, or "tunics": the outer fibrous tunic, the middle vascular tunic, and the inner nervous tunic.

Fibrous Tunic

The fibrous tunic is the outer coat of the eyeball and is composed posteriorly of the sclera, and anteriorly of the transparent cornea. The sclera, or "white of the eye," is leathery, white, and relatively thick, and is composed of connective tissue. The cornea, or "window of the eye," is a continuation of the sclera and forms a transparent rounded bulge through which light passes.

Vascular Tunic

The vascular tunic is the eye's middle layer and is composed of three portions: the posterior choroid, the anterior ciliary body, and the iris. Collectively, these three structures are called the uveal tract. The choroid carries the blood vessels for the eyeball and contains a large amount of pigment, thus preventing internal reflection of light. Around the edge of the cornea the choroid forms the ciliary body, a thickened structure containing smooth muscle. A thin diaphragm of mostly connective tissue and smooth muscle fibers with an opening in the center is attached around the anterior margin of the ciliary body. The muscles of the ciliary body serve to change the shape of the lens, allowing changes in the focal distance of the eye. The third portion of the vascular tunic is known as the iris, and contains the pigment responsible for the color of the eye. The hole in the iris is the pupil, which permits light to enter the eye. Some of the smooth muscle fibers in the iris encircle the pupil and others radiate from it. Contraction of the radial muscle dilates the pupil and contraction of the circular muscle constricts the pupil. By their control of pupil diameter, these muscles regulate the amount of light entering the eye.

Nervous Tunic

The third and innermost tunic of the eye, the retina, translates light waves into neural impulses. An extremely complex structure, the retina contains several layers of nerve cells and their processes, including two types of receptors, the rods for vision in dim light, and the cones for daytime or color vision. Cones are most densely concentrated in the central fovea, a small depression in the center of the macula lutea. The macula lutea, or yellow spot, is in the central part of the retina. The fovea is the area of sharpest vision because the highest concentration of cones are located there. Rods are absent from the fovea and macula, but they increase in density toward the periphery of the retina. The optic disk, where the optic nerve exits the eye, is a weak spot in the fundus (posterior wall) of the eye because it is not reinforced by the sclera. The optic disk is also called the blind spot, because it lacks photoreceptors and light focused on it will not be detected.

The interior of the eyeball contains an anterior and posterior chamber separated by the lens. The anterior chamber is filled with a watery fluid called the aqueous humor, which maintains intraocular pressure, provides nourishment, and helps maintain the shape of the eyeball. The posterior chamber is filled with a jelly-like substance called the vitreous humor, which maintains the spherical shape of the eye and supports the inner structures. Both substances are transparent, thus allowing light to pass through the eye to the retina (Figure 26-4).

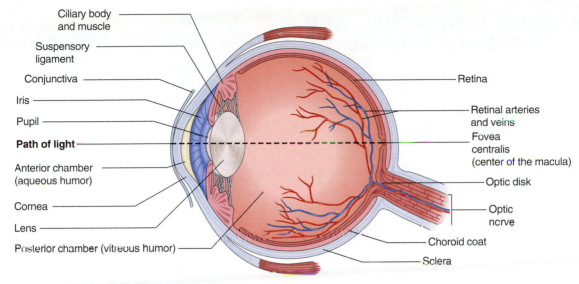

Figure 26-4 Lateral View of the Interior Eyeball

The lens, located in the anterior chamber of the eye, is a transparent biconvex crystalline body enclosed in an elastic capsule held by suspensory ligaments. The shape of the lens changes to focus the image.

External Structures

The eyeball is protected from the external world by the eyelid, which contains a thin protective layer of epithelium, the conjunctiva (Figure 26-5). The conjunctiva covers the anterior portion of the eyeball and lines the eyelid. Projecting from the border of each eyelid is a row of eyelashes, which protect the eye from foreign particles. The lacrimal gland produces a secretion called tears, which contain a lysozyme, muramidase, to destroy pathogens.

COMMON DIAGNOSTIC TESTS

Commonly used diagnostic tests for clients with problems in hearing and vision are listed in Table 26–2. See Chapter 12, Diagnostic Tests, for explanation/normal values and nursing responsibilities.

Table 26–2 COMMON DIAGNOSTIC TESTS FOR SENSORY ALTERATIONS
• Weber test (tuning fork)
• Rinne test (tuning fork)
• Audiometric testing (audiogram)
• Speech audiometry (Spondee threshold)
• Caloric test
• Brainstem auditory evoked response (ErA and BAER)
• Tympanometry
• Computed tomography (CT)
• Magnetic resonance imaging (MRI)
• Romberg test
• Otoscopic exam
• Past-point testing
• Color vision tests
• Tonometry
• Slit lamp examination
• Perimetry
• Visual acuity
• Electroretinogram (ERG)
• Ocular ultrasonography
• Ophthalmoscopic examination
• Orbital computerized tomography
• Fluoresce in angiography

Temporal side   **Nasal side**

Lacriminal gland (under eyelid)   Upper lid
Pupil
Eyelashes
Outer canthus
Inner canthus
Palpebral fissure
Lower lid   Caruncle
Iris
Conjunctiva Limbus Sclera

Figure 26-5 External View of the Right Eye

SENSORY, PERCEPTUAL, AND COGNITIVE ALTERATIONS

An individual usually experiences discomfort and/or anxiety when subjected to a change in the type or amount of incoming stimuli. A person can become confused as a result of either overstimulation or understimulation. According to the individual's ability to process the stimuli, confusion (or disorientation) may occur. **Disorientation** is a mentally confused state in which the person's awareness of time, place, self, and/or situation is impaired. When awareness of these four factors is accurate, a person is said to be "oriented × 4".

A person admitted to a health care agency experiences stimuli that are different from those usually encountered. A change in environment can overwhelm one's ability to perceive and interpret sensory input. As a result, the treatment setting itself can become a stressor that negatively affects sensory, perceptual, and cognitive functions. If one or more of the factors just discussed causes an alteration in sensation, perception, or cognition, the client may experience problems with perceiving and interpreting stimuli. These problems are manifested by three types of alterations: sensory deficit, sensory deprivation, and sensory overload.

SENSORY DEFICIT

A **sensory deficit** is a change in the perception of sensory stimuli. This deficit can affect all five senses. Examples of sensory deficit are vision and hearing losses such as those caused by cataracts, glaucoma, and presbycusis (steady loss of hearing acuity that occurs with aging).

The client's response to these losses usually depends on the time of onset and the severity of the condition. If the problem occurs suddenly and without warning, the client may have difficulty adjusting to the loss of sensory and perceptual function. If these alterations occur gradually, the client may be able to accommodate the change and actually compensate for it by strengthening one or more of the other senses.

The effects of hospitalization or intensive medical treatments can exacerbate the problems related to sensory deficit. For example, a client with acute hearing loss can feel alone and vulnerable when faced with an environment that does not provide an effective means, such as interpreters who sign, through which communication can occur. Because of these responses, clients with sensory deficit are at serious risk of experiencing either sensory deprivation or sensory overload.

SENSORY DEPRIVATION

Sensory deprivation is a state of reduced sensory input from the internal or external environment, mani-

GERONTOLOGICAL CONSIDERATIONS

Effects of Aging

Sensory, perceptual, and cognitive function begins to be diminished as the effects of aging, such as decreased visual or auditory senses or impairments in memory, are experienced. These changes can have a profound effect on a client's self-esteem and response to life.

fested by alterations in sensory perception. Individuals can experience sensory deprivation as a result of illness, trauma, or isolation. A person experiencing sensory deprivation misinterprets the limited stimuli with a resultant impairment of thoughts and feelings. Factors that contribute to sensory deprivation include:

- Visual or auditory impairments that limit or prohibit perception of stimuli
- Drugs that produce a sedative effect on the CNS and interfere with the interpretation of stimuli
- Trauma that results in brain damage and decreased cognitive function
- Isolation (either physical or social) that results in the creation of a nonstimulating environment

Some contributing factors (such as brain damage or blindness) result in chronic sensory deprivation. Other factors lead to acute, transient states of deprivation (such as receiving analgesic medications).

Individuals who are sensory-deprived may exhibit any of the following characteristics:

- Inability to concentrate
- Poor memory
- Impaired problem-solving ability
- Confusion
- Irritability
- Emotional lability (mood swings)
- Hallucinations
- Depression
- Boredom and apathy
- Drowsiness

SENSORY OVERLOAD

Sensory overload is a state of excessive and sustained multisensory stimulation manifested by behavior change and perceptual distortion. The individual experiencing this alteration is unable to process the amount or intensity of stimuli being received. Factors contributing to sensory overload are:

- Pain originating from a heightened quality or quantity of internal stimuli

- Invasive procedures that result in an increased amount of external stimuli
- Activity-filled, busy environment that contributes to the amount of stimuli being perceived
- Medications that stimulate the CNS and prohibit the client from ignoring selective stimuli
- Presence of strangers (both health care professionals and others) who contribute to the quantity of stimuli
- Diseases that affect the CNS and maximize the perception of stimuli

DISORDERS OF THE EAR

Disorders of the ear include impaired hearing, Ménière's Disease, otosclerosis, acoustic neuroma, otitis media, otitis externa, and mastoiditis.

IMPAIRED HEARING

Hearing loss is the most common chronic disability in the United States, affecting nearly 30 million adults (Spencer, 1998). It can be seriously debilitating by limiting the ability to socialize and work, or respond to the telephone or alarms, yet relatively few individuals who experience impaired hearing actually seek help. Some may deny the problem and others may feel that a hearing aid is a sign of old age. Often family members are the first to be aware of a hearing deficit.

TYPES OF HEARING LOSS

Hearing loss is generally categorized in two ways, conductive and sensorineural. Mixed hearing loss, both conductive and sensorineural, is possible, but far less likely. Either may occur at birth (congenital), develop later in life, be genetic, or be caused by injury or trauma.

Conductive hearing loss indicates an inability of the sound waves to reach the inner ear. This may be due to cerumen buildup or blockage, perforated tympanic membrane, or fixation of one or all of the ossicles.

In **sensorineural hearing loss**, the inner ear or cochlear portion of cranial nerve VIII may be abnormal or diseased. A tumor, infection, trauma, or exposure to loud noises may cause destruction of the nerve and result in sensorineural hearing loss.

Sensorineural hearing loss associated with aging is termed **presbycusis**. Higher frequency sounds like women's voices become especially difficult to hear, and distinguishing words may be a problem. According to Spencer (1998), 95 percent of the people with sensorineural hearing loss can be helped by hearing aids.

BEHAVIORS INDICATING HEARING LOSS

A hearing impairment is a serious disorder that is often debilitating and embarrassing to the client. Hearing is part of the communication process, so the inability to hear may cause the person to do or say the wrong thing in response to a question or command. Persons with hearing impairment may withdraw from conversation or seem indifferent to their surroundings or to those around them.

Oftentimes alterations in hearing are manifested by changes in speech habits and patterns. Individuals with hearing impairments may not notice the changes in their own speech pattern until someone constantly asks them to repeat themselves or to speak clearly. Indifference and withdrawal are common behaviors in response to hearing loss. If left undiagnosed and untreated, the person may truly regress, become unhappy, lonely, and possibly even paranoid. Some individuals overcompensate for the hearing loss by becoming very loud and aggressive.

Research on hearing impairment has created many devices to aid speech and sound discrimination. Early diagnosis, treatment, and rehabilitation are essential to help hearing impaired persons enjoy and appreciate the world they live in.

HEARING AIDS/ ASSISTIVE DEVICES

Hearing aids today come in a variety of designs and sizes. Some are quite small and tinted to a person's skin color so as to be virtually unnoticeable. Some are worn in the ear, behind the ear, or are part of eyeglasses frames. Persons with bilateral hearing loss may need binaural (worn in both ears) hearing aids.

A hearing aid converts environmental sound and

PROFESSIONAL TIP

Hearing Specialists

An audiologist evaluates hearing and determines the extent and type of hearing loss, and also provides nonmedical treatment such as the fitting of hearing aids, advice about assistive listening devices, and communication/aural rehabilitative training. An otolaryngologist (ear, nose, and throat physician) provides medical evaluation of hearing disorders and medical and surgical interventions. A hearing aid specialist is licensed to dispense hearing aids but does not have a medical background or training.

speech into electronic signals that are amplified and converted to acoustic signals. It makes speech and sound louder, but not necessarily clearer. Depending on the extent of hearing impairment and preference, the client may need to experiment with several different types of hearing aids. In addition, speech therapy, lip reading, and auditory training may be necessary to help discriminate speech and develop better listening skills.

Many other assistive hearing devices are available for the hearing impaired. Numerous television programs are closed-caption. Advanced technology allows telecommunication through a device called Telecommunication Device for the Deaf (TDD), also called TTY Typewriter, which sends a printed message onto a small screen. Both sender and receiver must have the typewriter/telephone device. Many businesses offer this option to conduct transactions.

Alarm clocks offer strobe lights or vibrators to awaken clients. State of the art receivers give instant access to radio, television, computer, and stereos to enhance receiving and listening systems. For travelers, complete kits are available to provide ready access for smoke alarm, clock, TDD, and door knock alert in hotels or inns.

Hearing guide dogs are also available. The animals are specially trained to meet the needs of the hearing impaired. At home, the dog responds to alarms, knocking on doors, and babies crying. In public, the dog takes a position between owner and a potential threat. Special identifiers, such as a collar for the dog and ID card for the owner are available. The dogs are trained to go wherever their master goes including restaurants, grocery stores, and on public transportation.

Medical–Surgical Management

Medical

It is important to identify the type of hearing loss and underlying etiology to determine the best medical or surgical management. The client should undergo a complete physical examination as well as thorough diagnostic hearing tests. Once the etiology is determined, the client and doctor can decide upon the best course of therapy.

Surgical

The cochlear implant as a possible treatment for persons with profound deafness. Studies thus far indicate better success with the implant in children than in adults. In this procedure, a receiver/stimulator is implanted in the skull and a group of electrodes are planted in front of the round window in the inner ear. The client wears a microphone near the ear that picks up and translates sound into electrical signals. These signals are then transmitted to the brain via the cochlear implant and cranial nerve VIII.

▶ NURSING PROCESS

▶ Assessment

▶ Subjective Data

Subjective data may be obtained by asking the client to describe the initial onset of symptoms and possible familial traits. The nurse should ask the client about recent infections of the ears, nose, or upper respiratory system. Recent trauma and past surgery as well as medical history such as diabetes, heart disease, or cancer should be determined. The nurse should note allergies to food, drugs, or environmental factors. The client's work history may reveal exposure to loud noises. The client should be asked about associated symptoms such as **tinnitus** (ringing sound in the ear), **vertigo** (dizziness), nausea, and vomiting.

▶ Objective Data

Objective data may be obtained by listening closely to the client and noting any deterioration of speech, slurring, or dropping of word endings. Current and recent medication use should be documented.

The outer ear should be inspected for abnormalities, lesions, or cerumen. The mastoid process, neck, jaw, and temporal regions of the head should be palpated for swelling or tenderness to touch. The nurse should note the degree of hearing loss as reported by the client and compare it to the diagnostic tests such as the speech audiogram. The client's perception of hearing loss may be significantly different from the diagnostic findings.

A nursing diagnosis for a client with impaired hearing may be:

Nursing Diagnosis	Planning/Goals	Nursing Interventions
▶ *Social Isolation related to hearing impairment*	The client will participate in conversations and other social situations.	Take time to engage client in conversation. Speak slowly and distinctly. Make sure you have the client's attention and be at eye level.

continues

Nursing Diagnosis	Planning/Goals	Nursing Interventions
		Give the client time to respond.
		Provide the client and family members written information regarding the availability, variety, and quality of assistive hearing devices.
		Encourage client to participate in social situations.

Evaluation The goal must be evaluated to determine how it has been met by the client.

MÉNIÈRE'S DISEASE

Ménière's disease, also known as endolymphatic hydrops, is a state of hearing loss characterized by tinnitus and vertigo. Although the exact etiology is unknown, it is postulated that the cause is an excessive accumulation of endolymph in the cochlear duct and possible leakage of endolymph into the perilymph due to increased capillary permeability. Mixing of the two fluids chemically alters the homeostasis of the perilymph and endolymph and can be responsible for the symptoms associated with Ménière's disease.

The major symptoms are the classic triad of vertigo, tinnitus, and unilateral fluctuating hearing loss. The vertigo is often associated with nausea and vomiting. Tinnitus may either be a preceding aura or occur simultaneously with the vertigo. Initially, tinnitus is intermittent, but as the disease progresses, it may be a constant, low-pitched roaring sound. The fluctuating, unilateral hearing loss becomes more profound with each attack.

PROFESSIONAL TIP

Assisting the Hearing Impaired Client

- Speak slowly and distinctly after getting the client's attention.
- Face the client and sit or stand to be at eye level with the client.
- Use short, simple sentences and give the client time to respond. Repeat or rephrase if necessary.
- Use written materials when possible to communicate information.
- Keep a notepad and pen or pencil available to write down new or unfamiliar words and concepts.
- If sign language is the client's preferred method of communication, locate a person who understands sign language.
- If the client wears a hearing aid, make sure that the battery is functional, it is turned on, and adjusted to a comfortable level.

The symptoms are frequently at their worst during the first attack, which may last from a few minutes to six hours. **Nystagmus**, repetitive and involuntary movement of the eyeballs, and diaphoresis may occur during an attack. Subsequent attacks are less severe, but over time may involve both ears and cause permanent bilateral hearing loss. Clients report many different precipitating events such as stress, weather changes, menstruation, or pregnancy, and various dietary influences including caffeine, alcohol, and salt. Smoking has also been implicated.

Medical–Surgical Management

Medical

Medical management is the preferred treatment and most helpful to about 80 to 85 percent of persons affected with this disease. Diagnosis is not difficult and is usually made based on the client's report of symptoms. Diagnosis may also be confirmed with caloric stimulation (though this test is primarily conducted on comatose clients) and an MRI to rule out a tumor. Medical management is symptomatic.

Surgical

Surgical intervention is usually needed only when the attacks are frequent and debilitating, or when the disease severely impacts the quality of life and the ability for self-care. Surgical treatment includes endolymphatic, subarachnoid shunt placement to drain excessive endolymph. With this procedure, hearing is preserved in 60% to 70% of the clients. With a vestibular neurectomy, the vestibular portion of cranial nerve VIII is severed; hearing is preserved in 90% of the clients having this procedure. In surgical destruction of the labyrinth, hearing is destroyed but the incapacitating vertigo is completely relieved.

Pharmacological

A number of medications are useful to help control the symptoms such as antihistamines, antiemetics, benzodiazepines, diuretics, tranquilizers, vasoactive agents, and oral niacin. The medications may be prescribed for long-term use or at the onset of symptoms. Since the cause of Ménière's disease is unknown, there is no cure.

Diet

Dietary interventions include strict salt restriction and avoidance of those foods or beverages that precipitate or aggravate an attack. Examples are beer, wine, soda, salty food or snacks, chocolate, and caffeinated coffee and tea.

Activity

Activity is not limited in a normal daily routine. However, during or after an attack, clients may require prolonged bed rest and restriction of activities that may be unsafe, such as driving or operating heavy equipment.

▶ NURSING PROCESS

▶ Assessment

▶ Subjective Data

The history should begin with identifying significant contributory data. Subjective data may be obtained by asking the client to describe the initial onset of symptoms including, but not limited to, the classic triad of tinnitus, vertigo, and fluctuating unilateral hearing loss.

Questions should be related to recent viral illness; upper respiratory infections; past medical, surgical, and dental history; and any problems related to the neck and face. Food, drug, or environmental allergies should be documented. Current or recent long-term medications should be recorded. The client's occupation and hobbies that may contribute to hearing loss should be identified.

▶ Objective Data

Objective data may be obtained with a thorough physical examination that includes looking at the ear for abnormalities, lesions and cerumen blockage, or unusual drainage. The neck, jaw, and mastoid process should be palpated for possible lymph node enlargement and tenderness. The nurse may assist with the otologic examination as needed. Audiological testing determines unilateral or bilateral hearing loss.

Nursing diagnoses for a client with Ménière's disease may include the following:

Nursing Diagnoses	Planning/Goals	Nursing Interventions
▶ *Activity Intolerance related to severe vertigo*	The client will be able to tolerate activities of daily living.	Provide adequate periods of bed rest. Keep the room dim and quiet when possible. Avoid jarring the bed and caution client to avoid sudden movements. Administer antiemetic before symptoms become too severe. Provide assistance with ambulation and encourage increased activity as tolerated.
▶ *Deficient Knowledge related to abrupt onset and unknown progression of the disease*	The client will verbalize understanding of the disease process and potential precipitating factors and how to manage or control the symptoms.	Assess the client's current knowledge of the disease process. Review the disease process and underlying etiology of Ménière's disease with the client. Ask the client to identify possible precipitating factors such as stress or dietary habits. Discuss health promotion programs for stress management and healthy cooking classes. Suggest consultations with dietary and social services. Review follow-up appointments, medications, dietary management, activity, and rest parameters. Evaluate client's readiness to discuss progressive hearing loss and current assistive hearing devices available.
▶ *Risk for Injury related to vertigo*	The client will not fall or be injured because of vertigo.	Keep side rails up. Teach client to move or turn slowly. Reiterate need to call for assistance when ambulating. Keep call bell within client's reach. Administer medications for vertigo prior to worsening of symptoms. Avoid glaring, bright lights. Instruct client to sit or lie down when vertigo occurs.

Evaluation Each goal must be evaluated to determine how it has been met by the client.

OTOSCLEROSIS

Otosclerosis is a conductive hearing loss secondary to a pathologic change of the bones in the middle ear. The exact cause is unknown. The ossicles are normally hard, but over time and without warning, the bone becomes softened, spongy, highly vascular, and partially or totally fixed. This fixation reduces or prevents transmission of source waves to inner ear fluids. Although all three bones may be affected, the stapes, which must vibrate on the oval window in order to transmit sound waves, is most commonly afflicted.

Otosclerosis is more common in adults, women are affected more often than men, and it is familial in some cases. It is the most common cause of conductive hearing loss.

The primary clinical manifestations are subtle changes in hearing and low-pitched tinnitus. It becomes more difficult to distinguish a whisper, or to hear in crowded places or understand conversation. Individuals affected by otosclerosis often blame others for speaking too softly or mumbling. Frequently, rather than asking others to speak up or to repeat themselves, the person will be irritable and withdrawn.

Diagnostic testing begins with the Weber and Rinne tuning fork tests. In addition, audiometric testing should be performed. Schwartz's sign, a pink blush, is seen on otoscopic examination. Tympanometry shows stiffness in the sound conduction system.

Medical–Surgical Management

Medical

Treatment for otosclerosis is limited to three options. The individual may choose to do nothing and obtain periodic audiometry to evaluate progression of the disease. The second choice is to use a hearing aid and the third choice is surgical management with an outpatient procedure known as a stapedectomy.

Surgical

A stapedectomy is the preferred surgical technique for improving hearing loss due to otosclerosis. A stapedectomy may be done under local or general anesthesia and routinely requires a surgical incision in the posterior ear canal, removal of the stapes, and implantation of a plastic prosthesis. A new technique, laser stapedectomy, may be performed through the ear canal without an incision. The stapes tendon is vaporized, chards are removed with delicate micro instruments, and an opening is made allowing the surgeon to implant a prosthetic piston. This restores normal vibration against the inner ear.

▶ NURSING PROCESS

▶ Assessment

▶ Subjective Data

Subjective data will include a careful history to discover possible hereditary traits or acquired disease. The client should be asked about recent infections of the ears, nose, or upper respiratory system, and also about past surgery, trauma, or other illnesses such as diabetes, heart disease, or cancer. Associated symptoms such as dizziness, tinnitus, vertigo, and nausea should be identified.

The nurse should note allergies to foods, drugs, or any environmental factors. The client's work history may reveal exposure to loud noises. Current and recent medications should be recorded, especially those known to be ototoxic.

▶ Objective Data

Objective data includes a thorough physical examination. The nurse must inspect the outer ear for abnormalities, lesions, or impacted ear wax. The mastoid process, neck, jaw, and temporal regions of the head should be palpated for pain or swelling. The degree of hearing loss should be assessed. The client may be vomiting.

Nursing diagnoses for the client with otosclerosis may include the following:

Nursing Diagnoses	Planning/Goals	Nursing Interventions
▶ *Anxiety related to decrease or loss in hearing*	The client will show evidence of reduced anxiety and verbalize understanding of the disease process and treatment regimen.	Encourage the client to explore feelings of anxiety and to ask questions to clarify concerns. Provide honest and realistic feedback. Collaborate with the physician to provide thorough and clear explanations of the disease process, treatment options, and anticipated results.
▶ *Risk for Injury related to vertigo*	The client will not fall or be injured because of vertigo.	Keep side rails up. Instruct the client to move or turn slowly. Reiterate need to call for assistance when ambulating and keep call bell within client's reach. Administer medications for vertigo prior to worsening of symptoms. Keep room well lit when client is ambulating.

continues

Nursing Diagnoses	Planning/Goals	Nursing Interventions
▶ *Deficient Knowledge related to activities after surgery*	The client will demonstrate the ability to change dressing correctly and verbalize knowledge of self-care and follow-up.	Teach client how and when to perform dressing change and have client demonstrate the procedure.
		Instruct client to avoid pressure changes (such as flying in an unpressurized aircraft), avoid heavy lifting (60 lbs) for one month, avoid nose blowing for ten days and if sneezing occurs, keep mouth open.
		Advise client to keep water out of the ear and keep the ear exposed to air as much as possible for one month. There will be some drainage which is initially red, then pink, and then brownish.
		Tell client to report any greenish, yellowish, or foul smelling drainage.
		Instruct client to take all antibiotics as prescribed and complete the full course of treatment.
		Advise client there should be very little pain or discomfort but if there is, take prescribed analgesics and notify doctor if pain is prolonged or intense.
		Warn client that hearing may be decreased for three to four weeks after surgery until gel-foam packing dissolves.
		Inform client that audiometric testing will be conducted one month after surgery.
		Instruct client to schedule an appointment with the physician in one month but call physician if uncontrolled pain is experienced or a malodorous, greenish discharge comes from the ear.

Evaluation Each goal must be evaluated to determine how it has been met by the client.

ACOUSTIC NEUROMA

Acoustic neuroma is a slow-growing and usually benign tumor of the vestibular portion of the inner ear (cranial nerve VIII). Detection at the onset of symptoms is essential and may be accomplished with an MRI. Presenting symptoms of dizziness, tinnitus, and hearing loss are common to many dysfunctions of the ear and the possibility of acoustic neuroma must not be overlooked.

Clients who present with dizziness, tinnitus, and hearing loss should have a complete workup for auditory and vestibular (balance) function. Facial weakness may be caused by compression of the tumor on cranial nerve VII. The Vth cranial nerve may also be affected as the tumor grows, causing paresthesia of the face and loss of the corneal reflex. Large neuromas can cause increased intracranial pressure, papilledema, vomiting, and headache.

Medical–Surgical Management

Treatment is almost always surgical excision of the tumor. Although antihistamines may reduce the dizziness, the pharmacologic treatment is only temporary until diagnostic tests are completed and surgery is planned.

▶ NURSING PROCESS

▶ Assessment

▶ Subjective Data

Subjective data may be obtained through the client history of the chief complaint, reported signs and symptoms, and all contributing data.

▶ Objective Data

Objective data will be obtained with the physical examination and should include a complete cranial nerve evaluation performed by the physician or audiologist to determine the extent of cranial nerve involvement.

A nursing diagnosis for a client with acoustic neuroma may be:

Nursing Diagnosis	Planning/Goals	Nursing Interventions
▶ *Anticipatory Grieving related to diminished quality of life, loss of ability for self-care, or possible loss of life*	The client will express feelings of grief and demonstrate adaptive coping mechanisms.	Assist the client to express feelings about progressive hearing loss and changes in activities of daily living, employment, and quality of life issues.
		Collaborate with physician and other members of the health care team to provide thorough and clear explanations of the disease process, treatment options, and anticipated results.

continues

Nursing Diagnoses	Planning/Goals	Nursing Interventions
		Observe the client's coping styles. Support those that the client finds helpful and explore other coping mechanisms that may prove useful in time (e.g., hobbies and other diversional activities, prayer, reading, and so on).
		Include the family in all interventions that the client desires.
		Examine the family's feelings and ability to cope.
		Consult social services, pastoral care, or other hospital and community resources when appropriate.

Evaluation The goal must be evaluated to determine how it has been met by the client.

OTITIS MEDIA

Otitis media is an inflammation of the middle ear and a common cause of conductive hearing loss, though usually temporary. Presenting symptoms include ear pain, fever, redness of auricle and ear canal, and sometimes enlarged lymph nodes over the mastoid process, parotids, and upper neck. Otitis media occurs more frequently in children than in adults.

Fluid accumulates behind the eardrum due to blockage of the eustachian tube (Figure 26-6). This may be secondary to an upper respiratory infection, allergies, or acute bacterial infection. On physical examination the tympanic membrane may be retracted, normal, or bulging. A pneumatic otoscope allows the practitioner to blow soft puffs of air against the tympanic membrane to assess movement. A stiff, nonmoving, or bulging tympanic membrane may indicate inflammation or fluid accumulation in the middle ear. Visualization of the normal landmarks may be obscured. The Rinne tuning fork test and audiometry confirm a conductive hearing loss.

Medical–Surgical Management

Medical

Topical heat and systemic analgesics may be used to control pain. The client should lie on the affected side to facilitate drainage.

Surgical

Surgical management may be necessary for diagnostic or therapeutic reasons. A myringotomy may be performed, in which an incision is made in the eardrum and fluid is aspirated. A polyethylene tube may be placed in the eardrum to equalize pressure and allow drainage of fluid.

A tympanoplasty may be needed if the tympanic membrane is ruptured. If there is a large tympanic membrane perforation, the malleus, which is connected to the tympanic membrane, or other ossicles may be damaged. Ossicular chain reconstruction typically refers to the removal of the actual bones and replacement with a plastic prosthesis. Often the prosthesis and the tympanic membrane reconstruction result in a significant improvement in hearing.

Pharmacological

Medications used include decongestants such as pseudoephedrine hydrochloride (Sudafed), antihistamines such as diphenhydramine hydrochloride (Benadryl), and systemic antibiotics such as ampicillin (Omnipen).

Activity

Activity is not restricted unless surgical management is indicated.

▶ NURSING PROCESS

▶ Assessment

▶ Subjective Data

The nurse should ask about the onset, duration, and severity of pain and what home remedies have been used. Hearing loss and/or tinnitus and a deep throbbing pain in the ear may be reported.

▶ Objective Data

A watery or yellow discharge may be seen. It may have a foul odor. The client may have a fever.

Landmarks obscured

Hairline air-fluid level

Fluid (amber-colored)

Bulging red drum

Figure 26-6 The Tympanic Membrane in the Presence of Otitis Media

A nursing diagnosis for a client with otitis media may be:

Nursing Diagnosis	Planning/Goals	Nursing Interventions
▶ *Acute Pain related to inflammation in the middle ear*	The client will experience pain relief.	Administer antibiotics as ordered.
		Teach client and family the importance of administering medications as ordered and to complete full course of prescription.
		Administer analgesics as ordered.
		Apply heating pad, set on low, for 20 minutes every 2 hours. Do not use on small children.
		Teach client if pain is unrelieved in 48 hours, to contact physician.

Evaluation The goal must be evaluated to determine how it has been met by the client.

OTITIS EXTERNA

Otitis externa or "swimmer's ear" typically involves a bacterial infection of the external ear canal skin. The canal skin becomes red and edematous. If the swelling is severe enough, it will block the ear passage and cause a mild conductive hearing loss. Also, in most cases there is a discharge. If the discharge is copious and the canal size is constricted, a mild conductive hearing loss may result.

MASTOIDITIS

Mastoiditis (inflammation of the mastoid) is most often the direct result of chronic or recurrent bacterial otitis media. The recurrent infection may find its way into the bone and structures surrounding the middle ear and, if left untreated, can cause severe damage, sensorineural deafness, facial weakness, brain abscess, and meningitis. Other symptoms include earache, fever, headache, and malaise. Antibiotics are given for a trial period. If symptoms do not resolve, surgical intervention such as mastoidectomy or meatoplasty may be necessary.

DISORDERS OF THE EYE

Disorders of the eye include cataracts, glaucoma, retinal detachment, infections, refractive errors, injuries, impaired vision, and macular degeneration.

CATARACTS

A **cataract** is a disorder that causes the lens or its capsule to lose its transparency and/or become opaque (Figure 26-7). The lens is normally clear and transparent and allows light to pass through to the retina. As clouding develops, visual impairment occurs. Cataracts usually affect both eyes; however the degree of visual impairment is often different in each eye.

Cataracts are typically associated with aging; however, they may be congenital, caused by severe eye injury, or secondary to certain systemic diseases characterized by metabolic problems (diabetes mellitus) and chronic eye disease (uveitis). Ophthalmoscopic examination is the primary method of evaluation.

Medical–Surgical Management

Surgical

The only treatment for a cataract is surgical removal of the lens. However, the mere finding of a cataract is not an indication for surgery. Surgery is indicated when significant vision loss has occurred. The lens may be removed by the intracapsular or extracapsular approach. During the intracapsular cataract extraction, the ophthalmologist removes the lens within its capsule. Extracapsular cataract extraction is the procedure most commonly used (Figure 26-8). The ophthalmologist removes the anterior portion of the capsule and then expresses, or removes, the lens. An intraocular

Figure 26-7 A cataract results in the loss of transparency of the lens of the eye. *(Courtesy of the National Eye Institute, Bethesda, MD)*

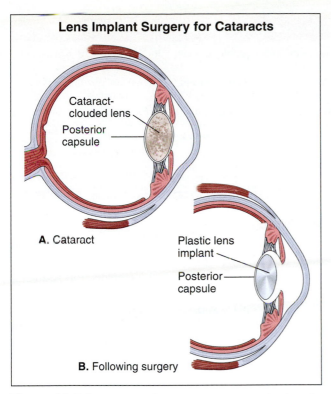

Lens Implant Surgery for Cataracts

Cataract-clouded lens
Posterior capsule

A. Cataract

Plastic lens implant
Posterior capsule

B. Following surgery

Figure 26-8 In extracapsular extraction to correct cataracts, the lens is removed, the posterior lens capsule is left intact, and a plastic intraocular lens (IOL) is placed.

PROFESSIONAL TIP

Eye Specialists

An ophthalmologist is a medical doctor who specializes in the diagnosis and treatment, both medical and surgical, of diseases of the eye, visual disorders, and eye injuries. An optometrist is a doctor of optometry and is licensed to examine, diagnose, manage and treat vision problems, diseases, and other abnormalities of the eyes and related structures.

The client is instructed to have a driver available to provide transportation postoperatively because driving is restricted for a few days. After the anesthesia wears off, the client is discharged.

Postoperatively, the client has a patch over the eye. The patch is removed and reapplied on the first postoperative day when miotic (makes pupil contract) eye drops are begun. Mild discomfort and scratchiness are expected. Atropine sulfate eye drops and cold compresses may be ordered to relieve these discomforts.

▶ NURSING PROCESS

▶ Assessment

▶ Subjective Data

A general medical history as well as a history of symptoms is needed. Symptoms may include: haziness, cloudiness, blurred vision, double vision, altered color perception, and glare when looking at lights, especially with night driving. Fear of losing one's eyesight can be very devastating. There is often a great deal of anxiety when the client seeks an eye examination.

▶ Objective Data

Upon inspection of the eye the usual black pupil appears clouded, progressing to a milky white appearance which is a characteristic finding of a mature cataract and indicates significant vision loss.

lens (IOL) is generally implanted. Glasses or special contact lenses may also be used.

Most eye surgery is done on an outpatient basis under local anesthesia. General anesthesia can be used at the client's request and for clients who are extremely anxious, deaf, or mentally retarded. A tranquilizer such as diazepam (Valium) is often given to reduce anxiety when receiving injections on the face and around the eye.

Preoperatively, the client can receive several types of eye medications to prepare the eye for surgery: mydriatic (makes pupil dilate) and cycloplegic (paralyzes ciliary muscle) eye drops, antibiotic eye drops as a prophylaxis against infection, and an intravenous infusion of an agent to lower intraocular pressure (mannitol or a carbonic anhydrase inhibitor).

Nursing diagnoses for a client with cataracts may include the following:

Nursing Diagnoses	Planning/Goals	Nursing Interventions
▶ *Disturbed Sensory Perception (Visual) related to ocular lens opacity*	The client will demonstrate improved ability to process visual stimuli and communicate visual limitations.	Assess and document baseline visual acuity. Elicit functional description of what the client can and cannot see.
▶ *Risk for Injury related to difficulty in processing visual images and altered depth perception*	The client will avoid activities associated with increased potential for injury.	Teach the client to change position slowly. Teach the client to avoid reaching for objects to maintain stability when ambulating, as depth perception is altered.

continues

Nursing Diagnoses	Planning/Goals	Nursing Interventions
▸ *Impaired Home Maintenance related to age, limited vision or activity restrictions imposed by surgery*	The client will perform self-care activities in home environment.	Discuss the client's ability to meet self-care needs and activities of daily living. Evaluate how the client's current functional ability will be affected by activity restrictions and postoperative care needs. Help the client decide on a realistic site for postoperative care needs.

Evaluation Each goal must be evaluated to determine how it has been met by the client.

GLAUCOMA

Glaucoma is a disorder characterized by an abnormally high pressure of fluid inside the eyeball (intraocular pressure, IOP). The aqueous humor does not return into the bloodstream through the canal of Schlemm as quickly as it is formed. The fluid accumulates and, by compressing the lens into the vitreous humor, puts pressure on the neurons of the retina. If the pressure continues over a long period of time, it destroys the neurons and brings about blindness.

There are two primary forms of glaucoma: open-angle glaucoma and closed-angle glaucoma. Open-angle glaucoma (chronic simple glaucoma) is characterized by a gradual rise in IOP, a slowly progressive loss of peripheral vision, and, if not controlled, a late loss of central vision and ultimate blindness. This is the most prevalent form of glaucoma and is usually bilateral. Closed-angle glaucoma (acute glaucoma) is characterized by attacks of suddenly increased intraocular pressure, exhibited clinically by a bulging iris, which is an emergency situation. Closed-angle glaucoma is usually unilateral with severe pain and loss of vision caused by acute obstruction of aqueous humor drainage within the eye.

Secondary glaucoma results from ocular or systemic disorders that are responsible for the elevation in IOP. These disorders or conditions indirectly disrupt the activity of the structures involved in circulation and/or reabsorption of aqueous humor. This can happen suddenly and without warning.

CLIENT TEACHING

Glaucoma Care
- Continue the use of eye medications as ordered.
- Continue to receive medical supervision for observation of intraocular pressure to ensure control of the disorder.
- Avoid exertion, stooping, heavy lifting, or wearing constrictive clothing as these increase intraocular pressure.

Medical–Surgical Management

Medical

Medical management for glaucoma is focused on drug therapy and the main objective is to reduce intraocular pressure. Two mechanisms for reducing this pressure are: (1) physically constricting the pupil so that the ciliary muscle is contracted, which allows better circulation of the aqueous humor to the site of absorption, and (2) inhibiting the production of aqueous humor.

Surgical

Surgical intervention to facilitate drainage of the aqueous humor is called an iridectomy. A surgical incision is made through the cornea to remove a portion of the iris to facilitate aqueous drainage.

A laser may also be used to treat various eye disorders. In open-angle glaucoma, a laser is used to create multiple scars around the trabecular meshwork (a supporting or anchoring strand that allows increased outflow of aqueous humor) thereby reducing intraocular pressure. In closed-angle glaucoma, laser energy is used to create a hole in the periphery of the iris, creating an opening between the anterior and posterior chambers for aqueous drainage.

Pharmacological

Drugs that enhance pupillary constriction are commonly used to treat glaucoma. Miotics and cholinesterase inhibitors such as pilocarpine hydrochloride (Isopto Carpine), carbachol (Carbacel), and demecarium bromide (Humorsol) are frequently used.

Beta-adrenergics such as timolol maleate (Timoptic Solution) are the drugs of choice for decreasing IOP. When used as eye drops, beta-adrenergics reduce aqueous humor production without pupil constriction.

Carbonic anhydrase inhibitors, such as acetazolamide (Diamox), reduce production of aqueous humor to help maintain a lowered IOP. Side effects reported are numbness, weakness, tingling of extremities, and rashes. Adrenergics such as epinephrine bitartrate (Epitrate) also reduce aqueous humor production. Osmotic agents such as mannitol and glycerin (Osmoglyn) may be administered systemically to the client with closed-angle glaucoma in an emergency as an effort to decrease IOP. The high osmolarity of these agents is used to draw fluid into the intravascular space, which lowers the IOP.

▶ NURSING PROCESS

▶ Assessment

▶ Subjective Data

The nurse should obtain a history noting the presence of risk factors: positive family history (believed to be linked in open-angle glaucoma), eye tumor, intraocular hemorrhage, intraocular inflammation, or contusion of the eye from trauma during cataract surgery.

Symptoms of open-angle glaucoma include gradual loss of peripheral vision, eye pain, difficulty adjusting to darkness, halos around lights and an inability to detect color. For closed-angle glaucoma, symptoms include sudden onset of severe pain in the eye often accompanied by headache, nausea, vomiting, malaise, rainbow halos around lights, and blurred vision.

▶ Objective Data

Assessment reveals acute increased intraocular pressure (21 to 32 mm Hg) as measured with a tonometer (normal range is 12 to 22 mm Hg).

A nursing diagnosis for a client with glaucoma may be:

Nursing Diagnosis	Planning/Goals	Nursing Interventions
▶ *Acute Pain related to closed-angle glaucoma*	The client will verbalize relief from discomfort.	Administer prescribed ophthalmic agent for glaucoma.
		Notify physician of the following: hypotension, urinary output less than 240 mL for 8 hours, no relief in eye pain within 30 minutes of drug therapy, and continual diminishing visual acuity.
		Monitor blood pressure, pulse, and respiration every 4 hours if not receiving osmotic agent intravenously and every 2 hours if receiving intravenous osmotic agent.
		Monitor degree of eye pain every 30 minutes.
		Monitor intake and output every 8 hours while receiving intravenous osmotic agent.
		Monitor visual acuity prior to each instillation of prescribed ophthalmic agent by asking if objects are clear or blurred and if the client can read printed material held at arm's length.
		Remind the client that miotics may cause blurred vision for 1 to 2 hours after use and that adaptation to dark environments is difficult because of the pupillary constriction.

Evaluation The goal must be evaluated to determine how it has been met by the client.

RETINAL DETACHMENT

In retinal detachment, there is an actual separation of the retina from the choroid (Figure 26-9). Partial separation becomes complete, if untreated, with the subsequent total loss of vision. A tear or hole in the retina can extend the separation as vitreous humor seeps through the opening and separates the retina from the choroid. The cause of retinal detachment may be from severe trauma to the eye or from intraocular disorders such as cataract extraction, perforating injuries, or severe **myopia** (nearsightedness). This condition is painless since there are no pain receptors in the retina.

Medical–Surgical Management

Medical

Early corrective intervention to reattach the retina may use one of several techniques. Three procedures can be used to create an inflammatory reaction that, once healing and scarring occur, result in the retina reattaching to the choroid. One such technique is electrodiathermy (heat therapy) which uses an ultrasonic probe to burn (seal) the scleral surface directly over the retinal break. Another technique is cryotherapy which uses an intensely cold probe applied to the scleral surface

Torn retina   Sclera   Choroid

Figure 26-9 Retinal Detachment

directly over the hole in the retina. Laser photocoagulation is also used to seal tears or holes in the retina.

Surgical

A surgical procedure called scleral buckling is sometimes used. This operation reduces the scleral surface and allows contact between the choroid and retina.

Pharmacological

Cycloplegic-mydriatic and anti-infective eyedrops are often ordered following the attachment procedure.

Activity

Bed rest and a patch on one or both eyes restricts activity. If air is injected into the vitreous humor, the client either lies prone or sits forward with the unaffected eye upward.

▶ NURSING PROCESS

▶ Assessment

▶ Subjective Data

Obtain a medical history for presence of causative factors: trauma, recent cataract surgery, eye tumor, severe myopia, uveitis. The client may describe sudden flashes of light (photopsia), floating spots (caused by bleeding into the vitreous cavity), blurred vision that becomes progressively worse, or complaints of a sensation of a veil in the line of sight.

▶ Objective Data

Ophthalmoscopic examination visualizes the detachment.

Nursing diagnoses for a client with retinal detachment may include the following:

Nursing Diagnoses	Planning/Goals	Nursing Interventions
▶ *Anxiety related to sensory visual impairment and lack of understanding about treatment*	The client will demonstrate reduction of emotional stress, fear, and depression; and an acceptance of surgery.	Assess degree and duration of visual impairment.
		Encourage conversation to determine client's concerns, feelings, and level of understanding.
		Answer questions, offer support, and assist client to devise methods for coping.
		Orient client to new surroundings.
		Explain surgery routines. Preoperative: Level of activity-ocular rest which includes bilateral eye patching and bed rest to facilitate settling of the retina and prevent detachment from worsening. The client will be NPO after midnight. The affected eye is maximally dilated before surgery to permit adequate visualization of the fundus. Intraoperative: Client must lie still during surgery or give surgeon warning if needs to cough or change position. Face covered with drapes. Air and oxygen provided. Monitoring, including frequent blood pressure measurements. Postoperative: Positioning (supine with a small pillow under the head), bilateral eye patches, activity restrictions, and need to call for assistance with ambulation until stable and vision is adequate.
		Explain interventions clearly.
		Announce yourself with each interaction; interpret unfamiliar sounds; use touch to assist with verbal communication.
		Encourage to carry out ADLs as ability allows.
		Order finger foods for those who cannot see well enough or do not have the coping skills to use implements.
		Encourage participation of family or significant others in client care.
		Encourage participation in social and diversional activities as allowed (visitor, radio, audio tapes, television, crafts, games).
▶ *Risk for Injury related to visual impairment or knowledge deficit*	The client will not have injury caused by visual impairment.	Assist client when able to ambulate postoperatively until stable and has adequate vision or coping skills (remember that clients with bilateral eye patches are unable to see).
		Assist client in arranging environment and do not rearrange furnishings without reorienting client.
		Discuss importance of wearing metal shield or glasses as ordered.
		Apply no pressure to the affected eye.
		Use proper procedure to administer eye medications.

Evaluation Each goal must be evaluated to determine how it has been met by the client.

INFECTIONS

Infections of the eye include keratitis, stye, chalazion, and conjunctivitis.

KERATITIS

Keratitis is inflammation of the cornea that may be caused by infection, irritation, injury, or allergies. Symptoms associated with keratitis include severe eye pain, red watering eye, photophobia, sometimes reduced vision, and sometimes rash (e.g., herpes simplex, herpes zoster, or rosacea).

Treatment of keratitis includes optical anesthetics to relieve pain and mydriatics to dilate the pupil. Dark glasses should be worn to relieve the photophobia. Antibiotic solutions are prescribed for the specific type of infection, since the microorganism may be bacterial, viral, or fungal.

STYE

A **stye** is also referred to as a hordeolum. It is a pustular inflammation of an eyelash follicle or sebaceous gland on the lid margin commonly caused by staphylococcal organisms. Symptoms include pain, redness, and swelling of a specific area of the eyelid. Treatment consists of warm compresses and topical antibiotic ointments. More severe cases may require incision and drainage. Once the pus drains, the pain is relieved and healing begins.

CHALAZION

A **chalazion** is a cyst of the meibomian glands, which are sebaceous glands located at the junction of the conjunctiva and inner eyelid margins. The hard cyst is filled with fatty material from the chronically obstructed meibomian glands. The inherent feature of a chalazion is painless localized swelling that develops over a period of weeks. Treatment usually involves surgical excision if the cyst is large, becomes infected, or interferes with vision or closure of the eyelids. The cyst remains when the inflammation subsides.

CONJUNCTIVITIS (PINK EYE)

Conjunctivitis is an inflammation of the conjunctiva (a membrane that lines the inside of the eyelids and covers the cornea) that results from invasion by bacterial, viral, or rickettsial organisms, allergens, or irritants. Symptoms include burning and itching of eyes, discharge, swelling, pain, and redness. Treatment consists of applying warm compresses using saline or boric acid solution and instilling antibiotic or antiviral

ointments. When caused by allergens, treatment includes avoiding the allergen, taking antihistamines, or being desensitized.

Conjunctivitis is contagious. Proper handwashing must be done by nurse and client. Gloves should be worn when applying compresses or instilling ointment. The client's linen should be disinfected to prevent spread of the infection.

REFRACTIVE ERRORS

Refraction is the deflection or bending of light rays when they pass from a medium of one density to a medium of another density. In the case of the eye, light waves pass through the air (less dense) into the fluids of the eye (more dense) so that they can be brought to focus on the retina.

Refractive errors result in changes in visual acuity or vision that is not 20/20. Refractive errors include myopia (nearsightedness), **hyperopia** (farsightedness), **astigmatism** (asymmetric focus of light rays on the retina), **presbyopia** (inability of the lens to change curvature in order to focus on near objects), and **strabismus** (inability of the eyes to focus in the same direction). Figure 26-10 shows a child with strabismus.

With myopia, parallel light rays come to focus in front of the retina because the refractive system is too strong or the eyeball is elongated. Near vision is normal but distant vision is poor.

With hyperopia, parallel light rays come to focus behind the retina because the refractive system is too weak or the eyeball is flattened. Vision beyond 20 feet is normal, but near vision is poor. Figure 26-11 illustrates where light rays focus for myopia and hyperopia.

Astigmatism is a visual defect due to unequal curvatures of the refractive surfaces of the eye. Light rays from a point do not come to focus on the retina, resulting in visual distortion.

Presbyopia is the loss of elasticity of the lens of the eye caused by aging that causes the near point of

Figure 26-10 Strabismus (*Courtesy of the Armed Forces Institute of Pathology*)

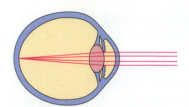

A. Normal eye
    Light rays focus on the retina

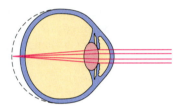

B. Myopia (nearsightedness)
    Light rays focus in front
    of the retina

C. Hyperopia (farsightedness)
    Light rays focus beyond
    the retina

Figure 26-11 Refraction: A. Normal eye; B. Myopia;
C. Hyperopia

vision to recede. The eye loses the ability to accommodate to near objects but remains accommodated for far objects.

Strabismus occurs when one eye is constantly deviated to the side.

Medical–Surgical Management

Medical

Refractory errors may be corrected by prescription glasses or contact lenses. The corrective lenses bend light rays to compensate for a client's refractive error.

Surgical

Radial keratotomy is a surgical procedure used to correct myopia and astigmatism. Under local anesthesia, incisions that resemble the spokes of a wheel are made in the cornea. These incisions start near the center of the cornea and extend outward to the edge. The incisions are made by a special knife that can be calibrated to cut at a predetermined depth. After the cuts are made, pressure in the anterior chamber of the eye reshapes the cornea to a normal or near-normal curvature.

▶ NURSING PROCESS

▶ Assessment

▶ Subjective Data

A general medical history should be obtained as well as a history of symptoms. Symptoms may include blurred vision, headache, or eye fatigue.

▶ Objective Data

The client is asked to view an eye chart while lenses of different strengths are systematically placed in front of the eye. The client is asked if the lenses sharpen or blur vision. The power or strength of the lens necessary to permit focusing of the image on the retina is expressed in measurements called diopters.

A nursing diagnosis for a client with refractive errors may be:

Nursing Diagnosis	Planning/Goals	Nursing Interventions
▶ *Anxiety related to impaired vision and having to wear glasses or contact lenses*	The client will accept wearing glasses or contact lenses.	Allow client to discuss impact of wearing glasses or contact lenses. Encourage client to wear the glasses or contact lenses as prescribed.

Evaluation The goal must be evaluated to determine how it has been met by the client.

INJURY

Injury to the eye or periorbital area can result from a variety of things such as chemical sprays, tree branches, slingshots, BB guns, flying debris from lawn mowers, and fireworks. Both children and adults are susceptible to eye injuries and the importance of protecting the eyes cannot be overemphasized. Injuries to the eyes require immediate attention by an ophthalmologist. Even a few hours delay in treatment may lead to permanent damage.

Corneal abrasion is the disruption of cells and the loss of the superficial epithelium. The outer surface is easily separated from the underlying layers and can be injured or destroyed by exposure (lack of moisture), chemical irritants that dissolve in the protective tear film, and abrasion from foreign bodies.

Safety: Avoiding Eye Injury
The eyes can be easily protected from injury by wearing protective goggles when performing tasks potentially hazardous to the eyes. Those who wear contact lenses should follow the manufacturer's recommendations for wearing them during certain activities such as swimming or when sleeping.

FOREIGN BODIES

Foreign bodies in the conjunctiva or on the cornea may cause excessive tearing, redness, and complaints of a foreign body sensation in the eye or under the eyelid, or just irritation in the eye. Foreign bodies often become embedded in the conjunctiva under the upper eyelid. The lid must be everted and the client instructed to look up to facilitate inspection and removal. If the particle is not located and removed, sterile fluorescein drops or strips should be instilled to visualize minute foreign bodies not readily visible with the naked eye.

CHEMICAL BURNS

Emergency treatment of chemical burns to the conjunctiva or cornea includes immediate lavage of the eye with tap water and referral to an emergency room or ophthalmologist. In the emergency room, a specially made lid speculum is placed directly on the eyeball and connected to a minimum of one liter of isotonic saline solution for irrigation. A topical anesthetic may be instilled to minimize pain during irrigation. No attempt should be made to neutralize the chemical, since the heat generated by the chemical reaction may cause further injury. Both eyes should then be patched to allow more comfort.

IMPAIRED VISION

The term blindness evokes an image of total darkness and is used for many legal purposes when central visual acuity is 20/200 or less with corrective lenses, in the better eye. Those who have visual acuity between 20/70 and 20/200 in the better eye, with the use of glasses, are often referred to as partially sighted.

The aids that follow are designed to make the most of the available vision (those in italics can also be used by persons who are blind): magnifying glasses; hand and stand magnifiers; telescopes; large print books, newspapers, magazines; talking books; *Braille* books; closed-circuit television which produces highly magnified images; *tactually marked watches and clocks; tactually modified table top games;* enlarged telephone dials, kitchen implements, tools, medication devices; talking clocks, timers, scales, calculators, computers; *text scanner which converts text to audio mode or Braille;* speech synthesizer; flashlight eye sonar devices; canes, laser canes, and seeing eye dogs.

MACULAR DEGENERATION

Macular degeneration is atrophy or deterioration of the macula, the point on the retina where light rays meet as they are focused by the cornea and lens of the eye. The person loses central vision, but still has peripheral vision.

The most common form of macular degeneration is associated with the aging process and is called age-related macular degeneration. Other forms of this disorder include exudative (wet) macular degeneration (sudden growth of new blood vessels in the area of the macula) and injury, infection, or inflammation that damages the macula.

Medical–Surgical Management
Medical

The treatment of age-related macular degeneration is geared toward assisting the client to maximize the use of the remaining vision. The loss of central vision may interfere with the client's ability to read, write, recognize safety hazards, and drive.

Management of clients with exudative macular degeneration is geared toward halting the initiating process and identifying further changes in visual perception. Fluid and blood may resorb in a small percentage of clients with exudative degeneration. Laser therapy to seal the leaking blood vessels in or near the macula may also limit the extent of the damage.

◗ NURSING PROCESS

◗ Assessment

◗ Subjective Data
A general medical history as well as a history of symptoms should be obtained. Symptoms would include blurred vision, disturbance in color vision (colors become dim), difficulty in reading or doing close work, distortion of objects (especially those with lines), and an empty area within the central field of vision.

◗ Objective Data
Coping mechanisms such as turning the head to use peripheral vision should be noted.

A nursing diagnosis for the client with macular degeneration may be:

Nursing Diagnosis	Planning/Goals	Nursing Interventions
▶ *Disturbed Sensory Perception (Visual) related to macular degeneration*	The client will discuss the impact of vision loss on lifestyle and use adaptive measures.	Allow client to express feelings about vision loss such as its impact on lifestyle. Convey a willingness to listen, but do not pressure client to talk.
		Provide a safe environment by removing excess furniture or equipment from client's surroundings.
		Orient client to surroundings and show how to use call light.
		Always introduce yourself or announce your presence upon entering the client's room; let client know when you are leaving.
		Provide sensory stimulation by using tactile, auditory, and gustatory stimuli to help compensate for vision loss.
		Suggest large print-books, talking books, audiotapes, or radio as preferred by client.
		Provide reality orientation if client is confused or disoriented.
		Give clear, concise explanations of treatments and procedures but avoid information overload.
		Make sure that health care personnel are aware of client's vision loss. Record information on the client's chart or post in room.
		Respond to call light quickly.
		Provide continuity by assigning same staff members to care for client when possible.
		Refer to appropriate community resources.

Evaluation The goal must be evaluated to determine how it has been met by the client.

SAMPLE NURSING CARE PLAN

THE CLIENT WITH MACULAR DEGENERATION

Mr. Datal is a 60-year-old high school Latin teacher. He describes having blurred vision in both eyes with a gradual loss of vision in only the right eye. He has trouble reading and is afraid to drive because he can no longer recognize safety hazards. He denies having pain. He also relates having fallen several times recently at home while going up and down the stairs. The family practitioner referred him to an ophthalmologist who diagnosed Mr. Datal as having macular degeneration in the right eye.

Nursing Diagnosis 1 *Disturbed Sensory Perception (Visual) related to macular degeneration as evidenced by his inability to recognize safety hazards when driving*

PLANNING/GOALS	NURSING INTERVENTIONS	RATIONALE	EVALUATION
Mr. Datal will discuss impact of vision loss on lifestyle.	Encourage Mr. Datal to express feelings about vision loss, such as the impact on lifestyle.	Allowing Mr. Datal to discuss the impact of vision loss aids in the acceptance of it.	Mr. Datal discussed the effects of vision loss on his lifestyle and contacted a local agency that provides assistance to the visually impaired.
	Convey a willingness to listen, but do not pressure Mr. Datal to talk. Discuss Mr. Datal's current ability to meet	Discussion can determine needs for assistance which will, in part, be based on current functional level.	

continues

self-care needs and activities of daily living.	Determine Mr. Datal's awareness of his limitations.		
Educate Mr. Datal in alternative ways of coping with vision loss; care of such adaptive devices as eyeglasses, magnifying glass, and contact lenses.	A knowledgeable client will be better able to cope with vision loss.		
Refer to appropriate community resources to help Mr. Datal and his family adapt to his vision loss.	Support from outside resources will help Mr. Datal and his family cope better with his vision loss.		

Nursing Diagnosis 2 *Risk for Injury related to difficulty in processing visual images and altered depth perception as evidenced by recent falls*

PLANNING/GOALS	NURSING INTERVENTIONS	RATIONALE	EVALUATION
Mr. Datal will not experience injury or visual compromise resulting from a fall.	Advise Mr. Datal that depth perception is changed with macular degeneration.	Information promotes understanding.	Mr. Datal has not fallen in two weeks.
	Teach Mr. Datal to avoid reaching for objects for stability when ambulating.	Objects may not be located where they are perceived. Excessive reaching alters the center of gravity which can precipitate a fall.	
	Advise Mr. Datal to go up and down steps one at a time.	Going up and down steps one at a time enhances the sense of balance.	

Nursing Diagnosis 3 *Impaired Home Maintenance related to limited vision, as evidenced by recent falls at home*

PLANNING/GOALS	NURSING INTERVENTIONS	RATIONALE	EVALUATION
Mr. Datal will develop a plan for self-care in the desired living environment.	Inform Mr. Datal about required self-care activities: personal care, eyedrop instillation, activities permitted, activity restrictions, medications, and how to monitor for complications.	Knowing what self-care activities are needed will help Mr. Datal plan for his care at home.	Mr. Datal is working on a plan so he can care for himself at home.

continues

Assist Mr. Datal to determine which activities will require assistance: personal care, meal preparation, eyedrop instillation, or shopping.	Helps Mr. Datal to plan for his care at home.
Evaluate sources of assistance: friends/family, home health care (skilled nursing care), or home care aids.	Determines availability of assistance.
Critique the safety of Mr. Datal's home: location of telephone, emergency plan, presence of loose rugs or carpets.	Changes can then be made to make Mr. Datal's home safer.

OTHER SENSES

Other senses include taste, smell, and touch.

TASTE

The sense of taste (gustation) serves as a protector from rotten or putrid food, and provides delightful sensations of creamy chocolate, crunchy carrots, chewy taffy, and fruitful pies. Taste sensors are most efficient at room temperature and respond only to substances in solution. The taste buds are located in four areas of the tongue that sense sweet, salt, bitter, and sour as shown in Figure 26-12.

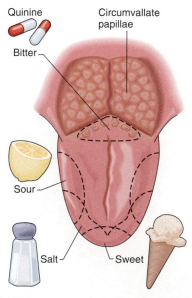

Figure 26-12 Taste Regions of the Tongue

GERONTOLOGICAL CONSIDERATIONS

Aging and Taste Sensation
The ability to taste sweetness remains as one ages, but the ability to taste bitterness declines.

Taste sensations can be altered secondary to neurological disorders or trauma. Clients who complain of food not "tasting good" should be evaluated for possible causes including dietary habits, medication use, smoking and caffeine use, as well as olfactory disturbances. The sense of taste works very closely with the sense of smell for identification of the taste sensations.

SMELL

The sense of smell (olfaction) also serves as a guardian from danger. Our nose warns us of impending danger from gas leaks, smoke, fires, rancid meat or fish, and sour dairy products. Body odors and halitosis are obvious clues regarding the need to maintain personal hygiene and dental care.

Disorders of the olfactory sense often go unnoticed. New tests such as the University of Pennsylvania Smell Identification Test (UPSIT) allow self-testing of smelling deficiencies. Early identification of the loss of the sense of smell may offer clues to alterations in dietary habits, weight loss or gain, anorexia, malnourishment, and changes in daily habits such as bathing and brushing teeth. The receptors for the sense of smell are located in the roof of the nasal cavity. If these cells are damaged, the sense of smell is impaired. The body cannot regenerate the olfactory cells.

TOUCH

The sense of touch (tactile) includes sensations pertaining to the skin. The tactile receptors are located throughout the integumentary system. Cutaneous sensations of touch, pressure, vibration, cold, heat, and pain are examples. Clients who are unable to sense temperature variations should be taught cautionary measures when applying heat or cold therapies, preparing bath water, cooking, or exposing self to hot or cold climates and environmental temperatures.

Clients with reduced or loss of tactile sensation risk injury when their condition confines them to bed. They are unable to sense pressure on bony prominences or the need to change position. The nurse's role in reducing or preventing impairment of skin integrity is crucial. Timely positioning, securing tubes or devices away from the client's body, and using products to minimize skin breakdown are a few of the interventions vital to excellent client care.

CASE STUDY

Katie Rollins is a 34-year-old nurse who was diagnosed with a right ear hearing impairment during a routine physical examination. She admitted to her doctor that she noticed she would only use her left ear to talk on the phone and that she had particular difficulty hearing her family or friends in a crowded restaurant or other public settings. She also noted that her husband asked her why she played the television so loud, yet if he turned it down to his normal hearing level, she could not hear it clearly. Her physician ordered an audiogram which showed a conductive hearing loss of 40% secondary to otosclerosis. Hearing in her left ear was normal.

Katie's doctor gave her three medical treatment options.

1. Do nothing and monitor her hearing impairment by audiogram every six months. If it were to worsen, other options would be considered.

2. Be fitted with a hearing aid.

3. Have a surgical procedure to correct the hearing loss.

Katie agreed to have surgery. She thought she would be too self-conscious to wear a hearing aid, after all she was only thirty-four, but she simply could not ignore the problem by doing nothing. Katie was scheduled for same-day surgery.

The following questions will guide your development of a nursing care plan for the case study.

1. How is a conductive hearing loss differentiated from a sensorineural hearing loss?

2. What does an audiogram tell you? What special things should Katie know before she has the audiogram?

3. Describe the surgical procedure that will most likely be used to correct the conductive hearing loss.

4. What will you teach Katie prior to her surgery about the procedure and expected postoperative course?

5. List four individualized nursing diagnoses and expected outcomes for Katie, and nursing interventions for each diagnosis.

6. Describe the expected discharge instructions that Katie must know related to diet, medications, activity restrictions, and follow-up care.

SUMMARY

- Hearing loss may be conductive, sensorineural, or a combination of the two. It may also be congenital.
- Ménière's disease is a result of excessive accumulation of endolymph causing severe vertigo, dizziness, and hearing loss. Treatment is primarily symptomatic.

- Otosclerosis is a conductive hearing loss resulting from fixation of the stapes, and may be treated medically with the use of a hearing aid, or surgically with a stapedectomy.
- Otitis media is inflammation of the middle ear. Treatment usually includes antibiotics, decongestants, and possibly a myringotomy.

- Cataract surgery is indicated when significant vision loss has occurred.
- Untreated retinal detachment results in total loss of vision.
- Many resources are available for the hearing impaired through community and national agencies.
- The senses of taste, smell, and touch are essential to our enjoyment of life and serve to protect us from danger or harm.

Review Questions

1. The three bones of the middle ear are:

   a. hammer, nail, and stirrup.
   b. malleus, incus, and cochlea.
   c. malleus, humorous, and stapes.
   d. malleus, incus, and stapes.

2. In a conductive hearing loss:

   a. the endolymph may cross the capillary membrane and mix with the perilymph resulting in severe vertigo.
   b. the ossicles of the middle ear fracture resulting in a tear of the eighth cranial nerve.
   c. sound waves are not transmitted through the ear canal to inner ear fluid.
   d. a tumor in the inner ear blocks the flow of fluid through the bony and membranous labyrinths.

3. A possible nursing diagnosis for a client with Ménière's disease is:

   a. activity intolerance related to impaired hearing.
   b. knowledge deficit related to surgical shunt placement to drain excessive endolymph.
   c. communication, impaired, verbal, related to tinnitus.
   d. injury, risk for, related to Ménière's disease.

4. Persons with hearing impairment or loss may benefit from:

   a. sitting in the middle of a crowded room so as to listen to all conversations at once.
   b. learning to lip read with family members.
   c. using a poorly fitted hearing aid with proper amplification.
   d. cupping the ear and turning the head toward the person speaking to them.

5. Chemical burns of the eye are initially treated with:

   a. local anesthetics and antibacterial drops for 24 to 36 hours.
   b. hot compresses applied at 15-minute intervals.
   c. flushing of the lids, conjunctiva, and cornea with water.
   d. cleansing of the conjunctiva with a small, cotton-tipped applicator.

6. Increased ocular pressure is indicated by a reading of:

   a. 0 to 5 mm Hg.
   b. 6 to 10 mm Hg.
   c. 11 to 20 mm Hg.
   d. 21 to 32 mm Hg.

7. A clinical symptom of a detached retina is:

   a. a sensation of floating particles.
   b. an area of vague vision.
   c. momentary flashes of light.
   d. pain in the eye.

8. Macular degeneration is characterized by:

   a. purulent periorbital drainage.
   b. pupil dilation.
   c. loss of central vision.
   d. ptosis (droopy lid).

Critical Thinking Questions

1. What would have to change in your life if you suddenly could not see?

2. What would change in your life if you suddenly could not hear?

3. Identify the rationale for each nursing intervention given for the possible nursing diagnoses in the chapter.

 WEB FLASH!

- What sites can you locate on the Internet that provide resources for individuals with sensory alterations? List self-help groups, books, media products, or other resources suggested at these sites.
- Identify Web addresses that are specifically designed to help the elderly and their families manage the sensory alterations that are a normal part of aging.

NURSING CARE OF THE CLIENT: ENDOCRINE SYSTEM

MAKING THE CONNECTION

Refer to the following chapters to increase your understanding of the endocrine system:

- Chapter 7, Wellness Concepts
- Chapter 10, Fluid, Electrolyte, and Acid-Base Balance
- Chapter 12, Health Assessment
- Chapter 17, Nursing Care of the Oncology Client
- Chapter 19, Nursing Care of the Client: Cardiovascular System
- Chapter 20, Nursing Care of the Client: Hemotologic and Lymphatic Systems
- Chapter 21, Nursing Care of the Client: Integumentary System
- Chapter 22, Nursing Care of the Client: Immune System
- Chapter 24, Nursing Care of the Client: Musculoskeletal System
- Chapter 25, Nursing Care of the Client: Neurological System
- Chapter 26, Nursing Care of the Client: Sensory System
- Chapter 29, Nursing Care of the Client: Urinary System
- Chapter 30, Nursing Care of the Client: Female Reproductive System
- Chapter 31, Nursing Care of the Client: Male Reproductive System
- Chapter 35, Nursing Care of the Older Client

LEARNING OBJECTIVES

Upon completion of this chapter, you should be able to:
- *Define key terms.*
- *Identify and locate the endocrine glands and list function(s) and hormone(s) secreted by each.*
- *Differentiate between type 1 and type 2 diabetes in terms of pathophysiology, presenting symptoms and treatment.*
- *Discuss the roles of diet and exercise in the management of diabetes mellitus.*
- *Identify signs, causes, and treatment of complications of hypoglycemia, diabetic ketoacidosis, and hyperosmolar hyperglycemic nonketotic syndrome.*
- *Discuss the major long-term complications of diabetes.*
- *Discuss rationale for the pituitary gland being traditionally called the "master" gland.*
- *Compare symptoms of the disease process resulting from a hyper- or hyposecretion of an endocrine gland.*
- *Discuss assessment techniques for a client suspected of having an endocrine disorder.*
- *Formulate a nursing care plan for the client with an endocrine disorder.*

KEY TERMS

agranulocytosis
autosomal
Chvostek's sign
cretinism
dawn phenomenon
endocrine
exophthalmos
glucagon
glycosuria
goiter
gynecomastia
hirsutism
hormone
hyperglycemia
hypoglycemia
hypovolemia
iatrogenic
insulin
ketonuria
lipodystrophy
myxedema
paroxysmal
polydipsia
polyphagia
polyuria
Somogyi phenomenon
tetany
Trousseau's sign

INTRODUCTION

The endocrine system is unique in that the components are not in direct physical contact but scattered throughout the body. The endocrine system provides the same general functions as the nervous system: communication and control; however, the endocrine system is generally slower and has longer lasting control over the various body activities and functions. It exerts this control through the secretion of hormones that circulate through the blood. A malfunction of any part of the endocrine system can result in a shift of homeostasis with far-reaching systemic reactions.

Assessment of the endocrine system is difficult. Not only are the components not in direct contact, but only the thyroid gland is close enough to the body surface for direct physical assessment. Still the nurse needs to be familiar with the normal functioning of the endocrine system. In assessing the client for endocrine dysfunction, the nurse must take note of negative findings as well as positive ones. Assessment includes results of diagnostic tests as well as any precipitating or aggravating factors.

ANATOMY AND PHYSIOLOGY REVIEW

The endocrine system is composed of a group of various glands scattered throughout the body. The term **endocrine** (endo-within, crin-secrete) indicates that the secretions formed by these glands directly enter the blood or lymph circulation, rather than being transported via tubes or ducts. These secretions, called **hormones**, are chemical substances that initiate or regulate activity of another organ, system, or gland in another part of the body. The level of hormone in the blood is regulated by the homeostasis mechanism called negative feedback. If the blood level for a specific hormone falls below normal, negative feedback causes the specific endocrine gland to produce more of the hormone, which when increased to the normal level causes a decrease in production.

The glands discussed in this chapter that comprise the endocrine system are: the pancreas, pituitary, hypothalamus, thyroid, parathyroid, and adrenals (Figure 27-1). Several endocrine glands such as the pineal, thymus, ovaries, and testes are of great importance; however, they will be discussed in other chapters in connection with the organ system in which they function.

The pancreas lies horizontally behind the stomach at the level of the first and second lumbar vertebrae. The head of the pancreas is attached to the duodenum with the tail reaching to the spleen. It has both exocrine and endocrine functions.

The pituitary gland consists of an anterior and a posterior lobe. It has traditionally been called the "master" gland because so many of its secretions influence other endocrine glands and body systems. It is

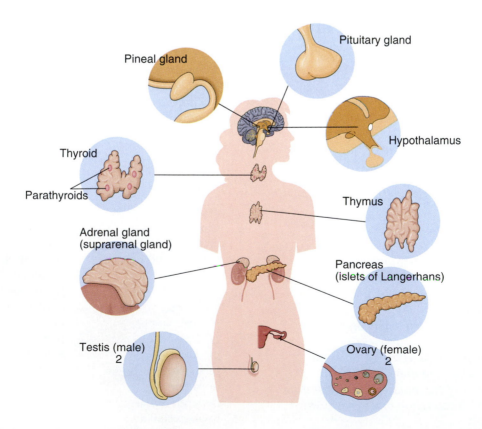

Figure 27-1 Structures of the Endocrine System

attached to the hypothalamus by a stalk called the *infundibulum*. The hypothalamus is located in the lower portion of the brain and produces secretions influencing the production and release of the anterior pituitary hormones as well as the production of the posterior pituitary hormones. Both the pituitary and hypothalamus are located in the head. The pituitary, about the size of a pea, is located in the sella turcica, a small depression in the sphenoid bone. The anterior pituitary, or adenohypophysis, produces and secretes the following 7 hormones:

- Thyroid-stimulating hormone (TSH)
- Adrenocorticotropic hormone (ACTH)
- Follicle-stimulating hormone (FSH)
- Luteinizing hormone (LH)
- Melanocyte-stimulating hormone (MSH)

- Growth hormone (GH)
- Prolactin or lactogenic hormone

The posterior pituitary, or neurohypophysis, releases two hormones—antidiuretic hormone (ADH) and oxytocin. The pituitary hormones have a variety of functions. Refer to Table 27–1 for specific endocrine hormones and functions.

The thyroid gland is butterfly-shaped and lies in the neck. It consists of two lobes—one on each side of the trachea connected by an isthmus. The gland sits saddlelike starting on the anterior surface of the trachea just below the larynx and surrounds it partway. The thyroid gland stores iodine. The thyroid gland produces thyroid hormones including thyroxine, which is the most abundant, and triiodothyronine. It regulates the metabolic rate for carbohydrates, protein, and fats.

Table 27–1 ENDOCRINE GLAND HORMONES

HORMONE	FUNCTION
Pancreas	
Glucagon	Raises blood glucose
Insulin	Lowers blood glucose
Somatostatin	Inhibits secretion of insulin, glucagon, and growth hormone from the anterior pituitary and gastrin from the stomach
Anterior Pituitary	
Thyroid-stimulating hormone (TSH)	Stimulates thyroid growth and secretion of the thyroid hormone
Adrenocorticotropic hormone (ACTH)	Stimulates adrenal cortex growth and secretion of glucocorticoids
Follicle-stimulating hormone (FSH)	Stimulates ovarian follicle to mature and produce estrogen; in the male, stimulates sperm production
Luteinizing hormone (LH)	Acts with FSH to stimulate estrogen production; causes ovulation; stimulates progesterone production by corpus luteum; in male, stimulates testes to produce testosterone
Melanocyte-stimulating hormone (MSH)	Causes increase in synthesis and spread of melanin (pigment) in skin
Growth hormone (GH)	Stimulates growth
Prolacting or lactogenic hormone	Stimulates breast development during pregnancy and milk secretion after delivery of baby
Posterior Pituitary	
Antidiuretic hormone (ADH)	Stimulates water retention by kidneys to decrease urine secretion
Oxytocin	Stimulates uterine contractions; causes breast to release milk into ducts
Thyroid Gland	
Thyroid hormone (thyroxine T_4 and triiodothyronine T_3)	Increases metabolic rate
Calcitonin	Decreases blood calcium concentration
Parathyroid Gland	
Parathyroid hormone	Increases blood calcium concentration
Adrenal Cortex	
Glucocorticoids (cortisol, hydrocortisone)	Stimulates gluconeogenesis and increases blood glucose; antiinflammatory; antiimmunity; antiallergy
Mineralocorticoids	Regulates electrolyte and fluid homeostasis
Sex hormones (androgen)	Stimulate sexual drive in females; in males, negligible effect
Adrenal Medulla	
Epinephrine (adrenalin)	Prolongs and intensifies sympathetic nervous response to stress
Norepinephine	Prolongs and intensifies sympathetic nervous response to stress

There are 4 parathyroid glands, although some individuals may have as many as 6. Two glands are embedded in the posterior portion of each thyroid lobe. They produce parathyroid hormone, parathormone, which regulates the concentration of blood calcium and phosphorus.

The adrenal, or suprarenal, glands are located on top of each kidney. The adrenal cortex secretes mineralocorticoids including aldosterone, glucocorticoids including cortisol, and androgens which are sex hormones. The adrenal medulla secretes epinephrine or adrenalin and norepinephrine or noradrenalin which help the body to function under stress.

It is important to understand the normal function of the endocrine glands and hormones. Most endocrine disorders are a result of either overactivity or underactivity of these glands.

COMMON DIAGNOSTIC TESTS

Commonly used diagnostic tests for clients with symptoms of endocrine system disorders are listed in Table 27–2. See Chapter 13, Diagnostic Tests, for explanation/normal values and nursing responsibilities.

DIABETES MELLITUS

Diabetes mellitus is a disorder of metabolism. When we eat, most of the food we eat is broken down by digestive juices into chemicals, including a simple sugar called *glucose*. Of the food we eat, 100% of carbohydrate and approximately 58% of protein and 10% of fat is broken down to glucose. For the glucose to get into the cells, insulin must be present (Figure 27-2).

Insulin is a hormone produced and secreted by the beta cells in the islets of Langerhans of the pancreas. Insulin stimulates the active transport of glucose into muscle and adipose tissue cells, making it available for cell use. For glucose to cross the cell membrane, insulin must connect with a receptor on the cell membrane. Some clients with diabetes mellitus have enough insulin, but too few functioning receptor sites. Others have inadequate or no insulin production. Blood glu-

---

Table 27–2 COMMON DIAGNOSTIC TESTS FOR ENDOCRINE SYSTEM DISORDERS

Pancreas Diagnostic Tests

Blood glucose, Fasting blood sugar (FBS)

2-hour postprandial glucose (2hPPG) or 2-hour post-prandial blood sugar (2hPPBS)

Glucose tolerance test (GTT)

Pituitary Gland Diagnostic Tests

Adrenocorticotropic hormone (ACTH), Corticotropin

Antidiuretic hormone (ADH), Vasopressin

Follicle-stimulating hormone (FSH)

Growth hormone (GH), Human GH (HGH), Somatotropin hormone (SH)

Growth hormone (GH) stimulation test, GH provocation test, Insulin tolerance test (ITT), Arginine test

Luteinizing hormone (LH) assay

Prolactin levels (PRL)

Thyrotropin-releasing hormone (TRH) test, Thyrotropin-releasing factor (TRF) test

Urine specific gravity

Long bone x-rays

Sella turcica x-ray

Computed tomography of head (CT scan of head), Computerized axial transverse tomography (CATT)

Thyroid Gland Diagnostic Tests

Antithyroid microsomal antibody, Antimicrosomal antibody, Microsomal antibody, Thyroid autoantibody, Thyroid anti-microsomal antibody

Calcitonin, HCT, Thyrocalcitonin

Serum free triiodothyronine (T_3)

Thyroid-stimulating hormone (TSH), Thyrotropin

Thyroid-stimulating hormone (TSH) stimulation test

Thyroxine index free, FTI, FT_4 Index

Thyroxine, T_4, Thyroxine screen

Triiodothyronine, T_3 radioimmunoassay, T_3 by RIA

Radioactive iodine uptake, (RAIU), Iodine uptake test, ^{131}I uptake

Thyroid scan, Thyroid scintiscan

Thyroid ultrasound, Thyroid echogram, Thyroid sonogram

Thyroid biopsy

Parathyroid Gland Diagnostic Tests

Parathyroid hormone (PTH), Parathormone

Calcium, total/ionized Ca^{++}

Phosphorus

Adrenal Glands Diagnostic Tests

Adrenocorticotropic hormone (ACTH) stimulation test, Cortisol stimulation test, Cosyntropin test

Cortisol, Hydrocortisone

Dexamethasone suppression test (DST), Prolonged/rapid DST, Cortisol suppression test, ACTH suppression test

Plasma renin assay, Plasma renin activity (PRA)

Progesterone assay

Aldosterone assay

17-Hydroxycorticosteroids (17-OHCS)

17-Ketosteroids (17-KS)

Urine cortisol, Hydrocortisone

Vanillylmandelic acid (VMA) & catecholamines, VMA & epinephrine, Norepinephrine, Metanephrine, Normetanephrine, Dopamine

Adrenal angiography, Adrenal arteriogram

Adrenal venography

Computed tomography of adrenals (CAT scan of adrenals), CT scan of adrenals

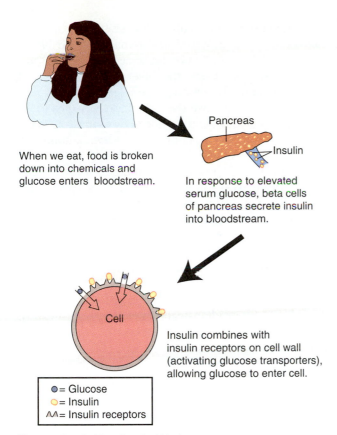

When we eat, food is broken down into chemicals and glucose enters bloodstream.

Pancreas

Insulin

In response to elevated serum glucose, beta cells of pancreas secrete insulin into bloodstream.

Cell

Insulin combines with insulin receptors on cell wall (activating glucose transporters), allowing glucose to enter cell.

● = Glucose
○ = Insulin
ᴧᴧ = Insulin receptors

Figure 27-2 How Insulin Works

cose can always be used by the brain and kidneys. Insulin is not needed for glucose to enter brain cells or cells of the glomeruli.

The amount of glucose in the blood regulates the rate of insulin secretion. When a meal is eaten, the blood glucose elevates and the beta cells of the islets of Langerhans release insulin. As the blood glucose level drops, insulin secretion diminishes. It is important to note that during times of fasting (overnight or between meals) a low level of insulin continues to be secreted along with **glucagon**. Glucagon secreted by the alpha cells of the pancreas stimulates release of glucose by the liver. The balance and interactions of insulin and glucagon serve to maintain a constant serum glucose level.

Other functions of insulin include:

- Promoting conversion of glucose to glycogen for storage in the liver and inhibiting conversion of glycogen to glucose
- Promoting the conversion of fatty acids into fat that can be stored as adipose tissue and preventing breakdown of adipose tissue and conversion of fat to ketone bodies
- Stimulating protein synthesis within tissues and inhibiting the breakdown of protein into amino acids

In summary, insulin actively promotes those processes that lower the blood glucose level and inhibits those processes that raise the blood glucose level. A deficiency of insulin results in **hyperglycemia**, or elevated blood glucose. Excess insulin results in **hypoglycemia** (low blood glucose). Diabetes mellitus is actually a group of disorders characterized by chronic hyperglycemia.

DIAGNOSIS AND CLASSIFICATION

The Expert Committee on the Diagnosis and Classification of Diabetes Mellitus (1997) presented to the American Diabetes Association (ADA) new criteria for diagnosis and new classifications for diabetes which the ADA approved.

Diagnosis

The Committee identified two precursors to diabetes, new screening criteria, and new diagnostic criteria, and it eliminated one diagnostic test.

The two precursors identified are:

1. Impaired glucose tolerance (IGT)—a glucose level of 140 to 199 mg/dL 2 hours after a glucose load
2. Impaired fasting glucose (IFG)—a fasting glucose of 110 to 125 mg/dL

The new criteria for who should be screened for diabetes include:

PROFESSIONAL TIP

Diabetes

According to the Centers for Disease Control and Prevention (CDC) (1998), there are 10.3 million Americans diagnosed as having diabetes mellitus. This is an increase from 8 million in 1995. Another 5 million are estimated to be undiagnosed. Diabetes was the seventh leading cause of death in the United States and is associated with many serious complications (CDC, 1999). Diabetes is the leading cause of new blindness among adults, the leading cause of new cases of renal failure, and is present in more than half of persons experiencing non-traumatic lower extremity amputations. Diabetes and its complications shorten a person's life span, create disability, and impose an economic burden on persons who have the disease (CDC, 1999).

Diabetes is seen in all age groups and races. One-third of clients with diabetes are over age 60. African American, Hispanic, and some Native American populations have a higher incidence of diabetes than the white population.

1. Anyone age 45 and older
2. Anyone, regardless of age, with one of the following risk factors:
    *   Obesity (body mass index of 27 or greater)
    *   Immediate family member with diabetes
    *   Member of high-risk ethnic group (African American, Hispanic American, some Native American groups)
    *   Having a baby weighing more than 9 pounds
    *   History of gestational diabetes mellitus (GDM)
    *   Hypertension
    *   High-density lipoprotein level of 35 mg/dL or less, or a triglyceride level of 250 mg/dL or more
    *   Have either of the two precursors of diabetes

The new diagnostic criteria identify when a physician can make a diagnosis of diabetes. The situations are:

*   A random blood glucose of 200 mg/dL or greater with the classic symptoms of polyuria, polydipsia, and unexplained weight loss
    or
*   A fasting blood sugar of 126 mg/dL or greater
    or
*   The 2-hour sample of the oral glucose tolerance test is 200 mg/dL or greater using a load of 75 grams of anhydrous glucose

The committee also recommended not using glycosylated hemoglobin to diagnose diabetes. Terminology is confusing, and there are many methods of measuring glycosylated hemoglobin.

Classification

The new system uses etiology, not insulin use, to classify diabetes into four categories: type 1 diabetes, type 2 diabetes, other specific types, and gestational diabetes mellitus.

Type 1 Diabetes

There are two forms of diabetes resulting from pancreatic beta-cell destruction or a primary defect in beta-cell function resulting in no release of insulin and ineffective glucose transport. There is usually an absolute insulin deficiency so the clients are insulin-dependent. The two subdivisions of type 1 diabetes are:

*   Immune-mediated—islet cell or insulin antibodies destroy beta cells. The rate of this destruction is usually higher in children than in adults. Children and adolescents may rapidly develop ketoacidosis. Adults seldom develop ketoacidosis unless they have an infection or other stressor. This is what used to be called type I, insulin-dependent diabetes mellitus (IDDM), or juvenile-onset diabetes.
*   Idiopathic—no evidence of autoimmunity; the individual just does not produce insulin and is prone to ketoacidosis.

In the absence of insulin, glucose from food eaten cannot be used or stored and remains in the bloodstream, resulting in hyperglycemia. In addition, glucose production from the liver goes unchecked, further elevating the blood glucose level.

As the blood glucose rises, the kidney begins to excrete excess glucose in the urine (**glycosuria**). Glucose eliminated in the urine pulls excessive amounts of water with it (osmotic diuresis), resulting in fluid volume deficit and producing symptoms of excessive thirst (**polydipsia**) and increased urination (**polyuria**).

Insulin deficiency also results in impaired metabolism of fats and proteins. Because of the impaired glucose, fat, and protein metabolism and the inability to store glucose, clients frequently experience protein wasting, weight loss, and increased hunger (**polyphagia**).

Metabolism of fat stores for energy leads to production of acid by-products called ketones, which can be detected in the urine (**ketonuria**). As ketones accumulate, the associated decrease in pH leads to metabolic acidosis, or more specifically a condition known as *diabetic ketoacidosis,* discussed later in this chapter.

Type 2 Diabetes

These clients have insulin resistance with relative insulin deficiency. Most of these clients are obese. When weight is lost, insulin resistance diminishes but reappears if the client regains weight. Age, lack of exercise, history of GDM, hypertension, dyslipidemia, and being of African American, Hispanic American, or Native American origin are all risk factors. A strong family history of diabetes is often evident. Many clients do not require insulin, but eventually one-third will need insulin to maintain a normal glucose level. This is what used to be called type II, noninsulin-dependent diabetes mellitus (NIDDM), or adult-onset diabetes.

Hyperglycemia results when the pancreas cannot match the body's need for insulin and/or when the number of insulin receptor sites are decreased or altered. Although available insulin may be insufficient to meet the body's metabolic needs and prevent hyperglycemia, there is a sufficient amount of insulin to prevent fat breakdown for energy and the resulting ketoacidosis. Extremely elevated glucose in the type 2 diabetic will result in development of hyperosmolar hyperglycemic nonketotic syndrome (HHNK), discussed later in this chapter. Table 27–3 compares the clinical manifestations of type 1 and type 2 diabetes.

Other Specific Types

This includes conditions such as beta-cell genetic defects, endocrinopathies, and drug- or chemical-induced diabetes. These are in a separate category because there are different disease etiologies.

Table 27–3 COMPARISON OF THE CLINICAL MANIFESTATIONS OF TYPE 1 DIABETES AND TYPE 2 DIABETES

	TYPE 1 DIABETES (Type I, IDDM, Juvenile, Brittle/labile)	TYPE 2 DIABETES (Type II, NIDDM, Adult Onset)
Etiology	Autoimmune	Genetic susceptibility associated. Usually associated with long duration obesity.
Age of onset	Rare before age 1	Incidence increases with age
Percent of diabetics	5–10%	85–90%
Onset	Abrupt, rapid	Gradual, over years
Body weight at onset	Normal or thin	80% are overweight
Insulin production	None	Less than normal, normal, or greater than normal
Insulin injection	Always	Necessary for approximately 30%
Ketosis	Occurs mainly in children and adolescents	Unlikely
Management	Insulin, diet, exercise	Diet and weight loss, exercise, possibly oral hypoglycemics or insulin

Gestational Diabetes Mellitus

Occurring during pregnancy, this may be controlled either with or without insulin. Generally the client's glucose tolerance returns to normal after the infant's birth. The client should be rechecked 6 weeks after the birth to see if the diabetes persists.

Contributing Factors

Persons with a family history of diabetes are at greater risk for developing diabetes. In addition to family history, factors associated with diabetes include obesity, aging, and ethnic group. The most powerful risk factor for type 2 diabetes is obesity. For persons with a family history of type 2 diabetes, maintenance of an ideal body weight may delay or prevent the onset of diabetes.

Aging can also be considered a contributing factor.

It is known that members of certain racial groups are more likely to develop diabetes. In the United States, there is a greater chance of developing type 2 diabetes for Hispanics, certain Native American populations, and African Americans.

Other groups at risk for development of diabetes include those with a history of gestational diabetes or impaired glucose tolerance (IGT).

Medical–Surgical Management

Medical

There is no known cure for diabetes. The goal of therapeutic management is aimed at the control of blood sugar, and the prevention and early detection of the complications associated with diabetes. Diabetes is considered under control if the client maintains ideal body weight and enjoys good health, preprandial glucose levels are less than 140 mg/dL, postprandial glucose levels do not rise above 180 mg/dL.

Treatment plans vary and are individualized for each client. Control of blood glucose generally involves a balance of a dietary prescription, an exercise plan, and medications. Ultimately, the client is the manager of the treatment plan and, therefore, must be very well informed about diabetes and involved in all aspects of care planning and decision making.

Since the advent of home glucose monitoring devices, urine testing for glucose is rarely used for the estimation of serum glucose levels in the management of diabetes. Testing urine for ketone (product of fatty acid oxidation) production, however, continues to be recommended when the blood glucose level is consistently ≥ 240 mg/dL or when any symptoms of ketoacidosis are present.

The client with type 1 diabetes will always require administration of insulin to lower the glucose level and prevent complications of diabetes. Diet and exercise regimens are also important for the control of the glucose level and maintenance of health.

Dietary management is the cornerstone of treatment for the person with type 2 diabetes. As the obese person loses weight, the body's insulin requirements decrease, resulting in improved glucose tolerance. Exercise can also play a valuable role in losing weight and lowering the blood glucose level. Type 2 diabetes not controlled by diet and exercise may necessitate administration of medications. Oral hypoglycemic agents or parenteral administration of insulin may be required for optimal control.

COMMUNITY/HOME HEALTH CARE

Glucose Monitoring

The availability and use of home glucose monitoring equipment to evaluate serum (blood) glucose has revolutionized self-care for the diabetic client (Figure 27-3). Also called "finger stick blood glucose" (FSBG), self-monitoring of blood glucose (SMBG) can be done quickly using capillary blood that provides fairly accurate reading of the current blood glucose. Most often, the glucose level is checked before meals and at bedtime, thus allowing the client to adjust the treatment plan accordingly. Self-monitoring of blood glucose is recommended for all clients requiring insulin and for clients with widely fluctuating glucose levels. Symptoms of hypoglycemia at any time warrant immediate evaluation of the blood glucose level.

Figure 27-3 Diabetic Blood Testing Equipment: Glucose Meter, Cotton Balls, Lancet, Alcohol, Blood Testing Strip, and Watch

Surgical

Pancreas transplantations have been performed and have successfully eliminated the need for exogenous insulin in some clients. At present pancreas transplants are being performed primarily on clients with type 1 diabetes who also need kidney or other organ transplants. This is because the serious side effects of the antirejection medications do not justify a pancreas transplant alone. Pancreatic islet cell transplants are also being done experimentally with limited success, but hold much promise for the future.

Pharmacological

Various pharmacological treatments that are used in the management of type 1 and type 2 diabetes are discussed in the following text.

Insulin Persons with type 1 diabetes always require insulin administration. Persons with type 2 diabetes often do not require insulin when initially diagnosed, but insulin therapy may become necessary over time, as endogenous insulin production decreases, or during times of stress or illness.

Historically, insulin has been obtained from beef or pork pancreas. Today, biosynthetic human insulin is used almost exclusively, but there are some clients still using pork or beef insulin. Human insulin is purer, more effective, and has a much lower incidence of causing insulin allergies and resistance. Insulin is available in short-, intermediate-, and long-acting forms that can be injected separately or mixed in the same syringe. Premixed insulins are also available. See Table 27–4 for descriptions of types of insulins and their actions. Insulin is routinely administered subcutaneously. Regular insulin (short-acting) may be administered in-

travenously when immediate response is desired, as in treatment of greatly elevated glucose levels occurring with diabetic ketoacidosis (DKA) or hyperosmolar hyperglycemic nonketotic syndrome (HHNK). Regular insulin, which is the only clear insulin, is the *only* insulin that can be given intravenously (IV).

The strength of insulin correlates to the number of units of insulin per cubic centimeter. The most common concentrations of insulin used today are U-50 and U-100 insulin (50 and 100 units of insulin per 1 cc respectively). U-500 insulin is also available for clients who have developed insulin resistance and require very high doses.

Insulin should always be measured in an insulin syringe which is marked in units. When mixing two types of insulin in the same syringe, it is important that the regular (clear, short-acting) insulin be drawn up first. The policy of many health care institutions requires that 2 nurses check insulin dosages prior to administration. Even if the facility does not have such a policy, checking the insulin dosage with another nurse will help protect against an adverse reaction due to error.

Insulin dosages are individually determined, usually requiring 2 or more injections per day and involving a combination of a short-acting and a longer-acting insulin. Various regimens of insulin administration can be used, each with its own advantages and disadvantages. In general, the more complex the regimen, the more normal the blood glucose level throughout the day. Clients can be taught to use the results of their self monitoring blood glucose to adjust their insulin doses, allowing more flexibility in their meals and schedules. Recent studies strongly support the theory that intensive insulin regimens that tightly control the blood glucose level delay the onset and progression of complications of diabetic retinopathy, nephropathy, and neuropathy.

Sliding Scale Insulin During times of surgery, illness, or stress, clients may have their glucose level managed with an insulin sliding scale in lieu of their regular regimen of insulin or oral hypoglycemics. A sliding scale determines insulin dosage based on fingerstick blood glucose level. Regular (short-acting) insulin is used and a dose is administered every 4 or 6 hours based on the blood glucose level. The sliding scale allows for much flexibility and ensures frequent monitoring of and response to changes in the client's glucose level. An example sliding scale might be:

- 4u Humulin R Insulin for glucose 151–200 mg/dL
- 6u Humulin R Insulin for glucose 201–250 mg/dL
- 8u Humulin R Insulin for glucose 251–300 mg/dL
- 10u Humulin R Insulin for glucose 301–350 mg/dL
- Call physician for glucose > 350 mg/dL

Insulin Injections Insulin injections are administered into the subcutaneous tissue. If an inch of skin can be pinched, the needle is injected at a 90-degree angle, otherwise, at a 45 degree angle. The 4 main areas for injection are the abdomen, arms, thighs, and hips (Figure 27-4). Factors affecting absorption should be considered when selecting an injection site. Absorption occurs most quickly in the abdomen, followed by the arms, thighs, and hips.

Rotation of sites for injection has traditionally been recommended to prevent **lipodystrophy** (atrophy or hypertrophy in the subcutaneous fat). More recently, some authorities are recommending that the abdomen,

Figure 27-4 Possible Sites and Rotation for Insulin Administration

which provides the most predictable absorption of insulin, be used exclusively for insulin administration.

If sites other than the abdomen are used, site rotation needs to be done in a systematic manner to prevent erratic absorption. One system of rotation is to always use the same area of injection the same time each day, e.g., always using the abdomen in the morning and the thigh in the afternoon. Another system of rotation is to use all available injection sites in one area before moving to another.

Areas of lipodystrophy should not be used for injection, as absorption may be diminished. Exercise will increase the rate of absorption, so diabetics planning

Table 27–4 TYPES OF INSULIN AND THEIR ACTIONS

TYPES OF INULSIN	APPEARANCE	ACTION IN HOURS		
		ONSET	PEAK	DURATION
Very short-acting insulin Lispro (Humalog)	clear	¼	1–1½	5 or less
Short-acting Humulin R	clear	½–1	2–4	6–8

Intermediate-acting
  Humulin U
  Humulin L
	cloudy
	cloudy
		1–1½
		1–2-½
			4–12
			7–15
				up to 24
				22

Long-acting Humulin U	cloudy	4–8	10–30	36+

Premixed
  Reg/Humulin N
  Humulin 70/30
  Humulin 50/50
	cloudy	½–1	4–8	24

to exercise should not inject insulin into the areas to be exercised.

Vials of insulin not being used should be refrigerated to prevent loss of potency. Vials in use may be kept at room temperature to decrease local irritation at the injection site, which can occur when cold insulin is used. When mixing a short-acting and a longer-acting insulin in the same syringe, the regular (clear) should always be drawn up into the syringe first, followed by the longer-acting (cloudy) insulin. Figure 27-5 illustrates mixing and administering insulin.

It is recommended that insulin syringes be used only once and then discarded.

The visually and/or neurologically impaired diabetic client may benefit from assistive devices available to facilitate drawing up the insulin and administering it. Clients dependent on others for drawing up their insulin may benefit from prefilled syringes, which are considered stable for up to 3 weeks when stored in the refrigerator.

The nurse should keep in mind that the most important factor in the administration of insulin is consistency in technique. Also, simplification of the procedure may have a major impact on a client's ability to comply and to maintain independence. It is important that the nurse understand the basic principles of insulin administration and thereby remain flexible when teaching new clients or assessing the skills of experienced clients.

Insulin Pumps A portable insulin infusion pump delivers insulin continuously through a subcutaneous needle, usually anchored in the abdomen (see Figure 27-6). A continuous, or basal rate, of regular (rapid-acting) insulin is programmed and delivered to closely imitate the body's natural insulin secretion. Additional boluses can be manually administered to coordinate with meal times. The injection site is changed every 24 to 48 hours. The use of the insulin pump prevents multiple injections and allows flexibility in meal size and time. Use of the pump requires a motivated and

The client may withdraw two different types of insulin into the same syringe. In this series of diagrams, a rapid-acting insulin (R vial) is combined with an intermediate-acting insulin (N vial).

1 After cleaning the rubber stopper on both vials with an alcohol wipe, inject the amount of air equal to the dose of the intermediate-acting insulin into the N vial.

2 Inject the amount of air equal to the dose of the rapid-acting insulin into the R vial.

3 Withdraw the correct amount of rapid-acting insulin.

4 Withdraw the correct amount of intermediate-acting insulin. (Note: Pull the plunger down to the unit mark that equals the dose of rapid-acting insulin plus the dose of intermediate-acting insulin. The insulins will mix immediately in the syringe. If too large an amount of intermediate-acting insulin is withdrawn, the entire contents of the syringe must be discarded.)

Figure 27-5 How to Mix Insulin (*Adapted from* Clinical Pharmacology and Nursing, 3rd ed., *by C. L. Baer & B. R. Williams, 1996, Springhouse, PA: Springhouse Corporation.*)

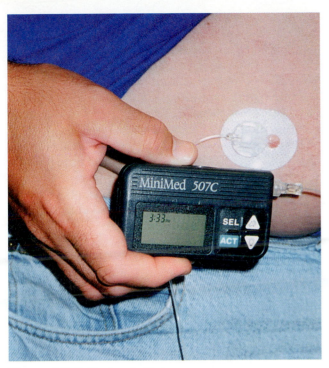

Figure 27-6 The Insulin Pump

educated client, because intensive self-monitoring of blood glucose is essential.

Complications of Insulin Therapy Complications of insulin therapy include hypoglycemia (discussed later in this chapter), insulin resistance (requiring more than 200 units/day), lipodystrophy, Somogyi phenomenon, and the dawn phenomenon. Lipodystrophy can be minimized by using human insulin, using room temperature insulin, and by rotating sites of insulin injection.

The **Somogyi phenomenon** occurs when a rapid decrease in blood glucose (hypoglycemia) generates the release of glucose-elevating hormones (epinephrine, cortisol, glucagon). The hypoglycemia usually occurs during the night, but manifests as an elevated glucose in the morning and may be inadvertently treated with an increase in insulin dosage. The Somogyi phenomenon can be diagnosed by checking the blood glucose during the night about 3 A.M. Adjusting the insulin regimen to avoid the peaking of insulin during the night will correct this effect.

The **dawn phenomenon** is an early morning glucose elevation produced by the release of growth hormone. Administering the evening insulin dose at a later time will coordinate the insulin peak with the hormone release.

Oral Hypoglycemic Agents Oral hypoglycemic agents are used in the treatment of persons with type 2 diabetes who are not controlled with exercise and diet. These agents are meant to supplement diet and exercise, not replace them. Oral hypoglycemics are not insulin and work by other mechanisms.

Sulfonylurea is the class of oral hypoglycemic medications most commonly used for diabetes therapy. The sulfonylureas work primarily by increasing the ability of the islet cells of the pancreas to excrete insulin. It is also believed that they have some effect by increasing the cells' sensitivity to insulin and decreasing glucose production by the liver.

All sulfonylureas can be taken with food, except for glipizide (Glucotrol) which should be taken 30 minutes before eating (Chase, 1997). Hypoglycemia can occur in any client taking a sulfonyluric oral hypoglycemic, but hypoglycemia is more common and more dangerous in the elderly. Recognition of hypoglycemia may be more difficult for the older adult because aging decreases the adrenergic mediated hypoglycemic responses of shaking, sweating, and nervousness. Older adults are also more likely to be taking medications for other chronic illnesses that may interact with the oral hypoglycemic. Various medications have the potential to interfere with or enhance the action of oral hypoglycemics.

Other side effects of sulfonyluric oral hypoglycemic agents are rare, but can include skin rashes and gastrointestinal disturbances. Clients should be warned that the oral hypoglycemics, especially chlorpropamide (Diabinese), are known to produce a disulfiram (Antabuse)-like effect in some clients when alcohol is ingested. Reaction may be severe and include symptoms of flushing, sweating, nausea and vomiting, palpitations, and hyperventilation.

Metformin (Glucophage), a biguanide, does not increase insulin release but works by making existing insulin more effective at the cellular level. Metformin may be given alone or in combination with other oral hypoglycemics. In some clients, Glucophage works more effectively if given with some dose of Diabeta. Because it does not stimulate increased insulin release, metformin is not associated with episodes of hypoglycemia. The major side effects of metformin are gastrointestinal and include anorexia, nausea, abdominal discomfort, and diarrhea.

 PROFESSIONAL TIP

Insulin Injection Practices

Fleming (1999) suggests:
- Rolling the insulin vial does not adequately mix lente or NPH insulins; the vial should be shaken carefully.
- Skin preparation with alcohol is unnecessary.
- The angle of injection may vary from 45° to 90°, depending on the client's weight.
- Aspiration before injection, for needle placement, has never been proven in clinical studies.
- Unrefrigerated insulin is effective for 1 month.

Oral hypoglycemics require some production of insulin by the pancreas and, therefore, are not useful in the treatment of type 1 diabetes. See Table 27–5 for a description of oral hypoglycemic agents available in the United States.

Diet

Nutritional therapy continues to be considered the cornerstone of diabetic management. Dietary prescriptions are individualized to meet client and family needs. Consideration must be given to usual eating habits and other lifestyle factors such as dietary likes and dislikes, cultural influences, who prepares the meals, and family finances. It is important that meals remain a social experience, and the diabetic person does not feel isolated or different.

The goals of nutrition are to maintain as near-normal blood glucose level as possible, achieve optimal serum lipid levels, provide adequate energy for maintaining or attaining a reasonable weight, prevent complications of diabetes, and improve overall health. Because of the complexity of nutrition issues, it is recommended that clients be referred early to a registered dietician for nutritional education.

Diabetes is a strong risk factor for atherosclerosis and cardiovascular disease. Therefore, reducing the serum lipid level is a goal of diabetic nutrition therapy. To reduce the risk of cardiovascular disease, the ADA recommendations incorporate a reduction in saturated fat and cholesterol consumption.

It is recommended that individuals taking insulin or oral hypoglycemic agents eat at consistent times synchronized with the actions of the medications used. Distribution of calories over 24 hours, with regular meals and snacks, helps to prevent extreme highs and lows in blood glucose.

Exchange System The diabetic exchange system, developed by the American Diabetes Association and the American Dietetic Association, is the most frequently used system for ensuring that the diabetic integrates all aspects of the dietary prescription. This system divides food into 4 categories according to the amount of protein, carbohydrate, fat, and calories supplied by the food. Clients are given meal plans or prescriptions, specifying the number of exchanges from each list that should be eaten at each meal. With the exchange group system, any food in the proper amount may be substituted for another food in the same exchange list. Table 27–6 shows a sample menu based on the exchange system. The diabetic exchange system continues to be widely used. Once it is learned, it is simple, flexible, and provides wide variety.

Other Diet Systems Many tools and plans for dietary compliance are available to diabetics. Another system gaining more popularity is one that monitors the amount of carbohydrate available in each meal. Insulin doses are then regulated according to total available carbohydrate.

Position Statement: American Diabetes Association According to *Nutrition Recommendations and Principles for People with Diabetes Mellitus, 1996,* there are five goals of nutrition therapy besides improved metabolic control. They are:

1. Maintain as near-normal blood glucose level.
2. Achieve optimal serum lipid levels.
3. Provide adequate calories to maintain or attain a reasonable weight (reasonable weight is determined by client and health care provider).
4. Prevent and treat acute complications of insulin-treated diabetes.

Table 27–5 ORAL HYPOGLYCEMICS

GENERIC (BRAND)	USUAL DOSE	ONSET TIME (HOURS)	DURATION (HOURS)
First-Generation Sulfonylureas			
tobutamide (Orinase)	500–2,000 mg divided dose	1	6–12
acetohexamide (Dymelor)	250–1,500 mg single or divided dose	1	12–24
tolazamide (Tolinase)	100–1,000 mg single or divided dose	4–6	12–24
chlorpropamide (Diabanese)	100–750 mg single dose	1	60
Second-Generation Sulfonylureas			
glipizide (Glucatrol)	2.5–40 mg single or divided dose	1–1½	10–16
glimepride (Amaryl)	1–4 mg single dose	1	24
glyburide (Diabeta, Micronase)	1.25–20 mg single or divided dose	2–4	24
Biguanides			
metformin hydrochloride (Glucophage)	500–2,500 mg two or three divided doses	24–48	6–12
Alpha-Glucosidase Inhibitors			
acarbose (Precose)	25–100 mg with meals (tid)	1	No data
miglitol (Glyset)	25–100 mg with meals (tid)	2–3	4–6
Thiazolidenediones			
troglitazone (Rezulin)	200–600 mg with a meal (qd)	2–3	No data

Table 27–6 SAMPLE DIET, USING EXCHANGE SYSTEM (2,200 CAL)

FOOD GROUP	TOTAL EXCHANGES	BREAKFAST	LUNCH	DINNER	SNACKS P.M.	HS
Carbohydrates						
Milk and milk products	3	1	1	—	—	1
Vegetable	4	—	2	2	—	—
Fruit	4	1	1	1	1	—
Starch/bread	9	3	2	2	1	1
Other carbohydrates	1	—	—	1	—	—
Meat and Meat Substitutes	7	1	2	3	—	1
Fat	5	2	2	—	1	—
Free Foods	—	1	1	2	—	—

Breakfast	Lunch	P.M. Snack	Dinner	Hour of Sleep (H/S) Snack
1 medium peach	½ c summer squash	5 crackers	3 oz pork chop	3 c popcorn, plain
½ c oatmeal	½ c broccoli	2 tsp peanut butter	⅓ c brown rice	1 oz cheese
1 poached egg on slice wheat toast	tuna sandwich (2 breads, 1 oz tuna, 2 tsp mayo)	1 orange	½ c green beans	1 c skim milk
1 bran muffin	1 medium pear		Tossed green salad with Italian dressing (¼ cup)	
1 tsp margarine	Diet soda		½ c applesauce	
1 c skim milk	1 c yogurt, nonfat		1 dinner roll	
coffee			½ c fat-free ice cream	
			iced tea	

5. Improve overall health through optimal nutrition (Dietary Guidelines for Americans and Food Guide Pyramid are examples to follow).

Protein intake of both animal and vegetable sources should make up 10% to 20% of the daily calorie intake. If nephropathy is present, protein should be 10% of the daily calorie intake.

Total fat intake depends on the goals set by the client and health care provider for desired levels of glucose, lipid, and weight. If lipid level is normal, 30% or less of calories should come from fat with less than 10% from saturated fat. If weight loss is a primary issue, reduction in fat intake is an efficient way to reduce calorie intake. When lipid level is a problem, a decrease of saturated fat intake to < 7% of the total calories, total fat to < 30% of total calories, and cholesterol to < 200 mg/day is recommended.

The remainder of the calorie intake comes from carbohydrates. The amount consumed is more important than the source of the carbohydrate.

Persons with diabetes should follow the same precautions regarding the use of alcohol as applied to the general public. Alcohol may increase the risk for hypoglycemia in people treated with insulin or sul-

fonylureas such as acetohexamide (Dymelor), chlorpropamide (Diabinese), or tolazamide (Tolinase).

Activity

The beneficial effects of regular exercise for the diabetic are multiple. Exercise decreases the blood glucose by increasing the uptake of glucose by body muscles and improving insulin usage. Exercise also increases circulation, improves cardiovascular status, decreases stress, and assists with weight loss.

Before starting an exercise program, the diabetic individual should have a complete physical and review the exercise plan with the physician or primary health care provider. Regular daily exercise rather than sporadic exercise should be encouraged.

Diabetics need to correlate exercise with their blood glucose, taking care to avoid periods of hypoglycemia or exercising when blood glucose is too high. Exercise potentiates the action of insulin, resulting in lower insulin requirements and an increased risk of hypoglycemia during and after exercise. On the other hand, in the diabetic who is insulin-deficient, exercise may cause a further rise in blood glucose and rapid development of ketosis. Diabetics must know they should not exercise at the peak of insulin activity,

CLIENT TEACHING

Guidelines for Exercising

- Try to exercise at the same time and in the same amount each day.
- Test blood glucose level before, during, and after exercise.
- Do not inject insulin into a limb that you will be exercising.
- Do not exercise at the peak of insulin activity.
- Do not exercise before meals unless trying to lower blood glucose level.
- Do not exercise with a blood glucose level over 250 mg/dL or with ketones in the urine. This indicates severe insulin deficiency and may predispose to hyperglycemia.
- Eat a snack (15 gm carbohydrates) prior to or during exercise if appropriate, based on blood glucose level.
- Always carry a source of carbohydrates and emergency cash, if away from home, in case hypoglycemia occurs while exercising.
- Always carry personal and medical alert identification.
- Watch for postexercise hypoglycemia. Individuals who have more than usual exercise during the day should increase their carbohydrate intake and test their glucose during the night to detect nocturnal hypoglycemia. (Hypoglycemia can occur 8 to 15 hours following exercise.)

CLIENT TEACHING

Fingersticks

- Use shallow skin penetration, just to get enough blood for the meter.
- Rotate sites; use sides of fingertips and thumb.
- Use alcohol sparingly or wash hands with warm soapy water before fingerstick *instead* of using alcohol. The warm water brings more blood into the fingers.
- Apply firm pressure *directly* over the puncture for 10 to 15 seconds; if area is still bleeding, apply pressure until it stops.

cose should be monitored 4 to 6 times per day and urine should be checked for ketones. Blood glucose greater than 300 mg/dL or ketones in the urine should be reported to the physician.

If the client cannot ingest the planned meal, carbohydrates in the form of soft foods and liquids can be substituted. Extreme nausea and vomiting or diarrhea should be reported to the physician because extreme fluid loss can be dangerous. Clients with type 1 diabetes who are unable to retain fluids may need to be hospitalized to avoid ketoacidosis.

Acute Complications of Diabetes

There are three major acute complications of diabetes related to blood glucose imbalance: hypoglycemia, diabetic ketoacidosis (DKA), and hyperglycemic hyperosmolar nonketotic syndrome (HHNK).

Hypoglycemia (Insulin Reaction)

Hypoglycemia (low blood glucose) occurs when a client's glucose level drops below 70 mg/dL with the most severe reactions occurring when it drops below 50 mg/dL. Hypoglycemia can occur any time of the day, but most often will occur before meals or when insulin action is peaking. Factors that can contribute to the development of a hypoglycemic reaction are skipping meals or eating late, unplanned exercise, and administration of excess insulin.

when blood glucose is greater than 250 mg/dL, or if they have ketones in their urine.

Health Promotion

The diabetic educator plays a pivotal role in assisting the diabetic client/family to understand diabetes and the necessary lifestyle changes. Some teaching is unique to an individual client and is done one-to-one, while some teaching applies to all clients with diabetes and is often done in a class setting. This also allows clients with diabetes to meet each other and share concerns, information, and ideas that have worked for them.

The diabetic educator nurse is part of a team including the client/family, physician, dietitian, and pharmacist who all work together to help the client understand and comply with the treatment plan.

Sick Day Management It is important that diabetics have a plan for managing their diabetes in the event of illness. They should know that it is important that they continue to receive their insulin or oral hypoglycemic medication when they are experiencing illness, as illness and fever can increase blood glucose and the need for insulin. Some diabetics who do not normally take short-acting insulin may require insulin coverage during times of fever or illness. Blood glu-

Hypoglycemic symptoms can occur suddenly and unexpectedly, and vary from client to client (Table 27–7). The cardinal rule is: *Always believe clients who tell you they are having an insulin reaction.* Most diabetics have had hypoglycemic reactions before, so they know the symptoms that precede an insulin reaction.

When a hypoglycemic reaction is suspected, the nurse must respond immediately according to the institution's protocol. Treatment involves assessing the client, checking blood glucose level, and administering glucose in the most appropriate form. Hutchison and Peppard (1998) suggest using glucose tablets or gel for hypoglycemia. The client taking acarbose (Precose), which slows digestion and absorption of most

Table 27–7 SYMPTOMS OF ACUTE COMPLICATIONS OF DIABETES

Symptoms of Hypoglycemia (Insulin Reaction)		Symptoms of Diabetic Ketoacidosis (DKA)
Mild hypoglycemia		• Same as HHNK plus symptoms of acidosis:
• Diaphoresis	• Palpitations	• "Fruity" odor to breath
• Pallor	• Tremors	• Kussmaul's respirations (deep, nonlabored)
• Paresthesias	• Anxiety	**Symptoms of Hyperglycemic Hyperosmolar Nonketotic (HHNK) Syndrome**
• Excess hunger		
Moderate hypoglycemia		• Polyuria
• Confusion, disorientation	• Behavior changes	• Polydipsia
• Slurred speech	• Irritability	• Skin hot, dry, decreased turgor
Severe hypoglycemia		• Dehydration—hypotension, increased pulse
• Seizures		• Blurred vision
• Loss of consciousness		• Weakness
• Shallow respirations		• Mental status changes, confusion to coma
• Nursing Alert: Severe hypoglycemia is a medical emergency. Administer some form of glucose immediately.		

carbohydrates—including hard candies and many fruit juices—but not gluocse, will not have the rapid response to fruit juice or sugar that other clients will have. Hypoglycemic reactions can be fatal, so *leaving the client untreated is more dangerous than causing mild hyperglycemia with overtreatment*. Figure 27-7 provides a sample hypoglycemic protocol.

Diabetics and their families must be instructed about the symptoms and treatment for hypoglycemia. Hypoglycemic episodes can be prevented by following a regular pattern of eating, exercise, and insulin administration. Between meals and bedtime snacks can be used to cover times of peak insulin action. Additional food should be eaten when engaging in greater than usual exercise. Blood glucose level should be checked at the first suspicion of hypoglycemia. All diabetics should wear an identification bracelet or tag indicating that they have diabetes, as hypoglycemic reactions can occur unexpectedly.

Diabetic Ketoacidosis

Diabetic ketoacidosis (DKA) is one of the most serious complications of hyperglycemia. Glucose is a hyperosmolar substance drawing fluid out of the cell and into the circulation where it is excreted by the kidneys. This oncotic diuresis results in polyuria (increased urine output), dehydration, and electrolyte imbalances. Increased fat metabolism results in accumulation of ketones, resulting in metabolic acidosis. Surgery, stress, or illness may trigger DKA, which usually develops in clients with immune mediated type 1 diabetes, although it can occur in clients with type 2 diabetes. The client with undiagnosed immune mediated type 1 diabetes may also present with DKA.

The onset of DKA may be gradual or sudden. Classic symptoms of hyperglycemia (polyuria, polyphagia,

polydipsia) usually precede DKA. Other symptoms include nausea and vomiting, abdominal pain from acidosis, headache, weakness, fatigue, and blurred vision. Assessment may reveal hot, flushed skin and signs of hypovolemia or shock. Acidosis will produce signs of hyperpnea (Kussmaul's breathing), fruity odor to breath from respiratory elimination of acetone, and decreased level of consciousness ranging from lethargy to coma.

Laboratory values will reveal blood glucose from 300 to 800 mg/dL and metabolic acidosis. Urine will be positive for glucose and ketones.

Hyperglycemic Hyperosmolar Nonketotic Syndrome

Hyperglycemic hyperosmolar nonketotic (HHNK) syndrome occurs when there is insufficient insulin to prevent hyperglycemia, but enough insulin to prevent ketoacidosis. HHNK occurs in persons with type 2 diabetes. Because symptoms of acidosis do not occur, hyperglycemia and oncotic diuresis can be much more severe.

HHNK occurs most often in the elderly client with undiagnosed type 2 diabetes. HHNK can also occur in the poorly controlled client and is usually precipitated by illness or other stressor.

Clinical manifestations of HHNK reflect dehydration and shock. Hyperosmolality eventually results in lethargy, seizures, and coma (refer to Table 27–7). Blood glucose level ranges from 600 to 2,000 mg/dL and serum osmolality > 350 mOsm/L.

Medical management of DKA and HHNK involves fluid and electrolyte replacement (particularly potassium), insulin, and treatment of any precipitating factors. DKA and HHNK are associated with significant mortality rates, and the client is usually acutely ill. Treatment will occur in the intensive care setting until the client is stabilized.

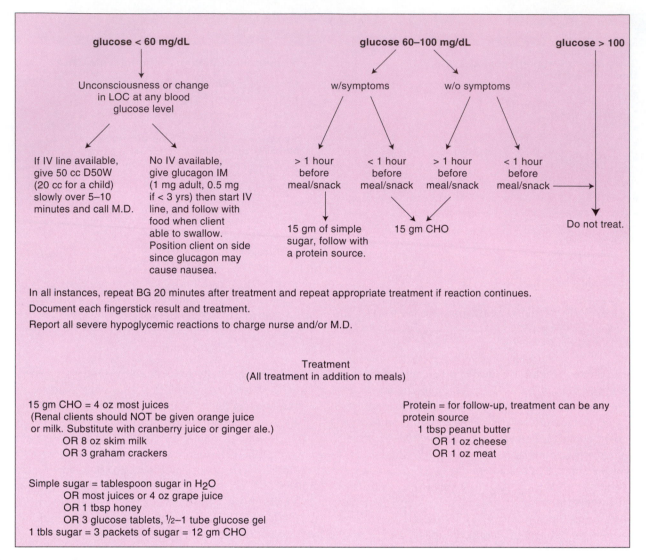

glucose < 60 mg/dL   glucose 60–100 mg/dL   glucose > 100

Unconsciousness or change   w/symptoms   w/o symptoms
in LOC at any blood
glucose level

If IV line available,   No IV available,   > 1 hour   < 1 hour   > 1 hour   < 1 hour
give 50 cc D50W   give glucagon IM   before   before   before   before
(20 cc for a child)   (1 mg adult, 0.5 mg   meal/snack meal/snack meal/snack meal/snack
slowly over 5–10   if < 3 yrs) then start IV
minutes and call M.D. line, and follow with
                       food when client   Do not treat.
                       able to swallow.   15 gm of simple   15 gm CHO
                       Position client on side sugar, follow with
                       since glucagon may   a protein source.
                       cause nausea.

In all instances, repeat BG 20 minutes after treatment and repeat appropriate treatment if reaction continues.

Document each fingerstick result and treatment.

Report all severe hypoglycemic reactions to charge nurse and/or M.D.

Treatment
(All treatment in addition to meals)

15 gm CHO = 4 oz most juices   Protein = for follow-up, treatment can be any
(Renal clients should NOT be given orange juice   protein source
or milk. Substitute with cranberry juice or ginger ale.)   1 tbsp peanut butter
    OR 8 oz skim milk   OR 1 oz cheese
    OR 3 graham crackers   OR 1 oz meat

Simple sugar = tablespoon sugar in H_2O
    OR most juices or 4 oz grape juice
    OR 1 tbsp honey
    OR 3 glucose tablets, 1/2–1 tube glucose gel
1 tbls sugar = 3 packets of sugar = 12 gm CHO

Figure 27-7 Sample Hypoglycemic Protocol

Chronic Complications of Diabetes

Long-term complications of diabetes occur 5 to 10 years after diagnosis in both type 1 and type 2 diabetes. The exact pathophysiology is not completely understood but is known to be related to effects of elevated blood glucose level. Recent studies have shown that intensive insulin therapy and tight glycemic control can reduce or delay the occurrence of many long-term complications associated with diabetes.

Infections

Diabetics, particularly clients who are poorly controlled, appear to be more prone than others to developing certain infections. Infections of particular concern to diabetics include diabetic foot infections, boils, cellulitis, necrotizing fasciitis, urinary tract infections, and yeast infections. Small cuts on the feet can become gangrenous (Figure 27-8) and require amputation.

Infections increase the need for insulin and can result in ketoacidosis. Infections, once they occur, can often be difficult to treat and heal slowly due to impaired circulation.

Figure 27-8 Gangrene of the toes and foot as a result of an infection often means eventual amputation.

CLIENT TEACHING

Guidelines to Healthy Feet

- Wash feet daily and dry them carefully, especially between the toes.
- Inspect feet and between toes for blisters, cuts, and infections. Use a mirror to see the bottoms of the feet. If your vision is impaired, have a family member examine your feet. Remember, because of decreased feeling in your feet, you may have an infection and not know it.
- Avoid activities that will restrict blood flow to the feet, especially smoking. Do not sit with legs crossed.
- Wear shoes that are comfortable, well-fitting, and closed toed. Wear new shoes for short intervals until broken in. Do not walk barefoot.
- Prevent cuts and irritations. Always wear stockings. Look inside shoes for rough edges, nail points, foreign objects.
- Avoid temperature extremes. Test bath water with hands before getting in. Do not use water bottles or heating pads on feet.
- See your physician regularly and make sure that your feet are examined each visit.
- When toe nails are trimmed, cut them straight across. When corns or calluses are present, see a physician or podiatrist. Do not cut them yourself.

Diabetic Neuropathies

Neuropathies are the most common chronic complication associated with diabetes. The incidence of peripheral neuropathies increases with age and duration of disease and is related to elevated blood glucose level. Neuropathies can affect all types of nerves but the two most common types of diabetic neuropathy are sensorimotor polyneuropathy and autonomic neuropathy.

Sensorimotor polyneuropathy, also called *peripheral neuropathy,* causes paresthesias and burning sensations, primarily in the lower extremities. Decreased sensations of pain and temperature coupled with decreased peripheral circulation place the client at high risk for injury and undetected foot injury.

Autonomic neuropathy can affect almost any organ system including: gastrointestinal (delayed gastric emptying,

GERONTOLOGICAL CONSIDERATIONS

Diabetic Neuropathy

Advancing age is the strongest risk factor regardless of disease duration and blood sugar control.

constipation, diarrhea), urinary (retention, neurogenic bladder), and reproductive (male impotence).

Nephropathy (Chronic Renal Failure)

Diabetic nephropathy develops slowly over many years, progressing eventually to kidney failure. Controlling hypertension and blood glucose level is the key to delaying renal damage. Good hydration before and diuresis following any dye study is valuable in preventing renal damage. Urinary tract infections can be prevented by encouraging the client to use the bathroom "by the clock" to reduce stagnant, residual urine (Hernandez, 1998).

Retinopathy

Changes in the small vessels of the retina result in diabetic retinopathy, which is a major cause of blindness among diabetics. Because of the insidious onset of type 2 diabetes, retinopathy is often present at diagnosis. The severity and progression of retinopathy appear to be closely related to glucose and blood pressure control. Diabetics also develop cataracts at an earlier age. Although the majority of clients develop some degree of retinopathy, most do not develop visual impairment. To facilitate early detection, diabetics should have ophthalmologic evaluations every 6 to 12 months.

Vascular Changes

Diabetes is an independent risk factor for atherosclerotic vessel disease. Atherosclerotic changes that occur in diabetics are similar to those that occur in nondiabetics, but they occur at earlier ages and progress at a more rapid rate.

Cardiovascular Hypertension is twice as common in diabetics and is an important factor in the progression of retinopathy, nephropathy, and vascular (large vessel) disease. The incidence of coronary artery disease, angina, and myocardial infarction is higher when compared to the nondiabetic population. Cerebral vascular disease and cerebral vascular accident are also more common in persons with diabetes.

Therapies aimed at lowering risk factors and effects of atherosclerosis are recommended for the diabetic client. These management techniques include weight control, low-fat diet, treatment of hypertension and hyperlipidemia, regular exercise, and control of blood glucose level.

CLIENT TEACHING

Retinopathy Prevention

- Refrain from straining to have a bowel movement.
- Use stool softener or laxative.
- Avoid postures that lower the head.
- Avoid lifting weight above shoulders.

Peripheral Vascular Disease Peripheral vascular disease (PVD) occurs most commonly in diabetics with hypertension or hyperlipidemia and in diabetics who smoke. Diabetics have 2 to 3 times the incidence of occlusive peripheral arterial disease when compared to the nondiabetic population. Diabetes is present in more than half of persons experiencing nontraumatic lower extremity amputations.

▶ NURSING PROCESS

▶ Assessment

▶ Subjective Data

This includes assessment of the health history, family history, diet, activity regimen, and the understanding of the disease and medical therapies. The client may describe fatigue, weakness, weight changes, mental status changes, polyuria, polyphagia, polydipsia, numbness or tingling of the extremities, blurred vision, and increased appetite.

▶ Objective Data

Objective data should focus on the symptoms of diabetes, the common acute and chronic complications, and the results of diagnostic tests. There may be dependent redness or cyanosis of the lower extremities as well as the absence of hair. A fasting glucose level greater than 126 mg/dL or a nonfasting (random) level greater than 200 mg/dL, on two separate occasions, suggests a diagnosis of diabetes (The Expert Committee on the Diagnosis and Classification of Diabetes Mellitus, 1997).

Nursing diagnoses, based on the assessment findings, may be varied and extensive due to the multiple problems and complications caused by diabetes mellitus. Nursing diagnoses may include the following:

Nursing Diagnoses	Planning/Goals	Nursing Interventions
▶ *Deficient Knowledge diabetes, medical regimen, diet, exercise, self-care management skills (insulin injection, SMBG) related to new diagnosis or changes in treatment*	The client will relate basic understanding of pathophysiology of diabetes, and relationship between insulin and hyper-/hypoglycemia.	Teach client about diabetes and the use of insulin to prevent hyper-/hypoglycemia or assist client to enroll in a formal diabetic education program.
	The client will verbalize how/when to take oral hypoglycemics and the side effects to report or will correctly demonstrate how to administer insulin and rotate sites.	Teach client about oral hypoglycemics or insulin, whichever the client will be using.
	The client will relate importance of an exercise program.	Discuss how exercise is related to diabetes management.
	The client will describe the relationship between dietary management and glycemic control; choose foods that comply with diet prescription.	Discuss how dietary management is related to the control of blood glucose and provide an exchange list of foods.
	The client will correctly demonstrate how to use SMBG to determine blood glucose level.	Teach client how to perform SMBG and have client return demonstration.
	The client will verbalize symptoms and treatment of hypoglycemia.	Provide client with a list of symptoms and treatment for hypoglycemia.
▶ *Risk for Deficient Fluid Volume related to hyperglycemia, polyuria, and dehydration*	The client will exhibit normal skin turgor, moist mucous membranes, and maintain oral fluid intake of 2,500–3,000 mL/day.	Measure client's intake and output, administer intravenous fluids as ordered, and encourage oral fluids.
	The client will have vital signs within normal limits.	Monitor vital signs and serum electrolytes.
▶ *Imbalanced Nutrition: Less than body requirements related to imbalance between insulin, diet, and activity*	The client will have weight within normal range for height and age.	Assist client to adjust dietary intake in order to maintain weight in normal range.

Evaluation Each goal must be evaluated to determine how it has been met by the client.

PITUITARY DISORDERS

Hyperpituitarism and hypopituitarism are discussed following.

HYPERPITUITARISM

Hyperpituitarism is most commonly diagnosed between the second and fourth decade of life but can appear in infancy and childhood. Although other pituitary hormones may be affected, the most common are the growth hormone and antidiuretic hormone.

Excess secretion of growth hormone (GH) produces different changes depending on the client's age when it occurs. When the excess secretion occurs in childhood before the epiphyses close, gigantism is the result; in adults, acromegaly is the result.

Syndrome of inappropriate antidiuretic hormone and pituitary tumors are also discussed.

GIGANTISM

Gigantism affects infants and children, causing proportional overgrowth of all body tissues. By the time these children reach adulthood, they may be more than 8 feet tall.

Hyperplasia of the anterior pituitary is usually the cause of GH oversecretion. This tissue may develop into a tumor causing other symptoms. Clients with gigantism do not have the strength their size implies.

Medical–Surgical Management

Medical

Irradiation of the anterior pituitary may be the treatment chosen. The child must then be observed for heart failure, hypertension, thickened bones, osteoporosis, and delayed sexual development.

Surgical

If the cause is a tumor, surgery may be performed to remove the tumor (explained under "Acromegaly").

Pharmacological

When the pituitary is either destroyed by irradiation or removed by surgery, pituitary hormone replacement is necessary.

▶ NURSING PROCESS

▶ Assessment

▶ Subjective Data

Listening to the child's description of the disease process may provide insight into the child's emotional responses.

▶ Objective Data

Frequent measurements of growth indicate a more rapid rate of growth than expected.

ACROMEGALY

Since acromegaly occurs after epiphyseal closure of bones, there is bone thickening with transverse growth and tissue enlargement. This occurs between 30 and 50 years of age. Photographs over years will reveal a progressive enlargement of the face and hands.

Acromegaly involves a gradual onset of clinical manifestations including: visual defects from pressure of the pituitary tumor on the optic nerve, soft tissue swelling, or hypertrophy of the face and extremities. The cartilaginous and connective tissue overgrowths result in a characteristic hulking appearance with thickened ears and nose, and marked projection of the jaw. The jaw can appear enlarged and the tongue may also thicken. The paranasal sinuses can become enlarged. Also laryngeal hypertrophy can occur. The client has thick fingers with tips that appear "tufted" (shaped like arrowheads on x-rays). The client exhibits a characteristic moist, weak, doughy handshake. The heart, liver, and spleen may enlarge. Some other characteristics are: diaphoresis (profuse perspiration), oily or leathery skin, fatigue, heat intolerance, weight gain, headache, joint pain, hirsutism (excessive hairiness especially in females), and sleep disturbance. The client may experience decreased libido or impotence, oligomenorrhea (scanty or infrequent menstruation), and infertility.

The client's history and clinical manifestations along with cranial x-rays and a CT scan make a diagnosis of acromegaly. Serum growth hormone levels are elevated.

Prognosis depends upon the causative factor, hyperplasia or a tumor; however, there is generally a reduced life span. Diabetes mellitus is a possible complication of hyperpituitarism because of glucose intolerance caused by the insulin-antagonistic character of the growth hormone.

Medical–Surgical Management

Medical

Medical treatment consists of either medication that affects the growth hormone or irradiation of the pituitary gland. Proton beam therapy uses a very low dose of radiation and is much less destructive to nearby tissue than conventional radiation therapy.

Surgical

Surgical treatment for hyperpituitarism is to remove the pituitary gland. Two surgical approaches to remove the pituitary are transfrontal or transsphenoid hypophysectomy. The transfrontal approach is rarely used because it has a high risk of mortality as well as permanent loss of smell and taste and causes severe diabetes insipidus. The transsphenoid approach

Figure 27-9 Transsphenoidal Approach to Hypophysectomy

(Figure 27-9) involves an incision in the superior maxillary gingiva. Surgery may be the treatment of choice or used after attempting medical treatment.

Postoperatively, nasal packing should be checked for clear colorless drainage. If it occurs, the drainage must be documented and reported to the physician. If this drainage is suspected of being cerebrospinal fluid, it should be checked for glucose, which is found in cerebrospinal fluid. The nurse should observe for infection which includes elevated leukocytes, sudden temperature elevation, or complaint of headache or nuchal rigidity. Analgesics are administered as needed. The client should avoid activities such as coughing, straining, vomiting, or sneezing. The client should be encouraged to use an incentive spirometer instead of coughing. The client should not brush teeth for 2 weeks to avoid problems with the incision. Mouthwash can be

used. The client should be instructed to avoid lifting and bending at the waist for 2 to 3 months after surgery.

Pharmacological

Two drugs may be prescribed for acromegaly. Bromocriptine mesylate (Parlodel) is a nonhormonal drug that activates dopamine receptors to inhibit the release of the growth hormone and prolactin. Bromocriptine mesylate (Parlodel) should be given with food to decrease gastric upset. Since it can cause drowsiness or dizziness, the client should be instructed to avoid activities that require mental alertness. If the client is on oral contraceptives, alternate contraceptive measures should also be used because bromocriptine can stimulate ovulation.

The other drug, octreotide acetate (Sandostatin), inhibits the growth hormone. Although octreotide is given by injection, it can still cause gastric distress. The injections should be given between meals and at bedtime. Clients with diabetes mellitus should closely monitor their blood sugar level.

▶ NURSING PROCESS

▶ Assessment

▶ Subjective Data

The nurse should obtain a thorough nursing history and ask about vision impairment, headache, muscular weakness, and psychological disturbances.

▶ Objective Data

Objective data includes gait changes, vital sign changes (tachycardia or hypotension which may indicate congestive heart failure), and dyspnea. The jaw is enlarged and projected, so the client may have difficulty in chewing.

Nursing diagnoses for a client with gigantism or acromegaly may include the following:

Nursing Diagnoses	Planning/Goals	Nursing Interventions
▶ *Risk for Disproportionate Growth related to increased level of growth hormone*	The client will comply with treatment to minimize hyperpituitarism and stop excessive growth with treatment.	Assist client with activities of daily living. Administer medications as ordered. Assist client with range of motion exercises. Remind client to carry medications on person.
▶ *Chronic Low Self-Esteem related to irreversible physical changes*	The client will acknowledge physical changes, express positive feelings about self, and exhibit ability to cope with altered body.	Encourage client to verbalize feelings. Offer emotional support and help client to develop coping strategies. Show respect and acceptance of the client as a person. Refer to professional counseling as needed. Assist client in setting achievable short-term goals. Provide a positive but realistic assessment of the situation.

Evaluation Each goal must be evaluated to determine how it has been met by the client.

SYNDROME OF INAPPROPRIATE ANTIDIURETIC HORMONE

Syndrome of inappropriate antidiuretic hormone (SIADH) results from an excess of ADH. This causes the kidneys to reabsorb excess water, which decreases urine output and increases fluid volume. The most common cause is bronchogenic lung cancer (Heater, 1999b). Other causes are lymphoid pancreatic, duodenal, thymus, and prostate cancer; lupus erythematosis; central nervous system trauma, infection, hemorrhage, or neoplasm; chronic obstructive pulmonary disease; acute respiratory failure; mechanical ventilation; and medications such as antineoplastic agents, tricyclic antidepressants, and anesthetics.

The client will have hyponatremia (< 130 mEq/L), water retention, weight gain, concentrated urine (urine osmolality > 1,200 mOsm/L; specific gravity > 1.020), muscle cramps, and weakness. The low osmolality of the blood allows fluid to leak out of vessels and causes brain swelling. If untreated, lethargy, seizures, coma, and death will result.

Medical–Surgical Management

Medical

The underlying disorder must be treated or medications stopped that may be contributing to SIADH. Water restriction will be implemented to prevent further hemodilution. Serious hyponatremia (< 120 mEq/L) will usually be treated with intravenous administration of 5% NaCl. The serum sodium level should be increased by 12 mEq/L or less per day.

Pharmacological

Furosemide (Lasix) is given to increase urine output, while demeclocycline hydrochloride (Declomycin) and fludrocortisone (Florinef) are given to enhance sodium retention.

Diet

Fluid restriction will be determined by the serum sodium level.

▸ NURSING PROCESS

▸ Assessment

▸ Subjective Data

The client may describe muscle cramps, weakness, anorexia, nausea, and headache.

▸ Objective Data

The client will have weight gain and fluid intake greater than output. The client may be irritable and disoriented, become progressively lethargic, and have seizures and diminished or absent deep tendon reflexes. Serum sodium and osmolality will be decreased. Urine osmolality and specific gravity will be increased.

Nursing diagnoses for a client with SIADH may include the following:

Nursing Diagnoses	Planning/Goals	Nursing Interventions
▸ *Excess Fluid Volume related to decreased urine output*	The client will have increased urine output.	Assess client's weight daily on same scale at same time. Assess vital signs. Accurately record I & O. Monitor laboratory reports. Administer medications as ordered. Maintain fluid restrictions.
▸ *Impaired Oral Mucous Membrane related to restriction of fluid intake*	The client will have moist, intact oral mucous membranes.	Provide frequent oral care, avoiding alcohol-based mouth washes and lemon-glycerine swabs. Allow client to rinse mouth with water, but not swallow any. Provide lubricant for client's lips. Allow client to choose fluids and times to drink them.

Evaluation Each goal must be evaluated to determine how it has been met by the client.

PITUITARY TUMORS

Pituitary tumors more often affect the anterior pituitary rather than the posterior portion. Adenomas of the pituitary, which are rarely malignant, replace glandular tissue and enlarge the sella turcica. The cause is unknown, but there may be a predisposition toward tumor formation from an inherited **autosomal** dominant trait, meaning it is a dominant characteristic carried on any chromosome other than the one determining sex.

Clinical manifestations frequently start with a headache unrelated to stress or other factors. The next obvious manifestation is visual problems caused by the tumor putting pressure on the optic nerve. Others include personality changes, dementia, amenorrhea, impotence, lethargy, and weakness. The client may complain of cold intolerance, increased fatigue, and constipation. The client may have seizures. Although the tumor is not malignant, damage is done by tumor invasion of normal tissue.

Treatment is removal of the tumor. Complications of pituitary tumors are endocrine abnormalities if there is no replacement therapy after removal of the tumor. If the hypothalamus is compressed, diabetes insipidus can result. If the tumor has eroded the base of the skull, the client may have rhinorrhea (thin watery nasal discharge). Prognosis depends upon the extent of invasion. In most cases, the tumor causes excessive secretion of the anterior pituitary hormones.

Medical–Surgical Management

Medical

Medical treatment of a pituitary tumor would be radiation therapy. This can be used for small tumors or if the client is a poor surgical risk. Radiation can also be used after surgery to shrink tissue remaining after surgical excision. Another alternative to surgery is cryo-hypophysectomy. This involves freezing the area with a probe inserted via the transsphenoidal approach.

Surgical

Large tumors, especially those impinging on the optic nerve, are generally removed by using the transfrontal approach. Smaller tumors can be resected via the transsphenoidal approach.

Pharmacological

After surgery, the client will need hormone replacement therapy.

▶ NURSING PROCESS

▶ Assessment

▶ Subjective Data

The nurse will obtain a thorough client history and assess for manifestations of a tumor such as visual problems, headache, impotence, lethargy, cold intolerance, fatigue, or constipation. The family may also provide insight into any personality changes.

▶ Objective Data

The client is assessed for tilting of the head to compensate for visual disturbances, axillary and pubic hair loss, a waxy appearance to the skin, and few wrinkles.

Nursing diagnoses for a client with a pituitary tumor may include the following:

Nursing Diagnoses	Planning/Goals	Nursing Interventions
▶ *Fatigue related to decreased ACTH and TSH levels*	The client will verbalize an understanding of the relationship between fatigue, the disease, and activity level, and express feeling of increasing energy as treatment progresses.	Explain relationship between pituitary tumor, fatigue, and activity level. Suggest alternating periods of activity with periods of rest. Administer medications as ordered. Encourage completion of all treatments.
▶ *Disturbed Sensory Perception (Visual) related to altered sensory reception, transmission, and/or integration due to pressure on optic nerve by the pituitary tumor*	The client will use adaptive devices and appropriate resources to compensate for visual changes, and regain normal vision with treatment.	Provide information about adaptive devices and resources for visual changes. Provide a safe clutter-free environment. Make certain that the bed is in the low position and the call signal in reach of the client. Use side rails as needed.

Evaluation Each goal must be evaluated to determine how it has been met by the client.

HYPOPITUITARISM

Hypopituitarism is a complex syndrome marked by metabolic dysfunction, sexual immaturity, and growth retardation when it occurs in childhood; Simmonds' disease and diabetes insipidus are examples of hypopituitarism. The most common cause of hypopituitarism is a tumor. Other causes are: congenital defects (hypoplasia or aplasia), pituitary infarction (from postpartum hemorrhage), pituitary surgery or irradiation, or chemical agents. Hypopituitarism can be primary (meaning there is no known cause) or secondary. Secondary hypopituitarism can be a result of a deficiency of hypothalamic releasing hormones. This deficiency can be idiopathic (without a known cause) or a result of infection, trauma, or tumor.

Clinical manifestations develop slowly and generally are not apparent until 75% of the pituitary is destroyed. Specific manifestations will vary with the specific hormone that is deficient.

Deficiency of the growth hormone results in dwarfism, which becomes apparent by 6 months of age as the infant exhibits growth retardation, with chubbiness in the lower trunk and a short stature. As it progresses, secondary tooth eruption is delayed and later there is a delay in puberty. Growth continues at about half the normal rate until the child reaches about 4 feet in height. Body proportions are normal as is mental development. Frequently in adulthood, sex organs may not develop normally unless treated with hormones. Clients experience an accelerated pattern of aging, resulting in the life span being shortened by as much as 20 years. If the deficiency occurs in adults, manifestations are not as apparent. There are subtle signs such as wrinkles near the mouth and eyes.

Deficiencies of follicle-stimulating hormone (FSH) and luteinizing hormone (LH) cause differences in clinical manifestations between female and male clients. In the female, symptoms include: amenorrhea, dyspareunia, infertility, decreased libido, breast atrophy, sparse or absent axillary and pubic hair, and dry skin. In the male, symptoms include: weakness, impotence, decreased libido, decreased muscle strength, testicular softening and shrinkage, and retarded secondary sexual hair growth.

In a child a deficiency of thyroid-stimulating hormone (TSH) will result in severe growth retardation even with treatment. Other deficiency manifestations include: cold intolerance; constipation; increased or decreased menstrual flow; lethargy; dry pale puffy skin, and bradycardia. Thought processes may also be slowed.

A deficiency of adrenocorticotrophic hormone (ACTH) results in fatigue, nausea, vomiting, anorexia, weight loss, and depigmentation of the skin and nipples. Vital signs taken during periods of stress would show fever and hypotension.

Prolactin deficiency results in absent postpartum lactation, amenorrhea, and sparse or absent axillary and pubic hair. There may also be manifestations of thyroid or adrenal cortex failure.

Findings of hypopituitarism depend upon the specific hormone, client's age, and severity of condition when detected. X-rays of the wrist determine bone age, and a skull series will rule out a pituitary tumor. Total failure of the pituitary without treatment is fatal; however, prognosis is good with treatment by the appropriate hormone(s). Treatment is primarily replacement therapy for the deficient hormone(s).

SIMMONDS' DISEASE

Simmonds' disease is defined as a total absence of all pituitary secretions. This is also called *panhypopitu-*

itarism. This disease results from surgery, infection, injury, or tumor. It may also occur after a difficult labor in childbirth due to thrombosis formation during or after delivery.

Clinical manifestations, which vary in intensity, include: extreme weight loss, general debility, lethargy, pallor, and dry yellowish skin. There is also a loss of libido, amenorrhea, and intolerance to cold. The disease leads to loss of axillary and pubic hair, and atrophy of genitalia and breasts. It progresses to bradycardia (slow pulse), hypotension, premature wrinkling of the skin, and atrophy of the thyroid and adrenal glands.

Treatment consists of administration of ACTH, TSH, or thyroid, adrenal, and sex hormones for a lifetime.

DIABETES INSIPIDUS

Diabetes insipidus is a deficiency of ADH, causing a metabolic disorder characterized by severe polyuria and polydipsia. Diabetes insipidus generally starts in childhood or early adulthood with a median onset of 21 years. It affects males more often than females. Although a deficiency of ADH is the most common cause (neurogenic), diabetes insipidus can also be caused by failure of the kidneys to respond to ADH (nephrogenic).

Neurogenic diabetes insipidus may be caused by injury or ischemia to the hypothalamus or pituitary gland, CNS infections, pregnancy, sickle cell disease, or medications such as lithium carbonate (Carbolith), amphotereicin B (Fungizone), furosemide (Lasix) or ethycrynic acid (Edecrin). Nephrogenic diabetes insipidus may be caused by pyelonephritis, chronic renal failure, polycystic disease, or renal transplantation (Heater, 1999).

Clinical manifestations have an abrupt onset. The client experiences extreme polyuria of 4 to 16 L of dilute urine daily. In some cases, there can be up to 30 L of urine per day. Serum osmolality is > 295 mOsm/L and urine osmolality is < 150 mOsm/L. Urine specific gravity is < 1.005 and serum sodium is > 145 mEq/L. The client also has extreme thirst, preferring cold beverages. Even though there is an extraordinary volume of fluid intake, weight is lost. Other manifestations include dizziness, weakness, constipation, slight to moderate nocturia, and fatigue that could be a result of inadequate rest due to frequent nighttime voiding and excess thirst.

Complications of untreated diabetes insipidus are **hypovolemia** (abnormally low circulatory blood volume), circulatory collapse, unconsciousness, and central nervous system damage. Prolonged urine flow can cause chronic urinary system conditions such as bladder distension, enlarged calyces, and hydronephrosis.

Prognosis is generally good with fluid replacement in uncomplicated cases. Prognosis also depends upon the underlying cause of diabetes insipidus.

Medical–Surgical Management

Pharmacological

In addition to intravenous fluids, several medications can be used to treat diabetes insipidus. For neurogenic diabetes insipidus, desmopressin acetate (Stimate), a synthetic antidiuretic hormone which can be given parenterally or nasally, is the drug of choice. Also vasopressin (Pitressin) may be given parenterally or nasally. The nurse needs to make certain that the nasal passage is clear before administering the medication. The nurse must also monitor intake and output and assess for hypovolemia and electrolyte imbalance.

For nephrogenic diabetes insipidus, a diuretic such as hydrochlorothiazide (Hydrodiuril) increases sodium excretion which increases fluid reabsorption in the kidneys.

▶ NURSING PROCESS

▶ Assessment

▶ Subjective Data

A thorough client history is needed, including severity of thirst, weakness, fatigue, and lethargy.

▶ Objective Data

The client must be assessed for weight loss, constipation, and signs of fluid volume deficit such as dry skin and mucous membranes, fever, dyspnea, and poor skin turgor. Urine is checked for color, amount, and specific gravity, and weight is assessed daily.

Nursing diagnoses for a client with diabetes insipidus may include the following:

Nursing Diagnoses	Planning/Goals	Nursing Interventions
▶ *Risk for Imbalanced Fluid Volume related to polyuria*	The client will have sufficient fluid intake to prevent dehydration.	Provide easy access to bedpan/bathroom. Answer call signal promptly.
		Monitor the client for dizziness and weakness. Record client intake and output.
		Provide fluids as ordered to cover output.
		Teach client and family how to record intake and output.
		Monitor weight daily.
		Provide oral care. Use a soft toothbrush, mild mouthwash, and lubricant for the lips.
		Assess condition of oral mucous membranes.
▶ *Risk for Impaired Skin Integrity related to altered hydration*	The client will maintain skin integrity.	Assess skin, especially pressure points, 3 times a day.
		Apply moisturizing lotion to skin.
		Prevent pressure on skin by turning or ambulating client.
		Use eggcrate mattress or sheepskin.
		Encourage adequate intake of fluids, protein, vitamin C, and calories.

Evaluation Each goal must be evaluated to determine how it has been met by the client.

THYROID DISORDERS

Worldwide, a deficiency of iodine is the most likely cause of thyroid disorders. However, in countries where idoine in food is plentiful, autoimmune thyroid disease is the most common thyroid disorder (Walpert, 1998). Thyroid disorders are classified as hyperthyroidism, hypothyroidism, tumors, cancer, or goiter.

HYPERTHYROIDISM

Hyperthyroidism is a collective term for a condition marked by increased thyroid activity and overproduction of thyroid hormones thyroxine (T_4) and triiodothyronine (T_3). The thyroid gland itself may be enlarged. Variations of hyperthyroidism are Grave's disease, Basedow's disease, Parry's disease, or thyrotoxicosis. Although these are different forms of hyperthyroidism, Grave's disease is the most common. It generally affects females more often than males; however, it tends to affect males more severely. The highest incidence is in the 20- to 40-year-old group (Walpert, 1998).

In this autoimmune disorder, the immune system triggers the formation of thyroid-stimulating immunoglobulins (TSIs). The TSIs bind with thyroid-stimulating hormone (TSH) receptors and abnormally stimulate thyroid functioning.

Figure 27-10 Hyperthyroidism with Exophthalmia *(From The Thyroid and Its Diseases, 4th ed., by DeGroot, 1975, John Wiley & Sons, Inc.)*

Clinical manifestations include two obvious physical changes. The thyroid can be palpated for asymmetry and size. It may enlarge 3 to 4 times its normal size. The enlargement of the thyroid gland is called **goiter**. This is generally a result of overactivity of the thyroid gland. If there is an accumulation of orbital fluid behind the eyeball forcing it to protrude, this is called **exophthalmos** (Figure 27-10). This occurs in about half the cases of hyperthyroidism. It produces a characteristic stare.

As a result of increased thyroid hormone production, the client has an increased metabolic rate. This leads to weight loss despite increased appetite, fatigue, poor tolerance to heat, and profuse perspiration. The client is very nervous, leading to restlessness, irritability, difficulty concentrating, emotional lability, mood swings, possible personality changes, and sleep disturbances. The client may have fine tremors of the fingers and tongue, shaky handwriting, clumsiness, trouble climbing stairs, or dyspnea on exertion and possibly at rest. The skin is warm and moist with a velvety texture. The skin may be a characteristic salmon color. The hair is fine and soft with premature graying and increased hair loss. The nails appear fragile with distal nail separation from the nail bed (onycholysis). There may be general or local muscle atrophy and acropachy (soft tissue swelling with underlying bone changes where new bone forms). There is a tachycardia with bounding pulse up to 160 beats per minute and down to 80 beats per minute during sleep. Pulse pressure is

widened. There can be muscular weakness and atrophy, osteoporosis, and paralysis. There may be vitiligo, which is characterized by milky-white patches on the skin surrounded by areas of normal pigmentation. There is decreased libido, impaired fertility, and **gynecomastia** (abnormal enlargement of one or both breasts in males).

Diagnostic tests generally include TSH, T_3, T_4, radioactive iodine uptake, and a thyroid scan.

One major complication is thyrotoxic crisis, also called *thyroid storm*. This is a medical emergency that can lead to cardiac, hepatic, or renal failure. Thyroid storm can be precipitated by stressful situations such as surgery, infection, or trauma. Less common causes are cerebrovascular accident (CVA), myocardial infarction, sudden discontinuing of antithyroid medications, subtotal thyroidectomy with excess intake of synthetic thyroid hormone, toxemia, or diabetic ketoacidosis. Any of these events can lead to overproduction of thyroid hormone which, in turn, causes an increase in systemic adrenergic activity. This causes an overproduction of epinephrine and severe hypermetabolism leading to rapid cardiac, gastrointestinal, and sympathetic nervous system decompensation. The client will exhibit severe and rapid clinical manifestations of hyperthyroidism.

If the nurse suspects that the client is experiencing thyrotoxic crisis, the physician must be informed immediately. The client will be transferred to intensive care for closer monitoring of vital signs, EKG pattern, and cardiopulmonary status. Antithyroid therapy will be initiated immediately. The client's temperature is monitored and cooling measures initiated as needed. Acetaminophen may be administered to lower the temperature, but aspirin will not be given since it could cause a further increase in the client's metabolic rate. Supportive care would be given until the client is out of the thyrotoxic crisis.

Medical–Surgical Management

Medical

The goal of managing hyperthyroidism is to decrease excessive thyroid hormone production. With treatment to decrease the thyroid production of its hormone, the prognosis is good. The client can live a nor-

GERONTOLOGICAL CONSIDERATIONS

Hyperthyroid Complications

The older client particularly develops cardiovascular problems such as arrhythmias (atrial fibrillation), cardiac insufficiency leading to cardiac decompensation, and resistance to the usual dose of digoxin.

mal life. There can be a combination of treatment methods. The first method is to administer antithyroid medications. This is usually a temporary solution.

Radiation therapy of the thyroid gland could consist of external radiation to the neck; however, the more accepted method is the oral administration of a radioactive iodine, either liquid or capsule, that targets the thyroid tissue. It is most commonly used for the woman past the reproductive years or clients who do not plan to have children. If the client is of reproductive age, the client must sign an informed consent form since small amounts of the radioactive iodine could lodge in the gonads.

The client should stop taking antithyroid medications 4 to 7 days prior to treatment. The physician needs to be informed if the client is receiving amiodarone hydrochloride (Cordarone), an antiarrhythmic, because it contains large amounts of iodine. The oral ^{131}I should not be given to the client with severe vomiting or diarrhea.

This method involves a single dose of ^{131}I orally. It will destroy some iodine concentrating cells that produce the thyroxine. Clinical manifestations decrease in about 3 weeks with the full effect in about 3 months. Some clients may require a second or third dose.

Safety: Radioactive Iodine

No pregnant nurse should care for the client. The client should expectorate carefully for the first day since the saliva is radioactive. The client should drink plenty of fluids for 2 days to help circulate and eliminate the radioactive iodine. The toilet should be flushed twice after each use for at least 2 days or throughout the hospitalization. Disposable eating utensils should be used by the client. Close contact with children or pregnant females should be avoided for a week after the administration. Females should avoid pregnancy for 6 months after treatment.

The client usually resumes the thyroid hormone antagonist 3 to 5 days after ^{131}I therapy until the physician determines the thyroid to be atrophic (decreased in size). The physician may have the client continue to take propranolol hydrochloride (Inderal) for tachycardia, tremor, and diaphoresis. The client requires continued monitoring of thyroid hormone blood levels and physical condition.

The most common complication is hypothyroidism, which occurs about 2 to 4 months after treatment. The client is placed on thyroid replacement therapy, generally for life.

Surgical

Generally just a portion of the thyroid gland is removed, but a total thyroidectomy may be performed. This is the most expensive option and has the most risks. A thyroidectomy may also be done for respiratory obstruction by a goiter or thyroid cancer. If a partial thyroidectomy is done, the remaining thyroid tissue should provide adequate amounts of thyroid hormones. If a complete thyroidectomy is done, the client will require thyroid hormone replacement for a lifetime.

Preoperatively, the client should be given explanations concerning activities after surgery. There will be a neck incision generally with some type of drain. The client may experience a sore throat and hoarseness. The client probably has taken propylthiouracil PTU for 4 to 6 weeks prior to surgery. Iodine preparations may have been prescribed 10 to 14 days before surgery to decrease thyroid vascularity and decrease bleeding. Depending upon the symptoms of hyperthyroidism, the client may also be taking propranolol hydrochloride (Inderal). Thyroid function tests and an EKG would be performed before surgery to provide baseline information. Informed consent must be obtained.

After surgery, the client is placed in high-Fowler's position to promote venous drainage. The client should support the head with a hand when moving the head to prevent strain on the incision. Respiratory problems may occur. Respiratory obstruction can be a result of tracheal collapse, tracheal mucous accumulation, or laryngeal or local tissue edema. A tracheotomy tray or endotracheal tubes and insertion tray must be kept readily available at the client's bedside in case of a respiratory emergency.

Since the thyroid is so vascular, the dressing must be checked frequently for drainage, especially at the back of the neck for bleeding. If there is a drain, approximately 50 cc of drainage is expected the first day. If there is no drainage, the drain must be checked for kinks or obstruction of the tubing. The nurse should encourage voice rest for 48 hours with voice checks every 2 to 4 hours as ordered to make certain there is no laryngeal nerve damage.

Because the parathyroid glands could be accidentally removed during the thyroidectomy, the client's blood calcium level must be monitored. The client is checked for Chvostek's sign or Trousseau's sign. (These will be discussed more fully in hypoparathyroidism.) Analgesics are administered as needed.

Complications of thyroidectomy are respiratory distress and hemorrhage. There can be damage to the laryngeal nerves affecting the voice. Manipulation of the thyroid gland during surgery can cause a release of large amounts of thyroid hormone causing thyroid storm, which is rare but may occur. Thyroid crisis usually occurs within the first 12 hours postoperative. Hyperthyroid signs and symptoms are exaggerated plus the client may vomit, have severe hypertenison and tachycardia, and sometimes have hyperthermia up to 106°F (41°C). The client may develop congestive heart failure and die. The client must be advised that tetany can occur up to ten days after surgery. **Tetany** is sharp flexion of the wrist and ankle joints, muscle twitchings, or cramps caused by decreased blood calcium level.

Pharmacological

Antithyroid therapy is used for children, younger adults, pregnant females, the client who refuses surgery, or clients following surgery. There are several drugs that can be used for antithyroid therapy. Propylthiouracil (PTU) is used frequently, especially in cases of thyroid storm. It reduces the production of the thyroid hormones. It should be given with food. The client must be instructed to avoid foods high in iodine such as shellfish and iodized salt. Over-the-counter preparations must be checked to see if they contain iodine. This drug requires several weeks to exert the full effect and it may be administered up to 2 years. This drug may cause **agranulocytosis** (a decreased number of granulocytes) so it is important to report signs and symptoms of infection immediately to the physician.

Methimazole (Tapazole) is another antithyroid preparation that interferes with thyroid hormone synthesis. It has a more rapid onset than PTU; however, it does not have as much consistency in effect. It should be administered at evenly spaced intervals with food to prevent gastric upset. This drug can also cause agranulocytosis, particularly in the client over the age of 40.

Iodide preparations may be given to the client with hyperthyroidism. Because iodides inhibit the release of thyroid hormones rather than the synthesis, they take effect in 2 days. Two common preparations are potassium iodide saturated solution, SSKI, and a solution of iodine and potassium iodide that is called Lugol's solution. When iodide preparations are administered orally, they should be mixed with milk, juice, or water and given after meals to decrease gastric upset. Drinking the preparations through a straw will decrease discoloration of the teeth. These drugs are contraindicated in the client with acute bronchitis or a known hypersensitivity to iodine.

Clients may be prescribed propranolol hydrochloride (Inderal) to counteract tachycardia and peripheral effects of hyperthyroidism. Clients should not smoke

PROFESSIONAL TIP

Hypersensitivity to Iodides
The first signs of hypersensitivity reactions caused by iodides are irritation and swollen eyelids.

while taking this medication. Abrupt withdrawal of the drug can cause hypertension, myocardial ischemia, or cardiac arrhythmias. Clients should rise slowly from a sitting or lying position in order to prevent orthostatic hypotension.

Topical medications such as isotonic eye drops may be ordered to protect the eyes of the client with exophthalmos. Care must be taken that the eyes are not injured or infected. Some physicians may order high doses of corticosteroids to help reduce exophthalmos.

During a thyrotoxic crisis, antithyroid drugs are given. Other medications that may be used are propranolol, corticosteroids, and iodine preparations. Individual client needs could indicate a need for vitamins, nutrients, fluids, or sedation.

Diet

Since the client has a greatly increased metabolic rate as well as weight loss, diet is a consideration. The client may require between 4,000 to 5,000 calories per day. There is a need for increased protein, vitamins (especially vitamins B and C), and minerals. In addition to 3 meals a day, the client will need additional meals or snacks. Fluids should be encouraged, but caffeine should be avoided.

▶ NURSING PROCESS

▶ Assessment

▶ Subjective Data

The nurse must obtain a thorough client history and ask about the ability to concentrate, nervousness, insomnia, jitteriness, excitability, emotional lability, or dysphagia.

▶ Objective Data

The nurse will assess for rapid pulse, elevated blood pressure, warm skin, elevated temperature, diaphoresis, or hand tremors. Female clients may cease to menstruate. Hair is fine and soft.

Nursing diagnoses for a client with hyperthyroidism may include the following:

Nursing Diagnoses	Planning/Goals	Nursing Interventions
Preoperative		
▶ *Imbalanced Nutrition: Less than Body Requirements related to increased metabolism*	The client will eat a nutritionally balanced diet with enough calories to prevent weight loss.	Arrange a consultation with the dietitian to assist in determining the client's increased nutritional needs. Provide snacks throughout the day. Encourage client to eat a well-balanced diet.
▶ *Risk for Injury related to exophthalmos*	The client's eyes will not be injured from exophthalmos.	Administer isotonic solutions or eye lubricants to keep the eye moist. At night, elevate head of the bed which may assist in keeping the eyelids closed, or the eyes may be taped shut to prevent drying. Suggest to client that dark or tinted wraparound glasses may protect the eyes from wind and airborne particles.
Postoperative		
▶ *Impaired Swallowing related to mechanical obstruction (edema)*	The client will have diminished problems with swallowing.	Ensure gag, cough, and swallowing reflexes are present before offering oral fluids. Encourage client to drink slowly and chew thoroughly. Maintain client in Fowler's position when drinking or eating.
▶ *Ineffective Airway Clearance related to edema and pain*	The client will be able to clear airway.	Keep suctioning equipment ready. Administer analgesic as ordered.

Evaluation Each goal must be evaluated to determine how it has been met by the client.

SAMPLE NURSING CARE PLAN

THE CLIENT WITH HYPERTHYROIDISM

Janey Jackson, 33 years old, has returned to her physician's office to find out results of her tests for hyperthyroidism. She continues to have multiple complaints. "I have lost fifteen pounds in the last month despite eating all the time. I am restless and can't sleep. I feel jittery and irritable. My family says my moods change so rapidly they don't know what to expect from me. I feel so hot most of the time and sweat a lot."

The office nurse notes Mrs. Jackson appears flushed and her eyes protrude slightly. Her vital signs, T.-100.6 orally, P.-120, R.-26, and B/P.-140/88, are slightly elevated from her previous office visit. Her test results confirm that she has hyperthyroidism.

Nursing Diagnosis 1 *Imbalanced Nutrition: Less than body requirements related to increased metabolism as evidenced by weight loss despite eating*

PLANNING/GOALS	NURSING INTERVENTIONS	RATIONALE	EVALUATION
Mrs. Jackson will eat a nutritionally balanced diet with enough calories to prevent weight loss.	Monitor amount of food ingested and caloric intake. Monitor weight daily. Provide a diet high in calories, protein, and carbohydrates.	Provides data to determine if diet is adequate to prevent weight loss. Determines weight gains or losses. Maintains or increases weight while preventing muscle mass break-	Mrs. Jackson gained or maintained weight.

continues

down, yet providing adequate energy.

Advise Mrs. Jackson to avoid highly seasoned or fibrous foods or foods causing flatulence.

Gas accumulation is common and could cause increased peristalsis resulting in diarrhea.

Provide small frequent meals spread over waking hours.

Provides adequate calories without extremely large meals.

Obtain nutritional consult as needed.

Assists with meal planning to ensure nutritional status while considering personal food preferences.

Nursing Diagnosis 2 *Hyperthermia related to increased metabolic rate as evidenced by complaints of feeling hot, flushing, and elevated temperature*

PLANNING/GOALS	NURSING INTERVENTIONS	RATIONALE	EVALUATION
Mrs. Jackson's body temperature will be within normal range.	Assess for elevated temperature, heat intolerance, and diaphoresis.	Indicates increased heat production from increased metabolic rate.	Mrs. Jackson maintained her temperature in a normal range.
	Provide a well-ventilated room with temperature controlled to coolness for comfort.	Promotes comfort if heat intolerant.	
	Suggest wearing cool loose-fitting lightweight clothing.	Provides comfort and prevents overheating.	
	Provide frequent bathing and changes in linens or clothing.	Promotes comfort if diaphoretic.	
	Provide fluids up to 3 liters per day.	Replaces fluid if diaphoretic.	

Nursing Diagnosis 3 *Risk for Impaired Skin Integrity related to diaphoresis as evidenced by excessive sweating*

PLANNING/GOALS	NURSING INTERVENTIONS	RATIONALE	EVALUATION
Mrs. Jackson's skin will remain intact and free of injury.	Assess skin for flushing and moisture.	Indicates heat intolerance.	Mrs. Jackson maintained an intact skin without impairment.
	Monitor skin for redness or breakdown, especially bony prominences.	Indicates potential for breakdown.	
	Keep Mrs. Jackson clean and dry.	Prevents skin breakdown.	

HYPOTHYROIDISM

Hypothyroidism is a condition in which the metabolic processes are decreased because of a deficiency of the thyroid hormone. It is termed primary if the problem arises from a dysfunction solely of the thyroid. It is secondary if the thyroid gland is not stimulated to produce normally or if the target cells fail to respond to normal thyroid functioning. This condition is more common in females than males. There is a significant increase in incidence between the ages of 30 to 60. Hypothyroid conditions include cretinism, myxedema, and Hashimoto's thyroiditis.

CRETINISM

A congenital condition due to a lack of thyroid hormones causes defective physical development and mental retardation. This is called **cretinism**. This occurs in about 1 of 4,000 live births. The child generally has a large head, short limbs, puffy eyes, thick and protruding tongue, excessively dry skin, and a lack of coordination. If untreated, the child will be permanently dwarfed, mentally retarded, and sterile. This condition is rare in the United States and is tested by the T_4.

MYXEDEMA

Myxedema is the term for severe hypothyroidism in adults. There are a variety of abnormalities that lead to decreased thyroid hormone production. The obvious ones are thyroid gland surgery such as thyroidectomy or irradiation of the thyroid gland. Some other causes are chronic autoimmune Hashimoto's thyroiditis, inflammatory conditions (sarcoidosis), pituitary failure to produce TSH, or hypothalamus failure to produce thyrotropin-releasing hormone. There may be an inability to synthesize thyroid hormones related to iodine deficiency (rarely from general diet deficiency) or as a result of taking antithyroid medications.

Clinical manifestations are vague and varied, developing slowly over a period of time, but are primarily related to the reduced metabolic rate. These include an energy loss, fatigue, forgetfulness, sensitivity to cold, unexplained weight gain, hypoventilation, and constipation. As the condition progresses, manifestations include reduced libido, menorrhagia, paresthesias, joint stiffness, and muscle cramping. There is a characteristic alteration in overall appearance and behavior including decreased mental stability and a thick and dry tongue, causing hoarseness and slow, slurred speech. The skin is flaky and inelastic, feels cool, dry, rough, and doughy. There is edema of the face, hands, and feet. The hair is dry and sparse, with patchy hair loss including loss of outer third of the eyebrow. The nails are thick and brittle with visible transverse and longitudinal grooves. The pulse is weak and bradycardic due to the decreased pumping strength of the heart. The thyroid gland may be so small that it may not be palpated unless there is a goiter. The blood pressure is generally lower than normal for the client.

Diagnostic tests generally include: TSH, T_3, T_4, radioactive iodine uptake, and a thyroid scan.

Complications affect almost every system. Cardiovascular complications include ischemic heart disease, poor peripheral circulation, enlarged heart, or pleural or pericardial effusion. Gastrointestinal complications include adynamic colon (decreased functioning of the colon), megacolon (massive and abnormal dilation of the colon), or intestinal obstruction. Other complications include conductive or sensorineural deafness, psychiatric disorders, carpal tunnel syndrome, or impotence or infertility. Prognosis depends upon the organs involved, duration, and severity of condition.

Myxedema coma or hypothyroid crisis is a serious complication of extreme hypothyroidism. It is life threatening. It is characterized by severe metabolic disorders, hypothermia, and cardiovascular collapse leading to coma. It has a gradual onset but is triggered by severe stress such as infection, exposure to cold, or trauma. Abrupt withdrawal of thyroid medication or the use of narcotics, sedatives, or anesthetics can also cause myxedema coma. If myxedema coma occurs, it must be reported to the physician immediately. The client would be moved to the intensive care unit. Intubation and mechanical ventilation are instituted (Young, 1999). The client will be monitored closely for vital signs, EKG changes, and cardiopulmonary status. Wrapping the client in blankets will warm the client, but a warming blanket should not be used as it could cause peripheral vasodilation and shock. Thyroid medications and possibly corticosteroids would be administered. Supportive care would be given until the client comes out of the myxedema coma. Myxedema coma is often fatal.

Medical–Surgical Management

Pharmacological

Thyroid replacement therapy lasts a lifetime. Thyroid (Armour Thyroid) is a natural form while levothyroxine sodium (Levothroid, Synthroid) is a synthetic. The physician will order thyroid hormone to begin slowly and increase the dosage every 2 to 3 weeks until the desired response is achieved. The medication should be given in 1 dose in the morning to prevent insomnia.

If the client has diabetes mellitus, insulin or oral hypoglycemic dosage might have to be adjusted. The blood sugar level must be monitored closely. If the

CLIENT TEACHING

Items Containing Iodine

Check the labels on multivitamins, dentrifices, and nonprescription medications; they may contain iodine.

client is on anticoagulant therapy, thyroid hormones potentiate the anticoagulant action. The client needs to be informed to watch for excessive bleeding or bruising. Digitalis preparations are also potentiated by thyroid hormone.

Because hypothyroidism impairs the metabolic rate, the client may have difficulty metabolizing medications. The client may have an increased sensitivity to hypnotics, sedatives, or opiates. Dosage may have to be adjusted appropriately. Synthesis of the thyroid hormone can be impaired by drugs such as lithium carbonate (Lithotabs) or aminoglutethimide (Cytadren).

Diet

The client should be instructed to avoid foods high in iodine and foods that interfere with thyroid hormone replacement. These include dried kelp, shellfish,

iodized salt, saltwater fish, cabbage, turnips, pears, and peaches. The diet is designed to increase weight loss and combat constipation. A high-fiber, high-protein, low-calorie diet is given. Sodium should be decreased to prevent fluid retention. A dietary consultation for meal planning and a list of foods to avoid should be provided to the client.

▶ NURSING PROCESS

▶ Assessment

▶ Subjective Data

Obtain a thorough client history and ask about lethargy, depression, irritability, impaired memory, and slowing of thought processes. The client may describe speech and hearing problems, anorexia, decreased libido, and constipation.

▶ Objective Data

Assess for hearing and speech deficits, thin hair, dry and thickened skin, enlarged facial features, masklike expression, low and hoarse voice, bradycardia, decreased blood pressure and respirations, and exercise intolerance.

Nursing diagnoses for the client with myxedema may include the following:

Nursing Diagnoses	Planning/Goals	Nursing Interventions
Activity Intolerance related to decreased metabolic and energy level	The client will express understanding for the need to increase activity level gradually.	Assist the client to gradually increase activity level but encourage rest between activities to avoid fatigue and decrease cardiac oxygen demands.
	The client will maintain blood pressure, pulse, and respirations within normal limits when active.	Measure the client's legs correctly so antiembolic hose, which help venous return, will fit properly when worn.
	The client will regain and maintain normal activity levels.	Reposition client every 2 hours and encourage client to continue activity when normal activity level is achieved.
Ineffective Tissue Perfusion (Cardiopulmonary) related to decreased cardiac output	The client will not have chest pain at rest.	Assess for chest pain and advise client to report any episodes of angina immediately.
	The client will have a normal heart rate and rhythm.	Monitor the client's vital signs.
	The client will avoid ischemic EKG changes.	Monitor cardiac status through EKG and assessment of heart and lung sounds plus checking for edema.
	The client will maintain adequate cardiopulmonary perfusion.	Restrict fluid and sodium during the time of cardiac decompensation as ordered. Monitor intake and output and weight.
Constipation related to decreased motility of the gastrointestinal tract	The client will have a regular bowel movement.	Provide high-fiber diet.
		Encourage intake of oral fluids.
		Assess frequency and character of stool.
		Administer stool softener, bulk laxative, or enema as ordered.

Evaluation Each goal must be evaluated to determine how it has been met by the client.

HASHIMOTO'S THYROIDITIS

Hashimoto's thyroiditis is an autoimmune disease characterized by the production of antiperoxidase antibodies which destroy an essential enzyme necessary for production of T_3 and T_4. The disease occurs more often in females than in males, between the ages of 30 and 50, and shows a marked hereditary pattern. There is an increased incidence in clients with Down syndrome and Turner's syndrome.

Clinical manifestations include a thyroid that is enlarged and has a lumpy surface. Generally the goiter is asymptomatic, but it could cause dysphagia and a feeling of local pressure. The thymus gland is also enlarged. Other clinical manifestations are similar to hypothyroidism.

Treatment of Hashimoto's thyroiditis is also similar to that of hypothyroidism. Thyroid hormone replacement is used. This is a chronic disorder that can be treated, but not cured. The client will be on lifetime thyroid hormone replacement.

THYROID TUMORS

There are several neoplasms of the thyroid gland. The benign thyroid cyst and adenoma are firm, encapsulated, noninvasive, slowly growing neoplasms of unknown etiology. Diagnosis of benign neoplasms is done by needle biopsy. These growths tend to be nonfunctioning (not affecting the functioning of the thyroid gland) so there is no treatment other than continued monitoring. If the adenoma is functioning (increasing the functioning of the thyroid gland), then it is treated by radioactive iodine or surgery.

CANCER OF THE THYROID

Cancer of the thyroid is rare and occurs in all age groups. Individuals who have had radiation therapy to the neck are more susceptible. There are 4 major types of thyroid cancer:

- Papillary carcinoma is the most common type. It can affect any age but is more common in females of childbearing age. It is well-differentiated, grows slowly, is usually contained and does not spread beyond the adjacent lymph nodes. Cure rate after thyroidectomy is excellent.
- Follicular carcinoma metastasizes to the regional lymph nodes and spreads through the blood vessels to the bone, liver, and lungs. It has a very low cure rate.
- Medullary carcinoma is a solid carcinoma associated with pheochromocytoma. It is curable if detected before signs and symptoms occur. Without treat-

ment, it grows rapidly, metastasizing to the bones, liver, and kidneys.
- Anaplastic or undifferentiated carcinoma resists radiation. It is almost never curable by resection. It metastasizes rapidly, generally causing death by invasion of the trachea and adjacent structures. It generally affects individuals over the age of 60.

Since there is no known cause of cancer, there are several risk factors. They are radiation exposure, especially in those children and adolescents who received radiation therapy to treat severe cases of acne vulgaris, or to shrink enlarged tonsils, adenoids, and thymus tissue; prolonged secretion of TSH resulting from radiation or heredity; familial disposition; or chronic goiter.

The first clinical manifestation is a painless lump. As it enlarges, it destroys the thyroid which leads to clinical manifestations of hypothyroidism. Although rare, the tumor could trigger excessive thyroid hormone production causing the client to display the clinical manifestations of hyperthyroidism. There can be dysphagia, hoarseness, and vocal stridor. There may be a detectable, disfiguring thyroid mass with a firm nodule on palpation.

The thyroid scan shows a "cold" nodule (decreased uptake of ^{131}I) for papillary carcinoma. Follicular carcinoma and benign adenomas show a "hot" nodule. Thyroid function tests are usually normal. A needle biopsy may be done to confirm diagnosis.

Medical–Surgical Management

Surgical

All carcinomas can be treated with surgery (discussed previously). Radioactive iodine or external radiation therapy may also be used. Response of the tumor will depend upon early diagnosis and treatment. These methods of treatment may be used individually or in combination. Client care is the same as for hyperthyroidism.

Pharmacological

Exogenous thyroid hormone may suppress thyroid activity. To increase tolerance to surgery or radiation therapy, the physician may prescribe simultaneous exogenous thyroid hormone and adrenergic blocker such as propranolol hydrochloride (Inderal). If there is widespread metastasis, the cancers will be treated with neoplastic chemotherapy.

Nursing Management

The nurse will monitor the client's level of anxiety and encourage the client to discuss feelings about the diagnosis and possible surgery. The nurse will also assist the client in identifying previously successful coping methods, and teach new coping methods if needed.

GOITER

A goiter is an enlargement of the thyroid unrelated to inflammation or neoplasm. There are three types of goiter. One type is a diffuse toxic goiter found in hyperthyroidism. This type of goiter may be moderate to massively enlarged. The consistency varies from soft to firm and rubbery. It generally feels smooth. Frequently it is associated with exophthalmos.

Another type of goiter is a simple nontoxic goiter. It develops when the thyroid is unable to utilize iodine properly or in response to a low iodine level in the blood. These goiters are more common in females. They develop during times of great metabolic demands such as adolescence or pregnancy. A deficiency of iodine can cause goiter formation. Clinical manifestations depend upon the size of the goiter. There is an obvious enlargement of the thyroid gland. A large goiter can compress the esophagus or trachea causing dysphagia, a choking sensation, or respiratory difficulty. If the goiter impairs venous return from the head and neck, the client may experience dizziness and syncope.

Diagnosis is based on history, clinical manifestations, and results of thyroid function tests. T_3 is generally very low. Treatment concentrates on the underlying cause. This may involve thyroid hormone replacement therapy or prescribing iodine supplements or increasing dietary iodine sources. Surgery is done when respiration or swallowing is impaired or for cosmetic effect.

The third type of goiter is the nodular goiter. It is similar to the simple goiter except that palpation reveals multiple nodules causing the enlargement. It is found frequently in females over 40. It usually is asymptomatic. Treatment varies with the client's age and clinical manifestations.

PARATHYROID DISORDERS

Disorders discussed include hyperparathyroidism and hypoparathyroidism.

HYPERPARATHYROIDISM

Hyperparathyroidism is a condition resulting from overactivity of one or more of the parathyroid glands. It results in increased secretion of parathyroid hormone (PTH), which causes calcium to leave the bones and accumulate in the blood. This cannot be compensated by renal excretion or uptake into the soft tissues. It occurs twice as often in postmenopausal females than males. It occurs frequently between the ages of 35 and 65. Hypercalcemia may also be caused by excessive intake of thiazide diuretics, vitamin D, or calcium supplements.

X-rays will show skeletal decalcification. Blood PTH and alkaline phosphate levels are increased. Serum calcium level is elevated.

It is termed primary if there is an enlargement of one or more of the parathyroid glands increasing secretion of PTH and thus increasing the blood calcium level. The most common cause is adenoma, but other primary causes include genetics or multiple endocrine neoplasms.

The condition is termed secondary if there is excess compensatory production of PTH stemming from a hypocalcemia-producing abnormality other than the parathyroid gland. Some of these abnormalities are rickets, chronic renal failure, vitamin D deficiency, or osteomalacia due to laxative abuse or phenytoin (Dilantin).

Many clients are asymptomatic; however, there are several clinical manifestations. The client may have polyuria, chronic low back pain, bone tenderness, or renal calculi. The client may also experience nausea, vomiting, anorexia, constipation, lethargy, or drowsiness. There can be changes in level of consciousness, disorientation, stupor, coma, or personality changes with a loss of initiative and memory. There may be marked muscle weakness and atrophy especially of the legs, joint hyperextensibility, long bone skeletal deformity, or hyporeflexia.

Without treatment, there can be permanent damage to the skeleton or kidneys. There can be bone and articular problems including pathologic fractures. Renal complications include colic, nephrolithiasis, urinary tract infection, and renal insufficiency leading to chronic renal failure. Other complications may be stone formation in various organs, cardiac or vascular problems, or central nervous system changes.

Medical–Surgical Management

Medical

Medical management is aimed at decreasing overactivity of the parathyroid glands. This may be accomplished by medication therapy or surgery. If there is severe renal involvement, the client may require dialysis.

Surgical

Primary hyperparathyroidism can be treated by surgical removal of three and one-half of the four parathyroid glands. Surgery can relieve bone pain in 3 days but may not reverse renal damage.

Preoperative care includes explanations, encouraging fluids, limiting calcium intake, and administering medications to lower the blood calcium level.

Postoperative care involves administration of magnesium or phosphate. The client may receive calcium supplements for several days. The nursing care is similar to that provided to the client with thyroidectomy (refer to hyperthyroidism). A major complication is airway obstruction.

Pharmacological

Pharmacological treatment is aimed toward correcting secondary hyperparathyroidism. This involves treating the underlying cause. Since hypercalcemia is a major manifestation, medications are geared to decrease the calcium level in the blood. This includes the use of diuretics such as furosemide (Lasix) and ethacrynic acid (Edecrin).

Other drugs that decrease the calcium level in the blood are calcitonin-human (Cibacalcin), plicamycin (Mithracin), and magnesium- or phosphate-based drugs. Phosphate-based drugs lower the calcium level based on the inverse relationship between phosphorus and calcium.

▶ NURSING PROCESS

▶ Assessment

▶ Subjective Data

The nurse should obtain a thorough client history and ask about muscle weakness, apathy, nausea, mental status, and pain (low back or renal). The client is assessed for increased calcium intake, either dietary or supplements.

▶ Objective Data

Fatigue, drowsiness, anorexia, constipation, personality changes, renal colic, skeletal deformity, output, hematuria, vomiting, weight loss, hypertension, bradycardia, or dysrhythmias should all be noted.

Nursing diagnoses for the client with hyperparathyroidism may include the following:

Nursing Diagnoses	Planning/Goals	Nursing Interventions
▶ *Activity Intolerance related to generalized weakness caused by neuromuscular dysfunction*	The client will regain and maintain normal muscle mass and strength, maintain maximum joint range of motion, and perform self-care activity as tolerated.	Alternate rest and activity periods. Assist client with prescribed, individualized activities. Assist client to identify factors that increase or decrease activity intolerance. Encourage client to perform self-care.
▶ *Pain related to musculoskeletal changes resulting from persistently increased serum calcium level*	The client will express relief after analgesics, use comfort measures to decrease pain, and be pain-free when serum calcium level reaches normal.	Administer analgesics as ordered. Provide comfort measures for bone pain, and include turning and repositioning every 2 hours. Assess pain level and compare to serum calcium level. Assess environment for hazards and eliminate them. Assist the client to ambulate. Maintain the bed in a low position with siderails up and call light in reach. Lift and move the client gently to prevent pathologic fractures.

Evaluation Each goal must be evaluated to determine how it has been met by the client.

HYPOPARATHYROIDISM

Hypoparathyroidism is a condition resulting from a deficiency of parathyroid hormone (PTH) secretion by the parathyroids or the decreased action of peripheral PTH. Since the parathyroids normally regulate the serum calcium level, hypoparathyroidism will result in a decreased serum calcium level. PTH normally maintains the serum calcium level by increasing bone resorption and gastric reabsorption. It also maintains the inverse relationship between calcium and phosphorus levels. Hypoparathyroidism can be acute or chronic.

If hypoparathyroidism is idiopathic, it may be the result of an autoimmune disorder or congenital absence of parathyroid glands. Acquired hypoparathyroidism is generally irreversible. The most common cause is accidental removal during thyroid or other neck surgery. It could also be a result of ischemic infarction during surgery, sarcoidosis, tuberculosis, neoplasms, trauma, or massive thyroid irradiation. Reversible hypoparathyroidism can result from hypomagnesemia-induced impairment of hormone synthesis, suppression of normal gland function because of hypercalcemia, or delayed maturation of the parathyroid glands.

The characteristic sign of hypoparathyroidism is tetany, which is muscle spasms and tremors caused by a lack of calcium. Other clinical manifestations include dry skin, brittle hair, alopecia (loss of hair or baldness), and loss of eyelashes and fingernails. The teeth are stained, cracked, and decayed due to weak enamel.

A. Positive Chvostek's Sign

B. Positive Trousseau's Sign

Figure 27-11 Signs of Hypocalcemia and Hypoparathyroidism: A. Chvostek's sign; B. Trousseau's sign

The client may have altered neuromuscular irritability, tingling and twitching of the face and hands, and increased deep tendon reflexes. There may be personality changes or EKG changes.

There are two diagnostic assessment tests that can be performed. One is the **Chvostek's sign**, which is an abnormal spasm of the facial muscles in response to a light tapping of the facial nerve. The other test is **Trousseau's sign**, which is a carpal spasm caused by inflating a blood pressure cuff above the client's systolic pressure and leaving it in place for 3 minutes (Figure 27-11).

Expected test results include: decreased serum calcium, increased urinary calcium, increased serum phosphorus, and decreased urinary phosphorus.

Complications are related to long-standing hypocalcemia. This leads to decreased heart contractility leading to cardiac failure. There can be cataract formation or papillary edema from increased intracranial pressure. There may be bone deformity. In cases of severe tetany, the client can experience laryngospasm, respiratory stridor, anoxia, paralysis of vocal cords, and death.

Medical–Surgical Management

Pharmacological

Calcium gluconate or calcium chloride may be given intravenously. Give very slowly since it is very irritating to the vessel wall. Too rapid IV calcium infusion can cause cardiac arrest. After the initial IV dose, calcium may be given orally.

Unless the hypoparathyroidism is reversible, the client will require lifelong calcium replacement. Vitamin D may also be given to assist in the absorption of calcium. The calcium supplements should be given 1 to 1½ hours after meals to increase absorption. If the client cannot swallow the large tablets, they can be dissolved in hot water and the suspension cooled before administering to the client. The best sources of calcium are from the diet. The client needs to take calcium as ordered and not abruptly stop taking the drug. The client must be advised that calcium may cause digitalis toxicity. Cimetidine (Tagamet) interferes with normal parathyroid functioning.

Diet

The diet should be high in calcium and low in phosphorus containing foods. Since many foods that are high in calcium are also high in phosphorus, the client should be given a list of foods that are high in calcium but lower in phosphorus. Foods on this list include vegetables such as asparagus, broccoli, collards, and tomatoes; fruits such as apricots, bananas, cantaloupe, and many berries; and other foods such as kidney beans, lima beans, and brown sugar. Foods that have a high phosphorus content and should be avoided include: most legumes, nuts, cheeses, and seafood.

▶ NURSING PROCESS

▶ Assessment

▶ Subjective Data

The nurse will obtain a thorough client history and ask the client about recent surgery or irradiation, use of alcohol, numbness or tingling of the skin, anxiety, headache, irritability, depression, or nausea.

▶ Objective Data

The nurse will assess for dysphagia, laryngeal spasm, stridor, cyanosis, or dysrhythmias, and also check for Chvostek's sign and Trousseau's sign.

Nursing diagnoses for the client with hypoparathyroidism may include the following:

Nursing Diagnoses	Planning/Goals	Nursing Interventions
▸ *Risk for Injury related to calcium deficiency*	The client will not exhibit signs and symptoms of tetany, and will prevent injury from hypocalcemia.	Monitor Chvostek's and Trousseau's signs, serum calcium and phosphorus levels, as well as EKG changes.
		Keep tracheotomy tray readily available and maintain seizure precautions.
		Support the client while walking to prevent injury.
		Monitor the client taking digoxin for toxicity.
▸ *Imbalanced Nutrition: Less than body requirements, related to calcium intake*	The client will have adequate calcium intake.	Provide diet with calcium-rich foods.
		Give calcium replacement as ordered. The client who is taking digoxin must be monitored for toxicity.

Evaluation Each goal must be evaluated to determine how it has been met by the client.

ADRENAL DISORDERS

Disorders in this category include Cushing's disease/syndrome, Addison's disease, and pheochromocytoma.

CUSHING'S DISEASE/SYNDROME (ADRENAL HYPERFUNCTION)

Cushing's *disease,* primary adrenal hyperfunction, is the result of increased pituitary secretion of ACTH which causes an increased production of cortisol by the adrenal cortex. Cushing's *syndrome* refers to symptoms of cortisol excess caused by other factors. One cause is a corticotropin producing tumor in another organ such as oat-cell carcinoma of the lung (secondary adrenal hyperfunction). The most common cause of Cushing's syndrome is prolonged used of glucocorticoid or corticotropin medications for chronic inflammatory disorders such as chronic obstructive pulmonary disease, Crohn's disease, and rheumatoid arthritis. This is **iatrogenic** (caused by treatment or diagnostic procedures) adrenal hyperfunction.

Cushing's syndrome occurs in females more than males, generally between 30 and 50 years of age.

Classic clinical manifestations are adiposity of the face, neck, and trunk which give rise to the moon-shaped face and buffalo hump (Figure 27-12). Others include purple striae on the abdomen, hirsutism, and thin extremities due to muscle wasting. Boys exhibit an early onset of puberty, while girls exhibit development of masculine characteristics. The client may complain of fatigue, muscle weakness, sleep disturbances, water retention, amenorrhea, decreased libido, irritability, and emotional lability. There could be petechiae, ecchymoses, decreased wound healing, or swollen ankles.

There are multiple complications of Cushing's syndrome, most of which are produced by the stimulating and catabolic effects of cortisol. There can be increased calcium resorption from the bone leading to osteoporosis and pathologic fractures. It can cause increased hepatic gluconeogenesis and insulin resistance causing glucose intolerance and diabetes mellitus. The client may have frequent infections and slowed wound healing. There is a suppressed inflammatory response that can mask severe infections. The client may have decreased ability to handle stress, which can lead to psychological problems from mood swings to psychosis. Other complications include hypertension, ischemic heart disease, congestive heart failure, menstrual disturbances, and sexual dysfunction.

Plasma cortisol level is elevated. Plasma ACTH level may be elevated or low. Adrenalangiography is done for adrenal tumor. Twenty-four-hour urine tests for 17-ketosteroids and 17-hydroxysteroids are elevated.

Figure 27-12 A Client with Cushing's Syndrome: Untreated *(Photo courtesy of Dr. Matthew Leinung, Head, Division of Endocrinology and Metabolism, Albany Medical College, Albany, NY)*

Prognosis depends upon early diagnosis, identifying the underlying cause, and effective treatment. Without treatment, about half of these clients will die within 5 years.

Medical–Surgical Management

Medical

The major goal is to restore hormone balance. Treatment is based on the causative factor. This is accomplished primarily by medications. If there is adrenal cancer, the client may either have radiation therapy to the adrenal gland or surgery on either the pituitary gland or the adrenal glands, or all three treatments.

Surgical

If the underlying cause of Cushing's syndrome is related to the pituitary gland, the client may have a hypophysectomy done. (Refer to hypophysectomy in the section on hyperpituitarism.)

For an adrenal tumor, an adrenalectomy is performed. This could be unilateral or bilateral. During the first 24 to 48 hours after surgery, the client is observed closely for hemorrhage and shock. Vital signs and urine output must be monitored. Glucocorticoids are administered with changing dosage until a maintenance dose is established. The client's blood glucose level must be monitored, especially for hypoglycemia.

Pharmacological

Aminoglutethimide (Cytadren) inhibits synthesis of adrenal steroids. It can cause dizziness or drowsiness. The client should be instructed to avoid activities requiring mental alertness or manual dexterity.

Ketoconazole (Nizoral), while classified as an antifungal, inhibits adrenal steroidogenesis and is used in Cushing's syndrome.

Mitotane (Lysodren) directly suppresses the activity of the adrenal cortex. This cytotoxic agent is generally used for inoperable adrenal cortex cancer. It is given for at least 3 months. The client should avoid situations that cause injury or exposure to infections.

If the client had pituitary or adrenal surgery, cortisol therapy may be given before and after surgery to decrease physical stress. Steroid therapy could be a lifetime situation. The client should take the drug with food or antacids to decrease gastric distress. Two-thirds dose of the steroids should be taken in the morning with the remaining one-third in the early evening to mimic the body's diurnal schedule. Steroids can lead to osteoporosis and the possibility of pathologic fractures. Females should be warned that steroid use can interfere with oral contraceptive effectiveness. There may be an adverse effect on the male's sperm production and count.

The client with diabetes mellitus may have to adjust insulin dosage because the steroids can affect the glu-

cose levels. Steroids can mask severe infections and cause some immunosuppression. Wounds are slower to heal. The client should be instructed to contact a physician before using over-the-counter preparations. The client should not abruptly discontinue the steroid drug; dosage should be tapered before discontinuing.

Diet

The diet should be high in protein and potassium but low in sodium. Foods high in protein include: eggs, milk, whole grains, legumes, and meat; however, milk, cheeses, and whole grains are also high in sodium, depending upon processing. Many foods high in potassium are also low in sodium. These foods are: legumes; fruits such as figs, oranges, bananas, prunes, and raisins; and vegetables such as avocado, potato, and spinach. The client should be advised to read labels for sodium content. Processed foods and many preservatives have high sodium content and should be avoided. Reduced carbohydrates and calories help control hyperglycemia.

▶ NURSING PROCESS

▶ Assessment

▶ Subjective Data

The nurse should obtain a thorough client history and ask about the use of steroids, stress, methods of coping with stress, irritability, depression, mood swings, loss of libido, and the possibility of suicide.

▶ Objective Data

The client is assessed for thin and fragile skin, petechiae, ecchymoses, delayed wound healing, weight gain, increased abdominal girth, purple striae, hyperglycemia, and hypokalemia. Women may have **hirsutism** (excessive body hair in a masculine distribution), deepening of the voice, and menstrual irregularities.

🏠 COMMUNITY/HOME HEALTH CARE

Cushing's Syndrome
- Carry Medic Alert medal indicating Cushing's syndrome.
- Avoid extreme temperature changes, activities that could result in trauma, and people with infections.
- Wash hands often.
- Protect skin with good care.
- Maintain medication regimen.
- Notify physician if weakness, fainting, fever, nausea, or vomiting occur.

Nursing diagnoses for the client with Cushing's syndrome may include the following:

Nursing Diagnoses	Planning/Goals	Nursing Interventions
▸ *Disturbed Body Image related to changes in physical appearance*	The client will verbalize feelings about changed appearance.	Encourage the client to verbalize feelings about changed body image.
		Offer emotional support and a positive realistic assessment of the condition.
▸ *Risk for Infection related to suppressed inflammatory response from excessive corticosteroid production*	The client will take precautions to avoid or decrease exposure to infection.	Advise client to avoid people with infections.
		Provide a private room with reverse or protective isolation as indicated.
		Monitor the client's vital signs, intake and output, and weight.

Evaluation Each goal must be evaluated to determine how it has been met by the client.

ADDISON'S DISEASE (ADRENAL HYPOFUNCTION)

Addison's disease, primary hypofunctioning of the adrenals, involves decreased functioning of the adrenal cortex and its secretions—mineralocorticoids, glucocorticoids, and androgens. It can also be called *adrenal hypofunction* or *insufficiency*. It is fairly uncommon, occurring in one per 100,000 people in the United States. Although it affects all ages and both sexes, it is less common among the elderly.

Addison's disease occurs when more than 90% of the adrenal gland is destroyed. It is an autoimmune disease in response to conditions such as tuberculosis, histoplasmosis, HIV, and meningococcal pneumonia. It can be caused by bilateral adrenalectomy, hemorrhage into the adrenal gland related to anticoagulant therapy, or cancer of the adrenal gland. It is termed secondary if it results from decreased pituitary or hypothalamus function or abrupt withdrawal of long-term steroid therapy.

A classical clinical manifestation of Addison's disease is a bronze coloration of the skin resembling a deep suntan, especially in the creases on the hands, elbows, and knees. There may be some areas of vitiglio. The client may complain of fatigue, muscle weakness, lightheadedness upon rising, weight loss, and craving for salty foods. The client may have decreased tolerance even to minor stress. The client is anxious, irritable, and may become confused. The pulse may be weak and irregular. There is hypotension and a variety of GI complaints.

The acute form is called adrenal crisis. It may occur when there is trauma, surgery, other physiologic stress, or abrupt withdrawal of steroids. The clinical manifestations are the same only more severe with a rapid onset. The crisis requires immediate treatment. The client will be placed on intravenous therapy and IV administration of hydrocortisone (Cortef, Hydrocortone). Measures to maintain a stable blood pressure and normal water and sodium levels are instituted. After the crisis, the client will be placed on a maintenance dose of hydrocortisone.

Expected test results include: low serum sodium, high serum potassium, low serum glucose, low cortisol and aldosterone serum levels, and decreased urinary 17-ketosteroid and 17-hydroxysteroid levels.

Medical–Surgical Management

Medical

Treatment is geared toward prompt restoration of fluid and electrolyte balance and replacement of deficient adrenal hormones.

Pharmacological

The client will require lifetime maintenance of steroids. Administration of glucocorticoids such as hydrocortisone (Hydrocortone) and mineralocorticoids such as fludrocortisone acetate (Florinef) are given two-thirds of the daily dose in the morning and one-third in the evening. In times of stress the dose may need to be doubled or tripled.

Diet

The diet should be high in sodium and low in potassium. It should contain adequate calories and protein. If the client is anorexic, six small meals may increase caloric intake. A late afternoon or evening snack should be available if there is a drop in the client's blood glucose level.

▸ NURSING PROCESS

▸ Assessment

▸ Subjective Data

The nurse should obtain a thorough client history and ask about recent synthetic steroid use, adrenal surgery, infection, salt craving, nausea, weakness, vertigo, headache, disorientation, emotional status, anxiety, and apprehension.

▶ Objective Data

Assess for postural hypotension, inability to perform normal activities, syncope, dark pigmented areas on skin and mucous membrane, weight loss, vomiting, diarrhea, and very low or very high temperature.

Nursing diagnoses for the client with Addison's disease may include the following:

Nursing Diagnoses	Planning/Goals	Nursing Interventions
▶ *Deficient Fluid Volume related to low sodium level, vomiting, diarrhea, and increased renal losses*	The client will regain normal fluid and electrolyte balance.	Monitor the client's vital signs, level of consciousness, intake and output, and weight. Administer IV fluids as ordered and encourage fluid intake.
▶ *Risk for Infection related to suppressed inflammatory response*	The client will maintain normal temperature and leukocyte count and differential and use precautions to avoid or reduce risks of infection.	Monitor temperature every 4 hours unless elevated, then every 2 hours. Provide a private room with reverse or protective isolation as needed. Screen personnel and visitors for infection. Teach proper handwashing. Monitor laboratory test results for WBC and differential.

Evaluation Each goal must be evaluated to determine how it has been met by the client.

PHEOCHROMOCYTOMA

Pheochromocytoma, sometimes known as *chromaffin cell tumor,* is a rare disease characterized by **paroxysmal** (a symptom that begins and ends abruptly) or sustained hypertension due to excessive secretion of epinephrine and norepinephrine. Some medical experts estimate that about one-half percent of clients newly diagnosed with hypertension have pheochromocytoma. Although the tumor is generally benign, it can be malignant in 5% to 10% of the cases. It affects all races and both sexes. It is most common in females ages 20 to 50 years.

It is caused by a chromaffin cell tumor of the adrenal medulla, more commonly on the right side. Extraadrenal pheochromocytomas can also occur. Epinephrine overproduction occurs with the adrenal pheochromocytoma; however, norepinephrine overproduction is associated with both adrenal and extraadrenal pheochromocytoma. It is associated with a familial history of pheochromocytoma or endocrine gland cancer. It is considered to be inherited on the autosomal dominant gene in about 5% of the cases.

The classic triad of clinical manifestations is hypertension with diastolic pressure above 115 mm Hg, unrelenting headache, and profuse diaphoresis. Other clinical manifestations include palpitations, visual disturbances, nausea, or vomiting. These attacks may be triggered by activities or conditions that displace the abdominal contents such as heavy lifting, exercise, bladder distention, or pregnancy. Severe attacks can be precipitated by administration of opiates, histamine, glucagon, and corticotropin. Some attacks may have no precipitating factor. Some other clinical manifestations are mild to moderate weight loss due to increased metabolism or orthostatic hypotension when arising to an upright position. The client will have tachycardia. The actual tumor is rarely palpable; however, palpation could trigger a hypertensive attack.

The complications are similar to those of severe and persistent hypertension. These complications are stroke, retinopathy, heart disease, or irreversible kidney disease. The client with pheochromocytoma has an increased risk of severe complications or death during invasive diagnostic tests or surgery.

Although pheochromocytoma can be potentially fatal, the prognosis is good with treatment. About 90% of the clients are cured.

GERONTOLOGICAL CONSIDERATIONS

Pheochromocytoma

Pheochromocytoma is frequently diagnosed during pregnancy when the enlarged uterus puts pressure on the tumor causing more frequent attacks. The attacks could prove fatal to both mother and fetus. Although there is an increased risk of spontaneous abortion, most fetal deaths occur during labor or immediately after delivery.

Medical–Surgical Management

Surgical

The treatment of choice is surgical removal of the tumor. Sometimes the adrenal gland is also removed. The blood pressure is monitored closely during the immediate postoperative period. The client may have hypotension, but hypertension is more common. About 10% of the cases are not surgical candidates. These would be treated with medications to lower the blood pressure. Some may be given neoplastic chemotherapy.

Pharmacological

During acute hypertensive attacks, the drugs of choice are phentolamine mesylate (Regitine) or nitroprusside sodium (Nipride). Phentolamine mesylate (Regitine) and phenoxybenzamine HCl (Dibenzyline) are alpha-adrenergic blocking agents. They are used to control hypertension before surgery or when surgery is contraindicated. The client's blood pressure and pulse should be monitored. The client should be warned about orthostatic hypotension and rise slowly from a supine position to an upright position. The client should not take over-the-counter drugs or alcohol.

Nitroprusside sodium (Nipride, Nitropress) acts on the vascular smooth muscle to cause peripheral vasodilation. The drug is given in an intravenous infusion. An electronic infusion device must be used to monitor the infusion rate. The client's blood pressure is used to titrate the infusion rate per the physician's orders.

Metyrosine (Demser) is used to block catecholamine synthesis. This drug must be continued for life if the tumor is inoperable. Ongoing medications include adrenergic blockers such as propranolol hydrochloride (Inderal), atenolol (Tenormin), prazosin HCl (Minipress), labetalol HCl (Normodyne), or nifedipine (Procardia), a calcium channel blocker. The client's blood pressure must be monitored frequently to determine the effectiveness of the medication.

Propranolol hydrochloride (Inderal) should not be stopped abruptly. The client should not smoke while taking this medication. Atenolol (Tenormin) may enhance the client's sensitivity to cold. Prazosin HCl (Minipress) should be taken on an empty stomach. The initial dose should be given at bedtime. The client should not use cough, cold, or allergy medications without the physician's knowledge. If the client is given parenteral labetalol HCl (Normodyne, Trandate), the client should remain supine for 3 hours to decrease the possibility of orthostatic hypotension. Nifedipine (Adalat, Procardia) should be protected from light and moisture and stored at room temperature. Over-the-counter medications should not be taken.

Diet

The diet should be high in protein with adequate calories. Stimulating foods such as aged cheeses and yogurt; caffeine-containing beverages such as coffee, tea, and soft drinks; and beer and red wine should be avoided (Smeltzer & Bare, 1996).

Nursing Management

The nurse will ask about heat intolerance, severe headaches during hypertensive crisis, anxiety, trouble sleeping, palpitations, nervousness, dizziness, paresthesias, and nausea. The client is assessed for dyspnea, tremors, diaphoresis, glycosuria, hyperglycemia, or dilated pupils. The nurse must frequently assess blood pressure, pulse, and respirations for elevations, and observe for signs of anxiety to prevent it from triggering a hypertensive crisis.

CASE STUDY

Mr. Carnes, a 44-year-old African American male, is admitted to the medical unit from his physician's office. He reports that he has lost 18 pounds over the last month and has been very tired. He also reports symptoms of thirst, frequent urination, and blurred vision. His vital signs are: BP 166/92, P 88, R 16, T 99.2°F. Physical assessment reveals hot, dry, flushed skin. Laboratory exams reveal a blood glucose 490 mg/dL and urine negative for ketones. Mr. Carnes is a truck driver and leads a fairly sedentary lifestyle. History reveals that he is usually 30 to 35 pounds overweight, but has otherwise been in good health. He reports that his mother died from diabetes and renal failure, and an older brother was diagnosed as having type 2 diabetes three years ago.

The following questions will guide your development of a nursing care plan for this case study:

1. List physical symptoms that Mr. Carnes is experiencing that are suggestive of diabetes.

2. Based on history and laboratory values, would you expect Mr. Carnes to be diagnosed with type 1 or type 2 diabetes?

3. Which nursing diagnoses would you identify as priority for Mr. Carnes right now? List two.

continues

CASE STUDY *continued*

4. Mr. Carnes is treated with IV fluids and insulin sliding scale until his blood glucose is stabilized. Describe what an insulin sliding scale is, and when it is used.

5. A 2,000 calorie ADA diet is ordered for Mr. Carnes. Mr. Carnes does not care to eat the apple that came on his breakfast tray and asks if he can exchange it for another serving of scrambled eggs. How would you respond to Mr. Carnes?

6. Mr. Carnes is being discharged and will continue to attend diabetic education classes at a local diabetic treatment center. Assuming Mr. Carnes is to continue on a diabetic diet and will be receiving mixed insulin injections, list the pertinent information Mr. Carnes will need to know about his disease and therapies related to:

   - Diabetes and symptoms of hyperglycemia
   - Role of exercise
   - Effects of diet
   - Self-monitoring blood glucose
   - Insulin injections/technique
   - Symptoms of hypoglycemia
   - Sick day care
   - Long-term complications

SUMMARY

- The endocrine system is composed of glands at various body locations producing secretions (hormones) that directly enter the blood or lymph circulation.
- The endocrine system provides slower and longer lasting control over various body activities and functions.
- A malfunction of any part of the endocrine system can result in a shift of homeostasis with far-reaching systemic reactions.
- Assessment of the endocrine system can be challenging since the glands are scattered. Negative findings are as important as positive findings.
- Diabetes is a complex chronic disease with multiple acute and chronic complications. It is a systemic disease caused by an imbalance between insulin supply and demand.
- A coordinated program of exercise, diet, and medications is used to achieve diabetic control. Persons with type 1 diabetes always require insulin therapy in addition to dietary control and an exercise program. Persons with type 2 diabetes are managed through diet and exercise, and may or may not require oral hypoglycemic agents or insulin.
- The goal of diabetes management is enabling the diabetic to manage the disease by maintaining a blood glucose level within an acceptable range and thereby minimizing the incidence of acute and chronic complications.

- Regardless of disorder, the client should wear a Medic Alert bracelet and be aware that the treatment generally lasts a lifetime.

Review Questions

1. Mrs. Gavin tells the nurse that she is surprised that she developed diabetes at 40 years of age. The nurse knows that the development of diabetes in middle-aged people is most directly the result of:
   a. atherosclerosis.
   b. eating too much sugar.
   c. obesity.
   d. viral infection.

2. When teaching the diabetic client about mixing short- and longer-acting (NPH) insulin in the same syringe, the nurse should teach that:
   a. regular insulin should be drawn up first.
   b. the NPH insulin should be drawn up first.
   c. it does not matter which insulin is drawn up first since they will be mixed anyway.
   d. the two insulins do not mix and should be drawn up and administered separately.

3. Which of the following principles is used when planning for a diabetic who is to undergo surgery?
   a. All insulin is withheld until surgery is over and the client is eating.

b. Insulin or oral hypoglycemics are given as usual.

c. Sliding scale insulin is used to regulate glucose levels during the operative period.

d. Hyperglycemia poses the most serious danger to the client during surgery.

4. Mr. Schultz and the nurse collaborate to establish a meal plan for his 1,800 calorie ADA diet. The principle used in the exchange system is based on the fact that Mr. Schultz:

a. may eat any food as long as he has 3 meals and limits his calories to 1,800 calories.

b. may substitute any food in the correct amount for another on the same exchange list.

c. can eat any food any time as long as it is on an exchange list.

d. must weigh all food before determining serving size.

5. Ms. Perez, who has type 1 diabetes, complains of weakness and shakiness. She is pale, diaphoretic, and her pulse rate is increased. The nurse should recognize these symptoms as indications of:

a. hyperglycemia.

b. hypoglycemia.

c. ketoacidosis.

d. potassium excess.

6. Mrs. Lally, age 24, is newly diagnosed with type 1 diabetes. If Mrs. Lally's husband comes home and finds her unconscious, what is the first thing he should do?

a. Place some easily absorbed glucose under her tongue (e.g., monogel) or give glucagon SC or IM

b. Call the doctor

c. Administer 20U regular insulin

d. Add sugar to orange juice and administer orally

7. Explanations prior to diagnostic tests for an endocrine disorder are most important to:

a. enable the client to collect a 24-hour urine specimen.

b. ensure client compliance with test instructions.

c. prevent taking medications that interfere with test results.

d. reduce stress that can interfere with test results.

8. Which of the following nursing diagnoses would be most appropriate for the client with diabetes insipidus?

a. Alteration in growth and development related to increased growth hormone production

b. Alteration in thought processes related to decreased neurologic function

c. Fluid volume deficit related to polyuria

d. Hypothermia related to decreased metabolic rate

9. Meticulous skin care is especially important for the client with hyperthyroidism because of:

a. diaphoresis from heat intolerance.

b. edema from sodium and water retention.

c. poor nutrition due to nausea and vomiting.

d. pressure from immobility due to paralysis.

10. The nurse would assess for which of the following clinical manifestations in the client with hypothyroidism?

a. Hypertension, diaphoresis, nausea, and vomiting

b. Tetany, irritability, dry skin, and brittle nails

c. Unexplained weight gain, energy loss, and cold intolerance

d. Water retention, moon-faced, hirsutism, and purple striae

11. The client with hyperparathyroidism should have extremities handled gently because:

a. decreased calcium bone deposits can lead to pathologic fractures.

b. edema causes stretched tissue to tear easily.

c. hypertension can lead to a stroke with residual paralysis.

d. polyuria leads to dry skin and mucous membranes that can break down.

12. Which of the following assessments would the nurse expect to observe in the client with pheochromocytoma?

a. Bradycardia and tetany

b. Nausea, vomiting, and diarrhea

c. Personality changes

d. Systolic pressure up to 300 mm Hg

Critical Thinking Questions

1. What kind of lifestyle changes are necessary for each endocrine disorder?

2. Prepare a teaching plan for a client with type 2 diabetes.

 WEB FLASH!

- After searching the Internet, share new information about lab tests or treatments for endocrine disorders discussed in this chapter. What new information was found that could be shared with a client?

- What information is available on the Internet from the various resources listed for the endocrine system at the end of the book?

- What electronic resources and information can you locate for clients with diabetes? Is the information grouped by type of diabetes?

UNIT
7

Digestion and Elimination

NURSING CARE OF THE CLIENT: GASTRO-INTESTINAL SYSTEM

MAKING THE CONNECTION

Refer to the following chapters to increase your understanding of the gastrointestinal system:

- **Chapter 7, Wellness Concepts**
- **Chapter 9, Loss, Grief, and Death**
- **Chapter 10, Fluid, Electrolyte, and Acid-Base Balance**
- **Chapter 12, Health Assessment**
- **Chapter 14, Pain Management**
- **Chapter 17, Nursing Care of the Oncology Client**
- **Chapter 22, Nursing Care of the Client: Immune System**
- **Chapter 27, Nursing Care of the Client: Endocrine System**
- **Chapter 33, Nursing Care of the Client: Mental Illness**
- **Chapter 35, Nursing Care of the Older Client**

LEARNING OBJECTIVES

Upon completion of this chapter, you should be able to:
- *Define key terms.*
- *Discuss diagnostic tests associated with the digestive system.*
- *Discuss components necessary for a complete assessment of the digestive system.*
- *List medical and surgical management for clients with digestive disorders.*
- *Describe nursing interventions for clients with digestive disorders.*
- *Assist with the formulation of nursing care plans for clients with digestive disorders.*

INTRODUCTION

Disorders and diseases of the gastrointestinal system and accessory organs can affect not only the digestive process and nutrient absorption, but the lifestyle of the individual as well.

KEY TERMS

adhesion	hematemesis
appendicitis	hemorrhoid
ascites	hepatitis
calculi (calculus, sing.)	ileostomy
cholecystitis	intussusception
cholelithiasis	jaundice
chyme	ligation
cirrhosis	melena
colostomy	occult blood test
constipation	(guaiac)
digestion	pancreatitis
diverticula	peptic ulcer
diverticulitis	peristalsis
diverticulosis	peritonitis
effluent	polyp
gastric ulcer	postprandial
gastritis	steatorrhea
glycogenesis	stoma
glycogenolysis	stomatitis
haustra	volvulus

ANATOMY AND PHYSIOLOGY REVIEW

The digestive system, also known as the *gastrointestinal (GI) tract* or the *alimentary system,* is responsible for breaking down the complex food into simple nutrients the body can absorb and convert into energy (see Figure 28-1). This process is known as **digestion**.

Mouth/Esophagus

Digestion begins in the mouth where the teeth mechanically break food down into smaller pieces by chewing and mixing it with saliva. The chemical breakdown of cooked starches is begun by the enzyme salivary amylase in the mouth. The food is then swallowed as a small ball or bolus and transported down the esophagus, a hollow, muscular tube approximately 10 inches long. **Peristalsis**, coordinated rhythmic contractions of the muscles, pushes the bolus through the esophagus. The cardiac sphincter, also called the *lower esophageal sphincter (LES),* located at the distal end of the esophagus relaxes and allows the food to pass into the stomach.

Stomach

Further mechanical and chemical breakdown of the food occurs in the stomach, a J-shaped muscular organ located beneath the diaphragm. The stomach secretes gastric juices that contain hydrochloric acid (HCl) and pepsinogen, a nonactive form of the enzyme pepsin. HCl and pepsin are responsible for beginning the breakdown of protein and continuing the breakdown of starches. Starch digestion in the stomach gradually stops due to the acid environment. Mucous is secreted to protect the lining of the stomach. The stomach also secretes an intrinsic factor, which is necessary for vitamin B_{12} absorption, and gastrin, which stimulates HCl release.

The peristaltic movement of the stomach mixes the partially digested food and digestive enzymes into a semiliquid mass called **chyme**. The chyme will not pass into the small intestine until it is the proper consistency and particles are 1 millimeter or less. On average, the stomach empties in 3 to 4 hours. Carbohydrates are digested most readily, followed by proteins, with fats taking the longest to pass from the stomach. When the chyme has reached the proper consistency, the pyloric sphincter relaxes, releasing a portion at a time of the chyme into the small intestine.

Small Intestine

The small intestine is approximately 20 to 25 feet long and is responsible for absorbing nutrients from the chyme. The small intestine also secretes digestive

Figure 28-1 The Digestive System

enzymes, mucous to protect the mucosa, and hormones to aid in the absorption of nutrients.

The chyme enters the duodenum, the first 10 to 12 inches of the small intestine. The duodenum is responsible for absorbing calcium and iron as well as neutralizing the acids in the chyme. Enzymes from the pancreas and bile from the liver enter the duodenum from the common bile duct by way of the ampulla of vater; it is here that fats are digested.

The jejunum, the middle of the small intestine, is 8 to 10 feet long. It is responsible for absorption of fats, proteins, and carbohydrates. Vitamin B_{12} and bile salts are absorbed in the ileum, which is the distal 12 feet of the small bowel.

Large Intestine

The chyme enters the large intestine, also known as the *colon,* through the ileocecal valve into the cecum, a small pouch to which the appendix is attached. The colon is approximately 4 to 5 feet long and consists of the ascending or right colon, the transverse colon, the descending or left colon, and the sigmoid colon, an S-shaped segment before the rectum. The colon is responsible for absorbing water, electrolytes, and bile salts.

The last 5 inches of the large intestine comprise the rectum. The distal end of the rectum forms the anal canal composed of muscles that control defecation. The opening to the anal canal is called the *anus.*

Accessory Organs

The digestive system is also comprised of accessory organs that aid in the digestion of food. The accessory organs include the pancreas, liver, and gallbladder (Figure 28-2).

Pancreas

The pancreas is a fish-shaped glandular organ 6 to 8 inches long extending from the duodenum across the abdomen behind the stomach. The pancreas has both endocrine and exocrine functions. The endocrine functions, which include the production of glucagon and insulin to regulate the blood sugar level, are presented in Chapter 27.

The pancreas produces 3 main groups of enzymes in pancreatic juice for its exocrine function. The enzymes are:

amylase—converts carbohydrates into glucose

lipase—aids in fat digestion

protease—breaks down protein

Liver

The liver is the largest glandular organ of the body. It is located in the right upper quadrant of the abdomen. The liver is one of the most vascular organs, filtering 1,500 cc of blood per minute. Some of the many functions of the liver are to:

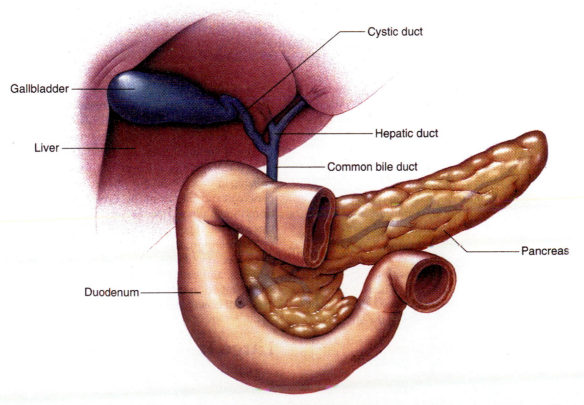

Figure 28-2 Accessory Organs. Bile travels from the liver to the gallbladder via the hepatic and cystic ducts. The bile is released into the duodenum via the common bile duct. The pancreas releases its digestive juice into the duodenum.

- Produce and secrete bile, which emulsifies fats
- Convert glucose into glycogen for storage (**glycogenesis**)
- Convert glycogen to glucose when blood sugar level drops (**glycogenolysis**)
- Metabolize hormones
- Break down nitrogenous wastes to urea
- Incorporate amino acids into proteins
- Filter blood and destroy bacteria
- Produce prothrombin and fibrinogen, which are necessary for blood clotting
- Manufacture cholesterol
- Produce heparin
- Store vitamin B_{12} and fat soluble vitamins A, D, E, and K
- Detoxify poisonous substances

Gallbladder

The gallbladder is a pear-shaped sac attached to the undersurface of the liver. The liver produces bile and transports the bile to the gallbladder by way of the hepatic and cystic ducts. The gallbladder stores and concentrates the bile until it is needed in the small intestine. When fats enter the small intestine, the gallbladder releases the bile through the cystic duct into the common bile duct and finally into the small intestine. The cystic duct, hepatic duct, and pancreatic duct combine to form the common bile duct.

Effects of Aging

As the body ages, several changes may occur in the digestive system (Table 28–1). It is important to educate clients about these changes and ways they can adapt their lifestyles.

GERONTOLOGICAL CONSIDERATIONS

The Aging GI Tract

- Loss of elasticity and slowed motility of the GI tract, accompanied by lack of exercise, make the elderly prone to constipation.
- As the intestinal wall weakens, diverticuli, or scars on the intestinal wall, can develop.
- Decreased liver mass and blood flow alter the pharmacokinetics of various drugs.

ASSESSMENT

As discussed in Chapter 12, a thorough assessment is necessary to collect data on which to make an accurate nursing diagnosis. For clients complaining of GI symptoms, the assessment should include:

1. History of the present complaint including length and frequency of symptoms, when symptoms occur, as well as aggravating factors.
2. Medication history including prescribed and over-the-counter (OTC) medications, and their effectiveness. Clients with GI symptoms frequently self-medicate with antacids, laxatives, suppositories, and enemas.
3. A complete nutritional history; a note should be made of any foods that increase or decrease symptoms. Also, assess if meals aggravate symptoms or if symptoms occur within a specific time period after a meal. Note the fiber and fat content of the diet as well as the amount of fluids typically consumed.

Table 28–1 CHANGES IN THE DIGESTIVE SYSTEM WITH AGING

COMMON CHANGES	RESULT	IMPLICATIONS FOR NURSES
Decrease in peristalsis	Food moves more slowly through digestive system. Bowel movements more infrequent. Increase in constipation. Feeling full and bloated and may eat less.	Increase fiber and fluid intake. Encourage smaller, frequent meals. Offer fiber supplements.
Oral changes	Dentures are common. Chewing is more difficult. Eating and drinking time may be prolonged. Number of taste buds decreases.	Make sure dentures fit. Cut food into small bites. Teach that softer foods may be better tolerated. Some clients may start using more salt and seasonings to compensate for less flavor; monitor salt usage.
Decrease in enzyme secretion	Food is harder to digest. Increase in indigestion. Intolerance to some food and seasonings.	Encourage water between meals. Avoid foods that are not tolerated while ensuring adequate nutrient intake.
Decrease in saliva	Food is more difficult to chew. Swallowing becomes difficult.	Encourage fluid intake with meals. Have clients chew food well and do two swallows with each bite of food. Have clients sit up to eat.

4. Psychosocial factors including compliance and noncompliance with health status. Meal patterns should be evaluated: note if the client eats alone, eats large meals at regular intervals, or snacks all day.
5. Physical examination including inspection, auscultation, percussion, and palpation of the abdomen. An evaluation of the client's ability to chew and swallow is also important.
6. Bowel elimination patterns including frequency, consistency, and amounts of bowel movements.
7. Evaluation of diagnostic data including laboratory analysis and radiologic and endoscopic examinations.

COMMON DIAGNOSTIC TESTS

Commonly used diagnostic tests for clients with digestive disorders are listed in Table 28–2. See Chapter 13, Diagnostic Tests, for explanation/normal values and nursing responsibilities.

DISORDERS OF THE GASTROINTESTINAL TRACT

Disorders of the gastrointestinal tract include: stomatitis, esophageal varices, gastroesphageal reflux disease, gastritis, ulcers, appendicitis, diverticulosis and diverticulitis, inflammatory bowel disease, intestinal obstruction, hernias, peritonitis, hemorrhoids, and constipation.

STOMATITIS

Stomatitis is a painful condition characterized by inflammation and ulcerations in the mouth. Stomatitis can be caused by infections, damage to the mucous membranes by irritants, or chemotherapy.

Medical–Surgical Management

Medical

Cultures may be done to determine if an infectious process is present.

Pharmacological

Because the client's mouth can be sore, topical anesthetics such as xylocaine may be used. Analgesics may also be ordered. If an infection is present, the appropriate medication will be ordered.

Diet

Dietary restrictions are based on what the client is able to tolerate. Bland, soft foods or liquids are usually tolerated best. As the sores heal, the diet may be advanced as tolerated. It is important to monitor dietary intake as caloric and fluid intake may be poor due to discomfort.

Table 28–2 COMMON DIAGNOSTIC TESTS FOR GASTROINTESTINAL DISORDERS

Laboratory Tests
- Complete blood count (CBC)
- Prothrombin time (PT)
- Partial thromboplastin time (PTT)
- Bilirubin
- Albumin
- Globulin
- Total protein
- Alkaline phosphatase
- Lactate hydrogenase (LDH-5)
- Gamma-glutamyl transpeptidase (GGT or GGTP)
- Aspartate aminotransferase (AST/SGOT)
- Alanine aminotransferase (ALT/SGPT)
- Cholesterol
- Triglycerides
- Amylase
- Carcinoembryonic antigen (CEA)
- HAA, now called hepatitis B surface antigen (HB$_s$AG)
- Stool O & P
- Stool occult blood (guaiac)
  Fecal occult blood Test (fOBT)
  Hemocult

Radiologic Studies
- Barium swallow
- Upper gastrointestinal tract (UGI) with small bowel follow-through
- Abdominal x-rays
- CT scans
- Ultrasound
- Barium enema
- Gallbladder series

Other
- Flexible sigmoidoscopy
- Esophagogastro-duodenoscopy (EGD)
- Endoscopic retrograde cholangiopancreatogram (ERCP)
- Colonoscopy
- Esophageal motility studies (manometry)
- Gastric secretion analysis
- Liver biopsy
- Peritoneal aspiration

▶ NURSING PROCESS

▶ Assessment

▶ Subjective Data

Clients usually complain of pain in the mouth and difficulty swallowing.

▶ Objective Data

Observations include inflamed mucosa of the mouth with ulcerations frequently present.

Nursing diagnoses for a client with stomatitis may include the following:

Nursing Diagnoses	Planning/Goals	Nursing Interventions
▶ *Acute Pain related to stomatitis*	The client will verbalize increase in comfort within 1 hour of initiation of treatment.	Assess the client frequently for discomfort. Administer medications such as topical xylocaine and analgesics as ordered. Allow for rest periods as indicated.
▶ *Imbalanced Nutrition: Less than body requirements related to inadequate caloric and fluid intake*	The client will be able to maintain caloric intake of 1,500 calories per day by 48 hours after initiation of treatment. The client will be able to maintain fluid intake at 2,000 cc per day by 48 hours after initiation of treatment.	Monitor daily caloric intake and consult with the dietitian to assist with food selection. Administer IV fluids as ordered and monitor I & O.
▶ *Impaired Oral Mucous Membranes related to stomatitis*	The client will have less inflammation and a decrease in the size of the ulcers by 36 hours after initiation of treatment.	Monitor the stomatitis every shift to assess status of condition. Provide oral care every 4 hours. Administer medications as ordered to combat the infection.

Evaluation Each goal must be evaluated to determine how it has been met by the client.

ESOPHAGEAL VARICES

A varix is an enlarged, tortuous vein or, occasionally, an artery. Although varices can occur in any part of the digestive system, they occur most frequently in the distal veins of the esophagus. The varices are often associated with cirrhosis of the liver or any other condition that causes chronic obstruction of drainage from the esophageal veins into the portal veins. Swelling of the veins causes the walls to weaken, making them prone to ulceration and bleeding. Anything that causes increased abdominal venous pressure such as sneezing, coughing, vomiting, the Valsalva maneuver, swallowing large, poorly chewed pieces of food, and the erosion of vessel walls by gastric acid can cause the varices to rupture.

Varices have no symptoms so clients may not be aware of them until they start bleeding. Death may ensue rapidly if the hemorrhaging varix is not treated immediately.

Medical–Surgical Management

Medical

The varices may be treated with sclerotherapy, ligation, or balloon tamponade. Sclerotherapy is a procedure in which a caustic substance is injected into the varix. An EGD is performed and a sclerosing agent is injected through a special needle. Several treatments are necessary to cause formation of scar tissue and to stop the bleeding. After the bleeding has stopped and the client has stabilized, the remaining treatments may be done on an outpatient basis.

Complications to sclerotherapy include mediastinal inflammation secondary to extra esophageal injection, perforation, ulceration, stricture secondary to scar formation, and rebleeding.

Esophageal **ligation**, also called *banding*, involves placing a rubber band, tie, or O-ring on the varix (Figure 28-3). An EGD is performed to guide the placement of the bands. The complications include rebleeding and stricture formation.

In a case where varices are actively bleeding, a 3 or 4 lumen balloon tamponade, known as a Minnesota or

Figure 28-3 Banding of an Esophageal Varix: A. Varix; B. Insertion of tube with O-ring; C. O-ring is placed around the varix.

Sengstaken-Blakemore tube, is passed into the esophagus. The balloon is then inflated in the esophagus to put direct pressure onto the bleeding varices. The balloon is periodically deflated to prevent necrosis of the esophageal tissue. Iced isotonic saline lavages may

also be done through the tube. During the procedure, the client must be kept NPO with the head of the bed elevated 30 to 45 degrees. Complications include perforation of the esophagus from pressure from the balloon and necrosis of the surrounding tissue.

Surgical

A portosystemic shunt eventually may be placed in clients with end-stage liver disease. The shunt relieves the pressure on the esophageal veins by redirecting blood from the portal vein to the inferior mesenteric vein. Some of the blood bypasses the liver and reenters the circulatory system (Figure 28-4).

A nonsurgical but invasive procedure, transjugular intrahepatic portosystemic shunt (TIPS), may also be performed. With this procedure, the right internal jugular vein is used to place a cannula into the hepatic and portal veins. A connection is made through the liver tissue between the hepatic and portal veins. A stent is placed in the connection. This allows some of the blood to bypass the liver and relieve pressure in the portal vein. This procedure is done in x-ray and is used with clients who are too unstable for surgery (also refer to Figure 28-11.)

Pharmacological

Octreotide (Sandostatin) may be given by IV to help control the bleeding by decreasing blood flow to the gut, thus lowering pressure in the portal system. Analgesics may be necessary following sclerotherapy

Figure 28-4 A. Normal Circulation of the Liver; B. An Example of a Portosystemic Shunt (may be performed in clients with elevated portal vein pressure that is resistant to medical management).

if clients have chest discomfort. Clients should avoid NSAIDs, aspirin, and all anticoagulants. Sucralfate (Carafate) liquid may be given to coat the esophagus, protecting it from erosion by gastric acid. IV rehydration as well as blood transfusions may be necessary for clients with active bleeding.

Activity

If varices are bleeding or have recently bled, the client should remain on bed rest. If no active bleeding is present, the client may be ambulatory but should avoid strenuous exercise.

▶ NURSING PROCESS

▶ Assessment

▶ Subjective Data

Assessment includes history of liver disease or alcohol abuse and nausea. With esophageal varices there is no abdominal pain. The symptom of abdominal pain helps distinguish esophageal varices from bleeding ulcers, which generally do cause pain (Giacchino & Houdek, 1998).

▶ Objective Data

Assessment includes testing stools for **occult blood** (**guaiac**) and **melena** (black, sticky, tar-like stools containing partially broken down blood), and assessing for **hematemesis**, or vomiting blood. The nurse reviews hemoglobin and hematocrit (H & H) to evaluate anemia and liver profile for elevated bilirubin and globulin levels and a decrease in albumin.

If cirrhosis of the liver is present, **jaundice**, a yellowing of the skin, mucous membranes, and sclerae of the eyes, is present. Jaundice results when the liver is unable to fully remove bilirubin from the blood. Nutritional status may be poor if the client abuses alcohol.

Nursing diagnoses for a client with esophageal varices may include the following:

Nursing Diagnoses	Planning/Goals	Nursing Interventions
▶ *Risk for Deficient Fluid Volume related to bleeding esophageal varices (if the varices are not actively bleeding)*	The client will maintain adequate fluid volume.	Monitor vital signs every 4 hours including orthostatic blood pressures. Orthostatic blood pressure is obtained by taking the blood pressure when the client is lying down and then when standing. A 20 mm Hg difference in blood pressures from lying to standing would indicate a change in fluid volume, possibly indicating varix bleeding.
		Monitor for nausea and dizziness.
		Monitor H & H every 4 to 8 hours as ordered. A decrease in H & H values would indicate bleeding.
▶ *Deficient Fluid Volume related to bleeding esophageal varices and gastric loss from vomiting*	The client will maintain an H & H within normal limits.	Monitor H & H.
	The client's blood pressure will be within 20 mm Hg of baseline with no orthostatic changes.	Frequently monitor vital signs. Administer IV fluids, electrolyte replacement, and blood transfusions as ordered.
▶ *Anxiety related to change in health status, threat of death*	The client will discuss concerns about health status.	Explain all tests and procedures to decrease anxiety. Allow client to express fears and concerns regarding condition.

Evaluation Each goal must be evaluated to determine how it has been met by the client.

GASTROESOPHAGEAL REFLUX DISEASE

Gastroesophageal reflux disease (GERD) is a disease in which the gastric secretions flow upward into the esophagus, damaging the tissues. An inability of the lower esophageal sphincter (LES) to close fully contributes to this condition. Environmental and physical factors may contribute to decreased pressure in the LES. Fatty foods, caffeine, nicotine, calcium channel blockers, and NSAIDs decrease the tightness of the sphincter. Symptoms include belching, dysphagia, esophagitis, epigastric pain, heartburn, flatulence, melena, and bleeding. Diagnosis is made by symptoms, a 24-hour pH monitoring, and an esophageal motility test. An endoscopy determines the extent of esophagitis and rules out a malignancy.

Medical–Surgical Management

Medical

GERD is generally treated conservatively with diet and medications. Clients are encouraged to lose weight if they are overweight.

Surgical

A fundoplication may be done to alleviate symptoms. A fundoplication is a laproscopic procedure in which the lower esphageal sphincter is tightened by wrapping and suturing the fundus of the stomach around the esophagus.

Pharmacological

GERD is treated conservatively with antacids, H2 receptor antagonists, proton pump inhibitors, cytoprotective agents, and gastrointestinal motility agents.

Diet

A low-fat, high-protein diet is recommended. The client is encouraged to avoid caffeine, milk products, alcohol, peppermint, licorice, and spicy foods.

▶ NURSING PROCESS

▶ Assessment

▶ Subjective Data

The nurse listens closely to the symptoms described by the client and obtains a dietary report from the client.

▶ Objective Data

The nurse observes for melena and signs of discomfort and pain.

GASTRITIS

Gastritis is an inflammation of the stomach mucosa occurring when the stomach has been exposed to irritating substances such as medications, smoke, food allergens, or toxic chemicals. Another contributing factor to gastritis may be impaired mucosal defenses, which occur when the epithelial cells of the stomach are not able to secrete adequate quantity or quality of mucous to protect the stomach. The presence of the bacteria *Helicobactor pylori* (*H. pylori*) has also been associated with gastritis.

Medical–Surgical Management

Medical

Diagnosis of gastritis is based on history and symptoms. An UGI or an EGD may be done to help diagnose the condition. If *H. pylori* is suspected, a biopsy is obtained during an EGD and a culture is performed.

CLIENT TEACHING

GERD
- Lose weight as needed.
- Avoid fatty foods, alcohol, nicotine, caffeine, and spicy foods.
- Take medications as instructed.
- Sleep with the head of the bed elevated 2 to 4 inches on blocks.
- Avoid wearing constrictive clothing.

Pharmacological

Treatment for gastritis is primarily pharmacological involving antacids and histamine (H_2) receptor antagonists (also call H_2 blockers). A proton pump inhibitor such as omeprazole (Prilosec) or prostaglandins may be used. If *H. pylori* is present, the use of bismuth preparations to inhibit *H. pylori* growth and antibiotics to eliminate the bacteria may be used (Table 28–3).

NSAIDs such as ibuprofen (Motrin) and indomethacin (Indocin) have been shown to compromise mucosal defenses and increase acid secretion. Clients who are on NSAIDs chronically, such as clients with arthritis, may need to be evaluated to determine if other analgesics would be effective or if a prostaglandin should be taken with the NSAIDs.

Diet

Although studies have shown that dietary modifications have little impact on the rate of gastritis healing, some modifications are indicated. Any foods that aggravate symptoms should be eliminated. Also, foods that increase acid secretions such as milk, coffee, decaffeinated coffee, tea, colas, and chocolate should be consumed only in small amounts or eliminated if possible. Bedtime eating should be avoided as it increases nocturnal acid secretions.

Health Promotion

Smoking and alcohol aggravate the mucosal lining of the stomach and significantly impair gastritis healing. Smoking and alcohol consumption should be minimized or eliminated if possible.

▶ NURSING PROCESS

▶ Assessment

▶ Subjective Data

Clients with gastritis may have no symptoms or may describe epigastric pain or burning, or nausea. They may also state that certain foods aggravate symptoms.

▶ Objective Data

Stools may test positive for blood.

Table 28–3 MEDICATIONS USED FOR ULCERS AND GASTRITIS

MEDICATION	PURPOSE	NURSING IMPLICATIONS
Antacids • aluminum hydroxide (Amphogel) • aluminum hydroxide and magnesium hydroxide (Maalox) • dihydroxyaluminum sodium carbonate (Rolaids)	Seal impaired mucosa. Neutralize acids.	Antacids containing aluminum hydroxide may cause constipation. Antacids containing magnesium hydroxide may cause diarrhea; monitor serum electrolytes; do not give with other meds.
H₂ Receptor Antagonists • ranitidine HCl (Zantac) • cimetidine (Tagamet)	Decrease gastric acid secretion.	Do not give within 1 hour of antacids.
Proton Pump Inhibitor • omeprazole (Prilosec)	Stop gastric acid secretion.	Give with food. Suspend granules in an acid liquid. Takes 4 days to achieve blood level.
Prostaglandins • misoprostol (Cytotec)	Decrease gastric acid secretion. Enhance mucosal defenses.	Give when NSAIDs need to be continued.
Bismuth Compounds • bismuth subsalicylate (Pepto-Bismol)	Enhance mucosal barriers. Inhibit *H. pylori* growth.	Do not give within 1 hour of H₂ blockers.
Antibiotics • ampicillin (Omnipen) • metronidazole (Flagyl)	Eliminate *H. pylori*.	Some antibiotics will cause N/V if taken with alcohol. Do not give with antacids or meals with the exception of Flagyl, which must be taken with food. Clients usually placed on two different antibiotics simultaneously.

Nursing diagnoses for a client with gastritis may include the following:

Nursing Diagnoses	Planning/Goals	Nursing Interventions
▶ *Acute Pain related to gastric acid on inflammation*	The client will experience less pain within 24 hours of onset of treatment as identified by pain scale.	Administer medications as ordered. Assess client for improvement of symptoms. Provide diet as ordered. Implement education about lifestyle changes.
▶ *Deficient Knowledge related to condition, therapy, and symptoms of potential complications*	The client will verbalize understanding of factors related to condition and symptoms of complications and comply with treatment regimen.	Educate regarding medication regimen and lifestyle changes. If the client smokes or drinks alcohol, provide information on smoking and drinking cessation. Discuss dietary modifications.

Evaluation Each goal must be evaluated to determine how it has been met by the client.

ULCERS

Peptic ulcers are erosions that form in the esophagus, stomach, or duodenum resulting from acid/pepsin imbalance. **Gastric ulcers** refer to erosions in the stomach and are correlated to exposure to irritants such as NSAIDs, smoking, alcohol, food allergens, toxic chemicals, *H. pylori* infections, and impaired mucosal defenses. Impaired mucosal defenses occur when the epithelial cells of the stomach are not able to secrete adequate quantity or quality of mucous to protect the stomach.

Clients with gastric ulcers frequently complain of pain 1 to 2 hours after eating. Eating may not relieve pain or may even increase pain. Weight loss is common. Risk factors include alcohol use, stress, and NSAID use.

Stress ulcers are a type of gastric ulcer that form when gastritis becomes erosive and starts bleeding. As the name implies, stress ulcers occur in clients whose bodies are experiencing stress, such as clients who have experienced major surgery, trauma, burns, chemotherapy, or radiation therapy. Clients with chronic respiratory disorders may also experience stress ulcers as hypoxia can lead to impaired mucosa. Bleeding may be massive resulting in significant blood loss or can be slow and insidious. Because of the multiple sites of bleeding, stress ulcers may be difficult to manage.

Duodenal ulcers refer to ulcers in the duodenum. Incidents of duodenal ulcers have been correlated to a high secretion of HCl. Clients with duodenal ulcers frequently complain of pain 2 to 4 hours after eating. Nocturnal pain may be present, occurring between midnight and 3:00 A.M. Eating frequently relieves symptoms. Weight gain is common. Risk factors include a history of pulmonary disease, cirrhosis, chronic pancreatitis, and/or chronic renal failure.

If an ulcer erodes through a blood vessel, the client may experience a life-threatening hemorrhage. A perforation occurs if the ulcer erodes through the wall of the stomach or small intestine resulting in gastric or intestinal contents entering the abdominal cavity and causing peritonitis.

Diagnosis of ulcers is based on symptoms, history, and an UGI or an EGD performed to visualize the ulcer. If an *H. pylori* infection is suspected, a biopsy is obtained during an EGD and a culture is performed.

Medical–Surgical Management

Medical

If an ulcer bleeds, an EGD may be performed and the ulcer is either injected with epinephrine to cause vasoconstriction or a special electrical probe is used to cauterize or burn the tissue that is bleeding. A naso-gastric (NG) tube may be inserted to remove gastric contents and blood, and iced isotonic saline may be instilled to help cause vasoconstriction and stop the bleeding.

Surgical

The most commonly performed surgery for peptic ulcers is a vagotomy in which a section of the vagus nerve is cut removing vagal innervation to the fundus of the stomach. This eliminates the production of hydrochloric acid, decreases function of the gastrin hormone, and slows motility of the stomach. A vagotomy eliminates the complications of the more aggressive surgeries, such as gastrectomies.

If the ulcer continues to bleed or if the ulcer has perforated, the client is taken to surgery and a gastrectomy is performed, in which the portion of the stomach or duodenum that is perforated is removed and the bowel is reconnected with an anastomosis (see Figure 28-5).

Complications from gastrectomies include gastric dumping in which the stomach experiences **postprandial** (after eating) rapid gastric emptying. Clients experience abdominal pain, nausea, vomiting, explosive diarrhea, weakness, and dizziness. Clients with gastric dumping have malabsorption of nutrients because the food passes too quickly to permit absorption, thus leading to malnutrition. In addition, many clients with significant symptoms may limit dietary intake to avoid symptoms, compounding the malnutrition and weight loss issues.

Management of gastric dumping includes small, frequent meals of high fiber and high protein and avoidance of simple carbohydrates.

A.

Billroth I
• Gastroduodenal hookup
• Used with vagotomy for duodenal ulcer

B.

Billroth II
• Gastrojejunal hookup
• Used with subtotal gastrectomy

C.

C-sendes Procedure (Roux-en-Y)
• Esophagogastrojejunostony
• Used in ulcers high in the stomach

Figure 28-5 Gastric resections are necessary when an ulcer perforates. The type of gastrectomy depends on the location of the ulcer.

Pharmacological

Treatment of ulcers is primarily pharmacological involving antacids, histamine (H_2) receptor antagonists (also called *H_2 blockers*), proton pump inhibitor, or prostaglandins. If *H. pylori* is present, the use of bismuth preparations to inhibit its growth and antibiotics to eliminate the bacteria are generally used (refer back to Table 28–3).

NSAIDs such as ibuprofen (Motrin) and indomethacin (Indocin) have been shown to compromise mucosal defenses and increase acid secretion. Clients who are on NSAIDs chronically, such as clients with arthritis, may need to evaluate if other analgesics would be effective or if a prostaglandin should be taken with the NSAIDs.

Diet

Although studies have shown that dietary modifications have little impact on the rate of ulcer healing, some modifications are indicated. Foods that aggravate symptoms should be eliminated. Also, foods that increase acid secretions such as milk, coffee, decaffeinated coffee, tea, colas, and chocolate should be consumed only in small amounts or eliminated if possible. Bedtime eating should also be avoided as it increases nocturnal acid secretions.

Health Promotion

Smoking and alcohol aggravate the mucosal lining of the stomach and duodenum and significantly impair ulcer healing. Smokers also experience a higher ulcer recurrence rate. Stress has been shown to increase the rate of peptic ulcers. Although the type or severity of stress may not be significant, the client's interpretation of the events as stressful is. Clients need to develop mechanisms for reducing stress such as exercise, biofeedback, and relaxation.

▶ NURSING PROCESS

▶ Assessment

▶ Subjective Data

Clients with gastric ulcers are often asymptomatic or may describe epigastric pain or burning one to two hours after eating, and nausea or bloating. Clients may experience an increase of symptoms when they eat and therefore may decrease dietary intake. When questioned about lifestyle, NSAID usage, stress, smoking, and alcohol use may be discovered.

Clients with duodenal ulcers may exhibit no symptoms or may complain of pain 2 to 4 hours after eating. Eating will frequently decrease symptoms so clients will often eat more frequently. When questioned about lifestyle, stress, smoking, and alcohol consumption may be discovered. The client may also have a history of pulmonary disease, cirrhosis, chronic pancreatitis, and/or chronic renal failure.

A client who is actively bleeding from an ulcer will experience an acute onset of epigastric pain, shortness of breath, and nausea.

▶ Objective Data

Clients with gastric ulcers may show a weight loss and stools may test positive for blood. An H & H may show anemia.

Clients with duodenal ulcers may show a weight gain and stools may test positive for blood. An H & H may show anemia.

The client who is actively bleeding from an ulcer will show signs of shock: pale clammy skin, an elevated pulse rate, and a drop in blood pressure. The client may also have hematemesis. Laboratory tests may show a low H & H. Stools may test positive for blood.

Nursing diagnoses for a client with ulcers may include the following:

Nursing Diagnoses	Planning/Goals	Nursing Interventions
▶ *Acute Pain related to gastric acid on ulcerated mucosa*	The client will experience less pain within 24 hours of onset of treatment as identified on pain scale.	Assess clients for decrease of pain. Administer medications as ordered. Assess for elevated BP.
▶ *Deficient Knowledge related to condition, therapy, and symptoms of complications*	The client will verbalize understanding of factors related to condition and symptoms of complications. Client will comply with treatment regimen.	Identify client's learning style and provide information in a manner compatible with the learning style. Educate regarding medication regimen and lifestyle changes. If indicated, provide client with smoking cessation information and stress reduction techniques such as exercise and biofeedback. Include signs and symptoms of possible complications.
▶ *Deficient Fluid Volume related to bleeding ulcer*	The client will exhibit normal fluid volume as evidenced by stable H & H and blood pressure within 20 mm Hg of baseline.	Check vital signs every 4 hours and PRN including orthostatic blood pressure. Administer IV fluids, electrolyte replacement, and blood transfusions as ordered. Monitor for dizziness and nausea. Check stool for blood.

Evaluation Each goal must be evaluated to determine how it has been met by the client.

APPENDICITIS

Appendicitis is the inflammation of the vermiform appendix, a 10-cm small, slender tube attached to the cecum. The appendix may be inflamed, gangrenous, or ruptured. If the opening to the appendix becomes blocked with feces, the *E. coli* multiply in the appendix and infection develops with pus formation. If it ruptures, fecal content spills into the abdominal cavity causing peritonitis. Peritonitis may be fatal.

A barium enema or an ultrasound may be ordered to confirm inflammation in the appendiceal area.

Medical–Surgical Management

Early diagnosis and treatment are necessary for the best client outcome. A white blood count and differential are usually ordered. Most clients will have a WBC above 10,000/mm^3, neutrophils over 75%, and an elevated temperature, which indicates infection. Sometimes an appendectomy may be performed along with other abdominal surgeries as a preventive measure.

Surgical

A surgical procedure called an *appendectomy* is necessary before the appendix ruptures. Appendectomies are the most common emergency surgery and require a hospital stay of 2 to 7 days. If no rupture has occurred, a laparoscopic appendectomy, in which the appendix is removed through a scope, may be done. A laparoscopic appendectomy requires only a small incision and allows the client to be discharged 24 hours after the surgery.

Pharmacological

Preoperatively, no analgesics are given so that symptoms will not be masked by the medication. Fluids and electrolytes may need to be replaced prior to surgery. Antibiotics are usually given preoperatively. Postoperatively, analgesics are administered for the relief of inci-

sional discomfort. Antibiotics are usually given postoperatively, especially if a perforation is present.

Diet

Preoperatively, the client is to be NPO. Initially postoperatively, the client is again NPO. If a perforation with peritonitis has occurred, the client will be kept NPO longer and an NG tube may be inserted until bowel sounds have returned. The client is first started on clear liquids and advanced to full liquids and finally, to a regular diet as normal bowel function returns.

Activity

Initially postoperatively, the client is encouraged to turn, cough and deep breathe every 2 hours. Next, the client should be encouraged to leave bed and increase ambulation gradually. Activity restrictions will depend on the severity of the appendicitis. Driving, exercise, and lifting will be limited for a few weeks to allow for incisional healing.

▶ NURSING PROCESS

▶ Assessment

▶ Subjective Data

Clients with appendicitis describe abdominal pain, typically located in the right lower quadrant around McBurney's point (halfway between the umbilicus and the right iliac crest). Clients also complain of anorexia (a loss of appetite) and nausea.

▶ Objective Data

Clients may have vomiting and a fever. Bowel sounds may be diminished or absent. Rebound tenderness, or pain that occurs when fingers are pressed into the right lower quadrant and then released suddenly, may also be present. A CBC will be done and WBCs will be elevated above 10,000/mm^3 with neutrophils over 75%.

Nursing diagnoses for the client with appendicitis may include the following:

Nursing Diagnoses	Planning/Goals	Nursing Interventions
▶ *Acute Pain related to appendicitis/appendectomy*	The client will experience a decrease in pain as evidenced by improved mobility and as identified on pain scale.	Preoperatively, monitor client's pain.
		Check abdomen for rigidity.
		Provide an ice pack to help relieve pain as ordered; never use heat.
		Postoperatively, give analgesics as ordered and medicate prior to activities such as ambulation.
		Teach client to use a pillow to splint the incision when coughing.
		If client is having difficulty passing flatus, administer enemas or a rectal tube as ordered, and encourage ambulation.

continues

Nursing Diagnoses	Planning/Goals	Nursing Interventions
▶ *Impaired Skin Integrity related to the abdominal incision*	The client will verbalize signs and symptoms of infection and factors that enhance wound healing, by discharge.	Administer antibiotics as ordered.
		Educate the client that incision may be left open to the air after 24 hours and that showers may be taken, per physician instruction.
		If adhesive strips are present, leave in place until they no longer cover the incision (approximately 10 days to 2 weeks).
		Educate client regarding signs and symptoms of infection and activity restrictions.

Evaluation Each goal must be evaluated to determine how it has been met by the client.

DIVERTICULOSIS AND DIVERTICULITIS

Diverticula are saclike protrusions of the intestinal wall. **Diverticulosis** refers to a condition of the colon in which multiple diverticula are present (see Figure 28-6). The exact cause of diverticulosis is not known. However, a diet low in fiber is felt to contribute to the formation of the pouches. Diverticulosis affects 30% to 40% of the elderly population (Cameron, 1998). It is asymptomatic unless perforation or hemorrhage occur.

Diverticulitis refers to the inflammation of one or more diverticula generally in the sigmoid colon. It is a complication of diverticulosis and is thought to be caused by stool impacted in the diverticula.

Medical–Surgical Management

Medical

Diverticulosis is typically asymptomatic and needs no intervention. Most cases of diverticulitis are treated with analgesics, antibiotics, bed rest, NPO to rest the bowel, and IV fluid hydration.

A barium enema or abdominal ultrasound is usually ordered when diverticulitis is suspected. A flexible sigmoidoscopy may also be performed.

Surgical

If bleeding or perforation of the diverticula has occurred, or if an abscess has formed, surgery is required to remove the portion of the bowel affected. A colon resection is performed. A colostomy may also be required. A **colostomy** is a surgically created opening from the colon through the abdominal wall to relieve either a disease or functional problem in the large intestine.

Stool consistency depends on the placement of the **stoma** (surgical opening between a cavity and the surface of the body) in the colon. A colostomy is named for the part of the colon where it is located. An ascending colostomy takes its name from the ascending colon and would be on the right side of the abdomen. It has a liquid output. A transverse colostomy would be more toward the midline of the abdomen, and the output would be a pasty liquid. A descending colostomy or sigmoid colostomy would have solid output. Figure 28-7 shows the different colostomy sites.

If a large amount of inflammation is present, a temporary colostomy may be performed to allow the colon to heal. The colon will be reconnected at a later time. In rare cases, a permanent colostomy may need to be performed.

STOMAL/OSTOMY MANAGEMENT

Assessment

Assessment includes giving the client an opportunity to ask questions and begin coping with a possible altered body image. Before ostomy surgery, the surgeon and the enterostomal (ET) nurse talk with the client and explain the reason for the surgery and the possibilities of ostomy surgery. Choosing the site or placement of the stoma will depend on the type of ostomy being created, the lifestyle of the client, and the contours of the client's abdomen.

On return from surgery, the new stoma will be edematous and range from deep red to dusky in color. The color of the stoma is checked with a penlight and

Figure 28-6 Diverticula in the Sigmoid Colon. Diverticulosis is almost always located in the descending or sigmoid colon.

Ascending colostomy

Transverse colostomy

Descending colostomy

Sigmoid colostomy

Figure 28-7 Colostomy Sites

documented at least once a shift. Color is important because it reveals the status of the blood supply to the stoma. If blood supply to the stoma is inadequate, the stoma will turn black. The physician should be called if the stoma becomes black.

Immediately after surgery there may be a small amount of serosanguineous drainage in the appliance. When the appliance is changed and the stoma is cleaned or touched when swollen, a small amount of bleeding may occur. The nurse must reassure the client that the small amount of bleeding is normal.

Bowel function is checked every shift to monitor for any obstruction or ileus. Bowel sounds, distention, and abdominal tenderness are checked every four hours.

Complications

Hemorrhage

Bleeding or hemorrhage may occur at the incision site or stoma site. It is important for the nurse to check the incision and stoma site for bleeding and to check the blood pressure and pulse frequently after surgery.

Infection

The risk of infection around the stoma is great due to the presence of stool around the new suture line.

Hernia

A hernia is the most frequent complication of an ostomy and is caused when a loop of bowel pushes up through the muscle next to the stoma and under the skin.

Obstruction

Obstruction of the bowel ostomy may occur as a complication after surgery. Ileostomy clients are instructed to chew their food well before swallowing because large pieces of food such as an olive or large piece of meat may get caught at the opening of the ostomy.

Prolapse

In prolapse, the bowel will sometimes telescope out, resembling an elephant's trunk. If the bowel continues to work, this is not an emergency. The physician or ET nurse may be able to replace the bowel back into the abdomen. If the doctor is not able to push the bowel back into the abdomen, the mucosa of the bowel may become injured if left outside of the body so the prolapse is corrected surgically. Prolapse can be frightening for the client, and the possibility of this occurring is discussed in postoperative teaching.

Electrolyte Imbalance

An ileostomy with a high output of effluent can cause electrolyte imbalances by loss of large amounts of potassium and protein. The client will have difficulty learning to cope with an appliance that is always filling and the need to take in enough fluid, protein, and potassium to replace the lost nutrients.

Skin Excoriation

The skin around a high output ostomy is in danger of becoming excoriated if an appliance that protects the skin cannot be found. Ileostomy effluent contains digestive juices that, if left on the skin, will start to digest the skin, resulting in red, open areas. To prevent this problem, correct appliance fitting that will stay in place is important for these clients.

DISCHARGE TEACHING OF THE OSTOMY CLIENT

Assessment

As the client prepares to go home, it is important to assess the client's or the family's ability to handle the care of the ostomy at home. The client still may be dealing with an altered body image and not want to look at or touch the stoma. The family may have to help with care and be supportive until the client can assume the care.

Appliances

If the client has only one bowel movement a day, a closed appliance that is taken off and emptied once a day will be all that is needed. If the client has several stools a day, an open-ended drainable appliance would be best.

For ileostomies, the one- or two-piece open-end appliance offers ease in emptying. Effluent usually varies from liquid to pasty, so the drainage will have to be emptied several times during the day. An appliance that can be drained without taking it off is important. A skin barrier is also necessary for the ileostomy or any ostomy with liquid output. (Refer to Figure 28-8 for instructions on applying an ostomy appliance.)

Irrigation

Colostomy irrigation is a means of regulating some colostomies. Descending or sigmoid colostomies may be irrigated daily or every other day for control of evacuation. After irrigation, the client may wear a small security appliance or a gauze pad over the stoma the rest of the day. The disadvantage of irrigation is that it takes about an hour or more to perform. The decision to irrigate is made by the client, with the consent of the surgeon, after healing has taken place. To irrigate a colostomy a cone tip is needed on the end of the irrigation catheter. Using the cone on the tip of the tubing prevents the end of the tube from poking into the side of the bowel and injuring the bowel and helps hold the fluid in the bowel. The cone will need to be lubricated liberally with lubricating jelly.

Support Person

Upon discharge, the client and family receive the telephone number of the hospital and unit where treatment was received so they may call if questions arise. Seeing the ET nurse again in 4 to 6 weeks is sometimes recommended to check how the client is doing with ostomy care. If there is a local stoma support group, a person from the group may call or visit the client at home and invite the client and family to come to the group sessions.

Having ostomy surgery is no reason to stop any life activity. People with ostomies live full, active, productive lives.

Pharmacological

Clients who have been identified as having diverticulosis are usually placed on fiber supplements or stool softeners. Clients with diverticulitis will be treated with sulfa antibiotics and other antimicrobial agents. Analgesics may also be ordered for discomfort.

1. Cut the center hole approximately the same size as the stoma, using the guidelines on the release paper. Do not cut beyond the last line.

2. Remove the release paper from the picture-frame support adhesive by bending the slit edges sharply backward. Do not remove the release paper from the side edges until later.

3. When Stomahesive® Paste is indicated, apply a bead of paste to the adhesive side of the skin barrier, around the stomal opening. Allow the paste to set for around 60 seconds prior to applying the pouch to the skin.

4. Press the disc against the skin, paying particular attention to the area closest to the stoma. Maintain gentle pressure on the disc to improve adhesion. Make sure the picture frame support adhesive is smooth and wrinkle free.

5. To attach the tail closure on drainable pouches, fold the pouch outlet spout over the "knife" edge of the closure only once. Press firmly on the closure, especially at the center, until it snaps and is securely closed.

Figure 28-8 How to Apply an Ostomy Appliance. *(Courtesy of Convatec, Skillmah, NJ)*

Diet

A diet high in fiber is believed to help reduce the occurrence of diverticulosis and diverticulitis. Clients experiencing diverticulitis will be NPO to rest the bowel. Once the diverticulitis begins healing, the client will be placed on clear liquids and then advanced to a bland, low-residue diet while the diverticulitis heals.

The client will be NPO, if surgery is performed, until bowel sounds return. The client will then be started on clear liquids, advanced to full liquids as more bowel function returns, and then finally advanced to a regular diet. A high-fiber diet should be encouraged for clients once the diverticulitis episode has resolved.

Activity

For clients experiencing diverticulitis, bed rest and decreased mobility are encouraged to allow the bowel to rest. In clients who have had a bowel resection, activity will gradually be progressed postoperatively.

▸ NURSING PROCESS

▸ Assessment

Diverticulosis often has no symptoms, and therefore, clients may not be aware they have it.

▸ Subjective Data

Clients with diverticulitis frequently complain of left lower abdominal pain, constipation or diarrhea, bloating, anorexia, and nausea.

▸ Objective Data

Assessment shows abdominal distention with tenderness on palpation, decreased bowel sounds, fever, vomiting, and stools that test positive for blood. A CBC will show an elevated WBC and, if bleeding is present, a low H & H.

Nursing diagnoses for clients with diverticulosis or diverticulitis may include the following:

Nursing Diagnoses	Planning/Goals	Nursing Interventions
▸ Acute Pain related to diverticulitis	The client will verbalize a decrease in pain within 24 hours after intervention as measured by the pain scale.	Encourage bed rest to allow healing. Maintain client as NPO. Administer analgesics and antibiotics as ordered.
▸ Risk for Infection related to abscess formation or perforation	The client will verbalize understanding of signs and symptoms of possible complications.	Monitor vital signs and pain level every 4 hours. Assess abdomen every 4 hours for increased tenderness and distention. Educate the client to notify staff of chills, shortness of breath, or increasing pain.
▸ Anxiety related to possible surgery	The client will verbalize fears related to surgery and exhibit decreased anxiety regarding the procedure and follow-up treatment.	Explain all tests and treatments to decrease the client's anxiety level. Allow the client to verbalize fears and concerns. Answer all concerns and questions. If a colostomy is planned, arrange a consult with an enterostomal therapist to help answer concerns.

Evaluation Each goal must be evaluated to determine how it has been met by the client.

SAMPLE NURSING CARE PLAN

THE CLIENT WITH DIVERTICULITIS

Mr. W. is a 67-year-old male admitted to the hospital with abdominal pain that started 2 days ago. The pain has been increasing in intensity and is now accompanied by nausea and anorexia. A physical assessment includes temperature 101.7, pulse 96, respirations 24, and blood pressure of 162/90. Mr. W.'s abdomen is tender on palpation. Mr. W. is in obvious discomfort and is unable to lie on his back. Mr. W. states he has not been eating any food or drinking adequate fluids for 24 hours. Skin turgor is poor. An abdominal ultrasound is ordered and demonstrates diverticulitis. An IV of D5 1/2 NS with 20 mEq KCl, droperidol (Inapsine) IV for nausea, meperidine (Demerol) IM for pain, and IV antibiotics are ordered. Mr. W. is placed on I & O, bed rest with bathroom privileges, and is made NPO. Mr. W. states that he does not understand why all this is being done. His first two voidings are 50 cc each and very concentrated (dark gold colored).

continues

Nursing Diagnosis 1 *Deficient Knowledge related to diagnosis and treatment regimen as evidenced by statement that he does not understand why all this is being done*

PLANNING/GOALS	NURSING INTERVENTIONS	RATIONALE	EVALUATION
Mr. W. will verbalize understanding of treatment plan.	Assess Mr. W.'s knowledge level of diverticulosis/diverticulitis.	Building on present knowledge helps client relate new information and integrate it into his behavior.	Mr. W. verbalizes understanding of the disease process and treatment regimen.
	Assess Mr. W.'s learning style and present information in a manner compatible with his style.	Presenting information in a learning style compatible with the client's increases understanding and retention.	
	Monitor for signs of pain and fatigue.	Pain and fatigue impair learning.	
	Answer questions and reinforce information.	Following up and clarifying information reinforces the new information learned.	

Nursing Diagnosis 2 *Acute Pain related to diverticulitis as evidenced by tender abdomen*

PLANNING/GOALS	NURSING INTERVENTIONS	RATIONALE	EVALUATION
Mr. W. will verbalize a decrease in pain within 24 hours of pain intervention.	Assess pain utilizing a scale of 1 (no pain) to 10 (extreme pain).	Using the pain scale to assess pain is an objective measure of the client's perceived discomfort and the effectiveness of the analgesics.	Mr. W. demonstrates adequate pain relief as demonstrated by a decrease in pain scale.
	Medicate with analgesics as ordered.	Provides pain relief.	
	Encourage Mr. W. to request analgesics when pain is increasing rather than waiting for pain to get intense.	Provides better control of pain.	
	Monitor effectiveness of pain medication by reassessing pain utilizing the pain scale 45 minutes after administration of medication.	Provides a measure of analgesic effectiveness.	

continues

Nursing Diagnosis 3 *Deficient Fluid Volume as evidenced by low urine output and poor skin turgor*

PLANNING/GOALS	NURSING INTERVENTIONS	RATIONALE	EVALUATION
Mr. W. will demonstrate adequate hydration by I & O being nearly equal, normal skin turgor, and electrolytes within normal limits by 24 hours after intervention.	Monitor I & O every shift.	Provides information on the hydration level of Mr. W.	Mr. W. demonstrates adequate hydration by nearly equal I & O, normal skin turgor, and electrolytes within normal limits.
	Administer IV fluids as ordered.	Provides needed hydration.	
	Assess skin turgor every shift.	Provides information on Mr. W.'s hydration.	
	Monitor laboratory reports for electrolyte levels.	Provides information on electrolyte balance.	

INFLAMMATORY BOWEL DISEASE

Inflammatory bowel disease (IBD) is the term used to describe Crohn's disease and ulcerative colitis (UC). Crohn's disease and UC are diseases characterized by inflammation and ulcerations of the bowel (Table 28–4).

Crohn's disease is characterized by lesions that affect the entire thickness of the bowel and can occur anywhere throughout the colon and small intestine. Symptoms include abdominal pain, diarrhea that usually does not contain blood, fever, anorexia, weight loss, and **steatorrhea** (fatty stools). Electrolyte imbalances, iron deficiency anemia, and amino acid malabsorption may occur when the disease involves the jejunum and the ileum. Long-term complications of Crohn's disease include bowel obstructions, fistulas, abscesses, and perforation. The risk for colorectal cancer, while not as high as in UC, is still elevated. There is malabsorption of fat and fat-soluble vitamins.

UC is characterized by mucosal lesions occurring typically in the rectal area and sigmoid colon and progressing throughout the colon. The lesions may progress from pinpoint hemorrhages to abscesses, ulceration, and necrosis (Martin, 1997). Symptoms include fever, anorexia, weight loss, cramping, spasms, abdominal pain, and bloody diarrhea. Long-term complications include fissures, abscesses, and an increased risk for colorectal cancer. Toxic megacolon, a severe, acute dilation of the colon, may occur in severe cases.

Tests to diagnose Crohn's disease and UC include barium enema with small bowel follow-through, and

Table 28–4 COMPARISON OF CROHN'S DISEASE AND ULCERATIVE COLITIS

PARAMETER	CROHN'S DISEASE	ULCERATIVE COLITIS (UC)
Involvement	Patchy areas. Can involve small and large intestine.	Starts in lower colon and spreads progressively throughout colon.
Tissue affected	Affects entire thickness of bowel.	Affects mucosal lining of bowel.
Major complication	Malabsorption.	Toxic megacolon.
Long-term complications	Intestinal obstruction, fistulas, abscesses, perforations; cancer risk increases with age.	Fissures, abscesses, increased risk for colorectal cancer.
Surgical intervention	Usually needed at some point to repair structural damage. Does not cure or limit the progress of the disease.	Ileostomy performed in approximately 20% of cases to remove the colon. Cures the disease.
Cause	Unknown: possibly altered immune state.	Unknown: possibly enteric bacterium *E. coli.*
Stools	3 to 4 semisoft/day; rarely bloody; steatorrhea and mucus present.	15 to 20 liquid/day; blood present; no steatorrhea.

colonoscopy with biopsies. Early symptoms for Crohn's disease and UC are similar and can make early diagnosis difficult.

Medical–Surgical Management

Medical

Treatment for Crohn's disease and UC is similar. Crohn's disease, however, is more debilitating since it involves more of the GI tract. UC is more limited, but can still produce significant symptoms.

A sigmoidoscopy done on a UC client will reveal continuous mucosal inflammation and ulceration, loss of mucosal vascularity, diffuse erythema, and often purulent exudate. A barium enema and x-rays may show stricture, pseudopolyps, and loss of **haustra** (the saclike pouches of the colon) (Martin, 1997).

The goals of treatment are to control inflammation, relieve symptoms, maintain fluid and electrolyte balance, provide adequate nutrition, and prevent complications (Martin, 1997).

Surgical

In severe cases of UC resistant to medical management, the colon is removed and an ileostomy is performed, curing the disease. An **ileostomy** is an opening created in the small intestine (ileum). The output from an ileostomy is a thin liquid, usually of a yellowish-green color. This thin output is called **effluent**. It generally has no odor, and may get thicker in time as the body adapts to the need to retain moisture. Many ileostomies have almost constant effluent output. The Kock continent ileostomy has a pouch made inside the abdomen to hold the effluent until the client is ready to empty the pouch. Figure 28-9 illustrates a Kock continent ileostomy.

Most clients with Crohn's disease need surgery at some point to repair the structural damage caused by scarring. Intestinal obstructions and perforations may also occur in Crohn's disease, necessitating further surgery. Surgical intervention, however, does not cure the disease.

Pharmacological

Treatment for both UC and Crohn's disease includes 5-ASA compounds such as sulfasalazine (Azulfidine) or salicylates such as mesalamine (Rowasa) or olsalazine sodium (Dipentum). If inflammation is severe, corticosteroids may also be administered. In cases resistant to the 5-ASA compounds and corticosteroids, immunosuppressors may be used. If an infection is present, antibiotics will be administered. According to Martin (1997), clients are seldom given antidiarrheal medications since they may precipitate colonic dilation.

Clients may need IV fluid and electrolyte replacement during severe flare-ups. In the most severe cases, clients may be placed on total parenteral nutrition (TPN) to allow for complete bowel rest and to improve nutritional status.

Figure 28-9 A Kock Continent Ileostomy

Diet

Malnutrition is a particular concern in clients with IBD. Because of the severe cramping, pain, and diarrhea brought on by foods, these clients typically put themselves on a very restrictive diet that is not nutritionally balanced. Clients with Crohn's disease may also have malabsorption of iron, vitamin B_{12}, and amino acids, and may develop lactose intolerance.

Nutritional support includes modifying the diet to eliminate foods that exacerbate symptoms while maintaining a balanced diet. A high-calorie, low-residue, nonspicy, caffeine-free diet that uses few milk products is recommended (Martin, 1997).

Health Promotion

Although stress has not been shown to exacerbate the symptoms of Crohn's disease or UC, the impact on the client's lifestyle can be significant, especially with Crohn's disease. Support groups can be beneficial. Clients should be encouraged to develop mechanisms to help them cope with the disease process and reduce stress. Exercise, meditation, and biofeedback are often helpful.

▶ NURSING PROCESS

▶ Assessment

▶ Subjective Data

Clients may complain of mild abdominal spasms and cramping, which may increase to severe abdominal pain, nausea, and anorexia. Clients with UC may have an urge to defecate with the cramping.

 CLIENT TEACHING

IBD

- Schedule a colon cancer screening regularly.
- If taking oral corticosteroids, strictly adhere to the prescribed schedule for taking medication.

▶ Objective Data

Clients show abdominal tenderness on palpation, guarding, distention, weight loss, diarrhea, an elevated WBC count, and fever. In clients with Crohn's disease, steatorrhea and iron deficient anemia may be present.

In clients with UC, stools may be positive for blood and the H & H may be low. The serum potassium, magnesium, and albumin levels are usually low. Because Crohn's disease is so debilitating, clients may become depressed.

Nursing diagnoses for clients with Crohn's disease or UC may include the following:

Nursing Diagnoses	Planning/Goals	Nursing Interventions
▶ *Imbalanced Nutrition: Less than body requirements related to post-prandial pain, bowel hypermobility, and decreased absorption*	The client will demonstrate adequate nutritional status as exhibited by maintaining weight within range for height and body type.	Monitor I & O every shift; caloric count and weight daily. Administer IV fluid and electrolyte replacement as ordered. Provide high-calorie, high-protein supplements as ordered along with small, frequent meals. Administer TPN, a high-calorie and nutrient-dense IV solution, as ordered. If TPN is administered, closely monitor lab reports for electrolytes and glucose level.
▶ *Risk for Deficient Fluid Volume related to diarrhea and altered intake*	The client will exhibit adequate hydration as evidenced by electrolytes within normal range, moist mucous membranes, and I & O nearly equal within 48 hours of start of intervention. The frequency and amount of diarrhea will decrease within 48 hours of start of intervention.	Administer 5-ASA compounds, corticosteroids, and immunosuppressors as ordered. Monitor I & O every shift. Administer IV fluid and electrolyte rehydration as ordered.
▶ *Powerlessness related to impairment in lifestyle secondary to disease process*	The client will verbalize a plan to seek support, by discharge.	Provide client with information on national organizations and local support groups. Allow client to verbalize feelings. Arrange social work consult if needed.

Evaluation Each goal must be evaluated to determine how it has been met by the client.

INTESTINAL OBSTRUCTION

An intestinal obstruction, sometimes called an *ileus,* occurs when the contents cannot pass through the intestine. Obstructions may occur in the large or the small intestine, with most occurring in the ileum. Obstructions may be mechanical, neurogenic, or vascular in origin.

A mechanical obstruction may be a partial or complete obstruction caused by a tumor; fecal impaction; hernia; **volvulus,** a twisting of the bowel on itself; **intussusception,** a telescoping of the bowel where the bowel slides inside itself; (Figure 28-10); or **adhesions,** scar tissue in the abdomen from previous surgeries or disease process such as Crohn's disease.

A neurogenic obstruction, known as a *paralytic ileus,* occurs when nerve transmission to the bowel is interrupted by trauma, infection, or medications, resulting in a portion of the bowel being paralyzed.

A vascular obstruction occurs when blood flow to a portion of the bowel is interrupted, as in atherosclerosis, and that portion of the bowel becomes necrotic.

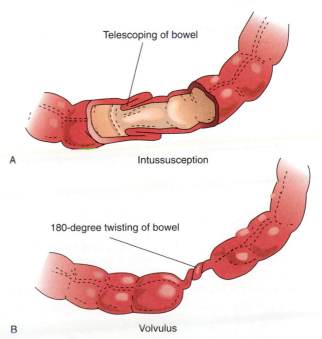

Figure 28-10 Bowel obstructions can be caused by: A. An intussusception; B. A volvulus

When the small intestine becomes obstructed, large amounts of fluid, bacteria, and swallowed air build up in the bowel proximal to the obstruction. The normal process of secretion and absorption of the electrolyte-rich fluid is interrupted. Distention and poor absorption occur when water and salts move from the circulatory system to the lumen of the intestine.

An abdominal x-ray and a barium enema or UGI with small bowel follow-through may be ordered when a bowel obstruction is suspected.

Medical–Surgical Management

Medical

Treatment of the obstruction is dependent on the cause and location. Some can be treated medically by inserting an NG tube for decompression, providing IV fluids for rehydration, and treating the cause, such as the use of enemas for fecal impaction.

Surgical

Most bowel obstructions require surgery. A bowel resection is performed to remove the portion of the bowel affected by the obstruction.

Pharmacological

Nonnarcotic analgesics are used to avoid the intestinal motility decrease caused by narcotic analgesics. Antibiotics may also be ordered.

Activity

In cases of paralytic ileus, ambulation should be encouraged to help bowel function return. Clients who have had a bowel resection should be encouraged to turn, cough, and deep breathe every 2 hours initially postoperatively. Activity should be progressed the next day.

▶ NURSING PROCESS

▶ Assessment

▶ Subjective Data

Clients may state symptoms of colicky abdominal pain, nausea, constipation, and bloating.

▶ Objective Data

Objective assessment includes abdominal distention and tenderness on palpation. Vomiting temporarily relieves the abdominal pain. The vomitus may include fecal material.

Laboratory analysis demonstrates decreased levels of sodium and potassium on electrolytes, elevated BUN, elevated amylase, and elevated H & H due to hemoconcentration.

Nursing diagnoses for a client with an intestinal obstruction may include the following:

Nursing Diagnoses	Planning/Goals	Nursing Interventions
▶ *Deficient Fluid Volume related to vomiting, shift in fluids, and NPO status*	The client will exhibit adequate hydration within 48 hours of initiation of treatment as evidenced by moist mucous membranes, electrolytes within normal limits, and I & O approximately equal.	Monitor I & O every shift. Administer IV fluid and electrolyte replacements as ordered. Allow limited ice chips to prevent further electrolyte imbalance in clients with NG tubes. Assess weight daily.
▶ *Acute Pain related to distention, edema, or ischemia*	The client will verbalize increased comfort within 1 hour of analgesic administration as measured on pain scale.	Administer nonnarcotic analgesics as ordered. In clients with a paralytic ileus, encourage ambulation to encourage return of bowel function. Maintain and monitor NG tube as ordered for abdominal decompression. Check bowel sounds every 4 hours or PRN.
▶ *Deficient Knowledge related to disease process, treatment regimen, and possible surgery*	The client will verbalize treatment course, possible complications, and possible need for surgery.	Identify client's learning style and present information in a manner compatible with learning style. Include intestinal decompression, need for ambulation, need for good oral care due to fecal drainage, and surgery.

Evaluation Each goal must be evaluated to determine how it has been met by the client.

HERNIAS

A hernia occurs when the wall of a muscle weakens and the intestine protrudes through the muscle wall. Hernias that do not return to the abdominal cavity with rest or manipulation and cause complete bowel obstruction are said to be *incarcerated*. If the blood supply to the hernia is cut off, the hernia is said to be *strangulated*. Immediate surgery is required to restore the blood supply. If this is not done, gangrene will develop and the situation may be fatal.

Several types of hernias exist. In an umbilical hernia, a portion of the bowel protrudes through the umbilicus. In children, these generally resolve on their own once the child begins to walk. Umbilical hernias most commonly occur in a multiparous female or in adults having cirrhosis with **ascites** (abnormal accumulation of fluid in the peritoneal cavity). Due to a high risk for strangulation in adults with umbilical hernias, surgery is usually performed.

Abdominal hernias occur in the midline of the abdomen between the umbilicus and the xyphoid process. Most are asymptomatic with a few causing pain on exertion that resolves with reclining and rest.

Inguinal hernias, the most common hernia, occur in the groin area. Inguinal hernias frequently occur after activities, such as lifting, that increase intraabdominal pressure; they subside with relaxation. Pain is located lower than in the abdominal hernia.

Femoral hernias occur when the intestine pushes into the passageway carrying blood vessels and nerves to the legs, and are more common in women than in men.

A hiatal hernia occurs when a portion of the stomach protrudes into the mediastinal cavity through the diaphragm. Symptoms of hiatal hernias include indigestion and heartburn, especially after eating a large meal.

Upon evaluation and recommendation of a physician, some hernias can be reduced or pushed back into place. This can be accomplished by having the client recline, applying direct pressure to the hernia and, in some cases, having the client exhale to decrease intraabdominal pressure. The nurse should never try to reduce a hernia.

Medical–Surgical Management

Medical

Because some hernias have no symptoms or have minimal symptoms, clients may not be aware they have one or may simply learn to live with it by reducing it when needed. Clients who are a poor surgical risk may use a truss, a device that applies pressure to the hernia, thus keeping it in the abdominal cavity.

Surgical

Hernias can be repaired with a surgery called a herniorrhaphy. The surgery is typically performed on an outpatient basis with clients going home the same day. If the surgery is more complicated because the hernia is incarcerated, the client may stay overnight.

If the hernia is strangulated, surgery is required to restore the blood flow; a bowel resection may even be required.

Surgical repair of a hiatal hernia involves reinforcing the esophagus with a portion of the stomach. The surgery is performed laparoscopically with the client remaining in the hospital 3 to 5 days postoperatively. Initially, the client will have an NG tube. The NG tube is removed 24 to 48 hours later and the diet gradually progressed to a soft diet.

Diet

Clients with hiatal hernias may need to modify their dietary patterns to include small frequent meals, and to avoid eating after supper, lying down for 2 hours after eating, and aggravating foods.

▶ NURSING PROCESS

▶ Assessment

▶ Subjective Data

Clients may complain of pain at the site of the hernia.

▶ Objective Data

Assessment may show a bulge through the abdominal wall. If the hernia is strangulated, the client will have the symptoms of a bowel obstruction.

Nursing diagnoses for a client with a hernia may include the following:

Nursing Diagnoses	Planning/Goals	Nursing Interventions
▶ *Acute Pain related to tissue edema*	The client will experience less pain within 1 hour of intervention as measured on the pain scale.	Administer analgesics as ordered. Evaluate aggravating activities (e.g., straining to have a bowel movement) and provide information on modification if indicated. Educate regarding signs of complications and when to notify staff of symptoms.

continues

Nursing Diagnoses	Planning/Goals	Nursing Interventions
▶ *Ineffective Tissue Perfusion (Gastrointestinal) related to strangulation*	The client will have minimal tissue necrosis.	Assess abdomen for bowel sounds every 4 hours. Insert NG tube to decrease abdominal distention as ordered. Prepare client for surgery as ordered. Keep client NPO. Administer IV hydration as ordered.

Evaluation Each goal must be evaluated to determine how it has been met by the client.

PERITONITIS

Peritonitis is the inflammation of the peritoneum, the membranous covering of the abdomen. Peritonitis is caused by irritating substances such as feces, gastric acids, bacteria, or blood in the abdominal cavity. A ruptured portion of the digestive system (such as a the appendix) a ruptured tubal pregnancy, or invasion of tumors through the gastric wall, can lead to peritonitis. Peritonitis can be a serious, life-threatening condition. Complications following peritonitis include adhesions (scar tissue), ileus, and pneumonia.

Medical–Surgical Management

Surgical

Treatment is primarily surgical with repair of the cause and irrigation of the abdominal cavity with saline and antibiotic solutions. Drains may be left in the abdomen for several days postoperatively to allow any remaining fluid to drain. Since bowel function usually stops due to the irritating substances, an NG tube is placed to decompress the abdomen and relieve nausea.

Pharmacological

Analgesics will be ordered postoperatively for discomfort. If an ileus develops, nonnarcotic analgesics will be ordered. Antibiotics will also be ordered preoperatively and postoperatively.

Diet

Clients will be NPO preoperatively and postoperatively until bowel sounds return. Clients will then be placed on a clear liquid diet and slowly progressed to a regular diet as more bowel function returns.

Activity

Preoperatively, clients will be placed on bed rest. Postoperatively, clients need to be encouraged to turn, cough, and deep breathe. Because clients tend to breathe shallowly with peritoneal inflammation, pulmonary hygiene is important. Activity should be progressed postoperatively, as soon as tolerated, to increase lung expansion and to encourage bowel function return. Exercise, lifting, and driving will be restricted until the incision heals.

▶ NURSING PROCESS

▶ Assessment

▶ Subjective Data

Clients may describe abdominal pain, nausea, and constipation.

▶ Objective Data

Assessment may reveal vomiting, absent bowel sounds, a tense or distended abdomen with tenderness on palpation, shallow and rapid respirations, weak and rapid pulse, dry mucous membranes, low urine output, fever, and limited mobility because of pain.

Laboratory analysis will include a CBC, which will show an elevated WBC. If bleeding is occurring, the H & H will be low. Electrolytes may show low sodium, potassium, and chloride.

Nursing diagnoses for a client with peritonitis may include the following:

Nursing Diagnoses	Planning/Goals	Nursing Interventions
▶ *Deficient Fluid Volume related to gastric losses and restricted intake*	The client will maintain hydration as indicated by an I & O that is nearly equal and electrolytes within normal limits.	Monitor I & O every shift. Monitor for signs of dehydration: dry mucous membranes, poor skin turgor, and low urine output. Monitor electrolytes as ordered. Administer IV rehydration and electrolyte replacement as ordered.
▶ *Hyperthermia related to inflammatory process and dehydration*	The client will maintain temperature within normal limits.	Assess VS including temperature every 4 hours. Administer antipyretics as ordered; probably rectal suppositories due to NPO status.

continues

Nursing Diagnoses	Planning/Goals	Nursing Interventions
		Monitor for dehydration: decrease in urine output, dry mucous membranes, and poor skin turgor.
		Provide comfort measures: cool cloth to the head or neck, assistance to turn, and a back rub with cooling lotion.
▶ *Acute Pain related to abdominal distention*	The client will have less pain and improved mobility within 1 hour of receiving analgesics as measured on the pain scale.	Administer analgesics as ordered.
		Encourage activity such as coughing and deep breathing after analgesics.
		Monitor NG tube to decompress abdomen. Maintain patency of NG tube.
		Teach splinting of incision for cough and deep breathing.

Evaluation Each goal must be evaluated to determine how it has been met by the client.

HEMORRHOIDS

Hemorrhoids are swollen vascular tissues in the rectal area. The hemorrhoids may be internal or external. Hemorrhoids may be caused by straining with constipation. Sitting on the toilet (reading) for an extended time may also be a cause. Hemorrhoids frequently occur with pregnancy. Hemorrhoids can cause burning, pruritis, and pain with defecation. At times, hemorrhoids can bleed, leading to anemia.

Medical–Surgical Management

Medical

Sitz baths or warm compresses on the rectal area for 20 minutes, 4 times a day, often helps decrease swelling.

Surgical

If bleeding continues despite medical intervention, or if discomfort is significant, the hemorrhoids can be surgically removed by a hemorrhoidectomy. If hemorrhoids are external, surgery is performed on an outpatient basis by placing a rubber band around the hemorrhoid, allowing it to necrose and fall off on its own. If hemorrhoids are internal, surgery can be done using sclerotherapy, cryotherapy, or laser. This usually requires an overnight stay in the hospital. Hemorrhoids can recur after surgical removal if the cause is not eliminated.

Pharmacological

Treatment includes creams and suppositories to decrease inflammation, some with cortisone to decrease swelling. Fiber supplements and stool softeners may be ordered to keep bowel movements soft.

Diet

Bowel movements can be kept soft with a high-fiber diet of 20 to 30 grams of fiber a day and at least 2,500 cc of fluid intake daily.

▶ NURSING PROCESS

▶ Assessment

▶ Subjective Data

Clients may complain of rectal burning, pain, and pruritis with bowel movements; constipation; and, occasionally, bright red bleeding. A dietary history should be obtained to determine fiber and fluid intake.

▶ Objective Data

If hemorrhoids are external, they can be visualized during a physical examination. If chronic bleeding is present, laboratory analysis may show a low H & H.

Nursing diagnoses for a client with hemorrhoids may include the following:

Nursing Diagnoses	Planning/Goals	Nursing Interventions
▶ *Acute Pain related to edema and inflammation of swollen vascular tissues*	The client will verbalize a decrease in discomfort within 48 hours of initiation of treatment.	Provide sitz baths or warm compresses for 20 minutes, 4 times a day.
		Administer creams and suppositories as ordered.
		Increase fiber and fluids in diet to keep stools soft to avoid straining.

continues

Nursing Diagnoses	Planning/Goals	Nursing Interventions
▶ *Deficient Knowledge related to diet, causes of condition, treatment, and potential complications*	The client will be able to verbalize treatment regimen and long-term management of hemorrhoids.	Determine client's learning style and present information in a manner compatible with learning style. Educate client about increasing fiber in diet to 20 to 30 grams per day, increasing fluid intake to 2,500 cc per day, causes of hemorrhoids, possible complications such as anemia, and modification of bowel habits (such as not sitting on the toilet for long periods).

Evaluation Each goal must be evaluated to determine how it has been met by the client.

CONSTIPATION

Constipation is characterized by hard, infrequent stools that are difficult and/or painful to pass. Constipation can be caused by tumors, low-fiber diet, inactivity, some diseases that interfere with the mechanical functioning of the bowel (such as multiple sclerosis), or some medications (such as narcotics, antidepressants, or anti-Parkinson drugs).

Medical–Surgical Management

Pharmacological

Fiber supplements and stool softeners may be ordered. Laxatives and enemas may be ordered, but long-term use should be avoided as they interrupt normal bowel function. If constipation is caused by medications the client is taking, the client should discuss with the physician other options such as modifying the dosage or changing medications.

Diet

Fiber should be increased to 20 to 30 grams a day. Fluid intake should be increased to 2,500 cc a day.

Activity

Activity level should be increased if possible as exercise, such as walking, increases motility in the colon.

▶ NURSING PROCESS

▶ Assessment

▶ Subjective Data

Clients complain of infrequent, difficult to pass stools. Dietary assessment of fiber and fluids usually reveals inadequate intake. Activity/exercise levels should also be assessed.

▶ Objective Data

Bowel movements will be hard-formed.

GERONTOLOGICAL CONSIDERATIONS

Constipation in the Older Client

The slowing of peristalsis, which is part of the aging process, may lead to constipation in the older client. An increase in dietary fiber and fluid intake (water) will help prevent constipation. A regular schedule for bowel evacuation is also helpful.

Nursing diagnoses for a client with constipation may include the following:

Nursing Diagnoses	Planning/Goals	Nursing Interventions
▶ *Constipation related to inadequate intake of fiber and fluids*	The client will have soft stools every other day by one week from start of intervention.	Encourage client to increase fiber in the diet to 20 to 30 grams a day and fluid intake to 2,500 cc a day. Administer fiber supplements and stool softeners as ordered. Determine fluid preferences of client and always have fluids at client's bedside within reach. Help the client establish a regular schedule for bowel movements, usually 30 minutes after a meal.
▶ *Deficient Knowledge related to dietary sources of fiber and the importance of adequate fluid intake and exercise*	The client will be able to select a menu high in fiber and fluids utilizing nutrients from the food pyramid within 48 hours and verbalize the need for adequate exercise.	Assess client's learning style and present information in a manner compatible with learning style. Teach client about foods that are high in fiber (fruits, vegetables, whole grains) as well as importance of fluid intake. Discuss with client importance of exercise in maintaining bowel function.

Evaluation Each goal must be evaluated to determine how it has been met by the client.

DISORDERS OF THE ACCESSORY ORGANS

Disorders of the accessory organs include: cirrhosis, hepatitis, pancreatitis, and cholecystitis/cholelithiasis.

CIRRHOSIS

Cirrhosis refers to the chronic, degenerative changes in the liver cells and thickening of surrounding tissue that result from the liver repairing itself after chronic inflammation. Causes of cirrhosis include chronic hepatitis, repeated exposure to toxic substances, disease processes (such as sclerosing cholangitis and hemochromatosis), cancer, and chronic alcohol abuse. Alcohol abuse accounts for most cases of cirrhosis.

Because the liver is responsible for so many functions, complications can be significant. Complications include: malnutrition, hypoglycemia, clotting disorders, jaundice, portal hypertension, ascites, hepatic encephalopathy, and hepatorenal syndrome.

Liver dysfunction causes several organ-related complications. Malnutrition results from the liver's inability to absorb fat and fat soluble vitamins, and leads to muscle wasting, weight loss, and fatigue. Hypoglycemia occurs when the liver is unable to perform glycogenolysis efficiently. Clotting disorders result when the liver is not able to produce sufficient amounts of prothrombin and fibrinogen.

Portal hypertension results when blood flow through the cirrhotic liver is inhibited, resulting in blood backflowing in the portal vein. Portal hypertension leads to distention of the esophageal veins, resulting in esophageal varices.

Because the liver is responsible for metabolizing medications, clients frequently become intolerant to some medications. Jaundice, a yellow discoloration of the skin, is usually present. Jaundice occurs when the liver is unable to convert bilirubin, an end product of red blood cell breakdown, into a water soluble form that can be excreted in the bile. The extra bilirubin collects in areas that contain elastin such as the sclera of the eyes, the skin, and the nail beds.

When blood flow through the cirrhotic liver is inhibited, blood backs up into the portal system. Congestion of blood in the portal system causes distention of the esophageal, gastric, mesenteric, splenic, and portal veins. The backflow of blood in these vessels increases the pressure in the vessels, causing portal hypertension. The distended esophageal veins cause esophageal varices (see the earlier section on esophageal varices in this chapter), and the distended rectal veins result in hemorrhoids. The distended splenic vein causes splenomegaly.

Fluid may accumulate in the pleural cavity in the form of pleural effusions. Fluid may also accumulate in the peritoneal cavity. This condition is called ascites. The cause of ascites is the congestion of blood in the portal system.

Hepatic encephalopathy is a condition in which too much ammonia accumulates in the bloodstream from the liver's inability to filter proteins and protein byproducts. Confusion, lethargy, and/or coma may occur. Symptoms of impending hepatic encephalopathy are disorientation and asterixis (liver flap), a flapping tremor of the hands. When the client extends the arms and hands in front of the body, the hands rapidly flex and extend.

Hepatorenal syndrome is a complication of cirrhosis in which the client goes into renal failure. Symptoms include oliguria (diminished production of urine), azotemia (excess nitrogen in the blood), anorexia, fatigue, and weakness.

Cirrhosis is a form of end-stage liver disease for which there is no cure. The process of cirrhosis can be slowed by removing the cause (i.e., abstaining from alcohol), but the damage cannot be reversed. Clients in end-stage liver disease may be evaluated to determine if they qualify for a liver transplant.

Medical–Surgical Management

Medical

The physician may perform a paracentesis to remove the fluid from the abdomen and relieve pressure on the diaphragm and lungs. A paracentesis is done by making a small incision and inserting a trochar into the abdomen to drain the fluid. Albumin may be infused at the same time to pull excess fluid back into the vascular system.

Surgical

If the client continues to develop ascites after medical treatment, a LeVeen or Denver peritoneal venous shunt may be used. The pressure-regulated shunt is implanted in the peritoneal cavity and threaded through the subcutaneous tissue into the superior vena cava, returning the fluid back to the vascular system. As fluid pressure builds in the peritoneal cavity, a valve opens and drains the fluid into the superior vena cava.

If esophageal varices are present, an EGD with sclerotherapy or banding will be done to prevent hemorrhage (refer back to Figure 28-3).

If portal hypertension cannot be controlled with medications, a portosystemic shunt or a transjugular intrahepatic portosystemic shunt (TIPS) may be performed. The purpose of the shunt is to redirect the blood flow, thereby relieving the portal hypertension and decreasing the risk of rupturing distended veins in the esophagus (Figure 28-11).

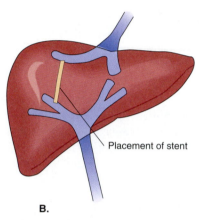

Figure 28-11 A. Blood Flow Prior to TIPS; B. TIPS is performed in radiology on clients deemed too unstable for the surgery necessary for a portosystemic shunt. A stent is placed to redirect the blood flow.

Pharmacological

A potassium sparing diuretic, such as spironolactone (Aldactone) is used to decrease ascites and pleural effusion. Lactulose (Cholac) is used to eliminate the ammonia from the blood into the bowel. The lactulose acts as a laxative and causes the body to excrete the stool containing ammonia. Tap water enemas may also be ordered to help the body eliminate the ammonia.

Propranolol hydrochloride (Inderal), an antihypertensive medication, may be ordered to lower portal hypertension. All unnecessary medications should be avoided since the liver cannot metabolize them.

Diet

Clients with cirrhosis are placed on a low-protein diet, usually 40 grams per day. If ascites is present, sodium will also be restricted to 2 grams or less a day to decrease the amount of fluid retained by the body. Fluids may also be restricted to 1,000 cc to 2,000 cc a day depending on the severity of fluid accumulation.

Activity

Safety: Cirrhosis

If hepatic encephalopathy is present, precautions should be taken to ensure the client's safety, such as elevating bedrails and allowing the client to ambulate only with assistance, especially if the client's gait is unsteady.

Because fatigue is such a common symptom of cirrhosis, the client's tolerance for activity will be diminished. Rest periods should be planned during the day, and activities should be scheduled between rests.

▶ NURSING PROCESS

▶ Assessment

▶ Subjective Data

Clients describe fatigue, nausea, anorexia, weakness, and indigestion.

▶ Objective Data

Assessment shows ascites, jaundice, enlarged liver and spleen, petechiae (small bruises on the skin), vomiting, weight loss, fever, epistaxis, and decreased breath sounds. Lethargy, confusion, or coma may be present if encephalopathy has occurred.

Laboratory analysis includes a CBC, which will demonstrate low WBCs, RBCs, Hgb, and platelets. A liver panel will show an elevated bilirubin, alkaline phosphatase, GGT, ALT, and AST. Albumin will be low. PT, PTT, and clotting times will be delayed.

Nursing diagnoses for a client with cirrhosis may include the following:

Nursing Diagnoses	Planning/Goals	Nursing Interventions
▶ *Disturbed Thought Processes related to elevated serum ammonia levels and hepatic coma*	The client will experience an improved level of orientation within 48 hours of initiation of treatment.	Administer tap water enemas and lactulose as ordered to eliminate ammonia-rich stools. An NG tube may be placed to give lactulose if client is comatose.
		Elevate bedrails to prevent injury.
		Monitor ammonia levels.
		As coma lessens, reorient client frequently.
		Provide low-protein diet.

continues

Nursing Diagnoses	Planning/Goals	Nursing Interventions
▶ *Excess Fluid Volume related to ascites*	The client will have less ascites by discharge.	Weigh daily.
		Measure abdominal girth daily.
		Restrict fluid to 1,000 to 2,000 cc per day depending on the severity of the ascites.
		Educate client to notify physician of weight gain of 1½ lbs or more in 1 week.
		Provide low-sodium diet of 500 to 2,000 mg a day depending on severity of the ascites.
		Teach client how to measure fluids and calculate sodium in diet.
		If a paracentesis is done, check vital signs every 15 minutes during the procedure and after the procedure until the vitals are stable. The amount of fluid removed from the abdomen should be measured and sent to the laboratory.
▶ *Risk for Impaired Skin Integrity related to accumulation of bile salts in skin, poor skin turgor, ascites, and edema*	The client will not experience skin breakdown while hospitalized.	Provide egg crate mattress.
		Turn client every 2 hours.
		Monitor skin closely for redness and skin breakdown.
		Apply lotion to skin frequently, especially to pressure areas. Assist with ADLs to promote good hygiene and conserve client's energy.
▶ *Imbalanced Nutrition: Less than body requirements related to inadequate diet, anorexia, or vomiting*	The client will eat a balanced diet of 1,500 calories a day.	Offer small, high-calorie meals frequently.
		Assist and encourage client to eat.
		Offer high-nutrient supplements if client is unable to maintain adequate caloric intake.
		Provide frequent oral hygiene.
		Observe for changes in mental status that would interfere with caloric intake (e.g., increased lethargy).

Evaluation Each goal must be evaluated to determine how it has been met by the client.

HEPATITIS

Hepatitis is a chronic or acute inflammation of the liver caused by a virus, bacteria, drugs, alcohol abuse, or other toxic substances. There is a diffuse inflammatory reaction with liver cells degenerating and dying. The functions of the liver slow down. Since viral infections are the most common cause of hepatitis, emphasis will be placed on viral hepatitis.

Researchers are still learning about the viruses that cause hepatitis. Five viruses are known to cause hepatitis: A, B, C, D, and E. The viruses are similar and have almost identical signs and symptoms. Incubation period, mode of transmission, and prognosis vary. See Table 28–5 for a summary of the hepatitis viruses.

Medical–Surgical Management

Treatment is focused on resting the liver and early detection of complications. The liver is rested by modifying the diet so that less bile is needed to digest the food. Treatment is related to the signs and symptoms present and the prevention of transmission.

Pharmacological

Antiemetics such as hydroxyzine hydrochloride (Atarax, also Vistaril) or trimethobenzamide hydrochloride (Tigan) may be given before meals if nausea is present. IV hydration with vitamin C for healing may be ordered. Vitamin B complex may also be ordered to help client absorb fat-soluble vitamins. Vitamin K may be ordered if clotting time is prolonged. All unnecessary medications, especially sedatives, should be avoided.

Those exposed to hepatitis B by needle puncture or sexual contact should have hepatitis B immunoglobin (HBIG). A vaccine for hepatitis A (HAV) is available and provides protection for up to 10 years or more. HAV is recommended for people at risk for exposure to hepatitis A such as homosexuals, IV drug users, travelers to countries with poor sanitation conditions, and laboratory workers who handle live hepatitis A virus.

Diet

Diet modifications may include decreasing fat intake to decrease the amount of bile needed in the digestive tract. A low-protein diet may be needed if the liver is no longer able to metabolize the protein. Anorexia is a common symptom that can be treated with small, frequent, high-calorie meals. Fluids may be restricted if the client is starting to retain fluids. No alcoholic beverages are recommended for at least 1 year or longer.

Table 28–5 COMPARISON OF DIFFERENT TYPES OF VIRAL HEPATITIS

	A	B	C	D	E
Etiologic Agent	hepatitis A viris (HAV)	hepatitis B virus (HBV)	hepatitis C virus (HCV)	hepatitis D virus (HDV)	hepatitis E virus (HEV)
Trans-mission	Fecal-oral; contaminated water or food; person to person	Blood; sexual; perinatal; breast milk	Blood	Only persons with hepatitis B can get hepatitis D; blood and blood products; needle sticks; seldom sexual; rarely perinatal	Oral-fecal route; contaminated water; person to person uncommon
Risk Groups	Household/sexual contact with infected person; international travelers	Injection drug users; Sexual/household contact with infected person; infants born to infected mothers; health care workers multiple sex partners	Blood transfusions or organ transplants prior to 1992; sharing needles; exposure to blood and blood products	Needle sharing; needle sticks	Mainly travel to countries where endemic
Incubation Period	15–50 days	45–160 days	14–180 days	15–60 days	15–60 days
Infectious Period	Usually less than 2 months	Before symptoms appear; lifetime if carrier	Before symptoms appear; lifetime if carrier	Not determined	Not determined
Diagnostic Tests	IgM anti-HAV	HBsAg	Anti HCV; serum ALT increased 10x; HCVRNA	IgG anti-HDV	None available
Symptoms	Flu-like; jaundice; dark yellow urine; light colored stools	Flu-like; may have jaundice; dark yellow urine; light colored stools	Many have no symptoms; flu-like	Flu-like; may have jaundice; dark yellow urine; light colored stools	Abdominal pain, anorexia; dark yellow urine; jaundice, fever
Prevention	Standard Precautions; enteric precautions; Hepatitis A vaccine (entire series); Immune globulin (for short term)	Standard Precautions; reduce risk behaviors; Hepatitis B vaccine (entire series); Immune globulin (for short term)	Standard Precautions; reduce risk behaviors; no vaccine	Standard Precautions; reduce risk behaviors; Hepatitis B vaccine; if client already has hepatitis B no prevention for hepatitis D	Standard Precautions; be sure water safe when traveling; no vaccine
Treatment	Immune globulin within 2 weeks of exposure	Immune globulin (HBIg) Alpha interferon	Alpha interferon; ribavirin (Virazole)	Alpha interferon	None given
Prognosis	Rarely fatal; not a carrier	No cure; may become a carrier	85% or less have chronic infection; 70% develop chronic liver disease	Chronicity uncommon	No evidence of chronicity

Data from: Centers for Disease Control and Prevention (CDC) (2000). Viral hepatitis A. [On-line] Available: www.cdc.gov/ncidod/diseases/hepatitis/a/index.htm; CDC (2000). Viral hepatitis B. [On-line] Available: www.cdc.gov/ncidod/diseases/hepatitis/b/index.htm; CDC (2000). Viral hepatitis C. [On-line] Available: www.cdc.gov/ncidod/diseases/hepatitis/c/index.htm; CDC (2000). Viral hepatitis D. [on-line] Available: www.cdc.gov/ncidod/diseases/hepatitis/d/hep00051; CDC (2000). Viral hepatitis E. [On-line] Available: www.cdc.gov/ncidod/diseases/hepatitis/e/hep00058; Lau, D. T., Kleiner, D. E., Park, Y., DiBisceglie, A. M. & Hoofnagle, J. H. (1999). Resolution of chronic delta hepatitis after 12 years of interferon alpha therapy. *Gastroenterology, 117*(5), 1229–33; National Institute of Diabetes and Digestive and Kidney Diseases (NIDDK) (1997). What I need to know about hepatitis A [On-line] Available: www.niddk.nih.gov/health/digest/pubs/hep/hepa/hepa.htm; NIDDK (1998). What I Need to Know About Hepatitis B. [On-line] Available: www.niddk.nih.gov/health/digest/pubs/hep/hepb/hepb.htm; NIDDK (1999). What I Need to Know About Hepatitis C. [On-line] Available: www.niddk.nih.gov/health/digest/pubs/hep/hepc/hepc.htm; NIDDK (2000). Chronic hepatitis C: Current disease management. [On-line] Available: www.niddk.nih.gov/health/digest/pubs/chrnhepc/chrnhepc.htm; NIDDK (2000). The digestive diseases dictionary: E–K. [On-line] Available: www.niddk.nih.gov/health/digest/pubs/dddctnry/pages/e-k.htm.

Activity

Bed rest is usually recommended for the first several weeks, generally at home unless the serum bilirubin is greater than 10 mg/dL or the PT is prolonged. If either occurs, hospitalization is usually recommended.

Once bed rest is no longer necessary, activity should be increased gradually as fatigue will be present for up to several months. Rest periods should be included throughout the day.

▶ NURSING PROCESS

▶ Assessment

▶ Subjective Data

Symptoms may include fatigue, anorexia, photophobia, nausea, headaches, abdominal pain, generalized muscle aches, chills, pruritis, and bloating.

▶ Objective Data

The client may have weight loss, hepatomegaly, fever, jaundice, dark amber urine, and clay-colored stools.

Laboratory analysis will show an elevated bilirubin, GGT, AST, ALT, LDH, and alkaline phosphatase. Clotting time and PT will be prolonged. Specific hepatitis test will be elevated (refer back to Table 28–5).

Nursing diagnoses for the client with hepatitis may include the following:

Nursing Diagnoses	Planning/Goals	Nursing Interventions
▶ *Deficient Knowledge related to disease process, treatment regimen, and mode of transmission*	The client will be able to explain disease process, incubation period, and mode of transmission, by discharge. The client will practice precautions to prevent spread of disease. The client will be able to select a menu using foods from the food guide pyramid and maintain a low-fat, low-protein diet.	Assess client's learning style and present information in a manner compatible with learning style. Educate about disease process and incubation period. Teach proper handwashing technique and emphasize importance of washing hands after using the bathroom. Emphasize that client cannot donate blood. Emphasize importance of follow-up laboratory analysis. Instruct in selection of low-fat, low-protein diet. For clients with hepatitis A, teach client to disinfect articles contaminated with feces (such as the toilet), not to prepare food for others, and not to share articles such as eating utensils or toothbrushes. For clients with hepatitis B, teach to avoid sexual contact until they test negative for HBsAg or their partners are immunized with the HBV vaccine. For clients with hepatitis C, teach that it is unknown whether it can be transmitted through sexual contact, so precautions are recommended until more is known.
▶ *Imbalanced Nutrition: Less than body requirements related to inadequate caloric intake, fat intolerance, nausea, and vomiting*	The client will maintain a caloric intake of 2,000 calories/day.	Monitor daily calorie count. Monitor I & O every shift. Weigh daily. Offer small, frequent, high-calorie, low-fat meals. Encourage low-protein diet of 40 gm of protein. Offer largest meal in morning, as food tends to be tolerated better in the morning. Note color and consistency of stools and color of urine. Encourage fluid intake of 2,500 to 3,000 cc daily. Administer antiemetic 30 minutes before meals as ordered.
▶ *Fatigue related to decreased energy production and altered body chemistry*	The client will verbalize plan to modify activity, by discharge.	Educate client regarding reasons for fatigue and that fatigue may be present for several months. Encourage client to maintain bed rest for several weeks. Advise client that when resuming normal activity, rest periods should be included until stamina returns.

Evaluation Each goal must be evaluated to determine how it has been met by the client.

PANCREATITIS

Pancreatitis is an acute or chronic inflammation of the pancreas caused when pancreatic enzymes digest the lining of the pancreas. Pancreatitis occurs when obstruction of the pancreatic duct occurs as a result of gallstones, tumors, exposure to chemicals or alcohol, or injury to the pancreas. In severe cases, the pancreas can hemorrhage resulting in a life-threatening condition.

Medical–Surgical Management

Medical

Treatment is dependent upon the cause of the pancreatitis. If the pancreatitis results from exposure to chemical or alcohol abuse, treatment is primarily medical. An NG tube is inserted to rest the bowel and relieve abdominal distention.

Surgical

If the pancreatitis is caused by structural changes such as gallstones, an ERCP with stone removal may be performed. Surgery to relieve the pancreatic duct obstruction may be necessary in cases where tumors or injury are the causes of the pancreatitis.

Pharmacological

Insulin may be given if the pancreas is unable to secrete enough to maintain normal blood sugar level. If nausea and vomiting are present, antiemetics may be ordered. Meperidine (Demerol) will be ordered for analgesia as morphine sulfate may cause spasms of the sphincter of Oddi. Atropine sulfate or propantheline bromide (Pro-Banthine) may be ordered to decrease pancreatic activity. Antacids or an H_2 receptor antagonist may be ordered to prevent stress ulcers.

Diet

Clients are kept NPO while the serum amylase level is elevated to decrease the demand for digestive enzymes in the bowel. An NG tube may be inserted to decrease pancreatic activity, and to prevent nausea, vomiting, and abdominal distention. As the serum amylase level begins to decrease, clients will be started on clear liquids and slowly advanced to a bland, low-fat, high-protein, high-carbohydrate diet. No coffee or alcohol is allowed.

IV rehydration is necessary while the client is NPO. If the pancreatitis is severe and the client must be NPO for a prolonged period, TPN, a high-calorie, high-nutrient IV solution, may be administered.

Activity

Clients are frequently placed on bed rest to decrease metabolic rate. Activity can be increased as the serum amylase decreases.

▶ NURSING PROCESS

▶ Assessment

▶ Subjective Data

Clients complain of excruciating epigastric pain that radiates to the back. Pain may decrease by leaning forward or lying in a fetal position. Nausea and anorexia are also present.

▶ Objective Data

Assessment includes steatorrhea, vomiting, low-grade fever, tachycardia, and jaundice. Laboratory analysis includes an elevated serum amylase followed by an elevated urine amylase and serum lipase, leukocytosis, and an elevated Hct. Glucose, alkaline phosphatase, and bilirubin may also be elevated.

Nursing diagnoses for a client with pancreatitis may include the following:

Nursing Diagnoses	Planning/Goals	Nursing Interventions
▶ Acute Pain related to inflammation and edema of the pancreas	The client will verbalize a decrease in pain as evidenced by pain scale by 1 hour after initiation of interventions.	Monitor NG tube to decompress the abdomen.
		Administer analgesics as ordered and monitor for relief.
		Position client in most comfortable position.
		Assess pain for increasing severity that would indicate worsening pancreatitis.
		Monitor serum amylase, WBCs, and H & H for signs of increasing severity of pancreatitis or hemorrhage.
▶ Imbalanced Nutrition: Less than body requirements related to NPO status, nausea, vomiting, and altered ability to digest nutrients	The client will experience no further weight loss during hospitalization.	Monitor I & O every shift.
		Weigh client daily.
		Maintain bed rest to decrease the metabolic rate.
		Insert NG tube to decompress the abdomen as ordered.
		Administer IV rehydration or TPN as ordered.
▶ Risk for Deficient Fluid Volume related to vomiting, NG tube, or hemorrhage	The client will maintain adequate hydration as evidenced by I & O that is nearly equal, electrolytes within normal limits, and moist mucous membranes.	Monitor I & O every shift.
		Administer IV hydration or TPN as ordered.
		Monitor electrolyte levels and H & H as ordered.

Evaluation Each goal must be evaluated to determine how it has been met by the client.

CHOLECYSTITIS AND CHOLELITHIASIS

Cholecystitis is an inflammation of the gallbladder. In more than 90% of the cases, gallstones are present. **Cholelithiasis** is the presence of gallstones or **calculi** (concentration of mineral salts) in the gallbladder. Not all gallstones cause cholecystitis. Some gallstones may pass out of the gallbladder and into the duodenum with the client being unaware of the stones. Sometimes gallstones migrate into the cystic or common bile duct causing an obstruction that, in turn, leads to cholecystitis. The exact cause of the formation of these stones is not known.

These two diseases are more common in multiparous women, age 45 and older; obese people; those who use birth control pills or control cholesterol with gemfibrozil (Lopid); and people with a history of a disease of the small intestine such as Crohn's disease. Also, clients on sudden weight reduction diets that are low in fat will cause the bile to pool in the gallbladder, increasing the risk for gallstone formation.

Ultrasound of the gallbladder is ordered if gallstones are suspected.

Medical–Surgical Management

In asymptomatic clients, no intervention is necessary.

Medical

If stones are lodged in the common bile duct, an ERCP may be performed.

Surgical

A sphincterotomy, an incision in the ampulla of vater, may be performed to enlarge the opening of the common bile duct. Stones may then be removed or crushed. If the stones are too large or for clients with repeated episodes of cholelithiasis, a cholecystectomy, the surgical removal of the gallbladder, may be performed. The cholecystectomy may be performed laparoscopically or by making a large abdominal incision.

Laparoscopic cholecystectomies, while having been performed for less than 10 years, have become the surgery of choice for cholelithiasis and cholecystitis. The gallbladder is removed by making 4 small incisions and extracting the gallbladder through an endoscope. If the cholecystectomy is performed laparoscopically, it is more difficult to perform an exploration of the common bile duct, especially in clients with cholecystitis. An ERCP may need to be performed if stones remain in the common bile duct (CBD). Clients are ready for discharge 24 hours after the surgery.

The cholecystectomy can also be performed by making a large abdominal incision. A cholangiogram can be performed easily and therefore this type of procedure is more common in clients with much inflammation of the gallbladder. If damage has occurred to the CBD due to severe inflammation or from a stone, a T-tube will be left in place to allow the bile to drain into a collection bag. This allows the CBD to heal. Clients are typically ready for discharge 3 to 7 days after surgery. Exercise, lifting, and driving will be restricted to allow for incisional healing.

Pharmacological

In acute cholecystitis, analgesics will be ordered to relieve the discomfort. Meperidine (Demerol) is preferred over morphine sulfate as morphine sulfate is believed to increase sphincter spasms. IV hydration may also be ordered if clients are unable to maintain hydration. Antiemetics will also be ordered if nausea and vomiting are present.

In clients who have surgery, analgesics will be ordered after surgery to control discomfort.

Diet

In clients with mild or moderate symptoms, a clear liquid diet to rest the bowel, followed by small frequent meals low in fat, may resolve the symptoms.

If clients are to have surgery, they will be NPO before surgery and initially after surgery until bowel sounds return. They will then be started on clear liquids first and then advanced, as tolerated, to a regular diet.

Activity

In acute cases of cholecystitis, bed rest is recommended to decrease metabolic rate. If surgery is performed, the client will be encouraged to turn, cough, and deep breathe every 2 hours initially after surgery. On the day following surgery, the client should be helped out of bed and encouraged to gradually increase activity. Clients who have had a laparoscopic cholecystectomy may be ambulated the evening of surgery. Clients can typically return to previous activity level 2 weeks after surgery. Clients who have an incision must restrict lifting, driving, and exercise until incisional healing is complete, usually 4 to 6 weeks.

▶ NURSING PROCESS

▶ Assessment

▶ Subjective Data

Clients describe pain in the right upper quadrant radiating to the right scapular area that occurs 2 to 4 hours after a meal containing significant amounts of fat; nausea; flatulence; and indigestion.

▶ Objective Data

Assessment may show vomiting, occasionally a fever, jaundice, steatorrhea, clay-colored stools, and dark amber urine. Laboratory analysis may show elevated alkaline phosphatase, GGT, WBCs, and bilirubin.

Nursing diagnoses for a client with cholecystitis and cholelithiasis may include the following:

Nursing Diagnoses	Planning/Goals	Nursing Interventions
▶ Acute Pain related to inflammation or blocked bile duct	The client will experience less pain as evidenced by pain scale within 1 hour of initiation of treatment.	Keep client NPO or on a clear liquid diet as ordered. Administer analgesics as ordered. Monitor NG tube to decompress the abdomen as ordered. Observe for jaundice and bile flow obstruction.
▶ Ineffective Breathing Pattern related to decreased lung expansion because of pain	The client will demonstrate appropriate breathing pattern and will not have respiratory complications while hospitalized.	Assist client to cough and breathe deeply every 2 hours. Teach splinting techniques for comfort and to facilitate breathing. Turn client every 2 hours and ambulate as soon as indicated. Teach use of incentive spirometer.
▶ Risk for Deficient Fluid Volume related to nausea, NG tube, NPO, or bile drainage	The client will maintain adequate hydration as evidenced by I & O that is nearly equal and moist mucous membranes.	Monitor I & O every shift including NG drainage and T-tube drainage if present. Administer IV hydration as ordered. Maintain patency of NG tube.

Evaluation Each goal must be evaluated to determine how it has been met by the client.

NEOPLASMS OF THE GASTROINTESTINAL SYSTEM

Neoplasms of the gastrointestinal system include oral cancer, colorectal cancer, and liver cancer.

ORAL CANCER

Oral cancer refers to cancers of the lips, tongue, oral cavity, and pharynx. According to the American Cancer Society, the occurrence of oral cancer is several times more frequent in people who use tobacco. The 5-year survival rate is low, primarily because the early symptoms are ignored. Symptoms include a mouth sore that does not heal, a sore throat, or difficulty swallowing. On the lips, the cancer may be a growth.

Medical–Surgical Management

Surgical

Treatment is primarily surgical and involves removal of the cancer with excision of tissue and lymph nodes surrounding the cancer. In cases of cancer involving the pharynx, a radical neck dissection is performed, which requires reconstruction of the pharynx. Clients undergoing radical neck dissection frequently have a tracheostomy.

Pharmacological

Chemotherapy is not effective against most oral cancers and is, therefore, used only in the most severe cases with metastases. Medications ordered will be based on the client's symptoms. If the client is experiencing side effects from the radiation such as nausea, antiemetics will be ordered.

If a client has surgery, analgesics will be ordered postoperatively. Analgesics may also be ordered if the cancer has progressed and is causing discomfort.

Diet

Because the surgery is in the oral area, it may be difficult to maintain adequate nutrition. Depending on the extent of the surgery, clients may require a soft diet or, in some cases, nutritional supplements to allow the surgical area to heal. Tube feedings, either by a feeding tube or by a gastrostomy tube (a special tube inserted through the abdomen into the stomach), are frequently needed in clients who have undergone a radical neck dissection.

Activity

If the surgery is minor, no activity restrictions will be necessary. If surgery is extensive, postoperatively, the client will need to turn, cough, and deep breathe. Activity will need to be progressed postoperatively. Clients receiving radiation treatments frequently experience fatigue and must have scheduled rest periods.

Other Therapies

In cases where the lesion cannot be surgically removed, radiation or radium implants may be used. High-energy radiation is used to destroy cancer cells. Clients may experience irritated skin, swallowing difficulties, dry mouth, nausea, diarrhea, hair loss, or fatigue. If radiation is done, the client will receive radiation daily for a specified period of time. If radium implants are used, the client will have a radioactive capsule implanted into the area.

▶ NURSING PROCESS

▶ Assessment

▶ Subjective Data

Clients may complain of a sore throat, difficulty swallowing, or a painful area in the mouth.

▶ Objective Data

Assessment may include a sore or lesion of the lips or in the oral cavity, and hoarseness.

Nursing diagnoses for a client with oral cancer may include the following:

Nursing Diagnoses	Planning/Goals	Nursing Interventions
▶ *Fear related to diagnosis and long-term prognosis*	The client will verbalize fear and express plan to cope with diagnosis.	Allow client time alone and with significant others. Answer questions. Allow client and family to express fears and concerns. Encourage contact with support system (e.g., clergy). Discuss past experiences with stress and individual responses to those situations.
▶ *Imbalanced Nutrition: Less than body requirements related to oral surgery or radical neck dissection*	The client will maintain weight while hospitalized.	Monitor I & O every shift. Weigh client daily. Administer tube feedings and IV rehydration as ordered. When indicated, introduce fluids. Monitor for aspiration.
▶ *Disturbed Body Image related to disfiguring surgery*	The client will verbalize feelings regarding surgery and altered body image.	Allow client time to verbalize feelings. Discuss options (e.g., plastic surgery or makeup). Answer questions. Provide information on support groups.

Evaluation Each goal must be evaluated to determine how it has been met by the client.

COLORECTAL CANCER

Colorectal cancer is the third most common cancer in the United States. Almost all colorectal cancers arise from **polyps**, an abnormal growth of tissue that protrudes into the colon. Risk factors for colorectal cancer include age 45 or older, history of polyps, family history of polyps and/or colorectal cancer, a history of ulcerative colitis, and a diet high in fat and low in fiber.

Prognosis is very good if caught in the early stages. Recommended routine screenings for early detection are outlined in Table 28–6.

A colonoscopy or barium enema may demonstrate the disease. A CBC may show anemia if the cancer is bleeding. A CEA may be effective in detecting recurrent cancer, but is not a valid screening test. Signs and symptoms include a change in bowel habits, guaiac positive stools, and abdominal pain.

Medical–Surgical Management

Surgical

Treatment is surgical to remove the cancer (see Table 28–7). In class A tumors, a colonoscopy is performed with a polypectomy, the removal of the polyp. In class B or C tumors, a colon resection will be done (Figure 28-12). In some cases a colostomy, either temporary or permanent, may be performed. In class D tumors, surgery will be done only to relieve symptoms (e.g., bowel obstruction).

Follow-up colonoscopies must be done throughout the client's life to monitor for recurrence of the disease.

Pharmacological

In cases of class B, C, and D tumors, chemotherapy will be given following the surgery. Side effects of chemotherapy include nausea, vomiting, weight loss,

Table 28–6 RECOMMENDED SCREENINGS FOR COLORECTAL CANCER

RISK	DEFINITION	RECOMMENDATIONS
Average Risk	No personal or family history of colorectal cancer or polyps.	Fecal occult blood testing (FOBT) age 40. Sigmoidoscopy every 3 to 5 years after age 50.
Mild Risk	Blood relative with colorectal cancer.	Begin above testing 5 to 10 years prior to age relative diagnosed or, at minimum, the above guidelines.
Moderate Risk	Client with previous colorectal cancer.	Colonoscopy at 6 months, 1 year, and 2 years after diagnosis, then every 1 to 3 years.
High Risk	Familial polyposis syndrome.	FOBT age 10 with sigmoidoscopy. Colonoscopy every 1 to 3 years.
Ulcerative Colitis	UC 8 years throughout colon or 14 years in sigmoid colon.	Colonoscopy every 2 years with biopsies.

Table 28–7 COLORECTAL CANCER CLASSIFICATION AND TREATMENT

CLASS	INVOLVEMENT	TREATMENT
Class A	Limited to the inner lining of the colon.	Polypectomy during colonoscopy removes cancer.
Class B	Involves from 2 layers to entire thickness of colon wall.	Colon resection, chemotherapy.
Class C	Class B with invasion to lymph nodes.	Colon resection, chemotherapy, and immunotherapy.
Class D	Metastases to other organs (lung and liver most common).	Colon resection as a palliative measure only. Chemotherapy, radiation, and immunotherapy.

hair loss, fatigue, and dry skin. Medications to combat some of the side effects of the chemotherapy will be ordered.

Immunotherapy as an adjunct therapy for class C and D tumors may also be ordered to boost the immune system.

Diet

Preoperatively, the client will be NPO. Postoperatively, the client will be NPO and an NG tube will be in place until bowel sounds return. The client will then be started on a clear liquid diet and progressed to a high-fiber, low-fat diet.

Activity

Postoperatively, the client will need to be encouraged to turn, cough, and deep breathe every 2 hours. The client will be ambulated the next day and activity will need to be progressed.

Other Therapies

No significant benefits have been found with the use of radiation on colorectal cancer. However, radiation may be used on metastatic sites in class D tumors.

▶ NURSING PROCESS

▶ Assessment

▶ Subjective Data

Clients may complain of a change in bowel habits and possibly abdominal pain.

▶ Objective Data

Stools may be guaiac positive for blood. An H & H may show anemia.

Class A colorectal cancer

Class B colorectal cancer

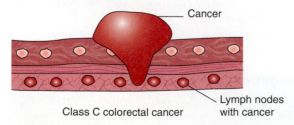

Class C colorectal cancer

Figure 28-12 Classes of Colorectal Cancer

Nursing diagnoses for a client with colorectal cancer may include the following:

Nursing Diagnoses	Planning/Goals	Nursing Interventions
▶ *Fear related to diagnosis and long-term prognosis*	The client will verbalize fear and express plan to cope with diagnosis.	Allow client time alone and with significant others.
		Allow client and family to express fears and concerns.
		Answer questions.
		Encourage contact with support system (e.g., clergy).
		Discuss past experiences with stress and identify individual responses to those situations.
▶ *Deficient Knowledge regarding disease process, treatment options, and follow-up*	The client will be able to explain disease process, treatment, and follow-up care.	Determine client's learning style and present information in a manner compatible with the learning style.
		Educate client regarding disease process.
		Discuss treatment options.
		Recognize that information may need to be presented more than once.

Evaluation Each goal must be evaluated to determine how it has been met by the client.

LIVER CANCER

Primary liver cancer is rare. Most liver tumors are metastatic from other sites in the body. Most cases of primary liver cancer are asymptomatic until later stages. Risk factors for primary liver cancer include a history of cirrhosis, hepatitis B, and exposure to toxic chemicals.

A primary liver tumor can be removed surgically if the disease is not extensive. Metastases cannot be surgically removed and are usually treated with chemotherapy and radiation.

CASE STUDY

Ms. R. is a 52-year-old female admitted to the hospital with acute abdominal pain. Ms. R. complains of right upper quadrant pain radiating to the back. She has had prior episodes, usually occurring about two hours after eating. This episode, however, is not resolving. Ms. R. also complains of nausea. Her vital signs are BP 152/88, pulse 92, and respirations 24 and shallow. Ms. R. is a slightly obese female who states she has recently been dieting to lose weight. Laboratory analysis includes a CBC with slightly elevated WBCs; elevated bilirubin; and elevated alkaline phosphatase. An IV is started and Ms. R. is given meperidine (Demerol) IM for pain. Ms. R. has been made NPO. An ultrasound of the gallbladder is ordered.

The following questions will guide your development of a nursing care plan for this case study.

1. List subjective and objective data a nurse would want to obtain about Ms. R.
2. List risk factors other than those Ms. R. has that would put a client at risk for developing cholecystitis.
3. List two nursing diagnoses and goals for Ms. R.
4. The ERCP is successful in removing the CBD stone. The decision is made to perform a laparoscopic cholecystectomy. What teaching will Ms. R. need?
5. Why is meperidine (Demerol) the medication of choice for pain control?
6. List at least 3 successful outcomes for Ms. R.

SUMMARY

- The gastrointestinal system is a complex system composed of the digestive tract as well as accessory organs.
- Disorders of the GI tract affect the breakdown and absorption of nutrients, breakdown of wastes and by-products, and the lifestyle of the individual.
- Because the liver is responsible for so many functions in the body, disorders of the liver can affect other systems significantly.
- Peptic ulcers may be either gastric or duodenal. *H. pylori* is a common cause of ulcers and can be treated with antibiotics.
- Diverticulosis is a commonly occurring disorder in the United States and is believed to be caused by a low-fiber diet.
- Inflammatory bowel disease includes both Crohn's disease and ulcerative colitis. IBD can lead to nutritional imbalances, bowel obstructions, alterations in the structure of the intestine, and affected lifestyle.
- Bowel obstructions have multiple causes and can lead to electrolyte imbalances, dehydration, and possibly sepsis.
- Viral hepatitis is a concern for health care professionals at risk for exposure. Standard precautions must be used to prevent the transmission of the virus.
- Colorectal cancer is one of the most preventable forms of cancer if routine screenings are performed.

Review Questions

1. A client with a bleeding esophageal varix:

    a. should be encouraged to vomit the blood so as to decrease abdominal distention and pressure.
    b. should have an NG tube placed to suction blood from the stomach.
    c. should have the Minnesota tube deflated every 4 hours.
    d. will not need follow-up once the bleeding has stopped.

2. A client with a perforated duodenal ulcer:

    a. requires an EGD to repair the perforation.
    b. may need to modify his or her diet after surgery.
    c. will have a vagotomy performed.
    d. may experience an increased risk for cholecystitis.

3. Clients with hepatitis C:

    a. should be instructed that all the mechanisms of transmission are not known.
    b. will have a negative HCV if they are a carrier.
    c. should be instructed that recombinant interferon alpha-2b will cure the hepatitis C.
    d. are not contagious until symptoms develop.

4. Changes in the gastrointestinal system caused by aging:

    a. are minimal and have little impact on clients.
    b. include an increase in digestive enzymes leading to an increase in the occurrence of ulcers.
    c. require clients to eat larger, fewer meals.
    d. may require the client to swallow 2 to 3 times with each bite.

5. Crohn's disease:

    a. can be cured by removing the colon.
    b. usually causes clients to gain weight from the slower metabolism of nutrients.
    c. can be a debilitating disease leading to depression.
    d. is cured as long as the clients remain on 5-ASA compounds.

6. Hernias are a protrusion through the muscle wall and:

    a. can be easily reduced by the nurse applying gentle pressure.
    b. are benign occurrences that do not need any intervention.
    c. can lead to bowel obstructions.
    d. are caused by a lack of exercise.

Critical Thinking Questions

1. What lifestyle changes are needed with a diagnosis of hepatitis A, B, C, and D?

2. List rationale for nursing interventions that would be effective for a client with an NG tube in place.

3. Compare and contrast the symptoms, treatments, and nursing interventions of Crohn's disease and ulcerative colitis.

4. Identify and discuss the rationale for each nursing intervention given for the nursing diagnoses in this chapter.

⚡ WEB FLASH!

- Locate support groups or resources on the Web for clients with GI disorders and their families? What resources are available for purchase?
- Visit the CDC's Web site. What information do they offer on the infectious disease hepatitis?
- What sites can you locate that specialize in GI cancer?

NURSING CARE OF THE CLIENT: URINARY SYSTEM

CHAPTER 29

MAKING THE CONNECTION

Refer to the following chapters to increase your understanding of the urinary system:

- **Chapter 7, Wellness Concepts**
- **Chapter 12, Health Assessment**
- **Chapter 19, Nursing Care of the Client: Cardiovascular System**
- **Chapter 30, Nursing Care of the Client: Female Reproductive System**
- **Chapter 31, Nursing Care of the Client: Male Reproductive System**
- **Chapter 35, Nursing Care of the Older Client**
- **Chapter 36, Rehabilitation, Home Health, Long-Term Care, and Hospice**

LEARNING OBJECTIVES

Upon completion of this chapter, you should be able to:
- *Define key terms.*
- *Describe the anatomy and physiology of the urinary system.*
- *Relate diagnostic test results to urinary disorders.*
- *Discuss the pros and cons of peritoneal dialysis/hemodialysis and kidney transplantation, including lifestyle changes for the client receiving dialysis.*
- *List four drug classifications and two examples of each used in the treatment of urinary disorders.*
- *State two changes in the urinary system related to the normal aging process.*
- *Compare and contrast acute and chronic renal failure, including nursing care.*
- *Assist in formulating a nursing care plan for clients with urinary disorders.*

KEY TERMS

anasarca	micturition
azotemia	nephrotoxic
cachectic	nocturnal enuresis
calculus(i)	overflow incontinence
cystitis	pyelonephritis
dialysate	pyuria
dialysis	renal colic
dysuria	residual urine
erythropoiesis	retroperitoneal
fulguration	stress incontinence
ileal conduit	urge incontinence
intravesical	urinary incontinence
litholapaxy	urinary retention
lithotripsy	urolithiasis

INTRODUCTION

Urology is the study of disorders of the urinary system. The National Kidney Foundation estimates that approximately 20 million Americans have kidney or urinary tract related diseases and millions more are at risk (National Kidney Foundation [NKF], 1997). Disorders of the urinary system may seriously affect an individual's health and, thereby, affect the lives of family members. Clients are treated by a urologist, specialist in urinary tract disorders, or a nephrologist, specialist in structure, function, and diseases of the kidney.

According to the National Kidney Foundation (1999b), the warning signs of kidney disease are:

- Burning or difficulty during urination
- Increase in the frequency of urination, especially at night
- Passage of bloody appearing urine
- Puffiness around the eyes, or swelling of the hands and feet, especially in children
- Pain in the small of the back just below the ribs (not aggravated by movement)
- High blood pressure

ANATOMY AND PHYSIOLOGY REVIEW

The urinary system consists of two kidneys, two ureters (upper urinary tract), a urinary bladder, and a urethra (lower urinary tract) (Figure 29-1). The kidneys manufacture urine. Urine normally consists of 95% water; the nitrogenous waste products of protein, which are urea, uric acid, and creatinine; the excessive electrolytes sodium, calcium, potassium, and phosphates; bile pigments; hormones; and metabolized drugs and toxins. Urine moves steadily by peristalsis through the ureters into the urinary bladder. The urine remains in the urinary bladder until capacity has been reached (about 500 mL) or until a desire to empty the urinary bladder (about 250 mL) is felt. The urine is then expelled from the bladder through the urethra, which is shorter in females than in males. **Micturition**, the process of expelling urine from the urinary bladder, is also called urination or voiding.

The kidneys are located beneath the false ribs, in the **retroperitoneal** space (behind the peritoneum outside the peritoneal cavity) of the abdominal cavity. The kidneys also assist in acid-base balance, raise blood pressure by secreting the enzyme renin, and produce the hormone erythropoietin which is responsible for **erythropoiesis** (the production of red blood cells and their release by the red bone marrow).

Within the kidneys are microscopic units called nephrons, which are responsible for urine formation. The nephron winds into the cortex and medulla of the kidney. Each nephron includes a renal corpuscle, which consists of a glomerulus, a ball-like network of capillaries formed from an arteriole and held within a cuplike Bowman's capsule. The Bowman's capsule is attached to a long, intricate, ultrathin looped and coiled tubular structure called the renal tubule. Continuing on from the glomerulus is an arteriole that forms a capillary network around the tubule. Blood flowing through this system is collected by venioles. The inset in Figure 29-1 illustrates a nephron.

Most of the contents of the blood, except for large molecules and blood cells, are forced out of the blood from the capillaries of the glomerulus and into the Bowman's capsule (glomerulofiltration). This occurs because of the high capillary blood pressure within the glomerulus. The glomerular basement membrane assists with the process of filtration. The material filtered from the blood is called glomerular filtrate, which contains water, electrolytes, glucose, various toxic substances, waste products (urea and creatinine), and just

Figure 29-1 The Urinary System with Inset of a Nephron

about everything else in the blood except large protein molecules and blood cells. As the filtrate passes through the first parts of the tubular structure, various substances such as necessary amounts of electrolytes, glucose, and water are reabsorbed (tubular reabsorption) back into the circulatory system through the capillaries or into the interstitial fluid. Tubular secretion then removes certain ions, nitrogen waste products, and drugs from the blood in the capillaries and adds it to the filtrate. The remaining filtrate—water, urea, excess electrolytes, toxic substances, and wastes, all of which constitute urine—continues through the tubules into the collecting duct, which collects urine from many nephrons. The urine passes from the collecting duct into the pelvis of the kidney, then through the ureter into the bladder and out of the body through the urethra.

ASSESSMENT

Assessment of the urinary system is included in the baseline data for all clients. The client may be reluctant to discuss urinary problems. The nurse can assist the individual to relax by asking open-ended questions, using familiar terms, and making sure the client understands the medical terms.

A more in-depth assessment is performed when the client is at high risk for renal disease because of exposure to nephrotoxins; an altered health state such as diabetes mellitus, pregnancy, or hypertension; trauma, dehydration, or fluid retention, which can compromise renal function; and those with suspected or active renal disease.

Subjective Data

The client is asked to describe how the symptoms developed and progressed. Is there pain? Is it sharp or a dull ache? Constant or intermittent? Does it radiate to the groin, genital area, or leg? Is the pain associated with urination? Have headaches been experienced?

Next, the client can describe the urine and urination pattern. Is there difficulty starting the stream? Is there urgency, frequency, incontinence, or hematuria? Does the bladder feel empty after voiding? Does the client have pruritis or dry skin?

Objective Data

If edema is present, the nurse asks the client whether it is always present or whether it disappears during the night. Refer to Figure 19-6, Grading Edema. I & O and vital signs are monitored, and the bladder palpated for retention. The client is weighed. Mucous membranes are assessed for moisture and the skin for dryness and uremic frost. Urine is evaluated for color, clarity, and odor. Diagnostic tests are assessed.

Changes with Aging

Needham (1993) identifies the following changes in the urinary system due to aging:

1. Nephrons decrease, resulting in decreased filtration and gradual decrease in excretory and reabsorptive functions of renal tubules.
2. Glomerular filtration rate decreases, resulting in decreased renal clearance of drugs.
3. Blood urea nitrogen (BUN) increases 20% by age 70. The creatinine clearance test is a better index than the BUN of renal function in the elderly.
4. Sodium-conserving ability is diminished.
5. Bladder capacity decreases, causing increased frequency of urination and nocturia.
6. Renal function increases when the client is lying down, sometimes causing a need to void shortly after going to bed.
7. Bladder and perineal muscles weaken, resulting in inability to empty the bladder. This results in residual urine and predisposes the elderly to cystitis.
8. Incidence of stress incontinence increases in females.
9. The prostate may enlarge, causing frequency or dribbling in males.

COMMON DIAGNOSTIC TESTS

Commonly used diagnostic tests for clients with symptoms of urinary system disorders are listed in Table 29–1. See Chapter 13, Diagnostic Tests, for explanation/normal values and nursing responsibilities.

Table 29–1 COMMON DIAGNOSTIC TESTS FOR URINARY SYSTEM DISORDERS

Urine Tests
Urinalysis
  Color
  Odor
  Albumin (protein)
  Acetone (ketone)
  RBCs
  WBCs
  Bilirubin
  Glucose
  Specific gravity
  Bacteria
  Casts
  pH
Culture and sensitivity (C & S)
Creatinine clearance *continues*

Table 29–1 COMMON DIAGNOSTIC TESTS FOR URINARY SYSTEM DISORDERS *continued*

Blood Tests
Blood urea nitrogen (BUN)
Serum creatinine
Antistreptolysin O titer (ASO titer)
Serum electrolytes
  Sodium
  Potassium
  Chloride
  Calcium
  Phosphorus

Radiographic Tests
Voiding cystrourethrography
Kidney-ureter-bladder (KUB) x-ray
Computed tomography (CT)
Magnetic resonance imaging (MRI)
Intravenous pyelogram (IVP)
Renal angiography
Renal scan
Ultrasound

Urodynamic Tests
Uroflowmetry
Cystometrogram (CMG)
Urethra pressure profile (UPP)

Endoscopic Exam
Cystoscopy

ALTERED URINARY ELIMINATION PATTERNS

Disorders in this category include urinary retention and urinary incontinence.

URINARY RETENTION

A person who is unable to void when there is an urge to void has **urinary retention**. This creates urinary stasis and increases the possibility of infection. The urine may overflow the bladder's capacity, causing incontinence.

There are a variety of causes such as a response to stress; obstruction of the urethra by **calculi** (concentration of mineral salts, known as stones), tumor, or infection; interference with the sphincter muscles during surgery; or as a side effect of medications or perineal trauma.

The client may experience discomfort and anxiety from urinary retention. Frequency of urination and voiding small amounts may also occur. The distended bladder can be palpated above the symphysis.

Treatment may include urinary analgesics and antispasmodics to help the client relax. A urinary catheter may be used to empty the bladder, or surgery may be performed to remove any obstruction.

When the client is able to void, a check for residual urine should be done. Immediately after the client voids, catheterization should be performed. The urine left in the bladder, **residual urine**, should be less than 50 mL.

URINARY INCONTINENCE

Urinary incontinence is the involuntary loss of urine from the bladder. The incontinence may be a complication of urinary tract problems or neurologic disorders and may be permanent or temporary. Medications such as sedatives, hypnotics, diuretics, anticholinergics, antipsychotics, and alpha antagonists may be associated with incontinence.

More than 13 million men and women in the United States experience incontinence, 11 million of whom are women (National Institute of Diabetes and Digestive and Kidney Diseases [NIDDK], 1998). This is not just a physiological problem but also affects the client's emotional, psychological, and social well-being. Incontinence can occur in clients of any age but is more common in the older adult. All types of incontinence can be treated at any age. At least 1 out of 10 persons age 65 or older has incontinence (National Institute on Aging, 1996). Incontinence is classified as stress, urge, overflow, total, or nocturnal enuresis.

STRESS INCONTINENCE

Stress incontinence is the most common type of incontinence. It is not a disease or a natural, inevitable effect of aging. Anyone can be affected; however, women are more likely to have this condition than men. In **stress incontinence** there is leakage of urine when a person does anything that strains the abdomen such as coughing, laughing, jogging, dancing, sneezing, lifting, making a quick movement, or even walking.

Medical management depends on the underlying cause. Stress incontinence often can be cured and nearly always can be substantially alleviated (Sasso, 1998). Treatment may include bladder retraining, medicines such as conjugated estrogens (Premarin Vaginal Cream), or surgery. Surgery may be necessary to restore the support of the pelvic floor muscles or to reconstruct the sphincter but is used after other treatments are unsuccessful. Another possible treatment is having collagen injected into the tissues surrounding the urethra. This closes the urethra enough to prevent urine from leaking out. The procedure is done in a nonsurgical outpatient setting. Several support prostheses and external barriers are now available (Sasso, 1998).

The client can be taught pelvic floor exercises (Kegel) to strengthen the muscles, thereby preventing or minimizing stress incontinence. Kegel exercises involve having the client tighten the pelvic floor muscles to stop the flow of urine when urinating, and then releasing the muscles to start the flow of urine again. Once the client can do this, the exercise may be done anytime, anyplace. Practicing the exercise 10 times, 7 or 8 times a day strengthens the muscles.

Bladder retraining begins with assessing the client's voiding pattern and encouraging the client to void 30 minutes before the projected time of incontinence. The schedule is extended until the client can stay dry for 2 hours, gradually increasing the time between voidings until a 3- to 4-hour schedule is achieved.

URGE INCONTINENCE

Urge incontinence occurs when a person is unable to suppress the sudden urge or need to urinate. Sometimes urine may leak without any warning. An irritated bladder is often the cause. Infection or very concentrated urine may irritate the bladder.

Treatment includes clearing up an infection, if present, and encouraging the client to have a fluid intake of 3,000 mL/day. This prevents the urine from becoming concentrated. Less fluid does not prevent incontinence but may promote infection.

OVERFLOW INCONTINENCE

When the bladder becomes so full and distended that urine leaks out, it is called **overflow incontinence**. This occurs when a blocked urethra or bladder weakness prevents normal emptying. The blockage may be an enlarged prostate. The distended bladder cannot contract with enough force to expel a stream of urine. Bladder weakness occurs most often in persons who have diabetes, drink a large quantity of alcohol, and have decreased nerve function. Bladder retraining may alleviate the situation.

TOTAL INCONTINENCE

When no urine can be retained in the bladder, it is termed total incontinence. The client may be able to manage with an indwelling catheter. A neurologic problem is usually the cause. Surgery to make a temporary or permanent urinary diversion may be required.

NOCTURNAL ENURESIS

Incontinence that occurs during sleep is called **nocturnal enuresis**. Limiting fluid intake after 6 P.M. will help the client remain continent during the night. However, the total fluid intake for the 24 hours should remain the same. The bladder should be emptied immediately before going to bed.

INFECTIOUS DISORDERS

Infectious disorders of the urinary system are called urinary tract infections (UTIs). There are two types: lower UTIs affect the bladder (cystitis) and urethra, while upper UTIs affect the kidneys (pyelonephritis, and acute and chronic glomerulonephritis) and ureters.

CYSTITIS

Cystitis is an inflammation of the urinary bladder. It is more common in females because of their short urethra, which allows bacteria to ascend through the urethra from the vagina or rectum to the urinary bladder. Also, bacteria from an infected kidney can descend through the ureter into the urinary bladder. The majority of urinary tract infections are caused by *Escherichia coli*, but some are caused by *Candida albicans*. Other common causes of cystitis are coitus, prostatitis, and diabetes mellitus.

As women age, pelvic floor muscles relax, leading to a decreased ability to empty the bladder completely. This contributes to stasis of urine and promotion of bacterial growth, as in pregnancy or benign prostatic hypertrophy. In men, cystitis usually occurs secondary to another infection such as epididymitis or prostatitis.

Once bacteria enter the bladder, they multiply, causing redness and swelling of the wall of the bladder. These changes give rise to urinary frequency, dysuria, pyuria, hematuria, and sometimes burning and urgency with urination. These symptoms increase as the bladder distends with even a small volume of urine.

A clean-catch midstream urinalysis showing a bacteria count greater than 100,000 organisms/mL confirms

GERONTOLOGICAL CONSIDERATIONS

Elderly Clients and UTIs

- Ten percent to 20% of people over age 65 have bacteriuria (Marchiondo, 1998).
- Elderly clients are more prone to UTIs because of incomplete emptying of the bladder, fecal incontinence with perineal soiling, and a decrease in urine acidity.
- Incomplete emptying of the bladder in women is caused by bladder or uterine prolapse or loss of pelvic muscle tone; in men it is caused by an enlarged prostate gland.

the diagnosis. The microscopic examination of the urine will also show hematuria and pus.

Medical–Surgical Management

Medical

Treatment of cystitis includes medication and fluids. Recurrence of a urinary tract infection usually occurs when the bacteria are not effectively treated. Obtaining and sending a urine specimen for C & S before the administration of any urinary antimicrobial is necessary to determine the most effective medication. A repeat urinalysis after 2 or 3 days on medication will confirm its effectiveness. Chronic lower urinary tract infections are often a factor in the development of pyelonephritis.

Pharmacological

Cystitis treatment entails the use of antimicrobial medication in conjunction with urinary tract analgesics. Cystitis is generally treated with norfloxacin (Noroxin), nitrofurantoin (Furadantin), ciprofloxacin (Cipro), or sulfonamides such as sulfisoxazole (Gantrisin) or trimethoprim-sulfamethoxazole (Bactrim, Septra). It is necessary to determine whether the client is allergic to sulfonamides or penicillins before administering the medication. The antimicrobial ordered is determined by the results of the urine culture and sensitivity. The length of treatment is related to the type of cystitis, acute or chronic. Some physicians may order a single dose or short course (3 or 4 days) of antimicrobial therapy rather than the traditional 7- to 10-day course. A single-dose medication, fosfomycin (Monurol), is indicated exclusively for UTI treatment. Its antibacterial effect is sustained for up to 3½ days (Marchiondo, 1998). **Dysuria** (difficult or painful urination) related to a burning sensation when voiding can be alleviated with the use of the urinary tract analgesic phenazopyridine hydrochloride (Pyridium), which causes red-orange urine and stains clothing and toilets.

Diet

Fluids are to be encouraged. Clients are usually asked to drink between 3 and 4 liters of noncaffeinated fluid per day. The intake of meats and whole grains makes the urine more acid and may discourage the growth of bacteria in the urinary bladder. Drinking cranberry juice has been advised for years, but how it worked was not understood. It is now believed that the concentration of tannins in the juice prevents *E. coli* from sticking to cells lining the urinary tract (NKF, January, 1999).

Activity

Since cystitis causes frequency of urination, clients on bed rest or those in need of assistance to the bathroom must have the call light answered promptly. Clients on bed rest are generally not able to empty their bladder completely when using a bedpan. Orders for bathroom privileges or using a commode chair are encouraged. The nurse can help allay the client's fears of being incontinent with proper and timed bladder management.

▶ NURSING PROCESS

▶ Assessment

▶ Subjective Data

The client will usually describe having frequency or urgency of urination or nocturia. This becomes annoying and embarrassing, regardless of age or sex. Burning and pain when voiding are common reasons clients seek medical care. Even clients with an indwelling catheter may complain of dysuria, burning, and frequency. Clients often just do not feel well.

▶ Objective Data

Perineal irritation may be noticed when the client with a catheter pulls on it in hopes of alleviating the bladder pain. The urine will smell foul and appear cloudy. Hematuria may be present. The elderly population in particular may become anorexic and develop a low-grade fever. The urinalysis will indicate the presence of bacteria and the C & S will identify the specific microorganism causing the urinary tract infection and the medication to which the pathogen is most sensitive.

Nursing diagnoses for a client with cystitis may include the following:

Nursing Diagnoses	Planning/Goals	Nursing Interventions
▶ *Impaired Urinary Elimination related to urinary tract infection*	The client will return to usual pattern of urinary elimination.	Encourage a large amount of fluid intake, at least 3,000 mL each day, especially water and cranberry juice.
		Administer urinary tract analgesics and antimicrobial medications as ordered.
		Alert the client, if Pyridium is being taken, that the urine will be red-orange and will stain clothing.

continues

Nursing Diagnoses	Planning/Goals	Nursing Interventions
▶ *Deficient Knowledge related to treatment regimen and prevention of recurrence*	The client will comply with treatment regimen and practice preventive habits.	Discuss the importance of taking all medication ordered even after the symptoms are relieved.
		Teach or reinforce the following preventive measures.
		Clean the perineum from front to back.
		If nylon undergarments are worn, they should have a cotton crotch.
		Wearing tight-fitting jeans and taking long bike rides may be irritating to the perineum.
		Perfumed perineal products such as menstrual products, douches, powder, or bubble bath may also be contributing factors to bladder infections.
		Spermicidal contraceptive products can be irritating, thus encouraging a lower UTI.
		Advise the client to void more frequently and not keep urine in the bladder.
		Advise women to void after sexual intercourse.
		Teach the elderly person who uses incontinence control products, such as Attends®, to change the product frequently to prevent cystitis.
		When this client is hospitalized, plan time for frequent ambulation to the bathroom or commode chair.

Evaluation Each goal must be evaluated to determine how it has been met by the client.

PYELONEPHRITIS

Pyelonephritis is a bacterial infection of the renal pelvis, tubules, and interstitial tissue of one or both kidneys. This condition is also known as pyelitis or nephropyelitis. Bacteria generally ascend from the urinary bladder through the ureter and enter the kidney in the area known as the renal pelvis. The bacteria can also enter from the blood and lymph. Pyelonephritis can be secondary to ureterovesicular reflux (back flow of urine from the bladder into the ureters) or when urine cannot drain from the pelvis of the kidney because of an obstruction blocking the kidney or ureter. Pyelonephritis may also occur during pregnancy, with prostatitis, when bacteria are introduced during a cystoscopy or catheterization, or from trauma of the urinary tract. Pyelonephritis can be an acute illness or a chronic condition leading to the development of high blood pressure and/or chronic renal failure.

Escherichia coli is the microorganism most often cultured. The inflamed kidney becomes edematous and the renal blood vessels become congested. Sometimes abscesses form in the kidney. The urine is usually cloudy, containing mucus, blood, and pus.

Medical–Surgical Management

Medical

Diagnostic tests that may be ordered include an IVP, a urinalysis with a C & S, CBC, BUN, and serum creatinine. Urine specimens should be collected prior to the administration of the antimicrobial medication. Medical treatment and care are focused on preventing pyelonephritis from becoming chronic. Follow-up care and treatment may be necessary for up to 6 months.

Pharmacological

Pyelonephritis is generally treated with sulfonamides, such as trimethoprim-sulfamethoxazole (Bactrim) or the antimicrobial ciprofloxacin hydrochloride (Cipro). Cipro may not be indicated if the client has renal damage. Antipyretics are necessary for fever reduction and analgesics for pain management.

Diet

As with infections in general, the individual's diet should be light during the febrile stage. Fluids must be increased to 3,000 mL/day by mouth and supplemented intravenously when indicated.

Activity

The disease process will cause fatigue. Bed rest should be maintained during the acute phase of pyelonephritis. Diversionary activities are important while bed rest is ordered. When the client is allowed to be ambulatory, dizziness related to the analgesic medication taken for pain may be a problem.

▶ NURSING PROCESS

▶ Assessment

▶ Subjective Data

In acute pyelonephritis the client is acutely ill with malaise, urgency in urination, and pain during voiding and in the flank area. **Renal colic**, severe pain in the kidney that radiates to the groin, may occur, impairing urination. The client may complain of being hot, with or without chills. In chronic pyelonephritis, only a general symptom of nausea may be present. The client may be very anxious that this kidney infection will cause permanent kidney damage.

▶ Objective Data

Physical assessment may find the client tender on one or both sides of the lower back. Temperature, pulse, and respiratory rate may all be elevated. The urine is foul smelling and cloudy. The urinalysis results show bacteria and **pyuria** (pus in the urine), and the CBC indicates leukocytosis. The client with chronic disease will have the systemic signs of vomiting, diarrhea, and elevated blood pressure. Some clients with pyelonephritis may be asymptomatic.

Nursing diagnoses for a client with pyelonephritis may include the following:

Nursing Diagnoses	Planning/Goals	Nursing Interventions
▶ *Anxiety related to unknown prognosis*	The client will verbalize fears and concerns to family and health care team.	Encourage the client to verbalize fears and concerns. Use active listening and observe for behavioral signs of anxiety. Answer questions honestly.
▶ *Impaired Urinary Elimination related to urinary tract infection*	The client will regain normal urinary pattern.	Encourage drinking cranberry juice. Encourage 3,000 mL fluid intake per day, especially water. Monitor intake and output. The intake of fluids is important to maintain function of the urinary system. Evaluate kidney function by measuring and observing urine output and monitoring the results of blood and urine tests.
▶ *Deficient Knowledge related to disease process, treatment regimen, and prevention*	The client will verbalize understanding of disease process, treatment regimen, and preventive measures.	Teach or reinforce the hygiene measure of cleansing the perineum from front to back and practice this when doing perineal care on any client. Instruct the client on the importance of taking all the antimicrobial medication as prescribed in order to eliminate the bacteria. Teach the client to refrain from using perfumed perineal products such as menstrual pads, tampons, or douches, and avoid bubble baths and hot tubs because they can be irritating to the tissues of the genital area. Encourage the client to empty the bladder frequently to avoid distention. Promote rest periods, which aid the healing process. Inform the client to call the physician immediately if there is a decrease in urine output or signs of infection (elevated temperature, chills, flank pain, urgency, fatigue, nausea, and vomiting). Teach client to weigh daily and report sudden weight gain (2 pounds/week) to the physician. Emphasize the importance of keeping all appointments with the physician for follow-up care and when signs of infection appear. Teach the client the importance of long-term treatment and monitoring for chronic pyelonephritis.

Evaluation Each goal must be evaluated to determine how it has been met by the client.

ACUTE GLOMERULONEPHRITIS

Glomerulonephritis is a condition that can affect one or both kidneys. In both acute and chronic disease, the glomerulus within the nephron unit becomes inflamed. It is predominantly a disease of children and young adults when the cause is bacterial. The viral form can affect all ages. The prognosis for most clients is a full recovery; however, some may develop chronic glomerulonephritis. Approximately 1 to 2% of people having acute glomerulonephritis will develop end-stage renal failure (Beare & Myers, 1998). Acute glomerulonephritis during childhood is known as Bright's disease.

Most clients develop symptoms 1 to 3 weeks after an upper respiratory infection (tonsillitis or pharyngitis with fever) or skin infection caused most commonly by group A β-*hemolytic streptococcus*. The infection triggers an autoimmune response and the glomeruli are attacked by antibodies at the site of the glomerular basement membrane, resulting in inflammation. Some clients are asymptomatic.

Immunologic effects on the body are not completely understood. Direct effects on the glomeruli result in the reduced ability of the glomeruli to function. The glomeruli become more permeable, resulting in the loss of red blood cells and protein from the blood. These substances escape from the body in the urine. The inflammatory process causes thickening of the membrane of the glomeruli and potential scarring.

Diagnostic tests on blood and urine as well as KUB x-rays will be performed. BUN, serum creatinine, potassium, erythrocyte sedimentation rate (ESR), and antistreptolysin O titer (ASO titer) will be elevated. Urinalysis will show protein and red blood cells.

Medical–Surgical Management

Medical

Medical treatment must start as soon as the client is diagnosed in order to restore the kidneys to normal functioning. Management includes drug therapy, diet, and rest. Treatment is correlated with the blood pressure and the results of urine testing for red blood cells and protein. The client is not considered to be free from the disease until the urine tests negative for protein and red blood cells for 6 months. Prevention of renal complications as well as complications to cardiac and cerebral functioning is the focus of care.

Pharmacological

Prophylactic antimicrobial therapy may be administered. The drug of choice is penicillin. Diuretic and antihypertensive medication furosemide (Lasix) may be ordered. Corticosteroids, chemotherapeutic drugs such as cyclophosphamide (Cytoxan), and/or immunosuppressive agents such as azathioprine (Imuran) may be ordered to control the inflammatory response.

Plasmapheresis may be indicated if there is no response from other treatments. Between 150 and 400 mL of blood is removed from the client and put in a cell separator. Here the blood is divided into plasma and formed elements. The formed elements are mixed with a plasma replacement and returned to the client through a vein. Another technique filters the client's own plasma to remove a specific disease mediator (antibody) and then returns the plasma to the client.

Diet

Fluid retention often requires fluid restriction. The restriction is adjusted according to the client's intake and output record and daily weight. Protein in the client's diet will be regulated according to the BUN and the creatinine blood levels. The kidneys need to

rest; however, particularly in children, it may not be necessary to restrict protein. Potassium will need to be replaced if the diuretic promotes its excretion. Sodium may be restricted to prevent fluid retention. Strict intake and output are necessary to monitor kidney function.

Activity

Physical and emotional rest are essential. Compliance with bed rest may be difficult, especially for a child or the client who feels well. Bed rest is indicated until the inflammation subsides, urinary flow increases, and as long as the client has hematuria or proteinuria. During this time a strict turning schedule needs to be followed, as skin breakdown is more likely in the presence of edema. Once bed rest restrictions are lifted, the client may feel weakened from the effects of anemia and inactivity.

▶ NURSING PROCESS

▶ Assessment

▶ Subjective Data

The health history will likely reveal a recent sore throat, skin infection, flulike symptoms, and a headache. The client describes flank pain as the kidneys become congested. Other symptoms the client may describe are headache, malaise, anorexia, cola-colored "smokey" urine (hematuria), and a marked decrease in the amount of urine (oliguria). Facial edema may have been the first sign noticed, may impair vision, and may cause the client to have negative feelings about body image.

▶ Objective Data

Vital signs will generally show an increase in body temperature and blood pressure. Facial (periorbital) edema is present. The edema will progress to dependent areas such as the sacral area and the legs. The location and degree of edema is monitored daily. Ascites may also develop. The general condition of the skin and skin integrity should be assessed, and the client weighed to establish a baseline weight. Heart and lung sounds are assessed for signs of congestive heart failure

COMMUNITY/HOME HEALTH CARE

Sodium Restriction

Advise to use low-sodium bottled water in cooking and for the drinking allowance when water supplies are naturally high in sodium or if water is chemically softened.

and pulmonary edema (unusual heart sounds and crackles in the lungs). Neck veins may be distended. Dyspnea on exertion or when recumbent, and shortness of breath, may both be noted. Urine output is decreased and hematuria is present (cola-colored to red).

The nurse monitors results of diagnostic tests: urine for red blood cells and protein (albumin) and blood for BUN, serum creatinine, potassium, ESR, ASO titer, and specific gravity, all of which will be elevated.

Nursing diagnoses for a client with acute glomerulonephritis may include the following:

Nursing Diagnoses	Planning/Goals	Nursing Interventions
▶ *Fear related to potential permanent damage to the kidneys*	The client will communicate fears of kidney damage to the family and the health care personnel.	Provide client and family with ongoing support and understanding.
		Encourage the client to discuss fears.
		Explain the importance of protecting the client from other infections.
		Allow no one with an upper respiratory infection to visit the client.
		Discuss the importance of compliance with medications, bed rest, and diet to prevent permanent damage to the kidneys.
		Emphasize the importance of keeping the follow-up visits to the laboratory for tests and to the physician's office.
		Arrange consultation with social services to assist the client in arranging time off from work and to help the client and family with their financial needs.
▶ *Excess Fluid Volume related to compromised regulatory mechanism secondary to renal dysfunction*	The client will have decreased edema and adequate urinary output.	Fluids will be restricted with specific amounts designated throughout the day. For example, 900 mL of fluids for a day might be divided in the following manner: 7 A.M. to 3 P.M. 600 mL; 3 P.M. to 11 P.M. 200 mL; 11 P.M. to 7 A.M. 100 mL.
		Encourage compliance to the fluid amounts.
		Maintain accurate intake and output records hourly.
		Provide oral hygiene several times a day. This is extremely important when water intake is restricted.
		Advise that thirst may be relieved by sucking on hard candy or, if allowed, a few ice chips.
		Provide eye care with normal saline to promote comfort from the periorbital edema.
▶ *Impaired Social Interaction related to changes in body image*	The client will resume social interaction.	Encourage client to keep in contact with friends and relatives by telephone.
		Encourage keeping appointments with the physician and laboratory.
▶ *Imbalanced Nutrition: More than body requirements related to the disease process*	The client will comply with nutritional restrictions.	Once the client's condition warrants solid foods, provide diet with complex carbohydrates instead of foods with concentrated sugar.
		If hematuria and/or proteinuria are still present, provide a diet with mild to moderate protein restriction to rest the kidney tissue. Protein foods that may be restricted include meats, fish, poultry, eggs, milk products, and whole grains.
		If edema persists, provide low-sodium diet. Processed, canned, or frozen foods will be substituted with foods made with fresh ingredients.
		If a restricted sodium and protein diet are ordered, arrange a dietary consultation to incorporate food preferences and religious and/or cultural needs. Finances may be an issue if the family has to incorporate foods that are not usually part of its budget.
		Teach client to plan menus and to read food labels in order to comply with the dietary restrictions.
		Before discharge, teach client and family about diet, fluids, and activity restrictions and measuring fluid intake and urine output.
		Provide client with guidelines listing reasons to call the physician.

Evaluation Each goal must be evaluated to determine how it has been met by the client.

CHRONIC GLOMERULONEPHRITIS

The prognosis for acute glomerulonephritis is often good when treatment is begun early; however, chronic glomerulonephritis generally leads to permanent kidney damage. Those who develop chronic glomerulonephritis may have neither symptoms nor a recent history of an infection. Chronic diseases, such as diabetes mellitus or systemic lupus erythematosus, often mask renal symptoms and the client does not seek medical care until kidney function is impaired. It may take up to 30 years for the signs of renal insufficiency to develop.

Chronic glomerulonephritis is a progressive but slow, destructive process affecting the glomeruli, causing loss of kidney function. The kidney will actually decrease in size as glomeruli are destroyed. If end-stage renal disease (ESRD) develops, the client may die quickly.

Nephrons lose their ability to filter nitrogenous wastes from the blood. Protein (albumin) and red blood cells escape into the urine and are present on a urinalysis. Nitrogenous waste remains in the blood, and the blood urea nitrogen (BUN) level increases. As glomeruli are destroyed, the serum level of creatinine also increases. BUN and serum creatinine are checked on a regular basis to monitor renal function and to assist with client care management. Serum electrolyte levels are also monitored. Anemia will be evaluated with a CBC.

Medical–Surgical Management

Medical

Medical treatment must begin immediately to limit further destruction of the glomerular tissue. Management includes drug therapy, diet, and bed rest. Exposure of the client to infection of any kind must be avoided. Blood transfusion may be required for severe anemia. The client may need to be transferred to a facility where dialysis and/or kidney transplantation can be performed. Prevention of further renal damage as well as heart or cerebral complications is the focus of care.

Pharmacological

Diuretic and antihypertensive medications are ordered. Antimicrobial therapy is generally given prophylactically. Side effects from all medications are monitored for and reported to the physician immediately.

Diet

Fluid intake is adjusted according to urinary output. Protein allowed in the diet will be regulated according to the BUN and the creatinine blood levels. As these levels increase, protein will be restricted to decrease the nitrogenous wastes. Sodium and potassium restrictions will be determined by the serum electrolyte levels. Carbohydrates are usually increased in the diet to provide adequate energy.

Activity

Bed rest is indicated when the client has hematuria or albuminuria.

◗ NURSING PROCESS

◗ Assessment

◗ Subjective Data

Clients may complain of a morning headache, pruritis, a decreased ability to concentrate, fatigue, and dyspnea making it difficult to perform ADLs. Facial edema and/or blurring of vision, due to retinal edema, may also be reported by clients.

◗ Objective Data

As chronic glomerulonephritis develops, fluid retention becomes evident, leading to shortness of breath, especially at night. Vital signs are monitored, and hypertension is usually present. Lung sounds need to be assessed every shift for crackles, a sign of fluid retention. Weight is monitored daily, after the baseline weight is obtained, and the degree of edema, its location, and if it is pitting or nonpitting is noted. **Anasarca** is generalized edema that appears as the client's condition deteriorates. The skin is assessed for color, presence of ecchymosis or rash, dryness, and evidence of scratching. Mental functioning, irritability, tremors, ataxia, or slurred speech is noted.

As nephrons lose their ability to concentrate urine, the urine becomes pale and dilute. Intake and output must be closely monitored because initially, polyuria develops, giving the client a false sense that recovery will be soon. Results of blood and urine tests are monitored.

Nursing diagnoses for a client with chronic glomerulonephritis may include the following:

Nursing Diagnoses	Planning/Goals	Nursing Interventions
▸ *Impaired Urinary Elimination related to the failing kidney function*	The client will have adequate urine output.	Measure urine output hourly, or every 4 or 8 hours as ordered, to determine kidney function. Parameters will be set by the physician for immediate notification.
		Assess and document the color and consistency of the urine.
		Measure intake to determine compliance with the amount of fluids permitted.
		Weigh client daily at the same time each day, on the same scale and with the same clothes.
▸ *Excess Fluid Volume related to compromised regulatory mechanism*	The client will have decreased edema.	Assess and describe the location of the edema.
		Administer medications as ordered for treatment of the edema.
		Monitor electrolyte values.
		Maintain fluid intake at restricted amount.
		Document I & O.
▸ *Anxiety related to threat to or change in health status (potential treatment with dialysis)*	The client will communicate less anxiety about possible treatment with dialysis.	Assist client to express concerns about possible treatment with dialysis.
		Arrange for a dialysis nurse to visit client.
▸ *Risk for Impaired Skin Integrity related to immobility and edema*	The client will maintain skin integrity.	Assess skin every time the client is repositioned.
		Cleanse the skin frequently, especially when crystals of urea form on the skin, causing itching and dryness.

Evaluation Each goal must be evaluated to determine how it has been met by the client.

OBSTRUCTIVE DISORDERS

Disorders of this type include urolithiasis, urinary bladder tumors, renal tumors, and polycystic kidney.

UROLITHIASIS

More than 1 million persons in the United States each year have kidney stones (NKF, 1998b). **Urolithiasis** is a calculus, or stone, formed in the urinary tract. A calculus (plural–calculi) is a solid mass of mineral salts occurring within a hollow organ such as the renal pelvis, ureters, bladder, or urethra (Figure 29-2). A urinary calculus can range in size from microscopic to 10 to 20 mm in diameter.

Calculi are formed from minerals that precipitate out of solution and collect within hollow areas. The reason stones form has not yet been identified, but individuals who are immobile, hyperparathyroid, or have recurrent UTIs are predisposed. When a person is immobile for long periods, calcium is pulled from the bones into the blood. The nephrons filter the excess calcium out of the blood into the urine. Calculi can also lodge in and obstruct an indwelling catheter. The size and location of the stone within the urinary system greatly affects the degree of pain and other

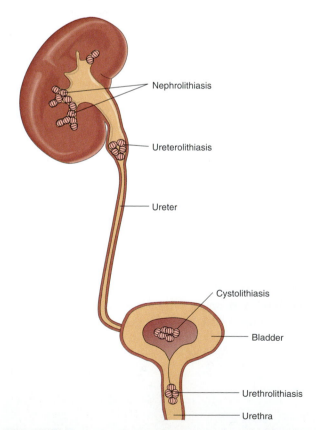

Figure 29-2 Common Locations of Urinary Calculi Formation

symptoms present. When the stone is in the kidney, the pain is dull and constant mainly in the back just below the ribs near the spine. Stones in the ureter often cause ureteral colic, an excruciating, intermittent pain that begins in the flank and radiates into the groin, inner thigh, or genitalia. It is caused by spasm of the ureter as the calculus moves down the ureter. The client often has nausea and vomiting also.

If a calculus becomes lodged any place along the ureter, the urine cannot pass and a condition called hydronephrosis and/or hydroureter occurs. The kidney and/or ureter become enlarged with the accumulated urine, as illustrated in Figure 29-3.

Tests to confirm the diagnosis and determine the size and location of the stone include KUB, IVP, cystoscopy, and ultrasound. A BUN and serum creatinine indicate whether the calculus has damaged kidney function. A urinalysis with a culture and a CBC may be ordered to determine whether an infection is present. A 24-hour urine may be sent to the laboratory to determine whether there is abnormal excretion of calcium oxalate, phosphorus, and uric acid.

Medical–Surgical Management

Medical

All urine must be strained whether voided or from an indwelling catheter drainage bag. Urine from a catheter drainage bag must be drained and strained every 2 to 4 hours. All strained particles are saved for the physician or sent to the laboratory.

A very small calculus may be flushed out by peristalsis and fluids. The client is encouraged to drink at least 4,000 mL of fluid/day, unless contraindicated by other health problems. The urologist may insert a small, pliable catheter into the ureter or urethra to allow temporary drainage of urine around the calculus.

Extracorporeal shock wave **lithotripsy** (ESWL) is a method of crushing a calculus any place in the urinary system with ultrasonic waves. The client is placed in a warm water bath and ultrasonic waves aimed at the stone break the stone into small pieces. An alternate method is to appropriately place a fluid-filled bag on the client's body and aim the ultrasonic waves at the stone through the bag. There is some discomfort and the client may be bruised where the ultrasonic waves hit the body. The urine will be slightly bloody for 24 to 48 hours and must be strained. The client should drink large amounts of fluids (3,000 mL to 4,000 mL/day) unless contraindicated. Clients should avoid taking aspirin and other drugs that affect blood clotting for several weeks before the procedure (NIDDK, 1998a).

Surgical

There are several surgical procedures, depending on the location and size of the calculus, from which the surgeon may choose. These include nephroscopic

Figure 29-3 Hydronephrosis and Hydroureter Resulting from a Stone in the Ureter

removal, pyelolithotomy, nephrolithotomy, or ureterolithotomy (Figure 29-4).

Percutaneous nephrolithotomy is the endoscopic procedure in which a small incision is made in the fleshy area on the client's side between the ribs and the hip. A catheter is inserted and an ultrasonic probe is inserted through the catheter. Ultrasound waves directed at the stone break it into small pieces that can be withdrawn through the catheter. The catheter is left in place until the edema subsides, usually 1 or 2 days.

A bladder calculus may be crushed with special surgical instruments and the fragments washed out through a catheter. This is called a **litholapaxy**.

Pharmacological

Narcotic analgesics are generally prescribed for the severe pain often called renal colic. Antispasmodics such as propantheline bromide (Pro-Banthine) or belladonna preparations may be ordered to relieve ureteral spasms. Antibiotics may be ordered prophylactically.

Drug therapy is specific to stone composition. Allopurinol (Zyloprim) reduces the serum urate level, thus preventing calcium oxalate stones. Sodium cellulose phosphate (Calcibind) binds with calcium in the bowel and facilitates excretion of calcium. Aluminum hydroxide gel (Amphojel) binds with excess phosphates in the gastrointestinal tract. The phosphates are then excreted.

Diet

Individuals who form calcium calculi may need to reduce their intake of dietary calcium, mainly dairy products, to no more than 600 mg/day. When the stones

Figure 29-4 Methods of Removing Urinary Stones: A. Nephroscopic removal (percutaneous nephrolithotomy); B. Pyelolithotomy, removal through the renal pelvis; C. Nephrolithotomy, removal through incision into the kidney; D. Ureterolithotomy, removal through the ureter

contain uric acid, purine-rich foods (meat, fish, and poultry) are restricted, and organ meats, anchovies, and sardines avoided. Foods rich in oxalic acid (broccoli, asparagus, chocolate, tea, rhubarb, and spinach) are restricted when oxalate stones form. A deficiency of pyridoxine, thiamin, and magnesium may also contribute to the formation of oxalate stones.

Sometimes an effort is made to change the pH of the urine and thus prevent the formation of calculi. Acid-ash or alkaline-ash diets are used. Acid-ash foods are meats, fish, poultry, eggs, cereals, cranberries, and plums. Alkaline-ash foods are vegetables and all other fruits. These diets are often difficult for the client to maintain.

Drinking large amounts of fluid, at least half of it water, dilutes the urine and helps move any micro-

scopic calculi through the system. Up to 4,000 mL/day of fluid is indicated for a client with renal calculi, unless contraindicated by another health problem such as congestive heart failure.

Activity

Exercising regularly helps reduce the formation of calculi and keeps calculi moving through the urinary tract. Clients on bed rest should perform active range-of-motion exercises daily in addition to frequent turning and positioning.

▶ NURSING PROCESS

▶ Assessment

▶ Subjective Data

Some individuals may be asymptomatic until the calculus begins to move or becomes too large. When the stone moves, the client usually describes intractable pain, that is, pain that is not relieved by ordinary measures. Nausea and vomiting are often reported also. The pain is often described as beginning in the flank and radiating down to the groin and inner thigh. Nonverbal client behaviors may indicate pain, such as tossing and turning when in bed or the inability to sit still when out of bed. If the calculus is not moving, the client may describe symptoms of infection such as lethargy, frequency of urination, dysuria, burning on urination, or feeling very warm. The client may express feelings of frustration related to the inability to complete daily tasks.

CLIENT TEACHING

Urinary System Calculi

A person with a family history of stones or who has had more than one stone is at risk to develop another stone. These clients can be instructed to:

- Drink plenty of fluids—water is best—to prevent stone formation,
- Avoid immobility,
- Take medications and modify diet as prescribed,
- Keep a record of intake and output, and
- Learn how to strain urine.

▶ Objective Data

Hematuria, vomiting, intake and output, and vital signs are assessed. Elevated pulse and blood pressure may indicate pain. Urine should be checked for stones when it is strained.

Nursing diagnoses for a client with urolithiasis may include the following:

Nursing Diagnoses	Planning/Goals	Nursing Interventions
▶ *Acute Pain related to irritation of the urinary tract and the mobility of calculi*	The client will verbalize a reduction in pain.	Develop a pain management plan. Inquire about intensity, location, duration, and alleviating factors of pain. Provide comfort measures and diversionary activities. Administer analgesics and antispasmodics as ordered. Observe for nonverbal signs of pain.
▶ *Impaired Urinary Elimination related to blockage of urine flow by the calculi*	The client will return to normal urine elimination.	Monitor urine for color and amount. Encourage fluids to dilute the urine and flush out the calculi. Assist client to ambulate, if able. Accurately monitor intake and output. If a ureteral catheter is in place, measure and record the urine output from it separately from the urine output from the bladder.

Evaluation Each goal must be evaluated to determine how it has been met by the client.

URINARY BLADDER TUMORS

According to the American Cancer Society estimates indicate approximately 54,200 new cases of urinary bladder cancer (ACS, 1999b). Men are affected 4 times more often than women. Bladder cancer occurs most frequently after the age of 50. The only early warning signs are increased urinary frequency and painless, intermittent hematuria. The main risk factor is cigarette smoking. Those individuals who smoke nicotine products have twice the risk of developing bladder cancer as do nonsmokers. Other risk factors are working with dyes, rubber, or leather products; caffeine intake; and the use of certain artificial sweeteners.

Benign papillomas are the most common urinary bladder tumor. Although the papillomas are quite small, they should be treated aggressively because they are considered to be premalignant. Cancer cells develop mainly in the area where the ureters enter the urinary bladder. The primary sites for metastasis are the liver, lungs, or bones. Symptoms resulting from ob-struction of the ureters is a frequent reason for the client seeking medical care. Diagnostic studies done usually include a urinalysis, a cystoscopic visualization and biopsy of the lesions, an IVP, and CT scan.

Medical–Surgical Management

Surgical

Surgical removal of small tumors is generally done by **fulguration** (a procedure to destroy tissue with long, high-frequency electric sparks) to burn the lesions off the internal bladder wall. Other surgical procedures used are laser surgery or snaring of the lesion. These procedures are usually performed with cystoscopic visualization. Several times a year, the client who has had bladder lesions should be monitored for recurrence of the lesions. A cytologic examination is done on any lesion(s) noted during a cystoscopic examination.

A cystoscopic examination is performed with either local anesthesia and sedation or general anesthesia. After the procedure, the client's legs may be sore as a lithotomy position is used. Analgesics will be prescribed for use as needed. After a cystoscopic procedure, the client may experience urinary frequency, burning on urination, and the presence of pink-tinged urine.

When the pathology of tissue specimens indicates a need for more extensive surgery, either a partial or total cystectomy may be performed. The surgery may be done in conjunction with radiation therapy or chemotherapy.

CULTURAL CONSIDERATIONS

Bladder Cancer

Caucasians are twice as likely to have bladder cancer as African Americans (ACS, 1999b).

When the urinary bladder is completely removed, a urinary diversion is necessary. Consideration is made for age, extent of the disease, and the prognosis. One option is a bilateral cutaneous ureterostomy, in which the ureters are implanted directly into the abdominal wall. Another option is for the ureters to be implanted into a piece of the ileum, which is then attached to the abdominal wall as a stoma. This is known as an **ileal** ("wet") **conduit**.

Other methods of urinary diversion are the implantation of the ureters into the sigmoid colon (ureterosigmoidostomy) and the creation of a continent stoma with a pouch of bowel. This urinary diversion is known either as a Kock (Figure 29-5) or Mainz pouch or a Gilchrist ileocecal reservoir, depending on which surgical procedure was used.

Pharmacological

One chemotherapy treatment is the instillation of an antineoplastic drug within the urinary bladder (**intravesical**). Systemic chemotherapy may also be used for cystectomy clients. Medications to relieve symptoms such as pain and nausea are important for the client's well-being.

Diet

If proctitis (inflammation of the rectum and anus) or diarrhea occurs, a low-residue diet is ordered to facilitate normal bowel elimination.

Activity

When the client is on bed rest, turning and positioning are important to maintain skin integrity because the client may be emaciated due to significant weight loss. Activity should be encouraged as the client's condition warrants. During the intravesical instillation of

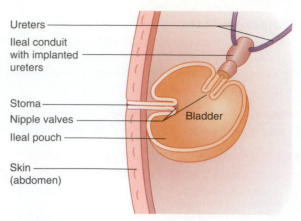

Figure 29-5 Urinary Diversion—Kock Pouch

an antineoplastic drug, the client will have to change positions every 15 minutes, for a period of several hours, to evenly distribute the chemotherapeutic drug around the urinary bladder.

▶ NURSING PROCESS

▶ Assessment

▶ Subjective Data

The client will describe having painless, intermittent hematuria and changes in voiding patterns. Fatigue may also be mentioned.

▶ Objective Data

Weakness will be noted if the client has become anemic from the hematuria. The nurse should check urine specimen with a reagent strip for blood, review results of diagnostic tests, and assess the client's understanding of current health situation.

Nursing diagnoses for a client with urinary bladder tumors may include the following:

Nursing Diagnoses	Planning/Goals	Nursing Interventions
▶ *Deficient Knowledge related to surgery and treatment regimen*	The client will describe surgical changes and treatment regimen.	If surgical removal of bladder lesions is done as an outpatient procedure, teach the client to observe for pink-tinged urine and to notify the physician if bright red urine is seen.
		Discuss the use of analgesics as ordered for pain of bladder spasms.
		Encourage adequate fluid intake.
		For urinary diversions: Refer the client with a stoma to the enterostomal therapist for specialized care and teaching. The therapist will assist the client with the appliance and skin care protocol.
		Monitor the color and integrity of the stoma daily to ensure that the tissue is receiving adequate circulation. The stoma is normally red and edematous for a time postoperatively. The stoma will remain red in color but will shrink in size during the healing process.
		If the stoma color changes, notify the physician.
		Refer to a local ostomy group for ongoing support and assistance or to the United Ostomy Association, which provides support and literature.
		Teach the signs and symptoms related to potential problems that should be reported to the physician.

continues

Nursing Diagnoses	Planning/Goals	Nursing Interventions
		Encourage the intake of fluids, up to 3,000 mL per day, unless contra-indicated.
		Teach about the medications to be taken at home.
		Encourage the client to attend all scheduled follow-up visits.
		Assist the client to plan the gradual return to the routines of driving, lifting, sexual activities, and work.
▶ *Impaired Urinary Elimination related to surgical procedure*	The client will maintain adequate urinary elimi-nation.	Accurately monitor urine output because this is the major postoperative concern.
		Assist client to discuss feelings about the altered urinary elimination method.
		Assist the client with a bilateral cutaneous ureterostomy to use leg bags for easier ambulation.
		Change the leg bag tubing back to straight bag drainage to promote uninterrupted sleep.
		Teach the client how to use both a leg bag and a straight bag drainage system.

Evaluation Each goal must be evaluated to determine how it has been met by the client.

RENAL TUMORS

The American Cancer Society estimates there will be approximately 30,000 new cases of kidney cancer in 1999 (ACS, 1999a). A unilateral renal adenocarcinoma is the most common tumor and is seen more often in men between the ages of 50 and 70. Risk factors include smoking, familial incidence, and preexisting renal disorders.

Intermittent, painless hematuria is often ignored by the client, and medical attention is not sought until the malignancy is quite advanced. By this time, the client usually has experienced weight loss, dull flank pain, gross hematuria, and a mass that may be palpable in the flank area. Lymph nodes in the area of the kidney, the renal vessels, and/or the inferior vena cava may become involved. The primary sites for metastases are the lungs, liver, brain, and bone. A pathological fracture may be the reason for admission of the client, resulting in the diagnosis of kidney cancer.

An IVP will detect a renal mass. Other diagnostic studies used to evaluate the kidney or the status of other body systems possibly involved are renal sonography or arteriogram, MRI, CT scan, or a needle biopsy. The

painless hematuria contributes to a decreased hematocrit.

Medical–Surgical Management

Medical

The physician may insert a nephrostomy tube into the renal pelvis of each kidney to evaluate the function of each kidney. Chemotherapy and/or radiation therapy have proved to be of minimal benefit.

Surgical

Usually a radical nephrectomy is performed if the other kidney is healthy and the disease is localized. The surgeon may enter the thoracic as well as the abdominal cavity during this procedure. If the chest is opened, the client will have a closed chest drainage system postoperatively. A nasogastric drainage tube may be in place and attached to suction. Hemorrhage and compromised respiratory effort are the postoperative problems for which to observe.

Pharmacological

If the client is receiving radiation therapy treatments, antiemetics or antispasmodics may be ordered. Analgesics are ordered to control pain and facilitate respirations and client activity. An antiemetic will usually be ordered to promote comfort and to encourage eating.

Diet

The client having a nephrectomy will have intravenous fluids until food can be tolerated. A well-balanced diet is then ordered. Fluid intake of at least 2,000 mL/day is needed to maintain adequate hydration. The use of alcohol should be avoided. If the client is **cachectic** (in a state of malnutrition and wasting) because of the cancer's pathology, parenteral nutrition may be indicated.

CULTURAL CONSIDERATIONS

Renal Cell Carcinoma

Those most at risk are:
- Hispanic men,
- Those exposed to leather, cadmium, asbestos, lead, and petrochemical products at their job, and
- Those with a family history of bilateral kidney disease (McKinney, 1996).

Activity

Ambulation is to be encouraged during the client's recovery. Frequent rest periods are also necessary even after discharge.

▶ NURSING PROCESS

▶ Assessment

▶ Subjective Data

The client will mention having a dull pain in the flank area and noticing blood in the urine intermit-tently. However, the client often comments that there is no difficulty in urinating. Fatigue and weight loss are also described.

▶ Objective Data

Weight is compared with usual weight. Vital signs and diagnostic test results are monitored. The client's lung sounds are assessed for possible respiratory distress resulting from metastases. Hematuria may be seen. A mass may be palpated in the client's flank area.

Nursing diagnoses for a client with renal tumors may include the following:

Nursing Diagnoses	Planning/Goals	Nursing Interventions
▶ *Fatigue related to disease process and treatment*	The client will understand reason for fatigue and not feel guilty for taking rest periods.	Discuss with client that fatigue is a result of blood loss in the urine and growth of the tumor.
		Because there is increased fatigue following any surgery, plan nursing care so the client will have several periods of uninterrupted rest each day.
▶ *Anticipatory Grieving related to diagnosis, treatment, and prognosis*	The client will maintain open communications with family and health care members.	Actively listen to what the client says.
		Encourage the client to express feelings about the diagnosis and treatment.
		Observe for signs of grieving such as crying, denial, anger, or withdrawal.
		Answer questions honestly.
		Assist client in identifying strengths and coping skills.
		Make referrals to other professionals as needed.
▶ *Deficient Knowledge related to limited information of disease process and treatment regimen*	The client will verbalize understanding of information taught.	Inform the client of the assessments to be done: neurological status, lung sounds, the incision, Homans' sign, peripheral pulses, vital signs, and serum electrolyte values.
		Teach the importance of accurate intake and output records.
		Provide routine preoperative teaching.
		Encourage the client to eat a well-balanced diet to enhance healing.
		Instruct the client not to wash off the skin markings if radiation therapy is being used.
		Teach the name, purpose, dosage, schedule, and side effects of all medications and the importance of drinking plenty of fluids and ambulating as tolerated.
		Inform the client and family of community resources and support groups.
		Point out the importance of following the instructions for care when discharged and keeping physician appointments.

Evaluation Each goal must be evaluated to determine how it has been met by the client.

POLYCYSTIC KIDNEY

Polycystic kidney disease (PKD) may be inherited or acquired. Acquired cystic kidney disease (ACKD) is associated with dialysis and end-stage renal disease. Approximately 90% of clients on dialysis for 5 years develop ACKD (NIDDK, 1998a). In PKD, multiple grape-like clusters of fluid-filled cysts develop in and greatly enlarge both kidneys. They compress and eventually replace functioning kidney tissue. PKD has an insidious onset that becomes obvious between 30 and 50 years of age.

Early symptoms include hypertension, polyuria, and urinary tract infections. Flank pain and headache are common. Recurrent hematuria and proteinuria develop. Diagnosis is made by x-ray or sonogram showing the cysts. BUN and creatinine are used to monitor kidney function.

The goal of medical management is to preserve kidney function, prevent infections, and relieve pain. Hypertension is carefully managed with antihypertensive medications, diuretics, and fluid and dietary modifications. Eventually, dialysis or renal transplantation may be needed.

RENAL FAILURE

According to NIDDK (May, 1999), any acute or chronic loss of kidney function is called renal failure and is the term used when some kidney function remains. Total, or nearly total, and permanent kidney failure is called end-stage renal disease (ESRD). It may take only a few days or weeks to lose renal function or it may deteriorate slowly over decades. Disorders of renal failure are either acute or chronic.

ACUTE RENAL FAILURE

The rapid deterioration of renal function with rising blood levels of urea and other nitrogenous wastes (**azotemia**) is termed acute renal failure (ARF). The nephrons also are unable to regulate the fluid and electrolyte or the acid-base balance of the blood. Predisposing factors include acute glomerular disease; severe, acute kidney infection; decreased cardiac output; trauma; or hemorrhage.

There are three major forms depending on the location of the cause: postrenal ARF (disrupted urine flow), prerenal ARF (disrupted blood flow to the kidney), and intrarenal ARF (renal tissue damage). Both postrenal ARF and prerenal ARF are reversible situations if they are identified early and treatment is begun. Undiagnosed postrenal ARF and prerenal ARF lead to intrarenal ARF.

POSTRENAL ARF

Postrenal ARF is caused by an obstruction and makes up approximately 5% of all ARF cases (Kelley, 1997). It should be checked out first when a client has an unexplained decrease in urine output or has anuria. Kidney function can be easily restored by removing the obstruction. Urine volume will vary depending on the location and degree of obstruction. Catheterization, ultrasound, and retrograde pylogram are used to diagnose an obstruction. An obstruction may be caused by renal calculi, blood clots, edema, tumors, urethral strictures, benign prostatic hypertrophy (BPH), or pregnancy. Postrenal failure can be ruled out if there is no obstruction. If an obstruction is confirmed, relief of the obstruction is imperative to minimize renal

damage and resolve azotemia. When postrenal failure is prolonged, both blood creatinine and BUN will rise.

PRERENAL ARF

Any abnormal decline in kidney perfusion that reduces glomerular perfusion can cause prerenal failure. Fluid volume status does not indicate perfusion. Effective arterial blood volume (EABV) is the amount of fluid in the vascular space that effectively perfuses the kidneys. Even in fluid volume excess situations, such as low cardiac output due to heart failure, the EABV falls, causing prerenal failure. The kidney interprets a fall in EABV as fluid volume deficit.

The glomeruli are then unable to filter waste from the blood. The renal tubules are structurally intact, and the kidneys can resume normal functioning if perfusion is restored fairly quickly. Ischemia results from prolonged inadequate perfusion, which can cause acute tubular necrosis (ATN).

The client generally has pale, cool skin; orthostatic hypotension; and oliguria. The BUN-to-creatinine ratio rises from 10:1 to more than 20:1. This rise is because there is greater reabsorption of urea when fluids flow slowly through the tubules. A urinalysis shows a low sodium level (less than 20 mEq/L), high osmolality (more than 500 mOsm/L), and high specific gravity (more than 1.020). This results because the kidneys are retaining sodium and water in an attempt to correct the perceived fluid volume deficit.

When the client truly has a fluid volume deficit, treatment consists of intravenous fluids and albumin, plasma, or blood to restore the EABV. When the cause is inadequate cardiac output, inotropic agents such as dobutamine hydrochloride (Dobutrex) or amrinone lactate (Inocor) are ordered.

INTRARENAL ARF

Tissue damage of the glomeruli and/or tubules causes a loss of renal function known as intrarenal ARF. Glomerulonephritis and ATN are the main reasons for renal tissue damage. The antigen/antibody complexes formed in glomerulonephritis become trapped in the basement membrane where they cause inflammation. The glomeruli then become more permeable so red blood cells and protein are allowed to enter the filtrate and ultimately the urine.

The majority of all intrarenal failure cases is caused by ATN, and is the most common cause of nosocomial acute renal failure. ATN is the result of ischemia or toxic insult to the renal tubules. Ischemia may result from untreated prerenal failure or severe hypoxemia. Radiographic contrast dye, pigments (myoglobin and hemoglobin), aminoglycoside and cephalosporin antibiotics, and NSAIDs are all **nephrotoxic** (substances that causes kidney tissue damage) and can cause acute tubular necrosis.

The BUN-to-creatinine ratio in acute tubular necrosis is usually normal between 10:1 and 15:1; however, both the BUN and creatinine are greatly elevated. For example, the BUN may be 70 mg/dL and the creatinine 7 mg/dL. Urine sodium is more than 40 mEq/L, urine osmolality less than 300 mOsm/L, and specific gravity less than 1.010.

There are three phases to the clinical course of ATN: oliguric/nonoliguric, diuretic, and recovery. The first phase is either oliguric or nonoliguric depending on the causative factor.

Oliguric/Nonoliguric Phase

A nonoliguric phase is usually seen when nephrotoxic agents are the causative factor. When adequate urine output is maintained, dialysis is needed less often and the morbidity and mortality rates are lower.

An oliguric phase, which may last 1 to 2 weeks, is seen more often when ischemia is the causative factor. Oliguria, voiding less than 400 mL/24 hours, can cause fluid volume overload; electrolyte imbalance, specifically high potassium and phosphorus, and low sodium and calcium; metabolic acidosis; and uremia.

Diuretic Phase

The diuretic phase is seldom seen because early dialysis keeps extracellular fluid volume at a fairly normal level. If it were seen, there would be a tremendous increase in urine output.

Recovery Phase

As renal function begins to improve, the client's urine output returns to normal and serum and urine laboratory test values move closer to normal. There is usually a short period of rapid improvement and then a period (may be several months) of slower improvement. Some clients will have residual renal insufficiency and a few will require long-term dialysis.

Medical–Surgical Management

Medical

Acute renal failure is often reversible, and complications can be prevented with early diagnosis and treatment. The goal is to have kidney function stabilized and returned to normal. Problems to be alert for are fluid volume overload, electrolyte imbalances, metabolic acidosis, high rate of catabolism, uremia, hemotological abnormalities, and infection.

Dialysis is now an early treatment in ATN. Homeostasis is maintained while the cause of ATN is determined and treated. Permanent kidney damage may thus be averted. See the section on dialysis later in this chapter.

CLIENT TEACHING

Acute Renal Failure

Teach clients at risk for ARF (older clients; diabetic clients; and clients with renal, heart, or liver disease) to:

- Immediately report to health care provider signs of fluid retention, pain on urination, and changes in urine output (amount or appearance),
- Avoid chronic use of and high doses of NSAIDs,
- Follow sodium and fluid restrictions as prescribed, and
- Advise all health care providers of condition.

Surgical

The obstructions causing postrenal failure are often removed surgically. The exact procedure will depend on what type of obstruction is present and its location.

Table 29–2 DRUGS USED IN ACUTE RENAL FAILURE

DRUGS	NURSING RESPONSIBILITIES
Antihypertensives methyldopa (Aldomet) minoxidil (Loniten) clonidine HCl (Catapres) hydralazine HCl (Apresoline)	Monitor BP and pulse, weigh daily, monitor for postural hypotension and K, Na, Cl, and CO_2 levels, I & O.
Diuretics furosemide (Lasix) hydrochlorothiazide (HydroDiuril)	Monitor output, maintain fluid restrictions, weigh daily.
Cardiotonics/inotropics digoxin (Lanoxin) amrinone lactate (Inocor)	Assess apical pulse before giving, report blood level of digoxin, monitor BP and P, monitor blood level of potassium.
Phosphate-binding antacids aluminum hydroxide gel (Amphojel)	Administer wtih meals, assess for constipation.
Potassium exchange sodium polystyrene sulfonate (Kayexalate)	Monitor serum potassium, assess BP and P, and for constipation.
Electrolyte replacement calcitrol (Rocaltrol) calcifediol (Calderol)	Monitor blood calcium and phosphate levels, report metallic taste.

Pharmacological

Drugs used in the treatment of acute renal failure include antihypertensives, diuretics, cardiotonics (inotropics), phosphate-binding antacids, potassium-lowering agents, and electrolyte replacement. It is important to ensure that drugs used are not nephrotoxic. See Table 29–2 for drugs used in acute renal failure.

Diet

Restrictions generally include sodium, potassium, phosphorus, protein, and fluids. The amounts allowed are based on the laboratory tests results. Carbohydrates and fats are increased to be sure energy needs are met and protein will be spared as a source of energy. Clients with a high rate of catabolism often require total parenteral nutrition (TPN) to provide adequate nutrition.

Activity

Because the client is often weak and may also be confused, activity is restricted during the initial phase of acute renal failure. As recovery becomes evident, ambulation is begun.

▶ NURSING PROCESS

▶ Assessment

▶ Subjective Data

The client may have various complaints, including diarrhea; nausea, possibly with vomiting; swelling; loss of appetite; headache; increasing fatigue; and/or a change in mental alertness. Anxiety and fear related to "not knowing" what is happening is often expressed.

▶ Objective Data

Physical findings will depend on how far the disease process has progressed. Assess for hypertension, GI bleeding and/or bruising, reduction in urine output, anasarca, poor skin turgor, and dry mucous membranes because vomiting or diarrhea can cause dehydration. In a severe stage, the client may be drowsy and have muscle twitching and convulsions.

The BUN and serum creatinine will be elevated as are the serum electrolytes potassium and phosphorus. The serum electrolyte calcium will be low. Blood level of red blood cells will decrease as the production of erythropoietin decreases. Leukocyte level will increase in the presence of an infection.

Nursing diagnoses for a client with acute renal failure may include the following:

Nursing Diagnoses	Planning/Goals	Nursing Interventions
▶ *Excess Fluid Volume related to sodium and water retention*	The client will maintain a stable fluid volume.	Monitor BUN, creatinine, and serum electrolyte and protein levels.
		Accurately measure urine output, often on an hourly basis. Parameters are often set for notification of the physician.
		Weigh daily to identify weight gain related to fluid retention. One pound of weight gain is equivalent to 500 mL of retained fluid.
		Assess skin turgor, edema, BP, lung sounds, jugular vein distention, pulse and respiratory rate and quality.
		Provide fluids within the prescribed limits.
		Teach client about importance of fluid restrictions.
▶ *Impaired Nutrition: Less than body requirements related to anorexia, dietary restrictions, and increased catabolism*	The client will have stabilized weight within normal limits.	Arrange for a dietary consultation to provide food in keeping with the prescribed restrictions and client preferences, including cultural and religious factors.
		Suggest 6 small meals throughout the day.
		Offer antinausea medications before meals.
		Provide or assist with oral hygiene prior to meals.
		Monitor weight and serum albumin level weekly.
▶ *Anxiety related to the disease process*	The client will verbalize anxieties with the family and health care workers.	Establish rapport with the client.
		Maintain open communications to foster expression of anxieties.
		Listen to the client's concerns.

Evaluation Each goal must be evaluated to determine how it has been met by the client.

SAMPLE NURSING CARE PLAN

THE CLIENT WITH ACUTE RENAL FAILURE

Mr. Long, age 65, has had a history of heart trouble for several years. He is admitted because he has urinated very little for 2 days, he gets dizzy when he gets up from lying down, and he cannot get his shoes on because his feet are "fat." He states that he does not know what is happening to him. Results of laboratory tests are BUN 90 mg/dL, creatinine 4 mg/dL, urine sodium 15 mEq/L, and urine specific gravity 1.030.

Nursing Diagnosis 1 *Excess Fluid Volume related to sodium and water retention as evidenced by "fat feet," urine sodium 15 mEq/L, and urine specific gravity 1.030*

PLANNING/GOALS	NURSING INTERVENTIONS	RATIONALE	EVALUATION
Mr. Long will have reduced fluid volume excess.	Accurately measure and record intake and output.	Provides information about retention of intake.	Mr. Long's feet are no longer "fat." His urine sodium is 18 mEq/L and urine specific gravity is 1.027.
	Weigh Mr. Long daily—same time, scale, clothes.		
	Assess skin turgor, edema, BP, lung sounds for crackles.	Provides information related to presence of fluid in tissue, lungs, or vascular system.	
	Monitor BUN, creatinine, and serum electrolyte and protein levels.		
	Administer inotropics or cardiotonic medications as ordered.	Medications will strengthen heartbeat, which will give better perfusion to kidneys.	
	Provide fluids within prescribed limits.		

Nursing Diagnosis 2 *Anxiety related to disease process as evidenced by his statement that he does not know what is happening to him*

PLANNING/GOALS	NURSING INTERVENTIONS	RATIONALE	EVALUATION
Mr. Long will have less anxiety by understanding what is happening to him.	Establish rapport with Mr. Long.	Begins a nurse-client relationship.	Mr. Long says that he feels better knowing what is happening.
	Encourage him to express his fears and anxieties.	Some people need encouragement to express feelings.	
	Provide Mr. Long with information, at his level of understanding, about what is happening to his body, why I & O and weighing daily are	Understanding reduces anxieties.	

continues

important, and what the medications are supposed to do.

Nursing Diagnosis 3 *Impaired Urinary Elimination as evidenced by his urinating very little for 2 days and BUN–creatinine ratio of 22.5:1*

PLANNING/GOALS	NURSING INTERVENTIONS	RATIONALE	EVALUATION
Mr. Long will increase amount of urination to 1,200 mL/day.	Administer diuretics as ordered.	Diuretics increase water elimination by enhancing the excretion of sodium by the kidneys.	Mr. Long is urinating 1,000 mL/day. His BUN is 50 mg/dL and creatinine is 3 mg/dL.
	Accurately measure and record intake and output.	Provides information about movement of fluid through the body.	

CHRONIC RENAL FAILURE (END-STAGE RENAL DISEASE)

Chronic renal failure is a slow, progressive condition in which the kidney's ability to function ultimately deteriorates. This condition is not reversible. The kidneys have an amazing capability to perform effectively, even though most of the nephrons are destroyed.

Renal erythropoietin decreases, causing anemia. Hypertension, acidosis, and glucose intolerance usually are also present. Urea in the blood is extremely elevated. As the disease progresses, uremia develops.

There are three stages of chronic renal failure: reduced renal reserve, renal insufficiency, and end-stage renal disease (ESRD). Symptoms of reduced renal reserve are not apparent until more than 40% of the nephrons fail. A prolonged urine concentration test or a decline in glomerular filtration rate (GFR) may be the only evidence of reduced renal reserve. When 75% of the nephrons stop functioning, renal insufficiency occurs. BUN and creatinine are above normal, and the client may have nocturia and polyuria. The onset of ESRD occurs when at least 90% of the nephrons fail. BUN and creatinine levels rise, polyuria changes to oliguria, and severe fluid and electrolyte imbalances are evident.

When the kidneys become unable to filter blood, an alternate method for filtration is necessary. Lifetime dialysis becomes inevitable unless kidney transplantation is performed and is successful. Life expectancy varies with the initial cause of chronic renal failure and the person's overall health at the time of diagnosis.

According to the American Society of Nephrology, 361,031 persons in the United States have ESRD, with the number increasing approximately 8% each year (American Society of Nephrology [ASN], 1999). There are numerous causes of chronic renal failure. The 4 leading causes are diabetes mellitus 34%, hypertension 25%, glomerulonephritis 16%, and cystic kidney 4% (ASN, 1999). Nephrotoxic drugs, including some over-the-counter drugs, aggravate the situation.

The diagnosis is confirmed when the BUN is at least 50 mg/dL and the serum creatinine level is greater than 5 mg/dL.

 CULTURAL CONSIDERATIONS

End-Stage Renal Disease

- African Americans account for 30% of clients with ESRD but make up only 12% of the U.S. population.
- The leading cause of ESRD in African Americans is high blood pressure, accounting for approximately 40% of new cases in that population (NKF, 1998a).
- End-stage renal disease is 4 times greater in African Americans than in whites.
- ESRD is increasing rapidly among Native Americans because of the significant increase in the incidence of diabetes in this population (NIAID, 1998).

Medical–Surgical Management

Medical

Chronic renal failure is a multisystem disease process. See Table 29–3 for the effects of chronic renal failure on various body systems. Medical management focuses on preserving the remaining kidney function for as long as possible and preventing complications. This helps preserve the integrity of the person's life. Fluid retention increases the risk of complications such as edema (ascites), hypertension, and congestive heart failure. Electrolytes are monitored and regulated.

Table 29–3 EFFECTS OF CHRONIC RENAL FAILURE BY BODY SYSTEM	
SYSTEM	**EFFECT**
Urinary	Oliguria from renal insufficiency. Azotemia.
Blood	Anemia from decreased RBC production. Decreased platelet activity, causing bleeding tendency.
Cardiovascular	Hypervolemia and tachycardia. Hypertension and dysrhythmias from hyperkalemia.
Respiratory	Dyspnea, pulmonary edema. Hyperventilation from metabolic acidosis. Eventually Kussmaul respirations.
Gastrointestinal	Urea in the blood is converted to ammonia by the mouth, causing uremic halitosis. Hiccups, anorexia, and nausea from edema within the gastrointestinal tract.
Skin	Dry skin with pruritis from uremic frost (excretion of urea through the skin with an odor of urine). Pallor with anemia.
Nervous	Lethargy, headaches, confusion, impaired concentration with disorientation, depression, decreased level of consciousness, sleep disturbances, and uremic encephalopathy resulting in seizures and coma.
Sensory	Peripheral neuropathy with numbness and tingling of extremities with complaints of a prickly, crawling feeling in the feet and legs, especially at night.
Reproductive	Decrease in libido. Decreased sperm count. Amenorrhea. Impotence. Delayed puberty.
Musculoskeletal	Joint pain and muscle cramping. Bone demineralization from hypocalcemia.
Immune	Greater chance of infections from immunosupression. Decrease in antibody production.

Pharmacological

Antihypertensives such as methyldopa (Aldomet) and propranolol hydrochloride (Inderal) are used to control hypertension. Diuretics such as furosemide (Lasix) are used for treatment of fluid retention; anticonvulsants, phenytoin (Dilantin) to control seizures; antiemetics, prochlorperazine (Compazine) to control vomiting; and antipruritics, cyproheptadine hydrochloride (Periactin) to control itching may also be used. Calcium acetate (Phos-Lo) is used to lower the phosphate level in the blood; however, it can be constipating. A low renal erythropoietin level causing anemia is often treated with epoetin alpha (Epogen). An iron supplement is used to decrease the anemia-related symptoms. Multivitamins with folic acid are used because dialysis promotes the loss of water-soluble vitamins.

Diet

Diet restrictions are similar to those in acute renal failure. Sodium, potassium, phosphorus, and protein are restricted. Fluids are also limited. Modifications are made as kidney function deteriorates. With consistent compliance, symptoms decrease, resulting in fewer complications. Resources are available for clients to obtain assistance with dietary restrictions. Meal ideas are published in newsletters like *NephroNotes*. Long-term dietary compliance is a challenge, and daily activities as well as special events during the year are a continual reminder of the client's dietary restrictions. As with other chronic diseases, those with renal failure need to have all members of their family and their friends encouraging them to adapt to their restrictions. Dietitians can assist the family to incorporate religious and cultural dietary practices. The person with chronic renal failure may also have to incorporate dietary guidelines for additional diagnoses such as diabetes mellitus and/or coronary artery disease.

With the progression of chronic renal disease, dialysis becomes necessary. Fluid restrictions must be adhered to and the amount allowed divided throughout the day. The greatest amount of fluid should be allowed during the day, incorporating enough fluids with oral medications. Some fluids should be planned for the evening meal, with a small amount to be allowed during the night; for example, days—500 cc, evenings—200 cc, and nights—100 cc. Protein restriction is closely monitored and regulated with the blood albumin level. The development of hyperkalemia will lead to a diet restricted in potassium. Foods high in potassium include dried fruits or dried beans and peas, peanuts, bananas, sweet potatoes, spinach, products with tomatoes, oranges, chocolate, artichokes, avocados, pumpkins, and mushrooms.

Activity

The client is encouraged to participate in activities of daily living. Safety becomes a significant factor during periods when the client has weakness, fatigue, or mental confusion. Confusion is seen in clients who have uremic encephalopathy. When bed rest is required, turning, ROM activities, and skin care are important. As symptoms continue to become more severe, the client will need total assistance for all the ADLs.

▶ NURSING PROCESS

▶ Assessment

▶ Subjective Data

The nurse inquires about the client's past medical history including the treatments for maintenance of renal disease. A complete medication history is taken, including the use of over-the-counter drugs. Description of fatigue, joint pain, severe headaches, nausea, anorexia, some chest pain, intractable singultus (hiccups), decreased libido, menstrual irregularities, and impaired concentration will be given by the client. The client may feel uncomfortable talking directly to the nurse if uremic halitosis is a problem.

▶ Objective Data

Changes in the client's neurological status such as reduced alertness and awareness should be noted. Kussmaul respirations appear as coma develops. Halitosis with a urine odor and "uremic frost," a white powder on the skin, result from the accumulation of urates.

Nursing diagnoses for a client with ESRD may include the following:

Nursing Diagnoses	Planning/Goals	Nursing Interventions
Excess Fluid Volume related to compromised renal mechanism	The client will understand the importance of prescribed (restricted) fluid amounts.	Monitor daily weight, intake and output (maybe hourly), skin turgor, edema, blood pressure, respirations, and lung sounds.
		Provide prescribed amounts of fluids.
		Teach client to plan nutritional and fluid intake within the prescribed amounts.
		Monitor laboratory reports for serum albumin level and serum electrolyte levels.
Imbalanced Nutrition: Less than body requirements related to dietary restrictions, GI distress, anorexia	The client will stabilize weight within normal limits and participate in dietary plan.	Provide or assist with complete mouth care before meals because uremic halitosis leaves a metallic taste in the client's mouth.
		Provide a clean, quiet, odor-free environment for meals.
		Suggest 6 small meals throughout the day.
		Arrange a consultation with the dietitian to plan alternate ways to prepare foods allowed on the diet.
		Ask the family to bring favorite foods, within the dietary restrictions, from home.
		Encourage self-feeding.
		Administer antiemetics 30 minutes before meals to control nausea.
		Suggest using herbs for flavoring instead of salt or salt substitutes, which often contain potassium.
Risk for Impaired Skin Integrity related to altered metabolic state leading to pruritis from "uremic frost"	The client will maintain skin integrity.	Bathe skin frequently to remove "uremic frost."
		Encourage the use of emollients and lotions on the skin.
		Administer antihistamines, as ordered, for the temporary relief of itching.
		Assist the client to change position every 2 hours.
		Provide an eggcrate mattress or Clinitron bed.
Ineffective Individual Coping related to uncertainty of long-term compliance of the treatment regimen	The client will verbalize feelings and intention to comply with treatment.	Encourage the client to discuss feelings about long-term lifestyle changes.
		Refer client to the local office of the National Kidney Foundation for information about client services and treatments for diseases of the kidney.
		Include the client and family in rehabilitation and discharge planning to ensure compliance. Topics for these sessions include diet, rest, medications, fluid restrictions, intake and output, activities, dialysis, required lab tests, and frequent visits to the physician.
		Incorporate into the discharge planning and teaching the client's socioeconomic needs, cultural background, role in the family unit, accessibility to medical care, and anticipated follow-up care.

continues

Nursing Diagnoses	Planning/Goals	Nursing Interventions
		Complete referrals prior to discharge in order to lessen client anxiety.
		Consider future needs of a newly diagnosed client with end-stage renal disease and include the availability of dialysis, vocational rehabilitation, home health care, financial assistance with medical needs, and psychological therapy for the client and family.

Evaluation Each goal must be evaluated to determine how it has been met by the client.

DIALYSIS

As the kidneys continue to deteriorate, nitrogenous waste products accumulate in the circulatory system. These waste products then need to be removed artificially with dialysis. **Dialysis** is a mechanical means of removing nitrogenous waste from the blood by imitating the function of the nephrons. It involves filtration and diffusion of wastes, drugs, and excess electrolytes and/or osmosis of water across a semipermeable membrane into a dialysate solution. The **dialysate**, a solution designed to approximate the normal electrolyte structure of plasma and extracellular fluid, is prescribed specific to the individual client's needs.

There are two types of dialysis: hemodialysis and peritoneal dialysis. These treatments can be obtained throughout the country at dialysis centers or at hospital dialysis units.

Hemodialysis

Hemodialysis is performed by a machine with an artificial semipermeable membrane used for the filtration of the blood. This machine is often referred to as an artificial kidney. A graft or fistula is surgically prepared to access the client's circulatory system. Figure 29-6 illustrates several ways this can be done. Research and development is improving the quality of graft materials. With each hemodialysis treatment, a catheter is inserted into the graft or fistula. The client's blood is circulated through the semipermeable membrane. Excess fluids are removed by osmosis and by-products of protein metabolism, especially urea and uric acid, as well as creatinine, drugs, and excess electrolytes, are removed from the blood by diffusion or filtration. In return, the client receives fluids, electrolytes, and blood products, as necessary. The solution (dialysate) is especially prescribed to meet the client's metabolic needs.

For the entire process, Standard Precautions must be followed and strict asepsis maintained. The client should be weighed before and after each dialysis session to determine if fluid is being retained. It is important to keep the client comfortable and provide diversionary activities during the treatment. Hemodialysis is usually performed 3 times a week and takes 3 to 6 hours each time.

CLIENT TEACHING

Dialysis
Clients who are receiving dialysis need a significant amount of teaching. All clients should have the process thoroughly explained. Other teaching topics are the importance of doctor and laboratory visits, and observations for which the doctor needs to be notified. Clients undergoing dialysis should wear Medic Alert tags stating their condition.

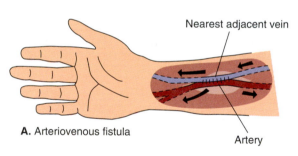

A. Arteriovenous fistula

Edges of incision in artery and vein are sutured together to form a common opening.

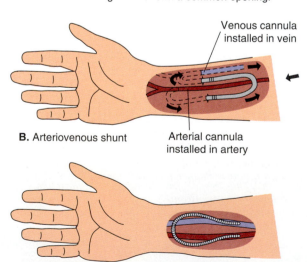

B. Arteriovenous shunt

C. Arteriovenous vein graft

Ends of natural or synthetic graft sutured into an artery and a vein.

Figure 29-6 Hemodialysis Access Sites

PROFESSIONAL TIP

Dialysate

To decrease client discomfort, the dialysate should be at body temperature and not instilled too rapidly.

PROFESSIONAL TIP

Nutrition for Dialysis Clients

- Optimal protein intake for maintenance adult hemodialysis clients is 1.2g/kg body weight/ day.
- Optimal protein intake for chronic peritoneal dialysis clients is 1.3g/kg body weight/day.
- Optimal energy intake (fats and carbohydrates) for adult dialysis clients 60 years old or less is 35 Kcal/kg body weight/day; clients over 60 years of age is 30–35 Kcal/kg body weight/day.
- Calories from peritoneal dialysis fluid must be taken into account when figuring the total energy intake for those clients (NKF, May 1999).

The graft or fistula site requires strict aseptic care and must be assessed daily for signs of infection: redness, swelling, or drainage. Circulation through the site is assessed by palpation or feeling the area and/or listening with a (Doppler) stethoscope. A thrill should be felt and/or a bruit should be heard. Lack of these may indicate a blood clot, which requires immediate surgical attention. Patency must be documented. Pulses peripheral to the graft site must also be assessed.

Blood pressure and blood draws should never be done on the extremity where the graft or fistula is placed. Also, restraints or intravenous solutions should never be applied to or inserted into that extremity. All health care personnel should be made aware of the location of the hemodialysis access site. These sites should not be used for any other purpose than dialysis.

Since most medications are removed during dialysis, they are generally not administered until after the dialysis session. Vancomycin hydrochloride (Vancocin) is not removed during dialysis and so is often used. If the client is hypertensive before dialysis, nifedipine (Procardia) is given because of its fast action.

Possible complications include hemorrhage, infection, and emboli formation. Some factors for the client and family to consider about hemodialysis are the distance they must travel to the dialysis center, the expense, the time involved, and the presence of a permanent arteriovenous (AV) line. Clients can be taught to do their own hemodialysis at a center. Portable units are being developed to make hemodialysis more usable in the client's home. This is a growing trend with home health care.

Peritoneal Dialysis

Peritoneal dialysis uses the peritoneal lining of the abdominal cavity as the membrane through which diffusion and osmosis occur instead of the artificial kidney machine. It is usually performed 4 times a day 7 days a week. A Tenckhoff or a flanged-collar catheter is placed by the physician, under aseptic conditions, into the client's peritoneal space. The client must void just before catheter insertion to prevent accidental puncture of the bladder. As with hemodialysis, the client should be weighed before and after each dialysis session. The nurse also checks bowel sounds.

The dialysate, held within a sterile soft container similar to an IV bag, is instilled aseptically through the catheter into the abdominal cavity. To decrease client discomfort, the dialysate should be at body temperature and not instilled too rapidly. Severe pain should not be experienced. The container, still connected to the catheter, is then rolled up and the dialysate remains in the abdominal cavity for a specified length of time. The client is free to ambulate during this time. The container is then unrolled and lowered below the abdominal cavity to allow the dialysate to drain, by gravity, back into the container. The dialysate now contains excess fluids, nitrogenous waste, and other impurities. The outflow of dialysate is inspected for color, sediments, and amount. The fluid should be light yellow and clear enough to read the printing on the bag when placed on a white towel. Usually 2 liters of dialysate are exchanged each time. If the outflow does not at least equal the inflow, the client is asked to turn from side to side to increase the outflow.

Peritoneal dialysis may be performed manually by the nurse, client, or family member as just described; by a cycler machine; or by continuous ambulatory peritoneal dialysis (CAPD). The cycler machine automatically completes dialysis after sterile setup and connection CAPD is performed by the client. After the dialysate is aseptically installed, the empty bag is rolled up under the clothing, and the client can go about normal activities. Every 6 to 8 hours, the solution is drained into the bag, which is then discarded following standard precaution guidelines. A new bag of dialysate is attached and instilled. This provides continuous dialysis 24 hours per day, 7 days per week. The client's lifestyle is only minimally disrupted. Peritoneal dialysis is less expensive, easier to perform, less stressful for the client, and almost as effective as hemodialysis.

The main complication of peritoneal dialysis is infection. Strict aseptic care of the catheter site is necessary. Standard Precautions are essential in caring for the dialysis client. Figure 29-7 shows a peritoneal dialysis setup.

Figure 29-7 Peritoneal Dialysis Setup

KIDNEY TRANSPLANTATION

According to the National Kidney Foundation (1998b) 11,460 kidney transplants were performed in 1997. Transplants are either from a live donor (usually a relative) or a cadaver. As of September 1998, there were 80,000 persons on the waiting list for a kidney transplant.

Prior to being placed on the nationwide donor waiting list, the client with ESRD must be tissue- and blood-typed to determine a compatible donor. Insurance coverage varies for this procedure. Lack of funds does not exclude anyone from needed care. Since 1973, an amendment to the Social Security Act allows Medicare to pay 80% of the cost for treating ESRD clients, regardless of age, including dialysis and kidney transplantation.

At the time a donor kidney becomes available, the client must be transported to the transplant medical center. The donor kidney can be preserved for 36 hours in solution or up to 72 hours if it is attached to an irrigating pump with perfusion maintained while en route to the recipient. Through a lower abdominal incision, the surgeon attaches the donor kidney to the client's blood supply. The donor kidney is usually placed in the iliac fossa anterior to the iliac crest. The donor ureter is anastomosed (surgical connection of tubular structure) to the client's ureter or surgically implanted into the client's urinary bladder. Generally, the client's nonfunctioning kidney is left in place to reduce the postoperative risk of hemorrhage.

After a couple days of bed rest, the client will be allowed increasing activities and, if no complications occur, will be discharged in 1 to 3 weeks. Routine nursing care includes monitoring urine output, blood tests, vital signs, and level of consciousness. Turning, coughing, and deep breathing are encouraged. The incision is assessed to ensure that wound closures are intact. In addition to these measures, the nurse must assess for rejection.

Organ Rejection

Signs of rejection include generalized edema, tenderness over the graft site, fever, decreased urine output, hematuria, edema (extremities or eyes), weight gain, oliguria or anuria, and/or an increase in feeling tired. The BUN and creatinine will be elevated.

Immunosuppressive drug therapy is begun to decrease the chance of organ rejection. These drugs include azathioprine (Imuran), cyclophosphamide (Cytoxan), cyclosporine (Sandimmune), and corticosteroids such as prednisone (Meticorten). The scheduling and dosage of these drugs vary with acceptance of the donor kidney and the side effects exhibited by the client. People continue to survive many years with a kidney transplant and maintain a quality life.

With the newly transplanted kidney, the recipient hopes to return to a normal life with enhanced energy and few dietary restrictions. However, a concern is organ rejection as the transplanted kidney is foreign tissue and can be rejected by the recipient's body.

Complications

The greatest complication in renal transplantation is infection. The immunosuppressive therapy to prevent rejection of the kidney increases the risk and masks the usual signs of infection. The client and family must learn how to recognize these signs of infection. There will be only a slight increase in temperature, development of a cough, low back pain, cloudy urine, or wound drainage. The client must always monitor urine output.

CASE STUDY

Ruth Andrews, 56, is a client in the extended care facility. She has amyotrophic lateral sclerosis (ALS) with muscle weakness that has progressed and involves her legs and arms. A hydraulic lift is used to transfer her out of bed. A student nurse and a classmate enter with the lift to assist Ms. Andrews OOB, when she asks to use the bedpan. As they help her on the bedpan, they recall that the staff nurse gave Ms. Andrews the bedpan about a half hour ago. Returning in a few minutes, they help Ms. Andrews off the bedpan and notice the urine is cloudy with a foul odor. Ms. Andrews is not on I & O; however, they notice that there is a very small amount of urine. She tells them that she does not know why she is going to the bathroom so often and why her urine smells bad.

The following questions will guide your development of a nursing care plan for the case study.

1. What subjective data should be gathered? What objective data should be gathered?
2. List diagnostic tests that may be ordered.
3. Write two nursing diagnoses for Ms. Andrews, related to her cystitis/UTI.
4. Write a goal related to each of Ms. Andrews' nursing diagnoses.
5. List pertinent nursing actions for the care of Ms. Andrews for each of the following areas as they relate to the cystitis/UTI:

   elimination-bladder
   diet and fluids
   safety, comfort, and rest
   teaching (client and nursing staff)

6. List two classifications of medications used for the treatment of an UTI.
7. List two successful client outcomes for Ms. Andrews.

SUMMARY

- The functions of the urinary system are reflected in their relationship with nearly all the systems in the body.
- Accurate intake and output is imperative for every client with a urinary system disorder.
- Teach proper perineal care, especially to females of all ages, about cleansing from front to back.
- Diet management is important for clients with renal calculi, glomerulonephritis, and renal failure.
- Encourage an adequate intake of fluids for clients unless fluids are restricted.
- Monitor laboratory test results for BUN, creatinine, and electrolytes.
- Level of consciousness, vital signs, lung sounds, and urine characteristics are important to monitor.
- Strict aseptic care is mandatory for dialysis clients.

Review Questions

1. A client states she has had pain when urinating for 3 days. This would be documented as:

   a. polyuria.
   b. dysuria.
   c. hematuria.
   d. oliguria.

2. A client has been admitted for chronic pyelonephritis. She is jittery and states she is concerned. Which of the following signs would indicate potential kidney damage?

   a. Urine output is 100 mL on your shift.
   b. Blood pressure is decreased with a rapid pulse.
   c. Blood pressure is elevated with a decreased pulse.
   d. BUN and creatinine clearance are within normal limits.

3. Georgia Smithson has glomerulonephritis. This condition affects her:

   a. kidney.
   b. ureter.
   c. bladder.
   d. urethra.

4. Mr. Ronald Osborne, 76, has had hematuria for several years and has been diagnosed with cancer of the kidney. His prognosis is poor. He told the nurse that he was too dizzy to go to the bathroom alone. Which of the following shows Mr. Osborne needs further teaching?

   a. Putting his bathroom call light on for assistance
   b. Holding on to the nurse's arm while walking
   c. Refusal to wait for the nurse to lower the side rail
   d. Saving his urine to be measured and tested

5. Jake Jones, 64, has had hematuria for several years. He is admitted to your same-day surgical unit scheduled for cystoscopic fulguration. Post-operatively, which of the following would you anticipate?

   a. Blood in the urine
   b. An elevated temperature
   c. Hypotension
   d. Smoky urine

6. Lawrence Denny, 29, had impetigo two weeks prior to his noting a decrease in urine output and urine that "did not look right." His admission diagnosis is acute glomerulonephritis. He is on intake and output with fluid restriction. Which of the following comments indicates knowledge of his nursing care?

   a. "I had my wife empty my urinal."
   b. "My urine still looks pretty bad."
   c. "I put my call light on so you can empty my urinal."
   d. "My wife helped me out of bed, so I urinated in the bathroom."

7. Gael Dominich is a client with chronic glomerulonephritis. She is discharged home with home health care. As the LP/VN assigned to her case, you are planning Gael's A.M. care. While preparing the bath supplies, she says, "Please do not use any soap. My skin is so dry and flaky." The rationale for this would be:

   a. kidney failure leads to uremia.
   b. the bladder does not concentrate urine.
   c. her blood sugar is elevated.
   d. confusion leads to comments of this nature.

8. Mr. Diego Ochoa, in his 50s, is attending classes to be able to do his own peritoneal dialysis. He states he feels well and is eager to continue to learn. Mr. Ochoa asks if washing his hands before the procedure is important. The best response is:

   a. "Yes, only if you have not done so today."
   b. "Yes, as you want to keep the procedure as clean as possible."
   c. "No, since you just went to the bathroom."
   d. "No, because all the equipment is sterile."

Critical Thinking Questions

1. What are the pros and cons for peritoneal dialysis, hemodialysis, and kidney transplantation?

2. What can an individual do to prevent urinary disorders?

3. Compare the differences between acute and chronic renal failure?

4. State the rationale for each nursing intervention given for the nursing diagnoses in this chapter?

WEB FLASH!

- Search the Internet for information about the various diseases discussed in this chapter. What information would assist you in client care?
- Find the resources listed for this chapter in the back of this text on the Internet. What services do they have available for clients?

Reproductive and Sexual Disorders

NURSING CARE OF THE CLIENT: FEMALE REPRODUCTIVE SYSTEM

CHAPTER 30

MAKING THE CONNECTION

Refer to the following chapters to increase your understanding of the female reproductive system:

- **Chapter 7, Wellness Concepts**
- **Chapter 10, Fluid, Electrolyte, and Acid-Base Balance**
- **Chapter 12, Health Assessment**
- **Chapter 17, Nursing Care of the Oncology Client**
- **Chapter 19, Nursing Care of the Client: Cardiovascular System**
- **Chapter 27, Nursing Care of the Client: Endocrine System**

- **Chapter 29, Nursing Care of the Client: Urinary System**
- **Chapter 31, Nursing Care of the Client: Male Reproductive System**
- **Chapter 32, Nursing Care of the Client: Sexually Transmitted Diseases**
- **Chapter 35, Nursing Care of the Older Client**

LEARNING OBJECTIVES

Upon completion of this chapter, you should be able to:

- *Define key terms.*
- *Identify the components of the reproductive systems.*
- *Describe the hormonal mechanisms that regulate the reproductive functions, including the menstrual cycle.*
- *Describe diagnostic tests for disorders of the reproductive systems.*
- *Describe the changes in the female reproductive system that occur with aging.*
- *Differentiate between impotence and infertility.*
- *Discuss contraceptive methods, including actions, side effects, and client teaching.*
- *Utilize the nursing process to develop a care plan for a client with a reproductive system disorder.*

KEY TERMS

abortion	menorrhagia
amenorrhea	metrorrhagia
contraception	oligomenorrhea
cystocele	polymenorrhea
dysmenorrhea	prolapsed uterus
dyspareunia	rectocele
endometriosis	tenesmus
infertility	urethrocele
menopause	vasectomy

INTRODUCTION

Because of modern technology, current medical and nursing knowledge, and health education programs, laypersons have access to much information about their bodies and their reproductive systems.

However, individuals continue to be seriously affected by health disorders. In some instances they may lack knowledge of how to detect signs and symptoms of these conditions. Often they simply delay routine medical examinations or avoid seeking medical treatment. In addition, individuals may have difficulty discussing symptoms related to their reproductive system.

The nurse, as a member of a holistic health care team, actively participates in prevention, maintenance, and restoration for women experiencing reproductive system disorders.

For the majority of women, the reproductive system functions without problems throughout life. For others, minor and major disorders require treatment. Some of the problems are related to alterations in structure; others are related more to altered physiology of the reproductive system. This chapter discusses disorders of the female reproductive systems by applying the steps of the nursing process.

ANATOMY AND PHYSIOLOGY REVIEW

The female reproductive system consists of external and internal structures and organs.

External Female Structures

The area known as the vulva includes the external female structures, such as the mons pubis, labia majora, labia minora, and clitoris. The Bartholin glands and Skene's glands, located proximal to the vaginal opening, produce and secrete lubricating fluids. The labia majora and minora serve as protective barriers for the softer internal structures. The clitoris, located proximal to the mons pubis, and superior to the urinary meatus, plays a role in sexual arousal in the female and is considered analogous to the male penis. During foreplay, the clitoris engorges and stimulates orgasm or climax in the female. It is covered by a small hood called the prepuce. The perineum is the distal portion of the vulva, located below the vaginal opening and superior to the anus.

The breasts are also a part of the external female reproductive system (Figure 30-1). Their external structures include the nipple, areola, and Montgomery tubercles. The nipples have several openings, or ducts, that lead from the lactiferous glands inside the breast. Milk is ejected through the ducts when the infant sucks on the breast. The areola, or the darker area around the nipple, becomes darker in response to the increased hormone levels during pregnancy. Small, mole-like, raised areas around the areola are the Montgomery tubercles. These glands produce a lubricant that keeps the nipple soft and supple.

Internal Female Structures

The vagina is an elastic, tubelike structure leading from the outside of the female body to the cervix. Approximately 2 to 3 inches long, it contains many rugae that allow it to stretch during intercourse and also permit the passage of the baby during delivery. The pH environment of the vagina is normally acidic, providing protection from microorganisms that could cause infections.

The uterus is a 3-inch long, 2-inch wide, 1-inch thick hollow, muscular structure as seen in Figure 30-2. The top is the fundus, the middle is the body (corpus),

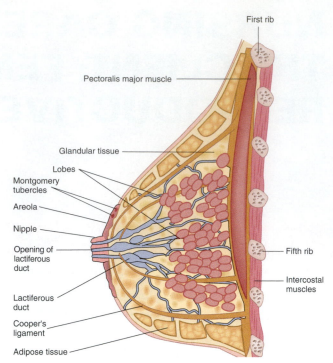

Figure 30-1 The Female Breast

and the lower portion is the cervix. Four sets of ligaments hold the uterus in its normal anteverted (forward) position and permit it the freedom to grow and move during pregnancy. The uterus has three distinct layers. The innermost layer is the endometrium, which sloughs with menstruation each month. The middle layer is the myometrium, which is constructed of many muscle fibers that are interwoven for strength, stretch, and contractility. The outer layer is the perimetrium, which is an external serous membrane covering.

The fallopian tubes are connected to the uterus on either side. They are continuous with the mucous membrane lining of the endometrium on the inside. Billions of cilia line each fallopian tube and make a sweeping motion toward the uterus, especially at the time of ovulation. This sweeping action moves the ovum along the path toward the uterus. The movement may also impede the progress of the sperm, which must swim upstream against the downward current produced by the cilia.

The cervix is the lower portion of the uterus and extends into the vaginal vault. Like the vagina, the cervix has muscle layers that allow it to stretch to a diameter of at least 10 cm (about 4 inches) during delivery.

An almond-shaped ovary, about 2 inches long and 1 inch wide, is located within the broad ligament on either side of the uterus, just below the fimbriae, the fingerlike projections at the distal end of the fallopian tubes. The ovaries contain all of the ova (eggs) that a woman will have from puberty until menopause. Each month, the ovary responds to hormonal signals from the anterior pituitary gland to ripen one or more ova. Follicle-stimulating hormone (FSH) is released by the

Figure 30-2 The Female Reproductive System

anterior pituitary and sends a message to the ovary to release estrogen, which causes the ovum to ripen and enlarge. The entire first part of the cycle is known as the proliferative phase.

Luteinizing hormone (LH) is then released. LH triggers a chain of events that stimulates the ovary to release the ovum. This point in the menstrual cycle is called ovulation. Another hormone, progesterone,

causes the glands and blood vessels of the endometrial lining to grow and thicken as they prepare for the implantation of a fertilized ovum. If fertilization does not occur, the progesterone level will decrease, the endometrium will be sloughed off, and the woman experiences menstruation. If fertilization does occur, the progesterone level remains elevated to ensure the optimal environment for implantation of the zygote about 6 to 8 days after fertilization. Figure 30-3 illustrates the menstrual cycle.

COMMON DIAGNOSTIC TESTS

Commonly used diagnostic tests for clients with symptoms of reproductive system disorders are listed in Table 30–1. See Chapter 13, Diagnostic Tests, for explanation/normal values and nursing responsibilities.

INFLAMMATORY DISORDERS

Inflammatory disorders discussed include pelvic inflammatory disease, endometriosis, vaginitis, and toxic shock syndrome.

PELVIC INFLAMMATORY DISEASE

Pelvic inflammatory disease (PID) is an inflammatory process involving pathogenic invasion of the fallopian tubes (salpingitis) or ovaries (oophoritis), or

Figure 30-3 Sequence and Approximate Time of Events in the Menstrual Cycle

Table 30–1 COMMON DIAGNOSTIC TESTS FOR REPRODUCTIVE SYSTEM DISORDERS

Laboratory Tests
- Alpha-fetoprotein (AFP)
- Cultures
- Human chorionic gonadatropin (HCG)
- Pap smear
- Serum calcium
- Segmented bacteriologic localization culture

Radiologic Tests
- Hysterosalpingogram
- Mammography

Surgical Tests
- Breast biopsy
- Dilatation & curettage (D&C)
- Endometrial biopsy
- Laparoscopy

Other Tests
- Colposcopy
- Pelvic examination
- Ultrasound

both, as well as any vascular or supporting structures within the pelvis, except the uterus. Pathogenic microorganisms such as gonococcus, streptococcus, and staphylococcus are frequent causes of PID. Infections are usually ascending by nature; that is, the pathogens are introduced into the reproductive system from outside and travel upward from the vagina to the fallopian tubes and then out into the pelvis. Risk factors associated with the incidence of PID include multiple sexual partners, frequent intercourse, IUDs (intrauterine contraceptive devices), and childbirth.

The symptoms of PID include a low-grade fever, pelvic pain, abdominal pain, a "bearing down" backache, a foul-smelling vaginal discharge, nausea and vomiting, **dysmenorrhea** (painful menstruation), **dyspareunia** (painful intercourse), and intense pelvic tenderness upon examination. Peritonitis or pelvic abscesses may develop as complications of PID if the pathogens spread into the pelvic cavity. Future **infertility** (inability or diminished ability to produce offspring) can be related to scarring and strictures of the fallopian tubes, which have developed as a result of a chronic inflammatory process within the pelvis. These problems have been associated with ectopic pregnancies because the fertilized ovum becomes trapped inside the fallopian tube before it can complete its trip to the uterus.

PID is often diagnosed during a pelvic examination. The nurse usually obtains a history of the client's symptoms. Frequently, vaginal and cervical cultures are obtained at the time of the exam to determine the causative agent. A pelvic ultrasound may be ordered to rule out other causes of pelvic pain. The nurse needs to instruct the client in the purpose of these procedures and any special preparations that may be required, such as having a full bladder.

Medical–Surgical Management

Medical

The client who is not acutely ill from PID may be treated as an outpatient at home with oral antibiotics and bed rest, unless the infection is herpes simplex virus II. Clients with herpes simplex II infections may require more intensive care in the hospital with IV antibiotic therapy. The physician may also order medicated vaginal suppositories for the vaginal discharge. The acutely ill client may require hospitalization for IV antibiotic therapy.

Surgical

If the inflammation is extensive, or if medical treatment is not successful, the client may require a hysterectomy.

Pharmacological

Antibiotics used may include doxycycline monohydrate (Vibramycin) or metronidazole (Flagyl). IV fluids are frequently administered to promote adequate hydration. A 5% dextrose in lactated Ringer's solution or a plain lactated Ringer's solution is often used.

Activity

During hospitalization, the client is placed on bed rest with bathroom privileges. A semi-Fowler's position is preferred because it will facilitate drainage of the pelvis. If vaginal suppositories are used, the client should lie in a supine position for 30 minutes.

 CLIENT TEACHING

Inserting Vaginal Suppositories
- Have the client wash her hands, then cleanse the vulva with a mild soap and warm water to remove any external discharge.
- Client should lie down in a supine position with her knees flexed.
- With one hand, the client can separate the labia and gently insert the suppository high inside the vagina.
- The client should remain supine for a minimum of 30 minutes to ensure adequate absorption of the medication through the vaginal mucosa.

▶ NURSING PROCESS

▶ Assessment

▶ Subjective Data

On the initial assessment, the nurse should inquire about the client's sexual activity, including the number of partners. Unprotected intercourse is the most frequent method of entry for the microorganisms that cause PID. The nurse should also include the client's history of **contraception** (measures taken to prevent pregnancy), previous vaginal infections and treatments, obstetrical history, and normal hygiene practices such as douching and tampon use. Complaints of nagging pelvic pain and a low-grade fever are often expressed.

▶ Objective Data

The nurse may note an elevated temperature, flushed, dry skin, the presence of a malodorous vaginal discharge, and positive vaginal or cervical cultures.

Nursing diagnoses for a client with pelvic inflammatory disease may include the following:

Nursing Diagnoses	Planning/Goals	Nursing Interventions
Acute Pain related to inflammation of the pelvic structures caused by invasion of pathogens	Using a pain rating scale of 0 to 10, the client will report that her pain has decreased.	Assess client's pain level every 4 hours, noting the location, duration, sensation, intensity, and factors that increase or decrease the pain. Administer analgesics as ordered.
Deficient Knowledge related to the etiology of the pelvic inflammatory process, treatment regimen, self-care, and preventive measures	The client will follow prescribed treatment regimen, self-care, and preventive measures.	Explain the importance of completing the entire course of antibiotics and other medications to ensure eradication of the pathogens from the pelvic organs. If suppositories are ordered, instruct the client in the proper method of insertion. Provide instructions to the client and partner (if available) about the causes of PID and ways to prevent the inflammation. Teach proper pericare and hygiene, especially handwashing before and after changing sanitary pads. Encourage the client to maintain a semi-Fowler's position to prevent the spread of inflammation to pelvic organs. Instruct client to change sanitary pads every 3 to 4 hours. Encourage client to make time for rest periods during the acute phase of the inflammation. Instruct client about pelvic rest, which includes no douching, tampons, or intercourse. Advise client to avoid strenuous activities such as straining or heavy lifting. Advise client to wear underpants with a cotton crotch. Teach client to cleanse the perineal area from front to back after each voiding or bowel movement. Discuss and encourage the use of safe sexual practices and the use of barrier contraceptives to prevent recurrence of PID symptoms. Make follow-up appointment.
	The client will contact her health care provider for follow-up and if her symptoms persist, worsen, or return.	Encourage client to notify the NP or physician at the first sign of PID symptoms. Advise client to monitor her own temperature, upon discharge, twice daily for 2 weeks and notify the physician or NP if the temperature increases or remains elevated.
Hyperthermia related to physiologic responses to the inflammatory or infectious process	The client's temperature will return to normal range after the initiation of therapy.	Monitor client's vital signs every 4 hours. Administer antipyretic and antibiotic as ordered by the physician.

Evaluation Each goal must be evaluated to determine how it has been met by the client.

ENDOMETRIOSIS

Endometriosis is the growth of endometrial tissue, the normal lining of the uterus, outside of the uterus within the pelvic cavity. The disease occurs most frequently in women 30 years and older and tends to be familial. It predominantly affects Caucasian females who have not given birth and is most common among the higher socioeconomic population. Endometriosis has been called the "career woman's disorder," because it is often diagnosed in the late twenties or thirties when the working woman makes plans for childbearing.

The endometrial tissue implants itself on other pelvic structures (Figure 30-4). Two of the most common areas for endometrial implants are the pouch of Douglas and the ovaries. The tissue implants respond to the monthly hormonal changes in the same way as the endometrial tissue inside the uterus does. Bleeding of the implants during the menses results in the formation of adhesions and scar tissue. The endometriosis appears as brownish or black "powder burns" or larger lesions. If the endometriosis becomes encapsulated in an ovarian cyst it is called a "chocolate cyst."

The disease appears to be progressive and has a tendency to be recurrent. Some women with minimal endometriosis experience severe monthly symptoms, such as lower backache, painful intercourse, a feeling of heaviness on the pelvis, and spotting. Other women have a more extensive disease but have minimal symptoms. Thus, the amount of endometriosis present may or may not be correlated with the severity of the symptoms experienced by the client.

Endometriosis is one cause of female infertility. Pregnancy inhibits the growth and bleeding of the endometrial implants because ovulation and menstruation are suppressed. Often it is difficult for the client to become pregnant because of the amount of scar tissue and adhesions around the pelvic organs, ligaments, and fallopian tubes.

Medical–Surgical Management

Medical

Endometriosis may be tentatively diagnosed by palpation of endometrial implants within the pelvis, but this method is inconclusive for treatment. Further investigation is required to confirm the diagnosis. Laparoscopy, performed under general anesthesia, is the best method of diagnosis by direct visualization of the pelvic structures. Consideration for treatment is dependent upon the client's age and desire for future childbearing. Sometimes pregnancy relieves the symptoms even after delivery.

Figure 30-4 Common Sites of Endometriosis

Surgical

The older multigravida who is experiencing severe, debilitating symptoms that affect her lifestyle and normal functions, role, or activity, may desire a hysterectomy. If the lesions are large or extensive, a laparotomy may be performed for adequate removal. However, if the implants are small and scattered, cauterization or laser vaporization may be most desirable. Lysis of pelvic adhesions would be done at the same time.

Pharmacological

The goals of pharmacological therapy are to suppress ovulation and menstruation, reduce symptoms, and cause the implants to shrink. Medications used in the treatment of endometriosis must effectively suppress the monthly hypothalamic-pituitary-ovarian hormonal stimulation of ovulation. Some medications act on the body as "pseudopregnancy" agents that produce anovulation, breast tenderness, nausea, weight gain, and hirsutism. Other hormonal therapies cause a temporary medically induced menopause state. Oral contraceptives may be administered continuously. Nafarelin acetate (Synarel) is a nasally administered gonadatropin analog that inhibits cyclic hormone release. Danazol (Danocrine) is another androgen hormone that must be taken continuously for 6 to 8 months or longer. This medication inhibits the release of gonadotropin. The resulting **amenorrhea** (absence of menstruation) will suppress the growth of the endometrial tissue. This medication is used in moderate to severe cases of endometriosis. Occasionally, Danocrine is given after surgical removal or cauterization of the endometriosis to relieve symptoms from residual disease.

All medications used to treat endometriosis cause mild to moderate side effects that may affect the client's desire to take them or her compliance with continuous usage. Examples of problems that may be experienced include oily skin, fluid retention, weight gain, acne, hot flashes, metrorrhagia, mastalgia, and depression.

▶ NURSING PROCESS

▶ Assessment

▶ Subjective Data

The data to be gathered include a description of pelvic pain, which is especially worse around the time of menstruation. The client may also voice concerns about pelvic discomfort with intercourse. The nurse should be alert to what the client says as well as what is left unsaid. Dyspareunia may result in marital tension if the client avoids sexual intimacy to reduce her pain. Equally important to the client's pain is the occurrence of prolonged, excessive menstrual periods. The client may report that she is experiencing periods that are getting closer and closer together. Another sign, although not as significant, is pain with defecation during the menstrual period.

In obtaining a client history, the nurse should note the onset of menses, regularity of cycles, and any changes the client has noted in the frequency, comfort, duration, and amount of menstrual flow. It is important to note the onset of the client's symptoms in relationship to the menstrual cycle, the severity as reported by the client, any alterations in lifestyle related to the pain or other symptoms, and the client's future plans for childbearing.

▶ Objective Data

The nurse's role in caring for this client is usually focused on collecting subjective data from the client interview and assisting the physician during actual procedures.

Nursing Management

Nursing diagnoses for a client with endometriosis may include the following:

- *Chronic Pain related to bleeding from endometrial implants in the pelvic cavity*
- *Anxiety related to treatment options, possible side effects, and infertility*
- *Sexual Dysfunction related to altered body function of structure (painful intercourse)*
- *Situational Low Self-Esteem related to functional impairment of the ability to conceive*

VAGINITIS

Several common types of vaginitis are caused by bacteria, protozoa, viruses, and yeasts. The vaginal mucosa is normally protected by an acid mantle. The acidic (pH less than 5.0) environment inhibits the growth of many pathogenic microorganisms. Because the vaginal opening is close to the external environment, microorganisms have an opportunity to invade the reproductive tract. Some organisms that cause vaginitis are transmitted to the female from the male partner during sexual contact. Natural protective barriers may vary with the fluctuating hormonal levels during the woman's monthly cycle because the hormones affect the vaginal pH. At ovulation, the vaginal pH becomes slightly less acidic owing to the high level of estrogen. Periods when the woman's system has lower estrogen levels, such as immediately after the menses and after menopause, are also times when there is a higher risk for infection because the epithelium is less active, no glycogen is present, and the pH may reach as high as 7.0. Occasionally, superinfections may develop during or after a course of antibiotic therapy to treat another problem. These usually result from a decrease in the presence of the normal flora along with pathogens, which allows an overgrowth of yeast (fungus).

Diagnosis is made after performing a vaginal examination and obtaining a sample of the vaginal discharge. When the client contacts the physician or nurse practitioner to report symptoms of vaginitis, the nurse should instruct her to avoid douching or using tampons before being examined because douching will wash away the discharge needed to be examined and tampons will absorb it.

Common types of vaginitis include candidiasis caused by *Candida albicans* (a fungus), trichomoniasis caused by *Trichomonas vaginalis* (a protozoan), *Gardnerella vaginalis* (a bacterium), and *Chlamydia trachomatis* (a parasite). Other causes of vaginitis symptoms may include streptococcus, staphylococcus, gonococcus, and herpes simplex II. Usually the symptoms depend upon the causative agent. The client's description of her symptoms along with the examination of the discharge help confirm the diagnosis. Most infections have a characteristic discharge and irritation with burning or itching that may be internal, external, or both.

Predisposing factors for candidiasis, also called monilia, may include obesity, diabetes, pregnancy, oral contraceptives, antibiotics, and frequent douching. Many of these factors alter the pH of the vagina. Symptoms of this fungal infection include a thick, white, cheesy or curdlike discharge with a musty, sweet odor, accompanied by vaginal or vulvar itching and irritation. Upon examination, the vaginal mucosa will have patches of white discharge present. If the

CLIENT TEACHING

Ways to Decrease Risk of Vaginitis

- Wear cotton-crotch underwear.
- Avoid sitting in a wet bathing suit in warm weather for long periods.
- Seek prompt medical attention at the first signs of infection.
- Eat an 8-oz container of yogurt with active cultures daily while taking antibiotics.

patches are scraped off, the tissue underneath will appear reddened and may bleed. Externally, the vulva may be reddened and edematous. The client may have scratches from attempting to ease the itching.

The preferred treatment is vaginal application of antifungal creams or suppositories such as miconazole (Monistat), clotrimazole (Mycelex-G, Gyne-Lotrimin), or nystatin (Mycostatin). The length of treatment is usually 7 days. Alternative therapies include douching with white vinegar solution (1 tablespoon/1 pint of water) twice a day for a week. This treatment restores the acid balance of the vagina and washes away the *Candida albicans.* Eating cultured yogurt with active acidophilus or applying the yogurt directly to the labia helps restore the normal bacteria and protective mechanisms in the vagina.

Trichomonasis is frequently passed from partner to partner during intercourse. A copious green-yellow, foul-smelling, frothy vaginal discharge is characteristic of this type of vaginal infection. It may produce itching or external burning and irritation. Metronidazole (Flagyl) is taken orally by both partners as a treatment of choice for this infection.

Flagyl is normally contraindicated in the first trimester of pregnancy, so obtaining a menstrual history or a pregnancy test may be needed before administration of this medication. It is also essential to inform the client and her partner to avoid any alcohol intake during therapy. Flagyl causes a strong antabuse-like effect which results in severe nausea and vomiting. Clients should read labels on over-the-counter medications being taken concurrently with the Flagyl because many preparations contain alcohol bases.

The nurse should instruct the client and her partner to abstain from intercourse during therapy and to finish all of the medication.

Gardnerella vaginalis often produces a gray-white vaginal discharge with a strong fishy odor or is asymptomatic. If itching or burning is present, it may suggest another microorganism. For the treatment of *Gardnerella,* and other bacterial vaginitis, the physician may order Flagyl or an oral antibiotic such as tetracycline hydrochloride (Achromycin) or ampicillin (Om-

nipen). Sulfa-based creams such as Sultrin, Triple Sulfa, and AVC may be used vaginally in conjunction with the oral medications once or twice a day for 6 to 14 days to completely treat this type of infection.

Chlamydial vaginitis infections are often asymptomatic but have been associated with infertility problems. A culture of vaginal secretions is necessary to specifically identify the organism. The treatment is usually oral antibiotics for at least 7 days. A repeat culture is recommended following treatment to ensure that the parasites have been eradicated.

Postmenopausal vaginitis (atrophic) is caused by a decreased level of estrogen in the vaginal tissue. The client may complain of painful intercourse (dyspareunia), itching, burning, or irritation. Estrogen replacement therapy often relieves the symptoms of this type of vaginitis. The medication may be administered orally, vaginally, or by transdermal patch.

▶ NURSING PROCESS

▶ Assessment

▶ Subjective Data

The nurse should obtain information from the client regarding the nature of her symptoms, the onset, menstrual history, contraceptive methods, recent or current use of antibiotics or other medications, recent illness, diabetes mellitus, sexual history, pregnancy history, usual hygiene practices such as douching, deodorant sprays, bubble baths, wearing of panty hose, type of underwear, and use of deodorized tampons or pads.

▶ Objective Data

The vaginal discharge is observed and any odor noted. Vaginal or vulvar irritation and possible scratches may be seen.

Nursing Management

Nursing diagnoses for a client with vaginitis, regardless of the etiology, may include the following:

- *Deficient Knowledge related to the origin of the infection, prevention, and treatment options*
- *Impaired Tissue Integrity related to the presence of vaginal discharge, itching, or irritation*
- *Sexual Dysfunction related to discomfort during intercourse or fear of transmitting the infection to the sexual partner*
- *Risk for Impaired Skin Integrity related to internal and external irritation from discharge and itching*

TOXIC SHOCK SYNDROME

Toxic shock syndrome (TSS) is a condition most often associated with *Staphylococcus aureus,* which enters the bloodstream. A strong relationship has been found between the use of tampons (especially super-absorbent) during menstruation and the onset of TSS symptoms. It has been hypothesized that the fibers from the tampon lower the level of magnesium in the woman's body and, therefore, produce a favorable environment for the growth of pathogenic micro-organisms. The condition was first diagnosed in the mid-1970s and the incidence increased throughout the 1980s. A high percentage of women who are affected by toxic shock syndrome are under 30. TSS can also occur in nonmenstruating women and men.

The client may present with a temperature of 102°F or greater, vomiting, diarrhea, and progressive hypotension. The client may also experience flulike symptoms of malaise, muscle soreness, sore throat, and headache. There may be a macular erythematous (flat, red) rash that is followed in 1 to 2 weeks by the peeling of the palms and soles. Disorientation may occur from the release of toxins and dehydration.

Medical–Surgical Management

Medical

Blood, urine, genitourinary, and throat cultures may be obtained and are usually negative except for *Staphylococcus aureus*. The goals of treatment are focused on the control of the falling blood pressure, fluid volume replacement, halting the infectious process, and maintaining adequate ventilation efforts. IV fluids are administered per the physician's order. The client may require mechanical ventilation and CPAP (continuous positive airway pressure).

Pharmacological

Broad-spectrum antibiotic therapy is recommended. Culture and sensitivity tests will indicate which type of

CLIENT TEACHING

TSS and Tampon Use
Instruct client to avoid tampon use for several cycles. If she chooses to use tampons in the future, they should be changed every 2 to 3 hours, especially the superabsorbent types.

antibiotic is best against the staphylococcus organism. Examples may include dicloxacillin sodium (Dynapen), clexacillin sodium (Tegopen), nafcillin sodium (Nafcil), and methicillin sodium (Staphcillin). The medication regimen is continued for at least 2 weeks to ensure control of the pathogens.

Activity

Bed rest is usually prescribed.

▶ NURSING PROCESS

▶ Assessment

▶ Subjective Data

Data to be obtained include recent use of tampons, length of time tampon is left in before changing, sore throat, headache, myalgia, and fatigue.

▶ Objective Data

Erythematous rash, edema, peeling of palms and soles, hypotension, level of consciousness, nonpurulent conjunctivitis, and hyperemia of vagina and oropharynx are all assessed.

Nursing diagnoses for a client with toxic shock syndrome may include the following:

Nursing Diagnoses	Planning/Goals	Nursing Interventions
▶ *Hyperthermia related to inflammatory process*	The client will have normal-range temperature within 48 hours.	Administer antipyretics as ordered. Give cooling sponge bath. Encourage oral fluids as tolerated.
▶ *Deficient Fluid Volume related to diarrhea, vomiting, fever, and decreased intake*	The client will have fluid and electrolyte balance within 24 hours.	Administer intravenous fluids as ordered. Encourage oral fluids if client is not vomiting. Administer antiemetic and antidiarrheal medications as ordered. Assess skin turgor and mucous membranes. Monitor I & O.
▶ *Risk for Impaired Skin Integrity related to dehydration and effects of circulating toxins*	The client will maintain skin integrity.	Encourage or assist with position change every 2 hours. Provide or assist with personal hygiene, especially after diarrhea. Assess bony prominences for reddened areas.

Evaluation Each goal must be evaluated to determine how it has been met by the client.

BENIGN NEOPLASMS

Benign neoplasms include fibrocystic breast disease, and fibroid tumors.

FIBROCYSTIC BREAST DISEASE

Fibrocystic breast disease (FBD) is also called chronic cystic mastitis or lumpy breast syndrome. It is the most common breast lesion in females and usually occurs between 35 and 50 years of age. Many cases will subside after menopause. The incidence of the potential for developing breast cancer is increased 3 to 4 times with fibrocystic breast disease. There appears to be a familial tendency toward the development of breast cancer.

Lumps may occur as single or multiple cysts that are frequently fluid-filled. It is difficult to differentiate fibrocystic tissue changes from other breast lesions because the dense fibrocystic areas may mask areas of breast cancer. Figure 30-5 shows the differences among cysts, fibroadenomas, and carcinomas of the breast.

The pathophysiology of fibrocystic breast disease is found in the formation of fibrous tissue caused by hyperplasia of the epithelial cells in the breast lobules and ducts. The proliferation of the fibrous tissue deviates from the expected normal cyclic response to female hormone shifts during the menstrual cycle. Research on fibrocystic breast disease has indicated that there may be a link between caffeine intake and the growth of the abnormal tissue. The caffeine may keep the hormonal triggers in an "on" position, and they foster the hyperplasia.

Routine mammograms may be ordered to provide baseline information and to differentiate the palpable breast lumps between benign and malignant types. A computer-directed biopsy may also be performed. The method of biopsy is more specific because the lesion can be pinpointed by the computer, and guessing the location is eliminated.

Women should be taught breast self-examination (BSE) as adolescents and encouraged to practice it at the end of each menstrual cycle, when it is easier to palpate the breast tissue. Figure 30-6 provides specific information on how to perform a breast self-examination.

A yellow-greenish, sticky discharge from the nipple is occasionally present with fibrocystic breast disease. A Pap smear may be done on the discharge to rule out the presence of malignant cells. The presence of any breast discharge should be noted and reported to the health care provider as soon as possible. The physician or nurse practitioner (NP) may perform a biopsy or aspiration of the abnormal areas in the office. If fluid is obtained from the area, it is sent to pathology for examination. If no fluid is obtained, it may be a solid cyst or tumor, and biopsy may be required.

In the office, a breast biopsy may be performed with a local anesthetic. If there is any question of malignancy, or if the physician suspects that the lesion will be malignant on the basis of the mammography report, the biopsy may be performed in the hospital under general anesthetic so that additional tissue may be removed if necessary. A frozen section may be obtained and sent to the laboratory for a preliminary examination to rule out a malignant lesion.

Medical–Surgical Management

Surgical

Aspiration or surgical excision may be indicated for diagnostic or therapeutic reasons. The cystic tissue may be aspirated with a small-gauge needle and syringe. The nurse prepares the client for the procedure and assists the doctor or NP with the procedure. The nurse assists the client into a supine position on the examination table and sets up the equipment and instruments needed. The area to be biopsied is cleansed. Upon completion of the aspiration or biopsy, the nurse labels the specimen and sends it to the pathology department.

If the areas of fibrocystic tissue are extensive and have not responded to conservative treatments and methods, or if the risk of cancer is high, the tissue may be excised completely. Removal of fibrocystic tissue does not guarantee that the client will not develop breast cancer in the remaining tissue, and she must continue to perform monthly BSE.

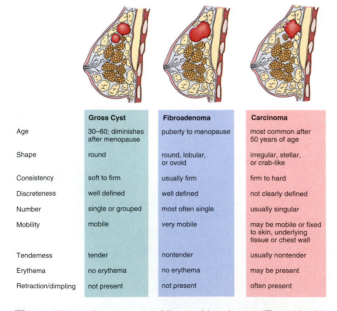

	Gross Cyst	Fibroadenoma	Carcinoma
Age	30–60; diminishes after menopause	puberty to menopause	most common after 50 years of age
Shape	round	round, lobular, or ovoid	irregular, stellar, or crab-like
Consistency	soft to firm	usually firm	firm to hard
Discreteness	well defined	well defined	not clearly defined
Number	single or grouped	most often single	usually singular
Mobility	mobile	very mobile	may be mobile or fixed to skin, underlying tissue or chest wall
Tenderness	tender	nontender	usually nontender
Erythema	no erythema	no erythema	may be present
Retraction/dimpling	not present	not present	often present

Figure 30-5 Comparison of Breast Neoplasms (*From* Health Assessment & Physical Examination (2nd ed.), *by M. E. Z. Estes, 2002 Albany, NY: Delmar. Copyright 2002 by Delmar. Reprinted with permission.*)

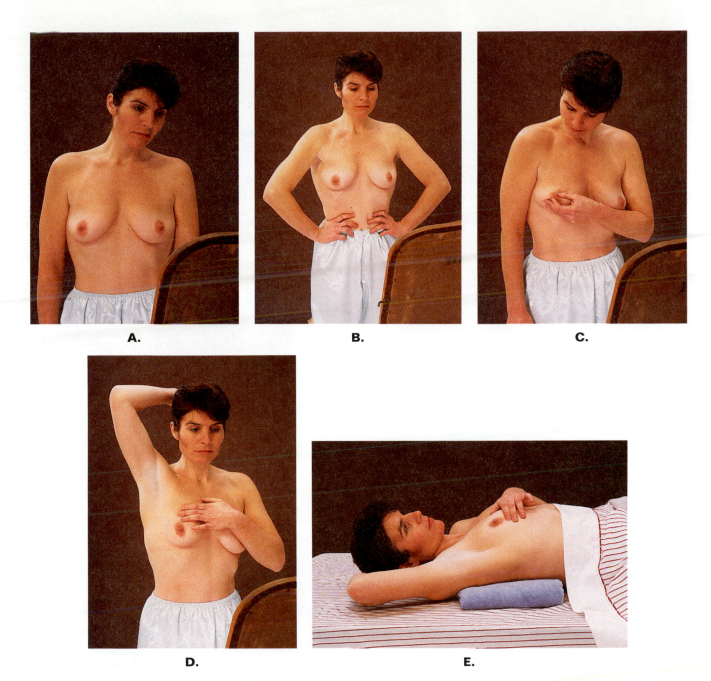

Figure 30-6 Performing a Breast Self-Examination: A. Standing in front of mirror, check breasts for puckering, dimpling, scaliness, or discharge from nipples. B. Clasp hands behind head and press hands forward, watching for changes in the shape or contour of breasts. Press hands on hips and bend toward mirror while pulling shoulders and elbows forward (shown). C. Gently squeeze each nipple, looking for discharge. D. Raise one arm and use fingers of other hand to check breast for lumps or masses under skin. Use a pattern of motion (circular, up-and-down, etc.) to cover entire breast. E. Repeat "D" while lying flat on back with one arm over head and a towel under the shoulder.

Pharmacological

Some physicians recommend up to 600 units of vitamin E daily. It is believed that the vitamin supplement helps to break down the fibrocystic tissue because it reacts with the polyunsaturated fats in the membrane of the cell. It may also have some effect on the balance of female hormones.

Diet

Most health care providers recommend limiting or completely eliminating caffeine-containing products from the woman's diet. This would include teas, colas, coffee, and chocolate. These products are all available in caffeine-free forms.

▶ NURSING PROCESS

▶ Assessment

▶ Subjective Data

The client may report that the lumps are more tender as she approaches her menstrual period and that there is a greenish, sticky discharge from one or both breasts. The nurse should inquire about the client's dietary habits, especially caffeine intake, frequency of BSE, and the date of the most recent mammogram, if applicable. Since FBD lumps are more tender near the menses, the client should be seen for an exam the week after her menstrual period. The tissue contains less fluid during that time and palpation is easier and less uncomfortable.

▶ Objective Data

When examined, single or multiple lumps may be palpated in one or both breasts. The lumps are not always discrete but should be freely movable.

Nursing diagnoses for a client with fibrocystic breast disease may include the following:

Nursing Diagnoses	Planning/Goals	Nursing Interventions
▶ *Deficient Knowledge related to the cause of fibrocystic breast disease and method of breast self-examination*	The client will verbalize and demonstrate her understanding of the cause of FBD and her role in treatment.	Demonstrate BSE for the client either in person or by video with a follow-up return demonstration by the client.
		Observe the client as she performs the BSE so that immediate feedback can be given. Explain the best timing for the BSE and the rationale for performing the procedure after the menses.
		Assist client with mammogram. Encourage mammography at regular intervals dependent upon the client's age and risk factors.
		Teach the client about dietary modifications, such as limiting caffeine.
▶ *Anxiety related to the underlying potential and risk of breast cancer*	The client will display behaviors of decreased anxiety related to the potential for breast cancer.	Explain the differences between malignant breast lesions and FBD to help alleviate the client's anxiety.

Evaluation Each goal must be evaluated to determine how it has been met by the client.

FIBROID TUMORS

Fibroids (leiomyomas) are benign tumors that grow in or on the uterus. A higher incidence is seen with nulliparous women and those who are over 30 years old. The fibroids may appear below the serosal membrane or the mucosa. An early symptom is often **menorrhagia**, an excessively heavy menstrual flow. Later, the client may experience increasing pelvic pressure as the tumors grow, along with dysmenorrhea, abdominal enlargement, and constipation. Growth of the fibroids is usually slow but can be stimulated by estrogen. During pregnancy, when the estrogen and progesterone levels dramatically increase, the tumors grow much faster. Concern arises for the fetus when the fibroids begin to enlarge and crowd the uterus. Overcrowding may compress the fetus or initiate the onset of preterm labor. With either situation, the pregnancy must be monitored carefully.

A medical diagnosis of uterine fibroids may initially be based upon the client's symptoms and the findings of the pelvic examination. If on palpation the uterus feels like an irregular mass or several masses, a pelvic ultrasound will be ordered to confirm the diagnosis.

Medical–Surgical Management

Medical

The physician may opt to wait and observe the growth pattern of the fibroids before advising the client to have surgery. This "wait and see" attitude may be swayed by the significance of the client's symptoms, size of the fibroids, amount of discomfort the client is experiencing, and amount of menorrhagia and/or **metrorrhagia**, vaginal bleeding between menstrual periods. Reexamination is encouraged at least every 6 months.

Surgical

If the menorrhagia is significant with each menstrual cycle, a dilatation and curettage (D&C) may be performed to determine the exact etiology of the bleeding. A myomectomy, a surgical procedure to remove the tumor, may be performed if the client desires future pregnancies. In the case of severe menorrhagia, with a dropping hemoglobin level or multiple tumors, the physician may recommend a hysterectomy as the option of choice.

Diet

A diet with many sources of iron helps prevent iron deficiency anemia, which may result from the extra blood loss.

❱ NURSING PROCESS

❱ Assessment

❱ Subjective Data

These would include the client's description of excessive menstrual flow, dysmenorrhea, and/or pelvic pain and pressure. The client may also report difficulty fitting into clothes because of abdominal enlargement, constipation, or urinary frequency or urgency.

CULTURAL CONSIDERATIONS

Fibroid Tumors

Fibroid tumors are most prevalent in African Americans and Mediterraneans with dark skin.

❱ Objective Data

These would include counting the number of sanitary pads the client saturates in an hour; observing the presence or absence of clots in the blood, and a hemoglobin level of less than 12 mg/dL. The nurse may observe that the client's skin color is pale. Her blood pressure may be slightly lower than normal and her pulse may be increased as a compensatory mechanism. When the pelvic examination is performed, irregularities in or on the uterus may be palpated.

Nursing diagnoses for a client with fibroids may include the following:

Nursing Diagnoses	Planning/Goals	Nursing Interventions
❱ *Risk for Deficient Fluid Volume related to excessive blood losses*	The client will have a hemoglobin above 12 mg/dL and will maintain fluid balance.	Assess client's blood loss for amount, color, and clots.
		Provide an accurate count of the saturated sanitary pads, along with the length of time taken to saturate a pad.
		Monitor vital signs at least every 4 hours, or more frequently if the client is having active blood loss.
		Monitor laboratory report for Hgb level.
❱ *Acute Pain related to pressure on pelvic structures caused by growing tumors and cramping during the menses*	The client will verbalize less discomfort and pelvic pressure.	Administer analgesics as ordered.
		Assess pain on 0 (least) to 10 (most) pain scale and note location, onset, and duration.

Evaluation Each goal must be evaluated to determine how it has been met by the client.

MALIGNANT NEOPLASMS

Malignant neoplasms include breast, cervical, endometrial, and ovarian.

BREAST CANCER

Breast cancer is the second major cause of cancer death among women. Statistics indicate that 1 woman in 10 will develop breast cancer sometime during her life. The American Cancer Society (ACS) estimates that 180,300 new cases were diagnosed in the United States in 1998. The 5-year survival rate is 97% for localized cancer, 76% for cancer that has spread regionally, and 21% for cancers having distant metastases (ACS, 1998). Elderly women (those over 65) have twice the inci-

dence of breast cancer as do younger women. Less than 1% of all breast cancers occur in men; in 1998, approximately 1,600 new cases of breast cancer were diagnosed in men.

The key to cure is early detection by physical examination, mammography, and breast self-examination. A painless mass or thickening is the most common presenting symptom.

Because it is so uncommon, breast cancer in men is all the more dangerous since it is not considered a threat. Late diagnosis is quite common; therefore, males need to be educated in the technique of and encouraged to do breast self-examination (BSE). Signs and symptoms of breast cancer include breast lumps, pain, or discharge from the nipple.

Women at greatest risk for developing breast cancer are those who:

- Had a mother or sibling with breast cancer
- Never had children or had their first child after the age of 30
- Never breast fed
- Have a history of fibrocystic breast disease
- Started menstruating before age 10
- Are obese
- Consume a high-fat diet and a moderate amount of alcohol
- Smoke
- Experienced a late menopause

A woman generally presents at the health care office after the discovery of a lump in her breast. If she has been performing BSE routinely each month, she is likely to be familiar with even minute changes in the breast tissue. Breast cancers often occur in the upper, outer quadrant of the breast and may extend into the tail of the breast and spread upward into the axilla. It is important to teach clients to examine the axillary region as well as the breast during BSE (refer to Figure 30-6).

Women also seek medical advice because they notice a discharge from the breast, dimpling of the skin, retraction of the nipple, pain, a unilateral change in breast size (Figure 30-7), or an orange-peel appearance (peau d'orange) of the skin. Dimpling and puckering are usually associated with the breast tissue or tumor attaching to the skin or the underlying muscle mass, which does not permit movement. The nurse should not be misled by the client's report of a tender lump or mass and assume it is fibrocystic breast disease (FBD). All new or enlarged lumps or masses in the breast require immediate assessment.

The presence of tiny, palpable clusters of calcium, or "microclusters," may be an early sign of breast cancer. These should be followed closely with mammography every 6 to 12 months to detect subtle changes in shape or size.

Figure 30-7 Asymmetry of Breasts Due to Cancer *(Courtesy of Dr. S. Eva Singletary, University of Texas, M. D. Anderson Cancer Center)*

The American Cancer Society (1998) recommends that women ages 20 to 40 perform BSE each month and have a clinical breast examination every 3 to 4 years. For women 41 to 49 years of age, BSE should also be performed monthly, a clinical examination every 1 to 2 years, and a mammogram every 1 to 2 years. Women 50 and older should follow the monthly routine for BSE and have a clinical examination and mammogram every year.

Mammography may be performed by the stereotactic computer guided technique. This advanced method allows needle biopsies to be taken at the same time if necessary. Often, the physician or nurse practitioner will recommend this method after an initial mammogram has shown suspicious areas. This technique is less costly than excisional biopsy and can be performed with little discomfort to the client. The client is placed in a prone position on the special examination table with the breast hanging down through the opening in the table. The operator moves the position of the table to visualize the entire breast area via computerized guidance.

After the breast has been biopsied and the tissue has been examined by the pathologist, if a malignancy is confirmed, the client may be advised to proceed with surgical removal of the affected tissue. This procedure is referred to as a lumpectomy or mastectomy. Figure 30-8 shows the staging of breast cancer.

Medical–Surgical Management

Medical

Radiation and chemotherapy may be used as adjuvant therapy, but surgery is the primary form of treatment.

Surgical

There is an abundance of lymphatic vessels proximal to the breast. Malignant cells can thus escape into the general lymphatic system and be spread throughout the body. A lumpectomy is surgical removal of the cancerous mass. A simple mastectomy removes the tumor mass and only a small portion of the adjacent tissue. In the modified mastectomy, the entire breast tissue and nearby lymph nodes are removed; the muscles of the chest wall are left relatively intact. With the radical mastectomy, the entire breast, lymph nodes, and underlying pectoralis muscle are removed. Figure 30-9 shows the various options in the surgical management of breast cancer. The greater the extent of the surgical removal, the longer the client's recovery process and the greater the need for rehabilitation in the use of the upper extremity on the affected side.

Reconstructive surgery after a mastectomy may be determined by the amount of breast tissue and muscle remaining after the initial procedure, the position of the mastectomy scar, and the probability of recurrent breast

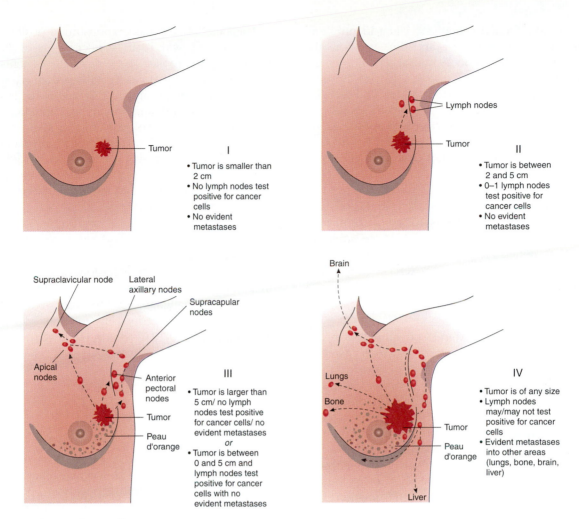

Figure 30-8 Breast Cancer Staging

cancer. Breast reconstruction can help the client deal with the disfigurement that results from the mastectomy.

The client's desire for reconstruction and her psychological status play an important role in determining the personal value of additional surgery. In the United States particularly, the breast is associated with child-

bearing and female sexuality. It may be difficult for the client to express her concerns to her partner regarding her sexuality and desirability after the mastectomy. She may have difficulty facing the physical alteration immediately after surgery and for some time in the future. The caring nurse with good interpersonal

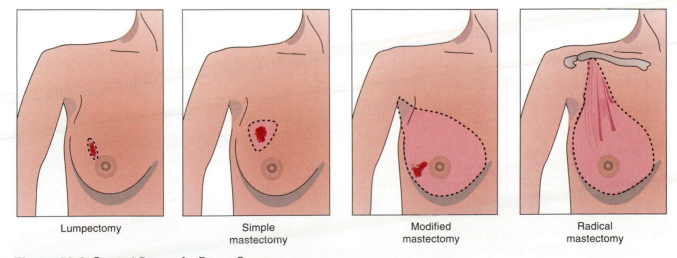

Figure 30-9 Surgical Options for Breast Cancer

communication skills can help the client identify and verbalize her feelings of loss and thus promote the psychological healing process and acceptance of the altered body image.

Breast prostheses constructed to look and feel like real breast tissue are available. The prosthesis fits into a special pocket inside the brassiere. Some types are available for swim suits and strapless tops. The construction of the prosthesis varies from sponge rubber to fluid- or air-filled.

Volunteers from the local cancer society often visit new mastectomy clients to assist them in the physical and psychological transition and adjustment after breast surgery. The American Cancer Society publishes a pamphlet entitled *Help Yourself to Recovery,* which includes simple postmastectomy exercises to perform as a part of the rehabilitation process.

Pharmacological

Some of the agents used in the treatment of breast cancer include antineoplastic drugs such as antiestrogens: megestrol acetate (Megace), medroxyprogesterone acetate (Depo-Provera), tamoxifen citrate (Nolvadex), and aminoglutethamide (Cytadren). Androgens for postmenopausal clients include testolactone (Teslac); methyltestosterone (Testred), or rotating combinations of chemotherapy agents such as cyclophosphamide (Cytoxan), an alkalating agent, doxorubicin hydrochloride (Adriamycin), an antitumor antibiotic; 5-fluorouracil (Adrucil) and methotrexate sodium (Rheumatrex); antimetabolites; and prednisone (Orasone), a glucocorticoid via intravenous or oral routes. These drugs may be initiated before or after surgery. These antineoplastic agents act in several ways to either inhibit cellular growth or interfere with DNA replication. A laboratory test called tissue assay determines if estrogen or progesterone stimulates the cancer cells to grow. If the cancerous growth is stimulated by estrogen, antiestrogen drugs are used to treat the breast cancer. When the tumors are not estrogen-dependent, estrogen is used as a chemotherapy agent to treat breast cancers. Examples of two estrogen medications are diethylstilbestrol diphosphate (Stilphostrol) and ethinyl estradiol (Estinyl).

Paclitaxel (Taxol) has demonstrated positive results in clinical trials with breast cancer therapies. It acts by prohibiting cell replication. One of the benefits of this agent is that it causes milder nausea than many of the other chemotherapy agents that are used. It has the potential to cause severe anaphylactic reactions due to a histamine release. To avoid this problem, the client should be medicated with the following medications before Taxol infusion therapy: a corticosteroid such as dexamethasone (Decadron), a histamine blocker such as cimetidine (Tagamet), and an antihistamine diphenhydramine hydrochloride (Benadryl).

Other Therapies

Breast tissue and lymphatic regions may be radiated before or after surgical excision of the tumor. This treatment may be done prophylactically to prevent the metastasis of malignant cells to other areas, or it may be done as a palliative measure to maintain the client's comfort. Figure 30-10 illustrates brachytherapy, the use of radioactive implants at the site of breast cancer.

▶ NURSING PROCESS

▶ Assessment

▶ Subjective Data

The client may come to the office concerned about a newly discovered breast lump and other changes in the breast, such as dimpling, puckering, or discharge. The nurse should ask how long the lump has been present, whether it is movable, whether it is tender, the frequency that BSE is performed, the date of the most recent mammogram, and current medications being taken. Pain should be assessed, using a pain scale to objectify data. Other questions should include the risk factors.

▶ Objective Data

The nurse should assess vital signs and weight and review the report of the last mammogram. Breasts should be examined for lumps and discharge from the nipples. During the postoperative phase, the client's vital signs and incisional site must be assessed, and the client's statements and behaviors monitored to determine emotional status.

COMMUNITY/HOME HEALTH CARE

After a Mastectomy
- Avoid carrying items in the affected arm or wearing purse straps over the affected shoulder.
- Have vaccinations and lab tests or blood draws done on the unaffected side only.
- Obtain immediate medical attention for all injuries and infections of the affected side to prevent complications.

PROFESSIONAL TIP

Tamoxifen

In October 1998, tamoxifen (Nolvadex) was approved to be used for prevention of breast cancer in healthy women who have a higher-than-normal risk factor for breast cancer ("Tamoxifen for breast cancer prevention," 1998).

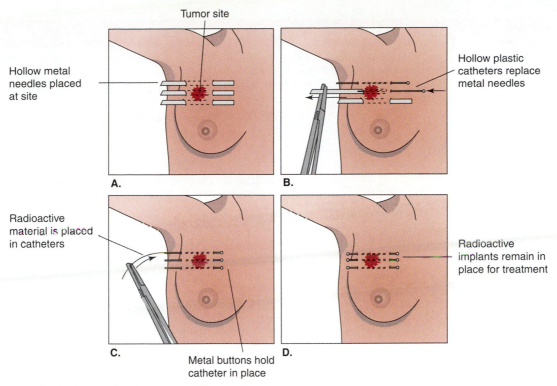

Tumor site

Hollow metal needles placed at site

Hollow plastic catheters replace metal needles

A.

B.

Radioactive material is placed in catheters

Radioactive implants remain in place for treatment

C.

D.

Metal buttons hold catheter in place

Figure 30-10 Brachytherapy for Treatment of Breast Cancer

Nursing diagnoses for a client with breast cancer may include the following:

Nursing Diagnoses	Planning/Goals	Nursing Interventions
▶ *Fear related to breast cancer, possible metastasis, surgery, and disfigurement*	The client will express fears. The client will state one positive method of coping.	Encourage client to express specific feelings of fear. Take extra time to clarify or explain procedures and treatments. Provide written information along with verbal information. Encourage support of family members and significant others. Encourage a preoperative visit by a member of the cancer society or Reach to Recovery.
▶ *Disturbed Body Image related to removal of the breast*	The client will discuss her feelings related to the loss of her breast and demonstrate acceptance of the change in physical appearance.	Remain attentive to signals from the client indicating readiness to look at the surgical site and encourage doing so when readiness is displayed. Be alert for client's comments regarding body changes. Encourage client recommended for chemotherapy to obtain a wig before therapy begins. Approximately 80% of clients undergoing chemotherapy will experience hair loss, and, if the client becomes accustomed to wearing a wig before hair begins to fall out, the client may feel more comfortable later. Inform client that she may have decreased sensation and lymphatic fluid retention in the arm on the affected side. Teach client to keep arm on affected side elevated above the level of the heart to promote lymph drainage. Encourage client to wear a properly fitting elastic compression sleeve on the affected arm that will help reduce the lymphedema. Anticipate the client's need to grieve the loss of her breast. Encourage use of rehabilitation services (Reach to Recovery).

continues

Nursing Diagnoses	Planning/Goals	Nursing Interventions
▶ *Ineffective Breathing Pattern related to the proximity of the surgical incision to respiratory muscles and pain with respiratory effort*	The client's breath sounds will remain clear to auscultation. The client will effectively cough and deep breathe every 2 hours.	Preoperatively, teach the client how to turn, cough, and deep breathe. Postoperatively, assess the client's breath sounds, rate, and quality of respirations every 4 hours. Monitor O_2 saturation with pulse oximeter. Encourage deep breathing or the use of incentive spirometry every hour. Provide O_2 as needed. Medicate the client or encourage use of the PCA pump before performing exercises or deep breathing.
▶ *Dressing/Grooming Self-Care Deficit related to limited use and range of motion on the affected side and postoperative discomforts*	The client will gradually regain ROM and provide self-care.	Begin passive range-of-motion exercises on the first or second postop day as ordered. Demonstrate postoperative exercises for the affected arm or request a consult from the physical therapy department. Observe the client as exercises are performed and reinforce correct performance. Encourage active ROM as soon as ordered by the physician to strengthen the operative side. This may be difficult at first due to tissue soreness from surgery. Encourage client to provide self-care as much as able.

Evaluation Each goal must be evaluated to determine how it has been met by the client.

SAMPLE NURSING CARE PLAN

THE CLIENT WITH BREAST CANCER

Claire Wilder, age 57, is married, with two children ages 24 and 22. During a bath, she noted a small, movable lump in her right breast, grew concerned, and went to see her health care provider. Family history is significant for fibrocystic breast disease and breast cancer on the maternal side (mother, aunt, sister). Personal history: onset of menses at age 10 with regular 28-day cycle, 5-day flow. She is 5 feet 5 inches tall and weighs 175 pounds. Her history is negative for alcohol use, but she smokes one to one-and-a-half packs of cigarettes daily. She did not breastfeed the children. Her last mammogram was 15 years ago. BSE is not practiced routinely. States: "I'm not sure just how to do the exam anyway."

Physical examination reveals a pea-sized lump in the upper right quadrant of the right breast and multiple clusters of lumps throughout each breast. Dimpling is present superior to the nipple. No nipple discharge was noted. The remainder of the exam was unremarkable. Vital signs were within normal limits. A mammogram revealed a suspicious mass, and a biopsy performed using stereotactic visualization was positive for cancer cells. A modified mastectomy was performed the next day with biopsies of adjacent lymph nodes. Six of ten nodes were also positive.

The morning after surgery, Claire displayed behaviors that the nurse interpreted as anxiety. She confided in the nurse that she was afraid she was going to die, as her mother had, from the cancer. Claire had a large chest pressure dressing with two Jackson-Pratt drains in place. She stated that she was glad she had the PCA pump to take care of the pain.

Nursing Diagnosis 1 *Bathing/Hygiene Self-Care Deficit related to temporary altered function of arm as evidenced by large chest pressure dressing and two drains in place*

continues

PLANNING/GOALS	NURSING INTERVENTIONS	RATIONALE	EVALUATION
Claire will meet her daily hygiene needs before discharge.	Assess Claire's ability to use affected arm to perform ADLs.	Assessment provides the nurse with baseline information related to Claire's abilities and limitations.	Claire's hygiene needs were met.
	Provide assistance as needed to complete hygiene tasks, such as bathing and grooming.	Assisting with tasks and encouraging Claire to participate will facilitate the return of function and self-esteem.	
	Encourage gradual resumption of activities as Claire indicates readiness.	By gradually increasing the use of the affected arm, Claire will regain strength and maintain the mobility of the extremity. Claire is empowered to help perform her own care, which validates her self-image and worth.	

Nursing Diagnosis 2 *Fear related to removal of the breast as evidenced by her fear of dying as her mother had*

PLANNING/GOALS	NURSING INTERVENTIONS	RATIONALE	EVALUATION
Claire will have less fear about breast removal.	Encourage Claire and family to verbalize their feelings and concerns related to the diagnosis and treatment.	Sharing feelings and concerns often relieves fear. Claire's and family's perceptions may differ from health care worker's and should be identified.	Claire verbalized having less fear about the removal of her breast.
	Assess Claire's normal or previously used coping behaviors	Identification of previous coping patterns enables the nurse to help the client use or change coping behaviors.	
	Involve Claire and her family in care planning.	Involving the client and the family in the planning of the care makes them more likely to feel a part of the team rather than simply accepting a passive "client role."	

continues

Nursing Diagnosis 3 *Acute Pain related to surgical manipulation of tissues and excision of tissue as evidenced by client statement that she was glad she had the PCA pump to take care of the pain*

PLANNING/GOALS	NURSING INTERVENTIONS	RATIONALE	EVALUATION
Claire will verbalize that pain is controlled.	Assess Claire's pain level and response to analgesia every 2 hours.	The nurse must be alert to increasing pain and how the client is tolerating the pain medication.	Claire reports pain is controlled at less than 2 on a 1–10 scale.
	Instruct Claire how to use the PCA pump.	Use of the PCA pump allows the client greater control over analgesia and provides consistent relief from pain.	
	Evaluate the effectiveness of analgesia q 2 hours.	Evaluating the client's response to medication allows the nurse to identify any untoward effects and effectiveness of the medication.	
	Reposition Claire q 2 hours.	Changing positions helps to improve vascular flow and relieves pressure on bony prominences.	
	Elevate the arm on the right side on pillows.	Increased venous flow decreases edema and discomfort due to pressure on nerves in the area.	

CERVICAL CANCER

An abnormal condition of the cervix known as dysplasia may be an early sign of developing cervical cancer. Dysplasia is a change in the size and shape of the cervical cells, and it is classified as mild, moderate, or severe. An abnormal Papanicolaou (Pap) smear may be the first indication of a problem. Pap smears are classified from 1 through 5. A 1 is considered a normal cervix, and a 5 would indicate a malignant condition.

Cervical cancer is the most preventable gynecological cancer. Sexual habits constitute a major factor in the development of cancer of the cervix. Sexually transmitted disease, particularly the human papillomavirus (HPV), is a particularly significant factor. According to Otto (1997), some 15% of all women who have genital herpes will develop dysplasia or cancer *in situ*. Other factors associated with cervical cancer include a history of multiple sexual partners and maternal use of diethylstilbestrol (DES) during pregnancy. The most common sign of cervical cancer is abnormal bleeding, which progresses from a thin, watery, blood-tinged discharge to frank bleeding. Contact bleeding may also occur after intercourse. Advanced disease is indicated by odor, pain in the lower back and groin, difficulty in voiding, hematuria, and rectal bleeding. The Pap smear is the key to early detection. Promotion of regular pelvic exams and education regarding risk are essential.

Although cervical cancer can occur at any age, it occurs most frequently in women between 35 and 55 years of age. It is usually insidious in its onset because it is asymptomatic. Cervical cancer has a high cure rate in the early stages, and it is easily detected by the routine annual Pap smear. The overall 5-year survival rate is 69% (ACS, 1998).

The nurse should immediately bring any abnormal Pap smear results to the attention of the physician or nurse practitioner so the client can be notified and the appropriate follow-up treatment initiated. A repeat Pap smear may be indicated after treatment with a vaginal antibiotic cream, or a colposcopy may be performed.

Staging of the cancer progresses from I to IV (Figure 30-11). Carcinoma *in situ* (CIS) means that the cancerous cells remain within the cervix and have not yet spread to adjacent areas. The higher the number on the staging table, the more the cancer has metastasized to other structures. Stages II through IV indicate that the cancer cells have invaded the bladder, vagina, or other pelvic organs.

STAGING SYSTEM FOR CANCER OF THE CERVIX		
Stage	Characteristics	
I	• Carcinoma is strictly confined to cervix (extension to corpus should be disregarded)	
IA	• Preclinical carcinoma	
IA1	• Minimal microscopically evident stromal invasion	
IA2	• Microscopic lesions no more than 5 mm depth measured from base of epithelium surface or glandular from which it originates, and horizontal spread not to exceed 7 mm	
IB	• All other cases of stage I; occult cancer should be marked "occ"	
II	• Carcinoma extends beyond cervix but has not extended to pelvic wall; it involves vagina, but not as far as lower third	
IIA	• No obvious parametrical involvement	
IIB	• Obvious parametrical involvement	
III	• Carcinoma has extended to pelvic wall; on rectal examination, there is no cancer-free space between tumor and pelvic wall; tumor involves lower third of vagina; all cases with hydronephrosis or nonfunctioning kidney should be included, unless they are known to be due to another cause	
IIIA	• No extension to pelvic wall, but involvement of lower third of vagina	
IIIB	• Extension to pelvic wall, or hydronephrosis or nonfunctioning kidney due to tumor	
IV	• Carcinoma has extended beyond true pelvis or has clinically involved mucosa of bladder or rectum	
IVA	• Spread of growth to adjacent pelvic organs	
IVB	• Spread to distant organs	

Figure 30-11 Cervical Cancer Staging

Medical–Surgical Management

Surgical

Treatment modalities may include conization, a surgical excision of a cone-shaped section of the abnormal cervical tissues. This procedure is desirable if the client is of childbearing age and wants to bear children in the future.

Laser surgery, cryosurgery (freezing of the cells with liquid nitrogen), or cauterization (burning) may be performed as alternative methods of treatment if the cervical lesions are easily visible for the procedure. A total hysterectomy or radical pelvic surgery may be required to eradicate the cancer. If the spread of the disease has become too extensive, treatment will be directed toward palliative measures.

Other Therapies

The physician may recommend the use of radium implants or radiation therapy before the surgical excision of the cervix. The nurse must be cautious in providing nursing care for the client with radium implants. Pregnant nurses or female nurses of childbearing age should not care for this client or spend extended periods of time at the bedside. Direct client care should be organized to optimize time spent at the bedside. A sign should be hung on the door to indicate that radiation is being used in the room and provide a warning for visitors to limit their visit time. With the implants in place, the client will remain on complete bed rest.

In addition, chemotherapy may be utilized as an adjunct therapy to help shrink the tumor or slow its growth.

▶ NURSING PROCESS

▶ Assessment

▶ Subjective Data

The client may complain of postcoital bleeding (bleeding after intercourse) or spotting between menstrual periods or after menopause and, occasionally, a foul-smelling vaginal discharge. Later, as the disease progresses, she may complain of increased or bloody discharge, weight loss, and pain that radiates down the lower back and legs.

▶ Objective Data

Objective data may include the presence and appearance of a vaginal discharge. The cervix may appear eroded or raw and may bleed easily when touched with a cotton-tipped applicator or Pap scraper. Necrotic tissue may be present and cause the foul odor. Pap smear results will probably indicate dysplasia or Class II through Class IV cell changes. Tissue samples obtained through colposcopic examination will also demonstrate cellular changes. In advanced disease, weight loss and anemia may be present. Laparotomy may be performed to stage the disease along with other laboratory and diagnostic testing to identify metastases. Areas most likely to be investigated will be proximal to the cervix, including the rectum, vagina, bladder, and pelvis.

Nursing diagnoses for a client with cervical cancer may include the following:

Nursing Diagnoses	Planning/Goals	Nursing Interventions
▶ *Anxiety related to unknown outcome and possible treatments*	The client will verbalize having less anxiety about treatment and possible outcome.	Be aware of the client's emotional state throughout the course of care and use effective interpersonal communication to facilitate the client's acceptance of her condition and the treatments.
		Explain diagnostic tests and procedures to client to decrease her anxiety.
		Provide therapeutic emotional support to client to help her cope with feelings.
▶ *Sexual Dysfunction related to vaginal bleeding, discomfort, and procedures*	The client will return to normal pattern of sexuality after recovery from treatment for cervical cancer.	Inform client that she may experience dyspareunia related to vaginal dryness after radiation therapy.
		Listen to client's concerns.
		Instruct client to use a water-soluble lubricant during intercourse or to use lubricated condoms to decrease irritation.
▶ *Impaired Urinary Elimination related to sensory motor impairment from radiation effects*	The client will regain normal urinary elimination.	Assess the function of the Foley catheter to ensure patency and drainage.
		Provide careful catheter care.
		Record I&O, including color of urine.
		Encourage the client to drink many fluids to flush the kidneys and decrease risk of UTI.
		Promote urination when catheter is removed.

Evaluation Each goal must be evaluated to determine how it has been met by the client.

ENDOMETRIAL CANCER

Postmenopausal women are at the greatest risk for endometrial cancer, especially if they have taken estrogen replacement therapy for several years (usually more than 5 years). Research has shown that unopposed estrogen stimulation of the endometrial lining has a strong relationship with the development of endometrial cancer. During the normal menstrual cycle, estrogen and progesterone rise and fall. These hormonal fluctuations affect the stimulation of the endometrial tissue to grow or to be sloughed off, in a sense in opposition to each other. Without the progesterone effects, the endometrial tissue is not sloughed off at regular intervals and may undergo cellular changes leading to a high risk for endometrial dysplasia or cancer. For this reason, many physicians and nurse practitioners recommend estrogen-progesterone therapy for clients who experience menopausal symptoms. The combination of the two hormones stimulates the normal menstrual hormonal cycle and causes monthly sloughing of the endometrium. Clients may resist this combination therapy because they are reluctant to continue having menstrual periods in their fifties and sixties.

Other risk factors associated with endometrial cancer may include never having borne a child, being Caucasian, being middle class, never having had sexual intercourse, or being of Jewish descent.

Cancer of the endometrium usually does not produce symptoms until it becomes relatively advanced. Routine Pap smear and pelvic examinations are inadequate for early diagnosis. An endometrial biopsy, which examines the tissue from the uterine lining under a microscope, is the best diagnostic tool to identify cellular changes. This may be done on an annual basis when the client has a routine examination. The medical follow-up treatment plan is dependent upon the biopsy results. D&C has a potential for spreading the cancer cells to adjacent tissues because the malignant cells may escape into the bloodstream at the time of the procedure. This is not usually a problem with the biopsy because the amount of tissue removed is so small and blood loss is minimal. A D&C is also more expensive, higher risk, and requires some type of anesthesia. The 5-year survival rate for endometrial cancer is 84% (ACS, 1998).

Medical–Surgical Management

Treatments for endometrial cancer may range from radiation, radium implants, chemotherapy, or surgery to a combination of any of the above. The choices of treatment are related to the staging of the cancer.

Medical

Intravenous fluid administration will be implemented to replace fluids lost by the excessive bleeding. A blood transfusion may also be ordered because of a low hemoglobin. A hemoglobin above 10 gm/dL is preferred before surgical intervention. The physician may order whole blood or packed red blood cells to increase the hemoglobin rapidly.

Surgical

Surgery for endometrial or cervical cancer includes hysterectomy. A total hysterectomy is the removal of the cervix and the uterus. In a subtotal hysterectomy, only the uterus is removed and the cervix remains. A radical or pan hysterectomy includes the removal of the ovaries, cervix, uterus, fallopian tubes, pelvic lymph nodes, and part of the vagina. Vaginal hysterectomy procedures have been refined with the laparoscopic approach so that many clients are released from the hospital within 24 to 36 hours postoperatively. If the cancer has spread beyond the uterus into the pelvic region, an abdominal hysterectomy may be the best approach for visualization and maneuvering room during the surgical procedure. The physician may recommend a course of radiation therapy after surgery.

Pharmacological

Hormonal therapy with megestrol acetate (Megace), medroxyprogesterone acetate (Depo-Provera), or hydroxyprogesterone caproate (Prodrox) may be administered to suppress tumor growth when the cancer is considered inoperable or has metastasized, especially if the tumor receptors are estrogen-stimulated.

Other Therapies

There is a tendency for endometrial cancer to confine itself to the uterus, which increases the client's 5-year survival prognosis. Endometrial cancer is also one that usually responds well to the therapies available at this time, including radiation. Radiation may be delivered to the pelvic region via external sources, or it may be delivered via intracavitary devices or implants with radium or cesium. There is a potential danger for injury to adjacent pelvic structures during radiation therapy. The nurse should be alert for signs of complications, such as bleeding from the rectum, moderate to severe abdominal pain, constipation, or diarrhea. New therapies are being developed using protons that are capable of more direct application of radiation, which decreases the chance of injury to other organs or structures.

PROFESSIONAL TIP

Radiation Exposure Risk

Owing to the risk of radiation exposure to the caregiver from the radiation implant device, keep procedures that require exposure to the client's perineal area at a minimum.

Nursing Management

One of the earliest symptoms reported by many clients is vaginal bleeding. If the client is post-menopausal, it is imperative that all bleeding be investigated as soon as possible unless it is from hormonally induced periods. Late in the progression of the cancer, the client may experience symptoms similar to those discussed with cervical cancer. Pain is often associated with the spread of cancer to adjacent organs and is considered a late sign.

Objective data may be collected from the client's physical exam findings, biopsy reports, and a history of hormone replacement therapy with or without the estrogen-progesterone combination.

OVARIAN CANCER

Ovarian cancer most often originates in the epithelial tissue of the ovary, and, like cervical and endometrial cancer, does not produce symptoms until it is in an advanced, inoperable stage and is sometimes called "the silent killer." Its symptoms are vague and may be ignored for a long time before the client seeks medical attention.

Ovarian cancer causes more deaths than does any other gynecological cancer, an estimated 14,500 in 1998 (ACS, 1998). The incidence is greatest in women between 45 and 65 years of age. Nulliparity (never having borne a child), smoking, alcohol, infertility, and a high-fat diet are factors that place the client at higher risk for developing ovarian cancer. Metastasis occurs in over 75% of cases before diagnosis, and often the cancer has spread beyond the pelvis. The colon is the most frequent site of ovarian cancer metastasis, then the stomach, and diaphragm.

Unfortunately, medical research has not yet developed an early diagnostic or screening tool to detect ovarian cancer. It is believed, however, that there is an increased risk of ovarian cancer for clients with breast cancer and vice versa. A family history of two or more female relatives with breast or ovarian cancer provides a sound rationale for more frequent breast and pelvic examinations. Often the physician or NP palpates an ovarian mass on a routine bimanual examination. This finding is cause for further investigation by pelvic ultrasound or CT scan to determine the size, character, and consistency (solid or fluid-filled) of the mass and whether other pelvic structures are involved. Some experts believe that there is a link between the occurrence of ovarian cysts and the development of ovarian cancers in certain women.

General diagnostic studies, such as a lower GI series, chest x-ray, intravenous pyelogram (IVP), and laparoscopy may be useful in determining the extent of the primary and secondary lesions. A substance called CA-125 may be measured in the blood if ovarian cancer is suspected because this type of malignancy produces the CA-125. Used alone, this is not diagnostic of ovarian cancer because the CA-125 marker in the blood may be present in some benign conditions of the ovary, such as benign ovarian cysts. If the client develops peritoneal fluid or ascites as the cancer progresses, it may be removed by paracentesis for cytologic examination.

Recurrent disease is common and may occur in 2 years or less. Continued medical surveillance is recommended every 2 months for a period of 2 years for the earliest possible detection of new lesions. The 5-year survival rate is 46% (ACS, 1998).

Medical–Surgical Management

Surgical

Surgical excision of the ovary is rarely successful because of the extensiveness of the disease. A total abdominal hysterectomy with a bilateral salpingo-oophorectomy is performed for most stages of the disease. Most often a combination of radiation, chemotherapy, immunotherapy, and surgery produces the best results, even if they are only palliative for the client. The client must be actively involved and informed of her treatment options as well as her prognosis to enable her to make sound choices in the treatments chosen.

Pharmacological

Chemotherapy drugs that have been used with ovarian cancer treatment include cyclophosphamide (Cytoxan), doxorubicin hydrochloride (Adriamycin), mitomycin (Mutamycin), and paclitaxel (Taxol). These may be administered by regional or intraarterial perfusion techniques. These percutaneous modes direct the drugs to the lesion's vascular supply. If the cancer has not metastasized, a regimen of chemotherapy using a single drug, such as Cytoxan, may be administered over the course of 5 days and repeated again at regular intervals over the course of a year. A combination of the chemotherapy agents, used in a rotating series, is often more effective for reproductive cancers in the advanced stages. For example, the client would receive one drug over the course of 5 days, then switch to another drug for 5 days, and then a third drug for 5 days. This series may be repeated over the year in a similar pattern to that used with a single agent.

Sometimes two or three different medications are necessary to achieve pain control. Intravenous medications are often given by a PCA pump with continuous low-dose narcotics. This method seems more effective for the client than IV bolus doses every 4 hours. Medications may also be given slow IV push (an RN procedure), orally in tablets or liquids, intramuscularly, or by transdermal patches (Duragesic). A liquid mixture of syrup, cocaine, morphine, alcohol, flavoring, and water called "Brompton's mixture or elixir" may be ordered. The client may drink up to 20 cc every 3 to 4 hours for pain relief. Most of these methods of narcotic administration are equally effective and may be used in the home care or hospice setting. Other types of medication that may be given include tranquilizers, antiemetics, and laxatives.

▶ NURSING PROCESS

▶ Assessment

▶ Subjective Data

The client may describe fatigue, malaise, diarrhea or constipation, pelvic pressure, frequency of urination, loss of appetite, nausea, weight gain or loss, vaginal bleeding or spotting with intercourse, a foul-smelling vaginal discharge, and pain in the lower back. The list of symptoms is very vague and could be related to many reproductive and nonreproductive disorders.

▶ Objective Data

Objective data pertinent to all cancers of the pelvic reproductive organs may include information from the client's previous health history, reproductive history (onset of menses, pregnancies, contraceptives methods, infections, hormonal replacement therapy, and surgeries), the discovery of a palpable mass during a bimanual examination, an abnormal appearance of the cervix or adjacent tissues, abnormal Pap smear results greater than Class II dysplasia, abnormal cervical or endometrial biopsies, increased abdominal girth, or the presence of ascites and pleural effusion.

Diagnostic tests and laboratory studies may include all or some of the following: Pap smear, pelvic ultrasound, chest x-ray, IVP (intravenous pyelogram), kidney/ureters/bladder x-ray (KUB), CBC with differential, blood chemistry studies, bleeding and clotting time, endometrial biopsy, cervical biopsy, D&C tissue specimens, Schiller's test and colposcopy, laparoscopy, barium enema, and bone scan.

Nursing diagnoses for a client with endometrial or ovarian cancer may include the following:

Nursing Diagnoses,	Planning/Goals,	Nursing Interventions,
Preoperative		
▶ *Fear related to tentative diagnoses, pending surgical procedures, cancer treatment and its side effects, incapacitating or extended illness with resulting dependence, and possible death*	The client will verbalize fears and have behaviors consistent with reduced fear before and after surgery.	Facilitate the client's expression of fear by encouraging the client's open discussion of her concerns. Be alert for nonverbal cues as well. Arrange a consultation with a social worker or chaplain, if appropriate.
▶ *Chronic Pain related to the spread of cancer throughout the pelvis and adjacent structures*	The client will have pain controlled at a level that allows the client to continue to function in her activities of daily living as long as possible.	Administer analgesics as ordered. Provide comfort measures, such as position changes and back rub.

Nursing Diagnoses,	Planning/Goals,	Nursing Interventions,
Postoperative		
▶ *Impaired Skin Integrity related to surgical interventions, radiation, and chemotherapy side effects*	The client's skin integrity will be maintained.	Provide the client with proper skin care instructions during and after radiation therapy that may include avoiding soaps, creams, powder, deodorants, and other substances around the incision that may irritate the skin; not washing off the radiation markings; and avoiding tight clothing around the area. Teach the client to look for signs of reactions to radiation therapy, such as tenderness, flushed color (like a sunburn), delayed wound healing, and itching. Perform daily cleansing of the incisional area with water only. If the client is on complete bed rest due to radium implant therapy, provide a complete bedbath as well as morning and bedtime skin care.

continues

Nursing Diagnoses,	Planning/Goals,	Nursing Interventions,
		Organize time near the client's bedside to brief periods to avoid overexposure to radiation.
		Wear rubber gloves when disposing of soiled materials.
		Put soiled dressings in a biohazard waste container.
▶ *Impaired Urinary Bowel Elimination, Incontinence or Constipation, related to the proximity of surgical site to bowel and bladder, spread of cancer to adjacent structures, manipulation of organs during surgery, administration of narcotic analgesics, lack of activity, and changes in dietary intake*	The client will have adequate bowel and bladder function during the postoperative period.	Explain dietary modifications designed to reduce residue. The diet should be limited in dairy products, raw fruits, grains, and vegetables. Meats must be well cooked and possibly ground.
		If the client is not receiving radium implant therapy, weigh her daily on the same scale at the same time of the day.
		Review the client's normal elimination patterns from the baseline assessment data to help identify early changes in bowel or bladder elimination.
		Forewarn the client of radiation enteritis and cystitis, and common tissue responses to radiation therapy. Instruct her to report symptoms, such as diarrhea, cramping, frequency, urgency, and dysuria.
		Assess bowel sounds and abdominal distention at least every 4 to 8 hours.
		Carefully monitor the client's urinary pattern and maintain an accurate intake and output record.
		Observe urine and stool for color, consistency, amount, and the presence of blood.
		Monitor the client for other gastrointestinal problems, such as nausea, vomiting, and **tenesmus** (spasmodic contraction of the anal or bladder sphincter, causing pain and a persistent urge to empty the bowel or bladder).
▶ *Impaired Physical Mobility related to intracavity radiation*	The client will not develop deep vein thrombosis.	Accurately measure the client's legs to ensure the proper fit of the hose.
		Apply thigh-high antiembolitic stockings (TEDS) as ordered.
		Assist client to ambulate when allowed.

Evaluation Each goal must be evaluated to determine how it has been met by the client.

MENSTRUAL DISORDERS

Abnormalities of menstruation may be associated with an increase or decrease in secretion from any of the following glands: hypothalamus, pituitary, ovaries, adrenals, and thyroid. The normal menstrual pattern is controlled by a series of hormonal negative feedback mechanisms. The average menstrual cycle occurs every 28 to 30 days when the endometrial lining of the uterus sloughs off in the absence of a fertilized ovum.

DYSMENORRHEA

Painful menstruation, dysmenorrhea, also called "menstrual cramps," is more common in nulliparous women and in women who are not having intercourse. The exact pathophysiology is unknown, but it may be related to endocrine secretions such as prostaglandin F, which causes uterine cramping, irritation, and contractions. Other causes may include uterine anatomical anomalies, chronic illness, or psychological factors.

The primary symptom is pelvic pain before or at the onset of the menses that may be due to spasms of the uterus, narrowing of the cervical canal, emotional factors, endometriosis, pelvic inflammatory disease, or the presence of an intrauterine contraceptive device (IUD). The client may also state that the pain radiates across the lower back and downward into the legs.

The condition is diagnosed on the basis of the client's complaints and description of the timing of the onset of symptoms. The nurse should obtain information pertaining to the menstrual history and general health status of the client. A thorough physical exam will be performed by the physician, including a bimanual exam to rule out other possible causes. A pelvic ultrasound may be ordered.

One effective preventive intervention may begin before the young woman begins menstruation. A positive parental attitude toward the onset of menstruation can aid the young girl in adjusting to the physiologic and psychological changes that occur with puberty.

Certain medications have been used over the last 10 to 15 years that are effective in the treatment of dysmenorrhea. Analgesics such as acetaminophen (Tylenol) and ibuprofen (Motrin) are useful in relieving pain. Oral contraceptives have been used for some clients to inhibit ovulation, which appears to be an associated cause. Prostaglandin inhibitors such as naproxen sodium (Anaprox) and mefenamic acid (Ponstel) are useful if taken at the earliest sign of discomfort.

AMENORRHEA

Amenorrhea, the absence of menstruation, may be primary or secondary. Primary amenorrhea is defined as the absence of menstruation by the age of 17. Possible causes are related to anatomical or genetic abnormalities (Turner's syndrome). The treatment is dependent upon the cause. Secondary amenorrhea is defined as the absence of menstruation after 6 months of regular periods or after 12 months of irregular periods. Several etiologies are possible for secondary amenorrhea, including anatomic abnormalities, nutritional deficits (anorexia nervosa), excessive exercise with significant decreases in body fat, endocrine dysfunction, emotional disturbances, side effects of medications, pregnancy, and lactation.

This condition is diagnosed based upon the length of absence of menstruation. A complete physical examination should be performed, including a pelvic examination to rule out many factors discussed earlier. A progesterone challenge test may be administered in an attempt to force the body to respond hormonally. Medroxyprogesterone acetate (Depo-Provera) is taken orally for 5 to 10 days as ordered by the physician. When the medication is finished, the client should have a menstrual period within 3 or 4 days. A menstrual flow after taking the medication may be an indicator that the client has not been ovulating. If no bleeding occurs, further investigation may be necessary to uncover other causes. Hormonal imbalances, microscopic pituitary tumors, and nutritional deficits are common etiologies of secondary amenorrhea. A microscopic pituitary tumor will cause an elevation in the prolactin level and result in anovulation and amenorrhea. A serum prolactin level should be ordered, especially if the client has noticed any breast discharge. Normal prolactin level should not exceed 15 ng/dL. With pituitary tumors, the prolactin level may exceed 400 ng/dL. In these cases, the drug of choice is bromocriptine mesylate (Parlodel), which had been used in the past to suppress lactation in mothers who did not breastfeed their newborns. A careful examination of the client is needed before administration of Parlodel, because of an increased potential for cardiovascular problems recently associated with this medication. Because of this risk, the medication is no longer used for the postpartum client to suppress milk production. Other medical or surgical interventions will be dependent upon the cause of the amenorrhea.

OTHER DISORDERS

Other menstrual disorders include menorrhagia and metrorrhagia. Both types of abnormal bleeding can be problematic for the client and require further investigation. **Polymenorrhea** is a term used to describe short menstrual cycles of less than 21 days in length. The causes are similar to those of the other menstrual disorders. **Oligomenorrhea** is a diminished menstrual flow, but it is not classified as amenorrhea. It may be associated with low-dose oral contraceptives that inhibit the growth of the endometrium and result in minimal tissue sloughing at the end of the cycle. Other causes may be metabolic or hormonal. Again, treatment is specific to the etiology.

For conditions associated with heavy bleeding or bleeding between periods, a dilatation and curettage (D&C) may be performed. In this case, the procedure may be diagnostic and therapeutic. Tissue removed from the uterus will be examined microscopically and histologically to evaluate its stage in the menstrual cycle. A hysterectomy may be indicated if abnormalities are discovered or if the bleeding is so excessive that the client is significantly compromised. The client may require a blood transfusion to correct low hemoglobin and hematocrit levels before any other procedures. Supplemental iron generally is prescribed by the physician to also help correct the deficiency.

▶ NURSING PROCESS

▶ Assessment

▶ Subjective Data

The nurse should ask the client about the onset of the bleeding and its relationship to the timing of her normal menstruation, the color of the bleeding, amount, number of pads saturated, presence of clots, and presence of pain with the bleeding. A history of current medications, contraception, and the possibility of pregnancy are additional assessment data. Any pre-existing health problems that could affect bleeding and clotting times, as well as life stressors, should be explored by the nurse during the data-gathering process.

▶ Objective Data

Assessment of vital signs may indicate hypertension and tachycardia. Laboratory test results must be monitored.

Nursing Management

Possible nursing diagnoses for a client with any of the menstrual disorders discussed in this section may include:

- *Acute Pain related to uterine cramping or heavy bleeding*
- *Decreased Cardiac Output related to excessive blood loss*
- *Fatigue related to decreased hemoglobin and hematocrit levels*
- *Disturbed Body Image related to the absence of menstruation*

PREMENSTRUAL SYNDROME

One-third to one-half of women between 20 and 50 years of age experience some of the symptoms known as premenstrual syndrome (PMS). Once, this condition was thought by many physicians to be a psychological problem of women; however, recent research has supported data that there are many physiologic as well as psychological factors involved. PMS often occurs during the secretory phase of the menstrual cycle, after ovulation. Risk factors associated with the development of PMS include age (over 30), multiple life stressors, inappropriate nutritional status, a previous reaction to or side effects from oral contraceptive use, a sedentary lifestyle, marital status, a history of preeclampsia in pregnancy, and multiparity.

Over 150 symptoms have been reported that have been related to PMS. These include weight gain, bloating, irritability, edema, headache, mood swings, inability to concentrate, food cravings, acne, and numerous others. For many women, the PMS symptoms are merely a monthly nuisance, but for others, the symptoms are so incapacitating that they cannot function in their normal roles or responsibilities. The onset of symptoms is usually 7 to 10 days before the menstrual period starts; symptoms end after the menstrual flow begins.

Research has correlated hormonal imbalances of estrogen, progesterone, ACTH, and androgens with the symptoms of PMS. The presence of prostaglandin F in the tissue may also be a cause of some of the symptoms. Prostaglandins are associated with many inflammatory responses in the tissues.

The first step in identifying PMS is a physical examination to rule out other possible disorders of the reproductive system. The client may be asked to keep a monthly calendar of symptoms to see if there are patterns in severity, type, or onset. Blood tests may be ordered to assess estrogen and progesterone levels, as well as checking the glucose level. Low blood glucose level has been associated with irritability that sometimes accompanies PMS symptoms. The client should receive counseling, if needed, to facilitate coping with life stressors that may be complicating the complexity of the PMS symptoms.

Medical–Surgical Management

Pharmacological

Some physicians and NPs recommend medication such as acetaminophen (Tylenol), naproxen (Naprosyn), mefenamic acid (Ponstel), and ibuprofen (Advil) for the relief of minor discomforts of PMS. Tranquilizers and antidepressants have not proved to be effective for short-term use in PMS; however, in severe cases, they may be a last resort. Several PMS symptoms are thought to be related to a low progesterone level. For some clients, the use of progesterone suppositories or oral progesterone to supplement their own production during the secretory phase of the menstrual cycle has been useful.

Diet

A thorough diet history should be included in the assessment data collected. Certain nutritional deficits or cravings have been linked to the worsening of PMS. Items such as sugar, salt, caffeine, and chocolate are in this category. Many studies have shown that limiting intake of these substances may be helpful. Caffeinated beverages may increase anxiety, irritability, and deplete vitamin B stores in the body. Dairy products interfere with the absorption of magnesium, which helps stabilize the mood. Chocolates have been related to increased sugar cravings, mood swings, fluid retention, and increased vitamin B demands. Oranges and other fruits or vegetables that are highly acidic may worsen PMS. Foods that are recommended are whole grains, nuts, pasta, legumes, root vegetables, fruits like apples and pears, poultry, and seafood. A good vitamin supplement rich in vitamin B-complex, calcium, magnesium, and zinc should be taken daily, especially during the PMS period. Herbal tea formulas have shown some promise as alternative methods of relieving PMS.

Activity

As mentioned previously, a sedentary lifestyle and lack of exercise are associated with PMS. A regular exercise routine, coupled with the use of stress-management techniques such as deep breathing and relaxation exercises help the client cope with the increased sense of anxiety or irritability that may accompany the PMS. Meditation, positive affirmation, visualization, and imagery may be helpful. Other alternative therapies may include acupressure, neurolymphatic or neurovascular massage, and yoga.

▶ NURSING PROCESS

▶ Assessment

▶ Subjective Data

The client should describe her symptoms and the impact on her lifestyle. Many times, clients will seek medical attention for their PMS symptoms when the emotional impact has caused friction in the home, marriage, work, or family environment. Symptoms described may include weight gain, bloating, irritability, headache, mood swings, inability to concentrate, or food cravings. The client should be asked to relate symptoms to time of menstrual cycle.

▶ Objective Data

The client should be assessed for weight gain and edema. Results of all laboratory tests should be reviewed.

Nursing diagnoses for a client with premenstrual syndrome may include the following:

Nursing Diagnoses	Planning/Goals	Nursing Interventions
▶ *Excess Fluid Volume related to hormonal imbalance and increased sodium or sugar intake*	The client's intake and output will be balanced, and edema will be decreased.	Advise client that a certain amount of fluid retention is normal before the onset of the menstrual period and cannot be avoided, but by limiting sodium and sugar intake, she may be able to influence the amount of fluid retained.
▶ *Health-Seeking Behaviors related to finding methods to cope with symptoms of PMS*	The client will develop effective health-promotion skills to increase coping with PMS symptoms or to decrease symptom severity or frequency.	Teach client how to keep a monthly PMS calendar of events. Discuss prescribed medications with the client, including the dosage, expected effects, and side effects. Discuss relationship of foods to PMS.
▶ *Risk for Imbalanced Nutrition: More than body requirements related to cravings for sugar, sodium, and caffeine*	The client will modify her dietary intake of sugar, sodium, and caffeine to decrease PMS symptoms.	Advise the client in ways to modify her dietary intake and limit foods and beverages associated with PMS.
▶ *Situational Low Self-Esteem related to client's perception of appearance and relationship problems during PMS episodes*	The client's self-esteem will be maintained.	Encourage client to discuss her feelings about herself during PMS. Remind client that she is not alone in her condition but that millions of other women experience similar symptoms. This may help the client accept that she is not mentally ill but having a temporary problem associated with hormone imbalance.

Evaluation Each goal must be evaluated to determine how it has been met by the client.

COMPLICATIONS OF MENOPAUSE

Menopause, or climacteric, is the cessation of menstruation. It may occur as a natural hormonal decline or it may be surgically induced by removal of the uterus and ovaries. Some people may think of menopause as the "change of life." Many women will begin to experience signs and symptoms of approaching menopause around 50 years of age; however, the range of onset is from 45 to 60 years old. Menstrual cycles become further apart and the flow decreases. The onset is usually gradual, and it may take over a year before the woman has completely ceased menstruation. Reproductive capability is also lost with menopause. For some women this is a sad time perceived as the loss of womanhood; for others it is a welcome relief.

The decreasing level of ovarian hormone production affects women in a variety of ways, more than just the end of menstruation. There may be a relaxation of the pelvic support structures, loss of skin turgor and elasticity, and thinning of the hair on the head, axilla, and pubic regions. Other signs of decreasing hormones (estrogen and progesterone) are vaginal dryness, thinning of the vaginal mucosa, weight gain, dry skin, and stress incontinence. The estrogen level plays an important protective role in maintaining an adequate calcium balance in the bones and preventing coronary artery disease. Without calcium, bones become brittle, and there is an increased risk of fractures and osteoporosis. A baseline bone density study may be recommended before menopause.

Some women experience psychological responses to menopause, such as mild to moderate depression, nervousness, and insomnia. Consultation with a psychologist, minister, or counselor may be useful in facilitating the transition through this period for some women.

Women may also experience mild to moderate periods of profuse perspiration called hot flashes. These usually move from the waist upward. They are caused by the decreased estrogen level and its effect on the hypothalamus. The sensation may last from a few seconds to 2 to 3 minutes. It appears that many different things can trigger a hot flash—drinking hot beverages, eating spicy foods, smoking, and consuming caffeine and alcohol.

Medical–Surgical Management

Pharmacological

For some women, estrogen replacement therapy is recommended, especially if they are experiencing moderately uncomfortable symptoms. Estrogen replacement therapy (ERT) may help decrease some symptoms, such as insomnia, hot flashes, mood swings, and lack of concentration. Another positive benefit of taking estrogen is its protective nature against osteoporosis and cardiovascular disease. Estrogen elevates the high-density lipoproteins (healthy ones) and lowers the low-density lipoproteins (unhealthy) in the circulation. Estrogen may be administered orally, as a transdermal patch, or as a vaginal cream. The transdermal patch releases the hormone into the bloodstream percutaneously. This results in a bypass of the stomach and liver, which means less gastrointestinal tract irritation for the client. The patch is a good option of estrogen administration for clients with liver disease. Occasionally, the client may complain of a rash or skin irritation from the patch that is usually related to the adhesive.

Conjugated estrogen (Premarin), estradiol (Estrace), and estropipate (Ogen) are examples of oral estrogens available. Estrogen creams or water-soluble gels such as Lubrifax or K-Y, may be used to combat the vaginal dryness and resulting dyspareunia.

Many health care providers are concerned about the possible effects of unopposed estrogen's causing endometrial cancer. To alleviate some of this concern, a progesterone supplement may be added to the hormone regimen if the client still has a uterus. Progesterone, along with the estrogen replacement, will cause the woman to have some amount of endometrial sloughing every month, a menstrual period. This prevents the buildup of tissue inside the uterus, which has the potential to undergo cellular changes or mutation into cancerous cells. Some studies have suggested that a woman should be on ERT for approximately 10 to 15 years after menopause to reach the maximum benefits of the therapy.

Diet

The nurse should provide the client with instructions regarding the importance of an adequate daily intake of calcium-rich products, such as dairy products. Many low-fat, high-calcium products are available if the client has a concern about weight gain. Calcium supplements may also be taken in a tablet form. The woman should consult her health care provider before adding a calcium supplement because too much calcium increases the risk for other health problems. Herbal teas, vitamin E, magnesium, and primrose oil have been used as alternative methods to alleviate or decrease hot flashes and promote relaxation for some women.

Activity

One important way that the client can decrease the potential for calcium loss from weight-bearing bones is to exercise. A planned 30-minute program performed at least 3 times a week is adequate to maintain bone density. Exercises such as walking or swimming are excellent. Swimming provides good non-weight-bearing activity and promotes active movement of all extremities. Biking is a good exercise to maintain joint mobility in the lower extremities, but it does not require the use of the same muscle groups as walking.

▶ NURSING PROCESS

▶ Assessment

▶ Subjective Data

The client may present with concerns about decreasing regularity of menstruation or hot flashes. The nurse should obtain information from the client about gynecological and obstetrical history, including menstruation. It is helpful to know when the client began experiencing symptoms in predicting the length of time they may continue.

▶ Objective Data

These include a physical examination and Pap smear. The results of the Pap smear can indicate if there is less estrogen present in the cervical tissue than normal.

CLIENT TEACHING

Estrogen Transdermal Patch

- Rotate the application sites of the patch every 3 to 4 days.
- Hold the patch to the open air for 10 to 15 seconds before application to decrease the potential for skin irritation.
- The estrogen patch may provide less protection against bone and heart problems than oral estrogen does.

Nursing diagnoses for a client experiencing menopausal symptoms may include the following:

Nursing Diagnoses	Planning/Goals	Nursing Interventions
▶ Health-Seeking Behaviors related to perceived physiological and psychologic impact of decreased estrogen	The client will develop effective health promotion skills to increase coping with menopausal symptoms or to decrease symptom severity or frequency.	Encourage the client to continue to see her health care provider for annual Pap smears and breast examinations. Explain nutritional requirements for vitamins and calcium that increase with menopause. Encourage the client to begin a regular exercise program that includes weight-bearing activities such as walking to prevent loss of calcium from the bones.
▶ Impaired Tissue Integrity related to vaginal dryness and dry skin	The client will maintain skin integrity, and vagina will not be dry.	Advise the client to try estrogen creams or water-soluble gels such as Lubrifax or K-Y, to combat the vaginal dryness and resulting dyspareunia. Encourage the client to use body lotion to prevent dry skin.
▶ Stress Urinary Incontinence related to relaxation of the pelvic support structures	The client will not experience stress incontinence.	Teach client to perform Kegel exercises daily. Encourage client to empty bladder regularly.
▶ Decisional Conflict related to taking supplemental estrogen therapy	The client will make informed decisons about taking supplemental estrogen.	Discuss the advantages and disadvantages of estrogen replacement therapy with the client. Remind the client that if she has a uterus and takes hormonal replacements, she will continue to have monthly menstrual cycles.
▶ Deficient Knowledge related to factors causing symptoms and methods to prevent and to relieve symptoms	The client will verbalize an understanding of menopause, the effects of hormones, and treatment options.	Instruct the client in the normalcy of menopause and in the reasons for the physiologic changes resulting from decreased ovarian function. Explain nutritional requirements for vitamins and calcium that increase with menopause. Encourage the client to begin a regular exercise program that includes weight-bearing activities, such as walking, to prevent loss of calcium from the bones.

Evaluation Each goal must be evaluated to determine how it has been met by the client.

STRUCTURAL DISORDERS

Structural anomalies are separated into female and male disorders

CYSTOCELE, URETHROCELE, RECTOCELE, PROLAPSED UTERUS

Cystocele, urethrocele, rectocele, and prolapsed uterus are often associated with relaxation of the pelvic muscles that support the uterus, bladder, and rectum. A **cystocele** is a downward displacement of the bladder into the anterior vaginal wall. A **urethrocele** is a downward displacement of the urethra into the vagina, and a **rectocele** is an anterior displacement of the rectum into the posterior vaginal wall. **Prolapsed uterus** is a downward displacement of the uterus into the vagina (Figure 30-12). Possible causes for the four conditions are multiple pregnancies, third- or fourth-degree perineal lacerations with childbirth,

and weakening of the pelvic muscles as an aging process.

A prolapsed uterus is often accompanied by a cystocele and/or rectocele. Variations in the severity of uterine prolapse are described as first-, second-, and third-degree. With a first-degree prolapse, the cervix is visible at the vaginal introitus, or opening, without straining. With a second-degree prolapse, the cervix extends beyond the vaginal opening to the perineum. With a third-degree prolapse, the uterus protrudes outside of the vagina. This severe condition is called *procidentia uteri*.

Medical–Surgical Management

Medical and surgical interventions for the treatment of each of these conditions are focused on relief of the discomforts and restoration of the structure and function of the pelvic organs.

Medical

The pessary is a small molded plastic or rubber apparatus that fits into the vagina behind the pubic bone and in front of the rectum. Its function is to provide an

Figure 30-12 A. Cystocele; B. Urethrocele; C. Rectocele; D. Uterine Prolapse

artificial or mechanical support for the uterus. Pessaries are not uncomfortable and should not be felt by the client if properly fitted and in the correct position. The client should be taught how to insert and remove the pessary so it can be cleaned. The pessary may be washed in warm, soapy water once every 1 to 2 weeks. Prolonged use of a mechanical device such as a pessary may result in vaginal necrosis and ulceration. Periodic examination by a health care professional is recommended, especially with weight gain or loss of greater than 10 to 15 pounds.

Surgical

Surgery for a prolapsed uterus may require a hysterectomy. If the prolapse is accompanied by a cystocele or rectocele, an A&P repair may also be performed. An A&P repair (anterior/posterior colporrhaphy) may be performed vaginally to replace the bladder, urethra, or rectum in the correct anatomic position. Another pro-

cedure, the Marshall-Marchette-Krantz, may be performed to attach the bladder to the inferior surface of the pubic bone. Postoperatively, the client may be sent home with an indwelling Foley catheter because of the potential inability to void. This is a common postoperative situation that usually resolves itself spontaneously within 1 or 2 weeks after discharge.

Activity

Clients should be taught the Kegel exercise before childbearing. This exercise is performed by tightening and releasing the perineal muscles. An important muscle group, called the "levators," helps lift and support the organs inside the pelvis.

▶ NURSING PROCESS

▶ Assessment

▶ Subjective Data

The client often describes stress incontinence, which is a loss of urine when she coughs, sneezes, laughs, or jumps. She may describe it as "a leaky bladder." She may notice that her panties are damp or that she dribbles urine. Many women complain of frequent urination in small quantities with a feeling of urgency without burning or dysuria. The client may notice that she has been experiencing more constipation or a sense of bearing down pressure in the pelvis with a rectocele. Many of these symptoms will decrease or subside completely when she is lying down. The nurse should obtain information about the client's childbearing history, onset of current symptoms, and any other pertinent gynecological data.

▶ Objective Data

These include the visualization of a bulging of the bladder, urethra, or rectum into the vagina. The bulging increases when the client is asked to bear down. Urinalysis results should be evaluated.

CLIENT TEACHING

Kegel Exercises

- Suggest that the client practice when she has a full bladder. If she can successfully start and stop the flow of urine from the bladder, she is identifying and using the correct muscle groups.
- The muscles should be tightened and held for 5 to 10 seconds and then released slowly.
- Repeat the exercises at least 10 times.
- Kegel exercise can be practiced anytime and anyplace.
- A secondary benefit of increasing the strength and contractility of the pelvic and perineal muscles is seen in an improvement in pelvic sensations for both partners during intercourse.

Nursing diagnoses for a female client with a structural disorder of the reproductive system may include the following:

Nursing Diagnoses	Planning/Goals	Nursing Interventions
▶ *Stress Urinary Incontinence related to relaxation of the pelvic muscles*	The client will have less stress incontinence.	Teach the client Kegel exercise and encourage routine practice daily. Encourage client to empty bladder frequently.
▶ *Constipation related to relaxation of the anterior rectal wall into the vagina and decreased function*	The client will not have constipation.	Encourage client to defecate at same time each day. Encourage regular exercise. Encourage client to eat high-fiber foods and to drink plenty of fluids.
▶ *Risk for Infection related to exposure of internal tissues to external environmental factors*	The client will be free of signs and symptoms of infection.	Monitor the client's vital signs. Encourage client to practice proper personal hygiene and wear clean undergarments daily.
▶ *Sexual Dysfunction related to discomforts with intercourse*	The client will have a fulfilling sexual relationship without discomfort.	Be sensitive to client cues related to her sexual concerns. Encourage the client to openly discuss her feelings with her partner. Help the client set realistic goals during her recovery period to facilitate a new outlook on her relationship.

Evaluation Each goal must be evaluated to determine how it has been met by the client.

INFERTILITY

Approximately one in every six couples experiences infertility, the inability to produce offspring. Infertility may be primary or secondary. In primary infertility, the couple have never achieved a pregnancy or have never carried a pregnancy to viability. Secondary infertility involves problems that arise after the couple has had a successful pregnancy. Many factors may be investigated as causes of infertility in both female and male clients. Forty percent of infertility factors are female-related, 40% are male-related, and 20% are a combination of multiple factors that involve both partners. The more factors that are involved, the more difficult the infertility resolution.

The etiology of infertility may be related to anatomic or endocrine problems. The female anatomic or structural abnormalities may include blocked passages through the cervix or fallopian tubes caused by failed development or by past infections, such as PID, or STDs. Uterine and cervical abnormalities may also occur. The cervix may be too narrow or closed and sperm are unable to navigate through the passage. The uterus may have a partial or complete septum inside that limits the internal cavity space. Immune problems involve the development of antibodies by the woman's system to the male's sperm. These antibodies may be present in the cervical mucus and kill the sperm on contact. Hyposecretion or hypersecretion of FSH, LH, estrogen, or progesterone have been associated with infertility.

A basic infertility workup may be initiated when the client has been unable to conceive after 6 to 12 months of unprotected intercourse. One simple, non-invasive procedure is the use of a basal body temperature chart. The chart is kept for a minimum of 3 months and then reviewed for normal ovulatory fluctuations in the basal temperature. During the first half of the menstrual cycle, the body temperature may remain below 98°F. At ovulation, there is often a slight decrease in the temperature for a 24-hour period. This is the optimal period of fertility. After ovulation, the woman's basal body temperature should go above 98°F and remain in that range for a period of 14 days. The length of the luteal phase (secretory phase) of the cycle following ovulation is a critical factor in some infertility disorders. Variations in the temperature chart may indicate that the client has had an anovulatory cycle or has a shortened luteal phase. Since the fertilized ovum does not implant in the endometrium until 6 to 8 days after conception, the luteal phase is critical to maintain the blood-rich lining long enough for implantation to occur. A low progesterone level during the luteal phase may result in spontaneous **abortion** (ending a pregnancy before the age of viability) of the fertilized ovum before implantation. Diagnostic tests that may be ordered include the following:

- Endometrial biopsy to detect tissue responses during both phases of the menstrual cycle
- Endocrine imbalance testing which measures pituitary, gonadotropin, testosterone, estrogen, and progesterone levels

- Laparoscopy to discover conditions such as endometriosis, adhesions, or scar tissue that potentially immobilize the fimbriae or polycystic ovarian disease (Stein-Leventhal syndrome)

Medical–Surgical Management

There is no one treatment for infertility problems. The goal of treatment is successful achievement of a pregnancy that is carried to full term and produces a healthy offspring.

Medical

Infertility treatment may include artificial insemination with either the partner's sperm or donor sperm. This method is particularly useful if the male partner has a low sperm count, abnormal sperm, or no sperm production. With the procedure, the semen is placed directly into the cervix or uterus with a small flexible catheter and a syringe.

Surgical

Several methods can be used to accomplish a pregnancy, but each one is directed toward a different underlying cause of the infertility. One method is *in vitro* fertilization. This may be by GIFT (gamete-intra-fallopian transfer), or ZIFT (zygote-intra-fallopian transfer). With the GIFT technique, the female partner receives monthly cyclic hormone injections that cause ova to ripen. The hormones may cause more than one ovum to ripen during each cycle, which enhances the possibility that more than one ovum will be fertilized and implanted in the uterus. A semen specimen is collected from the male partner 1 to 2 hours before the GIFT procedure and the sperm placed into a special catheter. The ripened ovum is obtained from the female via laparoscopy or ultrasound aspiration and is loaded into the catheter in a sequential manner with the sperm and then injected through the fimbrial end of the fallopian tube, also by laparoscopy. This procedure takes approximately 1 hour to complete. Pregnancy is confirmed within 7 to 10 days with a blood hormonal test (Beta HCG) or an ultrasound, or both.

The ZIFT procedure is similar to GIFT. However, several ova are obtained just before ovulation and are placed in a special fluid for several hours while the sperm are prepared. The ova and sperm are then carefully mixed and closely observed for 2 to 3 days. The fertilized ova (now zygotes) are transferred into the fallopian tube or into the uterine cavity. Another name for the ZIFT procedure is IVF-ER (*in vitro* fertilization and embryo replacement), which more clearly defines what actually occurs.

Both GIFT and ZIFT are relatively expensive procedures (approximately $5,000 or more per cycle) and may or may not be covered by health insurance. For many couples, these are final efforts to conceive.

Pharmacological

Several medications are used in the treatment of infertility disorders, and most are focused on hormone imbalances or deficiencies. Clomiphene citrate (Clomid) stimulates release of follicle-stimulating hormone (FSH) and luteinizing hormone (LH) and is used to induce ovulation. Clomid is administered orally beginning on the fifth day of the menstrual cycle. If ovulation does not occur, the dosage will be increased for 5 days in the next cycle. If ovulation does not occur by the time the dose has been increased 4 or 5 times, it may be considered a Clomid failure. There is some chance of multiple gestation while the client is taking Clomid, and she should be informed of the potential. Most often it is a twin pregnancy, but occasionally triplets may be conceived.

Menotropins (Pergonal) mimics FSH and LH, causing follicular growth and maturation. It is administered by intramuscular injection. Although Pergonal is an expensive drug, it has been shown to increase the possibility for ovulation in clients who have not responded to other medications.

Human chorionic gonadotropin (Pregnyl) may also be administered with the Clomid or Pergonal therapy to help maintain the endometrial lining for implantation. It stimulates the production of progesterone from the ovary until the fertilized ovum implants and the placenta begins to function. Progesterone suppositories may be used vaginally 2 times a day to help correct a luteal phase defect by lengthening the time from ovulation until the onset of the menses or through implantation and pregnancy. Some clients continue with the progesterone suppositories throughout the first few weeks of the pregnancy to ensure that the endometrium remains intact. If the sperm count or motility is low, testosterone or thyroid extracts may be prescribed.

Health Promotion

Seeking prompt medical treatment for infections that involve the reproductive system is an essential means of preventing infertility problems, especially with STDs and PID. PID causes scarring of the outside of the fallopian tubes, and gonorrhea can result in scarring or strictures of the internal fallopian tube. Either cause can result in an ectopic pregnancy when the fertilized ovum cannot pass through the tube.

Other considerations may include wise choices in contraceptive methods. The use of oral contraceptives has been associated with primary and secondary infertility due to decreased pituitary function. This condition may resolve spontaneously, or medications may be required to stimulate ovulation in order to conceive.

Multiple sexual partners have also been associated with an increased risk of sexually transmitted disease, infections, and cervical cancer.

CONTRACEPTION

Contraception, or prevention of pregnancy, has been accomplished by many methods over the centuries. In weighing the options, safety, ease of use, effectiveness, and cost should be considered. Both partners' wishes should be considered in this decision-making process.

Contraception may be accomplished by natural means or medical interventions. This section of the chapter will discuss a basic overview of the types of contraceptive methods currently available, the advantages and disadvantages, the effectiveness of each kind, the mechanisms by which they work, and the client education that should accompany the methods (Table 30–2).

NATURAL METHOD

Natural methods of contraception may include what is called the "rhythm method." During the woman's fertile period of the month, usually lasting 7 days (3 days before ovulation to 3 days after), the couple should abstain from intercourse. The determination of the fertile period is based on the time of ovulation. Sperm can live up to 72 hours after ejaculation, and it is possible for sperm to still be in the cervix or uterus if the couple had intercourse 3 days before ovulation. The couple may also decide to maintain a basal body temperature chart to more accurately pinpoint ovulation each month. Another method to determine the approaching ovulation is to monitor the stretchiness of the cervical mucus. This is called "spinnbarkeit." As the woman nears ovulation, the hormones (estrogen) cause the cervical mucus to become clear, thin, and stretchy. This type of mucus provides a favorable environment for the sperm and helps their motility toward the ova. Immediately after ovulation, the cervical mucus becomes hostile to sperm. It becomes thick, cloudy, and more acidic. It also loses its stretchiness. Kits are available for purchase from the local drug store or pharmacy that react to chemicals in the cervical

Table 30–2 CONTRACEPTION: METHODS, EFFECTIVENESS, AND CONCERNS

METHOD	EFFECTIVE-NESS RATE	RISKS	SIDE EFFECTS	OTHER ADVANTAGES
Abstinence	100%	None known	Psychological reactions	Prevents infections including HIV
Barriers diaphragm cervical cap spermicide	 84% 73–92% 79%	Mechanical irritation, vaginal infections, toxic shock syndrome	Pelvic pressure, cervical erosion, vaginal discharges if left in too long	Protects to some degree against sexually transmitted diseases
Condoms	86%	None known	Decreased sensation, allergy to latex, less spontaneity in lovemaking	Protects against sexually transmitted disease, including AIDS; delays premature ejaculation
Oral contraceptives	97%	Cardiovascular complications such as stroke, blood clots, high blood pressure, and heart attacks with the higher-dose combined oral contraceptive	Possible nausea, headaches, dizziness, spotting, weight gain, breast tenderness, chloasma, cramping	Protects against PID, decreases risk of ovarian and endometrial cancer, decreases menstrual blood loss and dysmenorrhea (cramps), decreases benign breast disease, regulates irregular menses, protects bone density, decreases risk of atherosclerosis, lessens the risk of rheumatoid arthritis, decreases uterine fibroids, and decreases ovarian cysts
Norplant implants	99%	Infection at implant site	Menstrual changes, weight gain, headaches	May protect against PID, may decrease menstrual cramps and blood loss
Depo-Provera	98%	Pulmonary embolism	Headache, depression, hypertension, edema, nausea	Effective to treat obstructive sleep apnea
IUD	94%	Pelvic inflammatory disease, uterine perforation, anemia	Menstrual cramping, spotting, increased bleeding	None known except with progestin-releasing IUD, which may decrease menstrual pain and blood loss
Sterilization female male	 99.6% 99.8%	Infection	Pain at surgical site, psychological reaction with subsequent regret	None known

mucus and predict the time of ovulation. The kits are inexpensive and simple to use, much like home pregnancy tests.

BARRIER AND SPERMICIDE METHODS

Methods of barrier contraception include male and female condoms, the diaphragm, and the cervical cap. Barrier devices work by blocking the pathway of the sperm through the cervix into the uterus. Spermicides kill sperm before they can enter the cervix. This type of contraceptive requires some preplanning on the part of one or both of the partners and may reduce the spontaneity of the sex act.

Spermicides contain a chemical, nonoxynol-9, that kills sperm on contact. If used alone, spermicidal agents have a lower efficacy rate than if used with a condom. The nurse should advise the couple to use a spermicidal gel, foam suppository, or film in addition to another barrier method for the greatest effectiveness. Foam should not be used with the diaphragm because it can result in deterioration of the latex. These agents must be placed in the vagina at least 15 minutes before intercourse to promote the spermicidal reaction. This method is safe and inexpensive but requires a high level of compliance each time or the effectiveness of the method drops significantly.

HORMONAL METHODS

Oral contraceptives, Norplant, and Depo-Provera are discussed following.

Oral Contraceptives

The "pill" has been available as a contraceptive method for many years. Since its earliest form, it has been refined and the level of hormones reduced. Oral contraceptives work by suppressing ovulation. In a sense, the body thinks it is pregnant when the pill is used. Some oral contraceptives contain estrogen and progesterone; others contain only progestins.

In response to the pseudopregnancy state, the client may experience mild side effects and discomforts often associated with pregnancy such as, nausea, headache, breast tenderness, or weight gain. Major side effects from oral contraceptives may include cardiovascular accidents or thrombophlebitis.

There is approximately a 1 in 200 chance of becoming pregnant while taking the oral contraceptive. If the woman thinks that she might be pregnant, she should stop the pill immediately and contact her physician. When the woman and her partner decide that it is time for a pregnancy, she should discontinue the oral contraceptive for at least 2 to 3 cycles before having unprotected intercourse. This "rest period" will lessen the

possibility that pill effects will remain in her system and will allow her body to return to its own natural rhythm. Some women will find that they experience primary or secondary infertility problems after being on the pill for several years owing to pituitary suppression. The remedy is often fertility drugs such as clomiphene citrate (Clomid). Women who have never established a regular pattern of menstruation may not be good candidates for oral contraceptives, except as being used to regulate the cycle by artificial means. Other clients who should not take oral contraceptives include women with a history of hypertension, diabetes, cardiovascular disease, or thrombophlebitis. Some physicians may consider oral contraceptives in the newer low-dose combinations for clients who were previously in this high-risk group.

Norplant

Levonorgestrel (Norplant System) consists of six small progestin-filled pellets that are inserted under the skin of the upper arm under a local anesthetic. Theoretically, Norplant is effective for up to 5 years. Some clients will experience mild breakthrough bleeding during the first few months after the Norplant is in place. This usually subsides or lessens with time, but for some clients it is an inconvenience. This is a good option for the woman who is sure she does not desire a pregnancy for at least 5 years, although the pellets may be removed before the end of that time. Because of the expense of the Norplant and placement procedure, the nurse or physician should make sure the client has a clear understanding of the method before proceeding.

Depo-Provera

The medroxyprogesterone acetate (Depo-Provera) injection is administered intramuscularly every 12 weeks. It works like oral contraceptives to suppress ovulation. The client may experience breakthrough bleeding after the first injection, but this is not an indication that the hormone is not working. It usually requires about 3 weeks after the first injection before the contraceptive is effective, so the client should be advised to use a barrier contraceptive method during that period. The client must receive the injections at regular intervals to ensure effectiveness. Norplant and Depo-Provera are good options for the client who is approaching her forties or who smokes because they contain only progestins, which decreases the risk of cardiovascular problems.

INTRAUTERINE DEVICE METHOD

The intrauterine device (IUD) has been used for many years and has undergone several changes. The

Dalcon shield, which was used in the 1960s and 1970s, caused many problems from infection to infertility. The IUD works by causing an irritation inside the uterine cavity that results in a hostile environment for the fertilized ovum that causes it not to implant. It is then sloughed off with the menstrual flow. The intrauterine device is recommended for women who have had children because the cervix has been dilated. This allows for easier insertion of the device. The IUD is inserted or removed while the client is having her period because there is slight dilatation of the cervix at that time. A string attached to the distal end of the device hangs out of the cervix into the vagina. The client is instructed to check the string each month after the menstrual period to make sure the device has not been expelled. Some women experience more dysmenorrhea with the IUD in place and a heavier menstrual flow. Because there is an increased risk of infection with the IUD, a monogamous relationship is advisable for the client. The intrauterine devices that are currently available are effective for 1 year or 7 years.

STERILIZATION METHOD

Sterilization is considered a permanent and very effective method of contraception. In a rare incident, a woman will become pregnant after a tubal ligation or after her partner has had a vasectomy. The procedure interrupts the pathway through the fallopian tube. Sterilization may be performed on an outpatient basis in a surgical clinic or the outpatient department at the hospital. The tubal ligation is done under a general or epidural anesthetic with laparoscopy. The procedure takes about 30 to 60 minutes. The abdomen is distended with a gas to permit better visualization of the pelvic structures during the procedure.

The male sterilization, **vasectomy** (surgical resection of the vas deferens), is usually performed with local anesthesia on an outpatient basis. Rest, with ice to the scrotum, for 4 hours should follow. The client should not engage in strenuous activity or exercise for 1 week.

It may take up to 6 weeks for the semen to be clear of sperm. The client is instructed to return to the clinic for a sperm count after 20 ejaculations. If he is sexually active, during those ejaculations he should use a condom or some other form of contraception. At 6 months a sperm count should be repeated and then monitored annually thereafter.

The female sterilization is more expensive and, because it requires more anesthesia, carries a slightly higher risk than the male procedure.

Refined microsurgical techniques have made it possible to reverse sterilization procedures. The reversals are not always successful, and the couple need to consider the odds of success before venturing into the expense of this type of surgery.

CASE STUDY

Mrs. Mary Keiver, a forty-year-old, African-American school teacher, nullipara, was seen by her physician because of heavy menstrual bleeding. She stated that she had been saturating a sanitary pad every thirty minutes since early that same morning. She reported that her menstrual periods had been getting heavier for the past six months and were accompanied by severe cramping. She also noted that after her period she felt "physically drained." Other symptoms that Mary had observed included an increasing sense of heaviness in her pelvis and that her skirts and slacks were too tight around the abdomen, even though her weight had not changed significantly.

When Mary was examined by the physician, it was noted that her uterus was enlarged approximately equal to twelve weeks gestational size and it felt irregular in shape. Mary's skin was pale and cool to touch. Her mucous membranes and conjunctival sacs were pale pink. Her blood pressure was 100/60, pulse 90, temperature 98.8°F. The results of an H & H were as follows: Hbg-7.0 mg/dL and HCT-26. An ultrasound confirmed the findings of the pelvic exam for the presence of multiple uterine fibroids. The bleeding did not subside, and Mary was admitted for an outpatient dilatation and curettage (D & C) with a diagnosis of monorrhagia secondary to uterine leiomyoma.

The following questions will guide your development of a nursing care plan for the case study.

1. List the clinical signs and symptoms manifested by this client that suggest that the heavy bleeding may be related to uterine fibroids.

2. List two reasons why a hemoblobin and hematocrit were ordered.

3. Describe what other diagnostic tests were ordered and why.   *continues*

CASE STUDY *continued*

4. List the subjective and objective data the nurse should obtain during the assessment.

5. Write three individualized nursing diagnoses and goals for Mrs. Keiver.

6. Describe pertinent nursing actions/interventions to be taken in caring for this client prior to and following the D & C related to:
   - Bleeding
   - Cardiac output
   - Comfort/rest
   - Activity
   - Medications
   - Teaching

7. List a minimum of three specific topics the nurse should discuss when talking to this client regarding her condition.

8. Discuss discharge instructions or teaching necessary for this client.

9. List a minimum of three successful outcomes for this client.

10. Discuss how the nurse might evaluate the effectiveness of treatment and care for this client.

SUMMARY

- Potential complications from PID may include sterility or infertility from scarring of fallopian tubes.
- Toxic shock syndrome (TSS) occurs during the menses, and a strong correlation exists between the onset and use of super-absorbent tampons.
- A BSE is an important method for detecting breast changes and should be practiced each month. Breast cancer is the most common female cancer in the United States.
- Cervical cancer is most common in women with multiple sexual partners.
- Endometrial cancer often produces symptoms only after it is widespread. Any unusual vaginal bleeding should be investigated, especially if it occurs after menopause.
- Menstrual disorders are often associated with hormonal imbalances, increased or decreased function of the endocrine glands, or neoplasms.
- Menopause is a normal, gradual decline in the ovarian production of female hormones that occurs around age 50. Estrogen replacement therapy is recommended by many health care providers to decrease the symptoms of menopause and as a preventive measure against cardiovascular disease and osteoporosis.
- Infertility affects at least 1 in every 4 couples in the United States and is caused by hormonal imbalances, and structural or physiologic abnormalities in both male and female clients.

- Women who smoke and are over age 40 are at greater risk for major complications while using oral contraceptives. Major health risks include cardiovascular accidents and deep vein thrombosis.

Review Questions

1. The best method of screening for cervical cancer is:
   a. genitourinary cultures.
   b. cervical biopsy.
   c. Pap smear.
   d. ultrasound.

2. The female client should perform BSE (breast self-examination):
   a. just before the menstrual period.
   b. just after the menstrual period.
   c. at ovulation.
   d. any time of the month.

3. Which cancer is the "silent killer" of many women?
   a. cervical
   b. uterine
   c. breast
   d. ovarian

4. Heavy bleeding between a woman's normal menstrual cycles is:

   a. amenorrhea.

   b. polymenorrhea.

   c. metrorrhagia.

   d. menorrhagia.

5. Bowel and bladder complications that may follow pelvic radiation therapy for uterine cancer are often caused by:

   a. dehydration.

   b. lack of mobility.

   c. damage to the tissue from radiation effects.

   d. damage to tissues during surgery.

6. The most common cancer of the female reproductive system is:

   a. breast.

   b. ovarian.

   c. cervical.

   d. uterine.

7. An antiestrogenic drug used in the treatment of female reproductive cancers, especially in breast cancer, is:

   a. megestrol acetate (Megace).

   b. cyclophosphamide (Cytoxan).

   c. 5-fluprouracil (t-FU)

   d. testolactone (Teslac).

8. The primary microorganism associated with the occurrence of toxic shock syndrome is:

   a. *Escherichia coli.*

   b. *Streptococcus aureus.*

   c. *Staphylococcus aureus.*

   d. *Pseudomonas.*

9. A barrier method of contraception is:

   a. condom.

   b. the "pill."

   c. an IUD.

   d. Norplant.

10. A dietary element frequently associated with fibrocystic breast disease is:

   a. fats.

   b. protein.

   c. sodium.

   d. caffeine.

11. Which of the following are characteristic signs of a trichomonas vaginitis?

   a. Thick, white, "cheesy" discharge with itching

   b. Frothy, foul-smelling, yellow discharge with itching and irritation

   c. Creamy, thin, vaginal discharge with a musty or fishy odor

   d. Painful intercourse due to decreased lubrication

12. The drug of choice to treat PID (pelvic inflammatory disease) is:

   a. penicillin V potassium (V-cillin K).

   b. doxycycline hyclate (Vibramycin).

   c. erthromycin estolate (Ilosone).

   d. cyclophosphamide (Cytoxan).

13. When the cervix and the uterus extend out of the body past the vaginal opening, the degree of prolapse is:

   a. first.

   b. second.

   c. third.

   d. fourth.

Critical Thinking Questions

1. Prepare a teaching plan for a breast self-examination.

2. What is the rationale for each nursing intervention given for the nursing diagnoses in this chapter?

WEB FLASH!

- Search the Internet for the disorders discussed in this chapter. Share new treatments discussed for any of the disorders with other students.
- Visit the Web sites for the Resources listed at the end of the book for the reproductive systems. What type of information do these organizations have available for the client and family? For health care providers?

NURSING CARE OF THE CLIENT: MALE REPRODUCTIVE SYSTEM

CHAPTER 31

MAKING THE CONNECTION

Refer to the following chapters to increase your understanding of the male reproductive system:

- **Chapter 7, Wellness Concepts**
- **Chapter 10, Fluid, Electrolyte, and Acid-Base Balance**
- **Chapter 12, Health Assessment**
- **Chapter 17, Nursing Care of the Oncology Client**
- **Chapter 19, Nursing Care of the Client: Cardiovascular System**
- **Chapter 27, Nursing Care of the Client: Endocrine System**

- **Chapter 29, Nursing Care of the Client: Urinary System**
- **Chapter 30: Nursing care of the Client: Female Reproductive System**
- **Chapter 32, Nursing Care of the Client: Sexually Transmitted Diseases**
- **Chapter 35, Nursing Care of the Older Client**

LEARNING OBJECTIVES

Upon completion of this chapter, you should be able to:
- *Define key terms.*
- *Identify the components of the reproductive systems.*
- *Describe the hormonal mechanisms that regulate the reproductive functions.*
- *Describe diagnostic tests for disorders of the reproductive systems.*
- *Describe the changes in the male reproductive system that occur with aging.*
- *Differentiate between impotence and infertility.*
- *Discuss contraceptive methods, including actions, side effects, and client teaching.*
- *Utilize the nursing process to develop a care plan for a client with a reproductive system disorder.*

INTRODUCTION

Routine health care must be maintained and early diagnosis made in order to reduce the incidence and seriousness of male reproductive health disorders.

KEY TERMS

hematuria
hesitancy
impotence
nocturia
orchiectomy
post void residual
priapism
spermatogenesis
stent
urethrostomy

These goals can be facilitated with skilled nursing assessment and client education.

This chapter is designed to provide a review of anatomy and physiology of the male reproductive system to assist the learner in identifying key structures involved in the various disorders. The learner will also be provided with detailed descriptions of disorders of the male reproductive system along with explanations of related treatment and nursing care.

847

ANATOMY AND PHYSIOLOGY REVIEW

The male reproductive organs and associated structures are illustrated in Figure 31-1. The scrotum is a fleshy structure that is suspended below the perineum, anterior to the anus. It is divided into two parts, each of which contains a testis, an epididymis, and a portion of the spermatic cord (vas deferens). The left side of the scrotum is usually lower than the right because the left spermatic cord is often longer.

The testes, two smooth, oval endocrine glands, are suspended in the scrotum. This location helps to maintain proper temperature and also protects the testes from trauma. Certain cells of the epithelium lining the seminiferous tubules of the testes produce half a billion sperm each day (**spermatogenesis**). They also secrete the androgenic (causing masculinization) hormone testosterone. Spermatogenesis is regulated by the follicle-stimulating hormone (FSH), which is produced by the anterior pituitary gland. The production of testosterone is regulated by luteinizing hormone (LH), which is also produced by the anterior pituitary gland. After the sperm mature in the epididymis, they travel through the vas (ductus) deferens, a long tube that is attached to the epididymis. The vas deferens, along with associated nerves and blood vessels, forms the spermatic cord.

The vas deferens travels up and around the bladder and carries sperm from the epididymis to the seminal vesicle. The seminal vesicle is a small pouch that produces secretions that, when mixed with sperm and prostatic fluid, form semen.

The prostate is an encapsulated gland that encircles the proximal portion of the urethra. The prostatic fossa, a depression on the cranial border of the prostate, allows entry of the ejaculatory ducts. Within the prostate is a cluster of 30 to 50 tubuloalveolar glands that secrete prostatic fluid. The prostate gland is of clinical significance because as men age, it is a common site for malignant disease or benign enlargement that can cause urethral obstruction.

The penis is a cylindrical organ through which urine is passed and semen is ejaculated. Half of the penis is located within the body. The external half of the penis is flaccid, unless the male is sexually aroused, at which time it becomes erect owing to engorgement with blood. There are three cylindrical columns of erectile tissue: two corpora cavernosa and the corpus spongiosum. A fold of skin, the prepuce, surrounds the tip of the penis in the uncircumcised male.

COMMON DIAGNOSTIC TESTS

Commonly used diagnostic tests for clients with symptoms of reproductive system disorders are listed

Figure 31-1 The Male Reproductive System

GERONTOLOGICAL CONSIDERATIONS

Circumcision

Circumcision is performed on many Western society infants to remove the prepuce, or foreskin. In 1975 the American Academy of Pediatrics (AAP) did not support any medical need for routine circumcision. In 1988 they reversed their position on the basis of increased evidence that circumcision reduces the incidence of urinary tract infections. Circumcision is also performed for cultural or religious reasons.

in Table 31–1. See Chapter 13, Diagnostic Tests, for explanation/normal values and nursing responsibilities.

INFLAMMATORY DISORDERS

Inflammatory disorders discussed include epididymitis, orchitis, and prostatitis.

EPIDIDYMITIS/ORCHITIS/ PROSTATITIS

Epididymitis can be a sterile or nonsterile inflammation of the epididymis. A sterile inflammation may be caused by direct injury or reflux of urine down the vas deferens. Urinary reflux that is related to strain exerted by a male while his bladder is full can be caused by lifting heavy objects or doing strenuous exercises. Nonsterile inflammation may occur as a complication of gonorrhea, chlamydia, mumps, tuberculosis, prostatitis, or urethritis. Prolonged use of an indwelling catheter or an invasive procedure can also lead to nonsterile inflammation.

Signs and symptoms of epididymitis include sudden, severe pain in the scrotum, scrotal swelling, fever, dysuria, and pyuria. Treatment includes bed rest, antibiotics, scrotal support (Figure 31-2), and ice compresses to the area. Bilateral epididymitis can cause sterility. Untreated epididymitis leads quickly to testicular tissue necrosis, septicemia, and death.

Orchitis is an inflammation of the testes that most often occurs as a complication of a bloodborne infection originating in the epididymis. Other causes of orchitis include gonorrhea, trauma, surgical manipulation, and tuberculosis and mumps that occur after puberty. In most instances, both testes are involved, and often sterility results. In orchitis, unilateral involvement does not cause sterility. Orchitis signs and symptoms include sudden scrotal pain with pain radiating to the

Table 31–1 COMMON DIAGNOSTIC TESTS FOR REPRODUCTIVE SYSTEM DISORDERS

Laboratory Tests
- Alpha-fetoprotein (AFP)
- Cultures
- Human chorionic gonadatropin (HCG)
- Prostate-specific antigen (PSA)
- Prostatic smear
- Serum alkaline phosphatase
- Serum calcium
- Semen analysis
- Segmented bacteriologic localization culture

Radiologic Tests
- Dynamic infusion cavernosometry and cavernosography (DICC)

Surgical Tests
- Prostatic biopsy
- Testicular biopsy

Other Tests
- Nocturnal tumescence penile monitoring

inguinal canal, scrotal edema, chills, fever, nausea, and vomiting. Treatment includes bed rest, scrotal support, and ice to the area.

Prostatitis, an inflammation of the prostate, is a common complication of urethritis caused by chlamydia or gonorrhea. Infecting organisms may reach the genital tract by direct spread through the urethra or may be borne by blood or lymph. The condition may be acute or chronic, with the chronic form leading to development of fibrotic tissue. This fibrotic tissue

Figure 31-2 A Bellevue Bridge for Scrotal Support

causes the prostate to harden, so prostatitis may be difficult to differentiate from prostate cancer. It may take 3 to 6 months for the granulomatous form to resolve. Signs and symptoms of prostatitis include perineal pain, fever, dysuria, and urethral discharge.

Medical–Surgical Management

Medical

When it is suspected that the client currently has urethritis, he should not be catheterized. The infection spreads rapidly to the genital organs because of the trauma of catheterization and the possible spread of bacteria from the nonsterile distal part of the urethra. The physician may order that segmented bacteriologic localization cultures be obtained.

Pharmacological

Treatment of epididymitis and orchitis includes antibiotics and injection of procaine around the spermatic cord. Pharmacological treatment of prostatitis includes antibiotics, analgesics, and stool softeners.

Activity

Treatment of prostatitis includes bed rest. While the client is in bed, his scrotum should be elevated and cold packs applied to the area. The client should be encouraged to drink a large amount of fluids and use sitz baths for comfort. These interventions are used to reduce inflammation, swelling, and discomfort. Periodic digital massage of the prostate by the physician increases the flow of infected prostatic secretions.

▶ NURSING PROCESS

▶ Assessment

▶ Subjective Data

The nurse should question the client about the presence of urethral discharge or dysuria as well as the nature and location of the pain. A description of pain may include arthralgia, low-back pain, and myalgia. In addition, a careful medical history is obtained. A positive history of recent bacterial or viral infection is of special significance. Ongoing nursing assessment should include monitoring for pain, using a pain scale to objectify data. The nurse asks the client if he is experiencing nausea, as this could be a sign that his condition is deteriorating. The client also needs an assessment of his educational and emotional needs as he may be worrying needlessly about possible sterility or impotence.

▶ Objective Data

The client's vital signs, especially his temperature, is monitored. An increase in temperature may be an indicator that the client's condition is worsening. Scrotal edema and purulent urethral discharge may be present. Intake and output are monitored. The client also is monitored for constipation.

Nursing diagnoses for the male client with an inflammatory disorder may include the following:

Nursing Diagnoses	Planning/Goals	Nursing Interventions
▶ *Risk for Injury related to worsening of the inflammatory process*	The client will not experience worsening of his condition.	Monitor the client's vital signs, especially his temperature.
		Report hyperthermia, hypotension, nausea, and tachycardia to the physician immediately.
▶ *Risk for Deficient Fluid Volume related to nausea and vomiting*	The client will maintain fluid balance.	Monitor the client's intake and output. Encourage him to drink plenty of fluids when not nauseated.
▶ *Acute Pain related to inflammation*	Using a pain scale of 0 to 10, the client will report pain has decreased to 2 or less within 48 hours after treatment initiation.	Assess client's pain level every 4 hours.
		Administer analgesics as ordered.
		Encourage the client to maintain bed rest.
		Provide diversional activities to increase compliance.
		Encourage the client with prostatitis to take a sitz bath, but never the client with epididymitis or orchitis as local heat may increase destruction of sperm cells.
		Fill a plastic glove with crushed ice and place it under the scrotum when heat is contraindicated.
		Remove the ice for short intervals every hour to prevent ice burns.
▶ *Anxiety related to concerns about possible sterility or impotence*	The client will verbalize decreased anxiety.	Reassure the client that with proper treatment, sterility and impotence are not likely complications of prostatitis.

Evaluation Each goal must be evaluated to determine how it has been met by the client.

BENIGN PROSTATIC HYPERPLASIA

Benign prostatic hyperplasia (BPH) is a progressive adenomatous enlargement of the prostate gland that occurs with aging. More than 50% of men over the age of 50 and 75% of men over the age of 70 demonstrate some increase in the size of the prostate gland (Martini, 1995). Although this disorder is not harmful, the urinary outlet obstruction that may be associated with the disorder is a problem.

Because the urethra is encircled by the prostate, common early symptoms of BPH are related to partial or complete obstruction of the urethra. Early symptoms include **hesitancy** (difficulty initiating the urinary stream), decreased force of stream, urinary frequency, and **nocturia** (awakening at night to void). However, a temporary reduction of these symptoms may occur as the bladder muscles hypertrophy in response to the increased work they must do to force the urinary stream past the obstruction.

Although this bladder muscle compensatory response may temporarily reduce symptoms, eventually the muscle decompensates, becoming noncompliant and hypotonic. This decompensation leads to atony of the mucous membranes between the muscle bands that causes stagnant urine to collect in the small compartments (cellules) of the membranes. In addition, the man is unable to completely empty the bladder when voiding (**post void residual**). Because these changes in urinary function promote urinary alkalosis by increasing the urine pH, a perfect environment for bacterial growth is created. This bacterial growth can cause a urinary tract infection (UTI), which may eventually lead to kidney damage.

Medical–Surgical Management

Medical

The physician will perform a digital rectal examination in order to identify any enlargement of the lateral lobes or nodular lumps on the surface of the prostate gland. Diagnostic tests will be ordered to learn more about the client's condition; these may include a prostate-specific antigen (PSA), measurement of residual urine, cystoscopy, intravenous pyelogram, and ultrasonography. The physician will also carefully monitor the client's condition to detect any exacerbation of symptoms such as increased hesitancy, urgency, hematuria, or repeated urinary tract infections.

Many alternatives to surgical treatment of BPH have been introduced over the past several years. Medical treatment methods have ranged from balloon dilation of the prostate to a prostate urethral **stent**, as shown in Figure 31-3, to thermotherapy. Balloon dilation of the

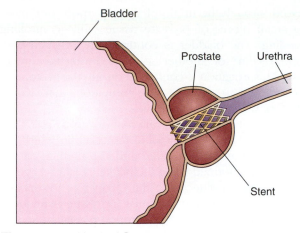

Figure 31-3 Urethral Stent

prostate during an endoscopic examination is done to break the prostatic capsule and facilitate decompression of the prostate. A stent is material that is used to hold tissue in place or, in this instance, to provide support to the urethra, which is being compressed by the prostate. Various types of thermotherapy that may be used are microwave thermotherapy and hyperthermia. Although these minimally invasive treatments are safe, they do not remove the urinary obstruction.

Surgical

The traditional surgical intervention for enlargement of the portion of the prostate that surrounds the urethra has been transurethral resection of the prostate (TURP). This surgery is performed via a resectoscope, an instrument that includes a cutting and cauterization device (Figure 31-4). The client receives either a general or a spinal anesthetic, and the resectoscope is

Figure 31-4 Transurethral Resection of the Prostate Gland Via Resectoscope

passed through the urethra for the purpose of removing small pieces of prostate tissue while controlling bleeding. The bladder is continuously irrigated with normal saline or another solution during the procedure. This irrigation is continued during the postoperative period to reduce clot formation that would interfere with urinary drainage.

The traditional surgical alternatives to a TURP are open operations. A suprapubic resection, in which the prostate is removed from around the urethra via the bladder, is performed when the prostate mass is large. In a retropubic prostatectomy, the bladder is not opened but instead is retracted and prostatic tissue is removed through an incision in the anterior prostatic capsule. Both of these alternatives involve an abdominal incision (Figure 31-5). In a perineal prostatectomy, a perineal incision is made and the prostatic tissue is removed through an incision in the posterior prostatic capsule.

Although these traditional surgeries successfully relieve bladder obstruction, they are costly, and postoperative complications can endanger or seriously affect the quality of a man's life. These complications include hemorrhage, water intoxication, infection, thrombosis, damage to surrounding structures, sexual dysfunction, and urinary incontinence.

Laser prostatectomy, the most recently developed surgical intervention for BPH, is based on thermal action. The transurethral ultrasound-guided laser-induced prostatectomy (TULIP) is performed with a probe that is passed transurethrally into the prostatic urethra. While the adjacent prostate area is visualized by ultrasound, the laser energy is directed at the prostate tissue, resulting in tissue necrosis and sloughing. The procedure is easy and quick to perform. However, the large amount of sloughing tissue necessitates having an indwelling catheter for several weeks to facilitate bladder drainage. The client is less likely to experience water intoxication because this surgical method allows blood vessels to seal rapidly, keeping irrigant fluid from being forced into the circulation.

Pharmacological

A pharmacological intervention that has been successfully used to treat BPH is the use of alpha blockers. These drugs relax the smooth muscles along the urinary tract without compromising normal urinary control reflexes. Because alpha blockers such as terazosin hydrochloride (Hytrin) and doxazosin mesylate (Cardura) are also used to treat hypertension, the side effect of orthostatic hypotension is possible. Belladonna and opium (B & O) suppositories are used to reduce postoperative bladder spasms, and narcotic analgesics are used to relieve postoperative pain.

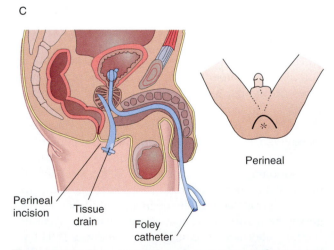

Figure 31-5 Three types of prostatectomies: A. Suprapubic; B. Retropubic; C. Perineal

▶ NURSING PROCESS

▶ Assessment

▶ Subjective Data

Urinary patterns are the primary focus of a preoperative nursing assessment of a client with BPH. The nurse should ask the client about the presence of urinary frequency, hesitancy, dribbling, number of times he gets up at night to void, and the force of the urinary stream. In addition to a careful general medical history, any information pertaining to a history of chronic urinary tract infections needs to be noted.

Postoperative nursing assessment should include assessing for pain (on a 0 to 10 scale) related to bladder spasms. The client's emotional needs should also be assessed as he may be experiencing anticipatory grieving, body image disturbance, anxiety, or concerns about alteration in sexuality patterns or possible sexual dysfunction. Behavioral or verbal cues from the client may indicate a need for further information or reassurance regarding his condition and related treatment.

▶ Objective Data

When assessing for hemorrhagic shock or postoperative infection, the nurse should monitor vital signs and avoid the use of a rectal thermometer. A bright red urine color persisting for more than a few hours after surgery may be a sign of hemorrhage. Hemorrhage, hyperthermia, hypotension (low blood pressure), and tachycardia should be reported to the physician immediately.

After a TURP, the client will have a three way Foley catheter and continuous bladder irrigation for at least 24 hours. Intake and output will need to be recorded to ensure that the client has adequate oral intake to promote urinary flow and reduce the infection risk. In measuring output, the amount of irrigant must be subtracted from the total output in order to determine the actual urinary output. After the catheter is removed, the client should be assessed for post void residual and incontinence. Palpating the abdomen for bladder distention, checking the bed linens and clothing for signs of incontinence, or asking the client if he is experiencing loss of urinary control are also assessments to be performed.

It is important for the nurse to assess for water intoxication, which may be the result of absorbing irrigating fluid in addition to the IV fluids. The most common early symptoms of water intoxication are changes in the client's mental status. These may be manifested by agitation, confusion, and, later, convulsions. The client may also have a slow bounding pulse with an increase in systolic and decrease in diastolic blood pressure.

A suprapubic or retropubic prostatectomy does not require a three-way Foley. Instead the client will have a urethral catheter, a tissue drain from the prostatic fossa, and an abdominal dressing (refer to Figure 31-5). The nurse needs to assess for incisional pain and do a dressing check, being careful to also check the linens underneath the client's back for drainage.

Nursing diagnoses for a postoperative client having a TURP for benign prostatic hyperplasia may include the following:

Nursing Diagnoses	Planning/Goals	Nursing Interventions
▶ Acute Urinary Retention related to obstruction secondary to TURP	The client will avoid urinary retention.	Monitor the client's urinary output, noting the amount, color, and presence of clots. After 24 hours, the urine should be a light pink color.
		Increase rate of flow of the bladder irrigant if the urine has clots, a darker color, or decreased output.
		Monitor the client's intake; encourage a fluid intake of 2500 to 3000 mL/day
▶ Acute Pain related to bladder spasms or incision	The client will state that pain has decreased.	Assess for pain using a pain scale every 2 to 4 hours.
		Maintain traction on the urethral catheter by anchoring the catheter to the leg with tape, taking care that accidental additional traction will not occur with leg movement.
		Monitor for signs of bladder spasm pain such as facial grimacing, nonflow of irrigating solution into bladder, and urinating around the catheter. Administer analgesics and antispasmodics as ordered.
		Teach deep breathing, relaxation techniques.
▶ Risk for Excess Fluid Volume related to postoperative irrigation	The client will not experience water intoxication.	Accurately record I&O including irrigation fluid.
		Monitor for changes in the client's behavior, especially confusion and agitation, which may be the first signs of cerebral edema.
		Monitor for hypertension, bradycardia, weakness, and seizures.

continues

Nursing Diagnoses	Planning/Goals	Nursing Interventions
▶ *Stress Urinary Incontinence related to poor sphincter control after catheter removal after surgery*	The client will achieve urinary control after removal of the catheter.	Advise the client that temporary urinary incontinence frequently occurs after surgery, and reassure him that this is normal. Teach the client perineal exercises that will help him regain urinary control. These exercises consist of tightening and relaxing gluteal muscles and are to be used each time the client urinates.
▶ *Sexual Dysfunction related to surgery*	The client will regain sexual function postoperatively.	Monitor the client's statements to determine if he has any misunderstanding of the surgery and sexual function. Instruct the client to avoid sexual intercourse until physician approval is given and that it may take time for his previous level of sexual function to return. Encourage the client to use a variety of forms of sexual expression, such as kissing, stroking, and cuddling. Provide the client with opportunities to voice his feelings and ask questions. Advise the client that it is normal and not harmful if his urine has a milky appearance due to retrograde ejaculation.

Evaluation Each goal must be evaluated to determine how it has been met by the client.

MALIGNANT NEOPLASMS

Malignant neoplasms include breast, prostate, testicular, and penile cancers.

BREAST CANCER

While males may have gynecomastia of breast tissue as a result of puberty, older age, or medication, breast cancer in the male is an uncommon disorder. Because it is so uncommon, breast cancer in men is all the more dangerous since it is not considered a threat. Late diagnosis is quite common; therefore, males need to be educated in the technique of and encouraged to do breast self-examination (BSE). Signs and symptoms of breast cancer include breast lumps, pain, or discharge from the nipple.

Medical–Surgical Management

Medical

The primary form of treatment is surgery, however, adjuvant therapy with radiation and chemotherapy are also indicated.

Surgical

Removal of the tumor is indicated. The surgery may be limited to the tumor or more may be extensive based on whether there are metastases involved.

▶ NURSING PROCESS

▶ Assessment

▶ Subjective Data

Preoperatively, the client's emotional and educational needs must be assessed. Preoperatively and postoperatively, the nurse should assess for pain, using a pain scale to objectify data.

▶ Objective Data

The nurse will examine the breasts for lumps and discharge from the nipples. During the postoperative phase, the nurse needs to assess the client's vital signs and incisional site, and to monitor the client's statements and behaviors to determine the emotional status.

Nursing diagnoses for the male client with breast cancer may include the following:

Nursing Diagnoses	Planning/Goals	Nursing Interventions
▶ *Risk for Injury due to hemorrhage and infection related to the surgery.*	The client will experience minimal bleeding and avoid infection.	Monitor the client's vital signs and incisional drainage. Report hyperthermia, tachycardia, hypotension, increased incisional drainage, and swelling or redness around the incision to the physician immediately. Maintain strict asepsis when handling wound dressings.

continues

Nursing Diagnoses	Planning/Goals	Nursing Interventions
▶ *Deficient Knowledge related to the surgery*	The client will demonstrate understanding of postoperative medical follow-up.	Provide the client with information concerning any follow-up treatments such as radiation or chemotherapy.

Evaluation Each goal must be evaluated to determine how it has been met by the client.

PROSTATE CANCER

Prostate cancer is the second leading cause of cancer deaths in men. According to 1998 estimates by the ACS, 184,500 new cases were diagnosed. Unfortunately, incidence and mortality are currently increasing. Incidence increases with age, as 80% of all prostate cancers are diagnosed in men over age 65, but it is much more lethal in younger men. Improved detection methods have greatly increased the number of individuals having positive outcomes. Diagnostic tests that may be performed are measurement of serum prostate specific antigen (PSA), transrectal ultrasonic examination, and prostatic biopsy. Studies indicate that the use of the PSA for routine screening is not necessarily useful because of the number of false-positive levels reported in men with benign prostatic hyperplasia (BPH) and the false-negative levels in men with prostate cancer. Therefore, the most useful screening method continues to be a rectal examination, which all men over the age of 40 should have annually.

Most prostatic cancers are adenocarcinomas, slow-growing tumors that spread through the lymphatics (Figure 31-6). Early symptoms include dysuria, a weak urinary stream, and increased urinary frequency. Later symptoms are related to complete urethral obstruction or hematuria. Blood in the urine (**hematuria**), which can lead to anemia, occurs because of the rupture of blood vessels that have been overstretched.

PROFESSIONAL TIP

Risk Factors for Prostate Cancer
- Advancing age (over 55 years)
- First-degree relative with prostate cancer
- African American heritage
- High level of serum testosterone (Estes, 2002)

Medical–Surgical Management

Treatment depends on the extent of the disease and the age of the client.

Medical

Radiation is the traditional alternative to surgical removal of the malignant prostate gland. However, radiation may fail to eradicate the tumor or may lead to diarrhea, bowel obstruction, lymphocele formation, edema of the extremities, pulmonary embolism, wound infections, infection, impotence, incontinence, or radiation cystitis. An alternative successful radiation treatment option for early stage prostate cancer is transrectal assisted radioactive seed implant. With the use of ultrasound, the physician is able to precisely position the rice-sized radioactive seeds inside the malignant prostate gland. With this procedure, men have reported no incontinence, and the impotency rate is less than half that reported with traditional surgical treatment.

Surgical

Surgical treatment of prostatic cancer involves removal of the entire prostate gland, including the capsule and adjacent tissue. The urethra is then anastomosed to the bladder neck. Sometimes the retropubic approach is used, but the usual approach is perineal with the incision made between the scrotum and the rectum. Because of the proximity of the bladder sphincters to the prostate gland, urinary incontinence may be a complication. Other complications include sexual dysfunction and the universal surgical risks of hemorrhage, infection, thrombosis, and strictures. Removal of the testes (**orchiectomy**) may also be done as a palliative measure to help eliminate the androgenic effect that promotes tumor growth.

Another surgical alternative is cryosurgical ablation. This method was used in the 1960s but abandoned

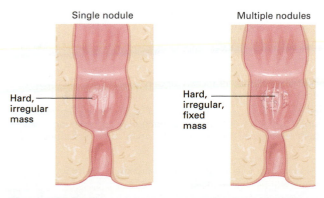

Single nodule   Multiple nodules

Hard, irregular mass

Hard, irregular, fixed mass

Figure 31-6 Cancer of the Prostate *(From Health Assessment & Physical Examination, 2nd ed., by M. E. Z. Estes, 2002 Albany, NY: Delmar. Copyright 2002 by Delmar. Reprinted with permission.)*

owing to the complications of tissue sloughing and fistula development. With the advent of the transrectal ultrasound and the transurethral warming device, cryosurgery has become a more viable alternative. The ultrasound allows the surgeon to selectively freeze prostate gland tissue while the temperature of the prostatic urethra is kept at 44°C by irrigation with heated water. This surgical approach is an option for those who cannot tolerate more extensive surgery, have a localized tumor, or do not have successful radiation treatment. It can be performed more than once, involves a shorter hospital stay, and produces fewer side effects.

Pharmacological

Hormonal agents such as diethylstilbestrol (DES), goserelin acetate (Zoladex), or leuprolide acetate (Lupron) may be used to counteract the production of androgen-dependent hormones. Although systemic chemotherapy has not proved very effective in the treatment of prostate cancer, it may be used for clients who fail to respond to hormone manipulation. Unfortunately, response is limited. Overall, the 5-year survival rate is 89% (ACS, 1998).

▸ NURSING PROCESS

▸ Assessment

▸ Subjective Data

The client may seek care for BPH, which often accompanies cancer of the prostate. The client may describe back pain or sciatica, frequency, dysuria, or nocturia.

▸ Objective Data

The client needs a complete physical assessment that includes palpation of the abdomen and skin assessment. The abdomen is palpated to determine if there is any bladder distention. Skin assessment is important because the client is at risk for skin breakdown. There may or may not be hematuria present. If the client has a perineal prostatectomy, he will return from surgery with an indwelling urethral catheter and Penrose or sump drain in place. With some prostatectomy surgeries, the client may have an indwelling catheter and also a suprapubic catheter in place. Vital signs, the incisional site, and intake and output must all be assessed. Hyperthermia, hypotension, tachycardia, or increased incisional drainage should be reported to the physician immediately.

Because a catheter is used postoperatively to maintain urinary drainage and as a splint for the urethral anastomosis rather than for hemostasis, there are minimal bladder spasms. Patency of the catheter can be monitored by assessing the drainage for color, amount, and presence of clots. If the tubing is not draining freely, it should be repositioned or milked. The nurse should call the physician if these measures fail to restore patency. During the first week of the postoperative period the client also needs to be monitored for fecal incontinence related to relaxation of the perineal sphincter. This is a complication that occurs when a perineal surgical approach is used because the incision is made between the scrotum and the rectum.

Nursing diagnoses for a client (postoperative) with prostate cancer may include the following:

Nursing Diagnoses	Planning/Goals	Nursing Interventions
▸ *Urinary Retention related to urethral obstruction, secondary to urethral anastomosis*	The client will not experience urinary retention.	Monitor the client's urinary output, noting the amount, color, and presence of clots. The urine should not appear bright red for more than a few hours postoperatively, after which time it should be dark red.
		Reposition or milk the catheter tubing if not patent. If these interventions fail, notify the physician.
		Monitor the client's intake, encouraging a fluid intake of 2,500 to 3,000 mL/day.
▸ *Functional Urinary Incontinence related to bladder sphincter trauma*	The client will achieve urinary control following removal of the catheter.	Advise the client that temporary urinary incontinence frequently occurs following surgery, and reassure him that this is normal.
		Teach the client perineal exercises that will help him regain urinary control. These exercises consist of tightening and relaxing perineal (Kegel exercises) and gluteal muscles and can be performed in a variety of ways.
▸ *Bowel Incontinence related to loss of rectal sphincter control because of perineal incision*	The client will achieve rectal sphincter control.	Advise the client that temporary fecal incontinence frequently occurs after a perineal incision.
		Teach the client perineal exercises that will help him regain bowel control.
		Avoid the use of rectal thermometers, rectal examinations, and enemas.

continues

Nursing Diagnoses	Planning/Goals	Nursing Interventions
▶ *Risk for Impaired Skin Integrity related to incontinence*	The client will not experience skin breakdown.	Keep the client clean and dry, especially if he is experiencing fecal or urinary incontinence. Reposition client every 2 hours.

Evaluation Each goal must be evaluated to determine how it has been met by the client.

TESTICULAR CANCER

Although testicular cancer accounts for only 1% of all cancer in men, it is the most common cancer in young men between the ages of 15 and 35. According to the ACS (1998), advances in treatment have made the 5-year survival rate 95%. The etiology is unknown, but the incidence is highest in men with undescended testicles and those whose mothers had taken hormones during pregnancy. A small, hard, painless lump is usually the first symptom noted (Figure 31-7).

Because early diagnosis of testicular cancer is so essential for a positive surgical outcome, men need to be taught how to perform a testicular self-examination (TSE) and be encouraged to routinely perform that examination (Figure 31-8).

TSE is performed as follows:

- Perform TSE after a bath or shower when scrotum is warm and most relaxed.
- Grasp testis with both hands and palpate gently between thumbs and forefingers.
- The testis should feel smooth, egg-shaped, and firm to the touch.
- The epididymis, located behind the testis, should feel like a soft tube.
- Any abnormal lumps or changes in the testes should be reported to a physician.

Figure 31-7 Testicular Tumor (*From* Health Assessment & Physical Examination, 2nd ed., *by M. E. Z. Estes, 2002 Albany, NY: Delmar. Copyright 2002 by Delmar. Reprinted with permission.*)

Figure 31-8 Performing a Testicular Self-Examination

Medical–Surgical Management

Medical

Testicular ultrasound is used to study the testes for enlargement or lesions. In addition to a testicular ultrasound, the client may have a serum acid or alkaline phosphatase test done. They are both elevated in malignancies.

Surgical

Biopsy of the testis is contraindicated because of the increased potential for metastases. Surgical removal of the testis, spermatic cord, and inguinal canal contents, with examination of the nodes, is indicated for testicular cancers. If unilateral removal of a testis is indicated, the remaining healthy testis will continue to maintain sperm and androgen production.

Pharmacological

Although chemotherapy and radiation are used as adjuvant treatments, radical inguinal orchiectomy remains the primary intervention. Combination chemotherapy with cisplatin (Platinol), vinblastine sulfate (Velban), and bleomycin sulfate (Blenoxane) is effective.

▸ NURSING PROCESS

▸ Assessment

▸ Subjective Data

The client may describe a feeling of heaviness in the scrotum, and may mention weight loss. During the postoperative phase, the client needs to be assessed for pain, using a pain scale to objectify data. He also needs to have emotional and educational needs assessed. For example, the client should be able to accurately describe his activity restrictions and how to provide scrotal support postoperatively. His behaviors and statements need to be monitored for signs of anxiety or depression.

▸ Objective Data

Physical examination should include palpation of the abdomen and assessment of the scrotum. Positive findings in the scrotum include a firm, painless mass in the testis and an enlarged scrotum. As gynecomastia (breast enlargement) is another symptom of testicular cancer, the client's breast tissue should be assessed for enlargement. Postoperative assessment includes monitoring vital signs to detect signs of hemorrhage or infection. Also, the incisional site should be monitored for excess drainage, swelling, or redness.

Nursing diagnoses for the client with testicular cancer may include the following:

Nursing Diagnoses	Planning/Goals	Nursing Interventions
Risk for Injury due to infection and hemorrhage related to surgery	The client will experience minimal bleeding and avoid infection.	Monitor the client's vital signs and incisional drainage. Report hyperthermia, tachycardia, hypotension, increased incisional drainage, and swelling or redness around the incision to the physician immediately. Maintain strict asepsis when handling wound dressings.
Disturbed Body Image related to surgery	The client will maintain or regain a positive body image.	Provide the client with opportunities to voice concerns and ask questions. Monitor the client for statements and behaviors that indicate concern about loss of masculinity. Suggest sexual counseling if he does not appear to be resolving these issues. Advise the client that unilateral removal of a testis will not cause him to be sterile or demasculinized.
Deficient Knowledge related to surgery and postoperative care	The client will demonstrate understanding of postoperative activity restrictions and medical follow-up.	Advise the client that he needs to be on bed rest for 12 to 24 hours postoperatively. Instruct the client to wear tight-fitting underwear or an athletic supporter when ambulating and to avoid heavy lifting for 4 to 6 weeks.

Evaluation Each goal must be evaluated to determine how it has been met by the client.

PENILE CANCER

Penile cancer is rare and has a high correlation with poor hygiene and delayed or no circumcision. The bacteria harbored in the foreskin of the uncircumcised male are irritants to the glans penis and the prepuce. The chronic nature of this irritation is thought to be carcinogenic. Males with a history of STDs are also predisposed to developing penile cancer. Symptoms of penile cancer include a painless, nodular growth on the foreskin, fatigue, and weight loss. Metastases are common in the inguinal nodes and adjacent organs.

Medical–Surgical Management

Medical

The primary penile cancer treatment is surgery. Treatment with radiation alone is ineffective, and chemotherapy alone is used only for palliative treatment of penile cancer with deep distant metastases. However, the client may receive adjuvant therapy with either radiation or chemotherapy.

Surgical

If the tumor is not extensive and no metastases are involved, the remaining penis should be long enough for the client to void standing and avoid soiling himself. If a penectomy is necessary, a permanent fistula opening into the urethra will be made between the scrotum and the anus (**urethrostomy**).

▶ NURSING PROCESS

▶ Assessment

▶ Subjective Data

Although the tumor is painless, the client should be asked if he is experiencing any pain, to rule out other possible diagnoses. The client also needs to be asked if he is experiencing fatigue or weight loss. Preoperatively, the client needs an assessment of his emotional and educational needs. He needs to be asked questions that can be used to determine his understanding of the surgical procedure and the need for counseling. Postoperative assessment also includes monitoring for pain and using a pain scale to objectify data.

▶ Objective Data

The client needs a physical assessment that includes inspection of the penis for the presence of painless, nodular growths. During the postoperative phase, monitoring of vital signs, incisional site, and intake and output must be done. Hypotension, tachycardia, excessive incisional drainage, redness or swelling around the incision, or bright red or low urinary output, could be signs of complications.

Nursing diagnoses for a client with penile cancer may include the following:

Nursing Diagnoses	Planning/Goals	Nursing Interventions
▶ Risk for Injury due to infection and hemorrhage related to surgery	The client will experience minimal bleeding and avoid infection.	Monitor the client's vital signs and incisional drainage. Report hyperthermia, tachycardia, hypotension, increased incisional drainage, and swelling or redness around the incision to the physician immediately. Maintain strict asepsis when handling wound dressings.
▶ Disturbed Body Image related to surgery	The client will maintain a positive body image.	Provide the client with opportunities to voice his concerns and ask questions. Keep in mind the typically young age of the client and the associated self-image and sexuality issues.
▶ Anxiety related to surgery	The client will discuss anxieties.	Provide the client with information about the operative procedure, postoperative and discharge care. When available, a video may be used to present this information, with the nurse being available to answer the client's questions.
▶ Ineffective Sexuality Patterns related to the altered body function or structure	The client will maintain satisfactory sexuality patterns postoperatively.	Advise the client to seek sexual counseling for both himself and his partner if he is unable to maintain normal sexuality patterns.
▶ Impaired Urinary Elimination related to surgery	The client will achieve urinary control postoperatively.	Monitor the client's intake and output. Report low urinary output to the physician immediately.

Evaluation Each goal must be evaluated to determine how it has been met by the client.

STRUCTURAL DISORDERS

Cryptorchidism is a condition in which one or both testicles fail to descend into the scrotum by the time of birth. The cause is usually unknown. Decrease or loss of sperm production may occur because of the damage that occurs to the seminiferous epithelium. When the testes are within the normal path and do not descend or cannot be pulled into the scrotum, surgery (orchiopexy) is usually done between 5 and 7 years of age. Even with the corrective surgery, as adults, these males have a 10 to 30 times higher incidence of testicular cancer.

A hydrocele is a benign, nontender collection of clear, amber fluid within the space of the testes and the tunica vaginalis or along the spermatic cord. This collection of fluid may result in scrotal swelling, which can be painful if it develops suddenly. Inflammation of the epididymis or testis or a lymphatic or venous obstruction may cause this condition. Congenital hydrocele in the newborn occurs when the canal between the peritoneal cavity and the scrotum does not close completely during fetal development. Aspiration of the fluid serves only as a temporary measure and can lead to secondary infection. Therefore, treatment for the condition is surgery.

Hypospadias is an abnormal placement of the urethral opening on the ventral surface of the penis. Epispadias is the opening of the urethra on the dorsal surface of the penis. The treatment is determined by the position of the urethra on the penis. Infants with either condition should not be circumcised before a urology consultation is obtained, because the foreskin is used in the repair.

A spermatocele is a benign nontender cyst of either the epididymis or the rete testis. It contains milky fluid and sperm. Usually this condition is painless and does not require medical treatment.

A varicocele is dilation of the veins of the scrotum that occurs when the venous system that drains the testicle lengthens and enlarges. This dilation occurs when incompetent or absent valves in the spermatic venous system permit blood to accumulate, resulting in increased hydrostatic pressure. This condition is most commonly found on the left side because of the increased retrograde pressure of the renal vein, the length, and fewer competent valves. It is theorized that the hyperthermia that occurs with this condition decreases spermatogenesis, resulting in decreased fertility. Symptoms may include a bluish discoloration of the scrotal skin or palpation of a wormlike mass when the male bears down. This condition seldom requires treatment.

Torsion of the spermatic cord occurs when the vascular pedicle of the testis twists, resulting in partial or complete venous occlusion. The three forms of this disorder are (1) rotation of the spermatic cord, (2) torsion of a testicular appendage, or (3) torsion of the spermatic cord and epididymis. Testicular torsion may be related to recent trauma, and the onset of symptoms often occurs quite suddenly. Symptoms of testicular torsion may include abdominal and scrotal pain, scrotal edema, nausea and vomiting and, possibly, a slight fever. The pain caused by testicular torsion is not relieved by bed rest or scrotal support.

Medical–Surgical Management

Medical/surgical management of male structural disorders is specific to the condition. Cryptorchidism may be treated with hormonal therapy. If this is not successful, surgery should be done within the first 18 months of life, in order to avoid possible sterility. In some newborns a hydrocele may resolve without medical intervention. Clients of all ages may have aspiration performed to reduce the swelling caused by fluid or a hematoma. However, this solution is usually only temporary, and surgical removal of the sac provides the only permanent solution to the problem. Although a spermatocele usually does not require treatment, sometimes surgical aspiration or excision is necessary.

Hypospadias and epispadias are surgically repaired (urethroplasty) before the child is 1 year of age. Usually, successful repair requires more than one surgery and often results in scarring of the penis.

Because a common complication of a varicocele is male infertility, ligation of the spermatic vein may be performed if infertility is a concern. Sometimes this does not resolve infertility problems because varicoceles may recur after surgery. When fertility is not a concern, the varicocele may be treated simply with scrotal support.

Torsion of the spermatic cord is one disorder that does require immediate surgery to perform surgical detorsion (untwisting) and suturing of the testicle to the scrotum.

▶ NURSING PROCESS

▶ Assessment

▶ Subjective Data

Diagnostic assessment for all structural disorders should include asking the client about the type and location of his pain. He should also be asked about related symptoms such as alteration in urinary patterns, warmth, fatigue, nausea, or vomiting. Postoperative assessments include monitoring for pain and using a pain scale to objectify data. The client's knowledge of his condition, treatment, and follow-up care also need to be assessed, as do the implications of sterility and impotence to the client's life.

▶ **Objective Data**

Physical assessment should include inspection and palpation of the genitals to detect the presence of scrotal swelling, testicular enlargement, scrotal immobility, redness, and warmth of the scrotum. Small varicoceles may be diagnosed by the presence of a wormlike mass in the scrotum when the client stands or is asked to bear down. Large varicoceles may be visible through the scrotal skin as a bluish discoloration. Bilateral palpation of the newborn's scrotum will determine the bilateral presence of testes.

Nursing diagnoses for a male client with a structural disorder of the reproductive system may include the following:

Nursing Diagnoses	Planning/Goals	Nursing Interventions
▶ *Risk for Injury related to inflammation and hemorrhage*	The client will experience minimal bleeding and avoid infection.	Monitor the client's vital signs and incisional drainage.
		Report hyperthermia, tachycardia, hypotension, increased incisional drainage, and swelling or redness around the incision to the physician immediately.
		Maintain strict asepsis when handling wound dressings.
▶ *Deficient Knowledge related to the condition and possible complications*	The client will demonstrate understanding of the possible complications of his condition.	Monitor statements made by the client to determine if there is any misunderstanding about how the surgery will affect his masculinity and fertility.
		Provide the client with opportunities to voice his feelings and ask questions.

Evaluation Each goal must be evaluated to determine how it has been met by the client.

FUNCTIONAL DISORDERS AND CONCERNS

Included in this category are impotence, infertility, and contraception.

IMPOTENCE

Impotence is defined as the inability of an adult male to have an erection firm enough or to maintain it long enough to complete sexual intercourse. There are three types of impotence: functional, atonic, and anatomic. Psychological factors that lead to concerns about sexual performance may contribute to functional impotence. These factors include aging and difficulty with communication or relationships.

Atonic impotence may be the result of medications such as antihypertensives, sedatives, antidepressants, or tranquilizers. For example, antihypertensives lower blood pressure in all arteries of the body, and reduction of the blood pressure to penile arteries may lead to failure of the penis to fill sufficiently to achieve erection. The use of alcohol, cocaine, and nicotine can also decrease potency. Disease processes leading to atonic impotence include diabetes and vascular and neurological disorders. Diabetic clients are at increased risk for impotence owing to their tendency to develop atherosclerosis and autonomic neuropathy. Vascular and neurological disorders include atherosclerosis, hypertension, spinal cord injuries, and multiple sclerosis. End-stage renal disease and chronic obstructive pulmonary disorders can also decrease potency.

Peyronie's disease causes development of nonelastic, fibrous tissue just beneath the penile skin, leading to anatomic impotence. The resulting loss of elasticity leads to a decreased ability of the penis to fill with and store blood during an erection. Peyronie's disease often causes the penis to bend upward, possibly leading to pain and an inability to penetrate the vagina (Figure 31-9).

Figure 31-9 Peyronie's Disease: A. Fibrous Plaque Causes a Curvature of the Penis; B. Cross Section of the Penis Showing Plaque

Medical–Surgical Management

Medical

The first step in treating impotence is to determine whether the client's lifestyle is a factor. Further assessment may include nocturnal penile tumescence monitoring or dynamic infusion cavernosometry and cavernosography (DICC). Treatment will be based on the assessment findings and test results. Treatment may include changes in lifestyle to reduce the need for medications, manage stress, lose weight, and exercise. These changes often help to improve the client's physical health, self-image, and attitude about his ability to function sexually.

External devices can be used to promote an erection. A vacuum constriction device (VCD) may be used to increase the blood supply to the penis, causing engorgement and rigidity (Figure 31-10). The client inserts his penis into a plastic cylinder and squeezes a pump to withdraw the air from the cylinder, creating a vacuum that draws blood into the penis. Once an erection has been achieved in this manner, a rubber ring is moved from the bottom of the cylinder to the base of the penis. This permits the blood to be safely trapped in the penis for up to one-half hour. Advantages of the VCD over surgical intervention are decreased expense and fewer complications.

Surgical

Surgical interventions for impotency include revascularization and penile implants. For clients with impotence related to blocked arteries, revascularization is done to bypass blocked arteries and remove veins that are causing excessive drainage. For clients who are not candidates for revascularization, penile prostheses are another option (Figure 31-11). One type is a semirigid implant, which is a silicone cylinder that may be flexible or inflexible. Another type is a hydraulic implant that has a cylinder that can be inflated by squeezing a pump located in the scrotum or at the end of the penis. Because of its ability to fill and empty, the hydraulic implant, unlike the silicone implant, which is always semirigid, most closely mimics flaccidity and erection. The disadvantages of surgical interventions are expense and postoperative complications, the most serious being postoperative infection.

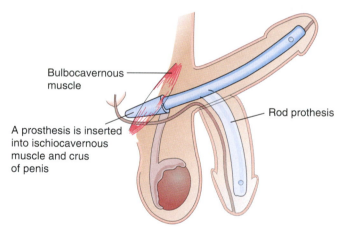

A. Semirigid implant in place

B. Hydraulic implant, pump in scrotum

Figure 31-11 Penile Prostheses

Figure 31-10 Vacuum Constriction Device

Pharmacological

Medications that promote erections are available. The one most widely used is sildenafil citrate (Viagra). One side effect of drug therapy is prolonged erection that does not occur in response to sexual stimulation (**priapism**). Oral neurotransmitters have been used with variable success, and sublingual apomorphine shows some promise as an erectogenic agent. When administered sublingually rather than subcutaneously, as was done in the past, there are fewer side effects. Self-injections of vasodilators or other drugs may result in serious complications.

▶ NURSING PROCESS

▶ Assessment

▶ Subjective Data

A complete assessment includes a history of illicit and prescribed drug use, alcohol consumption, previ-ous diagnoses, lifestyle, sexual functioning, and family disorders. The client's emotional and educational needs must be assessed to determine whether anxiety about sexual performance or lack of knowledge are contributing factors to impotence.

▶ Objective Data

If the client has surgery, the nurse needs to monitor vital signs, incisional site, and intake and output.

Nursing Management

Nursing diagnoses for a client who is impotent may include the following:

- *Sexual Dysfunction, related to altered body function or structure*
- *Sexuality Patterns, Altered, related to altered body function or structure*
- *Body Image Disturbance, related to impotence*
- *Knowledge Deficit, related to impotence*

SAMPLE NURSING CARE PLAN

THE CLIENT EXPERIENCING IMPOTENCE

Mr. Parry is a fifty-five-year-old, married male with diabetes and atherosclerosis. He recently also has been diagnosed as being impotent. He has trouble making eye contact as he discusses his condition and says he has told no one of his diagnosis, not even his wife. He tells you he doesn't understand why this is happening to him now when things have been going so well for him.

Nursing Diagnosis 1 *Disturbed Body Image related to his condition, as evidenced by Mr. Parry's lack of eye contact and statement that he has not told his wife.*

PLANNING/GOALS	NURSING INTERVENTIONS	RATIONALE	EVALUATION
Mr. Parry will achieve a positive self-image or seek counseling to assist him with that goal.	Provide Mr. Parry with opportunities to voice his concerns and ask questions in a private, comfortable atmosphere.	The related self-image and sexuality issues are often difficult to discuss.	Mr. Parry verbalizes that he is afraid that his wife will leave him if he is not able to perform sexually. He agrees to attend professional counseling with his wife to discuss these concerns.
	Monitor Mr. Parry for statements and behaviors that indicate he is experiencing a body image disturbance.	The nurse needs to observe Mr. Parry and listen to what he is saying in order to determine his concerns and needs.	
	Suggest that Mr. Parry seek sexual or marital counseling, if indicated.	If Mr. Parry does not appear to be meeting his goal, alternative resources may help him achieve his goals.	

continues

Nursing Diagnosis 2 *Deficient Knowledge related to his condition, as evidenced by Mr. Parry's statements that he does not understand why this is happening.*

PLANNING/GOALS	NURSING INTERVENTIONS	RATIONALE	EVALUATION
Mr. Parry will demonstrate an understanding of the health factors that are contributing to his impotency.	Monitor Mr. Parry's statements about his condition.	In order to determine Mr. Parry's educational needs concerning his condition and treatment options, the nurse needs to determine his current knowledge level.	Mr. Parry verbalizes that his impotency is caused by poor blood circulation to his penis.
	Educate Mr. Parry about how his diabetes and atherosclerosis are contributing to his impotency.	The nurse needs to build upon Mr. Parry's current knowledge level to increase his knowledge of his condition.	

INFERTILITY

The causes of infertility in males include varicoceles, cryptorchidism, impaired sperm, insufficient number of sperm, and hormonal imbalance. Tight-fitting undershorts will increase scrotal temperature, resulting in a reduced sperm count. Also, the use of hot tubs or saunas may decrease the sperm count.

The first step in treating an infertile couple is to obtain a history of sexual practices. In addition, a detailed health history needs to be obtained and physical examination performed.

Diagnostic tests that may be ordered include the following:

- Semen analysis, including sperm count, motility, and morphology
- Testicular biopsy (done when sperm are absent from the semen) to ascertain the presence of sperm
- Male-female interaction studies (Huhner test) to determine motility and number of sperm 2 to 4 hours after intercourse
- Testing of the sex chromosomes

Medical–Surgical Management

Medical

A treatment plan will be formulated based on these diagnostic tests. Vitamins and a well-balanced diet may be prescribed. The client may be advised to have intercourse every other day beginning 12 to 16 days prior to the woman's next menstrual period.

Surgical

With a diagnosis of cryptorchidism or varicocele, surgery may be advised.

Pharmacological

If the sperm count is low, testosterone or thyroid extracts may be prescirbed.

▶ NURSING PROCESS

▶ Assessment

The nurse should ask questions to determine the client's knowledge about the condition and treatment options. If surgery is necessary to correct a structural disorder, the nurse will be responsible for postoperative assessment. The nurse should ask the client questions to determine his emotional needs, as an infertility diagnosis may cause the client to experience guilt, grief, or a disturbance in self-image. Nursing diagnoses, goals, interventions, and evaluation will be based on the assessment findings.

CONTRACEPTION

When choosing a form of contraception, the male client has various options to consider. While weighing the options, safety, ease of use, effectiveness, and cost should be considered. The partner's wishes should also be considered in this decision-making process.

Contraceptive options available to males include abstinence, coitus interruptus, condoms, or voluntary surgical sterilization. Withdrawing the penis from the vagina before ejaculation (coitus interruptus) is not a very reliable method because sperm may have already been emitted in the lubricating fluids. Also, the man may experience difficulty in controlling the timing of his ejaculation.

Condoms are an inexpensive, readily available form of contraception. A condom is a latex or sheepskin sheath that is slipped over the erect penis before the penis is inserted into the vagina. The condom should be applied by holding it by the tip and unrolling it onto the penis. A space of about one inch should be left for semen at the tip. After ejaculation, the penis should be withdrawn carefully to prevent the condom from slipping off and spilling the contents. The condom should then be discarded, as it is designed for a single use. Condoms are available in a variety of colors, sizes, and other features. The 2% failure rate of condoms is probably related more to inconsistent use rather than actual product failure. Other problems associated with condom usage are allergic reactions to latex and reports of reduced sexual pleasure by both partners. Positive aspects of condom usage include protection against STD and HIV. It must be noted, however, that sheepskin condoms do not provide protection against HIV.

Vasectomy is a surgical form of sterilization for the male. Refer to Sterilization Method in Chapter 30, Nursing Care of the Client: Female Reproductive Disorders.

CASE STUDY

Mr. Able is a 70-year-old Caucasian male with a diagnosis of benign prostatic hyperplasia. Before his hospital admission for a TURP he had been in good health. He returned from surgery 3 hours ago with a three-way Foley catheter and continuous bladder irrigation. His vital signs 1 hour ago were as follows: temperature 98.9°F, apical pulse 68, blood pressure 130/84, and respirations 18. When the nurse enters his room to take another set of vitals, Mr. Able is restless and moaning and has cool, moist skin; his catheter is not draining properly. His pulse is now 120 and blood pressure is 88/50. The nurse calls the physician to report the change in Mr. Able's condition. The physician orders a STAT hematocrit and a bleeding and clotting time. An increase in the IV fluid drip rate is also ordered. The doctor is planning to arrive at the hospital within the next hour.

The following questions will guide your development of a nursing care plan for the case study.

1. List symptoms and clinical manifestations, other than Mr. Able's, that a client may experience after a TURP.
2. List reasons why the doctor has ordered the STAT blood work and the IV changes.
3. List other diagnostic tests that may have been ordered for Mr. Able.
4. Mentally do a head-to-toe or functional assessment on Mr. Able. List subjective and objective data a nurse would want to obtain.
5. Write three individualized nursing diagnoses and goals for Mr. Able.
6. Upon assessing Mr. Able, the doctor decides to inject additional fluid into the balloon that anchors the indwelling catheter and apply increased traction to the catheter. List pertinent nursing actions a nurse would do following these medical interventions:

   - Medications
   - Comfort/rest
   - Cardiac output
   - Intake and output
   - Activity
   - Teaching
7. List resources within the medical center and the local area that could assist Mr. Able with his postoperative recovery.
8. List teaching that Mr. Able will need before his discharge.
9. List at least three successful outcomes for Mr. Able.

SUMMARY

- Common male reproductive system inflammatory disorders include epididymitis, orchitis, and prostatitis. Bilateral epididymitis and orchitis can lead to sterility. Treatment includes antibiotic therapy.
- Benign prostatic hyperplasia is a common disorder in males over age 50. Early symptoms include hesitancy, decreased force of stream, urinary frequency, and nocturia.
- Male cancers related to the reproductive system involve the prostate, testes, breast, and penis. Emphasis should be placed on testicular self-examination and regular physical examinations in order to facilitate early diagnosis and treatment.
- Impotence may be caused by emotional or physical factors. Treatment includes counseling, medications, circulatory aids, and surgery.

Review Questions

1. Where is the most common site of cancer in the male reproductive system?
   a. breast
   b. testicles
   c. penis
   d. prostate

2. Which of the following factors predisposes males to penile cancer?
   a. Alcohol consumption
   b. Not being circumcised
   c. Advanced age
   d. Circumcision

3. Which of the following self-examinations should a young man be taught to do?
   a. Rectal
   b. Scrotal
   c. Prostate
   d. Testicular

4. Which of the following complications may occur after a TURP?
   a. Water intoxication
   b. Difficulty voiding
   c. Constipation
   d. Hypertension

5. Which method may be used to clear obstructed catheter tubing post-TURP?
   a. milking the tubing
   b. changing the catheter
   c. running the irrigation fluid faster
   d. releasing the traction from the catheter

6. What is a cause of male infertility?
   a. exercise
   b. hypospadias
   c. lack of sleep
   d. frequent hot tub or sauna usage

7. What is a cause of impotency?
   a. varicocele
   b. heavy exercise
   c. Peyronie's disease
   d. having multiple sexual partners

8. The purpose of post-TURP continuous bladder irrigation is to:
   a. decrease urinary output.
   b. reduce clot formation.
   c. decrease bleeding.
   d. increase urinary output.

9. Which of the following nursing interventions can help alleviate bladder spasms post-TURP?
   a. Increasing fluid intake
   b. Maintaining traction on the urethral catheter
   c. Administering B&O suppositories
   d. Applying ice to and elevating the scrotum

10. Which of the following is a method that can be used to assess the client's level of knowledge related to his inflammatory disorder of the reproductive system?
    a. Asking the client if he has any questions
    b. Asking the client to describe "safe sex" practices
    c. Asking the client if he has read the pamphlets about his disorder
    d. Asking the client to describe the symptoms of his disorder

Critical Thinking Questions

1. Prepare a teaching plan for testicular self-examination.

2. What is the rationale for each nursing intervention given for the nursing diagnoses in this chapter?

WEB FLASH!

- Search the Internet for the disorders discussed in this chapter. Are there any new treatments discussed for any of the disorders?
- Visit the Web sites for the Resources listed at the end of the book for the reproductive systems. What type of information do these organizations have available for the client and family? For health care providers?

NURSING CARE OF THE CLIENT: SEXUALLY TRANSMITTED DISEASES

MAKING THE CONNECTION

Refer to the following chapters to increase your understanding of sexually transmitted diseases:

- **Chapter 22, Nursing Care of the Client: Immune System**
- **Chapter 30, Nursing Care of the Client: Female Reproductive System**
- **Chapter 31, Nursing Care of the Client: Male Reproductive System**

LEARNING OBJECTIVES

Upon completion of this chapter, you should be able to:
- *Define key terms.*
- *List the most prevalent STDs, including causative agents.*
- *Describe currently used methods of prevention of STDs.*
- *Describe signs and symptoms, diagnostic aids, and treatment of the common STDs.*
- *Utilize the nursing process to plan the care of a client with an STD.*
- *Demonstrate the ability to teach self-care and reinfection prevention measures to the client with an STD.*

KEY TERMS

antibiotic resistance	incidence
chancre	incubation period
chlamydia	syphilis
cytomegalovirus	trichomoniasis
exposure	venereal disease
gonorrhea	

INTRODUCTION

Sexually transmitted diseases (STDs) can be defined as those diseases that are transmitted or passed from one person to another primarily through sexual contact. Another term that was used for STDs is **venereal disease**. Today the term *sexually transmitted disease* is preferred. The STDs covered in this chapter are chlamydia, gonorrhea, syphilis, genital herpes, cytomegalovirus, genital warts, trichomoniasis, and hepatitis B. Acquired immunodeficiency syndrome (AIDS) is not solely a sexually transmitted disease, although sexual activity is one of the primary modes of transmission (ways through which it is spread): AIDS is discussed in detail in Chapter 39.

The **incidence** (frequency of disease occurence) of STDs has been increasing worldwide, with trichomoniasis, chlamydia, and gonorrhea being the most widespread STDs today. Some diseases, such as syphilis, have been described as sexually transmitted diseases for centuries. Currently over 13 million Americans annually are diagnosed with an STD. Chlamydia, for example, affects over 3 million Americans every year, making it more than twice as common as gonorrhea (National Institute of Allergy and Infectious Diseases [NIAID] and National Institutes of Health [NIH], December 1998). Syphilis, although less common than either chlamydia or gonorrhea, still affects about 9,000 people each year in the United States (NIAID and NIH, December 1998).

The development of antibiotic treatment for STDs in the 1940s caused a dramatic decrease in the prevalence of STDs, and for a while it was predicted that STDs would be eradicated completely. But a variety of factors have contributed to the dramatic increase of STDs such as: casual sex, asymptomatic carriers of the disease, the use of nonbarrier methods of birth control, and lack of knowledge of methods of preventing STDs.

Another factor that has contributed to the vast increase in STDs in recent years is the increased consumption of alcohol and the use of illegal drugs. Not only is the sharing of needles among intravenous drug abusers a factor in the increased incidence of STDs, but so also is the lessening of inhibitions that occurs with drug and alcohol abuse. The trading of sex for drugs is also a factor in the spread of STDs.

Inadequate reporting of STDs may also cause statistics to be inaccurate. There is no great uniformity in the reporting requirements for STDs. Reporting regulations differ from state to state and from disease to disease. All states in the United States require that cases of gonorrhea and syphilis be reported to a health officer in that state. Only 35 states have mandatory HIV reporting (Sharts-Hopko, 1997). The Centers for Disease Control and Prevention (CDC) keep statistics on reportable diseases.

Public education regarding the causes, methods of transmission, and methods of prevention of STDs is the most important weapon in the battle against STDs. Although many STDs caused by bacterial infection are curable with modern antibiotics, the viruses are not.

Since sexual activity is beginning at earlier ages today, sex education, including information about STDs, is being presented in elementary schools. Many schools have comprehensive education programs already in place to teach about STDs and recommendations to prevent the spread of STDs. Television, especially educational programs, also has been helpful in informing the public of the dangers of having sex without protection against STDs.

Many messages have been disseminated to the general public regarding the best methods of prevention of STDs. The only 100% effective method of prevention of STDs is abstinence (refraining from sexual intercourse or mucous membrane to mucous membrane contact altogether). Couples who are mutually monogamous are also not at risk, unless one of them was previously infected. The popularity of the pill has decreased consistent condom use. Most current methods of birth control are not effective in preventing the transmission of STDs. Only a barrier method, the latex condom, has been effective in preventing the spread of STDs, although even this method only provides safer sex, not totally safe sex.

Once the diagnosis of an STD is made, identification of all sexual contacts is also important. Many people are reluctant to be candid regarding sexual activity and sexual contacts, since this is an area of life considered to be extremely private. One of the most difficult aspects in dealing with STDs is that many of the diseases are totally asymptomatic, especially in women. These asymptomatic partners can both transmit the disease to new partners and/or reinfect a treated partner, if they are not identified and treated.

An overview of the STDs covered in this chapter is presented in Table 32–1.

ANATOMY AND PHYSIOLOGY REVIEW

The major system affected by the sexually transmitted diseases is the reproductive system. Males are generally more symptomatic than females and will seek

Table 32–1 SEXUALLY TRANSMITTED DISEASES: AN OVERVIEW

DISEASE	CHARACTERISTICS	NURSING IMPLICATIONS
Chlamydia	*Male:* Painful urination Urethral discharge *Female:* Asymptomatic or may experience purulent discharge *Note:* If untreated, pelvic inflammatory disease (PID) can develop.	Instruct client to notify sexual partner(s) of past 2 months of their need for treatment. Instruct client to avoid sexual activity or to use condoms until both client and partner(s) are symptom free. Provide instruction regarding medications prescribed.
Cytomegalo-virus (CMV)	Often asymptomatic, occasionally fever, fatigue, and weakness Generally acquired during childhood or adolescence 80% to 100% of adults have antibodies to CMV.	Implicated in some spontaneous abortions or mental retardation. Congenital infection produces cytomegalic inclusion disease. May be life threatening in a client with a poorly functioning immune system.

continues

Table 32–1 SEXUALLY TRANSMITTED DISEASES: AN OVERVIEW

DISEASE	CHARACTERISTICS	NURSING IMPLICATIONS
Genital Herpes: Herpes Simplex Virus 2 (HSV-2)	Vesicles on penis, vagina, labia, perineum, or anus Can progress to painful ulceration Lesions may last up to 6 weeks Recurrence common *Note:* May be asymptomatic	Refer sexual partner(s) for examination. Teach that virus can be transmitted even when the person experiences no symptoms. Instruct in use of condoms. Teach females of need for annual Pap smear. Provide instruction regarding medications prescribed.
Gonorrhea	*Male:* Urethritis (inflammation of the urethra) Purulent discharge Urinary frequency Epididymitis (inflammation of the epididymis) *Female:* Often asymptomatic May lead to PID or salpingitis (inflammation of the fallopian tube) Can occlude the fallopian tubes, resulting in sterility	Instruct client to return if symptoms persist. Sexual partner(s) of past 60 days must be assessed. Instruct client to avoid sexual activity until symptoms subside in both client and partner(s). Provide instruction regarding medications prescribed.
Hepatitis B Virus (HBV)	Varies greatly from asymptomatic state to severe hepatitis to cancer	Partner(s) should receive medical prophylaxis within 14 days after exposure. For client and partner(s), recommend three-dose immunization series when this episode has abated.
Genital Warts (Human Papilloma-virus)	Fleshy, cauliflowerlike growth on genitalia	Inform and treat sexual partner(s). Provide instruction regarding medications prescribed.
Syphilis	Disease consists of 4 stages with distinct manifestations as follows: *Primary:* A painless papule on penis, vagina, or cervix (chancre) Usually negative serologic blood test Highly infectious during this stage *Secondary:* Rash, especially prevalent on palms and soles Low-grade fever Sore throat Headache *Early latency:* Possible infectious lesions, otherwise asymptomatic Reactive serologic tests *Late latency:* Possible lesions in central nervous and cardiovascular systems Noninfectious except to fetus of pregnant woman	Interview client to identify sexual contacts. All those exposed to the disease should be given penicillin. Educate client and sexual contacts about the disease. Provide instruction regarding medications prescribed. Counsel and educate client. Counsel and educate client.
Trichomoniasis	Petechial lesions Profuse urethral or vaginal discharge that is foul smelling, yellow, and foamy	Treat sexual partners simultaneously with metronidazole (Flagyl). Provide instruction regarding medication prescribed.

health care more readily since the signs of disease on the external genitalia are more visible. In females, the sex organs are internal; females, therefore, are more likely to suffer complications and increased severity of symptoms by the time the disease is identified.

In addition to the reproductive system, any area of sexual contact, such as oral and rectal areas, may also exhibit signs and symptoms of the disease process.

COMMON DIAGNOSTIC TESTS

Commonly used diagnostic tests for clients with symptoms of sexually transmitted diseases are listed in Table 32–2. See Chapter 13, Diagnostic Tests, for explanation/normal values and nursing responsibilities.

CHLAMYDIA

Chlamydia is caused by a spherical bacterial organism known as *Chlamydia trachomatis*. Outside the body, the organism has difficulty surviving, but inside the body, chlamydia reproduces rapidly inside host cells. The mode of transmission in chlamydia must be through intimate body contact, since the organism is so fragile that it cannot survive long when outside of the body.

Most chlamydia infections are asymptomatic. Chlamydia is known as the "silent STD" for this reason. If left untreated, chlamydial infections cause tissue inflammation, ulceration, and scar tissue formation in both women and men. Salpingitis (inflammation of the

fallopian tubes) or pelvic inflammatory disease (PID) can lead to scarring of the delicate fallopian tubes, ectopic pregnancy, or even infertility.

When symptoms of chlamydia appear in males, they are dysuria and genital discharge. Females may have a grayish white mucopurulent vaginal discharge, itching, and dysuria, although as many as 85% of women will be asymptomatic (NIAID and NIH, June 1998b).

Medical–Surgical Management

Pharmacological

The treatment of choice is doxycycline (Vibramycin). If compliance with an extended period of drug therapy is thought to be a problem, azithromycin (Zithromax) can be given orally in a single dose. Pregnant women may be treated with erythromycin estolate (Ilosone) or amoxicillin (Amoxil), but they should be cultured again after treatment is completed to confirm the absence of chlamydial infection. Retesting is not required after treatment with doxycycline or azithromycin. It is important that all sexual partners be tested and treated for chlamydia since reinfection is probable if only one partner is treated.

Health Promotion

Persons who have more than one sexual partner, especially women less than 25 years old, should regularly be tested for chlamydial infection even when there are no symptoms. The use of male or female condoms or diaphragms during sexual intercourse may help reduce transmission (NIAID and NIH, June 1998b).

GONORRHEA

Gonorrheal infections are often seen in combination with chlamydia. **Gonorrhea** is a serious bacterial infection, caused by the gram-negative bacterial organism *Neisseria gonorrhea*. An estimated 800,000 cases occur annually in the United States (NIAID and NIH, June 1998c). The organism multiplies quickly in warm, moist areas of the body including the oral cavity, reproductive tract, and the rectum. Mouth-to-mouth kissing does not transmit gonorrhea. It is spread during sexual intercourse—vaginal, oral, and anal. The cervix is the usual site of infection in women. The disease progresses in much the same manner as chlamydia and can cause many of the same complications, such as infertility from salpingitis and PID.

Symptoms of infection may occur within 2 to 10 days after **exposure** (contact with an infected person or agent). Again, men are more likely to exhibit symptoms such as burning on urination and a purulent discharge from the penis. Many women are asymptomatic, but the remainder may have pain or burning on urination and/or a yellow or bloody vaginal discharge.

Table 32–2 COMMON DIAGNOSTIC TESTS FOR SEXUALLY TRANSMITTED DISEASES

Blood Tests
- Enzyme-linked immunosorbent assay (ELISA)
- Western blot
- Venereal Disease Research Laboratories (VDRL)
- Rapid plasma reagin (RPR)
- Fluorescent treponemal antibody-absorption test (FTA-ABS)
- Reiter test

Culture
- Tissue: Male urethra, female endocervix
- Discharge
- Tzanck

Urine
- Urine specimen

Other
- Dark field examination of wart scrapings
- Microscopic examination

CLIENT TEACHING

Gonorrhea and HIV
- Infection with gonorrhea increases the risk of HIV infection.
- Prevention and/or early treatment of gonorrhea is critical.

If a woman is infected with gonorrhea when she gives birth, the infection may be transmitted to the newborn's eyes as the baby travels through the birth canal. In the United States, all infants are treated with an antibiotic opthalmic ointment within 1 to 2 hours of birth to prevent the gonorrheal-induced eye infection known as opthalmia neonatorum.

Medical–Surgical Management

Once the presence of gonorrhea has been confirmed, both partners should be treated with a course of antibiotic therapy. One of the problems in treating gonorrhea is that new strains of gonorrhea have developed **antibiotic resistance** (resistance to a previously effective antimicrobial agent). Penicillin used to be the drug of choice when treating gonorrhea, but since penicillin has been so widely used against many types of infection, some strains of *Neisseria gonorrhea* have adapted and are no longer affected by penicillin. The current practice is to treat all cases of gonorrhea as though they were resistant to the traditional drug therapies.

Pharmacological

A variety of antibiotics are effective against gonorrhea. One of the most effective therapies includes a single dose of ciprofloxacin (Cipro), followed by a 7-day course of oral doxycycline (Vibramycin). Because almost half of all clients with gonorrhea also have chlamydia, doxycycline (Vibramycin) is an appropriate choice of drug therapy since it combats both infections effectively. For pregnant clients, or those under 16 years of age, an injection of ceftriaxone sodium (Rocephlin), followed by oral erythromycin estolate (Ilosone), is recommended. Follow-up cultures to determine the success of the course of treatment are recommended when the treatment has been completed.

SYPHILIS

Syphilis, an STD almost eradicated after the discovery of antibiotic therapy in the 1940s, is on the upswing again, with 8,550 cases reported in 1997 (NIAID and NIH, December 1998). The causative organism of syphilis is a spirochete, a spiral-shaped bacteria known as *Treponema pallidum,* which was first identified in 1905. Transmission of syphilis is either through sexual contact or congenitally (mother to child). Syphilis is often seen with human immunodeficiency virus (HIV) infection, just as chlamydia is often seen with gonorrhea.

Syphilis has 4 stages. In primary stage syphilis, the **incubation period**, or interval between exposure to an infectious disease and the first appearance of symptoms, can be 10 to 90 days, with the development of a **chancre** usually occurring within 2 to 6 weeks. A chancre is a clean, painless ulcer, which usually is present at the site of body contact (Figure 32-1). There is usually just one chancre present, but multiple chancres have been known to occur. Chancres may occur on the internal genitalia of women (for example, the cervix) and thus not be noticed. The chancre will heal within a few weeks, even without treatment, and either leave a thin scar or none at all. If not identified and treated, about one-third will progress to secondary syphilis.

In secondary syphilis, the client has a skin rash of penny-sized brown sores that appear approximately 3 to 6 weeks after the chancre. The rash may be on all or any part of the body, but almost always involves the palms of the hands and the soles of the feet. Active bacteria are in the sores so any contact, sexual or nonsexual, with the broken skin of the infected person may spread the infection. The rash heals within several months. Other symptoms such as low-grade fever, fatigue, headache, sore throat, and generalized lymph node swelling may occur. Occasionally a wartlike growth known as condyloma latum may be present in the genital area of both men and women (Figure 32-2). Since this is so close in appearance to the condylomata acuminata of human papillomavirus infection, it may be confused with genital warts. Symptoms of secondary syphilis may come and go for 1 or 2 years. Since many of these symptoms are also common to many other diseases, syphilis has often been called "the great imitator."

Figure 32-1 The chancre usually occurs at the point where the organism contacted the body.

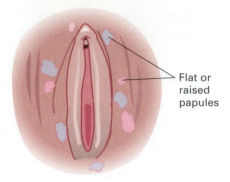

Flat or
raised
papules

Figure 32-2 Condyloma latum, a wartlike growth, may be present in the genital area of males and females in secondary syphilis.

When not treated, syphilis enters into a latent period when no symptoms are present and the disease is no longer contagious. Only about one-third of those clients with secondary syphilis will develop the symptoms of tertiary syphilis; that is, when the bacteria damages the heart, eyes, brain, nervous system, bones, joints, or any other part of the body. Tertiary syphilis can last for years or decades and may result in heart disease, blindness, neurologic problems, and death.

Approximately 3% to 7% of untreated persons will develop neurosyphilis (NIAID and NIH, July 1998c). Symptoms may range from none to headache, fever, seizures, and stroke symptoms. Sometimes it may take 20 years for this to occur.

Medical–Surgical Management

Pharmacological

Since the time that syphilis was first treated with antibiotic therapy, penicillin has remained the drug of choice, since no cases of penicillin-resistant syphilis have been identified. All types of penicillin are effective, but penicillin G benzathine (Bicillin L-A) is often preferred. Antimicrobial therapy will destroy *Treponema pallidum* at any stage, but any damage done to body organs is irreversible. If the client has a demonstrated allergy to penicillin, alternative medications may be administered, such as doxycycline (Vibramycin), tetracycline HCl (Achromycin V), or

CLIENT TEACHING

Testing for Syphilis
- Sexually active individuals with a suspicious rash or sore in the genital area should see a health care provider, and should avoid sexual contact.
- If treated for another STD, the client should also be tested for syphilis.

erythromycin estolate (Ilosone). For pregnant women who are allergic to penicillin, erythromycin is recommended as the best alternative therapy.

Clients being treated for syphilis must have periodic blood tests to ensure that the infecting agent has been completely destroyed.

GENITAL HERPES

Genital herpes affects an estimated 45 million persons in the United States with an estimated 500,000 new cases each year (NIAID and NIH, July 1998a). It is caused by the herpes simplex virus (HSV). There are two types of HSV. HSV type 1 commonly causes sores on the lips (fever blisters, cold sores). HSV type 2 causes genital sores. Either can infect the other area following oral-genital sex. Genital herpes is usually acquired through sexual contact with an infected person. That person may or may not be aware of having genital herpes. In fact, 80% of persons infected with genital herpes are unaware of their disease (NIAID and NIH, July 1998a).

When symptoms occur in the first episode, they usually appear in 2 to 10 days after infection and last an average of 2 to 3 weeks. Itching or burning sensations; pain in genital area, legs, or buttocks; vaginal discharge; or abdominal pressure are the early symptoms. Within a few days lesions (sores) appear at the infection site (perianal area), in the vagina or on the cervix of females, or in the urethra of females and males.

Small red bumps appear first, change into blisters (Figure 32-3), and then become open sores that crust over in a few days. Other symptoms with the first episode may include fever, muscle aches, headache, dysuria, vaginal discharge, and swollen glands in the groin.

With the first episode, the virus travels through the sensory nerves and remains inactive in nerve cells (Figure 32-4) until the virus travels back to the skin, causing a recurrence. Most people will have monthly recur-

Figure 32-3 Chronic Mucocutaneous Perianal Herpes Infection (*Courtesy of Centers for Disease Control and Prevention, Atlanta, GA 30333*)

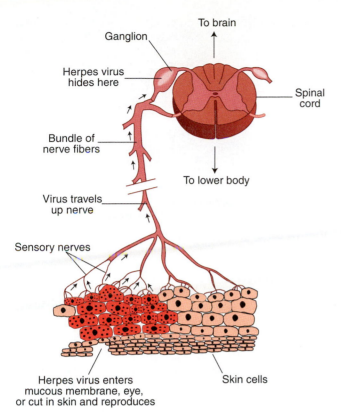

Figure 32-4 Herpes virus invades the nervous system from its portal of entry. (*Adapted from March of Dimes Birth Defects Foundation, White Plains, NY*)

rences (some only 1 or 2 a year), but new sores may or may not be apparent. Symptoms are usually milder than the first episode and last approximately 1 week.

The most accurate method of diagnosis is a viral culture, which takes several days. A blood test detecting HSV antibodies only indicates that the person has been infected at some time.

Medical–Surgical Management

Pharmacological

There is no known cure for the herpes simplex virus at this time. Treatment has been geared toward alleviating symptoms of the disease. Acyclovir (Zovirax) has been utilized in the treatment of herpes. A topical form may be applied to the lesions; the drug may also be taken orally to shorten the duration of the lesions in a primary outbreak. When taken daily, it prevents most recurrences. Famciclovir (Famivir) and valacyclovir (Valtrex) suppress viral activity and also prevent recurrences.

Cleansing the area of the lesions with mild soap and water, hydrogen peroxide, or Burow's solution often helps reduce the discomfort of the lesions and decrease the chance of secondary infections. The area should be blown dry with a hairdryer and then the dry skin may be dusted with a cornstarch powder, which aids in decreasing client discomfort.

CYTOMEGALOVIRUS

Another virus in the herpesvirus family is **cytomegalovirus** (CMV), which is found in saliva, urine, and often in semen and vaginal secretions. Figure 32-5 shows an electron micrograph of CMV. Unlike the more commonly recognized herpes viruses, CMV rarely produces noticeable clinical symptoms.

CMV is primarily transmitted from person to person through contact with body fluids like saliva, urine, and blood. The virus has been identified in semen and cervical mucus, so it can be spread by sexual contact. CMV is incurable. People are infected for life. The inactive virus may reactivate from time to time.

Most people acquire CMV during childhood or adolescence through contact with saliva and respiratory secretions, and by adulthood somewhere between 80% and 100% of adults will have developed antibodies to CMV. Most of these people will not notice any symptoms, but occasionally a client will present with fever, fatigue, and weakness. These symptoms may persist for several weeks and may lead to a tentative diagnosis of infectious mononucleosis, although the sore throat and swollen lymph nodes of "mono" are not present with CMV.

CMV has been implicated in some complications of pregnancy such as spontaneous abortion or mental retardation of the neonate. Congenital infection of an infant produces cytomegalic inclusion disease that ranges from an asymptomatic condition to a severely debilitating condition that may even result in death. The central nervous system damage to the infant may be profound, although it occurs rarely. An estimated 6,000 babies each year develop life-threatening complications of congenital CMV at birth or have mental retardation, blindness, or epilepsy (NIAID and NIH, June 1998c). CMV can also become a life-threatening illness in a client who has a poorly functioning immune system, such as a client with AIDS.

Figure 32-5 Electron Micrograph of CMV (*Courtesy of Centers for Disease Control and Prevention, Atlanta, GA 30333*)

There is no antiviral agent specifically utilized for this disorder, since most of the population will not have any symptoms.

GENITAL WARTS

Another virus that is sexually transmitted is the human papillomavirus (HPV), which causes genital warts, also called condylomata acuminata. These genital warts may occur in the urogenital, perineal, or anal areas, and may be either external or internal. The population at risk seems to be teenage girls or young women in their twenties. In the United States, it is estimated that there are approximately 1 million new cases of genital warts identified every year, and as many as 24 million already infected with HPV (NIAID and NIH, July 1998b). The incubation period for genital warts appears to be approximately 1 to 2 months, but may be up to 6 months. Unlike genital herpes, genital warts are usually painless, soft fleshy growths appearing most commonly in the genital area. Sometimes many warts may grow together to form a large cauliflower-shaped growth (Figure 32-6).

The greatest health threat that HPV poses to a female client is the predisposition to the development of cervical cancer. Although there are over 60 different types of HPV, only 6 of those have been associated with the development of cervical cancer. Cigarette smoking has been linked to the development of cancerous cervical changes in women with HPV. Women who have HPV should be advised not to smoke. HPV appears to play a role in the development of cervical cancer, along with many other factors. An abnormal Pap test may be the first indication of HPV.

Genital warts are less common in men. If seen, they are usually on the tip of the penis.

Medical–Surgical Management

Since genital warts are caused by a virus, there is no cure for the disease. The focus is on preventing the spread of the disease to sexual partners, and reducing the possibility of cancer. Use of a condom during sexual intercourse may provide some protection. Once the genital warts disappear, the disease may lie dormant for many years until there is a recurrence of the outbreak.

Surgical

The warts may be removed under local anesthesia. This is especially recommended if the warts have formed a large fleshy cauliflowerlike growth. Freezing the warts off with cryosurgery, or surgical use of extreme cold, is the treatment of choice for small warts. The warts may also be removed with laser surgery, or cauterized. Whatever treatment is recommended, it

Warts caused by
human papillomavirus (HPV)

Figure 32-6 Genital Warts (Condyloma acuminatum)

must be remembered that the treatment will not cure HPV, but only provide a palliative effect. The warts may recur after any treatment.

Pharmacological

A topical solution of podophyllum resin (Poddoen) may be applied to the genital warts. It is only recommended for treatment of 1 or 2 lesions at a time, since it can be toxic if applied to too large an area at one time. Most people report experiencing a good deal of pain from the treatment. After the solution has been in contact with the genital warts for a period of 4 to 6 hours, it is then washed off with soap and water. If not thoroughly washed off, podophyllum may cause chemical burns that heal very slowly and are very painful. This therapy must not be used on a diabetic client, a client with poor circulation, or a pregnant client.

A cream, imiquimod (Aldara), is applied before bedtime and washed off in the morning. It can be used 3 times a week for 16 weeks or less.

AIDS

AIDS, or acquired immunodeficiency syndrome, is not truly a sexually transmitted disease, but needs to be discussed briefly here since sexual contact remains one of the primary modes of transmission of this disease. AIDS is the end stage of the disease process caused by the human immunodeficiency virus (Chapter 23). Similar to the viruses previously discussed in this chapter, AIDS is not curable. Unlike the other viruses, herpes genitalis and genital warts, AIDS is ultimately fatal. AIDS results in a severe disorder of the body's immune system functioning, leading to an inability of the body to fight off disease. The client's failing immune system makes him vulnerable to opportunistic infections, such as *Pneumocystis carinii* pneumonia.

Persons at risk are those who have multiple sexual partners, IV drug users who share needles, and persons with hemophilia. There are three basic modes of transmission—sexual, bloodborne, and from mother to baby either prenatally, during the birth process, or when breast-feeding. When first identified in 1981, HIV infection was primarily found among homosexual men, but by 1990 the disease was moving into heterosexual populations with great rapidity. By the mid-1990s, cases of AIDS were occurring more frequently among women than among men. The greatest growth in AIDS rates among women occurred in African American and Hispanic women. Teenagers also have one of the fastest growing rates of HIV infection.

TRICHOMONIASIS

Trichomoniasis is caused by a parasitic protozoan called *Trichomonas vaginalis*. Trichomoniasis is a very common STD, with an incidence of approximately 3 million new cases every year (NIAID and NIH, June 1998d). It is seen frequently in combination with gonorrhea. The most common method of transmission is sexual, although the protozoa can survive for a period of time in water so other modes of transmission are possible.

The incubation period after initial exposure to trichomoniasis ranges from approximately 4 to 20 days. About 25% of women infected with trichomoniasis will have no symptoms, and men almost never have symptoms. In these clients, the *Trichomonas* organisms may remain dormant for years, without becoming an active infection. Precipitating factors that may encourage the growth of *Trichomonas* include pregnancy, sexual intercourse, menstruation, or illness. Vulval and vaginal pruritus is the most common symptom, with a vaginal discharge of a frothy, copious yellow-green mucus. Only 10% of women will present with the classic symptoms of a *Trichomonas* infection: severe itching of the vulva, redness, swelling of the vulva, pain on intercourse and urination, urinary frequency, and a grayish, malodorous discharge. Males most often have a watery, whitish discharge and difficult or painful urination, but may also have urethritis and an accompanying inflammation. In men, *Trichomonas* in the dormant state are usually harbored in the prostate or urethra.

Medical–Surgical Management

Pharmacological

Both partners should be treated with metronidazole (Flagyl) either given orally in a single dose or for a period of approximately 1 week. Metronidazole is effective against both protozoal and bacterial infections. If given vaginally, metronidazole (Flagyl) is not as effective. Pregnant women are usually treated after the first trimester to avoid the possibility of birth defects, since metronidazole is known to cross the placenta.

Adverse effects occur in about 10% of clients taking metronidazole (Flagyl) and usually affect the gastro-

CLIENT TEACHING

Metronidazole (Flagyl)

No alcohol should be consumed as it causes severe nausea and vomiting, flushing, palpitations, abdominal cramps, and headache.

intestinal system in the form of nausea, vomiting, diarrhea, and abdominal cramping. CNS effects, such as headache or dizziness, may also be seen.

HEPATITIS B

Hepatitis B, caused by the hepatitis B virus, is now recognized as an STD. Today it is primarily transmitted through sexual contact, as opposed to the oral-fecal or blood contact routes that were far more prevalent 20 years ago (Sharts-Hopko, 1997). An estimated 77,000 cases of sexually transmitted hepatitis B occur each year in the United States (NIAID and NIH, December 1998).

Clients with hepatitis B experience anorexia, vague abdominal discomfort, nausea, vomiting, fatigue, and jaundice. Fever may be mild or absent. Symptoms may progress to chronic liver disease, hepatic cancer, hepatic failure, and death.

Medical–Surgical Management

Medical

There is no specific therapy. Treatment is based on relieving symptoms.

Health Promotion

Hepatitis B is the only STD for which a vaccine is available. It is recommended that all newborn infants, 11- to 12-year-old children, and high-risk groups of all ages receive the vaccine (CDC, July 1999a).

▶ NURSING PROCESS

The following is a general nursing process for the client with an STD.

▶ Assessment

▶ Subjective Data

Data to be gathered from a client who presents with a suspected STD are very similar, regardless of the actual STD. Either the nurse or physician must take a thorough history. A relaxed, nonjudgmental attitude will help to elicit accurate information from the client, since pertinent questioning will deal with very private areas of the client's life. Confidentiality and privacy are extremely important when dealing with both the history and physical examination for STDs. Pertinent information must be gathered regarding the client's sexual orientation (homosexual, heterosexual, bisexual), any prior treatment for an STD, and the number of sexual partners that the client has had in the last 6 months.

Women will be asked about symptoms such as vulval or vaginal itching, vaginal discharge, pain or discomfort, skin rashes or pruritus, and any changes in the menstrual periods or other abnormal bleeding. Men will be questioned regarding the presence of symptoms such as pain or burning on urination, abnormal penile discharges, skin rashes or itching, or lesions on external genitalia. Both men and women will be questioned regarding urinary frequency or discomfort and systemic symptoms such as fatigue, malaise,

or sore throat. Homosexual men need to be questioned regarding rectal symptoms such as abnormal discharge, itching, lesions, or pain on defecation.

▶ Objective Data

The systems that need to be carefully evaluated include the reproductive, gastrointestinal, and integumentary systems. The presence or absence of skin rashes or lesions and abnormal discharges must be determined. Females need a speculum examination of the vagina and cervix to closely observe internal organs for changes consistent with STDs. The rectal area is examined to look for any abnormal discharge, lesions, or tenderness. Inguinal lymph nodes should be palpated to look for signs of infection.

Nursing diagnoses for the client with an STD may include the following:

Nursing Diagnoses	Planning/Goals	Nursing Interventions
▶ *Anxiety related to unknown procedures, embarrassment, or other factors (relates to nearly every client who presents with an STD)*	The client will admit lack of knowledge and embarrassment.	Provide a relaxed, nonjudgmental attitude which will aid in reducing client anxiety. The nurse must examine own attitudes toward STDs and the clients who suffer from them. Listen actively to both the spoken and unspoken concerns of the client.
▶ *Deficient Knowledge related to mode of transmission of the STD, prevention methods, and risk for spread of the STD*	The client will accurately discuss the mode of transmission of an STD and list appropriate measures to avoid reinfection or future infection.	Teach mode of transmission, prevention of further infection, and risk for spread. Take time to make sure the client has a thorough understanding of all necessary aspects of the disease.
▶ *Risk for Infection related to incomplete treatment or lack of precautions with untreated, infected partners*	The client will state the need for having all sexual partners notified and treated. The client will state understanding of the treatment regimen and of the importance of completing treatment. The client will explain appropriate use of latex condoms, including how and when to apply and remove the device.	Discuss the need for all sexual partners to be notified and treated. Discuss the importance of completing treatment regimen. Teach the importance of abstaining from sexual intercourse until the infection is resolved, or of using appropriate measures, such as latex condoms, to prevent reinfection.

Evaluation Each goal must be evaluated to determine how it has been met by the client.

SAMPLE NURSING CARE PLAN

THE CLIENT WITH GENITAL HERPES

Julie Blackwell is a single woman in her middle twenties who has been coming to the clinic for annual Pap smears and birth control for several years. She is a well-nourished, healthy-appearing young woman of medium height. She rescheduled her annual Pap smear to come into the clinic early because she noticed a

continues

cluster of small blisters on the inside of her left thigh that also involves the labia majora. She also reports that she has just gotten the flu as evidenced by headache, fever, and general achiness.

Ms. Blackwell has used birth control pills in the past, and reports satisfaction with this method of birth control. She reports that she and her new boyfriend became intimate about 2 weeks ago, so she wants to renew her birth control pill prescription. She also states that intercourse has been uncomfortable since the appearance of the lesions and that she does not feel comfortable with sexual activity while the lesions are present, since they make her feel "ugly."

The assessment determines the presence of a cluster of small blisters as well as swollen, tender inguinal lymph nodes. A Tzanck smear test is obtained.

Nursing Diagnosis 1 *Ineffective Sexuality Patterns related to lesions as evidenced by her comment that intercourse has been uncomfortable since the appearance of the lesions.*

PLANNING/GOALS	NURSING INTERVENTIONS	RATIONALE	EVALUATION
Ms. Blackwell will express her feelings about potential changes in her sexual behavior before leaving the clinic.	Provide a nonjudgmental atmosphere to encourage Ms. Blackwell to express her feelings about this perceived change in her sexual identity.	This demonstrates the caregiver's positive feelings toward Ms. Blackwell, and any concerns she may have regarding her future sexuality.	Ms. Blackwell states that she is still in shock, but thinks that she will be able to deal with her diagnosis. She also states that she will call back to the clinic in a few days with more questions after she has assimilated some of the information.
	Provide privacy and an uninterrupted amount of time to talk with Ms. Blackwell.	This demonstrates respect for Ms. Blackwell, and conveys reassurance that the caregiver will be comfortable discussing sexuality issues and concerns with her.	
	Provide accurate information to Ms. Blackwell about genital herpes, and include literature or videos that she can share with her boyfriend later.	This helps Ms. Blackwell focus on specific, necessary information and encourages her to ask questions.	
	Offer the names of local support groups such as HELP (Herpetics Engaged in Living Productively) or other support persons who will be able to provide information and group support to Ms. Blackwell.	This provides Ms. Blackwell with resources for support once she has returned home and the reality of her diagnosis has set in.	

continues

Nursing Diagnosis 2 *Anxiety related to threatened sexual identity as evidenced by her comment that she is not comfortable with sexual activity while the lesions are present since they make her feel "ugly."*

PLANNING/GOALS	NURSING INTERVENTIONS	RATIONALE	EVALUATION
Ms. Blackwell will be able to express feelings of anxiety and identify support systems to help her cope with these feelings before leaving the clinic.	Explain any procedures clearly and concisely before performing them.	This will help alleviate anxiety.	Ms. Blackwell expresses feelings of anxiety about the diagnosis of herpes. She states that she has a cousin with herpes whom she will use as a resource person. She states that she has a secure relationship with her boyfriend and will talk to him about herpes also. She states that she will continue to call the clinic for any further support or information that she may need.
	Listen attentively to any concerns or expressions of anxiety that Ms. Blackwell may offer.	This will identify any anxious behaviors that she may be exhibiting and the source of her anxiety.	
	Include Ms. Blackwell in as many decisions related to her care and follow-up as is possible.	Involving Ms. Blackwell in decision making regarding her care may reduce her feelings of anxiety and make her feel like she has regained some control.	

Nursing Diagnosis 3 *Risk for Infection related to break in skin integrity as evidenced by the presence of blisters.*

PLANNING/GOALS	NURSING INTERVENTIONS	RATIONALE	EVALUATION
Ms. Blackwell's herpes blisters will heal without secondary infection within 10 days.	Wear gloves when examining perineal area and when handling exudate from herpes lesions.	Gloves prevent secondary infection in herpes blisters from caregiver's hands and offer protection to the caregiver when dealing with wound exudate as part of a standard precautions policy.	Ms. Blackwell has been taught to keep blisters clean and dry and states that she will contact the clinic if the lesions develop any signs of a secondary infection. She makes an appointment to return to the clinic in 10 days for a follow-up evaluation.
	Teach Ms. Blackwell how to wash hands very thoroughly after using the toilet or handling the area around the herpes lesions.	Handwashing prevents the spread of herpes infection in the genital area to other areas of Ms. Blackwell's body or to another person.	
	Instruct Ms. Blackwell in the importance of keeping the herpes lesions clean and dry until they heal.	Keeping the herpes lesions clean and dry until they heal will help prevent the occurrence of a secondary infection that may delay healing for up to 6 weeks.	

continues

Instruct Ms. Blackwell to wear cotton underwear and loose-fitting clothing during occasions of herpes outbreaks.	These measures will provide for air circulation to promote healing and reduce further local irritation.

CASE STUDY

Noelle Landers, a 17-year-old student, has come to your clinic seeking treatment. Noelle is complaining of pain and burning on urination, as well as pain during intercourse. She states that she is infrequently sexually active with her 17-year-old boyfriend, and is also seeking a form of birth control. She has not used any form of birth control in the past and neither has her boyfriend. She also complains of a yellowish vaginal discharge, and has been wearing a panty liner to deal with this. Upon examination, Noelle complains of some abdominal tenderness, but denies that she has had any tenderness prior to this time. Noelle is screened for chlamydia and gonorrhea. She denies having had sex with any other partners, but does admit that she and her boyfriend had a fight and broke up temporarily about a month ago. They went back together about a week later. She does not know if he had any other sexual contacts during their period of separation. Noelle is concerned that she has contracted an STD, and states, "I'll die of embarrassment!"

The following questions will guide your development of a nursing care plan for the case study.

1. What other information should be elicited from Noelle?

2. What other sexually transmitted diseases will Noelle most likely be tested for in addition to chlamydia and gonorrhea?

3. Write 3 nursing diagnoses and goals for Noelle.

4. List the medications that Noelle will be most likely to receive to treat a chlamydial infection.

5. List some complications that Noelle may experience if she does not receive treatment for an active chlamydial or gonorrheal infection.

6. What information will you include when you counsel Noelle regarding sexual activity and forms of birth control? (See Chapter 30, Nursing Care of the Client: Female Reproductive System, for additional information.)

SUMMARY

- Sexually transmitted diseases are among the most common infections occurring in the United States today.
- Despite massive education efforts, the number of new STD cases identified each year continues to grow.
- Early, intensive education regarding STDs is being utilized to help combat the high incidence of STDs,

virtually an epidemic among young, urban dwelling populations.

- Many STDs, such as gonorrhea, syphilis, and chlamydia, are treatable with antibiotics, but many others are caused by viruses and are not curable.
- Identification of groups at risk for STDs and appropriate prevention teaching are the most effective weapons in the ongoing battle against STDs.

Review Questions

1. The two most effective medications commonly used to treat chlamydia are:

   a. doxycycline and azithromycin.
   b. penicillin and podophyllum.
   c. erythromycin and acyclovir.
   d. doxycycline and penicillin.

2. If a female client with chlamydia fails to complete treatment, complications that may arise in the future include:

   a. fever and headache.
   b. nausea, vomiting, and diarrhea.
   c. infertility and ectopic pregnancy.
   d. urinary retention.

3. When instructing a client with gonorrhea regarding medication, the nurse will be sure to tell the client:

   a. to take the medication until it is gone.
   b. to take the medication until symptoms subside.
   c. to take the medication at bedtime.
   d. to avoid sunlight while taking the medication.

4. When obtaining a health history from a client, the nurse asks the client to report on the presence of which of the following common symptoms of syphilis?

   a. Nausea and vomiting
   b. Fever, cellulitis, and diarrhea
   c. Dysuria and mucopurulent discharge
   d. Painless sore or ulcer in the genital area

Critical Thinking Questions

1. Develop a teaching plan for a client with multiple sexual partners. Consider the sensitivity of the information to be shared and the client's receptivity.

2. What is the rationale for each nursing intervention given for the nursing diagnoses in this chapter?

 WEB FLASH!

- Search the Internet for information about sexually transmitted diseases. What type of information is available? For whom is it intended?
- What information do you find about syphilis and gonorrhea specifically? How can a client become part of a clinical trial?

Physical and Mental Integrity

NURSING CARE OF THE CLIENT: MENTAL ILLNESS

MAKING THE CONNECTION

Refer to the following chapters to increase your understanding of mental illness:

- **Chapter 5, Communication**
- **Chapter 7, Wellness Concepts**
- **Chapter 22, Nursing Care of the Client: Immune System**
- **Chapter 34, Nursing Care of the Client: Substance Abuse**
- **Chapter 35, Nursing Care of the Older Client**

LEARNING OBJECTIVES

Upon completion of this chapter, you should be able to:
- *Define key terms.*
- *Identify and describe the components of a therapeutic nurse–client relationship.*
- *Cite nursing interventions for working with clients who are angry, aggressive, homicidal, and/or suicidal.*
- *Detail nursing interventions for working with clients who are experiencing anxiety.*
- *Identify and explain the potential side effects associated with anti-anxiety medications.*
- *Recount nursing interventions for working with clients who are depressed.*
- *Identify and explain the potential side effects associated with antidepressant medications.*
- *Detail nursing interventions for working with clients who have schizophrenia.*
- *Identify and explain the potential side effects associated with antipsychotic medications.*
- *Detail nursing interventions for working with clients who have bipolar disorder.*
- *Identify and explain the potential side effects associated with mood stabilizers.*
- *Cite nursing interventions for working with clients who have attention-deficit/hyperactivity disorder.*
- *Recount nursing interventions for working with clients who have been neglected or abused or who have been exposed to domestic violence.*

KEY TERMS

abuse
actively suicidal
affect
anger-control assistance
anorexia nervosa
anxiety
anxiolytic
auditory hallucination
brief dynamic therapy
bulimia nervosa
cognitive behavior
  therapy
command hallucination
confidentiality
crisis
cycling
delusion
depression
domestic violence
electroconvulsive
  therapy
empathy
euphoric
flashback
genuineness
hallucination
hypersomnia
hypervigilant

hypomania
insomnia
lethargy
libido
mania
mental disorder
mental illness
mood
neglect
paradoxical reaction
physically aggressive
pressured speech
psychoanalysis
psychosis
psychotherapy
rapport
respect
seclusion
serum lithium level
startle response
suicidal ideation
suicide
tolerance
toxic
trust
verbally aggressive
visual hallucination
word salad

INTRODUCTION

Because they will encounter clients who are emotionally disturbed and/or mentally ill, it is imperative that nurses understand and feel comfortable working with such individuals—not just on psychiatric units, but in all types of circumstances and settings. This chapter is designed to give licensed practical/vocational nurses (LP/VNs) a beginning knowledge base regarding mental health and illness and to better prepare them for working with individuals who are in a state of crisis or who have emotional needs and/or psychiatric problems.

As the nurse becomes more knowledgeable about mental illness, opportunities arise to increase self-awareness and to examine any personal experiences, preconceived ideas, or prejudices that might negatively affect the nurse's ability to work effectively with clients. For example, the nurse who has some unresolved issues regarding sexuality or becomes embarrassed when discussing sexuality will probably be uncomfortable talking about the potential problems in sexual functioning secondary to antidepressant therapy (McEnany, 1998). Examining personal ideas and prejudices prior to working with clients will facilitate a positive nurse–client relationship.

MENTAL HEALTH AND ILLNESS

In general, a person is considered mentally healthy when he possesses knowledge of himself; meets his basic needs; assumes responsibility for his behavior; has learned to integrate thoughts, feelings, and actions; can successfully resolve conflicts; maintains relationships; communicates directly with others; respects others; and adapts to change. **Mental illness** occurs when an individual is not able to view self clearly or has a distorted view of self; is unable to maintain satisfying personal relationships; and is unable to adapt to the environment (Frisch & Frisch, 1998). The American Psychiatric Association defines **mental disorder** as "clinically significant behavior or psychological syndrome or pattern that occurs in an individual and is associated with present distress (i.e., negative response to stimuli that are perceived as threatening) or disability (i.e., impairment in one or more important areas of functioning) or with a significantly increased risk of suffering, death, pain, disability, or an important loss of freedom."

One of the ways to conceptualize psychiatric disorders is to think of a continuum, with mental health being situated at one end and mental illness at the other (Figure 33-1). Between these two extremes lie a variety of psychiatric disorders ranging in nature from mild to severe. The fourth edition of the *Diagnostic and Statistical Manual of Mental Disorders* (better

Figure 33-1 Mental Health Continuum

known as the *DSM-IV*) (American Psychiatric Association [APA], 1994) is the reference tool used to identify and establish psychiatric diagnoses. The psychiatrist is the individual most often involved in this process, although other mental health care practitioners may give input and make recommendations for diagnoses.

One of the primary roles of the nurse in working with clients who have mental illness is that of teaching. The nurse is responsible not only for teaching clients about their illnesses, including the probable courses of their given disorders, but also for adequately preparing and educating the client's family. The nurse is usually the first individual to have contact with the family and is most often the one with whom family members maintain consistent contact.

RELATIONSHIP DEVELOPMENT

Psychiatric nursing differs from some of the other fields of nursing in that the primary skill that the nurse employs is what is referred to as "the therapeutic use of self" (Sundeen, Stuart, Rankin, & Cohen, 1998). Many theorists such as Rogers and Peplau have been instrumental in identifying and exploring the factors that significantly influence the development of therapeutic relationships. Townsend (2000) identifies five components necessary to the development of a therapeutic working relationship and of particular importance in the therapeutic nurse–client relationship. These five components are trust, rapport, respect, genuineness, and empathy.

Trust

Trust is the ability to rely on an individual's character and ability. Trust must be present for help to be

PROFESSIONAL TIP

Confidentiality

Because of the highly personal and sensitive nature of mental disorders, the concept of **confidentiality**, which is the nondisclosure of the identity of or personal information about an individual, is vitally important in psychiatric nursing.

Table 33–1 ESSENTIAL FACTORS OF TRUST		
CONSISTENCY	**RESPECT**	**HONESTY**
Follow through on plans	Call client by name	Ask client about personal preferences
Adhere to schedule	Provide clear explanations	Keep any promises
Seek out client for extra time to interact	Recognize own strengths and limitations	Maintain confidentiality
Be straightforward/ no hidden motives	Listen to client	Be flexible in responding to requests

From Fundamentals of Nursing: Standards & Practice, *by S. DeLaune and P. Ladner, 1998, Albany, NY: Delmar. Copyright 1998 by Delmar.*

Figure 33-2 Spending time with the client one-on-one helps to promote a trusting relationship.

given and received. A therapeutic relationship is firmly rooted in trust. How does the nurse promote a trusting relationship? Three major activities facilitate the development of trust: consistency, respect, and honesty. Table 33–1 lists actions that facilitate the development of trust. Being consistently trustworthy is an expression of the nurse's personal integrity and builds the foundation for nursing effectiveness (Figure 33-2).

Many clients with emotional and/or psychiatric problems have great difficulty trusting and having confidence that others will be good to their word. They may have been lied to or hurt in the past, and this makes it difficult for them to trust again, even with health care professionals who are trying to help them. It is very important, therefore, that the nurse fulfill any promise made to the client.

Rapport

Rapport is a bond or connection between two people that is based on mutual trust. Such a bond does not just happen spontaneously; it is planned by the nurse who purposefully implements behaviors that promote trust. The nurse sets the tone of the relationship by creating an atmosphere wherein the client feels free to express feelings. When seeking to develop trust, the nurse acts in a manner that indicates recognition of the client as a unique individual and reinforces that individuality. Such actions, which serve to humanize the client, are therapeutic. To establish rapport, the nurse must show that the client is considered important. Actions are implemented to boost the level of the client's self-esteem. Nonverbal interventions are of utmost importance in helping establish rapport. Interacting with family and significant others is also helpful in establishing rapport with the client. Recognizing the importance of the family and its influence on the healing process allows the nurse to bond with those who will encourage and support the client during recovery.

Respect

Respect is the acceptance of an individual as is and in a nonjudgmental manner. The concept of respect is an integral component of the nurse–client relationship. Respect means caring for clients whose value system may differ greatly from that of the nurse (Figure 33-3). To show respect, the nurse must not react with shock, surprise, or disapproval toward a client's lifestyle, dress, or behaviors. The nurse must respect the client's choices and actions while setting limits on unhealthy or undesirable behavior.

Genuineness

Genuineness (sincerity) is an attribute easily perceived by the client and can be the most significant aspect of the nurse–client relationship. Nurses are often

Figure 33-3 The nurse must show acceptance of the client, even if the client has values and beliefs that differ from her own.

concerned about whether they will say the right thing to a client; though saying the right thing is important, more important is that the nurse be honest and genuine in communications with the client.

Empathy

Empathy (the ability to perceive and relate to another's personal experience) is an important quality necessary to successful nurse–client interactions. The empathic nurse understands that the client's perception of the situation is real to him. By perceiving the client's understanding of his own needs, the nurse is better able to assist the client in determining what will work best. Empathy enables the nurse to assist the client to become a fully participating partner in treatment, rather than a passive recipient of care. Through empathy, the nurse validates the experiences of the client (Figure 33-4).

Figure 33-4 Through empathetic listening, the nurse can reach an understanding of the client's experience and help the client see the positive aspects of the experience.

THE CLIENT EXPERIENCING A CRISIS

In psychological terms, a **crisis** is a stressor that forces an individual to respond and/or adapt in some way. Emotions may intensify during a crisis situation or serious illness, and any situation or illness can potentially become a crisis if the stressors are severe enough. The understanding of crisis is particularly important in psychiatric and mental health nursing. A crisis taxes the individual's coping resources, and each person responds differently to seemingly identical situations. Crisis requires that an individual call on all of her personal skills as well as on the outside social and familial supports that she has built through her life (Frisch & Frisch, 1998). Each individual has personality strengths, interpersonal networks, and socioeconomic resources that offer some protection against the threat of crisis. When any (or all) of these protections are weak, however, a person's response to crisis may be dysfunctional, and the result may be one or more symptoms of mental illness. While theories differ in their definitions of crisis and stress, it is generally accepted that most psychiatric problems result from or are strongly influenced by the interaction of stress and overwhelmed coping mechanisms (Frisch & Frisch, 1998). The client experiencing crisis may be anxious, angry, aggressive, homicidal, suicidal, psychotic, or any combination of these.

THE CLIENT WHO IS ANXIOUS

Anxiety is a state wherein a person feels a strong sense of dread frequently accompanied by physical symptoms of increased heart and respiratory rates and elevated blood pressure in the absence of a specific source or reason for these emotions or responses. Nurses frequently encounter clients and family members who are anxious due to alterations in or threats to health and physical well-being. Peplau (1963) identifies four escalating stages of anxiety beginning with mild anxiety, moving to moderate anxiety, followed by severe anxiety, and, finally, to the stage of panic anxiety, if not effectively treated. Intervention can occur at any point along the continuum, preferably before the stages of severe or panic level anxiety are reached. Some of the most common psychiatric diagnoses related to anxiety are Generalized Anxiety Disorder, Panic Disorder, and post-traumatic Stress Disorder.

MILD ANXIETY

The mildly anxious client is beginning to experience some of the signs and symptoms of anxiety, such as irritability and restlessness; at this phase, however, the person is still able to concentrate and focus on the task at hand. In fact, *mild* anxiety can actually benefit an individual as far as enhancing performance ability (Townsend, 2000).

MODERATE ANXIETY

The individual with moderate anxiety experiences additional physiologic and cognitive symptoms. Blood pressure, pulse, and respirations increase, and the client becomes diaphoretic. The moderately anxious individual begins to have difficulty concentrating or learning new material. This is important to recognize before teaching a client about a medication or test, or performing a procedure. Before teaching can be effective, the client must be assisted in lowering the level of anxiety (Townsend, 2000).

SEVERE ANXIETY

Severely anxious clients are significantly impaired in a number of areas. Their ability to cognitively process material may drastically diminish, they may experience tunnel vision, their focus may become very limited, and the physiologic symptoms of anxiety become much more pronounced. Clients at this high level of anxiety are often very fearful and may be irrational in their thought processes (Townsend, 2000).

PANIC ANXIETY

The individual experiencing panic anxiety may begin to manifest symptoms of **psychosis** (losing touch with reality), such as **delusions** (false beliefs that misrepresent reality) and/or **hallucinations** (perceptions that something is present when it is not, e.g., hearing voices that are not really there). The individual with this level of anxiety requires constant reassurance, monitoring, and supervision to maintain safety (Townsend, 2000).

THE CLIENT WITH GENERALIZED ANXIETY DISORDER

The client with generalized anxiety disorder (GAD) exhibits symptoms of excessive anxiety or dread. Clients usually realize that their symptoms are out of proportion to any real threat. The symptoms include three or more of the following: restlessness, easy fatigue, difficulty concentrating, irritability, muscle tension, and sleep disturbance. For anxiety to be termed excessive, clients must experience symptoms frequently over a period of 6 months or more.

THE CLIENT WITH PANIC DISORDER

Panic disorder is a condition wherein the client experiences periods of intense anxiety that begin abruptly and peak within 10 minutes. These episodes are characterized by a set of any four of the following symptoms: palpitations or rapid heart rate, sweating, trembling, shortness of breath, sensation of choking, chest pain, nausea, dizziness, fear of losing control, fear of dying, numbness or tingling, chills or hot flushes, and some sense of altered reality. The client has a strong desire to run away or escape from the situation that triggered the attack. In some individuals,

the attack is brought about by specific stimuli or a particular setting, for example the dentist's office. In others, the attacks come on "out of the blue."

THE CLIENT WITH POST-TRAUMATIC STRESS DISORDER

Clients suffering from post-traumatic stress disorder (PTSD) have experienced a serious trauma. The client who has been severely beaten or emotionally, physically, or sexually abused or who has lived through or witnessed a catastrophic event or natural disaster such as a flood, earthquake, hurricane, or plane crash might be suffering from PTSD. "The traumas that cause the disorder range from a single loss of control over one's life ([such as] during a tornado, rape, mugging, or car accident) to repeated traumatization over time ([such as] in combat, abusive relationships, being held hostage, or [being] in a physically or psychologically unsafe work environment)" (Clark, 1997). The response to the trauma must have been one of fear or helplessness, and the event is persistently re-experienced through recurrent recollections, dreams, or hallucinatory-like flashbacks. Individuals with this disorder exhibit impairment of social functioning, the presence of specific anxiety symptoms, and "persistent avoidance of stimuli associated with the trauma, and numbing of general responsiveness" (American Psychiatric Association, 2000).

Medical–Surgical Management

Medical

Psychotherapy (the treatment of mental and emotional disorders through psychological rather than physical methods) continues to be widely used in the treatment of anxiety disorders. Psychotherapy can be viewed as falling into two general categories: those therapies based on helping individuals achieve insight into *why* they feel anxiety and those that emphasize behavioral means of controlling the anxiety.

Psychotherapy based on insight into symptoms may sometimes be valuable, especially for highly motivated individuals whose symptoms are not disabling. **Psychoanalysis** (therapy focused on uncovering unconscious memories and processes) is among the best known of the insight therapies and has been widely employed to assist persons with anxiety.

In contrast, there is strong empirical evidence that behaviorally based treatments are effective in treating at least some anxiety disorders. Cognitive-behavior therapy often results in significant benefit for persons suffering from panic attacks. **Cognitive-behavior therapy** assumes that clients can learn to identify the common stimuli that give rise to their anxiety, develop plans to respond to those stimuli with nonanxious responses, and problem solve when unanticipated anxiety-provoking situations arise. While insight is very much involved in this process, it is not insight into deep psychological causes, as in psychoanalysis, but, rather, practical, commonsense problem solving. Treatment appears both to be effective during the relatively brief course of therapy and to remain effective for some months after therapy finishes. Sometimes medical and psychological follow-up are important to ensure satisfactory improvement.

Pharmacological

The drugs of choice for treating clients with anxiety are usually the **anxiolytics**, or antianxiety agents (Table 33–2). Some of the antianxiety medications such as alprazolam (Xanax) and lorazepam (Ativan) may also be helpful in alleviating the symptoms of anxiety, nervousness, and sleeplessness frequently associated with panic disorder and PTSD.

Most of these medications can be used on either a routine or as needed (PRN) basis, and the majority of these medications belong to the family of benzodiazepines. Onset of action for the benzodiazepines usually occurs within 30 minutes after oral administration, and most individuals respond favorably to these medications, that is, a reduction or cessation of the symptoms of anxiety is experienced.

Clients should be warned about the potential risk of addiction associated with the antianxiety medications. These particular medications should be used with extreme caution, as long-term use can lead to an increased **tolerance**, or acquired resistance to the effects of the drug. Tolerance results in the need to increase the frequency and amount of medication in order to achieve the same benefit. Over time, this may cause a dependency on the medication, actually creat-

CLIENT TEACHING

Antianxiety Medications

Be sure to instruct each client taking an antianxiety medication in the following:

- Do not increase the dose or frequency of the medication without consulting your physician.
- Tolerance develops quickly with the medication and unsupervised use can lead to addiction.
- Do not drink alcohol while on the medication.
- Do not take any other medications unless prescribed by your physician.
- Do not stop taking the medication abruptly.
- Do not drive or operate heavy machinery while on the medication.

ing another serious problem for the client. Therefore, the antianxiety agents are usually indicated for short-term management of anxiety rather than for long-term use. The benefits of a particular medication for the client must always be weighed against the possible risk of addiction, particularly if long-term use is or may be indicated. The one exception is buspirone hydrochloride (BuSpar), a nonbenzodiazepine antianxiety medication, which does not appear to have any addictive potential. However, the therapeutic effectiveness of BuSpar is not reached for approximately 7 to 10 days; thus, although it can be given as a regularly scheduled antianxiety agent, BuSpar has absolutely no value as a PRN medication. When initiating therapy with BuSpar, another antianxiety medication such as alprazolam (Xanax) or lorazepam (Ativan) may be given concurrently until the therapeutic level is reached; the other medication can then be gradually decreased.

Table 33–2 ANTIANXIETY MEDICATIONS

GENERIC NAME	TRADE NAME	TYPE	POTENTIAL SIDE EFFECTS
alprazolam	Xanax	Benzodiazepine	Dizziness, drowsiness, lethargy, physical and psychological dependence, tolerance
buspirone hydrochloride	BuSpar	Nonbenzodiazepine	Blurred vision, chest pain, clamminess, dizziness, drowsiness, excitement, fatigue, headache, insomnia, nasal congestion, numbness, myalgia, nausea, nervousness, palpitations, paresthesia, skin rashes, sore throat, syncope, tachycardia, tinnitus, incoordination, weakness
clonazepam	Klonopin	Benzodiazepine	Ataxia, behavioral changes, drowsiness, physical and psychological dependence, tolerance
diazepam	Valium	Benzodiazepine	Dizziness, drowsiness, fatigue, hypotension, hypertension, CV collapse, dependence, tolerance
lorazepam	Ativan	Benzodiazepine	Agranulocytosis, CV collapse, dizziness, drowsiness, lethargy

Data from PDR Nurses Handbook, *by G. Spratto and A. Woods, 2001, Albany, NY: Delmar.*

PROFESSIONAL TIP

Achieving a State of Relaxation

Clients who are anxious and feeling overwhelmed will often require assistance in achieving a state of relaxation. Nurses can help the client identify a number of activities that are relaxing, such as listening to favorite music, watching television, reading a book, playing a game, drawing a picture, working a puzzle, or whatever is calming to the client. Nurses can also teach the client a variety of stress-management techniques such as deep-breathing exercises, progressive deep-muscle relaxation, and guided imagery (Figure 33-5). All of these will assist the client in reaching a greater state of relaxation. Wilkinson (1996) states that becoming more centered or balanced is done by an "acquired ability to focus and channel emotional energy in a healthy and deliberate manner." The nurse can explore with the client the possibility of enrolling in a martial arts course such as Tai Chi, TaeKwondo, Karate, or Kung Fu as a means of stress reduction (Wilkinson, 1996). In addition to providing physical activity, the martial arts assist in achieving a state of balance and increasing one's ability to focus.

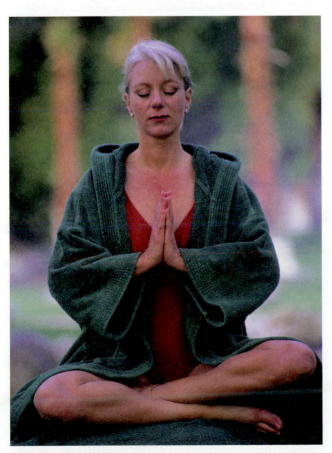

Figure 33-5 Clients may find relief from anxiety through meditation. *(Courtesy of Photo Disc)*

Activity

The anxious client's activity level may be negatively affected by both the anxiety disorder itself and the side effects of the prescribed medication. The side effects of sedation and drowsiness can pose safety hazards for certain activities and must be emphasized to the client.

▶ NURSING PROCESS

▶ Assessment

▶ Subjective Data

Clients experiencing anxiety report problems concentrating, and fear that something dreadful is about to happen. They may verbalize an overwhelming feeling of impending doom. They may also report that the anxiety is very frightening to them and that they are afraid of losing control. Table 33–3 lists questions that may help in identifying a client's anxiety.

Clients with PTSD "may complain of unwanted memories of an event, express suicidal ideation, or express

Table 33–3 ASKING CLIENTS ABOUT SYMPTOMS OF ANXIETY DISORDERS	
Following are questions that have proven useful in eliciting information from clients about symptoms of anxiety disorders. You may find that you prefer to word these questions somewhat differently, but the important thing is to ask them. Many clients experience anxiety symptoms for years before a doctor, nurse, or psychologist takes the time to ask about these symptoms.	
Generalized anxiety disorder	Do you find yourself worrying frequently about a number of different things, such as the way things are going for you at home, work, or school?
	Do you find yourself feeling anxious or tense much of the time without any obvious reason?
Panic disorder	Have you ever experienced sudden, intense fear for no reason?
	Have you found yourself experiencing intense physical symptoms of chest pain, shortness of breath, dizziness, or sweating, along with a sense that something terrible or life threatening was happening to you?
Post-traumatic stress disorder	Have you ever had a particularly traumatic experience such as witnessing or experiencing violence or a catastrophic event (such as a flood or fire)?
	Have you ever found yourself re-experiencing a violent or catastrophic event through dreams or waking "flashbacks"?

From Psychiatric Mental Health Nursing, *by N. Frisch and L. Frisch, 1998, Albany, NY: Delmar. Copyright 1998 by Delmar.*

fantasies of retaliation toward the identified source of trauma" (Clark, 1997). The client with PTSD may describe feeling extremely fearful and "on guard" at all times and may report having **flashbacks** (reliving of the original trauma as if currently experiencing it) along with recurrent dreams and/or nightmares.

▶ Objective Data

The anxious client may manifest changes in vital signs, such as an increase in blood pressure, pulse, and respirations. In addition, restlessness, irritability, pacing, and agitation may become more pronounced as anxiety level increases.

Clients with PTSD may exhibit an exaggerated **startle response** (overreaction to minor sounds or noises), or they may be **hypervigilant** (constantly scanning the environment for potentially dangerous situations). Clients with PTSD "may react under stress with survival responses appropriate for the trauma that they survived. For example, abused children may seek to placate adults, female incest victims may be-

PROFESSIONAL TIP

Flashbacks

The client experiencing a flashback is usually not aware of current surroundings and often does not recognize familiar individuals. For the duration of the flashback, the client is actually re-experiencing and reliving the original trauma once again. For this reason it is extremely important to never touch a client during a flashback, as the client may perceive you as dangerous and react to you as if you are trying to inflict harm. Talk to the client in a soft, calm voice and gently let the client know who you are, where the client is, and what is happening.

come flirtatious or seductive with men, and war veterans may become threatening or aggressive" (Clark, 1997).

Nursing diagnoses for the client with anxiety may include the following:

Nursing Diagnoses	Planning/Goals	Nursing Interventions
▶ Anxiety related to a subjective sense of uneasiness and tension	The client will learn how to demonstrate and utilize new and more effective methods of managing anxiety.	Teach the client relaxation exercises. Explore with the client those things that are calming and relaxing. Encourage physical movement or participation in some type of recreational or sporting activity to release excess energy.
▶ Fear related to a specific object (e.g., hospitals)	The client will report feeling less fearful.	Remain with the client while level of fear is high. Talk to the client in a calm, soothing voice. Reassure the client that he is in a safe place.
▶ Post-Trauma Syndrome related to anxiety felt following a significant life-threatening event	The client will experience a decrease in frequency and intensity of symptoms.	Orient the client to reality, if the client is confused, disoriented, or experiencing flashbacks. Do not touch the client without permission. Teach the client, family, and significant others about the symptoms of PTSD, including flashbacks, amnesia, memory loss, and nightmares.

Evaluation Each goal must be evaluated to determine how it has been met by the client.

THE CLIENT WHO IS DEPRESSED

Depression is the state wherein an individual experiences feelings of extreme sadness, hopelessness, and helplessness. A number of symptoms may be seen with depression, which can range anywhere from mild to severe and be manifested in many different ways.

One of the first symptoms seen with depression is often a change in the usual pattern of sleeping. Individuals with depression experience symptoms uniquely, for example, a client may have **insomnia** (difficulty in falling asleep initially or returning to sleep once awakened) or **hypersomnia** (excessive sleeping). Other possible symptoms of depression include a change in the usual pattern of eating indicated by either an increase or decrease in appetite, **lethargy** (decreased energy level), decreased **libido** (sexual energy), frequent crying spells, racing thoughts, difficulty concentrating, forgetfulness, and **suicidal ideations** (thoughts of hurting or killing self). Clients can experience mild, moderate, or severe depression with varying degrees of symptomatology. Some of the psychiatric diagnoses associated with depression include Major Depressive Disorder and Dysthymic Disorder.

MILD DEPRESSION

Individuals with a mild depression may notice a difference in the way they are feeling and their ability to function in certain situations, but they may not be able to identify the problem at this point in time. Although they are still able to function and carry on their daily routines, doing so may put quite a strain on them both physically and mentally.

MODERATE DEPRESSION

Moderate depression interferes with the individual's life in a variety of ways. A decrease in the ability to perform on the job may be noticed. Relationships are affected as the individual becomes increasingly withdrawn and isolated and disinterested in things that previously were pleasurable, such as hobbies and leisure-time activities. Interventions performed at this stage are most effective in arresting the depression before the individual's mental health deteriorates any further.

SEVERE DEPRESSION

When depression progresses to a severe state, the individual becomes seriously impaired. The individual with severe depression may experience psychosis, or a loss of contact with reality, in addition to the symptoms of depression.

THE CLIENT WITH MAJOR DEPRESSIVE DISORDER

To qualify for the diagnosis of Major Depressive Disorder, DSM-IV requires the presence of at least one Major Depressive Episode. This episode must (1) last at least 2 weeks, (2) represent a change from previous functioning, and (3) cause some impairment in a person's social or occupational functioning. During an episode, it is also required that five or more symptoms be present. One of these symptoms *must* be either depressed mood or loss of interest in previously enjoyable activities. The individual must also experience at least four additional symptoms, which may include changes in appetite or weight; sleep disturbance (usu-

ally trouble staying asleep); fatigue or loss of energy; feelings of worthlessness or guilt; difficulty concentrating, thinking, or making decisions; or recurrent thoughts of death or suicide.

A person experiencing a depressive episode may express feelings of sadness and hopelessness or may express the sense of feeling empty or having no feelings. Some persons express somatic symptoms such as bodily aches and pains rather than sadness. Also, some individuals, particularly adolescents, exhibit irritability or crankiness rather than sadness. Family members or close friends will notice a change in the individual, most commonly a social withdrawal and a neglect of activities that previously brought the person pleasure

Major depressive episodes frequently develop over a few days or weeks, and without treatment commonly last for longer than 6 months (Frisch & Frisch, 1998).

THE CLIENT WITH DYSTHYMIC DISORDER

Whereas the essence of Major Depressive Disorder is discrete episodes of depression, persons with Dysthymic Disorder feel depressed nearly all of the time. The DSM-IV criteria for Dysthymic Disorder include "depressed mood for most of the day, for more days than not . . . for at least 2 years." A person with Dysthymic Disorder must also have at least two of the following symptoms: appetite disturbance, sleep disturbance, fatigue, low self-esteem, poor concentration or difficulty making decisions, and feelings of hopelessness. As with Major Depressive Disorder, the symptoms must cause clinically significant distress or impairment in social or occupational functioning. Dysthymic Disorder is somewhat rarer than Major Depressive Disorder, occurring during a lifetime in approximately 6% of persons (Frisch & Frisch, 1998).

Medical–Surgical Management

Medical

Psychotherapy refers to any of over 250 types of largely verbal techniques designed to help individuals surmount psychological stresses including depression. Psychotherapy based on psychoanalytic interventions emphasizes helping clients gain insight into the causes of their depression. This approach is long term and requires much motivation on the part of the client to invest considerable time, effort, and money (Frisch & Frisch, 1998).

Brief dynamic therapy focuses on core conflicts that derive from personality and living situations. The goal is to resolve depressive symptoms by improving these conflicts and resolving stresses. The therapist in this approach takes an active role to direct sessions

PROFESSIONAL TIP

Journaling

Suggest to depressed clients that they keep personal journals in which they write down their thoughts and feelings. Putting thoughts and emotions down on paper may help clarify issues relating to depression and is an excellent way of venting or releasing pent-up feelings.

toward resolution of conflicts. Techniques of confrontation and interpretation of behaviors and events are frequently used. Conflicts, their meanings, and individuals' choices are emphasized. This type of therapy can be done either with individuals or in a group format.

Cognitive therapy focuses on removing symptoms by identifying and correcting perceptual biases in clients' thinking and correcting unrecognized assumptions. The therapy concentrates on changing negative thoughts and behaviors into alternatives that do not sustain depression.

Electroconvulsive therapy (ECT) is a procedure wherein the client is treated with pulses of electrical energy sufficient to cause a brief convulsion or seizure (Bolwig, 1993). Electroconvulsive therapy is carried out under anesthesia. Muscle-depolarizing agents are also given so that no actual convulsive movements occur; the primary effect of ECT is on the brain itself. Studies show that clients do not find the actual ECT treatment frightening, painful, or unpleasant. Although deaths have occurred from ECT, particularly in elderly clients or those with heart disease, the risk is quite low. Side effects depend on the specific technique used but are mostly limited to memory deficits (Frisch & Frisch, 1998).

Pharmacological

The main classification of medications usually prescribed for treatment of depression is the antidepressants. Within this classification are several groups including the tetracyclic and atypical antidepressants (Table 33–4), the selective serotonin reuptake inhibitors (SSRIs) (Table 33–5), the tricyclic antidepressants (Table 33–6), and the monoamine oxidase inhibitors (MAOIs) (Table 33–7). These antidepressant families have unique properties, as do the individual medica-

---

Table 33–4 TETRACYCLIC AND ATYPICAL ANTIDEPRESSANTS

GENERIC NAME	TRADE NAME	TYPE	POTENTIAL SIDE EFFECTS
mirtazapine	Remeron	Tetracyclic	Agranulocytosis, drowsiness, dry mouth, impotence, nausea
nefazodone hydrochloride	Serzone	Antidepressant	Constipation, dizziness, dry mouth, insomnia, nausea, NMS, weight loss
venlafaxine hydrochloride	Effexor	Antidepressant	Abnormal dreams, altered taste, anorexia, constipation, diarrhea, dizziness, dry mouth, dyspepsia, headache, nausea, nervousness, paresthesia, rectal hemorrhage, rhinitis, seizures, sexual dysfunction, visual disturbances, vaginal/uterine hemorrhage, weakness, weight loss

Data from PDR Nurses Handbook, *by G. Spratto and A. Woods, 2001, Albany, NY: Delmar; and "Depression and Your Patient," by A. Isaacs, 1998, AJN 98(7), 26–31.*

Table 33–5 SELECTIVE SEROTONIN REUPTAKE INHIBITORS (SSRIs)

GENERIC NAME	TRADE NAME	POTENTIAL SIDE EFFECTS
fluoxetine hydrochloride	Prozac	Abnormal dreams, anxiety, diarrhea, drowsiness, excessive sweating, headache, insomnia, nervousness, palpitations, pruritus, seizures, tremors, visual disturbances, weight loss
fluvoxamine maleate	Luvox	Constipation, convulsions, diarrhea, dizziness, dry mouth, drowsiness, dyspepsia, headache, heart failure, insomnia, MI, nausea, nervousness, weakness
paroxetine hydrochloride	Paxil	Anxiety, constipation, diarrhea, dizziness, drowsiness, dry mouth, ejaculatory disturbance, headache, insomnia, nausea, seizures, sweating, weakness, tremors
sertraline hydrochloride	Zoloft	Diarrhea, dizziness, drowsiness, dry mouth, fatigue, headache, increased sweating, insomnia, nausea, palpitations, sexual dysfunction, tremors, vomiting

Data from PDR Nurses Handbook, *by G. Spratto and A. Woods, 2001, Albany, NY: Delmar.*

Table 33–6 TRICYCLIC ANTIDEPRESSANTS

GENERIC NAME	TRADE NAME	POTENTIAL SIDE EFFECTS
amitriptyline hydrochloride	Elavil	Arrhythmia, blurred vision, constipation, dry eyes, dry mouth, heart block, hypotension, lethargy, MI, sedation, stroke
clomipramine hydrochloride	Anafranil	Arrhythmia, blurred vision, constipation, dry eyes, dry mouth, heart block, lethargy, male sexual MI, dysfunction, nausea, sedation, stroke, vomiting, weakness
imipramine hydrochloride	Tofranil	Arrhythmia, blurred vision, constipation, drowsiness, dry eyes, dry mouth, fatigue, hypotension, seizures, urinary retention

Data from PDR Nurses Handbook, *by G. Spratto and A. Woods, 2001, Albany, NY: Delmar.*

Table 33–7 MONOAMINE OXIDASE INHIBITORS (MAOIs)

GENERIC NAME	TRADE NAME	POTENTIAL SIDE EFFECTS
isocarboxazid	Marplan	Arrhythmia, blurred vision, diarrhea, dizziness, headache, orthostatic hypotension, insomnia, restlessness, seizures, weakness; these medications usually have the side-effect of lowering blood pressure. A potentially fatal hypertensive crisis can result when MAOIs are taken in combination with certain foods and drugs such as broad beans, certain cheeses (e.g., brie, cheddar), liver, caffeine, figs, dry sausage (pepperoni), tea, yogurt, amphetamine, cocaine, dopa, and many OTC cold products, hay fever medications, and nasal decongestants.
phenelzine sulfate	Nardil	
tranylcypro-mine sulfate	Parnate	

Data from PDR Nurses Handbook, *by G. Spratto and A. Woods, 2001, Albany, NY: Delmar.*

tions within each. It is the responsibility of the nurse to adequately educate the client and family about the prescribed medications.

Diet

The client experiencing depression often has a disturbance in eating patterns. Some individuals will not be hungry and will eat very little or sometimes not at all, whereas others will overeat. A nutritional assessment should be done as part of the health history obtained by the nurse, and if any significant problem areas are identified, a dietary consult may be indicated.

When a client is started on antidepressant therapy, the client and family must be educated regarding any special dietary needs, depending on the type of medication prescribed. The client receiving SSRI therapy may experience an initial loss of appetite during the first part of therapy, because of the gastrointestinal (GI) side effects frequently associated with these medications (refer to Table 33–5). Anorectic clients or those at risk for weight loss must be closely monitored. The client receiving MAOI therapy must be especially alert to the dietary restrictions associated with this particular type of medication (refer to Table 33–7).

PROFESSIONAL TIP

Antidepressant Therapy

Prior to initiating antidepressant therapy, a baseline electrocardiogram (EKG) is needed to determine whether any pre-existing underlying cardiac problems are present. If the client develops cardiac difficulties during antidepressant therapy, another EKG can then be obtained and reviewed against the original to assist in ascertaining whether the administration of the antidepressant has exacerbated the cardiac condition.

CLIENT TEACHING

Potential Adverse Drug–Drug Reactions with MAOIs

A serious drug–drug reaction can occur when a MAOI is taken concurrently with certain other medications. The combination of a MAOI and some common prescription or OTC medications can result in a hypertensive crisis that is often fatal. Some of the most dangerous reactive medications include meperidine (Demerol), stimulants, decongestants, and weight-reduction aids.

Activity

Clients suffering from depression often experience a significant decrease in level of activity and report feeling tired and lethargic. Clients experiencing depression will often require encouragement to engage in any type of physical activity (Figure 33-6).

Figure 33-6 Exercise was found to be an effective antidepressant in a meta-analysis of 77 studies on exercise and depression (North, 1989). *(Courtesy of Photo Disc)*

CLIENT TEACHING

Tricyclic Antidepressants

Be sure to instruct each client taking a tricyclic antidepressant medication in the following:

- Do not drink alcohol while on the medication.
- Do not take any other medications unless prescribed by your physician.
- Drowsiness and sedation may impair the ability to drive and operate heavy machinery.
- Some of the side effects may diminish in intensity once your body adjusts to the medication.
- Do not stop taking the medications without physician approval.
- Increase fluid intake to assist in combating dry mouth and constipation.
- Sugarless candy and gum can help decrease the side effect of dry mouth.
- Increase dietary fiber to decrease the side effect of constipation.
- Rise slowly from a lying position to prevent dizziness and a sudden drop in blood pressure.

CLIENT TEACHING

Tetracyclic and SSRI Antidepressants

Be sure to instruct each client taking a tetracyclic, atypical, or SSRI antidepressant medication in the following:

- Take the medication *only* as directed by your physician.
- Do not take the medication unless prescribed by your physician.
- Do not take fluoxetine (Prozac), paroxetine (Paxil), or sertraline (Zoloft) on an empty stomach.
- Mirtazapine (Remeron) does not need to be taken with food.
- Ability to drive and/or operate heavy machinery may be impaired while taking the medication.
- Do not drink alcohol while taking the medication.
- If female, advise your physician if you are breastfeeding, suspect you are pregnant, or are planning a pregnancy while taking the medication.
- Wear sunscreen and protective clothing while outdoors, as fluoxetine (Prozac), paroxetine (Paxil), and sertraline (Zoloft) increase susceptibility to sunburn.

- The medications may cause drowsiness.
- If taking fluoxetine (Prozac), mirtazapine (Remeron), or nefazodone (Serzone), rise slowly from a lying position to prevent dizziness and a sudden drop in blood pressure.
- Utilize good oral hygiene in conjunction with sugarless candy or gum to minimize the discomforting side effect of dry mouth associated with fluoxetine (Prozac), mirtazapine (Remeron), nefazodone (Serzone), paroxetine (Paxil), and sertraline (Zoloft).
- Monitor weight, as mirtazapine (Remeron) may cause an increase in appetite.
- Do not take any over-the-counter (OTC) cold medications with mirtazapine (Remeron).
- If taking mirtazapine (Remeron), inform your physician of the medication regimen prior to surgery.
- If taking venlafaxine (Effexor), fluvoxamine (Luvox), or nefazodone (Serzone), inform your physician if signs of allergic reaction occur.

PROFESSIONAL TIP

MAOIs

MAOIs are most often used to treat depression that has proven resistant to other medications.

CLIENT TEACHING

MAOIs

Be sure to instruct each client taking an MAOI antidepressant medication in the following:

- *Do not take any other medications, including OTC medications,* unless prescribed by your physician.
- Take the medication exactly as prescribed.
- Do not drink alcohol while on the medication.
- Rise slowly from a lying position to prevent dizziness and a sudden drop in blood pressure.
- *Avoid all foods containing tyramine,* including alcoholic beverages, especially beer and wine; aged cheeses; avocados; bananas; caffeine; chocolate; and smoked or pickled meats (such as salami, pepperoni, smoked fish, and summer sausage).

▸ NURSING PROCESS

▸ Assessment

▸ Subjective Data

The client experiencing depression may verbalize any number of symptoms including overwhelming feelings of sadness, thoughts of suicide, a loss of interest and pleasure in activities that were previously enjoyable, and problems with memory, recall, and concentration. In addition, they may report a decreased libido, extreme lethargy, and having insufficient energy to complete activities of daily living (ADLs) and needed tasks. The depressed client who has become increasingly withdrawn and socially isolated may experience problems in intimate, personal, and social relationships.

▸ Objective Data

The client experiencing depression may manifest a noticeable decline in personal hygiene and grooming, possibly due to a lack of energy and an inability to perform even the simplest of tasks. Weight loss resulting from the client's failure to eat is also a symptom of depression.

Nursing diagnoses for the client with depression may include the following:

Nursing Diagnoses	Planning/Goals	Nursing Interventions
▸ *Social Isolation related to inability to engage in satisfying personal relationships*	The client will increase the number of interactions with other individuals.	Build rapport and develop therapeutic relationship with client. Spend time with client individually. Encourage client to interact with others. Encourage client to initiate conversation with others. Verbally praise client for increasing interactions and initiating conversation.
▸ *Bathing/Hygiene, Dressing/Grooming, and Feeding Self-care Deficit related to lack of concern or regard toward self*	The client will attend to own basic health care needs.	Encourage client to bathe and wear clean clothes. Teach client the importance of balanced nutrition. Praise client for each activity done on own.

Evaluation Each goal must be evaluated to determine how it has been met by the client.

THE CLIENT WHO IS POTENTIALLY VIOLENT

In today's society, violence has become increasingly common and widespread. The media routinely and graphically reports the numerous violent crimes and acts that occur on a daily basis (Aguilera, 1998). Upon occasion, nurses come face to face with angry clients and their families and significant others and, perhaps, even angry colleagues. When confronted by someone who is angry, the natural reaction is to respond in a like manner or, perhaps, to feel intimidated. In such difficult situations it is important to maintain objectivity and not get "hooked" into the client's anger and respond in an inappropriate manner.

Nurses may encounter clients who are **verbally aggressive** (prone to saying things in a loud and/or intimidating manner), **physically aggressive** (prone to threatening or actually harming someone), or a combination of the two. Mind-altering substances such as alcohol and phencyclidine (PCP) often increase the risk of aggression. **Anger-control assistance** is defined as a nursing intervention aimed at facilitation of the expression of anger in an adaptive and nonviolent manner (McCloskey & Bulechek, 1996). For the psychiatric nurse, anger control includes establishing a basic level of trust and rapport with the client and using a calm and reassuring manner. The nurse should use every means possible to learn from the client (or his family/friends) those situations that are likely to bring on anger. Further, the nurse should encourage the client to inform the nursing staff when he is feeling tension. While the nurse has a responsibility to help the client learn to deal with his anger, she also has a clear duty to assess for inappropriate aggression and to intervene before such aggression is expressed.

Some of the techniques used in anger control include limiting access to frustrating situations, providing physical outlets for expression of anger or tension (such as punching bags, large motor activities [sports], and anger journals), and ensuring that a client for whom anger is a problem is given enough personal space that he does not have to feel encroached upon by others when he is unable to tolerate environmental stimuli.

Two interventions commonly used in situations where the client is out of control are physical restraints and seclusion. These external controls may be used only when there is no other option for protecting the client and/or others.

THE CLIENT WHO IS HOMICIDAL

The client who is homicidal is planning or threatening to harm or kill another individual or individuals. It is the responsibility of health care personnel to attempt to ascertain the seriousness of the intent, that is, whether the individual is actually threatening someone else or just "blowing off steam." Once the nurse is aware of an individual's threat or intent to harm some-

PROFESSIONAL TIP

Assessing for Risk of Violence
- Be aware of those clients with past history of violence and poor impulse control.
- Observe the client's body language: Notice changes in behavior, words, or dress.
- Assess for aggressive behaviors, increasing tension, clenched fists, loud or angry tone of voice, narrowed eyes, and pacing.
- Remember that hostility tends to be contagious. Do not reciprocate with anger and hostility!

one else, she must inform the individual(s) at risk of the potential for harm and/or notify the proper authorities and enlist their help. The first step in such a situation is to contact the supervisor and offer an accurate appraisal of the situation.

THE CLIENT WHO IS SUICIDAL

Purposefully taking one's own life, or **suicide**, is the ultimate form of self-destruction. Clients who are suicidal often feel overwhelmed by life events and decide that the only relief will come from ending their own lives. Intense feelings of fear, loss, anger, or despair can drive individuals to commit suicide, and the effects of an attempted or completed suicide can be devastating and long lasting. Nurses must learn to recognize the danger signs of clients at risk for suicide and know the appropriate interventions to help clients preserve their health and dignity.

"Suicide is the eighth leading cause of death in the United States, claiming some 30,000 lives each year" (Badger, 1995). The populations at greatest risk are individuals with diagnosed mood disorders such as Major Depressive Disorder, elders, and those with serious or life-threatening medical illnesses such as cancer or human immunodeficiency virus (Badger, 1995).

THE CLIENT WITH SUICIDAL IDEATIONS

The client experiencing suicidal ideations has thoughts of hurting or killing himself but may or may not be planning to act on these thoughts. It is important to understand the difference between thoughts and actions; that is, having a thought does not necessarily mean that the behavior will follow. When confronted with a client's verbalization of possible suicide, however, it is always wise to take the client's expression of intent seriously. Because suicide is a leading cause of death in the United States, nurses must know how to evaluate a client for the likelihood of a completed suicide. It is critical that the nurse thoroughly assess the client and attempt to accurately ascertain the degree of danger the client is experiencing. Once this is done, the nurse must then take the precautions necessary to maintain the client's safety (Table 33–8).

THE CLIENT WHO IS ACTIVELY SUICIDAL

The **actively suicidal** client is intent upon hurting or killing himself and is in imminent danger of doing so. This situation requires immediate and appropriate action on the part of the nurse to protect the client

Table 33–8 ASSESSMENT OF RISK FOR SUICIDE

The following areas are to be assessed in all potentially suicidal clients:

1. Does the client have a *plan* to commit suicide?

Example: Client plans to "end it all" after wife leaves for work on a Monday.	***Rationale***: Some clients may be experiencing thoughts of wishing they were dead or killing themselves, but may not have a plan for doing so. *The client who has a plan for committing suicide is at increased risk.*

2. How *specific* is the plan to commit suicide?

Example: Client states he plans to overdose on sleeping pills.	***Rationale***: *A specific plan increases the risk of completing a suicide.*

3. Does the client have access to the *means* to commit suicide?

Example: Client states he will use his spouse's sleeping pills to overdose.	***Rationale***: *Easy availability of the means to kill oneself increases the risk of suicide.*

4. How *lethal* is the intended means to commit suicide?

Example: Client states he will "blow his brains out" with a gun.	***Rationale***: Some means of suicide are more likely to result in a completed suicide. *Gunshots are the most common cause of completed suicide.* The lethality of guns makes the potential for a successful intervention very slim. Intervention in light of means that are less lethal may yield a more favorable outcome (e.g., overdose, cutting of wrists).

from potentially fatal self-destructive behavior. If the client is in a supervised setting, it is the responsibility of the nurse to maintain the safety of the client and to inform other staff members of the client's suicidal intentions. The client at high risk for self-inflicted injury must be monitored closely (per institutional policy and the frequency as ordered by the physician). All pertinent observations such as verbalizations and behaviors that are indicative of self-harm potential should be documented in the client record. Any changes in the client's condition should be reported immediately to the physician. The conversation with the doctor as well as any new orders or changes in orders must also be documented in the client's record (Eskreis, 1998).

Medical–Surgical Management

Medical

The client who is severely agitated, aggressive, actively suicidal, and/or homicidal and who is exhibiting or threatening violent acts may need to be restrained

PROFESSIONAL TIP

Level of Observation

The frequency of client observation is determined by the degree of suicide risk and is written as a specific order from the physician. Observations of the client are documented. Some clients must be checked a minimum of once every 15 minutes. Other clients may require more frequent observation and monitoring. If the client is *actively* suicidal and/or homicidal and is indicating an imminent intent to harm self or others, a specific staff member will be assigned to that client at all times on a one-to-one basis.

or placed in seclusion in order to be safely contained. The physical holding of someone or use of mechanical restraints severely restricts movement and can constitute a violation of the client's rights unless sufficient clinical justification exists. Thus, all of the client's comments and behaviors plus any nursing interventions must be documented in the client record per agency policy. This documentation provides the necessary justification for the use of restraints or seclusion. In addition, the physician must write a specific, time-limited order that spells out the reason restraints or seclusion was indicated for use with the client.

Physical Restraints Physical restraints, usually leather straps, are used to immobilize a person who is clearly dangerous to self or others and who poses sufficient risk of harm. Physical restraints may be applied only under the direction and supervision of a registered nurse (RN) and must comply with state laws regarding their use. In almost all cases, there must be a

PROFESSIONAL TIP

Providing a Safe Environment

When a client verbalizes an intention to inflict self-harm, the nurse must take measures to ensure the client's safety. One way to do so is to provide and maintain a safe, secure environment for the client. This may require a change in the way a client's surroundings and living space are usually viewed. For example, a pencil or pen could be used as a dangerous weapon; an empty soda can could be used to deeply cut the wrists or to seriously injure someone else; and the glass from a bottle of make-up could cause great harm. These and all other potentially dangerous items must be removed from the client's immediate area.

PROFESSIONAL TIP

No-Suicide Contract

Obtaining a "No-Suicide Contract" from the client is one way to help reduce the risk of suicide attempts. There are several guidelines to follow in working through this process:

- Ask the client whether he is able to make a promise *to himself* that he will not do anything to harm himself. ***Rationale***: It is important for the client to make the contract with himself, because if the contract is made with someone else, such as a nurse, and the client later becomes angry or upset with that person, he may then harm himself in order to "get back" at that person.

- If the client is unable to commit to the No-Suicide Contract for the rest of his life, work with him on establishing a time frame to which he can commit, for example, 1 week, 24 hours, 8 hours, or some other time frame. Always meet with the client at the end of the allotted time frame and review/renew the contract at that time. ***Rationale***: The suicidal individual may feel overwhelmed at the thought of promising *never* to harm himself, but may be able to sincerely commit for a shorter length of time.

- Ask the client whether he is able to maintain the No-Suicide Contract *no matter what happens*. ***Rationale:*** Some clients will leave a way out of the contract. For example, the suicidal client may outwardly make a promise to not commit suicide but inwardly think "unless something really bad happens, like if my wife leaves me." If the wife then files for a divorce, the client may feel that he has "permission" to kill himself. Adding the *no matter what happens* clause blocks off this avenue of escape from the contract.

- Ask the client whether he can make a promise to himself that if thoughts of suicide return, he will talk to someone and let them know before taking any action. ***Rationale***: If the client talks to someone regarding his thoughts of suicide *before* he attempts suicide, a successful intervention and suicide prevention are more likely.

- Assist the client in developing a detailed plan of action regarding those persons he will contact in the event that he again experiences suicidal thoughts. Include names and phone numbers of all significant and supportive individuals. ***Rationale***: During a crisis, the suicidal individual is not able to think rationally and will behave and act in an impulsive manner. Having a well-developed plan of action increases the likelihood that the suicidal individual can follow these guidelines.

- At the bottom of the list put the name and phone number of the local suicide crisis hotline and/or local emergency number (911). ***Rationale***: Including these numbers ensures that there will always be someone available for the suicidal client to talk to 24 hours a day, 7 days a week, 365 days a year.

- Assist the client in putting the No-Suicide Contract in writing and in his own words. Give the client the original and put a copy in the client's chart. ***Rationale***: When the contract is in writing and the client has a copy, he will be more likely to follow through with his promise to not commit suicide.

---

physician's order to apply the restraints, and there must be clearly documented evidence that the restraints were needed. Some of the observable behaviors indicating that restraints are necessary include increased motor activity, verbal and/or physical threats, overresponsiveness to stimuli, and actual physical assault (Frisch & Frisch, 1998).

Seclusion Seclusion is the process of confining a client to a single room. The room may be locked or unlocked, and it may or may not have furnishings. The purpose of seclusion is to provide security, to remove the client from a situation of escalating anger and violence, and to remove the client who is hypersensitive to environmental stimuli from the stimulation of a hospital unit. Seclusion, like the use of physical restraints, can be used only when all other avenues for control have been exhausted. The client must be told what is

happening and why. He must not be left alone; a staff member should be assigned to observe the client, usually from the doorway. Seclusion is an enforced "time-out," where the client is removed from the situation only long enough to allow him to calm down, regain a sense of control, and then reenter the unit.

Therapy Psychotherapy is often indicated and initially may focus on personal and social conditions that bring about and/or perpetuate suicidal thoughts. Cognitive-behavioral therapy may be particularly useful, as may techniques to deal with frustration and anger. Substance use and abuse are often involved and may require separate outpatient or inpatient interventions.

Pharmacological

The severely agitated, aggressive, suicidal, and/or homicidal client who is violent or threatening violence may require a medication with strong anxiolytic (antianxiety) and/or sedative properties, such as one of the antianxiety agents or a sedative-hypnotic (refer back to Table 33–2). Additionally, the suicidal client who is depressed may be evaluated for treatment with one of the many available antidepressants such as fluoxetine hydrochloride (Prozac), sertraline hydrochloride (Zoloft), paroxetine hydrochloride (Paxil), fluvoxamine maleate (Luvox), mirtazapine (Remeron), or one of the many others (refer back to Tables 33–4, 33–5, 33–6, and 33–7).

Diet

Foods are not necessarily restricted for the client who is severely agitated, aggressive, actively suicidal, and/or homicidal; however, the food tray should be inspected for any potentially dangerous objects such as glassware or silverware. Even plasticware can be broken in such a way as to yield a very dangerous weapon for hurting self or others.

Activity

The activity level of the client who is severely agitated, aggressive, actively suicidal, and/or homicidal their may need to be restricted for a period of time in order to maintain the client's safety and the safety of others.

▶ NURSING PROCESS

▶ Assessment

▶ Subjective Data

The client who is severely agitated, aggressive, and/or homicidal may argue, yell, curse, and make numerous verbal threats in a loud voice. The suicidal client may indicate intentions verbally, nonverbally, or a combination of the two. The client contemplating suicide may verbalize his thoughts either directly or indirectly. A direct statement may be something as straightforward as "I am planning to kill myself." An indirect statement might be "I'm not going to be around here anymore" or "Everyone will be better off without me" (Gorman, Sultan, & Raines, 1996).

▶ Objective Data

The client who is severely agitated, aggressive, and/or homicidal may exhibit restlessness, pacing, and "poor impulse control"; may be physically intimidating; and may use or try to use a variety of available weapons such as books, furniture, or a coffee pot (Gorman et al., 1996). A nonverbal signal of possible intentions of suicide may be seen in the client who begins making arrangements for people and pets to be taken care of, putting personal affairs in order, and giving away personal possessions, especially treasured items.

Nursing diagnoses for the client who is severely agitated, aggressive, actively suicidal, and/or homicidal may include the following:

Nursing Diagnoses	Planning/Goals	Nursing Interventions
▶ Risk for Self-Directed Violence related to risk factors such as mental health, emotional status, or suicidal plan.	The client will not harm self.	Assess for the presence of suicidal thoughts and whether a specific plan is present.
		Evaluate the degree of risk associated with the client's verbalization of suicide intent.
		Contact the attending physician or psychiatrist and inform of the client's intentions and current condition (Isaacs, 1998).
		Assess and evaluate the client's surroundings and environment for any potentially dangerous items or objects that could be used for self-harm.
		Remove or secure any potentially harmful items after thoroughly evaluating the situation.
		Increase the level of observation so that the client is frequently monitored.
		Assist the client in developing a No-suicide Contract (Badger, 1995).
▶ Risk for Other Directed Violence related to risk factors such as history of violence against others, suicidal behavior, impulsivity.	The client will not harm anyone.	Assess for the presence of homicidal ideations.
		If the client is verbalizing a plan to harm someone, immediately notify the proper authorities so they can alert this individual.

Evaluation Each goal must be evaluated to determine how it has been met by the client.

SAMPLE NURSING CARE PLAN

THE SUICIDAL CLIENT WITH MAJOR DEPRESSION

Alice is a 27-year-old female who was brought to the emergency department of a county hospital by ambulance following a serious suicide attempt via ingesting a bottle of insecticide. After being treated in the emergency room, she spent 2 days in the intensive care unit (ICU) and then was transferred to a locked adult inpatient psychiatric unit for evaluation and treatment. Alice reports she became suicidal following the recent ending of a 4 year relationship with her boyfriend and decided to take her life because she felt "completely hopeless," that "there was nothing left to live for," that "no one would miss her" if she were dead, that she "would never be loved," and that she "could never be happy again." Prior to the suicide attempt, Alice reports that she had not been eating, had only been sleeping 1 to 2 hours per night, and had been crying almost continuously throughout the day. Since admission to the psychiatric unit, Alice has been started on sertraline (Zoloft).

Nursing Diagnosis 1 *Risk for Self-Directed Violence related to recent loss, feelings of abandonment, and impulsive behavior as evidenced by suicide attempt of drinking bottle of insecticide, verbalizations that "there was nothing left to live for" and that "no one would miss her" if she were dead*

PLANNING/GOALS	NURSING INTERVENTIONS	RATIONALE	EVALUATION
Alice will verbalize that she is no longer at risk of harming herself.	Assist Alice in developing a No-suicide Contract. Obtain in writing if possible, make a copy for her chart, and give her the original.	A written No-suicide Contract may help deter self-destructive behavior in the future.	At the time of discharge from the adult inpatient psychiatric unit, Alice was no longer actively suicidal or intent upon harming herself. She still had occasional suicidal ideations; however, she did not feel compelled to act on them. She had made a promise to herself that she would never try to kill herself again no matter what happened, and that if those thoughts returned, she would find someone to talk to before she did anything. She also had developed a written list of friends and relatives she could call if she again experienced thoughts of suicide.
	Explore with Alice factors that contributed to her becoming suicidal.	Knowledge of those things that led to the current suicide attempt can be the first step in preventing another.	
	Encourage Alice to verbalize her feelings related to the recent break-up and to explore any unresolved past issues that this loss might have triggered.	Current feelings of loss and abandonment are often magnified and intensified by unresolved past situations and circumstances that were never effectively handled.	
	Explore with Alice her usual methods of coping with stressful situations and whether these have been effective for her.	Looking at one's behaviors and their effectiveness or ineffectiveness can lead to a better understanding of those behaviors that must be changed.	
	Assist Alice in identifying and then developing stress-management	Identifying healthier behaviors is necessary before any changes can	

continues

methods as alternatives to attempting suicide.

be made. This assists the client in recognizing alternate methods of managing stressful situations.

Assist Alice in developing a suicide-prevention plan and in identifying supportive individuals and resources that she can turn to in the event that she begins to again have suicidal thoughts.

Plans to prevent suicide must be developed ahead of time, because individuals contemplating suicide are impulsive and unable to problem solve or think clearly. They may, however, be able to follow through with a previously defined plan of action.

Teach Alice about possible side effects associated with sertraline (Zoloft), such as nausea and GI upset, and encourage her to have something to eat prior to taking this medication.

Medication education is an integral part of treatment.

Emphasize the importance of taking this medication as prescribed and not stopping the medication on her own, even if she starts to feel better and thinks that she no longer needs it.

Clients often stop taking prescribed medications when their symptoms disappear, because they think that the medications are no longer needed. However, if medications are discontinued prematurely, symptoms usually reappear and are often much more serious.

Encourage Alice to keep a journal to reflect on her thoughts and feelings.

Writing in a journal can be a safe and effective method of identifying, expressing, and releasing feelings and emotions.

Encourage Alice to keep follow-up appointments for medication to monitor progress.

Follow-up appointments for medication are recommended to evaluate effectiveness and to monitor for any side effects.

Assist Alice in setting up an appointment for outpatient counseling/therapy upon discharge per recommendation from

Follow-up treatment with counseling and/ or therapy is recommended after a suicide attempt in order to ad-

continues

the treatment team.
Encourage Alice to keep
counseling
appointments.

dress the underlying
issues and to prevent
future attempts.

Nursing Diagnosis 2 *Hopelessness related to feelings of loss about her life and future as evidenced by verbalizations of feeling: "completely hopeless," that she "would never be loved," and that she "could never be happy again"*

PLANNING/GOALS	NURSING INTERVENTIONS	RATIONALE	EVALUATION
Alice will be less hopeless as indicated by verbalizations of plans for her future.	Develop a therapeutic nurse–client relationship with Alice utilizing the components of trust, rapport, respect, genuineness, and empathy.	Implementing the components of trust, rapport, respect, genuineness, and empathy will foster the development of a therapeutic nurse–client relationship.	Alice continued to have fleeting thoughts of hopelessness as far as ever having another significant relationship or being in love again; however, she now was beginning to catch herself and could identify these thoughts as being irrational and negative in nature and not helpful to her in any way.
	Encourage Alice to become involved in activities on the unit, for example, interacting with staff and other clients and attending and participating in therapy groups and recreational activities.	Being involved in some type of activity helps distract the mind from a preoccupation with losses, overwhelming feelings of depression, and suicidal ideations.	
	Provide things for Alice to do when she is feeling down, for example, go for a walk with the staff, read a newspaper or book, or play a game.	Clients who are severely depressed and suicidal have tunnel vision and are unable to see any other options or choices available to them. It is important to somehow buy enough time to allow for something to shift for them—for them to see the situation as not so utterly and permanently hopeless or for them to begin to feel better and think differently once they have started responding to medication.	
	Provide a message of hope for the future, for example, "Things might look a little different tomorrow."		
	Assist Alice in identifying the irrational beliefs or thoughts that she is having, for example, when she says no one	According to cognitive theory, it is the thoughts or messages that we tell ourselves in our heads that cause us to feel a	

continues

will *ever* love or want her again.

certain way. Therefore, if we change the way we are thinking by replacing irrational thoughts with rational or healthier ones, we will change the way we feel.

THE CLIENT WHO IS PSYCHOTIC

Psychosis is a state wherein an individual loses the ability to recognize reality. A psychotic person may experience hallucinations, wherein he hears voices or sees images of persons or things that others cannot see or hear. A psychotic person is frequently unable to care for basic needs of safety, security, nutrition, and so on. Such an individual is hospitalized for their own safety and to initiate treatment (usually involving some form of medication) to bring the symptoms under control. A psychotic person may slip into and out of reality.

Psychosis can be a component of several different psychiatric illnesses. In addition to Panic Anxiety and Major Depressive Disorder, other psychiatric diagnoses, including Schizophrenia and Bipolar Disorder, may involve psychosis.

THE CLIENT WITH SCHIZOPHRENIA

The client with schizophrenia can be very difficult to understand and treat. One of the reasons for this is that the symptoms of schizophrenia can be confusing and frightening to caregivers. Clients with schizophrenia frequently have belief systems that have become distorted in some manner, so that they hold firmly to false ideas or delusions, even when presented with evidence to the contrary. When confronted with an opposing belief system, they may become even more entrenched in their mistaken views and begin to believe others are "against them," when, in fact, they are not. Unfortunately, this makes them even more paranoid and suspicious, adding further to their already distorted views of reality. As a result, these individuals are often struggling to determine the difference between that which is real and that which is unreal or delusional.

Hallucinations can occur in relation to any of the five senses (hearing, sight, touch, taste, and smell), but the most common types of hallucinations are auditory and visual. Individuals experiencing **auditory halluci-**

nations think they are hearing someone talk to them, when, in reality, no one is. The voice may be that of someone the individual recognizes, or the voice may be unknown to the person. If the voice or voices are comforting, the individual will be very resistant to "giving them up." Most of the time, however, the voices are derogatory in nature, telling the person that there is something wrong with him. The most serious type of hallucination is referred to as the **command hallucination**, which occurs when the voice or voices tell the individual to harm themself or someone else in some manner. For example, the voices may tell the individual to jump off of a bridge or building, step in front of a moving motor vehicle, or take an overdose of medication. These hallucinations are extremely dangerous because the demands are so strong that the individual is very likely to act on them.

The individual experiencing a **visual hallucination** will perceive or see someone or something that is not actually there. Depending on the nature of the hallucination and whether the individual perceives it as threatening, the situation can be very frightening.

Medical–Surgical Management

Medical

At this time, there is unfortunately no cure for schizophrenia; however, it is possible for a number of these individuals to lead functional lives with minimally debilitating symptoms through psychosocial treatments.

The goals of psychosocial treatment interventions can be conceived in a number of different ways, but one useful approach has been to divide interventions into three categories: clinical and family support services, rehabilitative services, and humanitarian aid/public safety (Hargreaves & Shumway, 1989). The goal of clinical interventions is to reduce both positive and negative symptoms and to maximize functional outcome. Clinical support involves outpatient management and family/community services. Rehabilitation involves increasing clients' capacities, both for social interactions and for productive activity (including gainful employment, when feasible). Humanitarian interventions are those efforts that maximize an individual's independence and quality of life within the bounds of her mental disability. Public safety involves balancing personal liberty with the recognition that some social control may be needed to prevent harm, both to the individual and to society.

Electroconvulsive therapy (ECT) may be a consideration for the client in the acute phase of schizophrenia; however, ECT has not proven to be effective in cases of chronic schizophrenia (Townsend, 2000).

Pharmacological

The most commonly prescribed classification of medications for the client experiencing schizophrenia is the antipsychotics (Tables 33–9 and 33–10). This group of medications is given to reduce the signs and symptoms of psychosis, with a long-term goal of the client eventually being symptom free. If this is not possible, the goal is to reduce symptoms to a manageable level.

Because a number of side effects are associated with the antipsychotics, client teaching is an important part of the nurse's role. In addition to common side effects, some antipsychotic medications also have the potential for causing adverse reactions such as extrapyramidal symptoms (EPS), tardive dyskinesia (TD), and neuroleptic-malignant-syndrome (NMS).

One of the most important factors in symptom management for schizophrenia is medication compliance. In most cases, individuals who are schizophrenic must take some type of antipsychotic medication for the remainder of their lives. Clients suffering from schizophrenia are often extremely resistant to taking their

medications as prescribed and usually require multiple repeat hospitalizations for stabilization. Multiple reasons exist for noncompliance, one being the client's denial of the diagnosis or the illness itself or of the seriousness of the illness. As a result of denial, the individual with schizophrenia resists taking medication,

Table 33–9 ATYPICAL ANTIPSYCHOTICS

GENERIC NAME	TRADE NAME	POTENTIAL SIDE EFFECTS
clozapine	Clozaril	Agranulocytosis, angina, constipation, dizziness, orthostatic hypotension, increased salivation, leukopenia, NMS, drowsiness, seizures, tachycardia, weight gain
olanzapine	Zyprexa	Agitation, acute renal failure, amblyopia, constipation, CVA, dizziness, dry mouth, headache, NMS, orthostatic hypotension, restlessness, rhinitis, sedation, seizures, tachycardia, TD, tremors, weakness, weight gain
quetiapine fumarate	Seroquel	Dizziness, headache, NMS, seizures, TD, weight gain
risperidone	Risperdal	Acute renal failure, constipation, cough, decreased libido, diarrhea, dizziness, dry mouth, dysmenorrhea/menorrhagia, headache, increased dreams, increased sleep duration, insomnia, itching/skin rash, MI, nausea, NMS, pharyngitis, rhinitis, sedation, visual disturbances.

Data from PDR Nurses Handbook, by G. Spratto and A. Woods, 2001, Albany, NY: Delmar.

CLIENT TEACHING

Adverse Reactions to Antipsychotic Medications

- *Extra-pyramidal side effects:* a common adverse reaction of some antipsychotic medications (especially the older ones) involving muscle rigidity and involuntary muscle movements; reversible if the dose is lowered or an antiparkinson agent is administered
- *Tardive dyskinesia:* irreversible reaction to antipsychotics (usually associated with high doses over a long period of time) consisting of involuntary muscle and body movements
- *Neuroleptic malignant syndrome:* a rare and potentially fatal reaction to antipsychotic medications characterized by a very high fever, severe muscle stiffness, and changes in sensorium progressing to coma

Table 33–10 PHENOTHIAZINES (ANTIPSYCHOTICS)

GENERIC NAME	TRADE NAME	POTENTIAL SIDE EFFECTS
chlorpromazine, hydrochlorodine	Thorazine	Agranulocytosis, blurred vision, constipation, dry eyes, dry mouth, hypotension, laryngeal edema, NMS, photosensitivity, sedation, TD
fluphenazine hydrochloride	Prolixin	Agranulocytosis, EPS, photosensitivity, TD
thioridazine hydrochloride	Mellaril	Agranulocytosis, blurred vision, constipation, dry eyes, dry mouth, hypotension, NMS, photosensitivity, sedation, TD

Data from PDR Nurses Handbook, by G. Spratto and A. Woods, 2001, Albany, NY: Delmar.

CLIENT TEACHING

Phenothiazines

Be sure to instruct each client taking a phenothiazine medication in the following:
- Do not drink alcohol while on the medication.
- Do not take any other medications unless prescribed by your physician.
- Do not stop taking the medication abruptly.
- The ability to drive and/or operate heavy machinery may be impaired while taking the medication.
- Be aware of possible side effects of the medication.
- Increase fluid intake to minimize the side effects of dry mouth and constipation.
- Increase dietary fiber to minimize the side effect of constipation.
- Rise slowly from a lying position to prevent dizziness and a sudden drop in blood pressure.
- These medications are contraindicated during pregnancy and lactation. Female clients should advise their physicians immediately if they are either pregnant or planning to become pregnant.
- Wear sunscreen and protective clothing while outdoors, as the medication increases susceptibility to sunburn.
- Some of the side effects may diminish in intensity after an initial period of adjustment.
- The medication may increase your risk of developing EPS, TD, and NMS.

CLIENT TEACHING

Schizophrenia

Family involvement is important for all clients, but it is especially critical for the client with schizophrenia. Because the client may be too ill or confused to be trusted to take medications reliably, it becomes the responsibility of family members to help ensure medication compliance. Most hospital readmissions for the client with schizophrenia are due to noncompliance with the prescribed medication regimen. If the family understands the important role psychotropic medications can play in preventing decompensation (a return of the psychiatric symptoms) and subsequent hospital readmission, the client has a much better chance of remaining stabilized.

CLIENT TEACHING

Atypical Antipsychotics

Be sure to instruct each client taking an atypical antipsychotic medication in the following:
- Do not drink alcohol while taking the medication.
- Do not take any other medications, prescription or OTC, unless prescribed by your physician.
- Do not stop taking the medication without authorization from your physician.
- Do not stop taking the medication abruptly.
- The ability to drive and/or operate heavy machinery may be impaired while taking the medication.
- Rise slowly from a lying position to prevent dizziness and a sudden drop in blood pressure.
- The medication is contraindicated during pregnancy and lactation. Reliable contraception should be utilized while taking the medication. Female clients should advise their physicians immediately if they suspect they are either pregnant or planning to become pregnant.
- Be aware of the potential side effects of the medications.
- Notify your physician immediately of unexplained fever, sore throat, bleeding, bruising, or petechiae.
- Wear sunscreen and protective clothing while outdoors, as olanzapine (Zyprexa) and risperidone (Risperdal) increase susceptibility to sunburn.
- Avoid temperature extremes if taking olanzapine (Zyprexa), quetiapine fumerate (Seroquel), or risperidone (Risperdal), as the body's ability to regulate internal temperature is affected by these medications.
- Utilize good oral hygiene in conjunction with sugarless candy or gum to minimize the discomforting side effect of dry mouth associated most frequently with clozapine (Clozaril) and olanzapine (Zyprexa).
- Beware of associated risks including EPS, NMS, and a high risk of agranulocytosis and seizures with clozapine (Clozaril); EPS, TD, and NMS with olanzapine (Zyprexa), quetiapine (Seroquel), and risperidone (Risperdal); and seizures with olanzapine (Zyprexa) and quetiapine fumerate (Seroquel).
- Treatment with clozapine (Clozaril) requires *weekly* white blood cell (WBC) monitoring to assess for onset of agranulocytosis. Medication is dispensed in 7-day increments to maintain policy compliance and prevent this potentially life-threatening occurrence.

because to the client, taking medication equates to acceptance of having a serious mental disorder. Clients may also become noncompliant after a period of time on medication; once they start to feel better, they think the medication is no longer needed and stop taking it. After a short time of being off the prescribed medication, however, most individuals with schizophrenia will experience a return or significant worsening of their previous symptoms.

Probably the most common reason for medication noncompliance, however, is the number of troublesome side effects and potentially dangerous adverse reactions historically associated with antipsychotic medications. Fortunately, a number of newer antipsychotic medications are now available that have fewer side effects and are much better tolerated. Even with the advent of these newer and more effective medications, however, many individuals are unable to benefit from them due to the high cost and the difficulties sometimes associated with accessing these medications.

Diet

Some of the antipsychotics such as clozapine (Clozaril), olanzapine (Zyprexa), quetiapine fumerate (Seroquel), and risperidone (Risperdal) can cause weight gain over time. For the individual who has schizophrenia and its multiple associated problems, weight gain can constitute yet one more stressor. Teaching for the client who is at risk for gaining weight must therefore emphasize the importance of being cognizant of and conservative with regard to caloric and fat intake, avoiding a sedentary lifestyle, and increasing physical activity.

Activity

Clients with schizophrenia tend to be tired and lethargic, probably due to multiple factors including the disease process and, possibly, the sedative properties associated with some of the antipsychotics, especially some of the older ones such as chlorpromazine (Thorazine) and thioridazine (Mellaril).

PROFESSIONAL TIP

Refraining from Making Judgments

Sometimes nurses stereotype clients and may make judgments based on their own values, cultural biases, and personal beliefs. Such behavior can adversely affect their work with clients. The nurse's words can have a strong impact on the client, either favorable or unfavorable, even without the nurse's being aware of it. Something as simple as changing the words we use may help the client and family feel less defensive and may open the door for more effective communication. One example of an often-used term that carries negative connotations is *noncompliance*. Ward-Collins (1998) encourages nurses to consider using another term such as *nonadherence*, which does not carry the same degree of negative connotations.

▸ NURSING PROCESS

▸ Assessment

▸ Subjective Data

The client with schizophrenia may be very frightened, confused, and disorganized in thought process. The client may use a nonsensical combination of words that is meaningless to others (**word salad**), talk out loud even when no one is present, or respond to internal stimulation or hallucinations.

▸ Objective Data

The client with schizophrenia may be isolated, withdrawn, and experience great difficulty in any type of social interaction or situation. The client may be very lethargic and not want to do much of anything except stay in bed and sleep. Thus, the client may require a great deal of assistance and encouragement to perform ADL and complete basic hygiene needs.

Nursing diagnoses for the client with schizophrenia may include the following:

Nursing Diagnoses	Planning/Goals	Nursing Interventions
▸ *Disturbed Sensory Perception (Visual, Auditory) related to altered sensory perception*	The client will experience a decrease in the intensity and frequency of symptoms.	Assess for the presence of hallucinations. Assist the client in beginning to exert some control over the hallucinations. Educate the client about ways to decrease the intensity and power of the hallucinations.
▸ *Deficient Knowledge related to medication therapy*	Client will verbalize an understanding of the disorder and the ongoing need for medications.	Educate the client and family about the disorder of schizophrenia. Educate the client and family about the need for antipsychotic medications. Educate the client and family about the importance of continuing the prescribed medication regimen.

Evaluation Each goal must be evaluated to determine how it has been met by the client.

THE CLIENT WITH BIPOLAR DISORDER

Bipolar Disorder (previously known as manic–depressive disorder) is a psychiatric diagnosis characterized by wide fluctuations in **mood** (the way an individual reports feeling, e.g., depressed, elated, happy, sad) and **affect** (the objective or outward manifestation of the way an individual is feeling, e.g., avoids eye contact, smiles occasionally). In addition to having a wide range of both affect and mood, the individual with bipolar disorder may experience fluctuations between depression and **mania** (extremely elevated mood with accompanying agitated behavior). The client with bipolar disorder may experience these fluctuations in mood and affect in varying degrees and over varying time frames. For example, an individual may experience changes in mood and affect every few years, at certain times of the year, every few months, every few weeks, or even every few days. The alterations in mood between depression and mania are often referred to as **cycling**. Individuals who suffer what is known as rapid cycling may experience multiple swings between depression and mania in the same day. There are also several degrees of both depression and mania that the individual can experience. As is the case with depression, an individual can experience mild, moderate, or severe mania. The degrees of mania range on a continuum from **hypomania** (a mild form of mania without significant impairment) to severe or delirious mania (Townsend, 2000).

An individual in the depressed phase of bipolar disorder will manifest the same signs and symptoms as an individual with depression. The client in the manic phase of bipolar disorder may be very irritable and agitated and can be intimidating toward others, both verbally and physically. The client exhibiting manic behavior is often hyperactive, unable to sit down or remain still, and may display a **euphoric** (being elated out of context to the situation) affect and mood. Once in the manic phase of illness, clients will often exhibit behaviors incongruent with their usual personalities. For example, the manic client may dress in a flamboyant and provocative manner; spend money and buy things in a very lavish fashion; and become sexually promiscuous and engage in risky behaviors that would otherwise be out of character. After a while, the client in the manic phase of bipolar disorder can experience a great deal of conflict in social, familial, and personal relationships. It often becomes the responsibility of a significant other or family member to seek professional assistance for the individual. This already difficult situation is compounded by the fact that the client in the manic phase of bipolar disorder is frequently in denial about the illness, does not perceive the erratic behavior as problematic, and enjoys the "high" created by the disorder. As a result, the individual often refuses any type of help, and the family may be required to seek involuntary hospitalization in order to obtain the much-needed treatment.

Medical–Surgical Management

Medical

The severely agitated client in the manic phase of bipolar disorder may need to be secluded and/or restrained in order to protect against self-inflicted injury and/or the risk of injury to others.

Psychotherapy may be helpful to the client experiencing bipolar disorder, but it is not recommended as the only intervention. These clients typically require some type of medication management for the remainder of their lives in order to function adequately.

Pharmacological

The drug of choice for treatment of bipolar disorder is lithium carbonate (Lithonate) (Table 33–11). Lithium is a naturally occurring salt that has proven highly effective for many individuals in managing the severe mood swings associated with bipolar disorder. Lithium is referred to as a "mood stabilizer," meaning that it

---

Table 33–11 MOOD STABILIZER: ANTIMANIC

GENERIC NAME	TRADE NAME	POTENTIAL SIDE EFFECTS	SIGNS AND SYMPTOMS OF TOXICITY
lithium carbonate	Eskalith, Lithane, Lithonate	Abdominal pain, acneiform eruption, anorexia, arrhythmia, bloating, diarrhea, dizziness, drowsiness, EKG changes, fatigue, folliculitis, GI upset, headache, hypothyroidism, impaired memory, irritability, leukocytosis, muscle weakness, nausea, polyuria, seizures, tinnitus, tremors	Ataxia, change in level of orientation, confusion, diarrhea, drowsiness, excessive urination, lack of coordination, muscle weakness, tremors, vomiting

Compiled from Davis's Drug Guide for Nurses *(6th ed.), by J. H. Deglin and A. H. Vallerand, 1999, Philadelphia: F. A. Davis.*

Table 33–12 MOOD STABILIZERS: ANTICONVULSANTS		
GENERIC NAME	**TRADE NAME**	**POTENTIAL SIDE EFFECTS**
carbamazepine	Tegretol	Aganulocytosis, aplastic anemia, ataxia, drowsiness, drug-induced hepatitis, thrombocytopenia
valproic acid	Depakene	Aggression, depression, dizziness, indigestion, hepatotoxicity, leukopenia, nausea, thrombocytopenia, vomiting, weight gain

Data from PDR Nurses Handbook, by G. Spratto and A. Woods, 2001, Albany, NY: Delmar.

helps level or even out the wide mood swings associated with the disorder. However, some individuals either cannot tolerate lithium therapy or become resistant to its therapeutic effectiveness after a period of time. Fortunately, there are some other medications that are often prescribed for clients who cannot take lithium. These include the anticonvulsants valproic acid (Depakene) and carbamazepine (Tegretol) and the anxiolytic/anticonvulsant clonazepam (Klonopin) (Table 33–12).

Lithium has a very narrow range of therapeutic effectiveness. The amount of lithium the individual has available and whether this level is appropriate is measured by a blood test called **serum lithium level**. As a rule of thumb, the acceptable therapeutic range for the serum lithium level is 0.5 to 1.5mEq/L; however, the value may vary slightly depending on the laboratory that is performing the test (Deglin & Vallerand, 1999). A lithium level that is too low will not produce any benefit, and one that is too high may be **toxic**, or poisonous. It is therefore critical that the serum lithium level be obtained every 5 days until the client is stabilized on the medication. Blood should then be drawn at regular intervals, approximately every 12 to 16 weeks, for as long as the client is taking the medication (Bailey, 1998). Prior to initiating lithium therapy, a 24-hour urine creatinine clearance test is done to evaluate the functioning of the kidneys and their ability to adequately excrete the lithium.

Diet

Because lithium is a salt that is chemically similar to sodium chloride (table salt), lithium and sodium com-

CLIENT TEACHING

Lithium

Be sure to instruct each client taking lithium in the following:

- Do not drink alcohol while taking this medication.
- Do not take any other medications, prescribed or OTC, unless authorized by your physician.
- Do not stop taking this medication without authorization from your physician.
- Female clients should utilize a reliable form of contraception while taking this medication. Immediately inform your physician if pregnancy is suspected.
- Drink 2,000 to 3,000 cc of fluid (9–10 glasses) per day.
- Maintain a consistent level of salt in the diet.
- The ability to drive or operate heavy machinery may be impaired while on this medication.
- Serum lithium level must be checked at scheduled intervals throughout therapy.
- Be aware of signs and symptoms of lithium toxicity.

GERONTOLOGICAL CONSIDERATIONS

Creatinine Clearance

Because elders have reduced creatinine clearance, they are at a greater risk for developing toxicity while taking lithium (Andresen, 1998).

pete for absorption at receptor sites. This relationship is inversely proportional; thus, any changes in the body's sodium level will directly affect lithium level. Adequate fluid intake is very important for the client on lithium therapy. It is recommended that the client taking lithium consume a minimum of 2,000 to 3,000 cc of water per day. Due to the stimulating effects of caffeine, clients taking lithium should avoid any beverages containing caffeine.

Activity

The balance of sodium chloride to lithium can also be affected by the client's level of activity. An increase in activity, especially in hot and/or humid conditions when excessive perspiration is likely, can deplete the client's sodium level, thereby causing a drastic increase in lithium level and, potentially, lithium toxicity. A sudden increase in a client's activity level requires close monitoring and replacement of both fluid and electrolytes in order to prevent a sudden increase in the lithium level.

▶ NURSING PROCESS

▶ Assessment

▶ Subjective Data

The client with bipolar disorder may deny having a problem or may view the problem as residing in other people. The client may also be quite loud, flamboyant, and grandiose in verbalizations and manifest very quick and **pressured speech** (rapid, intense speech).

▶ Objective Data

The client may be sleeping very little or not at all and may not be eating or drinking, if in the manic phase. The client may at times be very irritable, agitated, quick to anger, and, possibly, violent. Clients with bipolar disorder often have extreme difficulty in interpersonal and social relationships, as they have no personal boundaries. They may also be very invasive and intrusive in their interactions with others, both verbally and physically.

CLIENT TEACHING

Anticonvulsants

Be sure to instruct each client taking an anticonvulsant medication in the following:

- Do not drink alcohol while taking the medication.
- Do not take any other medications, prescribed or OTC, unless authorized by your physician.
- Take the medication exactly as prescribed.
- Do not stop taking the medication without authorization from your physician.
- Do not stop taking the medication abruptly.
- The medications is contraindicated during pregnancy and lactation. Female clients should advise their physicians immediately if they are either pregnant or planning to become pregnant.
- Carbamazepine (Tegretol) can impair the effectiveness of hormonal forms of contraception. Female clients should practice an alternate form of birth control while on this medication.
- The ability to drive or operate heavy machinery may be impaired while on the medication.
- Laboratory tests monitoring complete blood count (CBC), platelet count, bleeding time, and hepatic functioning must be performed periodically throughout therapy.
- Notify your physician immediately of unexplained fever, sore throat, bleeding, bruising, or petechiae.
- Serum level must be checked at scheduled intervals throughout therapy.

Nursing diagnoses for the client with bipolar disorder may include the following:

Nursing Diagnoses	Planning/Goals	Nursing Interventions
▶ *Disturbed Sleep Pattern related to sensory alterations*	The client will sleep 6 hours per night.	Provide a quiet, peaceful environment.
		Decrease external stimulation and environmental distractions.
		Teach client relaxation exercises.
▶ *Noncompliance (medication and treatment regimen) related to health beliefs*	The client will demonstrate increased compliance with medication and treatment.	Educate the client and family about the disease process and the progression of the illness over time.
		Educate the client and family about prescribed medication, indications for use, dosage, times, and any possible side effects or untoward reactions.
		Educate the client and family about the importance of taking the medication as prescribed.
		Teach the client to continue taking medication and to not miss doses *even if the condition improves dramatically.*

Evaluation Each goal must be evaluated to determine how it has been met by the client.

THE CLIENT REQUIRING SPECIAL CONSIDERATION

Several categories of psychiatric disorders require special attention and consideration on the part of the nurse. These include disorders commonly associated with childhood and adolescence and with individuals who have been violated in some manner, such as via neglect and/or abuse.

THE CLIENT WITH ATTENTION-DEFICIT/HYPERACTIVITY DISORDER

The *DSM-IV* identifies 18 diagnostic criteria for Attention-Deficit/Hyperactivity Disorder (ADHD) that fall under the categories of *inattention, hyperactivity,* and *impulsivity* (APA, 2000). There are three varieties of Attention-Deficit/Hyperactivity Disorder listed in the *DSM-IV*: Attention-Deficit/Hyperactivity Disorder, Predominantly Hyperactive-Impulsive Type; Attention-Deficit/Hyperactivity Disorder, Predominantly Inattentive Type; and Attention-Deficit/Hyperactivity Disorder, Combined Type. The child with ADHD may exhibit one or more of these behaviors in any combination (inattention, hyperactivity, and impulsivity). The problematic behaviors associated with these disorders vary in severity for each individual. Once thought to be a disorder only of childhood, it is now known that ADHD may continue well into adulthood. Individuals with ADHD are extremely sensitive to their environments and surroundings and respond immediately to any type of stimuli or distraction that most individuals would not even notice.

PREDOMINANTLY HYPERACTIVE-IMPULSIVE TYPE

As the name suggests, hyperactivity is considered to be a hallmark feature of Predominantly Hyperactive-Impulsive Type ADHD, which is usually diagnosed in childhood when the symptoms first manifest. The pediatric client with ADHD may be referred for evaluation and treatment by parents or teachers because of impulsive and disruptive behavior in the classroom setting and/or at home. Research indicates that among the children with ADHD, the ratio of males to females ranges anywhere from 4 : 1 to 9 : 1 (APA, 2000). In many cases, there seems to be a familial or possible genetic link, as seen in health histories, which often reveal a parent or immediate family member as having had a similar problem as a child.

PROFESSIONAL TIP

Token-Economy System

A token-economy system is a form of behavior modification used to shape a client's behavior over time. The client receives a "token" (poker chips work well) each time an appropriate or desired behavior is exhibited. In the classroom, the desired behavior might be working 15 minutes on a math assignment; at home, it might be picking up dirty clothes off the bedroom floor. Receiving the token is a form of positive reinforcement for the client and provides immediate gratification. At the end of a designated period of time, the client may "cash in" earned tokens for a prize (game, puzzle) or a special privilege (going to get an ice cream). The cashing in of tokens emphasizes the concept of delayed gratification, which in turn teaches patience.

PREDOMINANTLY INATTENTIVE TYPE

In some children with ADHD predominantly inattentive type, the symptom of hyperactivity is not always present. This is the case in children who have problems primarily with attention span. The inattentive child cannot maintain attention on one task, does not appear to listen when spoken to, and is easily distracted and forgetful.

COMBINED TYPE

As the name suggests, children with ADHD of the combined type exhibit symptoms of hyperactivity, impulsivity, and inattention. The characteristics must typically be exhibited for a period of at least 6 months in order to qualify for the diagnosis.

Medical–Surgical Management

Medical

Counseling and therapy are often recommended to the client and family to assist in managing the child with this disorder. The parents will require assistance in developing an effective behavior-modification program, such as a token-economy system that rewards desired behaviors, to help manage some of the child's problematic behaviors (Glod, 1997).

Pharmacological

The central nervous system (CNS) stimulants, which include methylphenidate hydrochloride (Ritalin), pe-

Table 33–13 CENTRAL NERVOUS SYSTEM STIMULANTS

GENERIC	TRADE NAME	POTENTIAL SIDE EFFECTS
dextroamphetamine	Dexedrine	Anorexia, headache, hyperactivity, hypertension, insomnia, palpitations, physical and psychological dependence, restlessness, tachycardia, tolerance, tremors, urticaria, weight loss
dextroamphetamine/ amphetamine	Adderal	Anorexia, hyperactivity, insomnia, palpitations, physical and psychological dependence, restlessness, tachycardia, tremors
methylphenidate hydrochloride	Ritalin	Anemia, anorexia, hyperactivity, hypertension, insomnia, leukopenia, physical and psychological dependence, restlessness, skin rash, suppression of weight gain, tolerance, tremors
pemoline	Cylert	Anorexia, aplastic anemia, decreased growth, drug-induced hepatitis, insomnia, nausea, physical or psychological dependence, seizures, stomachache, tolerance, weight loss

Compiled from Lippincott's Need-to-know Psychotropic Drug Facts, *by K. P. Bailey, 1998, Philadelphia: Lippincott;* PDR Nurses Handbook, *by G. Spratto and A. Woods, 2001, Albany, NY: Delmar; and "Attention Deficit Hyperactivity Disorder throughout the Lifespan: Diagnosis, Etiology, and Treatment," by C. A. Glod, 1997,* Journal of the American Psychiatric Nurses Association, *3(3), 89–92.*

moline (Cylert), dextroamphetamine (Dexedrine), and, most recently, a combination of both dextroamphetamine and amphetamine (Adderal), is the class of medications usually prescribed to treat ADHD (Glod, 1997) (Table 33–13). As a rule, these medications have the tendency to stimulate an individual and therefore increase activity level often to the point of hyperactivity. When one of the CNS stimulants is given to someone with ADHD, however, it has the opposite effect, or **paradoxical reaction**. Thus, instead of making someone with ADHD more hyperactive, it actually helps calm him. Because most of the symptoms of the child with ADHD, such as hyperactivity and the inability to concentrate and remain on task, are manifested in the classroom, it is in this setting that any improvement will likely first be noted. When a child begins a new medication it is vitally important that the family communicate openly with the child's teacher to ensure close monitoring of the child's response to medication. The child with ADHD who has been hyperactive, unable to stay on task, or complete assignments before receiving medication may now be less disruptive in the classroom and better able to remain on task and complete assignments. In addition, the medication can be a useful adjunct to facilitate the child's ability to develop and strengthen internal mechanisms for improving behavior.

Teaching the client and family about the prescribed medication is very important, as there are some common side effects associated with the CNS stimulants, such as insomnia. To help decrease the risk of insomnia, these medications are usually given in the morning at breakfast, and if more is needed, another dose is given again at lunchtime. In some cases, a late-afternoon dose may be needed after school; however, this decision must be made very cautiously, because the later in the day that the dose is given, the greater the risk of insomnia that night for the child.

The client on CNS stimulants must be monitored for any vocal or motor tics, which might indicate the development of Tourette's syndrome. The CNS stimulant should be discontinued immediately if these symptoms are noted.

Diet

One potential problem associated with the CNS stimulants is that of decreased appetite, which can become serious if the child begins losing weight as a side effect of the medication. In such an instance, the medication may need to be given immediately after a meal to decrease the chance of suppressing the appetite. The family can be educated on the need to adjust the timing and amount of food intake. The child may have to eat larger meals later in the day, when the effects of the medication have worn off, or consume a larger snack in the evening prior to bedtime.

The role and importance of diet in the management of ADHD continues to be highly controversial; however, some data supports the restriction of certain foods as an effective method of managing this disorder. Foods that contain sugar and caffeine are sometimes recommended to be excluded from the diet of the child with ADHD. The theory behind this recommendation is that sugar and caffeine tend to energize and increase any child's activity level, and in the case of some children with ADHD, this effect seems to be even more accentuated. Another controversial issue surrounding the significance of diet is that of food sensitivities and allergies. Food allergies sometimes manifest in symptoms such as irritability and hyperactivity, which may then be confused or misdiagnosed as ADHD.

Activity

The child with ADHD will usually respond best to a highly structured environment, which includes clear

PROFESSIONAL TIP

CNS-Stimulant Abuse

Another consideration often overlooked in terms of the CNS stimulants is the risk for abuse due to the strong addictive potential of these medications. Not only is the client with ADHD at risk for abusing these medications, but sometimes the client "shares" prescribed medication with schoolmates and friends interested in drug experimentation. Another problem that may be encountered is abuse of the prescribed medication by a family member with a substance-abuse problem.

CLIENT TEACHING

CNS Stimulants

For each client taking a CNS-stimulant medication, instruct the client or, if the client is too young to understand or reliably carry out the instructions, the client's caregivers in the following:
- Take the medication only as prescribed.
- Do not take any other medications without physician approval.
- Be alert for decreased appetite and adjust meals and mealtimes accordingly.
- Do not take any doses after 5 P.M. as doing so will increase the risk of insomnia.
- Obtain periodic liver function tests if taking pemoline (Cylert).
- Obtain periodic CBC, platelet count, and differential if taking methylphenidate (Ritalin).
- Limit caffeine intake.

expectations and firm, consistent limits as well as appropriate consequences for unruly and disruptive behaviors. For example, a "time-out" may be used when the child must be temporarily removed from a setting or the environment.

▶ NURSING PROCESS

▶ Assessment

▶ Subjective Data

The child or adolescent with ADHD frequently verbalizes feeling "bad" about being unable to control hyperactive and disruptive behaviors. After numerous negative encounters with teachers and the principal, the child's esteem begins to erode, and he may verbalize feeling like a failure, especially in the classroom. After only a single dose of medication, however, the child sometimes states a noticeable difference in the ability to remain centered and focused.

▶ Objective Data

Although usually described as being hyperactive, unable to concentrate, unable to focus, and unable to remain on task, children with ADHD may sometimes be able to concentrate and remain quite attentive and focused. This usually happens in situations that the child enjoys, and sometimes in situations that are new to the child. It can be quite frustrating for parents to bring in their child for an evaluation or screening, only to have the child not exhibit any of the usual problematic behaviors. The knowledgeable practitioner or evaluator will be aware of what is happening and will obtain the necessary information from the parental report of the child's health history.

Nursing diagnoses for the child with ADHD may include the following:

Nursing Diagnoses	Planning/Goals	Nursing Interventions
▶ *Deficient Knowledge (medications and disease process), related to new diagnosis of disorder and treatment regimen*	The child and parents will verbalize an increased understanding of the disorder. The child and parents will verbalize an understanding about the role medications can play in treatment.	Educate the child and family about the disorder, including signs and symptoms. Educate the child and family about the medication, including indications for use, dosages, when to take the medication, and possible side effects. Educate the child and family about the benefits that can be expected with the particular medication. Emphasize the importance of taking the medication as prescribed.
▶ *Impaired Social Interaction related to unaccepted social behaviors*	The child will demonstrate an increase in appropriate peer interactions.	Explain to the child those behaviors that are expected. Observe the child in social situations with peers. Provide positive reinforcement for demonstration of appropriate behaviors. Immediately intervene when unacceptable behaviors are observed.

Evaluation Each goal must be evaluated to determine how it has been met by the client.

THE CLIENT EXPERIENCING NEGLECT AND/OR ABUSE

There are many types of **neglect** (a situation wherein a basic need of the client is not being provided) and **abuse** (an incident involving some type of violation to the client). Neglect can be quite evident, such as a lack of adequate food, clothing, or shelter, or less tangible, such as emotional neglect or an absence of nurturing. Abuse can be physical, emotional, psychological, financial, or sexual in nature, or any combination of these. Abuse can also take the form of **domestic violence**, which is aggression and violence involving family members. Oftentimes, neglect and abuse go hand in hand.

A client experiencing neglect or abuse is usually dependent on another individual for the meeting of basic care and needs. In many neglectful or abusive situations, the clients are vulnerable individuals such as children, adolescents, or elders. Others who are neglected or abused include individuals with some type of illness or incapacitation. Neglect and abuse can take many shapes and forms, ranging anywhere from mild cases to situations so severe that death is the end result.

ELDER ABUSE AND NEGLECT

Elder abuse became nationally recognized in 1981 after the House Select Committee on Aging issued its landmark report *Elder Abuse: An Examination of a Hidden Problem.* The committee found that elder abuse was simply "alien to the American ideal." Because it is such a difficult concept to come to grips with, even abused elders are reluctant to admit their loved ones have abused them.

The committee defined the following types of elder abuse: physical, passive physical, financial, psychological, sexual, and violation of rights. There is no federal legislation to protect elders from abuse, neglect, or exploitation. Forty-eight states, including the District of Columbia, have laws that offer some form of protection for elders or dependent adults. Adult abuse and protection laws are based on the legal premise that society (represented by the state) has the authority to act in a parental capacity for persons who are unable to care for and protect themselves and thus prevent them from suffering from abuse, neglect, or exploitation by those responsible for their care or from self-abuse (Frisch & Frisch, 1998). The purposes of adult protection service laws are to facilitate the identification of functionally impaired elders who are being abused, neglected, or exploited by others; to encourage expeditious reporting; and to extend protective services while protecting the rights of the abused. In most states, the adult protective services agency (APS) is the principal public agency that is designated to receive and investigate allegations of elder abuse and neglect. In most jurisdictions, the county departments of social services maintain the APS unit.

DOMESTIC VIOLENCE

Domestic violence occurs in relationships where intentional or controlling behavior is perpetrated by persons with whom a survivor has had or currently has an intimate relationship. The syndrome may include actual or threatened physical injury, sexual assault, psychological abuse, economic control, and/or progressive isolation (Medical Education Group Learning Systems, 1995).

Domestic violence occurs in relationships where conflict is the continuous result of power inequality between partners. One of the partners is afraid of and harmed by the other. This should not be confused with domestic strife, which is present in most relationships where neither partner has more power or control than the other and, thus, neither is victim or abuser. Domestic strife can be caused or made worse by many things, such as financial hardship, sexual infidelity, alcohol or other substance use, work pressure, jealousy, and differences in expectations about the relationship (Women's Issues and Social Empowerment [W.I.S.E.], 1997).

As of March 1994, all but five states have laws that, to varying extents, require nurses to report cases of domestic violence. Most states have general laws that mandate health care providers to report incidents when injuries are caused by a weapon (gun, knife, or other deadly weapon). Each state's statute has its definitions of terms, such as what constitutes "violence," "weapon," or "grave" injury, and when health professionals are mandated to report (Hyman, Schillinger, & Lo, 1995). Mandatory reporting laws have relieved some battered clients of the onus of reporting their batterers. However, some battered women are reluctant to seek medical care because they are afraid to admit that their injuries have been caused by abuse. They are ashamed or fear their partners will retaliate against them. They are also reluctant to call the police because they do not believe it will help their situation or they fear retaliation from their partners after the police leave or the abusers are released from jail. When nurses are required to report abused women to law enforcement, they should inform clients of their legal obligations and try to ensure the survivor's safety.

RAPE

Rape is a legal term, not a medical entity. It is a crime of violence. Rapists use sexual violence to dominate and degrade their victims and to express their own anger. It is not an act of lust or an overzealous release of passion done to satisfy a sexual urge (Frisch & Frisch, 1998).

According to Aguilera (1997), there are three basic types of rape: (1) rape by a person known to the survivor, for example, father, former and current friends (date rape), neighbors, partner or separated partner, dissatisfied clients of prostitutes; (2) gang rape; and (3) stranger-to-stranger rape. The latter, which women fear the most, follows an identifiable pattern. Such rapists look for women who are vulnerable, even though they differ on defining who is vulnerable. They might attempt to rape elders, people who are developmentally, physically, or mentally challenged, or intoxicated people. They might look for environments that are easy to enter and relatively safe (e.g., women's bedrooms) and where they will not be interrupted. They often select their victims long before they approach them and repeat the same pattern of victim selection over and over again. All types of rape can be an emotionally terrorizing experience for the survivors.

Medical–Surgical Management

Medical

Planning care for survivors of neglect and abuse and their families will require input from the clients and a survey of their resources to ensure that the targeted care is in line with their expectations and commitments. Nursing interventions directed at primary prevention of interpersonal violence are those that reduce or control the causative factors associated with interpersonal violence and sexual assaults. By identifying families at high risk for abuse, nurses can help the family plan efforts to modify those risk factors.

Health Promotion

Primary prevention includes empowering survivors of abuse by helping them learn to care for and protect themselves from the imposition by others. For example, children can be taught in health care settings or schools those things to do if they are being abused. It also includes changing the family's perceptions of violence as an acceptable mode of conflict resolution (Clark, 1999).

GERONTOLOGICAL CONSIDERATIONS

Abuse of Elders

Due to a loss of independence and a forced reliance on others, elders are vulnerable to being abused in a number of ways. Morris (1998) defines a vulnerable adult "as a person with a physical or mental condition—such as Alzheimer's disease or an infirmity related to aging—that substantially impairs his ability to care for himself." Laws have been developed to protect elders from abusive situations, and agencies such as APS have been established to facilitate this process.

Also included is providing anticipatory guidance. For example, by anticipating the challenges of toddlerhood, nurses can acknowledge that this can be a difficult period for parents and can provide practical advice about constructive discipline. They can teach college freshmen about date rape and to avoid vulnerable situations. They can encourage families with dependent elderly members to use respite care services and day care programs. Such support and anticipatory guidance can enhance the family's and client's competence and diminish the likelihood of violence or abuse.

▶ NURSING PROCESS

▶ Assessment

▶ Subjective Data

There is no comprehensive assessment tool that offers conclusive evidence that neglect, abuse, or violence has occurred. Nurses must act like detectives when assessing clients, given that clients or their abusers will rarely admit to abuse or violence. The nurse must make direct observations of the client and family members. For example, does the child seem afraid of the caregiver? Does the caregiver hit the child? These observations are clues that more probing is necessary.

PROFESSIONAL TIP

Caring for the Abused Client

When questioning clients about the possibility of interpersonal violence or sexual assault, the nurse must quickly develop a rapport and create an environment that indicates that their personal experiences are acceptable topics to discuss. This allows them the opportunity to express their fears and concerns. This can be done by:

- Treating them with dignity and concern,
- Giving priority to them over nonemergency clients,
- Placing them in quiet and private areas,
- Not leaving them alone,
- Speaking quietly and in a nonjudgmental manner,
- Using active and empathic listening skills,
- Not acting shocked or surprised at the details of their experiences,
- Reassuring them that the abuse was not their fault,
- Explaining any delays in treatment,
- Asking permission to call family members, friends, or in the case of rape, rape crisis advocates, and
- Providing information about community resources.

In order to properly assess survivors of abuse, nurses must know the symptoms that are commonly seen in interpersonal violence and sexual assaults and the common characteristics of the abusers. Many of the symptoms are subjective, so the nurse and the health care team must piece together the evidence to ascertain whether interpersonal violence has occurred or clients are at risk for violence. Psychological abuse is a particularly difficult area to assess, as emotional relationships are very culture bound, and words and emotions that may be harmful in one family are not necessarily so in another family.

▶ Objective Data

A more extensive examination is warranted when the history or behavioral symptoms indicate interpersonal abuse. Clients will need to have physical examinations to assess the extent of their injuries and to collect forensic evidence to prove who assaulted them. A traumagram, or body map (a drawing of the front and back of a nude human figure), is generally used to mark the location of all visible injuries. Each state has legally mandated procedures for collecting evidentiary material, and nurses must be sure that the legal "chain of evidence" pertaining to collection of forensic samples is unbroken. The medical record should document the injuries and nursing and medical treatment that may serve as legal evidence of the client's condition.

PROFESSIONAL TIP

Interviewing the Survivor of Abuse or Violence

The type of questions will depend on the type of violence and whether survivors have told you they have been abused. If they have told you they have been abused, you must ask specific questions about the abuse. If they have not, you must ask more open-ended questions to allow them to disclose sensitive information. Generally speaking:

- Inform the client that it is necessary to ask some very personal questions;
- Use language appropriate for the age and developmental level of the survivor;
- Use conversational language or street language;
- Keep questions simple, nonthreatening, and direct;
- Pose questions in a manner that permits brief answers;
- Indicate sensitivity to and acceptance of the client's state of confusion;
- Avoid using leading statements that can distort the client's report;
- Do not criticize the client's family; and
- Do not promise not to report the abuse; indicate that you are required by law to report the abuse.

Nursing diagnoses for the client experiencing neglect or abuse may include the following:

Nursing Diagnoses	Planning/Goals	Nursing Interventions
▶ *Interrupted Family Processes related to neglect*	The client will not experience any further neglect.	Provide support for the client.
		Document the evidence of neglect with which the client presents via written observations, laboratory reports, and/or pictures, if indicated.
		Report the case of neglect to the proper authorities: police, child protective services (CPS), APS, and any others that might be indicated.
▶ *Fear related to abuse*	The client will verbalize being less fearful.	Reassure the client that the client is in a safe place and that you are there to help in any way that you can.
		Provide emotional support to the client in a nonjudgmental manner.
▶ *Risk for Injury related to abusive home life*	The client will not experience any further injury or abuse.	Address the client's safety needs and attempt to assess whether abuse is occurring.
		If you suspect that abuse is occurring notify your supervisor so the proper authorities can be notified (Ladebauche, 1997).

Evaluation Each goal must be evaluated to determine how it has been met by the client.

THE CLIENT WITH AN EATING DISORDER

Eating disorders include anorexia nervosa and bulimia nervosa. **Anorexia nervosa** is characterized by self-imposed starvation by restricting caloric intake and compulsive exercising. **Bulimia nervosa** is character-ized by periods of binge eating of up to 10,000 calories at one time followed by self-induced vomiting and other forms of purging such as laxative and diuretic abuse. In bulimia nervosa, the client's weight is normal or above normal. In anorexia nervosa, body weight is low and keeps getting lower. Almost all clients with these disorders are female and below the age of thirty.

Complications can be serious and include cardiac

abnormalities such as bradycardia, hypotension, arrhythmias, CHF, and cardiovascular collapse; oral and esophageal erosions and dental caries from vomiting; renal abnormalities that affect the kidney's ability to filter urine; skin rashes from malnutrition; and bruising from vomiting.

Clients with anorexia nervosa tend to be high achievers, perfectionists, have a distorted body image in that they see themselves as fat, and are rigid and ritualistic.

Bulimia nervosa occurs more frequently than anorexia nervosa, with clients experiencing a fear of not being able to stop eating. Clients often experience guilt and depression after a binge.

Medical–Surgical Management

Diet

During severe cases, clients may be admitted for enforced feeding, including the placement of a feeding tube or TPN, IV fluid rehydration, and electrolyte replacement. Clients need to be monitored for refeeding complications such as pancreatitis and gastric dilation. Small quantities are given at first and very gradually the amount is increased.

Other Therapies

Treatment is primarily psychiatric, involving the client and family, and is typically done on an outpatient basis.

▶ NURSING PROCESS

▶ Assessment

▶ Subjective Data

Clients with both anorexia nervosa and bulimia nervosa may verbalize feelings of helplessness and being out of control, and may exhibit low self-esteem. They may also have overprotective parents. Clients with anorexia nervosa may also describe bad dreams and cold intolerance.

▶ Objective Data

Assessment of clients with anorexia nervosa may show low weight, usually lost over a short period of time, reluctance to eat with others, moving food around the plate without eating it, hypotension, heart irregularities, and altered thinking patterns.

Objective assessment of clients with bulimia nervosa may show normal weight, tooth erosions and dental caries, puffy face, callused knuckles, broken blood vessels in the eyes and face, reluctance to eat with others, and going to the bathroom immediately after eating.

Laboratory analysis will include a CBC, which may show low Hgb, Hct, and platelets; electrolytes, which may show low sodium, potassium, and chloride; an SMA-22 that shows low protein, phosphate, and magnesium; and elevated BUN.

Nursing diagnoses for a hospitalized client with anorexia nervosa or bulimia nervosa may include the following:

Nursing Diagnoses	Planning/Goals	Nursing Interventions
▶ *Imbalanced Nutrition: Less than body requirements related to psychological restriction of food intake, excessive activity*	The client will demonstrate increased consumption of nutrients as evidenced by weight gain daily and improved laboratory values.	Weigh daily. Monitor calorie intake. Monitor I & O every shift. Administer IV rehydration, electrolyte replacement, and TPN or tube feedings as ordered. Monitor behavior at and around meal time, such as going to the bathroom right after eating. Monitor exercise patterns.
▶ *High Risk for Deficient Fluid Volume related to inadequate intake of liquids, self-induced vomiting, laxative and diuretic use*	The client's intake and output will be approximately equal by the fourth hospital day. The client's electrolytes will be within normal limits, by the third hospital day. The client's fluid intake will be at least 2000 mL per day.	Monitor I & O every shift and bowel movements for diarrhea (a sign of continued laxative abuse). Monitor laboratory reports for electrolyte levels as ordered. Administer IV fluid and electrolyte replacement as ordered.
▶ *Ineffective Coping (Individual) related to maturational crisis and attempting to control environment*	The client will verbalize feelings regarding disease process and hospitalization, by discharge. The client will identify current coping strategies, by discharge. The client will identify personal strengths, by discharge.	Provide opportunities for the client to express feelings regarding hospitalization. Encourage client to identify coping mechanisms and strengths. Give positive feedback regarding identified personal strengths.

Evaluation Each goal must be evaluated to determine how it has been met by the client.

SUMMARY

- The components of a therapeutic nurse–client relationship include trust, rapport, respect, genuineness, and empathy.
- An individual's anxiety level may range anywhere from mild to panic level.
- The nurse often encounters clients and/or family members who are angry, aggressive, homicidal, and/or suicidal in the midst of a crisis situation.
- The depressed individual must be evaluated for risk of suicide.
- The individual with schizophrenia may be out of touch with reality and influenced by delusions and/or hallucinations.
- Individuals with bipolar disorder may experience wide mood swings ranging from depression to mania.
- Neglect and abuse can occur among any age group.
- Anorexia nervosa and bulimia nervosa are psychological disorders affecting mostly women. Severe nutritional imbalances can occur leading to serious effects on the cardiovascular system.

Review Questions

1. The client who is experiencing severe or panic level anxiety should:

    a. be left alone to calm down.
    b. be taught new information.
    c. never be left alone.
    d. be given an antidepressant immediately.

2. Two of the newest antidepressants are:

    a. pemoline (Cylert) and methylphenidate (Ritalin).
    b. mirtazapine (Remeron) and venlafaxine (Effexor).
    c. quetiapine (Seroquel) and olanzapine (Zyprexa).
    d. alprazolam (Xanax) and lorazepam (Ativan).

3. Clients receiving MAOIs must avoid foods containing which of the following?

    a. Thiamine
    b. Tyramine
    c. Tryptophan
    d. Thorazine

4. A nurse who is aware of a client's plan to kill someone else should do which of the following?

    a. Nothing; it is not her responsibility.
    b. Contact the physician and alert the proper authorities.

c. Discourage the client from following through with the plan.
d. Continue preparing the client for discharge per orders in the chart.

5. The client who is contemplating suicide may demonstrate which of the following behaviors?

    a. Giving away prized personal possessions
    b. Buying new personal items
    c. Purchasing an expensive item
    d. Purchasing an inexpensive item

6. Schizophrenia is usually treated with which of the following classification of medications?

    a. Antidepressants
    b. Antipsychotics
    c. Mood stabilizers
    d. CNS stimulants

7. Signs and symptoms of schizophrenia include:

    a. hyperactivity and decreased concentration.
    b. crying spells and decreased appetite.
    c. compulsive rituals.
    d. hallucinations and/or delusions.

8. Which of the following is the drug of choice for treating bipolar disorder?

    a. Librium
    b. Valium
    c. Thorazine
    d. Lithium

9. A client with bipolar disorder may manifest which of the following symptoms?

    a. Mood fluctuations alternating between mania and depression
    b. An addiction to drugs and alcohol
    c. Overwhelming feelings of fear and dread
    d. An over-exaggeration of physical symptoms

10. The child with ADHD will probably be prescribed a medication from which of the following classifications?

    a. Antipsychotics
    b. Antianxiety medications
    c. Mood stabilizers
    d. CNS stimulants

11. The client experiencing abuse will:

    a. always tell the truth about what is happening.
    b. often lie about what is happening in order to protect the abuser.
    c. always contact the authorities.
    d. never withhold significant information from health care providers.

Critical Thinking Questions

1. Consider your feelings after treating a client believed to be suffering from domestic abuse. What was your reaction to this client? Were you able to respond appropriately? How would you have felt if the client refused your attempts to help remove her from the abusive situation?

2. What actions would you take if you felt a co-worker was suffering from depression?

WEB FLASH!

- What resources can you find on the Web to help clients or families cope with schizophrenia?
- Can you find more information on the uses of ECT by searching the Web using *electroconvulsive therapy* as a key word?
- What research related to new drug treatments and psychiatric disorders can you find by searching the Web?

NURSING CARE OF THE CLIENT: SUBSTANCE ABUSE

MAKING THE CONNECTION

Refer to the following chapters to increase your understanding of substance abuse:

- **Chapter 3, Legal Responsibilities**
- **Chapter 4, Ethical Responsibilities**
- **Chapter 7, Wellness Concepts**
- **Chapter 12, Health Assessment**

- **Chapter 18, Nursing Care of the Client: Respiratory System**
- **Chapter 28, Nursing Care of the Client: Gastrointestinal System**
- **Chapter 35, Nursing Care of the Older Client**

LEARNING OBJECTIVES

Upon completion of this chapter, you should be able to:
- *Define key terms.*
- *Differentiate among dependence, abuse, and intoxication.*
- *Describe issues related to drug testing.*
- *Discuss substances frequently abused.*
- *Use assessment skills to identify possible substance abuse.*
- *Describe nursing interventions in working with substance abusers.*
- *Describe stages of alcoholism and the impact on the individual, family, and society.*
- *Discuss medications frequently used in the treatment of substance abuse.*
- *Describe an impaired nurse.*
- *Identify goals of programs for impaired nurses.*

KEY TERMS

abuse	misuse
addiction	opisthotonos
behavioral tolerance	relapse
codependent	reverse tolerance
confabulation	substance
cross-tolerance	synthesiasis
dependence	teratogenic
detoxification	tolerance
hallucination	withdrawal
intoxication	
Johnsonian intervention	

INTRODUCTION

Substance use has taken place for many centuries. It is not a new problem for society. A **substance** is a drug, legal or illegal, that may cause physical or mental impairment. With the great increase in world population there are more people involved in substance abuse. Today's speed of travel and communication has facilitated the broad distribution of substances.

Many street drugs are "cut" (mixed) with substances that should not be consumed, such as talcum powder, rodent exterminating powder, or even strychnine. The purity (strength) of the drug is then not known and overdose easily occurs. Fatalities can occur from the substance with which the drug is cut.

In the United States, substance disorders affect males and females, all ethnic groups, and persons of all levels of education and income. From the newborn to the elderly, all ages can be affected.

Substance disorders may be classified as intoxication, abuse, or dependence (addiction); definitions are based on the criteria presented in the American Psychiatric Association's *Diagnostic and Statistical Manual of Mental Disorders,* fourth edition (*DSM-IV*). The reversible effect on the central nervous system (CNS) soon after the use of a substance is termed **intoxication**. **Abuse** is the misuse, excessive, or improper use of a substance, the abstinence of which does not cause withdrawal symptoms. **Dependence (addiction)** is reliance on a substance to such a degree that abstinence causes functional impairment, physical withdrawal symptoms, and/or a psychological craving for the substance. The person has no control over use of the substance and feels pleasure only when using the substance. Table 34–1 shows diagnostic criteria for abuse and dependence.

HISTORICAL PERSPECTIVES

Nearly 6,500 years ago, ancient Egyptians used opium for pain relief. Later they used it for recreation when they discovered it provided anxiety relief, a pleasurable experience, and an escape from reality. Drug problems began in the United States with the Civil War in 1861. Wounded soldiers were given their own supply of morphine. Its use was uncontrolled. Dependence-producing drugs such as cocaine, heroin, and morphine were given freely to clients by doctors. Patent medicines, many containing alcohol, cocaine, and heroin, were said to cure almost any ailment a person might have.

The Pure Food and Drug Act of 1906, requiring accurate labeling of drugs, was the first measure designed to control drugs in the United States. In 1914, The Harrison Act made the use of certain narcotics illegal. Physicians then became unwilling to give individuals these drugs and drug use actually increased as those persons already using drugs turned to illegal markets for a supply. In 1919 Congress passed the 19th Amendment to the Constitution declaring the making and selling of alcohol illegal. Prohibition lasted until 1933 when the 19th Amendment was finally repealed because it had not controlled drunkenness or alcoholism as it was intended.

Many medical, law enforcement, and legislative efforts in the 1930s slowed narcotic abuse and addiction. Then marijuana flooded the market. The Marijuana Tax Act of 1937 was intended to raise revenue, identify the persons involved in its use, and discourage the recreational use of marijuana. Marijuana was removed in 1941 from the official list of drugs United States physicians could prescribe. World War II disrupted supply routes of drugs from Asia and Europe, and large-scale drug use disappeared in the United States.

Table 34–1 DIAGNOSTIC CRITERIA FOR SUBSTANCE ABUSE AND DEPENDENCE

SUBSTANCE DEPENDENCE

A maladaptive pattern of substance use, leading to clinically significant impairment or distress, as manifested by three (or more) of the following, occurring at any time in the same 12-month period:

(1) tolerance, as defined by either of the following:

    (a) a need for markedly increased amounts of the substance to achieve intoxication or desired effect

    (b) markedly diminished effect with continued use of the same amount of the substance

(2) withdrawal, as manifested by either of the following:

    (a) the characteristic withdrawal syndrome for the substance (refer to Criteria A and B of the criteria sets for Withdrawal from the specific substances)

    (b) the same (or a closely related) substance is taken to relieve or avoid withdrawal symptoms

(3) the substance is often taken in larger amounts or over a longer period than was intended

(4) there is a persistent desire or unsuccessful efforts to cut down or control substance use

(5) a great deal of time is spent in activities necessary to obtain the substance (e.g., visiting multiple doctors or driving long distances), use the substance (e.g., chain-smoking), or recover from its effects

(6) important social, occupational, or recreational activities are given up or reduced because of substance use

(7) the substance use is continued despite knowledge of having a persistent or recurrent physical or psychological problem that is likely to have been caused or exacerbated by the substance (e.g., current cocaine use despite recognition of cocaine-induced depression, or continued drinking despite recognition that an ulcer was made worse by alcohol consumption)

SUBSTANCE ABUSE

A. A maladaptive pattern of substance use leading to clinically significant impairment or distress, as manifested by one (or more) of the following, occurring within a 12-month period:

    (1) recurrent substance use resulting in a failure to fulfill major role obligations at work, school, or home (e.g., repeated absences or poor work performance related to substance use; substance-related absences, suspensions, or expulsions from school; neglect of children or household)

    (2) recurrent substance use in situations in which it is physically hazardous (e.g., driving an automobile or operating a machine when impaired by substance use)

    (3) recurrent substance-related legal problems (e.g., arrests for substance-related disorderly conduct)

    (4) continued substance use despite having persistent or recurrent social or interpersonal problems caused, or exacerbated by the effects of the substance (e.g., arguments with spouse about consequences of intoxication, physical fights)

B. The symptoms have never met the criteria for Substance Dependence for this class of substance.

Reprinted with permission from the Diagnostic and Statistical Manual of Mental Disorders, Fourth Edition. *Copyright 2000 American Psychiatric Association.*

The 1960s saw drug use move into the mainstream of life in the United States. Drugs were used as a form of relaxation. The Comprehensive Drug Abuse Prevention and Control Act was passed in 1970; it is commonly referred to as the Controlled Substance Act. This act regulates the manufacture, distribution, and dispensing of controlled substances. To enforce the provisions of this act, the Drug Enforcement Administration (DEA) was organized.

There are five classifications or schedules of controlled substances. The categories are based on the drugs' potential to cause psychological and/or physical dependence, and also on their potential for abuse. Table 34–2 identifies and explains the five schedules.

In the 1980s, marijuana and other drug use declined, especially among high school students. Cocaine and its derivative, crack, were the new drugs of choice. The increased supply hooked many people into heavy drug use. The 1990s have seen an increase in the use of all substances.

FACTORS RELATED TO SUBSTANCE ABUSE

There are many factors that interact to influence a person's substance abuse. Many people who have stopped substance abuse **relapse** (return to a previous behavior or condition) because of these same factors.

Table 34–2	SCHEDULES OF CONTROLLED SUBSTANCES
Schedule I (C-I)	High abuse and dependence potential. No accepted medical use in the United States. Includes heroin, mescaline, LSD, marijuana, and other hallucinogens and certain opiates. Can be obtained legally for limited research programs.
Schedule II (C-II)	High abuse and dependence potential. Have currently accepted medical use. Includes narcotics, barbiturates, and amphetamines. Obtained only with physician's prescription, nonrefillable.
Schedule III (C-III)	Less abuse potential, moderate dependence likely. Includes nonbarbiturate sedatives and some narcotics in limited doses. Prescription refills good for 6 months. Fewer controls than for Schedule II.
Schedule IV (C-IV)	Even less abuse potential, limited dependence likely. Includes some sedatives and antianxiety agents and nonnarcotic analgesics.
Schedule V (C-V)	Limited abuse potential. Includes cough medicines containing codeine and antidiarrheals. May be sold over-the-counter in pharmacies to persons over 18 years old. A record is kept of the buyer's name.

These factors may be categorized as individual, family, lifestyle, environmental, and developmental.

Individual Factors

Genetic factors are being researched as a possible reason for a person's susceptibility to substance abuse. According to Santomier and Hogan (1991), research has produced some evidence to suggest the presence of an abnormal chromosome in addicted individuals. This does not guarantee addiction but may predispose the person to addiction.

Other research suggests that variations in the intensity of the flow of neurotransmitters may cause certain individuals to be more susceptible to addiction. The personality traits of sensation seeking and being impulsive may make it easier for the person to experiment with substances.

Family Patterns

Substance abuse, especially in the adolescent, seems to be related to family relationships. Close family relationships, with the parents involved in their children's activities, appear to discourage substance abuse. Families with positive relationships between parents and children generally have less use of illicit drugs. Parent-child interactions that show a lack of closeness, lack of involvement in the children's activities, lack of or inconsistent discipline, and low aspirations for the children's education contribute to the prediction of substance abuse by the children.

Families of adolescent substance abusers generally have negative communication patterns. That is, there is a lack of praise and a great deal of blaming and criticism. Often there are unreal expectations of the children by the parents, inconsistent or unclear behavioral limits, and a pattern of self-medication by family members.

Lifestyle

All dimensions of a person's life that influence how that person lives are termed lifestyle. First is the physical dimension which includes food, clothing, shelter, and health care. The second is the social dimension, which includes friends, organizations, and activities with others. Third is the intellectual/emotional dimension, including education, parental support of education, self-esteem, and how the individual is treated by others. The fourth dimension is spiritual and includes a belief in a "higher being," caring and compassion for others, and being in touch with the inner self. Substance use, abuse, or dependence may be the coping mechanism used by an individual who has problems in any dimension of lifestyle.

Environmental Factors

There are many environmental factors that may encourage or predispose an individual to substance abuse. The social environment in which persons find themselves, the groups, clubs, gangs, sororities, fraternities, and other organizations influence the acceptance or rejection of substance abuse. The stresses in a person's life, including accidents, disabilities, illnesses, stressful family relations, frequent job changes, divorce, death, or precarious financial conditions may be too much for that person to handle. The maladaptive coping of substance abuse offers temporary relief. Because the symptoms of the stressors are reduced, substance abuse is reinforced.

Advertising can influence people in subtle ways to become involved in substance use and abuse. Landau (1995) describes how use of Camel cigarettes by the 18 to 24-year-old age group soared when the character Joe Camel was introduced in advertising promotions in 1988. It was "cool" to be associated with Joe Camel. Other advertising connects caffeine, nicotine, or alcohol with success, sexuality, and power.

Social traditions, especially in the use of alcohol, may open the door for abuse in certain individuals. Some examples of these social traditions include having wine with meals, making toasts at weddings and other celebrations, serving "holiday cheer," and going to "happy hour." For some individuals, these situations may predispose them to alcohol abuse or dependence.

Peer activities, especially during adolescence, may result in substance abuse. Even adults often feel they must go along with certain activities, such as drinks after work or cocktail hour, to get ahead in their career.

Some occupations, like health care, seem to be more associated with substance problems than others. Physicians and nurses, particularly, have access to many substances of abuse.

Developmental Factors

Many individuals have not had good role models in their life. They have not learned to identify with others and do not understand that their behavior affects others. Not learning the skills and attitudes of problem solving leaves the individual unable to apply personal resources to situations, and escape seems the only answer. Substances provide that escape.

Learning the intrapersonal skills of self-discipline, self-control, and self-assessment helps the individual to cope with tension and stress. These skills also work to prevent dishonesty with self, inability to defer gratification, and low self-esteem. A lack of interpersonal skills results in dishonesty with others, resistance to feedback, and inability to share feelings and give or accept help. Not learning to take responsibility or adapt one's behavior to a situation results in irresponsibility, not accepting the consequences of behavior, and seeing oneself as a victim of circumstances. Individuals who do not view themselves as empowered may choose substance use as a means of gratification.

PREVENTION

Prevention of substance abuse must be a proactive process to empower people to constructively confront stressful situations in their lives in adaptive ways. There are three levels of prevention. Primary prevention focuses on preventing the initial use or preventing further uses that may lead to abuse or dependence. This is usually aimed at school-age children. Children need to hear the message that drugs are not good for them. Education about substances and their effects must also emphasize personal, social, and health risks. Children need role models to teach them how to cope with life without drugs, to resist social and peer pressure, and to make effective decisions.

Secondary prevention focuses on preventing ongoing use from becoming a situation of abuse or dependence. If abuse is already evident, the focus is to return the client to a state of abstinence or at least reduced use.

Tertiary prevention focuses on returning the client to a drug-free state. If this is not possible, the goal is then to prevent physical and psychosocial problems from getting worse.

DIAGNOSTIC TESTING

Clients who have a problem with substance abuse or dependence often have abnormal liver function tests and electrolyte levels. Diagnostic criteria for specific substance-related disorders can be found in DSM-IV.

Tests may be done with either a blood or urine specimen. A positive test indicates only that the person has been exposed to the substance. It does not indicate abuse, addiction, or intoxication (except alcohol). Positive screening tests should be confirmed by a more specific test using a different process. Drugs for which tests can be done include alcohol, benzodiazepines, barbiturates, cocaine, crack, amphetamines, opiates, synthetic narcotic analgesics, cannabis, and PCP.

Urine is usually the body fluid tested because it is easily obtained and tested. When obtaining a urine specimen for drug screening, the client should be observed so as to prevent adulteration of the specimen by the client, such as substituting another person's drug-free urine. A "chain of custody" is maintained by having each person who handles the specimen sign an attached paper until the specimen has been tested.

Detection of a substance depends on the amount used and the time since last used. Most substances are detectable for less than 7 days. Chronic marijuana use, however, may be detected for up to 30 days. Cocaine, barbiturates, amphetamines, and opiates are detectable for less than 2 days and alcohol less than 1 day. A false negative may result if the client's drug level falls below the threshold of sensitivity for the test.

Positive results for reasons other than substance abuse can occur. This is called a false positive. Poppy seeds may give a positive result for opiates for up to 60 hours after ingestion. Using a Vicks® Inhaler or over-the-counter diet aids may give a positive result for amphetamines. The client should be asked about the use of these items.

Breath specimens can be used to determine alcohol levels. Law enforcement officials do this with the breathalyzer tests. If hair is not cut, hair analysis can detect substance use for up to a year after the person has used a drug for only 2 or 3 days. Testing meconium (first stools) from a newborn can detect illicit drug use by the mother during pregnancy.

TREATMENT/RECOVERY

Treatment depends on many factors, including the amount and frequency of substance use, age, health, diet, and overall lifestyle of the individual. Infection from the use of unsterile needles and/or tissue or organ damage caused by the substance used, such as lung damage from smoking crack or marijuana or using inhalants, will also require treatment.

Recovery requires abstinence along with intrapersonal and interpersonal changes. Most individuals need professional treatment and participation in a self-help program. Daley, Moss, and Campbell (1993) describe four areas of recovery: physical recovery, psychological and behavioral recovery, social and family recovery, and spiritual recovery.

Physical recovery means eliminating the substance from the body. This is termed **detoxification**. If the client cannot stop using the substance or if withdrawal symptoms are present, admission to a detoxification unit is usually necessary. After detoxification, treatment must focus on restoring the client's physical health and dealing with the cravings for the substance now removed from the client's body. It helps if environmental cues such as drug paraphernalia and alcohol bottles or cans are removed.

Psychological and behavioral recovery becomes evident when the client no longer denies the problem and accepts the inability to consistently control the substance abuse. The client will have developed a desire for abstinence and accepted the need for long-term recovery and support. Emotional stability will be restored when the client learns to cope with uncomfortable emotional states without the use of the abused substance.

Social and family recovery occurs when the client no longer denies the impact on the family and makes amends to family members and significant others who have been negatively affected by the substance abuse. The client works to improve family relationships and develops a recovery support system. Also, the client learns to resist social pressures to use alcohol or other drugs and participates in healthy leisure-time activities. The client's family should also attend a program for recovery. If a client returns to a dysfunctional family, it may be difficult for the client to maintain recovery.

Spiritual recovery is attained when the client has resolved the feelings of guilt and shame and developed a meaning for life and a relationship with a higher power.

SUBSTANCE USE PATTERNS

Patterns of substance use have changed throughout the years. Coffee (caffeine) and cigarettes (nicotine) are legal in our society and widely used. While many people still drink coffee, more and more are using decaffeinated coffee. Cigarette use has decreased in the older population as the addictive nature and negative effects of nicotine have become more evident. However, cigarette use has increased in the adolescent population.

The substance of choice is alcohol. It is legal and easily obtained. Many high school seniors have been drunk and some are already regular drinkers. There are still more alcoholic men than women, but the number of identified women alcoholics is increasing.

Elderly persons are more commonly addicted to prescription medications, especially minor tranquilizers and sleeping pills. Alcohol may be used by the elderly to soothe feelings of isolation and loneliness. Depression and paranoia may be misidentified as senility rather than a problem with alcohol.

Moderate consumption of alcohol may have been influenced by Mothers Against Drunk Driving (MADD) and Students Against Drunk Driving (SADD). Laws that make bars and individuals liable if they let guests leave and drive while drunk, and famous people like Betty Ford and Liza Minelli sharing with the public their illness and recovery, are other influences.

Johnston, O'Malley, and Bachman (1998) report on the ongoing study of illicit drug use among 8th-, 10th-, and 12th-grade students, which shows a decline in use. This is the second year of decline for 8th graders and the first year of decline for 10th and 12th graders.

CNS DEPRESSANTS

Central nervous system depressants usually decrease the heart and respiratory rates as well as voluntary muscle responses. Substances in this category include alcohol, benzodiazepines, and cannabis.

ALCOHOL

Low doses of alcohol depress areas of the brain that are inhibitory, causing diminished self-control and

Table 34–3 ALCOHOL CONTENT IN SELECTED BEVERAGES		
BEVERAGE	**PERCENT ALCOHOL**	**EQUIVALENT AMOUNTS**
Beer	4	12 ounces
Wine cooler	4	12 ounces
Wine	14	4 ounces
Hard liquor	40	1½ ounces

PROFESSIONAL TIP

Alcohol Use

According to the National Institute on Alcohol Abuse and Alcoholism (NIAAA) (1999b), 32% of all traffic crash fatalities were alcohol-related. The estimated cost of alcohol abuse for 1995 is $166.5 million (NIAAA, 1999c).

impaired judgment. Continued alcohol ingestion may cause unconsciousness and even death.

The active ingredient in alcoholic beverages is ethanol. Depending on the alcoholic beverage consumed, varying amounts of ethanol are ingested. It is metabolized at an average rate of 10 mL/hr. Table 34–3 shows the alcohol content in some beverages.

One ounce of alcohol provides 200 Kcal but no other nutrients. It is not converted to glycogen. The blood alcohol level depends on the size of the person, the amount ingested, and the time since ingestion. Most states have set the legal limit for blood alcohol while driving a motor vehicle at 100 mg/dL (0.1%), but some have reduced it to 0.08%.

Incidence

Several national surveys have found that approximately two-thirds of the population have more than an occasional drink. Men are likely to drink more frequently and in greater quantity than women. The vast majority of individuals with an alcohol problem are blue- or white-collar men and women. Some alcoholics drink little or nothing in public or with friends. They are "at home" or "hidden" alcoholics and are more likely to be women. It often takes a family quite awhile to realize that one of its members has an alcohol problem.

The individual with an alcohol problem often learns **behavioral tolerance**, a compensatory adjustment made by an individual under the influence of a particular substance. The person under the influence of alcohol learns how to compensate for the deterioration of motor performance and speech.

Signs and Symptoms

The ingestion of alcohol causes a feeling of euphoria, relaxation of skeletal muscles, changes in mental activity such as altered judgment, and reduced self-control. It has a diuretic effect that, in heavy drinkers, may cause increased loss of electrolytes, especially potassium, magnesium, and zinc. An increased level of alcohol depresses the cardiovascular and respiratory systems and produces a toxic effect on the intestinal mucosa, resulting in decreased absorption of thiamine,

folic acid, and vitamin B_{12}. Excess long-term consumption of alcohol often results in a severe lack of nutrient intake.

Psychosocial aspects include memory blackouts, secretive drinking, rationalization of drinking behavior, trouble with family and employer, loss of outside interests, neglect of food intake, impaired thinking, and moral deterioration. **Confabulation**, making up information to fill in memory gaps, is used by individuals abusing or depending on alcohol. Alcohol may be detected in the blood for 6 to 10 hours.

Potential for Addiction

The potential for addiction is high. Alcohol is not a scheduled or controlled drug.

Associated Problems/Disorders

Excessive and prolonged alcohol intake can affect numerous body systems.

Liver Deterioration

Chronic alcohol abuse causes three distinct diseases of the liver. They are fatty liver, an accumulation of triglycerides in the liver caused by obesity, excessive alcohol consumption, and certain drugs; alcoholic hepatitis, an acute toxic liver injury from excess alcohol consumption; and cirrhosis, a chronic degenerative liver disease that can be caused by alcohol consumption. Fatty liver is reversible, but alcoholic hepatitis and cirrhosis are not. Liver cells will not function once the scar tissue of cirrhosis develops. In 1995, 88.7% of deaths from cirrhosis of the liver were related to alcohol consumption (NIAAA, 1999a). Esophageal varices are associated with cirrhosis and could cause death if they bleed.

Gastrointestinal Disturbances

Alcohol damages the lining of the stomach and esophagus by irritating the mucosa and causing inflammation or ulcer formation. Aspirin with alcohol can result in greater irritation and bleeding in the gastrointestinal (GI) tract. Gastric pain, vomiting, and diarrhea are common in alcohol abuse and are often what brings the individual to the health care system.

Pancreatitis

An alcoholic has a higher risk of developing pancreatitis than an abstainer. Severe pancreatitis can result in death.

Wernicke's Encephalopathy

This inflammatory hemorrhagic and degenerative condition of the brain is caused by a thiamine deficiency. It is characterized by delirium, memory loss, unsteady gait, a sense of apprehension, and an altered level of consciousness. Thiamine intake improves the situation.

Korsakoff's Psychosis

Disorientation, amnesia, insomnia, hallucinations, and peripheral neuropathologies characterize this psychosis. Both thiamine and B_{12} deficiencies contribute to the degeneration of the brain and peripheral nervous system. Frequently, there is bilateral foot drop and pain over the long nerves. Thiamine and B_{12} intake may improve the situation.

Cardiovascular Disturbances

Moderate amounts of alcohol cause cutaneous vasodilation (flushed skin). This causes rapid heat loss, and the core temperature may drop to a dangerous level. Blood pressure decreases with intoxicating doses of alcohol. There may be irregularities in cardiac rhythm. Hematologic alterations such as bone marrow depression, anemia, leukopenia, or thrombocytopenia may also occur.

Fetal Alcohol Syndrome

Fetal alcohol syndrome is caused by the **teratogenic** (causing abnormal development of the embryo) effects of alcohol related to the amount of alcohol ingested and the stage of pregnancy when the alcohol is ingested. Even a small amount of alcohol can be detrimental and have lifelong consequences for the infant. For a diagnosis of FAS, the infant must meet certain criteria. Table 34–4 gives these criteria.

If only some of the FAS criteria are met, it is called fetal alcohol effects (FAE). The only treatment for FAS or FAE is prevention. Women who are pregnant or are trying to get pregnant should abstain from alcohol consumption.

Withdrawal

Withdrawal refers to the symptoms produced when a substance on which an individual has dependence is no longer used by that individual. Alcohol withdrawal syndrome (AWS) appears when the blood alcohol concentration of the alcoholic decreases. The onset of symptoms usually occurs 6 to 12 hours after drinking stops and may last up to 8 days. Chronologically, how long the drinking has occurred and the amount of alcohol consistently consumed are factors in the severity of the withdrawal symptoms. Figure 34-1 shows alcohol withdrawal patterns.

Alcohol withdrawal occurs in three stages:

- Stage 1 (minor withdrawal) includes restlessness, anxiety, sleeping problems, agitation, and tremors; other signs include low-grade fever, tachycardia, diaphoresis, and hypertension.
- Stage 2 (major withdrawal) includes stage 1 signs and symptoms plus visual and auditory hallucinations, whole-body tremors, pulse greater than 100, diastolic BP greater than 100, pronounced diaphoresis, and possibly vomiting.
- Stage 3 (delirium tremens) includes a temperature over 37.8°C (100°F); disorientation to time, place, and person; global confusion; and inability to recognize familiar objects or persons. This is a medical emergency with a mortality rate of 2% to 5% (National Institute on Drug Abuse [NIDA], 1997).

If alcohol abuse continues, symptoms of subsequent withdrawals are generally more severe. It is recommended that withdrawal be medically monitored to decrease the chance of fatality.

Table 34–4 INFANT CRITERIA FOR FETAL ALCOHOL SYNDROME

- Prenatal and/or postnatal growth retardation (weight, length, or head circumference below the 10th percentile)
- CNS involvement (signs of neurologic abnormality, developmental delay, or intellectual impairment)
- Craniofacial anomalies, at least two of the following (microcephaly or head circumference below 3rd percentile, microopthalmia or short palpebral fissure, poorly developed philtrum, thin upper lip, or flattening of maxillary area)

Figure 34-1 Alcohol Withdrawal Patterns

Treatment/Rehabilitation

Many treatment programs are based in hospital or residential treatment centers. These are generally called inpatient programs and last 30 days. Many insurance companies are encouraging clients to participate in lower-cost outpatient programs. Currently, there is no evidence that inpatient programs are more effective than outpatient programs.

Many outpatient programs have both day and evening sessions so clients can maintain their usual occupations. The programs usually consist of a 4-week intensive session with follow-up sessions for 6 to 24 months. The first part of either type of treatment program is detoxification.

Detoxification

The goal of detoxification (DETOX) is to halt or control the neuronal overactivity that occurs when the alcohol level is reduced or alcohol is no longer present in the client's body. This is done by substituting a pharmacologically similar drug and gradually reducing the dose given. The benzodiazepine drugs, chlordiazepoxide (Librium), diazepam (Valium), lorazepam (Ativan), and clorazepate dipotassium (Tranxene), are the most commonly used.

During DETOX, other problems such as malnutrition, vitamin deficiencies (B vitamins, especially thiamine), dehydration, and potassium and magnesium deficiencies must also be treated. A client with hypoglycemia should be given thiamine before administering dextrose to prevent Wernicke's encephalopathy. Ignoring these problems complicates the management of detoxification.

Psychologic Intervention

The classic psychologic intervention technique was originally described by Johnson (1973). Although several modifications have been published and used since then, the technique is still used and is known as **Johnsonian intervention**, which is a confrontational approach to a client with a substance problem that lessens the chance of denial and encourages treatment before the client "hits bottom." The client's significant others (spouse, teenage or older children, 1 or 2 close friends, possibly employer) meet with a professional addiction counselor. This group rehearses so that they may present a united front when confronting the client. They present specific examples of painful or embarrassing behaviors by the client while intoxicated that caused problems and concerns. It is difficult for the client to maintain denial in this situation. Then the group encourages the client to accept professional help. If the client refuses help, each individual of the group must plan to minimize codependent behavior in the future. This technique can also be used for substances other than alcohol. Examples of confrontations may be found in Johnson's books (1973, 1988). Codependency is discussed later in the chapter.

Education

The abuse of or dependence on alcohol is a maladaptive way to cope with life stressors. Learning basic life skills to improve personal competence and provide adaptive coping mechanisms helps the individual resist the use of alcohol.

One adaptive coping mechanism is exercise. Assist clients to become active in an exercise program and encourage them to participate. Exercise helps relieve feelings of stress and promotes feelings of well-being.

Teach clients about the Food Guide Pyramid for an adequate, balanced diet. Most alcoholics have, in the past, received the majority of their calories from alcohol. They must now learn how to maintain health by eating nutritious foods.

The interaction of alcohol with other drugs should also be taught. Some effects can be life-threatening. Table 34–5 shows the interaction of alcohol with some classifications of drugs.

Table 34–5 ALCOHOL INTERACTION WITH OTHER DRUGS

DRUG CLASSIFICATIONS WITH EXAMPLES	INTERACTION	DRUG CLASSIFICATIONS WITH EXAMPLES	INTERACTION
Narcotic analgesics • meperidine hydrochloride (Demerol) • proproxyphene HCl (Darvon) • hydromorphone HCl (Dilaudid)	• Loss of effective breathing (respiratory arrest) • Can be fatal	Antidepressants • imipramine HCl (Tofranil) • desipramine HCl (Pertofrane) • perphenazine and amitriptyline HCl (Triavil)	• Reduces CNS functioning • Chianti wine may cause hypertensive crisis
Nonnarcotic analgesics • aspirin (Bayer Aspirin)	• Stomach and intestinal bleeding	Antihistamines • Most cold remedies • pseudoephedrine HCl and triprolidine HCl (Actifed) • chlorpheniramine maleate and acetominophen (Coricidin)	• Increased calming effect • Person becomes very drowsy • Driving is hazardous
Anticoagulants • warfarin sodium (Coumadin, Panwarfin) • dicumarol	• Increases drugs' ability to stop blood clotting • May cause life-threatening or fatal hemorrhage		

continues

Table 34–5 ALCOHOL INTERACTION WITH OTHER DRUGS *continued*

DRUG CLASSIFICATIONS WITH EXAMPLES	INTERACTION	DRUG CLASSIFICATIONS WITH EXAMPLES	INTERACTION
Antihypertensives • reserpine (Serpasil) • methyldopa (Aldomet)	• Orthostatic hypotension	Antipsychotics • thioridazine HCl (Mellaril) • chlorpromazine HCl (Thorazine)	• Added CNS depression and impairs voluntary movements • Causes respiratory depression • Can be fatal
Antimicrobials • metronidazole (Flagyl) • cefotetan disodium (Cefotan) • rifampin (Rifadin)	• Possible disulfiram-like reaction, nausea, cramps, vomiting, headache, flushing or hepatotoxicity	Sedative-hypnotics • glutethimine (Doriden) • pentobarbital (Nembutal)	• Reduces CNS functioning • Sometimes causes coma and respiratory arrest • Can be fatal
CNS stimulants • Most diet pills • dextroamphetamine sulfate (Dexedrine) • caffeine (No Doz) • methyphenidate HCl (Ritalin)	• May reverse depressant effect of alcohol and give a false sense of security	Antianxiety agents • diazepam (Valium) • chlordiazepoxide (Librium)	• Reduces CNS functioning • Decreased alertness and judgment • Can lead to household and driving accidents
Diuretics • chlorothiazide (Diuril) • furosemide (Lasix)	• May reduce blood pressure and cause dizziness		

Self-Help Groups

Alcoholics Anonymous (AA), begun in 1935, is the model for other self-help groups such as AL-ANON for adults, AL-ATEEN for teenage children, and AL-ATOT for younger children in the family of an alcoholic. The holistic approach of AA to the individual with alcohol problems is described in the Twelve Steps (Table 34–6).

Disulfiram

Disulfiram (Antabuse) may be given to some alcohol abusers as a deterrent to drinking. It inhibits the enzyme needed to metabolize alcohol. Drinking alcohol with disulfiram in the body causes flushing of the neck and face, blurred vision, nausea, vertigo, anxiety, palpitations, tachycardia, and hypotension. Clients must be instructed not to use cologne, mouthwash, aftershave, over-the-counter cold preparations, cough syrups, vitamin-mineral tonics, as well as candies, sauces, and foods made with alcohol. These items will cause the same reaction as if the person took a drink of alcohol.

Therapy should not be started until at least 12 hours after the last drink of alcohol. The effects of disulfiram with alcohol can occur for 6 to 12 days after taking the disulfiram. As with any drug, there are side effects such as drowsiness, fatigue, and impotence. Garlic-like breath occurs frequently and is sometimes used as an indicator of compliance in taking the disulfiram. Disulfiram is contraindicated in clients with cardiovascular disease, hypothyroidism, suicide ideation, and in clients receiving antihypertensives or monoamine oxidase inhibitors (MAOI).

Table 34–6 ALCOHOLICS ANONYMOUS

1. We admitted we were powerless over alcohol—that our lives had become unmanageable.
2. Came to believe that a Power greater than ourselves could restore us to sanity.
3. Made a decision to turn our will and our lives over to the care of God *as we understood Him*.
4. Made a searching and fearless moral inventory of ourselves.
5. Admitted to God, to ourselves and to another human being the exact nature of our wrongs.
6. Were entirely ready to have God remove all these defects of character.
7. Humbly asked Him to remove our shortcomings.
8. Made a list of all persons we had harmed, and became willing to make amends to them all.
9. Made direct amends to such people wherever possible, except when to do so would injure them or others.
10. Continued to take personal inventory and when we were wrong promptly admitted it.
11. Sought through prayer and meditation to improve our conscious contact with God, *as we understood Him*, praying only for knowledge of His will for us and the power to carry that out.
12. Having had a spiritual awakening as the result of these steps, we tried to carry this message to alcoholics, and to practice these principles in all our affairs.

The Twelve Steps are reprinted with permission of Alcoholics Anonymous World Services, Inc. Permission to reprint the Twelve Steps does not mean that A.A. has reviewed or approved the contents of this publication, nor that A.A. agrees with the views expressed herein. A.A. is a program of recovery from alcoholism only—use of the Twelve Steps in connection with programs and activities which are patterned after A.A., but which address other problems, or in any other non-A.A. context, does not imply otherwise.

BENZODIAZEPINES AND OTHER SEDATIVE-HYPNOTICS

With the introduction in 1961 of chlordiazepoxide (Librium), the benzodiazepines have replaced most of the short-acting barbiturates and other nonbarbiturate sedative-hypnotics that were in use prior to that time. Examples of benzodiazepines include diazepam (Valium), secobarbital (Seconal), and paraldehyde (Paral). Street names include roofies, tranks, ludes, barbs.

Incidence

Benzodiazepines are not commonly used as recreational drugs but are widely prescribed and are thus available for abuse. Statistics are not available because some clinicians are still denying that addiction to these drugs occurs. Withdrawal symptoms are subtle and delayed, and the symptoms are not always connected to the benzodiazepines.

Barbiturates and other sedative-hypnotics are more abused but less prescribed. These are available on the illegal market.

Signs and Symptoms

Benzodiazepines in low doses produce drowsiness or sedation. Larger doses produce sleep, but surgical anesthesia cannot be induced. Respirations are not depressed and there is little effect on the cardiovascular system unless extremely large doses are taken. Then a decrease in systolic blood pressure and an increase in heart rate may result. Side effects may include motor incoordination, ataxia, increased hostility or rage, confusion, metallic-like aftertaste, headache, and blurred vision. **Tolerance** (a decreased sensitivity to subsequent doses of the same substance; an increased dose of a substance is needed to produce the same desired effect) to other benzodiazepines and **cross-tolerance** (a decreased sensitivity to other substances in the same category) to other CNS depressants occur with chronic use.

Barbiturates depress all areas of the CNS, some selectively according to the dosage. They do not reduce pain. Respirations are depressed but not significantly when therapeutic doses are taken. When a barbiturate is given to a client in pain, excitement rather than sedation may occur. Side effects may include drowsiness, residual effects on motor skills, and especially in the elderly, excitement, irritability, or delirium. An overdose of barbiturates causes decreased respirations, rapid and weak pulse, cyanosis, coma, and sometimes respiratory paralysis. Tolerance results from chronic use or abuse. Benzodiazepines may be detected for 1 to 6 weeks.

Potential for Addiction

The potential for addiction is high for all of these substances. Benzodiazepines are schedule IV drugs; barbiturates may be either schedule II, III, or IV drugs; and methaqualone is a schedule I drug.

Withdrawal

Symptoms of withdrawal for benzodiazepines, which may not manifest for a week or more, include cramping, sweating, disorientation, confusion, tremors, depression, hallucinations, and paranoia. Barbiturate withdrawal symptoms include anxiety, weakness, anorexia, insomnia, tremors, delirium, and seizures that occur within 72 hours of the last use. Withdrawal reactions related to other sedative-hypnotics include nausea, headache, cramping, toxic psychosis, insomnia, and convulsions.

The withdrawal pattern is the same as for alcohol.

Treatment/Rehabilitation

Ideally, treatment for benzodiazepine abuse is a gradual reduction in the amount taken until the client is no longer taking any. A cross-tolerant drug such as phenobarbital is sometimes given to control symptoms and then its dosage is reduced. Hospital treatment is likely to be needed. Treatment for barbiturate and other sedative-hypnotics overdose or withdrawal is symptomatic.

Rehabilitation that focuses on teaching clients alternative methods of coping with the anxiety and stressors in their lives is necessary. Supportive individual psychotherapy or a self-help recovery group is almost always advisable. The goal is to assist the client to identify the consequences of the behavior and to understand the risks of relapse.

CANNABIS

Marijuana is the most common type of cannabis used. It is composed of dried leaves, stems, and flowers of the plant *Cannabis sativa* and can be smoked or added to food. Hash or hashish is a potent concentrate of the resin from the flowers. Hash oil is extremely concentrated, made by boiling hashish in a solvent and filtering out the solid matter. Street names include grass, pot, reefer, smoke, weed, and Mary Jane. "Blunts" are cigars emptied of tobacco and refilled with marijuana.

Incidence

Use in the United States began in the early 1900s, peaked in the period 1978 to 1980, and has steadily decreased since. According to Johnston, O'Malley, and Buchman (1991 and 1998), the prevalence of marijuana use by high school seniors increased from 20% in the class of 1969 to 60.4% in the class of 1979 and fell to 50.2% in the class of 1987 and fell again to 40.7 percent in the class of 1990. Use increased between 1990 and 1997 but declined in 1998 to 49%.

Signs and Symptoms

Short-term effects of marijuana use include memory and learning problems; distorted perception; difficulty in thinking and problem solving; loss of coordination; and increased heart rate, anxiety, and panic attacks. Long-term use produces changes in the brain similar to those seen after long-term use of other major drugs of abuse (NIDA, 1999j). A **reverse tolerance** can develop whereby a smaller amount of marijuana will elicit the desired psychic effects. Marijuana may be detected for up to 5 weeks.

Potential for Addiction

The potential for psychologic addiction is moderate. More than 120,000 persons seek treatment each year for their primary marijuana addiction (NIDA, 1999j). Marijuana is a schedule I drug.

Associated Problems/Disorders

Critical skills related to attention, learning, and memory are impaired in heavy marijuana users even 24 hours after the last use. Also, persons below college age who use marijuana tend to be more accepting of deviant behavior, have more aggression and delinquent behavior, act more rebellious, and have poorer relationship with parents (NIDA, 1999j).

Withdrawal

Nausea, myalgia, restlessness, irritability, nervousness, insomnia, and depression may appear after ceasing marijuana use. Symptoms may not appear for up to 1 week after the last use.

Treatment/Rehabilitation

Treatment focuses on relapse prevention and the development of new coping mechanisms, ways of living, and means of having fun without drugs. Weekly group therapy sessions to maintain a commitment to abstinence and enhance interpersonal skills are often used. Participation in a self-help group is encouraged.

CNS STIMULANTS

Drugs that stimulate the CNS include cocaine, amphetamines, caffeine, nicotine, and methylphenidate hydrochloride (Ritalin). They increase cortical alertness and electrical activity in the brain and spinal cord. There is tachycardia and an increase in blood pressure.

COCAINE

Cocaine is extracted from the leaves of the coca plant, *Erythroxylum coca*. It may be heated and the fumes inhaled. This is termed *free-basing*. As a white powder, cocaine may be snorted by inhaling it through the nose. It may also be heated to a liquid state and injected intravenously. Crack is a crystallized form of cocaine that is melted in a water pipe and smoked. Street names include coke, crack, flake, rocks, snow, "C," and blow.

Incidence

Cocaine abuse and dependence was the major illicit drug problem for the United States in the 1980s. The introduction of crack dramatically increased cocaine abuse among the poor. Crack is low cost and gives an intense "high." It is estimated that 3.6 million persons in the United States are chronic cocaine users (NIDA, 1999c).

Signs and Symptoms

The immediate reaction, less than 10 seconds, is an intense euphoria that lasts 10 to 15 minutes. This short response time leads people to binge on cocaine. That is, they repeatedly use cocaine trying to maintain the euphoria.

The heart rate increases, blood pressure goes up, pupils dilate, peripheral blood vessels constrict, and temperature increases. Normal pleasures are magnified, anxiety decreases, self-confidence increases, social inhibitions are reduced, communication is facilitated, and sexual feelings are enhanced. Other psychological effects are inability to concentrate, insomnia, reduced sense of humor, antisocial behavior, hallucinations, and compulsive behavior.

An overdose may occur with the first use because there is little quality control of drug strength in the street drug culture. A client with an overdose may have arrhythmias, tremors, convulsions, respiratory failure, cardiovascular collapse, and death. Cocaine may be detected for up to 4 days.

Potential for Addiction

The potential for addiction is high. Cocaine is a schedule II drug.

Associated Problems/Disorders

Many types of heart disease are linked to cocaine use, especially ventricular fibrillation, heart attack, and hypertension. When cocaine is snorted regularly, respiratory problems occur, including loss of sense of smell, nosebleeds, hoarseness, and respiratory failure.

When cocaine is taken with alcohol, the two drugs are converted in the body to cocaethylene, which is more toxic than either drug alone (NIDA, 1999c).

Withdrawal

The crash, a period of exhaustion, occurs in the client; there are symptoms of depression, anxiety, and a great need for sleep. The depression may be to the point of suicidal behavior. The client has no energy, shows little interest in the surroundings, and seems to have little ability to experience pleasure. These symptoms are the most intense during the first 3 days but continue for 1 to 4 months. An intense craving for cocaine is felt, including dreaming about cocaine. Then there is a period of less intense craving for cocaine called extinction, which may last months or even years. Withdrawal does not result in a medical emergency as seen with alcohol.

Treatment/Rehabilitation

Treatment is aimed at reducing the craving and managing the severe depression. Careful monitoring of the client is necessary to identify and prevent actions aimed at carrying out the idea of suicide. An individual with a history of cocaine usage has an intense craving for cocaine and a strong denial that cocaine is addicting. This creates a problem in engaging an individual in treatment. Inpatient programs for some clients with cocaine dependence should therefore be recommended, while other clients can be effectively treated in outpatient programs.

Medications

Bromocriptine mesylate (Parlodel) in small doses seems to reduce the withdrawal symptoms. Amantadine hydrochloride (Symmetrel) also has some success in treating cocaine withdrawal. Desipramine hydrochloride (Pertofrane) seems to reduce the craving for cocaine.

Education

Individual or group therapy should focus on helping the client feel pleasure again, improve energy level, and reduce cocaine craving. Peer support groups and self-help groups, such as Cocaine Anonymous, may be very effective. Random and regular urine testing is an external support to promote abstinence.

AMPHETAMINES

Amphetamines (also called uppers, speed, bennies) include dextroamphetamine sulfate (Dexedrine), amphetamine sulfate (Amphetamine), and methamphetamine hydrochloride (Desoxyn). Medically they are used to treat attention deficit hyperactivity disorder (ADHD), narcolepsy, and obesity.

Incidence

Amphetamines have been abused since the early 1930s. World War II greatly increased use and abuse when military personnel used amphetamines to decrease fatigue and increase alertness. Today, abuse ranges from truck drivers and college students who want to ward off sleep and increase alertness to the heavy abuser who injects or smokes homemade methamphetamine, known as meth, chalk, ice, crystal, crank, and glass. An estimated 4.9 million people in the United States have tried methamphetamine at some time (NIDA, 1999k).

Signs and Symptoms

Besides suppressing fatigue and increasing alertness, amphetamines enhance psychomotor performance, induce a temporary state of well-being, and give an instantaneous euphoria. Like cocaine, after several days the person becomes exhausted and lapses into a long period of sleep and depression (crash). The action of amphetamines lasts much longer than that of cocaine and there is a greater potential for adverse reactions and severe toxicity.

High abuse doses may cause insomnia, tachycardia, headache, arrhythmias, hypertension followed by hypotension, nausea, vomiting, cramping, diarrhea, hyperreflexia, convulsions, and death. The psychologic effect is termed amphetamine psychosis and closely resembles paranoid schizophrenia. Symptoms include paranoid ideation, confusion, compulsive behaviors, and visual and auditory hallucinations. Tolerance does develop. Amphetamines may be detected for up to 2 days.

Potential for Addiction

The potential for addiction is high. Amphetamines are schedule II drugs.

Associated Problems/Disorders

Cardiovascular problems occur, including irregular and rapid heartbeat; hypertension; and irreversible, stroke-producing damage to small blood vessels in the brain (NIDA, 1999k). Injecting the drug may damage blood vessels and cause skin abscesses, and if injection equipment is shared, there is an increased risk of HIV/AIDS and hepatitis B and C transmission.

Withdrawal

There are no physical manifestations of withdrawal. Psychological changes include apathy, irritability, depression, disorientation, anxiety, paranoia, aggression, and an intense craving for the drug.

Treatment/Rehabilitation

Urinary acidifiers, such as ascorbic acid (vitamin C), increase the excretion of amphetamines. Diazepam (Valium) is given for sedation to ease the withdrawal crash. Bromocriptine mesylate (Parlodel) or levodopa (Dopar) may help decrease the craving. A quiet environment is also helpful.

Behavioral therapy is used to help the client recognize and accept the need to stop using amphetamines. Supportive individual or group therapy, and especially self-help groups, aids the client to stay abstinent and in treatment.

CAFFEINE

Caffeine is found in coffee, tea, cola beverages, cocoa, chocolate, and some nonprescription drugs.

Incidence

Caffeine is probably the best known and most frequently used and abused CNS stimulant.

Signs and Symptoms

Caffeine causes relaxation of smooth muscles in blood vessels and bronchi, diuresis, an increased gastric acid secretion, suppression of appetite, increased feeling of energy, and constriction of cerebral blood vessels. An increased level of caffeine intake causes jitteriness, restlessness, nervousness, excitement, flushed face, palpitations, and nausea.

Potential for Addiction

The potential for addiction is moderate. Caffeine is not a scheduled drug.

Withdrawal

Withdrawal produces headache, irritability, and tremulousness.

Treatment/Rehabilitation

A gradual reduction of caffeine intake can reduce or eliminate the withdrawal symptoms. The client can then drink decaffeinated coffee and tea and caffeine-free soft drinks. The intake of cocoa and chocolate should be greatly reduced or eliminated. Caffeine can be avoided by reading labels and not using nonprescription products that contain caffeine.

NICOTINE

Nicotine is found in tobacco in a 1% to 2% concentration. There is no therapeutic use for nicotine. Smoking and other uses of tobacco have been in and out of favor several times during the past 5 centuries. This century has seen the greatest degree of abuse. Reasons for this increase are related to the mass production of tobacco products, mass advertising campaigns, and the psychological dependence produced by the nicotine. Tobacco, even when used in moderation, will likely produce disease and death. Tobacco kills more than 430,000 U.S. citizens each year. That is more than alcohol, cocaine, heroin, homicide, suicide, car accidents, fire, and AIDS combined (NIDA, 1998b).

Incidence

About 29% of the population age 12 and over uses tobacco (NIDA, 1999b). In high school students, smoking increased from 27.5% in 1991 to 36.4% in 1997 (NIDA, 1998b).

Signs and Symptoms

Nicotine causes decreased skeletal muscle tone, decreased sensitivity of some receptor sites (pain, heat, taste buds), reduced appetite, vasoconstriction, decreased body temperature, and increased blood pressure. Tolerance develops so the daily intake must increase to continue the desired effect.

Potential for Addiction

The potential for addiction is high. Even first-time users can become dependent within weeks of their initial use. Nicotine is not a scheduled drug.

Associated Problems/Disorders

Other ingredients in the smoke (tar, carbon monoxide, and incompletely burned waste products) are largely responsible for the negative health consequences.

Respiratory

Chronic obstructive pulmonary disease is caused by the many changes tobacco use makes in the respiratory system. Smokers are more prone to developing pneumonia, and asthma is exacerbated by smoking. Chronic exposure to smoke inhalation gives children higher rates of otitis media and respiratory illnesses.

Cardiovascular

Ischemic heart disease is twice as likely to develop in a smoker than in a nonsmoker. Cerebrovascular accidents and peripheral vascular disease are strongly associated with smoking. Cessation of smoking, about 10 years, reduces the risks for these 3 vascular diseases to the nonsmoker's level. Nearly 20% of deaths due to heart disease are attributable to smoking (NIDA, 1998b).

Cancer

Many cancers—oral, pharyngeal, laryngeal, esophageal, lung, pancreatic, kidney, and bladder—are strongly associated with tobacco. Secondhand smoke causes lung cancer in nonsmoking adults. Cigarette smoking is linked to approximately 90% of all lung cancer cases (NIDA, 1998b).

GERONTOLOGICAL CONSIDERATIONS

Smoking

- Menopause generally occurs earlier in women who smoke.
- The older smoker is often less motivated to quit because of the feeling that "I've survived this long."

Withdrawal

Short-term effects of nicotine withdrawal include nausea, diarrhea, headache, drowsiness, insomnia, irritability, and poor concentration. Increased appetite along with an intense craving for tobacco may persist for 6 months or longer.

Treatment/Rehabilitation

Nicotine replacement therapy by patch, nasal spray, inhaler, or gum helps individuals break the habit. It is important that the client not smoke while using the patch. Serious adverse effects may be experienced with a high serum nicotine level. It can be toxic. Later, a gradual withdrawal of the nicotine patch can be accomplished. The first nonnicotine prescription drug to treat nicotine addiction, bupropion (Zyban), was approved by the Food and Drug Administration in 1996. The availability of these products has produced a 20% increase in successful quitting each year (NIDA, 1998b).

An exercise program will help with stress management and minimize possible weight gain. Relaxation techniques will also reduce stress. Support by family and significant others for the person quitting tobacco use may help the process. A lack of support may greatly increase the difficulty of quitting for the individual. The rate of relapse is highest in the first few weeks, and diminishes considerably after 3 months.

METHYLPHENIDATE HYDROCHLORIDE (RITALIN)

Currently, there is an increase in the use (misuse and overuse) of Ritalin that is becoming a growing problem. Ritalin is an accepted treatment for children with attention deficit hyperactivity disorder (ADHD). Although Ritalin is a CNS stimulant, there is a paradoxical calming effect on children with ADHD. Many children are being given Ritalin without thorough testing to eliminate other causes of attention deficit. These children have the potential for dependence. Ritalin is also used for narcolepsy. It can be detected for 1 to 2 days and is a schedule II drug.

HALLUCINOGENS

Hallucinogens refers to a group of naturally occurring and synthetic agents that produce essentially the same mind-altering effects.

Psilocybin and psilocin are naturally occurring organic compounds found in some mushrooms that grow in the United States and Mexico. These mushrooms have been used for centuries in southern Mexico, primarily in religious ceremonies. Fresh or dried mushrooms, sometimes mixed with food, are ingested orally.

Dimethyltryptamine (DMT) and diethyltryptamine (DET) are found in tropical plant leaves and seeds. For centuries they have been dried and powdered and used as snuff. They are not orally active. Sometimes the powder is added to tobacco or marijuana.

There are several amphetamine-like hallucinogens. Probably the two best known are 2,5 dimethyl-4-ethylamphetamine (DOM) and methylene-dioxyamphetamine (MDMA, ecstasy), which are chemically manufactured compounds. These are usually taken orally but may be injected intravenously or inhaled.

LYSERGIC ACID DIETHYLAMIDE

Lysergic acid diethylamide (LSD), a manufactured chemical compound, is perhaps the most widely known and used hallucinogen. In the past, LSD has been used as a legitimate medication and in research. In the 1960s when its abuse became so widespread, the manufacturer refused to supply it for research. It had already been discontinued as a useful medication. It is generally taken orally but can be injected intravenously.

Incidence

The use of hallucinogens declined throughout the 1980s. The early 1990s indicated that LSD was making a comeback. The 1990 and 1991 annual survey of high school seniors found that for the first time since 1976,

CULTURAL CONSIDERATIONS

Mescaline

Mescaline is the active ingredient in peyote cactus found growing in the southwestern United States and Mexico. It is the only legally used hallucinogen. Members of the Native American Church of the United States may use it for religious purposes. It is ingested orally. A cross-tolerance to LSD and psilocybin occurs.

more seniors had used LSD than cocaine in the previous 12 months. The 1998 survey showed a slight downward movement in LSD use (Johnston et al., 1998). Other names for LSD are acid and microdot.

Signs and Symptoms

The functioning of both the peripheral nervous system and the central nervous system is altered by LSD. Physical effects include hypertension, increased temperature, sweating, loss of appetite, dilated pupils, and dry mouth. Time and distance are distorted, rational judgment is impaired, and visual **hallucinations** (perceiving things that are not really there) and delusions along with **synthesiasis** (hearing colors and seeing sounds) occur. A state of either euphoria or depression is experienced. The depression with feelings of anxiety, panic, or suicidal tendencies is termed a "bad trip." Flashbacks occur suddenly days or years after LSD use. Their occurrence and frequency are unpredictable but seem to happen in times of high stress. LSD may be detected up to 8 hours.

Potential for Addiction

LSD is not considered an addictive drug, but it does produce tolerance. It is a schedule I drug.

Associated Problems/Disorders

Personality changes occur with LSD use and may happen after a single LSD experience. Acceptable social behaviors seem to diminish with use.

Withdrawal

There is no withdrawal seen.

Treatment/Rehabilitation

A person on a "bad trip" should be carefully watched to prevent self-injury. Reassurance, support, and "talking down" should be done in a quiet, pleasant manner. The person should be encouraged to sit up or walk. Closing the eyes intensifies the "bad trip." The person should be reminded that the drug is causing the effects, which will soon go away.

After cessation of chronic LSD use, long-term psychotherapy is usually required to determine what needs were fulfilled by the use of this drug. A 12-step program and family assistance are usually necessary to reinforce the decision to remain abstinent. If the client is upset by flashbacks or the fear of flashbacks, an anxiolytic drug such as diazepam (Valium) may be ordered.

PHENCYCLIDINE

Phencyclidine (PCP) was made for use as an anesthetic agent, but it produced such adverse reactions that it was withdrawn from clinical trials. However, it can easily be manufactured in an unsophisticated laboratory from simple materials. The degree of purity varies widely. It is often found as a contaminant in other street drugs. The anesthetic is used in veterinary medicine.

Incidence

PCP is primarily used by adolescents and young adults with the first use between the ages of 13 and 15 years. Approximately 3% of those between the ages of 12 and 17 years had used PCP in 1991. The use increased to approximately 4% in 1997 (NIDA, 1999l). Other names for PCP are angel dust, ozone, wack, and rocket fuel. Marijuana combined with PCP is called killer joints or crystal super grass.

Signs and Symptoms

There are usually four phases, with the symptoms dose related. Acute toxicity is characterized by visual disturbances, auditory hallucinations, combativeness, catatonia, convulsions, and coma, and lasts about 3 days. The toxic psychosis phase has visual and auditory hallucinations, agitation, paranoid delusions, and disturbed judgment, and lasts about 7 days. The third phase has psychotic episodes, including thought disorders, paranoid ideation, and affect disorders much like schizophrenia and lasts a month or more. Depression is the fourth phase that may end in suicide. The use of other street drugs may alleviate the depression. Behavior is highly unpredictable. Death can occur from respiratory depression. For 2 to 8 days PCP can be detected.

Potential for Addiction

Even chronic use does not produce physical dependence. Psychological dependence does develop as evidenced by a craving for PCP. It is a schedule I and II drug.

Associated Problems/Disorders

Seizures are a common occurrence with PCP. Hypertension and hyperthermia must be treated before they become a crisis situation. **Opisthotonos**, a complete arching of the body with only the head and feet on the bed, usually is relieved as the blood level of PCP decreases. Cardiac arrhythmias may need interventions by a cardiologist. Acute renal failure may result from the use of PCP. Strokes also have been reported.

Withdrawal

PCP is fat soluble and its effects are felt weeks after the last use as it is gradually released from the fatty tissue into the circulation.

Treatment/Rehabilitation

Treatment should begin in an inpatient setting because of the high risk of suicide. The goal is to keep the client from resuming drug use. Sedatives may be used and urinary acidifiers such as ascorbic acid may be given to increase excretion of PCP. Minimal confrontation should be used in a nonthreatening, nonstimulating, supportive environment. No effort should be made to "talk down" or calm the individual. Diazepam (Valium) may be ordered.

Vocational counseling and training may enhance self-esteem. Body awareness, yoga, and progressive relaxation help the client focus and improve attention span and concentration. Participation in a self-help group such as Narcotics Anonymous (NA) should be encouraged, though initial involvement is usually minimal.

OPIOIDS

Opioids is a term used to refer to naturally occurring opiates, semisynthetic opiates, synthetic opiates, and agonist-antagonists. Table 34–7 provides examples of these opioids. Heroin is the most abused and the most rapid acting of the opioids (NIDA, 1999g).

Incidence

Kleber (1994) described the 1990s as the decade of heroin. Cocaine addicts switched to heroin. Heroin was easily available, the purity was higher than in decades, and it could now be sniffed or smoked instead of injected (NIDA, 1999g). By 1998, the increase in heroin use by high school students had stopped (Johnston et al., 1998). Other names for heroin are horse, smack, "H," skag, and junk.

Signs and Symptoms

All of these drugs affect the central nervous system, causing mental changes, euphoria, drowsiness, analgesia, constricted pupils, and depressed respirations. These changes become more pronounced as the dose is increased.

Opioids increase stomach tone, decrease intestinal peristalsis, and increase the tone of the anal sphincter. This all adds up to constipation. Prolonged drug use may result in a fecal impaction.

Peripheral blood vessels are dilated by opioids, and orthostatic hypotension frequently occurs. The work of the heart is not changed by opioids, so they are frequently used to treat the severe pain of a myocardial infarction.

Tolerance may develop to one or more of the effects of opioids but not to others. For example, morphine addicts will always have pinpoint pupils even when the euphoric effects are not experienced. Tolerance to one opioid usually means tolerance to other

Table 34–7 OPIOIDS

TYPE	EXAMPLE
Natural Opiates	morphine sulfate codeine sulfate
Semisynthetic Opiates	heroin hydromorphone hydrochloride (Dilaudid) oxymorphone hydrochloride (Numorphan) oxycodone (in Percodan) hydrocodone (in Hycodan)
Synthetic Opiates	meperidine hydrochloride (Demerol) methadone hydrochloride (Dolophine) propoxyphene (Darvon)
Agonist-Antagonists	pentazocine (Talwin) nalbuphine hydrochloride (Nubain) butorphanol tartrate (Stadol)

opioids as well. Withdrawal symptoms from one opioid can be suppressed by using another opioid.

Potential for Addiction

The potential for addiction is high. Heroin is a schedule I drug; methadone, schedule II; morphine, schedule II or III; and codeine and opium are schedule II, III, or IV.

Associated Problems/Disorders

Chronic heroin injection may cause scarred and collapsed veins, bacterial infections of the heart valves and blood vessels, abscesses, and liver or kidney disease. Pneumonia may result from the respiratory-depressing effect of heroin. Additives to street heroin may clog blood vessels or cause immune reactions, leading to arthritis or other rheumatologic conditions. Sharing injection equipment can lead to infections of hepatitis B and C, HIV, and other blood-borne viruses, which can then be passed on to sexual partners and children.

Withdrawal

Withdrawal symptoms are dependent on drug purity, dose, and route of administration. Withdrawal is characterized by a rebound excitability of those functions that had been depressed. Symptoms include stomach cramps, nausea, vomiting, diarrhea, diaphoresis, hypertension, aching of bones and muscles, lacrimation, rhinorrhea, cold flashes with goose bumps, yawning, mydriasis, anxiety, irritability, restlessness, and sometimes paranoia, violence, fear, or depersonalization.

Morphine withdrawal symptoms begin within 8 to 12 hours after the last dose, and the acute phase is over in about 10 to 14 days. Figure 34-2 illustrates the signs and symptoms of morphine withdrawal. This is the basic pattern of withdrawal for all opioids.

Codeine withdrawal symptoms may be a little less severe than those of morphine withdrawal. Dilaudid and heroin withdrawal may begin slightly earlier than morphine withdrawal. Meperidine (Demerol) withdrawal begins within 3 hours and peaks in 8 to 12 hours. Propoxyphene (Darvon) withdrawal is considerably milder.

Methadone withdrawal is slower to develop and lasts longer. Symptoms may not occur for 1 to 2 days, with acute symptoms lasting 2 to 3 weeks but not disappearing until 6 weeks after abstinence begins. Symptoms of fatigue, sluggishness, and irritability may last up to 6 months.

Withdrawal from the agonist-antagonists begins in 6 to 8 hours and is usually over in 8 days. The symptoms are the same as for morphine only in a milder form.

Treatment/Rehabilitation

Initial treatment is symptomatic and supportive of vital functions until the acute phase is over.

Detoxification

Several methods currently used for opioid detoxification are methadone, LAAM, and naltrexone.

Methadone Methadone is given and the dose adjusted to keep withdrawal symptoms under control. The daily dose is gradually reduced over a period of 3 to 6 months. Routine and random urine testing is usually done to ensure no other drug use.

Levo-alpha-acetyl-methadol Levo-alpha-acetyl-methadol (LAAM) is a synthetic opiate, like methadone, used to treat heroin addiction. It blocks the effects of heroin for up to 72 hours, so it need be taken only 3 times a week.

Naltrexone Naltrexone (ReVia) blocks the effects of morphine, heroin, and other opiates. Its effects last 1 to 3 days depending on the dose. The pleasurable effects of heroin are blocked, making it useful to treat highly motivated individuals. It is also used to prevent relapse in former opiate addicts.

Counseling/Self-Help Groups

Individual and/or group counseling must go hand in hand with the detoxification to help the client learn new methods of coping with life's stresses. Participation

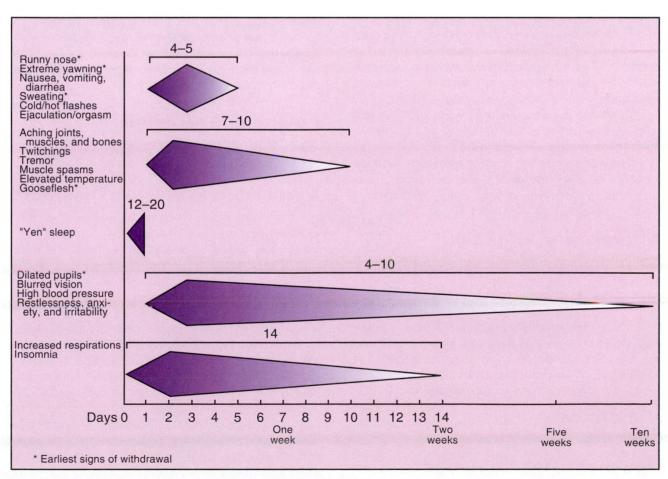

Figure 34-2 Duration of Morphine Withdrawal Signs and Symptoms

in Narcotics Anonymous (NA) helps the client maintain abstinence from drugs.

Behavioral Therapy

Contingency management therapy employs a voucher system. Clients earn "points" for having negative drug tests. These can be exchanged for items encouraging healthy living (NIDA, 1999g).

INHALANTS

Inhalants are inexpensive and easy to obtain. Examples are toluene (glues), gasoline, kerosene, isopropyl alcohol, lacquer thinner, acetone, benzene, naptha, carbon tetrachloride, fluorocarbons (aerosol propellants), correction fluid, and nitrous oxide. They are rapidly absorbed into the brain and stored in body fat.

Incidence

In 1997, 21% of 8th graders, 18.3% of 10th graders, and 16.1% of 12th graders reported using inhalants at least once (NIDA, 1999h). Inhalants are not scheduled drugs.

Signs and Symptoms

The desired effect of euphoria is followed by nausea, headache, and amnesia. Other effects of using inhalants include dizziness, unsteady gait, slurred speech, auditory and visual hallucinations, drowsiness, hypotension, heightened sexual response due to profound vasodilation, stupor, unconsciousness, and coma. Heavy use can lead to hypoxia, multiple organ damage, and death. Airway freezing and/or laryngospasm can be caused by nitrous oxide.

Behaviors that may indicate inhalant abuse include decreased school performance; loss of interest in extracurricular, family, and social activities; and the onset of legal problems.

Potential for Addiction

The potential for addiction is high for psychological dependence only.

Associated Problems/Disorders

Chronic pulmonary irritation and/or chemical pneumonitis may be caused by the use of inhalants. Toluene may cause renal tubular acidosis, hearing loss, and brain damage. Fluorocarbons sensitize the myocardium to catacholemines and may cause arrhythmias.

Withdrawal

There are no withdrawal symptoms.

Treatment/Rehabilitation

Initial treatment is to provide oxygen and respiratory support. Participation in a traditional chemical de-

pendency program is often needed. An adolescent 12-step group is very helpful. Individual and family counseling are essential.

ANABOLIC STEROIDS

Anabolic steroids are synthetic derivatives of testosterone. They cause both androgenic (masculinizing) and anabolic (tissue building) effects. Most people use anabolic steroids for their anabolic effects. Medically, they are used in the treatment of some anemias and in some cancer therapies. The use of anabolic steroids is banned by the International Olympic Committee and the National Collegiate Athletic Association.

Incidence

Primary users are athletes seeking to improve their performance. Other people use anabolic steroids to improve their physical appearance. In 1997, 1.8% of 8th graders, 2% of 10th graders, and 2.4% of 12th graders had used anabolic steroids (NIDA, 1999m).

Signs and Symptoms

The commonly perceived effects of anabolic steroids are an increase in skeletal muscle mass, enhanced physical performance of the skeletal muscles, and improved athletic ability. However, there is no conclusive evidence that these perceived effects are medically accurate.

Potential for Addiction

The potential for addiction is moderate. Anabolic steroids are schedule III drugs.

Associated Problems/Disorders

Other effects found when anabolic steroids are used include hepatocellular damage, cholestasis, hepatoadenoma, hepatocarcinoma, acne, hirsutism, male-pattern baldness, a deepening of the voice, increased cholesterol level, increased blood pressure, decreased glucose tolerance, mood swings, aggressiveness, depression, psychosis, and hepatitis or HIV infection if needles are shared. In males, there is also testicular atrophy, oligospermia, impotence, prostatic hypertrophy, prostatic carcinoma, and gynecomastia. In females, there is also amenorrhea, clitoromegaly, uterine atrophy, breast atrophy, facial hair growth, and teratogenicity.

These effects seem to be reversible when the anabolic steroids are no longer taken, except for the male-pattern baldness, liver tumors, and gynecomastia in males and clitoral enlargement, virilization, and male-pattern baldness in females. The increased aggressiveness and euphoria are probably beneficial during athletic competitions but otherwise may cause severe social problems.

Withdrawal

Symptoms of withdrawal include lethargy, abdominal muscle cramps, constipation, headache, and depression.

Treatment/Rehabilitation

Treatment of withdrawal focuses on providing symptom relief for the client and counseling to build self esteem and self-confidence in abilities without the use of anabolic steroids.

▶ NURSING PROCESS

Nursing care is an essential component of the multidisciplinary approach to substance abuse treatment.

▶ Assessment

The subjective and objective data given are related to substance abuse and dependence in general.

▶ Subjective Data

The client will often describe being very relaxed; feeling wonderful; or having a headache, fatigue, depression, sleep disturbance, suppression of appetite, dizziness, hallucinations, paranoia, anxiety, emotional lability, memory loss, heightened sexual desire (with early use), or loss of sexual desire (with continued use). Problems in various areas of life are common, such as frequent job changes; marital conflict, separation and/or divorce; work-related accidents, lateness, absenteeism; and legal problems, including arrest for driving while intoxicated. The client may describe having falls or fights and financial problems. Normal diet pattern and the presence of any disease conditions should be noted.

The client should be asked, "How often do you use drugs/alcohol? How much do you usually use? Have you ever used drugs/alcohol more than you use them now? When? Under what circumstances? What substance did you last use?" The information received from the client may not always be accurate. Validation with the family or significant other is helpful.

▶ Objective Data

Neglect of health and personal care is often evident. The client may have dental caries, bad breath, gingivitis, unkempt appearance, and be undernourished or malnourished. If substances have been inhaled, there may be irritation and bleeding of the nasal mucosa, destruction of the nasal mucosa and cartilaginous structures, or depression of respirations. If substances have been injected intravenously, there will be scarring of veins (needle marks, track marks), possibly skin infections, enlarged lymph nodes, and hematomas.

The client may appear older than the stated age and have chronic cough producing brown to black sputum, dilated or pinpoint pupils, tremors, slurred speech, lack of coordination, frequent episodes of sexually transmitted diseases, jaundice, or vomiting. There may be tachycardia, hypertension, ascites, or petechiae.

▶ Nursing Diagnoses

Nursing diagnoses for a client with substance abuse or dependence may include the following:

- *Imbalanced Nutrition: Less than Body Requirements*
- *Self-Care Deficit*
- *Risk for Injury*
- *Disturbed Sleep Pattern*
- *Activity Intolerance*
- *Impaired Physical Mobility*
- *Disturbed Sensory Perception*
- *Impaired Verbal Communication*
- *Risk for Infection*
- *Excess or Deficient Fluid Volume*
- *Disturbed Thought Processes*
- *Ineffective Coping (Individual)*
- *Situational Low Self-Esteem*
- *Risk for Violence (Other Directed or Self-Directed)*
- *Anxiety*
- *Impaired Social Interaction*
- *Hopelessness*
- *Powerlessness*
- *Ineffective Coping/Compromised Family Coping*

▶ Planning/Outcome Identification

There are several overall goals for the care of a client with a substance abuse problem. The client will do the following:

1. Abstain from using psychoactive substances
2. Adhere to the treatment plan
3. Make lifestyle changes to maintain abstinence
4. Engage in behaviors that foster good health

Other goals specific to nursing diagnoses must be formulated on an individual basis.

▶ Nursing Interventions

Nursing interventions include active listening, providing care in a nonjudgmental manner, teaching health promotion, and referral to self-help groups or individual counseling. Other nursing interventions must be specific for the goals and nursing diagnoses identified for the individual client. Examples might include the following:

1. Provide well-balanced diet. Monitor intake and lab tests results. Assess for GI bleeding.
2. Assist with personal hygiene. Encourage self-care.

GERONTOLOGICAL CONSIDERATIONS

Substance Misuse or Abuse

In the elderly:

- **Misuse** (using a legal drug for something other than intended or exceeding the recommended dose of a drug) is more common than abuse or dependence.
- Substances that decrease respirations can increase the frequency of mental confusion.
- Decreased coordination from alcohol or other substances is associated with falling more often and fracturing the wrist, back, and hips.
- Chronic medical conditions can be made worse from even minimal use of alcohol or other drugs as these substances can change the effect of prescribed medications.
- Unrealistic expectations of retirement may lead to use of mood-altering substances to relieve depression and boredom.

3. Administer medications as ordered to decrease or prevent symptoms of withdrawal. Keep call light in client's reach. Keep side rails up.
4. Provide warm milk at bedtime. Plan with client a time for bed. Encourage use of relaxation techniques. Reassure client that insomnia will improve.
5. Encourage client to do active ROM exercises.
6. Assist client to turn in bed. Assist client to ambulate as able. Answer call light promptly.
7. Do not argue with a client having hallucinations. Remind client of day, time, and place.
8. Watch client's nonverbal communication.
9. Encourage good personal hygiene. Inspect skin for integrity.
10. Administer antibiotics as ordered. Monitor vital signs. Monitor I & O. Monitor lab tests results.
11. Administer vitamins as ordered. Provide cues as needed. Encourage adequate diet intake.
12. Assess coping patterns to identify strengths and weaknesses. Actively listen to client. Refer to appropriate community agencies.
13. Assist client to identify areas of low self-esteem. Encourage client participation in group therapy. Refer to individual counseling as needed.
14. Monitor client closely. Use restraints as ordered. Keep bed in low position and side rails up.
15. Introduce client to other recovering persons. Encourage client to participate in self-help group.
16. Provide spiritual support if asked.
17. Involve client in decision making when possible. Give positive reinforcement for abstinence.
18. Encourage family to participate in treatment program.

▶ Evaluation

Each goal must be evaluated to determine how it has been met by the client.

CODEPENDENCY

Codependency was first recognized by those working with families of alcoholics. It is a learned pattern of feeling and behaving, a problem with relationships. In healthy relationships, people share love, concern, and respect for each other. There is equal give-and-take. This is termed interdependence. In unhealthy relationships, people are often out of touch with their own needs and feelings. They may be unwilling or unable to take care of themselves and have little self-esteem. Only by fulfilling the expectations of others do they feel good about themselves. This is termed codependence. **Codependent** persons live based on what others think of them. They always try to meet the needs of others, demand love from others, and manipulate and control the lives of others.

Serious family problems like addictions, abuse, family secrets, or other major stresses cause confusion and put a family at risk. Codependent behavior thrives when fear, guilt, blame, and low self-esteem become evident. When family members do not relate to each other in positive ways or when their interactions do not provide a healthy environment, the family is called dysfunctional. Many children grow up in dysfunctional families and learn to be codependent.

Codependency tends to run in families. Parents cannot teach their children how to cope in healthy ways if they do not know how themselves. Without intervention or a conscious change by the individual, a pattern of codependent behavior will continue in other relationships.

Characteristics

Persons who are codependent have specific characteristics or traits. They have low self-esteem, never feel they are good enough, and often feel shame. Emotions are denied. They are out of touch with their own feelings and deny their own needs. Their smile is phony much of the time. Problems with communication become evident as they have trouble expressing their needs and feelings. Often they say the opposite to hide their true feelings. They expect others to read their mind. Relationship problems occur because they are afraid of being hurt or that others might learn of their secret feelings and reject them. They cannot risk loving and losing. Relationships are desired but walls are always put up.

Codependent persons live through others. They are people pleasers who would rather give than take. The approval of others means they are "OK." They think they can fix others. The feeling of powerlessness occurs because they give power to others by looking to them for approval. They go to extremes. For a while they will try very hard for approval and then they will not try at all or they will keep negative feelings inside with a smile on their face and then blow up over some little thing. Table 34–8 lists some characteristics of the codependent person.

Treatment

Professional help is usually necessary to change codependent behavior. The goal of treatment is to help the codependent person feel happy and good about himself or herself. Therapy sessions focus on identifying and reconnecting with the true self, dealing with feelings, learning how to communicate feelings, learning to trust, setting boundaries for relationships, and taking charge of their own life.

THE IMPAIRED NURSE

Most states now have peer assistance programs to help nurses impaired by either alcohol or other substances. Substance abuse and dependence are greater problems among nurses than among the general public because nurses have access to many controlled substances. The impaired nurse often requests to give medications, makes medication errors, and "wastes" drugs frequently. This nurse may wear long sleeves and spend an extraordinary amount of time in the bathroom.

Peer assistance programs first appeared in 1980. They have been formed through the state nursing association or the state board of nursing, or through joint effort of both. The goals of the peer assistance programs are to assist the impaired nurse to receive treatment; protect the public from impaired nurses; help the recovering nurse reenter the nursing work force in a planned, safe manner; and monitor the nurse's recovery for a time. The state board of nursing may re-

Table 34–8 CHARACTERISTICS OF THE CODEPENDENT PERSON

Caretaking	"I always give to others. No one gives to me."
Obsession	"I can't stop worrying about __ problems."
Denial	"I pretend I don't have problems."
Poor communication	"No one understands me."
Lack of trust	"I don't trust myself."
Anger	"I resent feeling controlled and manipulated."

From Mental Health Concepts (4th ed.), by C. Waughfield, 1998, Albany, NY: Delmar. Copyright 1998 by Delmar. Adapted with permission.

strict access to controlled substances for the recovering nurse for some period of time.

Prior to the peer assistance programs, impaired nurses were generally just dismissed from employment. Then they would find employment at another health care agency where substance abuse or dependence would continue. This often went on for years.

As the name implies, peer assistance programs are staffed with nurses to help nurses. Many of the staff are volunteers who work in psychiatric nursing or substance abuse centers or who are themselves recovering from substance abuse. It is best not to cover up for a colleague with a substance abuse problem; rather, the nurse should report the situation to a supervisor who can arrange for the nurse to receive help. Some boards of nursing will discipline a nurse for failing to report a fellow nurse who is abusing drugs.

CASE STUDY

Joe, age 19, quit school 3 years ago. He has a part-time job at a fast-food place but has been tardy or absent quite often lately. Sometimes he is easy to get along with, and sometimes he is aggressive and difficult. His mother, with whom he lives, says he is a good boy and does not give her any trouble. Joe was brought to the emergency room by a friend after he passed out. His temperature is 99°F, respirations 10, and pupils are pinpoint. There are track marks on both arms.

The following questions will guide your development of a nursing care plan for the case study.

1. List signs and symptoms, other than Joe's, that a client may experience as a heroin addict.
2. List diagnostic tests that may be ordered.
3. List subjective and objective data the nurse should obtain.
4. Write three individualized nursing diagnoses and goals for Joe.
5. List resources within the medical center and local area that could assist Joe.
6. Describe the use of methadone in heroin addiction.
7. List teaching that Joe will need as a part of his rehabilitation.

SUMMARY

- Substance abuse and dependence have been problems for centuries.
- Factors related to substance abuse include individual, family patterns, lifestyle, environmental, and developmental factors.
- A false positive result on a drug screening test may be caused by ingestion of poppy seeds, use of a Vicks® inhaler, or use of over-the-counter diet aids.
- Detoxification is the first step in the treatment and rehabilitation of a substance abuser.
- Street drugs vary in strength and purity. Higher priced drugs are often mixed with cheaper or easier to obtain drugs.
- Neglect of health and personal care are often evident in substance abuse and dependence.
- Nurses have a higher incidence of substance abuse and dependence than the general public.
- Most states have peer assistance programs for impaired nurses.

Review Questions

1. Schedule II substances:
    a. can be sold as over-the-counter drugs.
    b. have high abuse and dependence potential.
    c. can have prescription refilled for 6 months.
    d. have no accepted medical use in the United States.

2. Substance use and abuse are:
    a. influenced by advertising.
    b. caused by a lack of education.
    c. rejected by all religious groups.
    d. caused by a chromosomal abnormality.

3. Prevention of substance abuse must be focused on:
    a. parents.
    b. children.
    c. teenagers.
    d. young adults.

4. Drug screening tests:
    a. are very accurate.
    b. indicate the level of abuse.
    c. indicate exposure to a substance.
    d. can test for all substances of abuse.

5. The substance most often chosen for abuse or dependence is:
    a. heroin.
    b. cocaine.
    c. alcohol.
    d. marijuana.

6. Alcoholics Anonymous is:
    a. the newest self-help group.
    b. a short-term temporary help group.
    c. a government agency to help those with an alcohol problem.
    d. a self-help group providing a holistic approach to abstinence.

7. Urinary acidifiers are used in the treatment of:
    a. opioids and LSD.
    b. amphetamines and PCP.
    c. alcohol and CNS stimulants.
    d. inhalants and benzodiazepines.

8. The use of inhalants:
    a. can be fatal.
    b. includes only glue and paints.
    c. has severe withdrawal symptoms.
    d. is a harmless activity of young male teenagers.

Critical Thinking Questions

1. Discuss your attitude toward substance abusers.

2. Should drug testing of all health care workers be required? How would you feel if requested to comply?

 WEB FLASH!

- Search the Internet for information about the various illicit substances. What type of information do you find? Will it be helpful in caring for a client with a substance abuse problem?
- Visit the resources for this chapter on the Web. What type of information or services do they provide?

Special Areas of Medical-Surgical Nursing

NURSING CARE OF THE OLDER CLIENT

MAKING THE CONNECTION

Refer to the following chapters to increase your understanding of the older adult:

- **Chapter 5, Communication**
- **Chapter 10, Fluid, Electrolyte, and Acid–Base Balance**
- **Chapter 16, Nursing Care of the Surgical Client**
- **Chapter 18, Nursing Care of the Client: Respiratory System**
- **Chapter 19, Nursing Care of the Client: Cardiovascular System**
- **Chapter 21, Nursing Care of the Client: Integumentary System**
- **Chapter 24, Nursing Care of the Client: Musculoskeletal System**
- **Chapter 25, Nursing Care of the Client: Neurological System**
- **Chapter 26, Nursing Care of the Client: Sensory System**
- **Chapter 27, Nursing Care of the Client: Endocrine System**
- **Chapter 28, Nursing Care of the Client: Gastrointestinal System**
- **Chapter 29, Nursing Care of the Client: Urinary System**
- **Chapter 30, Nursing Care of the Client: Female Reproductive System**
- **Chapter 31, Nursing Care of the Client: Male Reproductive System**
- **Chapter 33, Nursing Care of the Client: Mental Illness**
- **Chapter 34, Nursing Care of the Client: Substance Abuse**

LEARNING OBJECTIVES

Upon completion of this chapter, you should be able to:
- *Define key terms.*
- *Describe stereotypes associated with older adults.*
- *Discuss the biological and psychosocial theories of aging.*
- *Cite the normal physiologic changes that occur with aging.*
- *List the normal functional changes that occur with aging.*
- *Describe key factors of optimal health maintenance in the aging adult.*
- *Identify funding and policy changes that have influenced elder care.*
- *Identify common disorders related to aging.*
- *Detail nursing interventions for each disorder.*
- *Discuss areas wherein the nurse can advocate for older adults on the individual, community, state, and national levels.*

KEY TERMS

activities of daily living	gerontology
Balanced Budget Act	Health Care Financ-
delirium	ing Administration
dementia	Omnibus Budget
gerontological nursing	Reconciliation Act
gerontologist	polypharmacy

INTRODUCTION

Gerontology is the study of the effects of normal aging and age-related diseases on human beings. It is a general term used by all health care and social services disciplines. Aging (senescence) is a complex phenomenon that occurs on the continuum of human life, beginning with birth and continuing throughout the lifespan, and on into the end stages of life and death.

The phrase *older adult* is very subjective and has historically meant persons who are 65 years of age and older. However, there is a great deal of debate among **gerontologists** (gerontological specialists in advanced practice nursing, geriatric psychiatry, medicine, and social services) as to whether this specific age delineation should continue to be used. The practice of using 65 years of age as a dividing line for social welfare benefits began in the 1880s when Otto von Bismark randomly selected that age for benefits in Germany. It should be noted that there was no standardized clinical basis for establishing this age as the dividing line between young and old. Longer average life-expectancy rates (76.5 years for both genders, 73.6 years for men, and 79.4 years for women) (National Council on Aging [NCOA], 2000) along with a decline in the average number of children per family since the late 1960s have changed U.S. demographics. As a result, there is a great need to support and strengthen independence among older adults, and to value and utilize their life experiences in the areas of career, family, and community.

Retirement age is now less consistently determined by a mandatory age limit. Rather, retirement frequently is offered when the employee meets a formula of combined age and years of service. Since the 1990s, benefit penalties have been imposed on Social Security beneficiaries up to 70 years of age and who continue to earn incomes over a minimum amount. This was changed in April 2000 when the Senior Citizens' Freedom to Work Act of 2000 was signed into law by the president. This eliminates the Social Security retirement earnings test in and after the month in which a person is 65 years of age (the current full retirement age) (Social Security Administration [SSA], 2000).

Currently, the clinical delineation of an older adult is still someone who is 65 years of age or older; older-old adults are defined as those individuals 85 years of age or older. In 1900, there were a total of 3.1 million individuals over the age of 65 in the United States; by 1996, there were 33.2 million, 3.8 million of whom were over the age of 85 years (AARP, 1998). It is projected that by the year 2030, the number of older individuals in the United States will reach 69.4 million (Figure 35-1) including 8 million over the age of 85 (Administration on Aging [AoA], 2000). The most rapid increase is expected to occur in the years 2010–2030, when the "baby-boomers" reach age 65.

The aging of the United States and the world is a phenomenon that will impact all areas of society. The age range of 65 to 100+ years potentially comprises three generations: parents, grandparents, and great-grandparents. No other age group has the potential for as much diversity in both strengths and needs, both psychosocial and physical.

The future will also place demands on those who were born from the late 1950s to the late 1960s. Many in this age group chose to focus first on career, delay-ing marriage and childrearing until in their thirties. They have thus been labeled "the sandwich generation" to denote the challenges they will face in meeting social and financial responsibilities later in life as they work to provide for children entering college and for aging parents and, sometimes, grandparents and, in a few instances, great-grandparents.

This chapter presents an overview of influences on the older client, including the social impacts of aging. Also examined are theories of aging; myths and realities of aging; health promotion and aging; physiologic and functional changes that normally occur with aging; and some common disorders of aging along with nursing interventions to assist clients to achieve optimal outcomes related to those disorders.

As caregivers for older adults, nurses and other members of the client's health care team must also understand the budgetary and policy decisions that can affect the care they will provide to their clients. Thus, this chapter concludes with a short discussion on health care financing for elder care in the 21st century.

GERONTOLOGICAL NURSING

The acceptance of **gerontological nursing** as a separate nursing specialty that addresses and advocates for the special care needs of older adults has not been realized without a struggle. In 1961, gerontological nursing attained national recognition with the creation of its own division of nursing within the American Nurses Association (ANA). Nurses in the United States who were aware of the trends toward an aging population realized the importance of taking such a step. The charter members of the Division of Gerontological Nursing deserve a great deal of credit for their vision and commitment to developing gerontology education and recognizing the special nursing care needs of

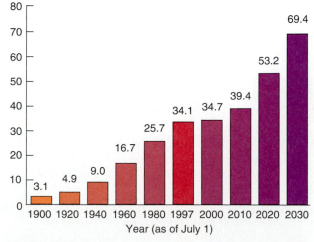

Number of persons 65+: 1900 to 2030

Figure 35-1 Number of Persons Over Age 65: 1900–2030 (*From* A Profile of Older Americans, *by The Administration on Aging and the AARP, 1998*)

older adults. The major topics addressed in the overview of the expanding scope of practice for gerontological nursing included (Bahr, 1994):

- The historical evolution of gerontological nursing practice based on population statistics;
- The way that ageism in U.S. society has affected the profession of nursing, the health care delivery system, and the care of older adults;
- Nursing education and care of older adults with a perspective derived from studies of the attitudes and interests of nursing personnel and nursing students;
- The delineation of various aspects of nursing care of older adults, including clinical practice based on the ANA Standards of Nursing Practice; select theories of nursing applied to the care of older adults; and the expanding scope of gerontological nursing, in general, and the roles of clinical nurse specialists and geriatric nurse practitioners, in particular; and
- Trends in gerontological nursing and long-term care.

The battle continues against the stereotyping of older adults, both in the health professions and in the community at large. There are many stereotypes or preconceived notions associated with aging and being old. Stereotypes are usually generated in an attempt to categorize people or to set standards that can be applied to large groups of people. They are often based on an individual's experience with persons in that group. Stereotypes may be true of some individuals, but not of a collective group.

Health professionals, in particular, must be diligent in avoiding age prejudice, as believing stereotypes can influence interactions between older adults and caregivers. The caregiver may treat the older adult as a child in an old body. This approach is demeaning to elders and strips individuals of their self-esteem and dignity. Clients with cognitive or expressive deficits cannot always process questions or comments quickly or follow through with responses. Nurses and caregivers must never make the mistake of believing that clients do not understand verbal and, especially, nonverbal messages. Elders are a diverse group; they deserve respect and, through their memories and life examples, can teach a great deal to younger persons about life and survival and coping skills. Learning from clients and their families and assisting clients to find activities that enhance the quality of life (regardless of state of health) make caring for older adults a rewarding and satisfying experience.

Aging is universal, progressive, and irreversible and eventually leads to death. The aging process itself, however, is very individualized and is independent of chronological age. The way whereby an individual ages is influenced by genetics; lifestyle; availability and quality of health services; cultural beliefs; and socioeconomic status. Certain physiologic changes are expected with aging (Figure 35-2), although there exists considerable variation in the time of onset, rate, and

Figure 35-2 The aging process is a normal and natural part of growth and development.

degree of these changes. In order to render effective and compassionate care to elderly clients, nurses working in gerontology must be familiar with the normal processes as well as the common disorders of aging.

THEORIES OF AGING

At this time, no single theory of aging has been universally accepted by practitioners in gerontology. Aging is a complex issue that must take into account the psychosocial, cultural, and experiential aspects of living. Several biological theories of aging have been proposed to explain the physiologic and functional changes that are observed in older adults. Psychosocial theories of aging strive to explain the behaviors and social interactions of older adults. These theories are summarized in Table 35–1. It should be noted, however, that each generation is unique and that biological and psychosocial theories of aging are thus unlikely to be universal. Also, as more knowledge is garnered from scientific studies (e.g., the study of the impact on cells of auto-oxidization by free radicals and the study of dietary chemical exposure) and gene sequencing efforts (e.g., the human genome project), it is likely that the biological theories of aging will change as well.

MYTHS AND REALITIES OF AGING

Myths are fictitious ideas. Myths about elders are abundant and do not reflect the reality of the aging population. Following are some common myths associated with aging, based (in part) on data from the United States Bureau of Census and *A Profile of Older*

Table 35-1 THEORIES OF AGING

BIOLOGICAL THEORIES

Title	Major Premise
Somatic mutation theory	Radiation or miscoding of enzymes causes changes in the DNA. Changes associated with aging are the result of decreased function and efficiency of the cells and organs.
Programmed aging theory	The life span is programmed within the cells. This genetic clock determines the speed at which the person ages and eventually dies.
Cross-linkage, or collagen, theory	Collagen is the principal component of connective tissue and is also found in the skin, bones, muscles, lungs, and heart. Chemical reactions between collagen and cross-linking molecules cause loss of flexibility, resulting in diminished functional mobility.
Immunity theory	The thymus becomes smaller with age. The ability to produce T-cell differentiation decreases. This impairs immunologic functions and results in increased incidence of infections, neoplasms, and autoimmune disorders.
Stress theory	Stress throughout the lifetime causes structural and chemical changes in the body. These changes eventually cause irreversible tissue damage.

PSYCHOSOCIAL THEORIES

Title	Major Premise
Activity theory	Roles and responsibilities change throughout the lifetime. Life satisfaction depends on maintaining an involvement with life by developing new interests, hobbies, roles, and relationships.
Disengagement theory	There is decreased interaction between the older person and others in his social system. The disengagement is inevitable, mutual, and acceptable to both the individual and society.
Continuity theory	Successful methods used throughout life for adjusting and adapting to life events are repeated. Characteristic traits, habits, values, associations, and goals remain stable throughout the lifetime, regardless of life changes.

 CULTURAL CONSIDERATIONS

Aging

At the same time that diversity continues to broaden in the United States, it remains important to understand the individual needs of clients. As with all clients, it is important to assess the older client's religious beliefs, traditions, and culture and to evaluate the ways that these may influence the client's health beliefs and health practices. Not only can caregivers make the mistake of not fully assessing the client's beliefs about health in elders, they can also be misled themselves by myths about aging that exist in U.S. society.

dementia, long-term memory can remain somewhat intact long into the disease process. Thus, nurses and caregivers find that interventions such as reminiscence, memory photo books, and activities that draw on the client's long-practiced skills provide positive client outcomes (Figure 35-3).

Myth: Incontinence is an expected result of aging.

Reality: Incontinence is not an expected outcome of aging and, in most cases, can be reversed through assessment and treatment. The challenge is that many people are embarrassed to discuss this problem with family or primary providers. Also, in long-term care settings, both the belief in this myth and the historically low staffing levels have served to dissuade clinical efforts at providing the needed nursing interventions (prompted voiding; consistent, nonhurried, timed voiding) to reverse urinary incontinence. In settings where care is provided to older adults, lack of funding, lack of policy support and education, and inconsistent enforcement of adequate staffing levels have often had a negative impact on client health outcomes. By developing

Americans developed by the American Association of Retired Persons (AARP) in 1998.

Myth: Senility is an expected result of aging.

Reality: Senility is an outdated term once used to refer to any form of dementia that occurred in older people. Dementia is a result of disease, can affect adults of all ages, and is not a natural consequence of aging. Although some slight declines are noted in short-term memory from the age of 40 on, most people adjust through the use of memory aids such as lists and calendars. Long-term memory can actually become clearer with age. Even for a client with

Figure 35-3 Sharing memories and photographs with younger family members is valuable for all generations.

urinary incontinence treatment programs, care facilities could improve clinical outcomes for clients and also reduce health care costs.

Myth: Older adults are no longer interested in sexuality or sexual activity.

Reality: Sexuality is a lifelong need. Elders can be and are sexually active, regardless of age. Although sexual function may be affected by changes in the reproductive systems, persons of both genders are capable of orgasm into old age. Despite interest and desire, physiologic or psychological problems and medication side effects may present barriers to intercourse. In such situations, sexuality without coitus can provide elders with love and intimacy. It is important to remember that human beings are social beings. Just as small babies can fail to thrive without human touch (hugs, nurturing, companionship, valuing of the individual), so can older adults fail to thrive without these same human interactions and support (Figure 35-4).

A national survey by NCOA in 1998 revealed that half of those age 60 and older were sexually active. Approximately 72% of those were as satisfied or more satisfied with their sex lives compared to when they were in their forties (NCOA, 2000).

The medication sildenafil citrate (Viagra) has proven beneficial to many older couples as they work to meet their sexual health needs. The debate over the acceptance and funding of this medication for erectile dysfunction sheds light on just how far U.S. society still has to go in debunking this myth and replacing it with the truth that normal human sexuality needs continue throughout the life span.

Myth: Most people spend the last years of their lives in nursing homes.

Reality: According to NCOA (2000), in 1996 only 4.2% of those over age 65 lived in nursing homes. The percentage rises steeply with age, however (1% of those 65 to 74 years of age, 4% of those 75 to 84 years of age, and 20% of those over 85 years of age). For many, that stay will involve rehabilitation following surgery, a fracture, or stroke before returning home after a short hospital stay. The late 1990s have seen a growing interest in the use of alternative care options for elders (retirement communities, assisted living centers, group homes, respite care, and partial hospitalization/adult day programs). However, the majority of older adults continue to live in communities with varying levels of assistive services or support as they age. The projected trends in long-term care needs are for continued use of alternate settings that will support interventions to meet residents' physical, psychosocial, cultural, spiritual, cognitive, and mental health needs.

Traditionally, elders in long-term care facilities have been taken from home environments where they have likely experienced the highest level of independence they have had in their lifetimes (to choose when to get up, eat, go to bed, and the like), and have been placed in settings where very few, if any, choices, including care decisions, are made based on their preferences. Gerontological nurses have an ongoing responsibility to help recreate the way care is provided to elderly clients and to advocate for individual choices for older clients in long-term care facilities. Nurse leaders must learn to think in new ways about long-practiced trends in elder care in the United States and to work with older clients and their families to envision and create better trends.

Myth: All elderly persons are financially impoverished.

Reality: Income range varies among those over 65 years of age, just as it does among those in younger groups. However, the high costs of medications does disproportionately affect those over age 65, who are more likely to have one or more chronic conditions that require management with medication. In the past, lack of reimbursement for preventive assessment, treatments, and medications led many elders to go without medications or to delay care until they were too ill to wait any longer. This resulted in increased use of acute care services in hospitals.

In 1996, families headed by persons over 65 years of age had a median income of $28,983, despite the fact that the median net worth of older households (assets over expenses) is $86,300 (AARP, 1998). The challenge for most elders below the median (especially older women, who often have lower retirement incomes) is that most of their assets are tied up in the family home or in other nonliquid holdings. Thus, when an acute illness strikes, there is little financial reserve to help cover costs.

Figure 35-4 Individuals of all ages benefit from intimacy and companionship.

HEALTH AND AGING

Like all age groups, elders can do much to adopt a healthy lifestyle that will enhance their remaining years.

Activities of Daily Living

Being well groomed enhances the self-esteem of all older adults. Adaptive devices and techniques are available for those who need assistance with the **activities of daily living** (ADLs), basic care activities that include mobility, bathing, hygiene, grooming, dressing, eating, and toileting.

Mobility

Many assistive devices are available to help the older client maintain mobility and independence. Handrails can decrease the risk of falls while the person is walking (Figure 35-5); they are also useful in the tub and, when used in conjunction with a plastic riser, can help the older adult get on and off the toilet safely.

Bathing

Skin dryness increases with aging; thus, it may be preferable for older adults to bathe or shower only two to three times per week and to take sponge baths in between. A gentle soap should be used sparingly for the bath, after which a moisturizing lotion should be applied. The individual or caregiver should be instructed to inspect the skin during bathing for any indication of skin breakdown, lumps, or changes in moles.

With aging oil secretion decreases in the scalp, and hair can thus become dry. Shampooing one or two times per week is usually adequate for most elders, and a simplified hairstyle may be helpful to those with limited mobility in the arms. The use of mild shampoos and conditioners can also enhance hair texture.

Figure 35-5 Handrails allow clients more independence when ambulating.

Hygiene

Fingernails may become more brittle with aging. Keeping the client's fingernails clean and short can prevent accidental injury or scratches to fragile older skin. Impaired circulation is common among older adults, and special attention should thus be given to care of the feet and lower extremities. Because toenails frequently become thick and tougher with aging, soaking the feet prior to trimming the toenails may ease the task. For clients with circulation or skin integrity problems of the feet and toes or for clients with diabetes, a referral to a podiatrist should be made for nail trimming. During bathing, the client's feet should be monitored for discomfort; inflammation; broken skin; color changes such as redness, pallor, or cyanosis (blue or purple discoloration resulting from lack of circulation); heat or coldness; cracking between toes; and corns or calluses.

The need for adequate oral care does not diminish with aging. Dental problems can result in poor eating habits and inadequate nutrition. Inadequate brushing and dental check-ups can lead to gingivitis (bleeding and edematous gums), which, if left untreated, can progress to periodontal disease that can destroy connective tissue, alveolar bone, and periodontal ligaments. The nurse must therefore monitor clients for proper oral care. For those clients with dentures, the nurse must inspect the dentures for cleanliness and proper fit. Clients with dentures must brush the dentures and the gums regularly with a soft brush and a mild cleanser. It is helpful to label dentures with the client's name to facilitate identification of the dentures in the event that the client is admitted to a hospital or an assistive care setting.

Grooming

Good grooming is important in promoting the older client's self-esteem and confidence. Keeping the hair neat and tidy, choosing attractive clothing and jewelry, and making decisions about makeup and other personal care practices will all contribute to the older client's sense of well-being and independence (Figure 35-6).

Male clients may feel much better with a clean shaven face. Infection-control principles demand that each razor (either electric or blade) be used for only one individual, and that that razor be marked with the client's name. Women may also require attention to facial hair, as estrogen levels decrease after menopause. It is not uncommon for older women to notice hairs on the chin or upper lip that were not there in younger days. Also, both men and women are likely to notice graying and diminished hair on legs, underarms, and pubic areas as they age.

Dressing

Dressing may be difficult for clients who have restricted joint movement, paralysis, or limited endurance

Figure 35-6 Good grooming for the older client includes choosing personal items such as jewelry and clothing.

Figure 35-7 Assistive devices such as these for panty-hose and buttons are available to help clients dress independently. (*Courtesy of Maddak, Inc.*)

due to health problems. Many choices are available to ease dressing, such as elastic waists, velcro fasteners, and assistive reaching and dressing devices (Figure 35-7).

Eating

Many older adults are able to maintain the ability to self-feed, thereby promoting independence and self-esteem. Neurological and musculoskeletal alterations may, however, affect ability to self-feed. Dysphagia, or difficulty swallowing, may place the older client at increased risk of choking, and diminished taste sensation may affect the desire to eat.

Toileting

Toileting habits also change with aging. Bowel elimination problems can often be prevented as clients age by:

- Ensuring adequate fiber intake,
- Ensuring adequate fluid intake,
- Ensuring regular daily exercise, and
- Developing regular elimination habits.

For the client in the hospital or a long-term care facility, it is helpful to:

- Maintain previously effective habits such as reading on the toilet or drinking warm liquids upon arising, and
- Assist the client to the toilet approximately 30 minutes after eating, to take advantage of the gastro-colic reflex.

As a result of the physical changes that occur with aging, increased frequency of urination may be noted in elders of both genders. It is not uncommon for older adults to self-limit fluid intake due to a fear of incontinence. This habit is unhealthy and should thus be discouraged. Cases of incontinence should be assessed to determine the cause and type, so that appropriate interventions and treatment can be implemented. Timing

the use of prescribed diuretics in the morning rather than the evening can prevent the increased need for urination at night, which is especially helpful to older clients who are being treated for congestive heart failure (CHF).

Exercise

What was once accepted as the normal deterioration of old age is now considered the result of disuse through sitting and bed rest. Research indicates that high-intensity, progressive resistance training can improve muscle strength and muscle size in frail elderly clients. Walking and all other maneuvers required for ADLs are also beneficial. Exercise programs should be individually planned and should take into consideration the older person's:

- General health status (Figure 35-8),
- Physiologic disorders (if present),
- Preference for solidarity or group activity,
- Physical environment, and
- Financial status.

▌ PROFESSIONAL TIP

Bowel Patterns in Elderly Clients

It is extremely important that caregivers of older adults monitor bowel patterns. Long periods of constipation (> than 2 to 3 days) should alert caregivers to the need for interventions to minimize the likelihood of bowel impaction, which can ultimately be life threatening if left untreated. Evacuation aids such as laxatives, lubricants, stool softeners, and enemas all have side-effects and should thus be avoided if at all possible. Dietary changes or an exercise regimen should be introduced first.

Figure 35-8 Exercise is important to all clients and should be tailored to interests and ability levels.

Nutrition

For many older adults, cultural heritage, religious rites, ethnic practices, and family traditions are linked to food. The physiologic, psychological, sociological, and economic changes of aging may compromise nutritional status. Elders must follow a balanced diet, often with lowered intakes of sugar, caffeine, and sodium. There are no universally accepted dietary guidelines specific to older adults. A dietitian can determine the needed food intake for a specific individual by taking into account the individual's height, ideal weight, activity level, and disease processes.

The National Institutes of Health (NIH) recommends 1,000 mg of calcium per day for both men and women over the age of 25. Postmenopausal women 50 to 65 years of age who are not receiving estrogen therapy have been reported to need 1,500 mg of calcium per day (Yen, 1995). It is important to note that calcium supplements should also contain vitamin D to provide for optimal metabolism by the body. The need for additional supplements depends on the older individual's nutritional status and ability to maintain an adequate diet. Growing discussion supports the needs for adequate protein intake, to maintain both skin integrity and bone density; moderate carbohydrates intake due to the metabolism of carbohydrates to sugars; and, whenever possible, the acquisition of needed calcium from dietary intake of unprocessed natural cheeses (Peskin, 1999).

It is important that nurses be knowledgeable about community services designed to help older clients meet their nutritional needs. Such services include grocery transportation and delivery services, homebound meals (e.g., Meals on Wheels), group meals at senior food sites, and the Food Stamp program. Nurses and caregivers should also realize that socialization and companionship are necessary components of adequate dietary intake, and should thus ensure that these areas are addressed as part of any food-assistance intervention.

Psychosocial Considerations

Older adults, like all individuals, have psychosocial and cognitive needs for lifelong learning. Many colleges have developed education program options for elder students (often at no tuition), and employers are beginning to recruit older workers for part-time positions (recognizing their historically good work ethic and experience). Many elders continue to volunteer countless hours each year, offering to help meet the social service needs of their communities. These efforts can result in feelings of productivity and self-worth for the older adult. Mental activity and emotional involvement are as necessary to the overall well-being as is physical activity. Older clients can benefit from building on their long-practiced skills to develop interesting and stimulating activities or hobbies. Such activities may be of an individual or group nature. Socialization with people of all age groups can help not only the older participants, but also the young and middle-age participants, by illustrating that aging is not a disease but, rather, a rich and natural part of the life process.

Strengths

Older adults generally have suffered many losses over the years. Some losses are slight and require only minor adaptation, whereas others may significantly affect the person. Physiologic changes or disease processes may result in losses, causing impairments in:

- Communication,
- Vision and learning,
- Mobility,
- Cognition, or
- Psychosocial skills.

If the impairment is severe, the individual could lose some degree of independence, and adaptations may be required. Furthermore, losses can cascade for the older client, as one loss contributes to another. For example, if an elderly person with diabetes were to lose her driver's license due to impaired vision related to diabetic retinopathy, socialization might be restricted, which in turn might increase her feelings of loneliness and diminished self-esteem. If, however, her spouse provides caregiving and transportation, these adaptations might allow her to remain active socially while still living in her home. If her spouse later dies, and her health continues to decline, a move to an assisted living facility may become necessary, if other community adaptations are unavailable. She would then be faced with adapting to the loss of both her home and her spouse.

Health care professionals should remember that persons who have lived for many years are survivors and can adapt to life changes better if they are allowed to utilize their existing strengths. They are often much stronger and more ingenious and enterprising than they are given credit for. The strengths of each individual (including past coping skills) must be identified and utilized when planning care and assisting the older client to find new ways to adapt and maintain optimal independence in a new setting.

Health Promotion and Disease Prevention

Older adults must be alerted to means of preventing disease and reducing risks. Being knowledgeable about self-care and participating in screening tests are important components of health maintenance. For older men, annual prostate examinations and a regular prostate specific antigen (PSA) level lab test, which can detect prostate cancer in the early stages, are recommended every 1 to 2 years. For older women, annual mammograms and Pap smears, and monthly breast self-examinations represent means of detecting breast and gynecological cancers in the early stages. Nurses can teach their clients habits for healthy living and inform them of signs and symptoms that require medical investigation. Older clients who have been exposed to environmental chemicals, tobacco, or extensive alcohol use over many years often experience serious health consequences as they reach older age. Older clients of any age can benefit from healthy lifestyles and from disease-prevention interventions such as being inoculated yearly against influenza and every 6 years against pneumonia; assessment of tuberculosis (TB) status; and adequate safe food and clean water intake.

In many cases, by the time a person reaches 65 to 70 years of age, that person has been prescribed medication to address at least one ongoing (chronic)

PROFESSIONAL TIP

Identifying Strengths of Older Adults as Part of Assessment

Assessment should include the identification of strengths as well as problems. Strengths are utilized to achieve or maintain optimal physical, mental, and emotional function. All of the following can be considered strengths:

- Cognitive health
- Freedom from or successful adaptation to deficits or impairments
- A history of healthy lifestyle with regard to diet, sleep, stress management, exercise, and chemical abuse (none)
- Adequate functional ability to carry out ADL
- Freedom from incapacitating physical discomfort and pain
- A physically safe living environment
- Feelings of security in present environment
- Realistic knowledge about capabilities
- Pattern of avoiding dangerous situations and unnecessary risks
- Compliance with health care regimen
- Capability with regard to managing own environment
- An intact support system
- Satisfying relationships with others
- Opportunities for sexual expression
- Access to transportation
- Adequate functional mobility
- Successful adaptation to life changes and crises
- History of relinquishing roles as phases of life require and replacing them with satisfying new roles
- A pattern of successful mourning for losses

- Participation in groups: religious, community, hobbies
- Membership in family whose members respect each other and are willing to give and receive help when necessary
- Successful problem-solving skills
- Willingness to seek information to improve situation
- Evidence of initiative and self-confidence in abilities and judgment
- Participation in self-care by making decisions and accepting responsibility for decisions
- A well-defined value system
- Acceptance of that which cannot be changed
- Successful use of assertive skills
- Strong spiritual beliefs and ability to find comfort and strength in spiritual and religious practices
- Enthusiastic appreciation for aging, with demonstrative embrace of the positive aspects and adaptation to the negative aspects
- Participation in healthy reminiscing; evidence of few regrets about life past
- Joyful appreciation for nature, art, music, hobbies, and activities
- A well-developed sense of humor

medical problem (e.g., hypertension, heart disease, diabetes, allergies, gastrointestinal disorders). The challenge many elders face is that side effects from one medication are often treated with another prescription medication. If the client then goes to different doctors, these doctors may prescribe even more medications to address the same or other health concerns. This is called **polypharmacy**, or the problem of clients taking numerous prescription and over-the-counter medications for the same or various disease processes, with unknown consequences from the resulting combinations of chemical compounds and cumulative side effects. In many settings, primary care providers, nurses, clinical pharmacists, and social workers collaborate on interdisciplinary teams to assist the older client and the family to oversee the client's medication management, as well as other health needs.

Among the biggest challenges facing older clients are shorter hospitalization stays and reduced time with physicians in the physician's offices. There is less time to ensure that the follow-up services the client will need are understood and in place and less time to educate client and family about medication regimens, including timing and possible interactions with other prescription and over-the-counter drugs or herbal remedies that the client may also be taking. The nurse, as part of the interdisciplinary team, plays a vital role as client advocate when ensuring that older clients have the teaching, services, and follow-up care they need.

PHYSIOLOGIC CHANGES ASSOCIATED WITH AGING

Although the aging process brings with it many physiologic changes, it should be remembered that aging and disease are not synonymous. Whereas the physiologic changes of aging described following are normal for most people, the medical disorders described are not considered normal.

Respiratory System

See Chapter 18 for an anatomy and physiology review of the respiratory system. The following respiratory changes result from the aging process:

- The muscles of respiration become less flexible, causing decreased vital capacity of the lungs.
- Decrease in functional capacity results in dyspnea on exertion or stress; usual activity does not affect breathing.
- Effectiveness of the cough mechanism lessens, increasing the risk of lung infection.
- The alveoli thicken and decrease in number and size, causing less effective gas exchange and, in individuals who also have chronic lung disease, intensifying respiratory deficits.

- Structural changes in the skeleton, such as kyphosis (seen in clients with osteoporosis as an often asymetrical convex curve of the spine) can decrease diaphragmatic expansion. Kyphosis in older clients can lead to a need for small, more frequent meals to balance nutritional requirements and respiratory function due to the restriction of adequate space for expansion and contraction of the diaphragm. It can also create skin integrity risks, as the bony prominences of the client's back press against the backs of chairs.

Common respiratory disorders related to aging include the following:

- Respiratory tract infection (RTI)
- Chronic obstructive pulmonary disease (COPD)
- Pulmonary tuberculosis (TB)

Nursing Interventions: Respiratory Tract Infections

1. Advise discussing the pneumovaccine with the primary care provider.
2. Advise obtaining annual influenza vaccine.
3. Assist the client to assume a position of comfort and assist with medications and respiratory treatments, as ordered.
4. Avoid distention of bowel, bladder, or stomach, any of which can increase breathing discomfort.
5. Allow adequate time for nursing care.
6. Administer humidified oxygen therapy, as prescribed.
7. Administer analgesics and antipyretics, as prescribed.

PROFESSIONAL TIP

TB in the Elderly Client

Elders can be vulnerable to TB because of:

- An ineffective cough reflex and the resulting inability to clear the lungs.
- An altered immune system and a reduced response to extrinsic antigens. Not only are elders at increased risk of infection via a new contagion, but older clients who contracted TB years ago and have been in remission since can experience reexacerbation. The risk of reexacerbation increases in cases where the initial infection was remote and healed (encapsulated) such that the immune system's memory of the T cells has been lost. Facilities where health care is provided to older clients and to immune compromised clients thus must regularly assess the TB status of both their clients and their employees.

8. Assess for signs of dehydration and ensure that fluids are accessible to the client, unless contraindicated.
9. Review diagnostic data and monitor lung sounds and intake and output every 8 hours or as needed given changes in the client's condition. Weigh the client daily, assessing for fluid retention.
10. Monitor for any signs of respiratory distress (cyanosis of lips, mucous membranes, or nailbeds) and obtain pulse-oximetry readings, as needed.

Nursing Interventions: Chronic Obstructive Pulmonary Disease

1. Assist the client to a position of comfort.
2. Teach the client to use pursed-lip breathing to avoid hyperventilation when short of breath.
3. Teach the client diaphragmatic breathing for use when active.
4. Teach proper use of inhalers. Steroid inhalers should be used first, with a full 60-second wait between puffs; after waiting 3 minutes, any bronchodilator inhalers that are prescribed should then be used, also with a 60 second wait between puffs.
5. Teach the client to cough and clear the airway.
6. Adminster chest physiotherapy (e.g., percussion, postural drainage), if prescribed.
7. Establish a schedule for ambulation, gradually increasing the distance ambulated.
8. Assist with active assistive range of motion exercises.
9. Monitor for signs and symptoms of infections (e.g., fever, blood-tinged or thick, greenish colored sputum, and diminished lung sounds) and immediately report same to the registered nurse and the primary care provider.
10. Monitor breathing and pulse rate and administer oxygen, if necessary, during periods of increased activity.

PROFESSIONAL TIP

COPD

Remember that in the client with COPD, breathing may not be triggered by a higher level of carbon dioxide as it would in clients without COPD, because the client with COPD always has a consistently high CO_2 level. The breathing impulse is instead triggered by a low level of oxygen. Increasing the oxygen level by more than 1 to 2 L/h in the client with COPD can shut shut down the trigger to breathe, and can drive the client into respiratory failure.

11. Suggest smoking cessation programs, if the client is a smoker.

Safety: Oxygen and Smoking
Ensure that no smoking is allowed around clients on oxygen therapy.

Nursing Interventions: Pulmonary Tuberculosis

1. Monitor clients for TB status and for symptoms including fever, night sweats, weight loss, and cough producing blood-tinged sputum.
2. Inform the client, family, and caregivers of the need for adequate isolation techniques.

Infection Control: TB
Remember that TB is spread through droplets when a client sneezes or coughs (direct and indirect contact). Consult the infection-control nurse on the client's interdisciplinary team and work to protect the client and others from transmission of *Mycrobacterium tuberculosis* and other infections.

3. Evaluate the client's risk for infection with the human immunodeficiency virus (HIV) and related pneumocystic pneumonia.
4. Monitor that the client's psychosocial needs are being adequately met while the disease is being pharmacologically addressed with medications like isoniazid (Laniazid). Tell the client and family that the entire course of medication must be completed.
5. Monitor the client's nutrition intake and provide supplements as necessary to maintain adequate body weight.
6. Provide for rest periods throughout the day. Encourage the older client with TB to monitor activity level and length of visits by family so as not to become overtired.

Cardiovascular System

See Chapter 19 for an anatomy and physiology review of the cardiovascular system. The following cardiovascular changes result from the aging process:

- Cardiac output and recovery time decline. The heart requires more time to return to a normal rate after a rate increase in response to activity.
- The heart rate slows.
- Blood flow to all organs decreases. The brain and coronary arteries continue to receive a larger volume than do other organs.
- Arterial elasticity decreases, causing increased peripheral resistance and, in turn, a rise in systolic blood pressure and a slight rise in diastolic blood pressure.
- Veins dilate, and superficial vessels become more prominent.

Common cardiovascular disorders related to aging include the following:

- Peripheral vascular disease (PVD)
- Hypertension
- Chronic CHF

Nursing Interventions: Peripheral Vascular Disease

1. Assess the lower extremeties, including the peripheral pulses, for signs of arterial or venous insufficiency.
2. Evaluate lifestyle factors that may aggravate or advance atherosclerosis, such as a high-carbohydrate, high-fat diet and little exercise.
3. Teach the client about the disease, including treatment, medication actions and side effects, and signs of thrombosis.
4. Educate the client and caregivers about the care and inspection of the lower extremeties.
5. Provide instructions on interventions specific to the client's type of PVD (arterial or venous).

Nursing Interventions: Hypertension

1. Evaluate food intake patterns, especially of cholesterol, fats, sodium, and carbohydrates. Make recommendations based on findings.
2. Evaluate for fluid retention.
3. Recommend a smoking cessation program, if necessary.
4. Advise the client to avoid alcohol use.
5. Recommend and facilitate a consistent and appropriate exercise program.
6. Discuss the relationship of stress to hypertension and provide resources from which the client can learn relaxation techniques.
7. Provide information on medications and the importance of taking daily blood pressure medications as prescribed, regardless of health status on any given day.
8. Arrange for and encourage regular blood pressure checks and teach the client or significant others proper use of blood pressure equipment, if applicable.

Nursing Interventions: Chronic Congestive Heart Failure

1. Frequently monitor serum digitalis level and monitor for any signs of digoxin toxicity, for which older clients are at increased risk due to the decreased rate of renal clearance of the drug. Withhold the digoxin and immediately contact the registered nurse and the physician if abnormal serum level or signs and symptoms of toxicity are present.

CLIENT TEACHING

Digoxin Toxicity

Possible signs and symptoms of digoxin toxicity include the following:
- Disturbances in cardiac rhythms
- Fatigue
- Listlessness
- Anorexia
- Nausea
- Visual disturbances (halos around lights)
- Shaking
- Unsteady gait
- Confusion

2. Take the apical pulse for a full 1 minute before administering digoxin. Withhold the medication if the apical pulse is below 60, and consult the registered nurse and the physician if this or any other significant changes in vital signs are noted.
3. Monitor the client's blood pressure and lung sounds.
4. Monitor electrolyte levels, blood urea nitrogen (BUN), and creatinine level to observe system changes including decreased kidney efficiency.
5. Monitor for signs of fluid retention such as intake and output (output too small), weight gain, shortness of breath, or coughing.
6. Encourage alternating periods of activity with periods of rest.
7. Encourage the client to maintain a level of exercise/physical activity appropriate to physical condition.
8. Teach the client and family about the safe use of the prescribed medications.
9. For clients on diuretics, which deplete potassium, monitor fluid intake and level of potassium, ensuring adequacy of each. Encourage administration of diuretics early in the day, unless contraindicated, to prevent increased urination at night.

Gastrointestinal System

See Chapter 28 for an anatomy and physiology review of the gastrointestinal system. The following gastrointestinal changes result from the aging process:

- Tooth enamel thins.
- Periodontal disease rate increases.
- Taste buds decrease in number, and saliva production diminishes.
- Effectiveness of the gag reflex lessens, resulting in an increased risk of choking.

- Esophageal peristalsis slows, and the effectiveness of the esophageal sphincter lessens, causing delayed entry of food into the stomach and increasing the risk of aspiration.
- Hiatal hernia may occur.
- Gastric emptying slows. Food remains in the stomach longer, decreasing the capacity of the stomach.
- Peristalsis and nerve sensation of the large intestine decreases, contributing to constipation.
- The incidence of diverticulosis increases with age.
- Liver size decreases after age 70.
- Liver enzymes decrease, slowing drug metabolism and the detoxification process.
- Emptying of the gallbladder lessens in efficiency, resulting in thickened bile, increased cholesterol content, and increased incidence of gallstones.

PROFESSIONAL TIP

Determining Alterations in Nutrition

- Height and weight: Record actual body weight, usual body weight, and ideal body weight. If usual weight has varied significantly from the ideal for several years, the use of height/weight tables may be meaningless. Compare actual body weight to usual body weight to determine present status.
- Review laboratory values: hematocrit, hemoglobin, total iron-binding capacity, total protein, BUN.
- Determine whether client is on a weight-loss diet.
- Determine whether client was edematous when initially weighed and has lost weight with treatment.
- Evaluate cognitive status. Cognitively impaired clients may be unaware of hunger or be unable to attend to the task of eating.
- In clients with central nervous system damage, evaluate the presence of sensory–perceptual deficits that interfere with eating.
- Evaluate ability to pick up utensils and glasses and to get items from table to mouth.
- Evaluate dental/oral status: status of teeth/dentures, gums, presence of oral dryness (xerostomia).
- Determine presence of impaired swallowing.
- Determine whether client has distaste for certain food groups.
- Assess knowledge in regard to nutrition and food purchase and preparation.
- Determine whether client is taking medications that interfere with taste or food absorption.
- Determine whether financial status interferes with food purchasing.
- Evaluate for history of compulsive eating.

Common gastrointestinal disorders related to aging include the following:

- Over-/undernutrition
- Constipation
- Dehydration
- Dental disorders

Nursing Interventions: Over-/Undernutrition

1. Assess nutritional status.
2. Provide nutritional instruction based on assessment findings.
3. Advise on community nutrition programs (e.g., Meals-on-Wheels, senior center food sites, food pantries, and Food Stamp program).

Nursing Interventions: Constipation

1. Assess food and fluid intake.
2. Make recommendations based on assessment findings (e.g., increase fiber intake, increase fluid intake).

COMMUNITY/HOME HEALTH CARE

Nutritional Status

Evaluate the following when assessing a client's nutritional status in the home:

- Ability to shop for and prepare meals (Figure 35-9)
- Mealtime environment, for unpleasant odors, noises, and visual stimuli
- Table setting, for appealing table cover, centerpiece, colorful dishes
- Appropriateness of food storage system (cabinets, refrigerator, freezer)

Figure 35-9 Cooking and preparing foods in the home are important skills to maintaining a nutritionally healthy lifestyle.

3. Discuss the relationship of exercise to bowel activity.
4. Discuss the importance of routine for regular bowel elimination.
5. Advise avoiding the overuse of laxatives.
6. Monitor adequate bowel elimination and provide interventions (e.g., prune juice, senna bars, milk of magnesia, as ordered) to assist the client in returning to a normal bowel elimination routine.

Nursing Interventions: Dehydration

1. Identify the reason for dehydration (i.e., inadequate fluid intake or excessive fluid output).
2. Identify the reason and corresponding interventions for inadequate fluid intake:
   - Fluids are inaccessible due to the client's physical limitations: offer fluids on a regular basis throughout the day.
   - The client dislikes water or other available fluids: identify fluid choices.
   - The client restricts fluids due to a fear of incontinence: explain the relationship of decreased fluid intake to bladder infections and arrange for assistance, as needed, for toileting.
3. Identify the reasons for any excessive fluid output and treat accordingly.

Nursing Interventions: Dental Disorders

1. Teach the oral hygiene procedures of brushing and flossing and facilitate and encourage brushing of the teeth and gums and flossing of the teeth, as tolerated.
2. Inspect the mouth regularly for signs of dental disorders.
3. Advise regular dental checkups.

Reproductive System: Female

See Chapter 30 for an anatomy and physiology review of the female reproductive system. The following reproductive changes result from the aging process:

- Estrogen production decreases with the onset of menopause.
- Ovaries, uterus, and cervix decrease in size.
- The vagina shortens, narrows, and becomes less elastic, and the vaginal lining thins. Secretions decrease and become more alkaline, resulting in increased incidence of atrophic vaginitis. These changes may result in discomfort during coitus, which can often be rectified with the use of a water-based lubricant. As at any age, protected intercourse (safe sex) through the use of a latex condom should be advised with new partners.
- Supporting musculature of the reproductive organs weakens, increasing the risk of uterine prolapse.
- Breast tissue diminishes, and nipple erection lessens during sexual arousal.

Figure 35-10 Sexuality and companionship remain important throughout the life span.

- Libido and the need for intimacy and companionship in older women remain unchanged (Figure 35-10).

Common female reproductive system disorders related to aging include the following:

- Breast cancer (the risk of which increases with age)
- Altered sexuality patterns related to physiologic changes, medications, changes in body image, or psychosocial changes such as the loss of significant other or a move to a setting that provides some level of assistive care (i.e., group home, assisted living center, or care facility)

Nursing Interventions: Female Reproductive System Disorders

1. Teach and encourage monthly breast self-exams and yearly mammograms for early detection and treatment of disorders.
2. Establish rapport and encourage the client to verbalize feelings and concerns related to sexuality, body image, and self-esteem.
3. Complete a sexual history and recommend interventions based on findings. Support the client's needs for companionship and intimacy throughout the life span.
4. Recommend that a bone density scan be discussed with the client's primary care provider to allow for early detection and treatment of osteoporosis.
5. Encourage annual gynecological examinations with the client's primary care provider.

Reproductive System: Male

See Chapter 31 for an anatomy and physiology review of the male reproductive system. The following reproductive changes result from the aging process:

- Testosterone production decreases, resulting in decreased size of the testicles.
- Sperm count and viscosity of seminal fluid decrease.
- Although more time is required to obtain erection, the older man often finds that he and his partner can enjoy longer periods of lovemaking (greater control) prior to ejaculation. As at any age, protected intercourse (safe sex) through the use of a latex condom should be advised with new partners.
- The prostate gland may enlarge.
- Impotency may occur. Medications and other medical interventions have been successful in reversing impotency problems in many older males. A thorough evaluation by the primary care provider and a urologist can provide clients with available options given health status and current medication regimen.
- Libido and the need for intimacy and companionship remain unchanged in older males.

Common male reproductive disorders related to aging include the following:

- Altered sexuality patterns related to physiologic changes, medications, changes in body image, or psychosocial changes such as the loss of significant other or a move to a setting that provides some level of assistive care (i.e., group home, assisted living center, or care facility)
- Benign prostatic hypertophy (BPH)

Nursing Interventions: Male Reproductive System Disorders

1. Establish rapport and encourage the client to verbalize feelings and concerns related to sexuality, body image, and self-esteem.
2. Complete a sexual history and recommend interventions based on findings. Support the client's needs for companionship and intimacy throughout the life span.
3. Provide client and family education regarding the signs and symptoms of prostate disorders (e.g., difficulty in starting the urine stream, a smaller urine stream, frequent urination, frequent nighttime awakening for the purpose of urinating, or, in severe cases, the failure or inability to urinate).
4. Teach and encourage monthly testicular self exam and yearly digital rectal examinations of the prostate gland by a primary care provider. The benefits of a PSA lab test performed every 1 to 2 years to facilitate early detection and treatment of prostate cancer are currently under research and debate.

Endocrine System

See Chapter 27 for an anatomy and physiology review of the endocrine system. The following endocrine changes result from the aging process:

- Alterations occur in both the reception and the production of hormones.
- Release of insulin by the beta cells of the pancreas slows, causing an increase in blood sugar.
- Thyroid changes may lower the basal metabolic rate.

The most common endocrine disorder related to aging is diabetes mellitus type 2.

Nursing Interventions: Diabetes Mellitus Type 2

1. Arrange for a consultation with a dietitian to assess nutritional status and to provide food-management instruction.
2. Teach the client, family members, or caregivers (as appropriate) the procedure for blood glucose monitoring specific to the equipment the client will be using.
3. Develop a personal exercise program with the client based on the client's physical condition, mental status, resources, and interests.
4. Provide information on prescribed oral hypoglycemic medications.
5. Teach the causes, signs, and treatment of hypoglycemia and hyperglycemia.
6. Advise on self-care and on careful monitoring of the extremities and of sores on the skin, to minimize threats to skin integrity.
7. Encourage the client to wear shoes and to have nails trimmed by a podiatrist, if unable to safely perform self-care.

Musculoskeletal System

See Chapter 24 for an anatomy and physiology review of the musculoskeletal system. The following musculoskeletal changes result from the aging process:

- Muscle mass and elasticity diminish, resulting in decreased strength, endurance, coordination, and increased reaction time.
- Bone demineralization occurs, causing skeletal instability and shrinkage of intervertebral disks. The flexibility of the spine lessens, and spinal curvature often occurs.
- Joints undergo degenerative changes, resulting in pain, stiffness, and loss of range of motion.

Common musculoskeletal system disorders related to aging include the following:

- Osteoporosis
- Degenerative arthritis
- Fractured hip

Nursing Interventions: Osteoporosis

1. Make dietary recommendations to ensure adequate intake of calcium, protein, and vitamin D.

2. Recommend a smoking cessation program, if necessary.
3. Advise the client to avoid alcohol.
4. Encourage the client to take a calcium supplement in conjunction with vitamin D, as ordered by the client's primary care provider.
5. Recommend consultation with the primary care provider regarding either estrogen replacement therapy (ERT) options for females, or the use of medications like alendronate sodium (Fosamax) to address bone density loss associated with osteoporosis.
6. Teach the client, family, and caregivers about measures to reduce the risk of falling and sustaining fractures.
7. Recommend evaluation (via x-ray) for the presence of stress, or compression, fractures of the spine in cases of severe back pain that occurs with or without a fall. In clients with osteoporosis, these fractures can occur more easily because the vertebrae are compacted by shrinkage of the intervertebral spaces as a consequence of aging.
8. Provide adequate pain control for back pain or other musculoskeletal discomfort.
9. Monitor for adequate dietary intake of calories and fluids and for effective elimination patterns.
10. Teach, encourage, and assist clients to establish exercise programs appropriate to their capabilities. Especially promote exercise programs that include walking or other weight-bearing activities, as tolerated (Figure 35-11).

Figure 35-11 This elderly client is able to ambulate and remain active with the help of an assistive device.

Nursing Interventions: Degenerative Arthritis

1. Suggest a schedule for alternating periods of activity and rest.
2. Advise a weight reduction plan, if necessary, to eliminate extra strain on affected joints.
3. Teach, assist, and encourage the client to establish an exercise program that emphasizes gentle stretching and movement of all joints. For those clients who are more independent, exercise programs in warm water can have positive outcomes.
4. Provide adequate pain control. Teach clients and caregivers to monitor for gastrointestinal distress related to arthritis medications such as nonsteroidal anti-inflammatory drugs (NSAIDs) and to be aware that enteric coated medications cannot be crushed, as they are designed to protect the stomach by dissolving in the duodenum.
5. Encourage the client to seek ongoing evaluation by the physician, as new arthritis medications such as celecoxib (Celebrex) are continually being developed and trialed.

Nursing Interventions: Fractured Hip

NOTE: Nursing interventions may vary depending on whether the older client has an open reduction/internal fixation fracture (ORIF) or total hip arthoplasty (THA).

1. Maintain postoperative positioning as appropriate to the client's form of treatment.
2. Provide adequate pain control prior to physical therapy and on an ongoing basis through the recovery process.
3. Prevent complications, including skin breakdown, RTIs, infections at the surgical site, and dislocation of the prosthesis or internal fixation device.
4. Facilitate and monitor with the registered nurse the client's consistent use of antiembolism stockings as ordered and the administration of anticoagulant medications and the related monitoring of lab values, to decrease the risk of pulmonary embolism (which can be a significant risk to older clients after hip fracture and/or hip replacement).
5. Teach the client about fall prevention. Evaluate the client's environment (home, room, bathroom) for safety with regard to mobility and make recommendations for rectifying any threats to safety.

Integumentary System

See Chapter 21 for an anatomy and physiology review of the integumentary system. The following integumentary changes result from the normal aging process:

• Subcutaneous tissue and elastin fibers diminish, causing the skin to become thinner and less elastic.

Figure 35-12 Hyperpigmentation is a normal result of the aging process.

Figure 35-13 Gray hair results from a reduction in melanin production.

- Ability of melanocytes to produce even pigmentation diminishes, resulting in hyperpigmentation or liver spots, typically on the hands and wrists (Figure 35-12).
- Eccrine, apocrine, and sebaceous glands decrease in size, number, and function, resulting in diminished secretions and moisturization and, thus, pruritis.
- Body temperature regulation diminishes due to decreased perspiration and, many times, decreased circulation.
- Capillary blood flow decreases, resulting in slower wound healing.
- Blood flow decreases, especially to lower extremities.
- Vascular fragility causes senile purpura.
- Cutaneous sensitivity to pressure and temperature diminishes.
- Melanin production decreases, causing gray-white hair (Figure 35-13).
- Scalp, pubic, and axillary hair thin, and women display increased facial hair on the upper lip and chin.
- Nail growth slows, nails become more brittle, and longitudinal nail ridges form.

Common integumentary disorders related to aging include the following:

- Pressure ulcers (alteration in skin integrity)
- Herpes zoster (shingles)
- Skin cancer (included because the risk of skin cancer increases with age)

Nursing Interventions: Alteration in Skin Integrity

1. Perform a pressure ulcer risk assessment upon the client's admission to the health care setting (Figure 35-14).
2. Implement pressure ulcer prevention protocol for clients at risk for pressure ulcer formation. It is important to consider and document pressure relieving interventions for all surfaces that the client will sit or lay on during the course of the day (Table 35–2).
3. Encourage adequate intake of protein and fluids to help ensure good skin integrity.

Infection Control: Skin Integrity

It is the nurse's responsibility to educate caregivers (including other staff members, as necessary) about the need to thoroughly wash and dry the client's perineal area, and to keep linens and clothing clean and dry, especially when incontinence is a problem. Such education may also include instruction on maintaining client privacy; properly retracting, cleansing, and repositioning the foreskin of an uncircumcised older male client; and proper cleansing of the skin folds of an older female client's perineal area. Clients and caregivers should also be instructed to cleanse front to back only and to not rinse and reuse washcloths again or use them on other body areas. These simple hygiene and infection-control guidelines can help maintain the client's skin integrity and can also prevent unnecessary infections.

Nursing Interventions: Herpes Zoster

1. Treat the pain.
2. Treat the ulcer with medications (e.g., acyclovir [Zovirax] topical cream), as ordered, to reduce the length of time of the outbreak.
3. Develop a plan to ensure continuity in meeting the client's psychosocial needs, and allow the client time to share concerns.

Infection Control: Herpes Zoster

Prevent cross-infection from drainage from the vesicular eruptions by practicing proper handwashing and implementing appropriate isolation procedures, especially if the client is in the hospital or another health care facility.

Date of assessment: _____   Nurse: _____

Pressure ulcer present on admission: No _____   Yes _____   Stage _____

A score of 11 or more places a client at risk for pressure ulcer formation. Preventive protocol should be established.

Activity		Total	Level of Consciousness		Total
Ambulant without assistance	0		Alert	0	
Ambulant with assistance	2		Slow verbal response	1	
Chairfast	4		Responds to verbal or painful stimuli	2	
Bedfast	6	_____	Absence of response to stimuli	3	_____
Mobility—Range of Motion			**Nutritional Status**		
Full range of motion	0		Good (eats 75% or more of required intake)	0	
Moves with minimal assistance	2		Fair (eats less than 75% of required intake)	1	
Moves with moderate assistance	4		Poor (minimal intake, consistent weight loss)	2	
Immobile	6	_____	Unable/refuses to eat/drink, emaciated	3	_____
Skin Condition			**Incontinence—Bladder**		
Hydrated and intact	0		None	0	
Rashes or abrasions	2		Occasional (fewer than 2/24 hours)	1	
Decreased turgor, dry	4		Usually (more than 2/24 hours)	2	
Edema, erythema, pressure ulcers	6	_____	Total (no control)	3	
Predisposing Disease Process			**Incontinence—Bowel**		
No involvement	0		None	0	
Chronic, stable	1		Occasional (formed stool)	1	
Acute or chronic, unstable	2		Usually (semi-formed stool)	2	
Terminal	3	_____	Total (no control, loose stool)	3	_____

Figure 35-14 Pressure Ulcer Risk Assessment

Table 35–2 PROTOCOL FOR CLIENTS AT RISK FOR PRESSURE ULCERS

OBJECTIVE	INTERVENTIONS	OBJECTIVE	INTERVENTIONS
Relieve pressure	• Establish positioning schedule. • Place pressure relieving mattress on bed, cushions on chair. • Teach client wheelchair exercises. • Stand and/or ambulate client in chair frequently. • Use wheelchair for transporting only. • Allow client to sit on bedpan, commode, or toilet for only brief periods. • Check areas of pressure under casts, braces, splints, slings, prostheses.	Prevent spasticity and contractures	• Avoid quick, rough movements. • Do range of motion exercises at least twice daily. • Assess for synergy patterns when positioning. • Administer oral antispasmodics if ordered.
Relieve friction and shearing	• Use turning sheet for positioning in bed and chair. • Keep head of bed lower than 30 degrees unless contraindicated. • Use supportive devices to prevent sliding in chairs. • Use appropriate transfer techniques. • Do not use powder on skin. • Place bed cradle under top covers.	Maintain hydration/ nutritional status	• Assess nutritional status. • Investigate causes of anorexia. • Correct underlying nutritional deficits. • Encourage additional fluids, unless contraindicated. • Give high protein supplement, if necessary. • Monitor weight weekly.
Prevent moisture/ maceration	• Implement scheduled toileting or bladder retraining program. • Use absorbent incontinent briefs or pads. • Check incontinent clients frequently. Wash and rinse thoroughly. Apply moisture barrier. • Avoid use of plastic/rubber sheets, protectors.		Continue with routine skin care. Do skin checks with each position change.

Nursing Interventions: Skin Cancer

1. Teach clients and caregivers both cancer prevention methods and skin self-examination to detect lesions early. Early detection and treatment of skin cancers are essential to optimal client outcomes.
2. Provide information in both verbal and written form and in collaboration with the client's multidisciplinary team, regarding treatment (surgery, chemotherapy, radiation, and other options).
3. Monitor for signs of infection at the lesion site.
4. Ensure that the client's psychological, psychosocial, spiritual, and dietary needs are also addressed.

Neurological System

See Chapter 25 for an anatomy and physiology review of the neurological system. The following neurological changes result from the aging process:

- Neurons in the brain decrease in number, resulting in decreased production of neurotransmitters and, thus, reduced synaptic transmission.
- Cerebral blood flow and oxygen utilization decrease.
- Time required to carry out motor and sensory tasks requiring speed, coordination, balance, and fine-motor hand movements increases.
- Short-term memory may somewhat diminish without much change in long-term memory.
- Night sleep disturbances occur due to more frequent and longer wakeful periods.
- Deep-tendon reflexes decrease, although reflexes at the knees remain fairly intact.

Many disorders that affect the neurological system are not unique to elders. However, the risk of acquiring one of these disorders increases with age. One of the most common diagnoses among elders in long-term care facilities is dementia, particularly one form of dementia called Alzheimer's disease (AD). **Dementia** is an organic brain pathology characterized by losses in intellectual functioning. The clinical manifestations associated with dementia are never considered normal aging changes.

It is important for care providers to assess the length of onset of confusion or cognitive changes in the client. Generally, dementia describes declines that have a slow onset of greater than 6 months, whereas **delirium** (or acute confusion) describes cognitive changes

that have a shorter onset of 6 months or less. Acute confusion can occur independently or as an exacerbation of a current dementia-related disorder in the client. Acute confusion can result from many stresses such as infections, medication side effects, drug interactions, metabolic imbalances, dehydration, or injuries from falls (e.g., subdural hematomas). Elimination of the causative factor can often turn the acute confusion around in a relatively short period of time to the pre-exacerbation level of functioning, unless further pathology to the brain has occurred.

PROFESSIONAL TIP

Mental Health in the Elderly
Mood disorders including depression, bipolar disorder, anxiety disorders, late onset psychosis, sleep disorders, substance abuse, schizophrenia (chronic and late onset), and other psychiatric diseases certainly occur among older clients and often go unaddressed or are ineffectively treated. Appropriate assessment, treatment, and clinical management of these clients require effective interdisciplinary teams comprising a geriatric psychiatrist; a neurologist; a clinical nurse specialist specializing in gerontology and mental health; a licensed social worker; a clinical pharmacist; other multidisciplinary team members (including direct care nurses and staff and activity therapists); and the client's family and, whenever possible, the client.

Nursing Interventions: Alzheimer's Disease

1. Before diagnosis, encourage a medical and psychological diagnostic workup including a mental status examination.
2. Facilitate orientation in the early stages of the disease with calendars, lists, and consistent schedules.
3. Arrange an environment that is therapeutic, consistent, calm, and safe and that alternates rest with activities that require the use of long-practiced skills.
4. Encourage and facilitate access for the client and family to support groups where they can independently share their feelings and concerns and have questions addressed.
5. When assistance is needed with ADLs, implement consistent routines with consistent caregivers but allow for delay of care if needed due to client stress or irritability. Encourage independence of the client while assisting with ADLs (e.g., offer a warm washcloth for client to wash the face and assist with those ADLs that the client cannot complete without assistance).

PROFESSIONAL TIP

Neurological System in the Elderly Client
In the absence of pathology, intellect and capacity for learning remain unchanged with aging.

6. Monitor general health status. Treat any underlying medical problems. Provide adequate pain control, as needed, and monitor for lack of sleep to minimize the risk of violent behavior (Andersen, 1999). Observe for the client's better times of the day, and plan activities or interventions accordingly.

7. Build a trusting relationship with the client. Use clear, simple directions and treat clients with respect and as individuals, building on their strengths and their unique interests and histories. Doing so demonstrates appreciation for the individual and can help build the client's self-esteem.

8. Be aware that as much is communicated to the AD client through the caregiver's nonverbal behavior and tone and volume of voice as is communicated through actual words. A calm attitude allows the client time to process and retrieve information when spoken to or asked a question.

9. Support the client's mobility within a safe environment, recognizing that as the disease progresses, baseline wandering often increases as a coping skill, whereas verbal communication often decreases (Fetters, 1994). Bean bag chairs, low mattresses, bed and chair alarms, positional (anti-sliding) wedges for chairs, merry walkers that support independent mobility, and assisted-ambulation programs to build leg strength are all therapeutic interventions for AD clients as the disease progresses and represent preferable alternatives to the use of restraints.

10. Monitor for changes in baseline behaviors and for intensity of wandering (both pacing or lethargy), as either often indicates underlying infections, metabolic imbalances, or stress. Encourage clients to alternate periods of activity and rest.

Nursing Interventions: Depression

1. Assess for signs of a physical basis for any fatigue (e.g., infection, pain, altered nutritional status, or shortness of breath upon exertion).

2. Administer treatment for underlying physiologic problems, if applicable.

3. If symptoms persist, encourage the client to have a medical diagnostic workup with a geriatric psychiatrist, if such a workup has not yet been done.

4. Monitor for verbal or nonverbal signs of suicidal thoughts/intent. Determine whether the client has a plan.

5. Provide one-on-one supervision of the client as needed and assure the client that the caregiver will keep him safe. If appropriate for the client, seek an agreement that he will not try to harm himself.

6. Administer antidepressant medication as ordered. Provide client and family education regarding medication, including length of time before therapeutic results should occur, and potential side effects. Report immediately to the registered nurse and primary care provider any extrapyramidal side effects (e.g., tremors, drooling, pin rolling of the fingers, shuffling gait) that are observed.

7. If the client is not assessed as being at risk for suicide but is isolating in his room, establish small goals with the client (e.g., coming out of the room and sitting safely in the hallway with the nurse for 5 minutes two times per day and for meals). Advance to more challenging goals as the client demonstrates increased tolerance for social interaction.

8. Facilitate the client's reintegration into a healthy support system and provide small community group time for the client to share his views.

Nursing Interventions: Transient Ischemic Attack

1. Assess for risk factors for stroke and for the existence of any previous carotid vascular tests for potential blockage (stenosis).

2. Provide client and family education explaining the relationship between risk factors and TIA and stroke.

3. Provide teaching to assist in reducing risk factors.

4. Monitor orthostatic blood pressure and encourage clients to change positions slowly to decrease the risk of falling.

Urinary System

See Chapter 29 for an anatomy and physiology review of the urinary system. The following urinary changes result from the aging process:

- Nephrons in the kidneys decrease in number and function, resulting in decreased filtration and gradual decrease in excretory and reabsorbtive functions of the renal tubules.
- Glomerular filtration rate decreases, resulting in decreased renal clearance of drugs.
- Blood urea nitrogen increases. The creatinine clearance test is a better indicator than is BUN of renal function in elders.
- Sodium-conserving ability diminishes.
- Bladder capacity decreases, causing increased frequency of urination, including nocturia.
- Renal function increases when the older client lies down, sometimes causing a need to void shortly after going to bed.
- Bladder and perineal muscles weaken, resulting in the inability to empty the bladder and predisposing the elderly client to cystitis.
- Incidence of stress incontinence increases in older females.
- The prostate may enlarge in older males, causing urinary frequency or dribbling.

Common urinary disorders related to aging include the following:

- Incontinence
- Urinary tract infections (UTIs)

Nursing Interventions: Incontinence

1. Complete an assessment for bladder management (Figure 35-15).
2. Identify the type of incontinence present (Table 35-3).
3. Implement an appropriate bladder management program (Table 35-4).
4. Frequently monitor for skin impairment.
5. Offer absorbent incontinent pads or briefs that draw the moisture away from the skin.
6. Teach all caregivers, the client, and the family the importance both of adequate cleansing of the genital area (proper retraction and cleansing of the foreskin in the older uncircumcised male and proper cleansing of the skin folds of the older female), legs, and back and of the use of clean linens, to ensure that the client's skin is kept clean and dry. Apply a moisture barrier cream as needed to prevent skin maceration from excessive exposure to moisture.
7. Teach and employ effective infection-control techniques (e.g., wipe and clean [from front to back only] after toileting and when bathing).
8. Encourage referral to discuss medical options (in addition to nursing interventions) for treatment of incontinence.
9. Allow the client to voice concerns over incontinence and assist to overcome any adverse effects on psychosocial functioning.

Table 35-3 TYPES OF URINARY INCONTINENCE

TYPE	CHARACTERISTICS
Functional	Bladder emptying is unpredictable but complete. Incontinence is related to impairment of cognitive, physical, or psychological functioning or to environmental barriers.
Urge	Incontinence occurs immediately after the sensation to void is perceived.
Reflex	Incontinence is related to neurogenic bladder and central nervous system or spinal cord injury. Bladder fills, and uninhibited bladder contractions cause loss of urine.
Stress	Increased abdominal pressure is higher than urethral resistance. Stress associated with coughing or laughing causes incontinence.
Total	Unpredictable, unvoluntary, continuous loss of urine.

Nursing Interventions: Urinary Tract Infections

NOTE: Elderly persons frequently do not present with the usual signs and symptoms of UTIs. Falling or signs of acute confusion (more than usual) may often be the major clinical manifestations.

1. Monitor fluid intake and output. Increase intake unless contraindicated. Offer cranberry juice frequently, per ordered diet.

To be completed and reviewed every 90 days or as frequently as needed based on outcome and response.

CLIENT_____ Adm No. _____ Date_____ Diagnoses_____ Birthdate_____

Bladder function: History of infection or other urinary problem._____ Urinalysis: Date_____

Protein___ Glucose__ Ketones__ RBC__ WBC__ Bacteria__ Crystals__ Sp.Gr.__ Culture: Date_____ Result_____

Treatment_____

BUN___ Ser.Creatinine___ Tot.Pro.___ FBS___ To be completed after 2-week assessment period

Frequency of voiding_____ Average amount_____ Is client aware of need to void?____ Urgency?____ Dribbling?____

Incontinence preceded by laughing, sneezing_____

Medications affecting bladder function/continence_____

Mental status: Short-term memory_____ Orientation_____ Able to express self_____

   Able to follow directions_____ Reaction to incontinence_____

Hydration baseline: Daily average fluid intake: Days_____ Eve._____ Night_____

Mobility/self-care skills: Ambulatory/self_____ Cane_____ Walker_____ Requires assist of one or two_____

   Weight-bearing_____ Propels self by w/c_____ Transfers self_____ Requires assistance_____

   Can manage clothing_____ Cleanses self after toileting_____ Washes hands_____

Figure 35-15 Assessment for Bladder Management

Table 35–4	BLADDER MANAGEMENT TECHNIQUES
PROGRAM	**DESCRIPTION**
Kegel exercises	Used for stress incontinence in cognitively alert persons. Exercises strengthen pelvic floor musculature.
Scheduled toileting	Client is on a fixed schedule of toileting—usually every 2 hours. Technique can be used to facilitate voiding and emptying of the bladder.
Habit training	Client is toileted according to individual pattern of voiding. Several days must be spent assessing pattern.
Bladder retraining	Restores normal pattern of voiding/continence. Requires accurate assessment before establishing schedule with progressive shortening or lengthening of toileting intervals. Client must be cognitively alert.
Prompted voiding	Client is prompted to toilet at regular intervals and is given social reinforcement for appropriate toileting behavior.

2. Teach and encourage client to empty the bladder every 3 to 4 hours.

3. Encourage the client to take all medication as prescribed.

4. Use proper infection-control techniques to minimize the risk of infection, including maintaining sterile technique for any urinary catheterization procedure (for urinalysis, assessment for bladder retention, or insertion of indwelling catheter), to prevent unnecessary introduction of bacteria into the bladder.

5. Teach female clients to wipe from front to back only; cleanse thoroughly after bowel movements; avoid bubble baths, colored toilet paper, douches, and vaginal sprays; and wear underwear made from cotton rather than synthetic fibers.

6. Teach the client and caregivers that hematuria (blood in the urine) and fever indicate the need for immediate assessment and intervention, as these signs and symptoms can signify a potentially serious infection or condition. Any signs and symptoms of bladder infection should be immediately reported to the registered nurse and the physician.

Sensory Changes

See Chapter 26 for an anatomy and physiology review of the sensory system. The following sensory changes result from the aging process:

Vision

- With aging, the lens becomes less pliable and less able to increase its curvature in order to focus on near objects, causing presbyopia (trouble seeing

objects up close) and decreased accomodation. The lens also yellows, causing distorted color perceptions, with greens and blues washing out and warm colors such as reds and oranges becoming more distinct. The incidence of cataracts also increases.

- Accommodation of pupil size decreases, resulting in both decreased adjustment to changes in lighting and decreased ability to tolerate glare. For instance, high-gloss tile floors in hallways can appear like hills and valleys to older clients, especially those with perceptual deficits; this may increase anxiety and safety risks.

- Vitreous humor changes in consistency, causing blurred vision. Changes in the anterior chamber may increase the pressure of the aqueous humor, resulting in glaucoma.

- Lacrimal glands secrete less fluids, causing dryness and itching. Entropion or ectropion (turning of the eyelids inward or outward) occasionally occurs in older clients. These conditions can not only impact vision, but can increase the risk of infection due to dryness and ineffective blinking. In these conditions, obtaining an order for artificial tears, lacrilube, and eye drop treatments for dryness or infection may be necessary.

 Infection Control: Eye Care

To decrease infection risks, remind all caregivers to wash from the center outward when washing clients' eyes.

Common vision disorders related to aging include the following:

- Presbyopia
- Cataract
- Glaucoma
- Age-related macular degeneration

Nursing Interventions: Visual Impairment

1. Teach visually impaired clients adaptive techniques for ADL, such as extra lighting.

2. Advise regular examination by an ophthalmologist.

3. Provide preoperative and postoperative care and teaching to clients undergoing cataract surgery, including lifting and bending restrictions as well as measures to prevent infection.

4. Teach proper eye drop administration techniques to all clients who are prescribed eye drops, including holding the drop in the eye with the lid closed for 30 seconds after administration.

5. Ensure that older clients have their glasses on when needed to decrease perceptual and spatial deficits.

Hearing

- As aging occurs, the pinna becomes less flexible, the hair cells in the inner ear stiffen and atrophy, and cerumen (earwax) increases.

- The number of neurons in the cochlea decrease, and the blood supply lessens, causing the cochlea and the ossicles to degenerate.
- Presbycusis, the impairment of hearing in older adults, is often accompanied by a loss of tone discrimination. High-frequency tones are lost first; thus, keeping the voice low and calm and decreasing any background noise can improve the client's comprehension of the caregiver's message.

Nursing Interventions: Hearing Impairment

1. Assess for ear pain; drainage; inflammation; abnormalities; surgeries; perforations; or impacted cerumen.
2. Evaluate medication regimen and assess for ototoxicity, if medication history reveals such a risk.
3. Advise hearing testing by an audiologist, if the previous assessments are negative.
4. Monitor the care and use of a hearing aid by the older client with unilateral or bilateral aids (Figure 35-16). Provide teaching and assistance as needed for cleaning the hearing aid(s) and replacing batteries.
5. Instruct caregivers and family about the communication and socialization needs of the client. For some older clients, either the use of a small erasable board to augment verbal questions or

Figure 35-16 Hearing aids help compensate for hearing loss that results from aging.

communication with written text represents a therapeutic intervention for hearing impairment. If writing dexterity or ability is also impaired, a story board that has pictures indicating the client's needs (e.g., bathroom, food, rest) can assist the client to independently communicate needs to caregivers.

SAMPLE NURSING CARE PLAN

THE CLIENT WITH ALZHEIMER'S DISEASE (AD)

Mrs. Jane Rodriguez, 64 years old, was admitted to the Alzheimer's unit of a long-term care facility. Last month, Mrs. Rodriguez was visiting her daughter in another state and wandered away from the daughter's home. Mrs. Rodriguez was found 60 miles away, unharmed but completely disoriented and agitated. Mrs. Rodriguez had worked as a nursing assistant before she retired. She is a widow and has two children in the same community where the nursing home is located, in addition to the daughter who she was visting in another state. Unless reminded, Mrs. Rodriguez does not shower or change clothes. She awakens at least once each night and asks for breakfast.

Nursing Diagnosis 1 *Disturbed Thought Processes related to progressive dementia as evidenced by disorientation to time and place, loss of short-term memory, inability to concentrate, and periods of agitation*

PLANNING/GOALS	NURSING INTERVENTIONS	RATIONALE	EVALUATION
Mrs. Rodriguez will remain calm and will not experience agitation and anxiety as a result of her disorientation and memory loss.	Provide Mrs. Rodriguez with clues for orientation: "Good morning, Mrs. Rodriguez. My name is Jean, and I will help you today." Avoid	People in the early stages of Alzheimer's disease may become agitated because their world is always unfamiliar to them. The	Mrs. Rodriguez remained calm and showed no signs of agitation or anxiety.

continues

putting her on the spot by asking questions she may not answer, such as "Do you know what day this is?"

issue is not whether individuals with a dementia are oriented, but whether they can cope with their environment.

Place a large sign on Mrs. Rodriguez's door with her name printed in large letters to help her find her room.

Short-term memory loss makes it impossible for Mrs. Rodriguez to remember where her room is or where the bathroom is. If she still recognizes her name, posting it on the door will help her find her way.

Have family bring in snapshots and photos to stimulate reminiscence.

Reminiscing can be a satisfying activity. It is especially helpful if the photos are from an earlier, happier time such as when her children were young. Long-term memory may still be intact, allowing her to recall these happier times.

Avoid changing Mrs. Rodriguez's room. Put items back in the same place all the time.

Consistency in the environment (as well as in routine and staff) reduces frustration.

Consult with activities staff in planning self-expressive, non-fail activities that require little concentration (e.g., painting with nontoxic paints, modeling with nontoxic clay).

Appropriate activities prevent boredom, which can lead to irritation. It is important to plan nonstressful, noncompetitive, failure-proof activities in order to prevent frustration.

If Mrs. Rodriguez is resistant to care, provide clear, simple, nonthreatening instructions and delay care as needed until she is calmer.

Persons with cognitive deficits often vary between combativeness and cooperation. Often, delaying care for even 10 to 15 minutes when resistance is encountered improves client outcomes. Also, exploring and understanding the antecedents to a client's combative behavior allows caregivers to intervene early and to change the environment or the approach to better ensure positive client outcomes (Andersen, 1999).

continues

Nursing Diagnosis 2 *Risk for Injury related to risk factors of mode of transportation and cognitive and affective factors as evidenced by wandering behavior, impaired judgment, and disorientation*

PLANNING/GOALS	NURSING INTERVENTIONS	RATIONALE	EVALUATION
Mrs. Rodriguez will remain free of injury while retaining as much independence and freedom as possible.	Lock up tools, medicines, and chemicals. Keep only nonpoisonous plants on the unit. Arrange furniture so that walkways are open. Pad sharp corners of tables and chests. Cover electrical outlets and hot radiators. Place electrical cords and telephone wires out of reach.	Persons with Alzheimer's disease do not recognize unsafe acts or conditions due to loss of impulse control and loss of judgment. They do not comprehend cause and effect.	Mrs. Rodriguez has experienced no injury.
	Provide assurance during fire drills.	Unusual activity of any sort increases agitation, especially when noise level is increased.	

Nursing Diagnosis 3 *Bathing/Hygiene and Dressing/Grooming Self-Care Deficit related to perceptual or cognitive impairment (memory loss and sensory–perceptual deficits) as evidenced by needing a reminder to shower and change clothes*

PLANNING/GOALS	NURSING INTERVENTIONS	RATIONALE	EVALUATION
Mrs. Rodriguez will complete ADL with minimal assistance now and with increasing assistance as the disease progresses.	Use verbal cues and hand-over-hand assistance with ADL. Instruct staff to avoid doing tasks that Mrs. Rodriguez can do by herself. Watch for signs of frustration and irritation and intervene when appropriate.	Using these simple techniques can minimize the need for assistance, thereby increasing feelings of self-esteem.	Mrs. Rodriguez participates in ADL.
	Ask family to bring in clothing that is easy to manipulate. Set clothing out in the order it is to be put on.	Dressing is one of the more difficult tasks to accomplish. Appropriate clothing can simplify the activity.	
	Consider tub baths rather than showers. Provide privacy, check the temperature of the bathroom, and do not leave the client alone.	Showers are frequently threatening or confusing to persons with Alzheimer's disease. Tub baths are also more relaxing.	

continues

Nursing Diagnosis 4 *Disturbed Sleep Pattern related to disorientation as evidenced by wakefulness at night*

PLANNING/GOALS	NURSING INTERVENTIONS	RATIONALE	EVALUATION
Mrs. Rodriguez will experience fewer periods of wakefulness during the night. If she awakens, she will remain calm and free of agitation.	Avoid stimulating activities prior to bedtime. Establish a consistent bedtime routine. Take Mrs. Rodriguez to the bathroom and allow sufficient time for complete bladder emptying.	Overstimulation prior to bedtime may increase anxiety, preventing sleep. Having the client participate in relaxation activities and repeating the client's long-practiced bedtime routine prior to bed may also be helpful.	Mrs. Rodriguez sleeps through the night several times a week.
	Help Mrs. Rodriguez with a sponge bath and with oral care; give her a back rub using warm lotion and slow, smooth strokes.	These activities are relaxing.	
	Provide a light snack of a warm, noncaffeinated beverage and a plain, easily digested cracker, cookie, or a piece of toast. Be patient and do not rush her.	Hunger or overeating can interfere with sleep.	
	Question family concerning previous bedtime routines and sleeping habits.	Individuals may have used specific sleep routines throughout their lifetimes, such as sleeping with a night light, having a window open, playing a radio, or wearing socks to bed.	
	Repeat bedtime routine when Mrs. Rodriguez awakens during night.	Mrs. Rodriguez will think it is time to go to bed.	
	Encourage a short nap early in the afternoon.	Sleep pattern disturbances may result from overfatigue.	
	Avoid the use of sleeping medications.	Sleeping medications are seldom effective and may increase confusion, disorientation, and restlessness.	

FINANCING ELDER CARE IN THE 21ST CENTURY

Since the 1960s, the U.S. Congress has developed and implemented a series of national entitlement programs to help ensure adequate income, housing, and access to medical care for older Americans. As the number of older clients (those over age 65, particularly those over age 85) continues to rise, caregivers and advocates for elder care should strive to understand the budgetary policies that have influenced and continue to influence the U.S. health care delivery system.

Medicare

Medicare (Title XVIII) is a nationwide health insurance program for Americans who are 65 years of age or older, for persons who are eligible for Social Security disability payments for longer than 2 years, and for certain workers and dependents who need kidney transplants or dialysis. The **Health Care Financing Administration** (HCFA) is the federal agency in charge of administering the Medicare program. The program was enacted as part of the Social Security Act of 1965 and became effective on June 1, 1966. It consists of two separate but coordinated programs: hospital insurance (called part A) and medical insurance (called part B), which covers physician's services, outpatient services, some medical supplies, and some skilled nursing and home health services. Medicare provides basic protection for the cost of health care but does not cover all expenses (U.S. Department of Health and Human Services, Social Security Administration, 1991). Among the expenses *not* covered by Medicare for older Americans are those associated with the following:

- Home health care that does not require skilled personnel (e.g., as of February 1998, expenses for a home health visit [skilled] for the purpose of obtaining a blood sample are not covered).
- Nursing home care (except for skilled care for a limited time)
- Some routine medical checkups and related tests
- Prescription drugs
- Eye and hearing tests and eyeglasses and hearing aids
- Routine dental care and checkups

In the late 1990s, many insurance policies were available to supplement at varying levels the benefits paid by Medicare. This led many older clients to "stack" insurance policies, or to buy numerous overlapping policies for fear of being underinsured. The insurance industry and Congress worked together to outlaw stacking of Medicare supplement policies.

Although there has been some improvement in insurance coverage for preventive screening tests such as mammograms, the lack of reimbursement for prescription drugs continues to significantly burden older Americans, many of whom must choose between costly medications and food.

Medicaid

The Medicaid program was also enacted as part of the Social Security Act of 1966 and is often referred to as Title XIX. This program, which is federally aided and state operated and administered, provides medical benefits to certain indigent, or low-income, Americans. Nursing home bills represent a staggering burden for many older Americans who require nursing care. In 1995, nursing home bills averaged $22,000 per person per year, and projections showed that two-thirds of elders who lived alone would run out of savings after 13 weeks in a nursing home (Gallo, Pulmer, Paveza, & Reichel, 1999). Medicaid takes into account government-determined poverty levels when providing benefits, with coverage being extended to persons who are at certain percentages of the poverty level (e.g., 200% of poverty level, 150% of poverty level, and 100% of poverty level). Long-term care facilities serve both private-pay clients (those whose expenses are paid by themselves, their families, or their long-term care insurance policies) and Title XIX- (Medicaid-) funded clients. Medicaid coverage for long-term care is not available until a person's assets have been depleted to a certain set level. Elder care advocates continue in their efforts to protect the assets of the spouse who is able to stay in the family home after the other spouse must be placed in a nursing home.

To some in the United States, the debate over Social Security, Medicare, and Medicaid financing is viewed as someone else's priority. However, the moral responsibility for providing access to quality services and care for our country's elderly is shared by all Americans. Elder care services should be developed to promote independence yet should provide assistance when needed.

Omnibus Budget Reconciliation Act

The **Omnibus Budget Reconciliation Act** (OBRA), first enacted in 1987 and reenacted in 1990, sought to ensure quality services for older Americans. The act included guidelines for services that were required to be made available to seniors, and promoted the rights of seniors. However, as was the case with all health care costs, elder care costs continued to rise in the United States, and discussions and proposed legislation for financial reforms intensified.

Balanced Budget Act of 1997

Among the most significant influences on the financing of elder care in the past decade is the **Balanced Budget Act** (BBA) of 1997. The BBA replaced cost-based reimbursement for care provided in skilled nursing facilities (SNFs) with a prospective payment system (PPS) based on client assessment within a resource utilization group system (RUGS). Reimbursement for home health services also shifted to a PPS.

The BBA also states that discharge from hospitals to SNFs or home care for 10 common but as yet unpublished diagnosis-related groups (DRGs) is to be considered as a transfer for payment purposes. Medicare's goal was to make a single blended payment that combined the traditional hospital DRG payment and the payment for postacute care services to be shared by the providers.

The intended implications for practice included reduced reimbursement to some SNFs, fewer discharges from hospitals to independent facilities for subacute care or home care, and, thus, encouraged the creation of integrated delivery systems and managed care. In reality, however, it has become more difficult to find placement in SNFs for clients with complex needs, because the new reimbursement system simply does not fund all their health care needs.

These reimbursement and regulatory changes surely represent only the beginning of such efforts to balance resources and need as the U.S. population continues to age. Certainly, significant work lies ahead for advocates of quality elder care in the United States and the world in the 21st century. Nurses will play a vital role in the ensuing debates, for they will see firsthand the positive and negative outcomes of their clients.

CASE STUDY

Mr. Jack Baroni, a 72-year-old male, was admitted to the skilled care facility for rehabilitation following an open reduction, internal fixation of the right hip. Mr. Baroni had fallen while going up the stairs of his home, suffering an intertrochanteric, comminuted fracture of the right femur. He has no recollection of what caused him to fall. He is married and, until his surgery, was working part time as a school-crossing guard. While in the hospital, Mr. Baroni exhibited mental status changes including disorientation and confusion. His wife reports that he never had this problem prior to the surgery. He is continent of bowel and bladder. Mr. Baroni was in relatively good health until the fall. He and his wife agree that he should return home after rehabilitation is complete.

The following questions will guide your development of a nursing care plan for the case study.

1. Identify specific admission assessments that would be required for Mr. Baroni because of his age and condition.
2. Identify complications for which Mr. Baroni is at risk.
3. List interventions to prevent each complication.
4. Cite possible reasons for Mr. Baroni's fall.
5. Describe methods for assessing Mr. Baroni's mental status.
6. Describe possible reasons for his altered mental status.
7. Write three individualized nursing diagnoses and goals for Mr. Baroni.
8. List nursing actions related to altered mental status.
9. List four successful outcomes for Mr. Baroni.
10. Develop a teaching plan for Mr. Baroni.
11. List the community resources Mr. Baroni may need after discharge.

SUMMARY

- The elderly population is rapidly growing.
- Although many stereotypes and myths are associated with aging, elders are in fact very diverse in their characteristics.

- Health maintenance is as important for older adults as it is for younger persons. A healthy lifestyle can enhance the quality of life.
- Many changes are associated with aging. The disorders commonly seen among elders are often the results of pathology and are thus not considered a

normal part of aging. However, the risk of acquiring these disorders increases with age.

- Nurses knowledgeable about aging can plan interventions that will prevent complications for which elders are at risk.

- Nurses have a responsibility to advocate for their older clients. Nurses should be active legislatively and should work collaboratively to develop elder-care services that are affordable, provide equal access for all older Americans, and promote optimal wellness and independence.

Review Questions

1. Which of the following is a true statement?

   a. All people eventually become senile if they live long enough.
   b. People lose interest in sex as they age.
   c. Most elders are financially impoverished.
   d. Incontinence is not an expected or normal change of aging.

2. The programmed aging theory states that:

   a. stress causes structural and chemical changes in the body, which, in turn, cause aging.
   b. a genetic clock determines the speed at which people age.
   c. changes in collagen are the cause of aging.
   d. the decreasing ability to produce T-cell differentiation causes aging.

3. The elderly individual can reduce the potential for acquiring RTIs by:

   a. obtaining an influenza vaccine each year.
   b. staying inside throughout the winter months.
   c. avoiding exercise.
   d. limiting fluid intake.

4. Research indicates that:

   a. weight-bearing exercise is not recommended for elders.

   b. high-intensity resistance training can improve muscle strength in elders.
   c. muscle deterioration in elders is to be expected.
   d. walking is the only healthy exercise for elders.

5. Integumentary changes associated with aging include:

   a. increased glandular secretions.
   b. increased capillary blood flow.
   c. increased melanin production.
   d. increased vascular fragility.

Critical Thinking Questions

1. What services are essential in a quality elder-care program?

2. How can you advocate as a nurse for your older clients?

3. If you were going to author an Older American client's bill of rights, what things would you include?

4. What myths or stereotypes have you observed that affect the elderly?

⚡ WEB FLASH!

- Search federal sites for some of the legislation and policies that are discussed in this chapter and affect elder care (e.g., OBRA and BBA).
- What clinical guidelines are available on the Internet from the government or other sources for the care of elderly clients (e.g., for urinary incontinence or pain treatment)?

REHABILITATION, HOME HEALTH, LONG-TERM CARE, AND HOSPICE

CHAPTER 36

MAKING THE CONNECTION

Refer to the following chapters to increase your understanding of rehabilitation, home health, long-term care, and hospice:

- **Chapter 3, Legal Responsibilities**
- **Chapter 4, Ethical Responsibilities**
- **Chapter 6, Cultural Diversity and Nursing**
- **Chapter 9, Loss, Grief, and Death**

- **Chapter 12, Health Assessment**
- **Chapter 14, Pain Management**
- **Chapter 35, Nursing Care of the Older Client**

LEARNING OBJECTIVES

Upon completion of this chapter, you should be able to:
- *Define key terms.*
- *List three reasons why there has been a significant change in the growth of nonacute care services.*
- *Discuss the legal/ethical implications of:*
  1. *Limiting aggressive health care services (such as rehabilitation or intensive care) for the elderly as a cost saving measure for the preservation of Medicare funds.*
  2. *Determining nurses' responsibility for accepting decisions made by individuals with questionable mental competency.*
- *Describe the differences between Medicaid and Medicare.*
- *Distinguish among licensure, certification, and accreditation.*
- *Describe the role of the LP/VN as a member of the interdisciplinary health care team in various health care settings.*
- *Discuss the types of clients that would benefit from participation in a rehabilitation program.*
- *Identify the responsibilities of the LP/VN in rehabilitation nursing, nursing in long-term care, in-home care, and hospice.*
- *List the various types of long-term care services.*

KEY TERMS

accreditation	Medicaid
adult day care	Medicare
assisted living	Medigap insurance
certification	rehabilitation
hospice	respite care
licensure	subacute care
long-term care facility	synergy

INTRODUCTION

There has been a strong emergence in the past decade of nonacute health care services. The growth of these services is a reflection of several changes occurring in the United States:

- The Tax Equity and Fiscal Responsibility Act of 1983 initiated the Medicare Prospective Payment system and the diagnosis-related group (DRG) system. This has resulted in the discharge of clients from acute-care hospitals much earlier. Clients, particularly elderly individuals, often require continuing care.
- Lives are being saved that would have been lost a few years ago. Ongoing health care services are often necessary for these individuals.

- The number of Americans over the age of 65 has tripled in this century. The risk of acquiring a chronic disease increases as individuals age, requiring health care throughout life.
- The cost of acute care has reached critical proportions. Case management is an attempt to contain costs by assisting people in defining their service needs, locating and arranging services, and coordinating the services of multiple providers. The cost of health care can be managed by controlling client access to services (General Accounting Office, 1994).

These changes have resulted in a vast increase in rehabilitation, home health, long-term care, and hospice services. There is an intermingling of services and settings under each of these categories of care. Rehabilitative services for example, may be provided in an acute-care setting, in a rehabilitation hospital, in a long-term care facility, or in the client's home. Home care may provide the same services that would be available in a subacute care nursing facility. Long-term care refers to both home and community-based services. Hospice care may be provided in the home or institution. While many of the clients requiring these services are elderly, there are an increasing number of services specializing in pediatric care.

LEGAL AND ETHICAL RESPONSIBILITIES

The legal basis for the provision of care in long-term care facilities is found in the Omnibus Budget Reconciliation Act (OBRA) of 1987. This act was legislated after a lengthy study of the care delivery in long-term facilities throughout the country. The major components of the act concern the issues of nursing assistant training, the regulation of the use of physical and chemical restraints, the Minimum Data Set (MDS) as an assessment tool, and the legal foundation for residents' rights. Many of the regulations found in OBRA also apply to home health nursing agencies.

The rights of the health care consumer are regulated for both long-term care and home health care. Before receiving services from either, the consumer must be given a copy of these rights and indicate an understanding of their content (Tables 36–1 and 36–2). In addition to OBRA, there are many other regulatory acts

Table 36–1 RESIDENT'S RIGHTS

This is an abbreviated version of the Resident's Rights as set forth in the Omnibus Budget Reconciliation Act. This document must be given to all residents and/or their families prior to admission to any long-term care facility.

1. **The resident has the right to free choice, including the right to:**
   - choose an attending physician
   - full advance information about changes in care or treatment
   - participate in the assessment and care planning process
   - self-administration of medications
   - consent to participate in experimental research
2. **The resident has the right to freedom from abuse and restraints, including freedom from:**
   - physical, sexual, mental abuse
   - corporal punishment and involuntary seclusion
   - physical and chemical restraints
3. **The resident has the right to privacy including privacy for:**
   - treatment and nursing care
   - receiving/sending mail
   - telephone calls
   - visitors
4. **The resident has the right to confidentiality of personal and clinical records.**
5. **The resident has the right to accommodation of needs including:**
   - choices about life
   - receiving assistance in maintaining independence
6. **The resident has the right to voice grievances.**
7. **The resident has the right to organize and participate in family and resident groups.**
8. **The resident has the right to participate in social, religious, and community activities including the right to:**
   - vote
   - keep religious items in the room
   - attend religious services
9. **The resident has the right to examine survey results and correction plans.**
10. **The resident has the right to manage personal funds.**
11. **The resident has the right to information about eligibility for Medicare/Medicaid funds.**
12. **The resident has the right to file complaints about abuse, neglect, or misappropriation of property.**
13. **The resident has the right to information about advocacy groups.**
14. **The resident has the right to immediate and unlimited access to family or relatives.**
15. **The resident has the right to share a room with the spouse if they are both residents in the same facility.**
16. **The resident has the right to perform or not perform work for the facility if it is medically appropriate for the resident to work.**
17. **The resident has the right to remain in the facility except in certain circumstances.**
18. **The resident has the right to personal possessions.**
19. **The resident has the right to notification of change in condition.**

(As determined by Omnibus Budget Reconciliation Act [OBRA] of 1987)

Table 36–2 CLIENT'S RIGHTS IN HOME CARE

Clients receiving home health care services or their families possess basic rights and responsibilities. These include:

The right to:

1. be treated with dignity, consideration, and respect.
2. have their property treated with respect.
3. receive a timely response from the agency to requests for service.
4. be fully informed on admission of the care and treatment that will be provided, how much it will cost, and how payment will be handled.
5. know in advance if they will be responsible for any payment.
6. be informed in advance of any changes in care.
7. receive care from professionally trained personnel, to know their names and responsibilities.
8. participate in planning care.
9. refuse treatment and to be told the consequences of this action.
10. expect confidentiality of all information.
11. be informed of anticipated termination of service.
12. be referred elsewhere if denied services solely based on ability to pay.
13. know how to make a complaint or recommend a change in agency policies and services.

The responsibility to:

1. remain under a doctor's care while receiving services.
2. provide the agency with a complete health history.
3. provide the agency all requested insurance and financial information.
4. sign the required consents and releases for insurance billing.
5. participate in care by asking questions, expressing concerns, stating whether information is not understood.
6. provide a safe home environment in which care is given.
7. cooperate with the doctor, the staff, and other caregivers.
8. accept responsibility for any refusal of treatment.
9. abide by agency policies that restrict duties the staff may perform.
10. advise agency administration of any dissatisfaction or problems with care.

that affect the delivery of care in the settings described in this chapter. These include the Self-Determination Act of 1990, which is a federal regulation, and legislation related to the reporting of client abuse (state regulations).

There is a fine line between what is a legal issue and what is an ethical issue. It is beyond the scope of this chapter to provide answers to the questions arising from such problems. However, these situations are examples of common legal and ethical issues.

1. An 80-year-old client in the third stage of Alzheimer's disease falls and fractures his hip. Should this client be transferred to a rehabilitation hospital for intensive rehabilitation? If not, what are the alternatives?
2. The staff of a long-term care facility suspects that a client was abused by her son before admission to the facility. The son wishes to take the mother home, and the mother is in agreement with this plan. The discharge planner learns that the local social services agency had investigated the client's living situation for abuse prior to the mother's admission. The case worker also suspects abuse but could find nothing objective upon which to build a case. Do the nursing staff and social workers of the facility have a legal or ethical obligation to attempt intervention? If so, what actions should be taken?
3. J.B. is a young adult (23 years old) receiving rehabilitation after suffering a traumatic brain injury

due to a motorcycle accident. He wishes to make decisions concerning his care and treatment. His mental competency is questionable. However, this has not been legally established, and his parents make decisions often in opposition to J.B.'s preferences. What are the legal and ethical responsibilities of the nurse in accepting the decisions of relatives versus client?
4. Mr. A. and Mrs. C. are both residents of a long-term care facility. Mr. A. is married and Mrs. C. is a widow. The two have developed an intimate relationship that appears to be mutually satisfying to them both. Both residents are mentally competent and consenting adults. Mrs. A. is troubled by this and expects the staff to intervene. Does the staff have the right to intervene? If so, does this conflict with the residents' rights?

SOURCES OF REIMBURSEMENT

Medicare and Medicaid have long been traditional sources of reimbursement for care. All health care providers must be certified by both Medicare and Medicaid to receive payment for services rendered. While virtually all hospitals are certified by both Medicare and Medicaid, many long-term care providers, including home health care and skilled care facilities, are not. Clients, families, and hospital discharge planners need to be aware of this when planning continuing care.

Medicare

In 1965, **Medicare** (Title XVIII) was signed into law as an amendment to the Social Security Act and is the source of payment for acute care services for 95% of persons over 65 years old and for permanently disabled individuals who receive Social Security disability benefits (Waid, 1998). Medicare is administered by the federal government through the Health Care Finance Administration (HCFA). Medicare Part A covers inpatient hospital care, home health care, and hospice care. Payment may be made for care in a skilled nursing facility. However, there are many restrictions, and criteria for coverage frequently change. Medicare Part B covers partial costs for physician services, outpatient hospital and rehabilitation care, and certain services and supplies not covered by Part A.

Medicare pays for limited skilled care and rehabilitation services in certified long-term care facilities if the client and the services provided meet specific criteria. Certified home health care agencies may be reimbursed for intermittent visits if the client requires skilled health care by a registered nurse. In 1998, Medicare spent $216.6 billion for the care of its 38.8 million enrollees (HCFA, 2000a).

Medicaid

Medicaid (Title XIX) pays for health services for the aged poor, the disabled, and low-income families with dependent children (Abrams, Beers, & Berkow, 2000). The program is financed by federal and state funds and is administered at the state level. Thus, services provided vary from state to state. Medicaid is currently the primary health financing program for low-income families and disabled individuals. It is a means-tested program, providing funds only when all other financial resources have been exhausted (Waid, 1998). Services covered include inpatient and outpatient hospital care, diagnostic services, physician services, skilled nursing care, and home health services. Medicaid spent $170.6 billion in 1998 (HCFA, 2000a). Medicaid is the principal source of financial assistance for long-term care. Medicaid pays for skilled home health care in all states, and 29 states also cover the optional benefit of personal care in the home. In 1997, home health care and personal care services cost Medicaid $157.1 billion (HCFA, 2000b).

Private Insurance

Sixty-six percent of beneficiaries of Medicare purchase **Medigap insurance** to pay for costs not covered by Medicare. These policies are purchased from private insurance companies. Medigap insurance has been restricted by Congress to a basic plan with nine possible expansions (Abrams, et al., 2000). Only 5% of all nursing home care costs are covered by private insurance (HCFA, 2000b). About 30% of costs are paid by the clients and their families, about 9% by Medicare, and 43.5% by Medicaid (HCFA, 2000b). Long-term care insurance is a relatively new concept and the benefits vary greatly depending on the insurance company.

LICENSURE, CERTIFICATION, AND ACCREDITATION

There are a number of processes that have been designed to assure the health care consumer that the facility, agency, or service meets minimal standards of care. **Licensure** is a mandatory system of granting licenses according to specified standards and is regulated by each state. **Certification** is a voluntary process that establishes and evaluates compliance with rules and regulations but is required for any provider who seeks reimbursement from government funds. Because government funding is regulated by the federal government, certification rules are generated by the federal government. **Accreditation** is an additional confirmation of quality and generally indicates that the provider has gone above the minimum standards in the delivery of care and service.

Licensure

All health care facilities must be licensed. Each state has a designated agency (often the Department of Public Health) that is responsible for licensing health care facilities. A team of surveyors visits each facility annually to determine whether the facility is in compliance with the rules and regulations of the state. Noncompliance in any area results in severe sanctions and financial penalties to the institution. The facility is given a limited amount of time to correct any deficiencies. In cases where residents' lives or well-being are threatened, the facility may lose its license to operate.

Certification

Certification is required for any facility that chooses to be reimbursed by government funds, Medicare, and Medicaid. There are regulations that must be met for certification to be granted. HCFA contracts with the state agencies to perform this function. In some states the long-term care survey for licensure and certification is done concurrently. Because there are two regulatory agencies (state and federal), the states have adopted the federal regulations and in some cases have exceeded federal regulations. Certification may not be granted if the facility is not in compliance with regulations. This means the facility will not receive any reimbursement from Medicare or Medicaid funds.

Accreditation

Seeking accreditation is voluntary (not required by law). Accrediting organizations issue standards whereas state/federal licensure and certification agencies issue rules and regulations. The Joint Commission on Accreditation of Healthcare Organizations (JCAHO) has long been accrediting hospitals and skilled nursing facilities. The Commission on Accreditation of Rehabilitation Facilities (CARF) has been accrediting comprehensive inpatient rehabilitation programs since 1966. Facilities like a subacute care unit specializing in rehabilitation may seek accreditation from both commissions.

REHABILITATION

Rehabilitation is a process designed to help individuals reach their optimal level of physical, mental, and psychosocial functioning. This goal is accomplished by preventing complications, modifying the effects of the disability, and increasing independence. By so doing, the individual's self-esteem is maximized, thus increasing quality of life. Rehabilitation is concerned with increasing the client's ability to complete the basic activities of daily living (ADLs) and the instrumental activities of daily living (IADLs). ADLs include grooming and hygiene, eating, dressing, toileting, and mobility. The IADLs include higher-level tasks such as household and money management, using the telephone, and driving a car. For persons who have limited potential for regaining total independence, the goal is to teach the client to manage his or her own care.

The Interdisciplinary Health Care Team

The interdisciplinary health care team (IHCT) is an essential component to any rehabilitation process. The client and family are the focus of the team and are encouraged to participate in the planning of care. The degree to which the family participates is determined by the client. The professional members of the team are selected based on the needs of the client. Physical and occupational therapists, a speech/language pathologist, recreational therapists, rehabilitation nurses, the physician, social workers, dietitians, and mental health professionals are usually required to provide services (Figure 36-1).

Each discipline completes an assessment and pools this information at the care planning conference so that a consensus among members (including the client and family) can be reached. The team process avoids both duplication of services and fragmented care. A holistic approach is utilized so that the client's physical, mental, and psychosocial needs will be identified.

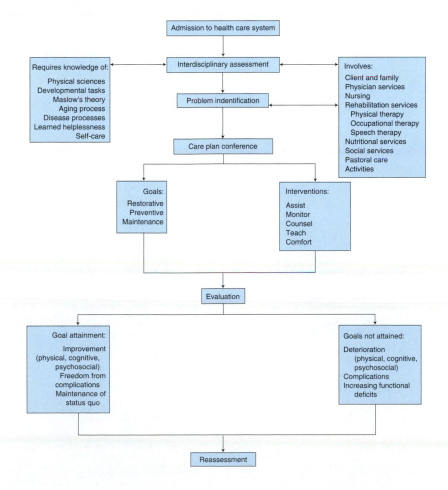

Figure 36-1 The Interdisciplinary Health Care Team Process

Role of the LP/VN

Rehabilitation nursing is a specialty practice and requires specialized knowledge, skills, and attitudes. A sound knowledge base in the anatomy and physiology of the neurological, musculoskeletal, gastrointestinal, and urological systems is a prerequisite. The nurse must have excellent clinical skills in the areas of therapeutic positioning, range of joint motion exercises, transfers, ambulation, and activities of daily living. The nurse is responsible for planning measures to prevent complications such as impaired skin integrity and contractures and to implement interventions for dysphagia, incontinence, and other identified problems.

The nurse is a member of the interdisciplinary team and as such may function as caregiver, counselor, coordinator of care, and client advocate. The nurse needs an understanding of the roles and responsibilities of each discipline and how the nurse interrelates with each discipline. There is a steady demand for rehabilitation nurses in all settings.

Functional Assessment and Evaluation for Rehabilitation

Clients who need rehabilitation are screened before admission to a program. Assessments are completed by health care professionals whose services may be required by the client (Figure 36-2). The purpose of screening is to select the best setting for services. Criteria for admission to a program usually require that the client be:

- Medically stable
- Able to learn
- Able to sit supported for at least 1 hour a day and to actively participate in the program

Interdisciplinary programs may stipulate that the client has disabilities in 2 or more areas of function:

- Mobility
- Performance of ADL
- Bowel and bladder control
- Cognition
- Emotional function
- Pain management
- Swallowing
- Communication

There are a number of standardized assessment instruments that are designed to evaluate motor function, cognition, speech and language, mobility, and the client's performance of activities of daily living. There are additional tools that identify the client's risk for pressure ulcer formation, and potential for bowel and bladder management for incontinence. Refer to the AHCPR publication *Post-Stroke Rehabilitation, Clinical Guideline Number 16,* for a complete description of assessment instruments (Gresham, et al., 1995).

Figure 36-2 Assessing Potential—Stroke Rehabilitation

Rehabilitation Settings

Rehabilitation can be conducted in a variety of settings. Rehabilitation begins during the acute stage of illness when the client's medical condition stabilizes. Continuing rehabilitative services are often needed after discharge from acute care, necessitating transfer to a hospital inpatient program, a skilled nursing facility, an outpatient rehabilitation program, or a home rehabilitation program. Decisions about entry into a rehabilitation program should reflect a consensus among the client, family or significant others, physician, and the rehabilitation program.

Hospital Inpatient Program

Hospitals may have a separate rehabilitation unit, or services may be available in a freestanding hospital specializing in the delivery of rehabilitation services. In either case, the hospitals are staffed by a full range of rehabilitation professionals. Registered nurses and a physician skilled in rehabilitation (physiatrist) are available 24 hours a day. Hospital programs are generally more intense and comprehensive than programs in other settings, requiring greater physical and mental effort from the client.

Skilled Nursing Facility

Skilled nursing facilities often offer rehabilitation services. The facility may be hospital based or community based. The programs are similar to those offered in hospital settings with a full range of services and health care professionals. Physician coverage varies, but professional nursing care is rendered 24 hours a day. The program is usually less intense than a hospital program; this may be a benefit to elderly clients with limited energy resources. Families should research the services available because they differ greatly from one facility to the next.

Outpatient Rehabilitation

Outpatient services are offered by hospital-based rehabilitation programs. The intensity may range from occasional visits to 3 or 4 visits per week. Day hospital programs are another form of outpatient services but require the client to spend several hours a day for 3 to 5 days a week at the hospital. Availability of transportation is a prerequisite for all outpatient programs.

Home Rehabilitation

Some home health agencies provide a full scope of services, including nursing, all therapies, and social services. Service is usually provided on an intermittent basis for medically stable clients. The accessibility of services varies greatly depending on the availability of therapists in the area.

HOME HEALTH CARE

Home care encompasses a number of services delivered to persons in their homes and is the fastest growing segment of health care delivery. The total number of home health care agencies increased by 26% between 1989 and 1994 (Millea, 1995). Clients are receiving intravenous therapy, ventilator care, parenteral nutrition, and chemotherapy at home. Many agencies have nurse specialists on staff for complicated cases involving care required for wounds, intravenous therapy, diabetes, and cardiac or respiratory problems.

Medicare certified agencies (7,747 in 1999) provide intermittent care to persons meeting the criteria for care (NAHC, 2000). A registered nurse may call on the client a specified number of times each week to assess the client's condition, supervise the work of LP/VNs and unlicensed workers, and deliver skilled nursing care. Nursing assistants are assigned to give personal care; check vital signs; and do positioning, transfers, and passive range-of-motion exercises. In addition to nursing staff, the agency may provide therapists and social workers to serve their clients, also on an intermittent basis. These services are time-limited by Medicare and are not reimbursable if the client is not deemed to require skilled care.

The home health agency may provide or arrange with other vendors for services needed by the client. This may include Meals-on-Wheels, homemaker services for light housekeeping tasks, companion services, transportation for outpatient care, intravenous therapy, pain management, and parenteral nutrition. The home health nurse needs to be aware of the availability of respite care because family members may need a break from the rigors of caregiving and may need encouragement from the nurse to do so.

Role of the LP/VN

Although the role of the LP/VN in home care is expanding, current (1994) statistics indicate that LP/VNs make up the smallest number of home health care professionals. There were 254,643 registered nurses, 34,757 LP/VNs, 171,346 home health care assistants, and 48,460 physical therapists working in home care (Millea, 1995). The responsibilities of the LP/VN vary among agencies. All nurses working in home care must have excellent assessment skills and a keen ability to identify actual and potential problems. Working with the family may be a greater challenge than meeting the needs of the client. Teaching the client and family is a major responsibility for the home health nurse. The educated client can assume more control. The client with a chronic health problem will have ongoing needs after the home health care is discontinued. Clients and their family caregivers must know the following:

The disease process
- Complications that may occur
- How to prevent the complications
- Signs and symptoms of the complications
- How to reduce risk factors such as dietary adaptations and exercise programs

Medications
- Actions of medications
- Special administration guidelines such as timing related to meals
- Side effects

Special skills
- Drawing up and administering insulin or other injectables
- Using a blood glucose monitor
- Changing dressings
- Monitoring vital signs
- Using special client care equipment, adaptive devices, and assistive devices

Documentation and communication
- How to keep records for nurse or physician visit; for example, blood glucose, blood pressure, and weight
- Communication with health care providers
- How and when to contact the home health nurse
- How and when to contact the physician
- How and when to contact emergency services

LONG-TERM CARE

Long-term care refers to a spectrum of services provided to individuals who have an ongoing need for health care. Long-term care has traditionally meant a community-based nursing home licensed for skilled or intermediate care. While there is a great demand for this type of care, there is also a market for other levels of health care. It is estimated that by the year 2030, more than 8 million seniors will be residing in nursing homes (American Health Care Association [AHCA], 1998). Currently 1.5 million persons live in 17,000 nursing homes. Of the residents, 90% are over age 65, but 24% are over age 85 (AHCA, 1998).

The increasing population of elderly persons has resulted in tremendous changes in health care delivery. Housing options are often a component of the package of services available. The least restrictive level of care that is appropriate for the client's needs will generally be the most cost effective.

Long-Term Care Facilities

A **long-term care facility** may be licensed for either intermediate care or skilled nursing care. Long-term care facilities provide services to individuals who are not acutely ill, have continuing health care needs, and cannot function independently at home. Intermediate care facilities (ICF) are not certified for reimbursement from Medicare but may be certified for

Medicaid funding. Skilled nursing facilities (SNF) are eligible for certification by both Medicare and Medicaid, but not all facilities choose to become certified. These facilities were formerly called nursing homes, rest homes, or convalescent centers. The term *extended care facility* (ECF) refers to any facility that renders care for a long period of time. It has no concrete definition and could refer to either an intermediate or skilled nursing facility. Facilities in every state that receive any government funds from any source are required by law to be in compliance with the OBRA regulations. It is estimated that 2 out of 5 persons in the United States will need long-term care sometime in their lives (AHCA, 1998).

Facilities of today bear little resemblance to those of the 1970s and 1980s. A restorative philosophy of care provides direction for the interdisciplinary team. Emphasis is placed on assisting the client (usually called resident) to attain and maintain the highest level of physical, mental, and psychosocial function. A holistic approach is utilized and families are important members of the care team.

A large number of facilities have special units devoted to the care of residents with specific problems. These units may care for persons with Alzheimer's disease, diabetes, respiratory disorders, wounds, and so on.

Subacute Care

Subacute care is a concept designed to provide services for clients who are out of the acute stage of their illnesses but who still require skilled nursing, monitoring, and ongoing treatments. The clients are not critically ill but do have complex medical needs. Subacute care is intended to fill the gap between the acute care hospital and the traditional long-term care facility (AHCA, 2000).

Subacute care facilities are usually housed in a section of a freestanding long-term care facility. The nurses may have a critical care background or are given additional training to equip them with the skills needed to provide care. Services may include intensive rehabilitation therapies, wound and pain management, care for clients with acquired immunodeficiency syndrome (AIDS), oncology care, postsurgical services, intravenous therapy, nutritional support, peritoneal dialysis, ventilator care, and cardiac monitoring. Many subacute care units specialize in 1 or 2 of these areas. Clients stay from 20 to 30 days. Efficient discharge planning and client teaching are essential components to the plan of care.

Continuing Care Retirement Communities

Continuing Care Retirement Communities (CCRC) are designed to provide continuing levels of care as the individual's health care needs change. These levels include:

- Independent living in apartments located on the campus—housekeeping services and meals are provided
- **Assisted living**—a combination of housing and services for persons who need help with the activities of daily living
- Health care—either short-term for persons recovering from a temporary disorder or permanent for long-term illnesses such as Alzheimer's disease. The health care facility of the CCRC may be licensed as either skilled or intermediate

CCRCs usually charge a fee upon entry to the system and a monthly fee thereafter. The client must give proof of adequate financial resources in order to be accepted into the system. In exchange, individuals have the security of knowing that they will receive care for the remainder of their lives. Most CCRCs stipulate that persons must enter the system when they are able to live independently in the apartments. The health care facility of the CCRC may be certified for Medicaid if clients exhaust their financial resources. The health care facility may be certified for Medicare for clients who are qualified to receive such services. Neither Medicare nor Medicaid will pay for the independent living or assisted living sections of a CCRC.

Assisted Living

Assisted living combines housing and services for persons who require assistance with activities of daily living. Nursing care is not provided. These are persons who cannot live alone but who do not need 24-hour care. It is a less restrictive environment than a long-term care facility and maintains the individual's independence and freedom of choice. This level of care may be offered in a freestanding facility or as a section of a long-term care facility or CCRC as previously described. A monthly fee is charged and covers rent, utilities, housekeeping services, meals, transportation, health promotion, exercise programs, and assistance with ADL (Assisted Living Federation of America [ALFA], 1999).

There are an estimated 30,000 assisted living residences in the United States with more than 1 million residents (ALFA, 1999). The typical resident is a female (single or widowed) 83 years old or older (ALFA, 1999). Assisted living residences are licensed by the state. Costs range from $1,000 to $3,000 per month and are mainly paid from personal funds (AHCA, 1998).

Adult Day Care

Adult day care centers may be located in a separate unit of a long-term care facility, in a private home, or be freestanding. They provide a variety of services in a protective setting for adults who are unable to stay

alone but who do not need 24-hour care. The centers are generally open from 7:00 A.M. to 6:00 P.M. 5 days a week and serve 2 or 3 meals a day. A daily or hourly fee is charged with an additional charge for meals. Services may be limited to socialization or may be comprehensive offering modest rehabilitation services and nursing care. Adult day care is often utilized by working persons who have a spouse or parent living with them who cannot be left alone. Fifty percent of clients in day care have some degree of cognitive impairment (NADSA, 2000).

Respite Care

Respite care may be offered by adult day care centers, long-term care facilities, or in private homes. It is intended to provide a break to caregivers and may be utilized a few hours a week, for an occasional weekend, or for longer vacations. Planned activities, meals, and supervision are included in respite care services.

Foster Care

Some states are investigating the use of foster homes for individuals who cannot live independently but who do not require the services of a health care facility. A person with Alzheimer's disease who is mobile but who is unable to stay alone because of cognitive impairment would be a candidate for foster care. The legal structure is similar to the foster home concept for children.

Role of the LP/VN

There are probably more career opportunities available for the LP/VN in long-term care facilities than in the other types of health care described in this chapter. In a small facility the LP/VN might act as supervisor during the night or evening shifts. In larger facilities the LP/VN might be in charge of one unit with a registered nurse as a house supervisor. The nurse needs sharp assessment skills and a sound ability to make nursing judgments based on assessment findings. The LP/VN may also be expected to supervise and coordinate the work of nursing assistants. The nurse may wish to seek additional course work to acquire supervisory skills. LP/VNs may take the Certification Examination for Practical and Vocational Nurses in Long-Term Care (CEPN-LTC™) given by the National Council of State Boards of Nursing (NCSBN). Those who pass the examination are certified in long-term care and may use the initials "CLTC" to signify their certification.

HOSPICE

Hospice is humane, compassionate care provided to clients who can no longer benefit from curative treatment and have 6 months or less to live. The special care is designed to provide sensitivity and support, allowing clients to carry on an alert, pain-free life with other symptoms managed so the last days are spent with dignity and quality of life at home or in a home-like setting. This is sometimes referred to as palliative care.

The first hospice in the United States began in 1974. Today, there are more than 3,000 programs that are estimated to serve 450,000 terminally ill clients and their families each year (National Hospice Organization [NHO], 1999).

The primary physician must refer the client to hospice. Care and support are provided to both client and family by a team consisting of the physician, nurses, counselors, therapists, social worker, aides, and volunteers. The team regards dying as a normal process and does nothing to hasten or postpone death. Relief of pain and other distressing symptoms is provided. The client is supported to live as actively as possible until death. The family is supported to help them cope during the client's illness and in their bereavement after the client's death. Health care workers may also need support as the task of caring for the dying is often quite stressful.

Benefits for hospice are included in most private

PROFESSIONAL TIP

Hospice Settings

Hospice care may be implemented in a variety of settings: the client's home, a special area of hospitals or nursing homes, or freestanding inpatient facilities. Most clients receive care at home. In 1995, 77% of hospice clients died in their home, 19% died in an institutional facility, and 4% died in other settings (NHO, 1999).

health care insurance, health maintenance organizations (HMOs), and managed care; Medicare; and in 43 states plus the District of Columbia by Medicaid. For hospice care in 1995, Medicare paid for 65.3% of the clients; private insurance, 12%; Medicaid, 7.8%; indigent (nonreimbursed) care, 4.2%; and other, 10.7% (NHO, 1999). As of 1999, 44 states had licensure laws for hospice programs. Some programs are certified voluntarily by Medicare and accredited by the JCAHO or Community Health Accreditation Program (CHAP) (NHO, 1999).

SAMPLE NURSING CARE PLAN

THE CLIENT REQUIRING REHABILITATIVE CARE

Mr. Jason, 65 years old, was admitted to a skilled nursing facility following hospitalization for a right cerebral hemisphere stroke. He is unable to purposefully change position without assistance. His gag reflex is weakened, swallowing is delayed, and there is coughing after swallowing. Mr. Jason has smoked for 50 years and is still doing so. Rehabilitation was initiated in the hospital. A feeding tube was put in place with the goal to assist Mr. Jason to regain his swallowing ability so the tube can be removed. Mr. Jason frequently expresses his discouragement with his dependency on the staff. He is married and lives in the community with his wife. Mr. Jason had been retired for 1 year before the stroke. Mrs. Jason works full time. Two adult children live in other states. Mrs. Jason hopes that her husband will regain adequate mobility skills so that she can eventually take him home.

Nursing Diagnosis 1 *Impaired Physical Mobility related to left hemiplegia and sensory/perceptual impairments as evidenced by inability to purposefully change position of body without assistance*

PLANNING/GOALS	NURSING INTERVENTIONS	RATIONALE	EVALUATION
Mr. Jason will maintain current level of range of motion in all joints.	Change position at least every 2 hours; place affected extremities out of synergy.	Prevent contracture formation and pressure ulcers. Hemiplegic limbs are flaccid immediately after stroke and then become spastic. **Synergy** patterns (abnor-	Range of joint motion is preserved. Complications related to immobility are prevented. Progress in mobilization is

continues

mal patterns of movement that result from an overactive stretch reflex due to CNS damage) may develop in response to spasticity, causing contractures. Positioning out of synergy avoids contracture formation.

achieved; movement in bed, transfers with 1 to 2 assists, transfer independently, and ambulation are noted.

PLANNING/GOALS	NURSING INTERVENTIONS	RATIONALE	EVALUATION
Mr. Jason will remain free of contractures.	Do passive range-of-motion exercises twice a day on affected extremities. Assist with active range-of-motion exercises on unaffected extremities. Teach to do self-range-of-motion exercises when condition permits.	Range-of-motion exercises maintain joint mobility and prevent contracture formation. Active and self range-of-motion exercises will also increase strength and endurance.	
Mr. Jason will begin program of progressive mobilization.	Teach Mr. Jason to move in bed: – Client begins in supine position with the knees bent and feet flat in bed. – Instruct client to raise the hips by pressing his heels down. – Stabilize the affected limb by exerting pressure downward through the thigh just above the knee while assisting the client to lift the pelvis clear of the bed (Galarneau, 1993). Consult with physical therapist about program for progressive mobilization.	Increases the client's bed mobility. The recovery of a client with a stroke is dependent on the cooperative efforts of several interdisciplinary team members. The physical therapist is an expert in mobility.	

Nursing Diagnosis 2 *Impaired Swallowing related to neuromuscular impairment as evidenced by weakened gag reflex, delayed swallowing, and coughing after swallowing*

PLANNING/GOALS	NURSING INTERVENTIONS	RATIONALE	EVALUATION
Mr. Jason will swallow without aspirating.	Consult with speech/language pathologist in regard to	A video-recorded fluoroscopy is used to make a definitive diag-	There are no signs of aspiration.

continues

video-recorded fluoroscopy for swallowing evaluation.

nosis of impaired swallowing. The results of the evaluation provide a basis for interventions suggested by the speech/language pathologist.

Serve semisolid foods of medium consistency. Use a commercial thickener for liquids. Avoid milk, citrus juices, and water.

These foods require less manipulation in the mouth and allow the client to concentrate on swallowing rather than chewing. Liquids are more manageable when thickened. Water provides minimal sensory stimulation, making it difficult for the client to manage water. Milk and citrus juices stimulate production of saliva.

Allow rest period before eating. Position client at 60°–90° angle before, during, and for 1 hour after eating.

Fatigue increases risk of aspiration.

Maintain head in midline with neck slightly flexed.

This position facilitates the passage of food through the pharynx.

Face the client, avoid haste.

Facing the client allows feeder to evaluate the eating process. If the feeder appears hurried, the client may try to eat faster.

Minimize distractions, keep conversation minimal.

The client's attention must focus only on eating.

Allow Mr. Jason to see and smell food. Give verbal descriptions. Use regular metal teaspoon, give one-half teaspoon at a time.

Sensory cues promote awareness of eating.

Place food on unaffected side of mouth. Teach to hold food in mouth, think about swallowing, and then swallow twice.

Buccal pocketing of food in the cheek on the affected side is common after a stroke.

continues

Nursing Diagnosis 3 *Situational Low Self-Esteem related to changes in functional abilities as evidenced by verbal expression of discouragement*

PLANNING/GOALS	NURSING INTERVENTIONS	RATIONALE	EVALUATION
Mr. Jason will verbalize acceptance of self, situation, and lifestyle changes.	Assess for signs of severe or prolonged grieving.	The client needs to grieve the loss of his former self. Prolonged grieving may indicate need for counseling.	Mr. Jason is progressing through all rehabilitation therapies and presents no signs of prolonged grieving.
	Assess client's interactions with significant others.	Other people may be reinforcing the concepts of helplessness and invalidism.	
	Listen in nonjudgmental fashion to comments about situation.	Each person responds differently to a crisis. Being nonjudgmental builds trust and encourages verbalization of thoughts.	

CASE STUDY

Mrs. Emma James, 72 years old, was admitted to Community Hospital for a left below knee amputation. Mrs. James has been an insulin dependent diabetic for 35 years. The amputation follows a long and unsuccessful period of treatment for venous stasis ulcers. Mrs. James was transferred from the hospital to a rehabilitation hospital on her fourth postoperative day. After 2 weeks at the rehabilitation hospital, she was transferred to a skilled care facility near her home for additional rehabilitation and regulation of the diabetes. She is now ready to be discharged to her home. Mrs. James has a prosthesis and is able to ambulate with a walker. She can perform her ADL with minimal assistance. She was on a sliding scale and blood glucose monitoring 4 times a day while in the long-term care facility. Her physician has now placed her on insulin twice a day with daily blood glucose checks. Her vision is somewhat impaired due to the diabetes. Mrs. James lives alone in a one-story home in a safe residential area. The discharge planner at the skilled care facility has arranged continuing care for Mrs. James through a local home health agency.

The following questions will guide your development of a nursing care plan for the case study.

1. Identify the assessment factors that are most important in planning Mrs. James's care.
2. List the nursing diagnoses that would be applicable to Mrs. James's assessment.
3. Describe the complications for which Mrs. James is at risk.
4. Describe nursing interventions for preventing the complications.
5. What specific actions would you take to prevent a recurrence of venous stasis ulcers?
6. What additional community services does Mrs. James need?
7. What nursing services (frequency of nurse visits, services from a nursing assistant, other home health services) would you plan to meet her needs? Which services would each person provide?
8. Describe the outcomes you would expect for Mrs. James.

SUMMARY

- There has been a significant increase in the growth of nonacute care settings.
- Medicaid (state and federal funds) and Medicare (federal funds) are major sources of health care payment, especially for the elderly and permanently disabled. The availability of these resources in the future is in jeopardy. Alternative funding sources are being explored by state and federal governments.
- Rehabilitation can be provided in a variety of settings.
- There is a need for the services and skills of the LP/VN in all of these health care services. Experience and additional education may be required for employment in special care settings.

Review Questions

1. One reason for the growth in nonacute care health services is:

    a. the diminishing supply of physicians.
    b. an increase in the number of hospitals in the country.
    c. the cost of acute care.
    d. the increase in Medicare reimbursement.

2. Medicare is a reimbursement system for health care providers that:

    a. is based upon the client's personal financial resources.
    b. is available to persons 65 years of age and over or who have been disabled for 2 or more years.
    c. pays the full cost of all medical care.
    d. is managed by each state.

3. Subacute care is most often provided:

    a. in a step-down unit of the hospital.
    b. in a special care unit of a skilled care facility.
    c. for clients who are terminally ill.
    d. for clients who require life support.

4. Which of the following clients would be most likely to benefit from rehabilitation services?

    a. Mr. J, 64 years old, had a stroke, is responsive and stable.
    b. Mrs. B, 89 years old, has Alzheimer's disease in the fourth stage.

    c. Miss Z, 26 years old, is recovering from pneumonia.
    d. Mr. K, 56 years old, has terminal cancer of the lung.

5. Which of the following is a legal requirement for health care facilities that is controlled by each state?

    a. accreditation
    b. certification
    c. licensure
    d. provision of free care

6. As a member of the interdisciplinary health care team, the LP/VN must be able to:

    a. participate in the planning of client care.
    b. plan the appropriate diet for clients.
    c. teach the new amputee how to walk with a prosthesis.
    d. provide alternative methods of communication for the client with recent stroke.

7. In the home health care setting, it is essential that the LP/VN possess skills in:

    a. advanced intravenous therapy.
    b. respiratory therapy treatments.
    c. physical assessment.
    d. planning and providing speech therapy.

8. In a long-term care facility, the LP/VN may serve as the:

    a. charge nurse of a unit.
    b. physical therapist.
    c. clinical nurse specialist.
    d. social worker.

Critical Thinking Question

1. What are the pros and cons related to working for a home health agency, a hospice, or a long-term care facility?

 WEB FLASH!

Search the Internet for the various types of health care discussed in this chapter. What information is available? Is it focused for consumer or provider?

UNIT
11
Integration of Body Systems

CHAPTER 37

NURSING CARE OF THE CLIENT: RESPONDING TO EMERGENCIES

MAKING THE CONNECTION

Refer to the following chapters to increase your understanding of emergency situations:

- **Chapter 2, Critical Thinking**
- **Chapter 3, Legal Responsibilities**
- **Chapter 4, Ethical Responsibilities**
- **Chapter 18, Nursing Care of the Client: Respiratory System**
- **Chapter 19, Nursing Care of the Client: Cardiovascular System**
- **Chapter 21, Nursing Care of the Client: Integumentary System**
- **Chapter 24, Nursing Care of the Client: Musculoskeletal System**
- **Chapter 25, Nursing Care of the Client: Neurological System**

- **Chapter 26, Nursing Care of the Client: Sensory System**
- **Chapter 28, Nursing Care of the Client: Gastrointestinal System**
- **Chapter 29, Nursing Care of the Client: Urinary System**
- **Chapter 30, Nursing Care of the Client: Female Reproductive System**
- **Chapter 31, Nursing Care of the Client: Male Reproductive System**
- **Chapter 33, Nursing Care of the Client: Mental Illness**
- **Chapter 34, Nursing Care of the Client: Substance Abuse**

LEARNING OBJECTIVES

Upon completion of this chapter, you should be able to:
- *Define key terms.*
- *Describe the emergency medical services.*
- *Explain the role of the nurse in emergency situations.*
- *List personnel needed to respond to an in-hospital emergency.*
- *Discuss the steps in assessing an emergency client.*
- *Cite the different levels of triage.*

KEY TERMS

chain of custody	Glasgow Coma Scale
emergency	paramedic
emergency medical technician (EMT)	shock
	trauma
emergency nursing	triage

INTRODUCTION

An **emergency** can be defined as a medical or surgical condition requiring immediate or timely intervention to prevent permanent disability or death. Emergency nursing has developed rapidly over the years in response to the changing environment and expectations of the community. Many advancements in emergency care can be attributed to the military. In order to manage vast numbers of injured soldiers, the military had to develop a systematic method of treating and responding to **trauma** (wound or injury). Casualties caused by wartime situations created the need for advancements in the care of large numbers of clients with injuries, wounds, and illness. Methods of caring for multiple clients were developed and implemented as a result of military influence.

In the U.S., trauma is the number one killer of those under the age of 37 and the fourth leading cause of death overall. Motor vehicle collisions kill more than 43,000 people each year, with over 4 million car crash victims cared for in the emergency departments (EDs) (Traum, 1998).

Emergency nursing is the care of clients who require emergency intervention. The emergency nurse must be capable of rapid assessment and history taking and immediate intervention formulation and implementation utilizing the nursing process. This role carries great responsibility. Throughout the assessment and care of the client, the emergency nurse must plan and teach prevention and health promotion, as well as rapidly develop rapport with the client and family, including assisting with emotional needs. Clinical knowledge, communication, client teaching, and empathy skills are essential to effective emergency care. Although licensed practical/vocational nurses (LP/VNs) are seldom hired for EDs, they may at times be required to float or help during emergency situations; therefore, a brief overview of emergency nursing is justified.

APPROACHES TO EMERGENCY CARE

There are three general approaches to emergency care: hospital triage, disaster triage, and the emergency medical services. To care for the emergent client, one must first determine the severity of illness.

Hospital Triage

Each hospital with an ED has an established "triage" system in effect (Figure 37-1). **Triage** refers to classification of clients to determine priority of need and proper place of treatment. Triage is typically utilized in the ED to establish priorities and levels of care needed by the clients. Although clients and their families define emergency according to their perceptions, it is the triage nurse's responsibility to sort and prioritize the clients as they arrive in the ED.

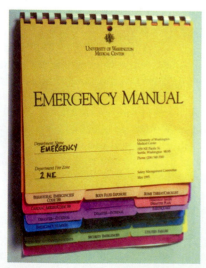

Figure 37-1 Hospitals have emergency manuals and procedures to guide personnel in caring for clients who present emergent conditions.

PROFESSIONAL TIP

Golden Rules of Emergency Care

1. Establish the safety of the scene
2. Remove the client from danger
3. Establish airway, breathing, and circulation
4. Manage shock
5. Attend to eye injuries
6. Treat skin injuries
7. Call for help

The simplest method of triaging clients is to utilize the American Heart Association's basic life support principles: Airway, Breathing, and Circulation (ABCs). By utilizing this method, those clients with airway problems would be immediately assessed and would become a top priority of care. If any of the ABCs were not functioning, either the Heimlich maneuver or cardiopulmonary resuscitation (CPR) would be initiated.

Infection Control: Mouth-to-Mouth Resuscitation

When delivering care to any client, the nurse should be careful to practice Standard Precautions. Direct mouth-to-mouth breathing should not be administered; instead, use of a bag-valve-mask for resuscitation is more effective in both protecting the health care worker and the client from possible infection and in administering respirations.

Most hospitals have a triage system established in order to provide expedient care to those requiring it first. Although the term *emergency department* implies emergency care, the client utilizing this department does not always require immediate care. The most commonly used triage classifications are emergent, urgent, and non-urgent (Table 37–1). Emergent clients require immediate care in order to sustain life or limb. Examples of emergent conditions include foreign bodies in the eye, shortness of breath, impending birth, and cardiopulmonary arrest. Urgent clients require care within 1 to 2 hours to prevent worsening of their conditions. Examples of urgent situations include acute abdominal pain and compound fractures. For non-urgent clients, care can be delayed without the risk of permanent consequences. Contusions and sprains are examples of non-urgent complaints.

Principles of first aid, developed for emergency medicine, are part of the triage process and include what are referred to as the golden rules of emergency care. The first of these rules cautions the health care worker to assess the physical environment for self protection. That is, safety at the scene must be established before rescue is attempted (Figure 37-2). The next rule is to remove the client from danger, such as that pre-

Table 37-1 TRIAGE CATEGORIES		
CATEGORY/ PRIORITY	**CLIENT NEEDS**	**EXAMPLES**
Emergent	Immediate intervention is required to sustain life or limb.	Cardiac arrest Multiple trauma
Urgent	Care is required within 1 to 2 hours to prevent deterioration of condition.	Compound fractures Persistent vomiting and diarrhea
Non-urgent	Care may be delayed without risk of permanent sequelae.	Contusions Minor sprains and fractures

Developed from Military Standard Operating Procedure (SOP) for General Hospitals.

Table 37-2 DISASTER TRIAGE		
CATEGORY/ PRIORITY	**CLIENT NEEDS**	**EXAMPLES**
Immediate	Simple injuries requiring immediate care	Chest wounds Crush injuries Burns
Delayed	Multiple injuries requiring extensive care	Open fractures of the long bones
Minimal	Minor injuries (the walking wounded)	Sprains Contusions Minor cuts
Expectant	Severe injuries likely leading to death	Massive head trauma Spinal cord injuries

Developed from Military Standard Operating Procedure (SOP) for General Hospitals.

sented by passing vehicles. These first two rules typically apply to emergencies occurring outside of an institutional setting.

Once the safety at the scene and of the client have been established, assessment turns to the ABCs—*airway, breathing, and circulation*. When these functions have been stabilized, the client should be assessed for shock. Eye and skin injuries should be evaluated next. The last thing to do is to call for help.

Disaster Triage

Disaster triage systems represent a second approach to emergency care. These systems are utilized in the event of a community disaster, either natural or man made, such as a train accident, hurricane, or tornado (Figure 37-3). Given the possibility of large numbers of casualties as a result of disasters, a different approach to triaging from that of the hospital system is utilized (Table 37-2).

Figure 37-2 Establishing the safety of the scene is the first priority in emergency care, as in this scene of a motor vehicle accident, where rescue workers may be in danger from oncoming vehicles. *(Courtesy of David J. Reimer, Sr.)*

Figure 37-3 Disaster systems are designed for response to community emergencies. *(Courtesy of John O'Connell.)*

Most communities have disaster/mass casualty committees. These committees include all hospitals, the emergency medical services (EMS) system, and citizens needed to alert the community of an impending or real disaster.

Emergency Medical Services

Prior to admission to the ED, the client may have been cared for by an **emergency medical technician** (EMT) or **paramedic** in the EMS (Figure 37-4). An EMT is a health care professional trained to provide basic lifesaving measures prior to arrival at the hospital. A paramedic is a more specialized health care professional trained to provide advanced life support to the client requiring emergency interventions. Both are part of the EMS and are essential to prehospital care of the emergency client.

SHOCK

Shock is a condition of profound hemodynamic and metabolic disturbance characterized by inadequate tissue perfusion and inadequate circulation to the vital organs (Table 37–3). Shock can result from trauma, injury, or insult. Recognizing and immediately treating shock are critical to the client's survival.

Hypovolemic shock is usually easily recognized. It results from severe fluid volume depletion through vomiting, dehydration, diarrhea, or blood loss. Severe external bleeding may be obvious, but internal bleeding, such as that from a gastric ulcer, is not readily observable.

Cardiogenic shock may be caused by several different heart conditions that result in loss of the contractile property of the heart muscle. The most common of these is acute myocardial infarction (heart attack). Severe heart failure and certain arrhythmias may also cause shock.

Septic shock is usually caused by overwhelming infection. Certain organisms may cause severe reactions resulting in collapse of the circulatory system. Toxic

Figure 37-4 Emergency medical technicians (EMTs) and paramedics are often the first to arrive at an emergency scene.

shock syndrome, gram-negative shock, and urogenic shock are types of septic shock.

Anaphylactic shock is a severe allergic reaction to a toxin to which a client has been exposed. Causes of anaphylactic reaction include insect bites and certain medications.

Neurogenic shock is the body's response to extreme pain or trauma to the spinal cord. As with the other forms of shock, it results in inadequate supply of oxygen, electrolytes, and other essential chemicals to the tissues.

Medical–Surgical Management

Medical

Management of shock is supportive in nature during initial resuscitation. The immediate priority is maintenance of the ABCs. Active bleeding should then be stopped. Blood may be administered in the event of major blood loss. After the client is stabilized, the underlying cause of shock must be identified and treated.

Pharmacological

Initial treatment involves the administration of oxygen and the insertion of two large-bore intravenous

Table 37–3	TYPES OF SHOCK		
TYPE	**CAUSES**	**SIGNS AND SYMPTOMS**	**EMERGENCY CARE**
Hypovolemic	Hemorrhage*, burns	Increased heart rate; hypotension; cold, clammy skin; profound thirst	Replace fluids
Cardiogenic	Myocardial infarction*	Increased heart rate; hypotension; cold, clammy skin	Initiate drug therapy for myocardial infarction; replace fluids; consider possible emergency coronary bypass surgery
Toxic	Overwhelming infection	Hot, dry, flushed skin; hypotension; increased heart rate	Locate source of infection and treat with broad-spectrum antibiotic; replace fluids
Anaphylactic	Medications*, insect bites or stings, foods	Throat edema in conjunction with increasing difficulty breathing; hypotension; increased heart rate	Manage ABCs; administer epinephrine (Adrenalin); administer diphenhydramine hydrochloride (Benadryl)
Neurogenic	Spinal cord injury	Slowed heart rate; hypotension	Replace fluids, administer drugs to increase blood pressure and heart rate

*Most common cause

(IV) lines. Intravenous lines must be instituted to establish lifelines through which life saving drugs and fluids may be administered. Fluid resuscitation and oxygen delivery are critical to management of the client in shock. Medications, including epinephrine, may be administered to improve circulation.

▸ NURSING PROCESS

▸ Assessment

▸ Subjective Data

Subjective assessment begins with determining whether the client is responsive and able to respond to questions, or is unconscious. After the client is alert and stabilized, assessment should include obtaining a history of the events leading to the injury or illness, including any food consumed or medication taken and any unusual event (such as a bee sting) that precipitated the shock state. The client should also be asked to describe any pain with regard to intensity, location, and duration.

▸ Objective Data

Immediate assessment involves evaluating the ABCs. Vital signs should be taken, because many clients in shock will present with hypotension, tachycardia, tachypnea, and pale, diaphoretic, clammy skin.

Nursing diagnoses for a client in shock may include the following:

Nursing Diagnoses	Planning/Goals	Nursing Interventions
▸ *Risk for Deficient Fluid Volume related to acute blood loss/vomiting/diarrhea*	The client will maintain adequate fluid balance.	Initiate and maintain fluid replacement with two large-bore IV access lines. Administer blood as ordered.
▸ *Ineffective Tissue Perfusion related to decreased oxygen-carrying hemoglobin secondary to blood loss and fluid depletion*	The client will maintain adequate tissue perfusion as manifested by stable vital signs.	Assess vital signs at least every 30 minutes. Administer oxygen per physician order.
▸ *Anticipatory Grieving related to grave nature of illness/injury*	The client will cope with illness/injury by cooperating with care provided by health care workers and will discuss outcomes with nurse and family.	Communicate with client and family. Explain all interventions as they occur, to decrease acute anxiety. Allow client and family to express their fears and worries about the situation. Answer questions about care.

Evaluation Each goal must be evaluated to determine how it has been met by the client.

CARDIOPULMONARY EMERGENCIES

Cardiopulmonary emergencies are those emergencies that jeopardize the function of the heart and lungs. These emergencies can result from trauma or illness. Cardiopulmonary emergencies such as drowning, foreign body obstruction of the airway, chest trauma, and chest pain are grouped together, because the effects, medical management, and nursing priorities are similar.

Near-drowning episodes occur most frequently in the summer months. Many clients will suffer other related injuries associated with drowning, such as head and spinal cord injuries (Table 37–4).

Foreign body obstruction of the airway most commonly occurs in the larger, right main bronchus. The most common source of airway obstruction is the tongue. Other sources of airway obstruction include hot dogs, candy, steak, and coins (especially in children).

Penetrating or blunt trauma to the chest can cause multiple injuries. Penetrating injuries are insults that puncture the chest, such as gunshot or knife wounds. Blunt trauma is more likely caused by falls or by forceful contact with a blunt object such as a baseball bat or steering wheel. Injuries associated with pneumothorax include cardiac tamponade, fractured ribs, fractured sternum, and flail chest.

PROFESSIONAL TIP

Flail Chest

A flail chest is defined as instability in the chest wall. This condition is caused by fracture of three or more ribs in two or more places. With a flail chest, breathing is unique: The flail segment moves inward during inspiration and outward during expiration. This is called paradoxical breathing.

Table 37–4 FRESH-WATER VERSUS SALT-WATER NEAR-DROWNING

TYPE	CLIENT SYMPTOMS	PATHOPHYSIOLOGY	SIGNS
Fresh-water	Fatigue, anxiety, difficulty breathing, fear	Water in lungs causes changes in surfactant, which in turn causes alveolar collapse.	Hypoxia, collapsed alveoli
Salt-water	Fatigue, anxiety, difficulty breathing, fear, rales, rhonchi	Hypertonic salt water pulls fluid into the alveoli.	Hypoxia, pulmonary edema

One of the most common complaints evaluated in the ED is chest pain. Those clients presenting with the symptom of chest pain must be clearly and carefully evaluated. Chest pain has a multitude of potential causes and can be frightening to the client until the cause is confirmed.

Medical–Surgical Management

Medical

Management of all cardiopulmonary emergencies is directed at maintaining the ABCs. If indicated, intubation is part of resuscitation in cardiopulmonary emergencies. Establishment of an IV line is essential for medical management, because the line provides access for administration of lifesaving medications.

After resuscitation has been achieved, other treatment modalities must be instituted. Chest x-rays, electrocardiograms (ECGs), and blood tests must be obtained. Pain control must be initiated. Morphine sulfate is the drug of choice for clients with these types of emergencies, because morphine decreases both pain and anxiety in the client, which, in turn, leads to improved breathing.

Pharmacological

With the near-drowning client, mannitol (Osmitrol) and furosemide (Lasix) are occasionally indicated in the event of fluid overload. Pain medication is essential for the client with chest injury, because hypoventi-lation may occur due to the pain associated with deep breathing. Pain control is also essential for the client experiencing chest pain. Pain medications can vary from sublingual nitroglycerine to IV morphine sulfate.

Activity

Most clients with cardiopulmonary emergencies are initially confined to bed and must be frequently rolled from side to side. In addition, deep breathing and coughing should be encouraged to prevent stasis of fluid and development of pneumonia.

▶ NURSING PROCESS

▶ Assessment

▶ Subjective Data

The client should be evaluated for restlessness, an early sign of hypoxia. Description of pain should be noted. Other areas to include in assessment are fatigue, anxiety, and level of consciousness. Ability to give a brief history of events prior to the cardiopulmonary emergency should be evaluated.

▶ Objective Data

Airway and breathing must be immediately assessed. Any cough, stridor, cyanosis, or inability to talk should be noted. Initial vital signs are essential to developing a baseline.

Nursing diagnoses for a client with a cardiopulmonary emergency may include the following:

Nursing Diagnoses	Planning/Goals	Nursing Interventions
▶ *Ineffective Breathing Pattern related to injury to the chest and inability to fully expand the lungs*	Client will regain spontaneous respiration within normal rate and pattern.	Initiate CPR, if indicated. Keep client medicated to alleviate painful respirations. Administer pain medications as ordered to ease the work of breathing. Note response to pain medications. Remain with the client during episodes of respiratory distress, because being left alone at these times escalates both the anxiety and breathing problems. Explain all procedures.

continues

Nursing Diagnoses	Planning/Goals	Nursing Interventions
▶ *Ineffective Airway Clearance related to accumulation of fluid and blood in the airway and to the client's inability to cough*	Client's lungs will be clear bilaterally to auscultation.	Maintain airway and breathing with suctioning, if secretions accumulate. Turn client frequently to mobilize secretions. Encourage deep breathing and coughing. Suction client as needed. Listen to lungs hourly or more frequently to evaluate secretions and suctioning.

Evaluation Each goal must be evaluated to determine how it has been met by the client.

NEUROLOGICAL/ NEUROSURGICAL EMERGENCIES

Head injuries are the most common type of neurological trauma. Spinal cord trauma can also occur as a result of injuries sustained in a head injury. Head trauma most often results from motor vehicle collisions (MVCs) (Figure 37-5). Head injuries vary from very minor contusions to major head trauma.

Clients experiencing a cerebrovascular accident, or stroke, must be immediately admitted to the health care system for prompt evaluation and care. Strokes are now considered "brain attacks" requiring the same initial consideration given to myocardial infarctions, or "heart attacks."

Medical–Surgical Management

Medical

As with all trauma, management is aimed at maintaining the ABCs. In addition, if head, neck, or spinal cord trauma is suspected, the client should be placed on a backboard, with the head and neck immobilized. Blood alcohol level should be determined. Intravenous access should be initiated early in the resuscitation phase. Radiological examination is necessary to determine the extent of damage. If the client does not have spontaneous respirations, the injury has probably occurred at C-4 or above, meaning that the client will not be able to independently maintain respirations. The client should be continuously monitored for increased intracranial pressure. Early signs of increased intracranial pressure include a headache; later signs include widened pulse pressure, dilated pupils, and spontaneous emesis without warning. Hiccoughs are an ominous sign and should thus be reported immediately. Utilization of the **Glasgow Coma Scale**, a neurological screening test that measures a client's best verbal, motor, and eye response to stimuli, is indicated (Figure 37-6).

Pharmacological

Increased cranial pressure and buildup of carbon dioxide will complicate the client's condition; oxygen will most often alleviate the resultant complications. Thus, oxygen should be administered immediately. Pain management should be accomplished through IV access.

Figure 37-5 Motor vehicle collisions are the most common cause of head trauma. *(Courtesy of David J. Reimer, Sr.)*

Figure 37-6 Neurological Flow Sheet, Including Glasgow Coma Scale

Activity

Clients with head injuries should be placed in semi-Fowler's position to decrease edema and intracranial pressure.

▶ NURSING PROCESS

▶ Assessment

▶ Subjective Data

Subjective assessment includes obtaining a history of the accident and the mechanism of injury. The client's perception of what has happened and the client's emotional response should also be evaluated. The client may describe having a headache and difficulty seeing.

▶ Objective Data

The client's vital signs and Glasgow Coma Scale level should be measured. Cerebrospinal fluid leaks, such as clear fluid coming from the nares or ear, should be noted. Unequal pupillary response, trouble making self understood, or difficulty swallowing should also be documented.

Nursing diagnoses for the client with a neurological/neurosurgical emergency may include the following:

Nursing Diagnoses	Planning/Goals	Nursing Interventions
▶ *Excess Fluid Volume (Cerebral) related to accumulation of fluid/blood in cranium*	The client will remain conscious, maintain a Glasgow Coma Scale score of 15, and experience no further increase in cranial fluid volume.	Monitor intracranial pressure. Maintain the client in semi-Fowler's position. Document vital signs hourly. Assess Glasgow Coma Scale score and record hourly. Administer oxygen.
▶ *Impaired Verbal Communication related to injury to speech center*	The client will be able to communicate with the nurse and family.	Orient the client frequently to date and time. Explain all nursing interventions. Modify communication methods, such as use of a message board, depending on the client needs. Allow the client choices about care when possible. Encourage client to verbalize feelings about condition; offer support.

Evaluation Each goal must be evaluated to determine how it has been met by the client.

ABDOMINAL EMERGENCIES

Abdominal emergencies can be diverse in nature. Trauma to the upper body and torso can result in multiple abdominal injuries, from a simple contusion and bruising to a ruptured spleen. Clients presenting to the ED with complaints of abdominal pain require careful evaluation. Illnesses causing abdominal pain range from gastroenteritis to gastrointestinal bleeding.

Abdominal injuries can result from blunt or penetrating trauma. It is important to determine the mechanism of injury, as certain causes, such as MVCs, often result in multi-system trauma. Blunt trauma, for instance from falling on the abdomen, usually results in injury to internal organs, such as the kidneys or spleen. Penetrating injuries such as gunshot wounds can affect any internal organ. Hemorrhage is a potential complication of both types of trauma.

Medical–Surgical Management

Medical

Initial management of abdominal emergencies is IV access with large-bore catheters. Oxygen should be administered immediately, and standard protocol calls for managing the ABCs. Blood products or plasma expanders may be administered in the event of large volume blood loss. Insertion of a nasogastric tube decompresses the stomach. A peritoneal lavage may be performed to check for blood in the abdominal cavity of clients with abdominal trauma. Presence of blood indicates a need for immediate surgical intervention. A computed tomography (CT) scan of the abdomen may be indicated as well. Blood work should be drawn, and a urinalysis should be done. Hematuria must be evaluated, and x-rays may be indicated.

Pharmacological

If the client is in severe pain and has been evaluated, narcotics may be indicated.

PROFESSIONAL TIP

Open Abdominal Wound

If loops of intestines are exposed to outside air, they should be covered with saline-soaked gauze.

▶ NURSING PROCESS
▶ Assessment
▶ Subjective Data

Assessment includes identifying the location, duration, severity, and radiation of pain. History of nausea, vomiting, and diarrhea must be obtained. In addition, the times of the client's last meal, bowel movement, and urination must be noted.

▶ Objective Data

Vital signs, active bleeding, abdominal girth, and weight should be assessed. The abdomen should be inspected for bruises, edema, and wounds.

Nursing diagnoses for the client with an abdominal emergency may include the following:

Nursing Diagnoses	Planning/Goals	Nursing Interventions
▶ *Deficient Fluid Volume related to active bleeding*	The client will stabilize, and vital signs and fluid balance will return to normal.	Establish IV access with at least two large-bore catheters. Monitor vital signs frequently, at least hourly. Evaluate abdominal girth and bowel sounds hourly.
▶ *Risk for Infection related to penetrating injury*	The client will not experience an elevated temperature or show signs and symptoms of infection.	Administer antibiotics as ordered to reduce the risk of infection. Monitor temperature at least every 2 hours. Change saturated dressings as needed. Note amount and quality of any drainage.
▶ *Activity Intolerance related to pain and bleeding*	The client will ambulate with assistance 1 day after surgical correction.	Turn client hourly from side to side. Assist client to ambulate when able to prevent stasis of fluid and to diminish the risk of infection.

Evaluation Each goal must be evaluated to determine how it has been met by the client.

GENITOURINARY EMERGENCIES

Rape is a legal term and is not considered a medical condition. It is defined as sexual penetration of a forceful and threatening nature with a nonconsenting person. Included under this legal term is penetration of persons who are unable to consent due to intoxication or mental illness. *Alleged sexual assault* is the terminology used by most centers for rape survivors. Due to the many legal implications and to the fact that there are not only physical symptoms, but also long-lasting psychological consequences of sexual assault, accurate and methodical care must be given to the survivors of sexual assault. Most communities have hospitals designated to care for rape survivors. These facilities are staffed with registered nurses and doctors familiar with the medical, psychological, and legal issues particular to caring for the client who has experienced a sexual assault.

Straddle injuries are another type of genitourinary emergency. These injuries occur when a client falls while straddling an object, such as a fence or metal bar, thereby injuring the perineum. Though not a very common injury, it is imperative to assess the client and promptly initiate treatment. These injuries can occur with multiple trauma or as a single injury.

Medical–Surgical Management

Medical

As with all emergencies, the ABCs must be managed first. Intravenous access should be established, and blood and urine specimens should be obtained. Rape crisis intervention is essential for the sexual assault victim. Those with straddle injuries must be evaluated for fractures. If blood is seen at the external

PROFESSIONAL TIP

Chain of Custody

Care should be taken in handling the clothing and belongings of a survivor of sexual assault, as these items may become valuable in legal proceedings. For purposes of potential future litigation, it is thus imperative to maintain a strict chain of custody of evidence. The **chain of custody** is the documentation of the transfer of evidence from one worker to the next in a secure fashion. This means that to follow the rape protocol, each person handling the client's clothing or lab work must sign the document used by the facility to indicate receipt and release of items. The fewer the names on the chain, the more secure the integrity of evidence.

urethral meatus, a urethral tear should be suspected, and catheterization should be avoided, as it will further damage the urethra. Radiological examination should be done to confirm injury.

Surgical

Certain injuries such as urethral or vaginal tears may require surgical repair.

Pharmacological

Douching and bathing for the sexual assault survivor should be delayed until all specimens are collected and all examinations are performed. For the sexual assault client, antibiotics are usually prescribed for possible sexually transmitted disease. Blood tests for baseline human immunodeficiency virus (HIV) and acquired immunodeficiency syndrome (AIDS) and a pregnancy test are usually part of the protocol. In addition, a "morning after" pill such as diethylstilbestrol diphosphate (DES) may be prescribed in the event of a possible pregnancy.

Diet

The client should be designated nothing by mouth (NPO) in case of the need to go to immediate surgery. Fluids can be given intravenously.

Activity

The sexual assault survivor may return to full activity as soon as able, though counseling may be needed before the client regains the desire to resume activities of daily living. Those with straddle injuries need bed rest and careful observation until testing is complete. Clients should be encouraged to resume sexual activities only when they feel physically and emotionally ready.

▶ NURSING PROCESS

▶ Assessment

▶ Subjective Data

Assessment of the sexual assault survivor includes obtaining a description of the rape or assault. A history of menstrual cycles, including date of last menstrual period, is vital in determining the potential for pregnancy.

▶ Objective Data

All bruises, scrapes, or abrasions caused by the assault must be assessed. A list of the client's clothing worn during the assault should be made, and the clothing should be kept for evidence in case of legal proceedings.

Nursing diagnoses for the client with genitourinary emergencies may include the following:

Nursing Diagnoses	Planning/Goals	Nursing Interventions
▶ *Impaired Urinary Elimination related to break in urethra*	Client will void clear urine before discharge and will regain normal pre-injury elimination patterns.	Closely monitor output. Test urine for blood using dipstick. Note and report hematuria. Offer bladder retraining and encourage client to resume pre-assault elimination patterns.
▶ *Risk for Infection (Sexually Transmitted Disease) related to alleged sexual assault*	Client will have negative outcomes on all lab specimens obtained.	Obtain all specimens as ordered. Teach the client how and when to obtain further specimens, as needed. Keep the client informed about all test results.
▶ *Rape-Trauma Syndrome related to alleged sexual assault and violence of event*	Client will state awareness of help groups for therapy and follow-up care.	Maintain open and nonjudgmental communication with the client. Call rape crisis center for immediate referral and assistance for the client. Refer the client to crisis help per community offerings. Teach the client that the trauma does not resolve overnight and that help is available at all times.

Evaluation Each goal must be evaluated to determine how it has been met by the client.

OCULAR EMERGENCIES

Most eye emergencies are urgent to emergent in nature. Foreign bodies can cause damage to vision very rapidly and thus require immediate attention. Clients with objects impaled in the eye must be immediately evaluated by an ophthalmologist. An eyeball may be avulsed, or forcibly torn out of its socket, either by blunt or penetrating trauma; such an injury requires immediate referral to and treatment by an ophthalmologist. Retinal detachment is a surgical emergency, as it is one of the leading causes of accidental blindness.

Medical–Surgical Management

Medical

The primary goal of care is restoring the health of the eye. The foreign body or impaled object must be removed as soon as the client's condition allows and the effects on the eye of removal of the object have been determined. The client's eye must be protected until definitive treatment is provided. Protective dressings are needed. In the event of ocular avulsion, the eyeball must be protected with a warm saline dressing. Because both eyes move together, patching of the opposite eye will help decrease movement of the affected eye, allowing it to heal more quickly.

Surgical

Immediate surgical intervention is needed for retinal detachment.

Pharmacological

As a prophylactic measure, all eye trauma must be treated with an antibiotic eye medication.

Diet

There should be no modifications to the diet of the client with a foreign body in the eye. Clients with avulsed eyes must be kept NPO in case immediate surgical intervention is needed.

Activity

Because sensory and depth perceptions may be altered when one eye is patched, activity should be limited initially. Clients are maintained in semi-Fowler's position to prevent or alleviate intraocular edema.

▶ NURSING PROCESS

▶ Assessment

▶ Subjective Data

Assessment includes obtaining both the client's perception of what has happened to the eye and a history of the accident, including the time it occurred. Care that has been given to an avulsed eye, such as placement in a plastic bag with water, must be documented.

▶ Objective Data

Assessment includes visual acuity testing and observation of tearing and/or redness of the eye.

Nursing diagnoses for the client with an ocular emergency may include the following:

Nursing Diagnoses	Planning/Goals	Nursing Interventions
▶ *Disturbed Sensory Perception (Visual) related to impaired vision*	The client will regain partial pre-injury vision.	Maintain the client in semi-Fowler's position in cases of ocular avulsion or retinal detachment.
		Assist the client to walk while wearing an eye patch and discuss problems that may be encountered and ways to accommodate decreased vision.
		Instruct the client to name one resource person to assist with decreased vision at home.
▶ *Risk for Infection related to trauma caused by foreign body*	The client will not develop ocular infection.	Instill initial eye medication and apply initial eye patch for the client.
		Teach the client to instill eye medication.
		Teach the client to apply eye patch.
		Instruct the client to immediately report any visual changes or drainage.
		Be alert and listen to the client's concerns.

Evaluation Each goal must be evaluated to determine how it has been met by the client.

MUSCULOSKELETAL EMERGENCIES

Musculoskeletal emergencies can vary from simple muscle strains to major trauma. A muscle strain is the overstretching of a muscle. A sprain is defined as a twisting of the joint with partial rupture of ligaments, which can cause injury to surrounding tissue. Sprains often occur in the wrist and ankle. A dislocation is the displacement of a bone from its joint. The most common sits of dislocation are the fingers and toes. A fracture is a break in the continuity of a bone. In the event of a long bone fracture, care must also be given to the cardiopulmonary system: Fat emboli from the fracture site can develop and cause severe respiratory problems if they settle in the pulmonary system.

Medical–Surgical Management

Medical

Initial treatment of simple strains and sprains can be managed utilizing the "RICE" formula, meaning *r*est, *i*ce, *c*ompression, and *e*levation. Fractures must be immediately immobilized, with attention also being given to body areas proximal to the fracture. Radiological examination is indicated to validate the diagnosis. Dislocations must be immediately reduced. Many fractures and dislocations can be reduced in the ED using conscious IV sedation. Tetanus toxoid should be given to any client presenting with an open injury.

Surgical

Some fractures require immediate surgical intervention. Most open, compound fractures fall into this category. Debridement is often indicated, because most fractures are trauma related, and dirt and other matter may imbed in the wound.

Pharmacological

Pain control is a major consideration in relation to musculoskeletal system injuries. Reduction and immobilization often significantly decrease pain. Those clients with minor sprains and strains respond well to anti-inflammatory medications such as ibuprofen (Advil, Motrin) and other nonsteroidal anti-inflammatory drugs (NSAIDs). Those with major or multiple fractures may initially require narcotic relief.

Diet

Clients with sprains, strains, and simple fractures do not need special diets. Those with major fractures and trauma must be kept NPO pending surgical intervention.

Activity

Depending on the site of the fracture, activity may be limited due to casting or immobilization. To help strengthen the muscles and minimize atrophy in cases of immobilization, the client must be taught to contract and release those muscles immobilized in the casting.

▶ NURSING PROCESS

▶ Assessment

▶ Subjective Data

The client will initially verbalize intense pain, tingling, and loss of use of the injured part.

▶ Objective Data

Obvious deformities, edema, cool skin, and decreased capillary refill will be present on the affected part. A break in the skin and visual bone fragments may also be noted.

Nursing diagnoses for the client with a musculoskeletal emergency may include the following:

Nursing Diagnoses	Planning/Goals	Nursing Interventions
▶ *Acute Pain related to traumatic fracture/dislocation*	The client's pain will decrease with immobilization and pain medications.	Administer pain medications as ordered.
		Immobilize affected body part.
		Elevate injured extremity.
		Apply ice packs, as directed.
		Listen attentively to the client's concerns and verbalizations of pain.
▶ *Ineffective Tissue Perfusion related to edema and fracture/dislocation*	The client's pulses will be equal bilaterally, and capillary refill will be less than 2 seconds at the affected site.	Assess the client's pulse, skin color, capillary refill, and ability to move the fingers and toes every 30 minutes.
		Ask the client about sensation in the injured body part.
		Instruct the client to move the toes and fingers.
		Apply an elastic bandage for compression in cases of a sprain.

continues

Nursing Diagnoses	Planning/Goals	Nursing Interventions
▶ *Impaired Physical Mobility related to limitations of pain and immobilization of fracture/dislocation*	The client will demonstrate the ability to mobilize with cast or other assistive devices.	Teach the client to care for the cast. Teach the client exercises to minimize muscle atrophy. Teach crutch walking, if needed.

Evaluation Each goal must be evaluated to determine how it has been met by the client.

SOFT-TISSUE EMERGENCIES

Most soft-tissue injuries are very common. Minor abrasions, lacerations, puncture wounds, contusions, bites of all varieties (human, insect, animal, and snake), and burn injuries fall into this category. Although most such injuries do not require emergency care, some are more severe than others and some are potentially fatal. Clients will seek medical attention for these injuries because of fear.

Medical–Surgical Management

Medical

Skin emergencies require prompt intervention. All injuries must be cleansed or debrided. Infection is a major consideration, and prophylactic treatment must therefore be initiated immediately. If a laceration is large, suturing may be necessary. Bites, unless extremely large, are usually not sutured due to the increased risk of infection presented by suturing these lacerations, which provide an excellent growth medium for bacteria. Burns can sometimes be treated in an ED, with follow-up care being provided at home. Cool water will decrease the pain associated with minor burns. Careful debridement using running cool water and antiseptic solution should follow. Because burns are painful, debridement should be performed after administration of pain medication. A silver sulfadiazine (Silvadene) dressing is usually applied after debridement.

Major burns may require client resuscitation with rapid EMS transport to a burn center. Initially, the ABCs must be established. "Packaging" the client for transport to a burn unit usually involves insertion of at least two large-bore IV lines, insertion of a nasogastric tube, intubation, Foley catheterization, sterile wrapping, and temperature regulation/monitoring.

Snakebites do not always result in envenomation (poisoning). A rubber band (not a tourniquet) above the site is the best intervention to control rapid spreading of the venom. Most snakebites occur in the foot, so a rubber band is easy to apply. In managing snake bites, it is best to establish the ABCs and, once the type of snake is identified, start antivenom treatment, as necessary.

Pharmacological

All clients with soft-tissue injuries, including those with burns, must be current with regard to immunizations, especially the diphtheria and tetanus (Td) immunizations. Pain medication should be given to alleviate pain related to lacerations, bites, and burns. Topical antibiotic agents must be applied to all injuries. Silver sulfadiazine (Silvadene) is the most widely used topical agent for burn injuries. Systemic antibiotics are often included in the treatment regimen.

Activity

Movement may be somewhat limited depending on the location of injury. Because muscle weakness and atrophy can occur rapidly, physical therapy must be initiated immediately for clients who are immobilized.

PROFESSIONAL TIP

Animal Bites

Many states require that all instances of clients seeking treatment in an ED for animal bites be reported to animal control officials. Know your state reporting rules and regulations.

PROFESSIONAL TIP

Snake Bites

In the event of snakebite, it is essential to note the location of the fang marks and the distance (in centimeters) between the marks. Doing so helps determine the size of the snake and, thus, the likelihood of envenomation, as smaller, younger snakes typically have not yet learned to control the amount of venom.

▶ NURSING PROCESS

▶ Assessment

▶ Subjective Data

In obtaining the health history, the nurse should elicit the client's report of the injury. Pain should be evaluated, and the client's level of pain should be documented.

▶ Objective Data

Vital signs must be measured. The wound or damaged area must be assessed with regard to depth, location, and size (in centimeters). In the event of a bite, the location and source of the bite must be noted.

Nursing diagnoses for the client with a soft-tissue injury may include the following:

Nursing Diagnoses	Planning/Goals	Nursing Interventions
▶ *Risk for Impaired Skin Integrity related to break/wound in skin*	The client's wound will heal.	Prepare client for cleansing and possible suturing of wound. Assist with possible suturing.
▶ *Risk for Infection related to imbedded dirt/bacteria in the wound*	The client's wound will heal without evidence of infection.	Cleanse wound thoroughly with soap and water. Administer tetanus intramuscularly (IM). Teach the client to keep the wound and sutures dry and clean. Apply a topical antibiotic and clean dressing, if indicated. Teach the client to remove and change the dressing if it becomes dirty or wet. Tell the client to return for additional care if wound becomes red, edematous, or painful or exhibits purulent discharge.

Evaluation Each goal must be evaluated to determine how it has been met by the client.

SAMPLE NURSING CARE PLAN

THE CLIENT WITH A SOFT-TISSUE INJURY

Mr. Perez, a 23-year-old Hispanic rancher, was brought to the ED after an accident at his ranch. He was riding his horse and fixing fences. The horse threw Mr. Perez over its head and stomped Mr. Perez's left upper abdomen with its right forefoot. Mr. Perez, who states that he has never been hurt or in the hospital before, presents with a large, 6-centimeter-by-3-centimeter-by-2 centimeter in depth, jagged laceration imbedded with dirt and other foreign material. There are no other associated injuries. A large pressure bandage that is saturated with bright-red blood is controlling the bleeding.

Nursing Diagnosis 1 *Deficient Fluid Volume related to active bleeding from traumatic abdominal laceration as evidenced by a large, jagged laceration measuring 6 centimeters by 3 centimeters and a large, bulky, saturated dressing.*

PLANNING/GOALS	NURSING INTERVENTIONS	RATIONALE	EVALUATION
Mr. Perez will lose no more blood.	Control bleeding with a pressure dressing.	The amount of blood loss will increase if pressure to the laceration is not maintained.	Mr. Perez's wound was sutured. The dressing that was applied after suturing was clean and dry and showed no

continues

| | Prepare Mr. Perez for suturing of the laceration. | To effectively stop the bleeding, the laceration must be sutured as quickly as possible. The physician will also be able to visualize the arteries and ascertain whether any have been severed and, if so, repair them. | further evidence of bleeding at discharge. |
| | Monitor vital signs. | Frequent monitoring of vital signs is necessary in order to ensure that the client is not going into shock from the blood loss. Hypotension and increased pulse and respiration require immediate attention and intervention. | |

Nursing Diagnosis 2 *Impaired Skin Integrity related to abdominal injury as evidenced by a jagged laceration measuring 6 centimeters by 3 centimeters and 2 centimeters in depth.*

PLANNING/GOALS	NURSING INTERVENTIONS	RATIONALE	EVALUATION
Mr. Perez will have regained skin integrity with sutures.	Prepare sterile environment for suturing.	The nurse is responsible for assisting the physician, who is suturing.	Mr. Perez had intact skin integrity, with 22 sutures in place.
	Assist physician with suturing of Mr. Perez's wound.	Maintaining a sterile field while suturing prevents additional bacteria from contaminating the wound.	

Nursing Diagnosis 3 *Risk for Infection related to laceration as evidenced by dirt and other foreign material imbedded in abdominal wound*

PLANNING/GOALS	NURSING INTERVENTIONS	RATIONALE	EVALUATION
Mr. Perez's wound will not become infected.	Administer tetanus booster.	All wounds require that the client be current with regard to tetanus booster.	Mr. Perez was given a tetanus booster because he remembered having received his last at the age of 15. He verbalized the need to take the complete course of antibiotics when he went home.
	Cleanse Mr. Perez's wound thoroughly after local anesthesia has been administered.	Because it has been exposed to an undetermined amount of dirt, including the horse's hoof, the wound should be thoroughly cleansed. This is done *after* the administration of anesthesia, because cleansing	

continues

	can cause the client a great deal of pain.
Demonstrate wound cleansing to Mr. Perez.	Mr. Perez should actually see the way the wound is cleansed so that he has no fear or questions about doing it himself.
Remove as much dirt and foreign material as possible.	All visible dirt should be removed because it can cause inflammation and infection at the wound site.
Cleanse sutured wound and demonstrate care to Mr. Perez.	Once sutured, the wound must be cleansed to remove old blood and other debris from the suturing. If foreign matter is left in the wound, inflammation and infection could occur. Mr. Perez must be taught the cleansing procedure, as he will be responsible for home care of the wound.
Give Mr. Perez explicit directions regarding taking oral antibiotics after discharge.	With the wound being very dirty, oral antibiotics will most likely be ordered by the physician. It is imperative that Mr. Perez takes the full course of the antibiotics in order to prevent infection.
Teach Mr. Perez to care for wound.	Because Mr. Perez has no prior experience with injury, it is imperative that he be taught to care for his wound, including being told to remove the dressing when it becomes wet or dirty. Application of a new and clean dressing should be taught to alleviate any fear he may have about the process and thereby encourage him to properly care for the wound and dressing.
Teach Mr. Perez the signs and symptoms that require a return visit to the doctor (redness, inflammation, increased pain, purulent drainage).	The signs and symptoms of infection should be taught, because Mr. Perez will need further care if the wound does become infected.

continues

Nursing Diagnosis 4 *Anxiety related to reaction to fall and large laceration as evidenced by client's verbalizing that he had never been injured before*

PLANNING/GOALS	NURSING INTERVENTIONS	RATIONALE	EVALUATION
Mr. Perez will demonstrate decreased anxiety as evidenced by his talking about his injury and participating in his care.	Allow Mr. Perez to talk about injury.	Allowing Mr. Perez to talk about his injury gives him the ability to verbalize his fears and thoughts about the injury.	Mr. Perez viewed his injury with the use of a mirror before and after suturing. He was amazed to see that the laceration was completely closed following suturing. He was concerned about the bruising and edema to the area.
	Provide explanations for all procedures.	Explaining all procedures assists Mr. Perez in understanding why certain things are being done.	
	Give Mr. Perez simple choices to make.	Giving Mr. Perez simple choices allows him to participate in his care and gives him some sense of control.	Mr. Perez was not able to assist with the care of his sutures. His wife was taught how to clean and dress the wound.

POISONING AND OVERDOSES

Poisoning and overdoses can be accidental or intentional. Poison control centers are the best source of antidote information for the client suffering from poisoning or overdose.

There are many types of poisonings and overdoses and several different entry routes. Ingested poisonings are most common. It is important to obtain a clear history of the route of entry: inhalation, ingestion, topical, or injection. In addition, the client must be evaluated for any associated injuries, such as lacerations from a fall.

Medical–Surgical Management

Medical

In treating overdoses, the ABCs must be managed. Oxygen must be immediately initiated, and IV access must be established. In addition, cardiac monitoring should be instituted. Blood and urine samples must be obtained for toxicology screening. After the client has been stabilized, efforts should be made to identify the substance so as to minimize or reverse the effects.

Pharmacological

If the substance has been ingested, and institutional protocol dictates, syrup of ipecac should be administered at 30 cc for a maximum of two doses in 20 minutes. Clients with caustic ingestions should not be given syrup of ipecac, as these products can damage the mucosal lining both from ingestion and emesis. Clients who have ingested caustic products should instead be given copious amounts of water to dilute the substance.

Diet

The client who has overdosed is typically kept NPO except for the water needed following the administration of syrup of ipecac.

▶ NURSING PROCESS

▶ Assessment

▶ Subjective Data

The client must be asked about the timing and the route of overdose. Mental status must be evaluated to establish whether the exposure was intentional. Other incidences related to the overdose, such as an altercation with a loved one, must also be documented.

▶ Objective Data

The client's vital signs are critical for baseline data. The substance involved, as well as the amount, must be identified.

Nursing diagnoses for the client with an overdose may include the following:

Nursing Diagnoses	Planning/Goals	Nursing Interventions
▶ *Risk for Poisoning related to ingestion of toxin*	The client will recover with no residual effects of poisoning.	Manage the ABCs and stabilize the client. Monitor baseline laboratory work and ECG. Administer antidotes to toxins. Document the client's response.
▶ *Risk for Self-Directed Violence related to harmful ingestion of toxic substance*	The client will not harm self and will participate in help groups to work through issues.	Encourage the client to share reasons for overdose. If overdose was accidental, discuss exposure to toxin and ways to avoid exposure in the future. Maintain a supportive, calm, reassuring environment for the client. Teach varying methods of coping. Refer to help groups.
▶ *Interrupted Family Processes related to ingestion of harmful toxin*	Client will begin to discuss problems with family.	Encourage client and family to discuss their problems openly and supportively. Assist the client in identifying different methods of coping. Encourage family counseling.

Evaluation Each goal must be evaluated to determine how it has been met by the client.

ENVIRONMENTAL/ TEMPERATURE EMERGENCIES

Exposure to extremes of heat and cold can be potentially life threatening. Severe cold, or hypothermia, can occur both in very cold weather and from prolonged submersion in cold water. Heart rate and metabolic rate fall, and cardiac arrest may follow. Frostbite is another potentially dangerous result of exposure to cold (Table 37–5). The most common sites of frostbite are the fingers, toes, ears, and nose. Initially, frostbite causes paleness and numbness to the affected areas. If exposure continues, frostbite can progress to blistering and loss of feeling. The client may lose voluntary control over the affected body part. Rewarming in an emergency setting is imperative.

Extreme heat can also cause potentially serious problems, especially in very young or elderly clients. As temperature rises, the body's ability to cool lessens. Table 37–6 compares heat injuries.

Medical–Surgical Management

Medical

For those exposed to extreme cold, rewarming is essential to resuscitation. The body's core (rectal) temperature must be taken. Gradual warming must be initiated using warm blankets, warmed oxygen, warmed IV fluids, warmed nasogastric tubes, and, in extreme instances, warmed enemas. Resuscitation should continue until the body has reached a core temperature of at least 34.4°C (94°F).

For frostbite, rewarming of the exposed body part is indicated. If the frostbite is severe, rapid rewarming is essential. This involves placing the frozen area in warm-water baths not exceeding 40.6°C (105°F). Tetanus should be administered. Acute pain should be treated with analgesics.

For heat injuries, rapidly reducing the body's temperature is vital. Supplemental oxygen may be administered. Pouring cool water over the client, chilling IV

Table 37–5 DEGREES OF FROSTBITE SEVERITY

DEGREE	SYMPTOMS	TREATMENT
Mild	Skin is cold to touch, pale, tingling, and numb, with a prickly sensation	Use blankets, warm clothing to warm cold flesh
Moderate	Affects deeper body tissue; skin appears waxy and is puffy to touch and itchy and burning with pain	Use gloves, blankets, warm clothing to warm cold flesh, observe closely for deeper injuries
Severe	Blistering, damage to all layers of soft tissue; flesh appears lifeless and is hard to the touch; no pain sensation in or ability to move frozen area	Initiate emergency rewarming in an ED using warm-water baths at 40.6° C (105°F); observe carefully for increased edema

Table 37–6 COMPARISON OF HEAT INJURIES

TYPE	SYMPTOMS	TREATMENT
Heat cramps	Muscle cramps in arms, legs, and abdomen	Move client to cool, shady area. Slowly administer copious amounts of water. Reevaluate.
Heat exhaustion	Diaphoresis, with pale, moist, cool skin, headache, weakness, dizziness; muscle cramps, nausea, chills, tachypnea, confusion, tingling of hands and feet	Move client to cool, shady area. Loosen/remove constrictive clothing. Pour water over client; place client near fan. Encourage client to slowly drink water. Elevate client's legs. Reevaluate.
Heat stroke (a medical emergency)	Red, flushed, hot, dry skin; no diaphoresis	Reduce client's body temperature by removing client's clothing and pouring cool water over client. Start two large-bore IV lines. Use fan to cool client. Place client on cardiac monitor. Elevate client's legs. Assess client's vital signs, especially core (rectal) temperature. Check for neurological signs (confused, combative, disoriented). Check client's core (rectal) temperature frequently.

Developed from U.S. Army Training Support Command Protocols.

fluids, and fanning the client will accelerate the cooling process.

Pharmacological

For heat and cold injuries, establishment of at least two large-bore IV lines is essential. Supplemental oxygen should be administered. Replacement of fluid and electrolytes is essential.

PROFESSIONAL TIP

Frostbite

Do not massage or rub frostbite injuries, as doing so can increase severity of damage to tissue. Caffeine, alcohol, and smoking should be avoided, as they decrease circulation to the damaged tissue.

Diet

In the event of heat injuries, fluids, especially water, should be encouraged, if the client is able.

▶ NURSING PROCESS

▶ Assessment

▶ Subjective Data

The client should be asked to give a history of both the heat/cold injury, if able, and any current medications.

▶ Objective Data

Core (rectal) body temperature and vital signs must be measured and documented. Skin color and temperature should be recorded. Cardiac monitoring should be initiated to track any cardiac response to the heat or cold stress to the body. Pupillary response must be evaluated because neurological problems may result from the heat/cold injury.

Nursing diagnoses for the client with a temperature/environmental injury may include the following:

Nursing Diagnoses	Planning/Goals	Nursing Interventions
▶ *Hypothermia related to exposure to cold environment/long submersion in cold water*	The client will regain normal core body temperature.	Administer supplemental oxygen. Monitor cardiac response carefully. If CPR is in progress, continue until the client's core temperature reaches 94° F and cardiac status is evaluated. Administer warmed IV fluids. Place warmed blankets on the client.
▶ *Hyperthermia related to environmental exposure to heat*	The client will regain normal core body temperature.	Remove the client's clothing. Pour cool water over the client. Use large fan to cool the client.

continues

Nursing Diagnoses	Planning/Goals	Nursing Interventions
		Administer chilled IV fluids.
		Administer supplemental oxygen.
		Initiate cardiac monitoring.
		Evaluate client's neurological status with reference to orientation to time, person, and place.
		Measure core temperature every 30 minutes to assess progress.

Evaluation Each goal must be evaluated to determine how it has been met by the client.

MULTIPLE-SYSTEM TRAUMA

Multiple-system trauma is injury sustained in more than one body system. During the initial care of the emergent client, the mechanism of injury is determined. Blunt injuries and penetrating trauma are most likely to result in multiple-system involvement.

Medical–Surgical Management

Medical

Immediate management of the ABCs is imperative. Bleeding must be stopped using pressure. Two to four large-bore IV lines should be started. All clothing must be removed for visualization of bleeding and injuries. Blood and urine specimens should be obtained. Radiographic studies must be done. Tetanus should also be administered.

▶ NURSING PROCESS

▶ Assessment

▶ Subjective Data

The client should be assessed for level of consciousness and orientation to time, person, and place. Verbalizations of pain should be evaluated. The client should be asked for an account of the accident.

▶ Objective Data

Airway, breathing, and circulation should be immediately assessed. Vital signs must be assessed, as must neurological status utilizing the Glasgow Coma Scale. Active bleeding must be assessed and controlled.

Nursing diagnoses for the client with multiple-system trauma may include the following:

Nursing Diagnoses	Planning/Goals	Nursing Intervention
▶ *Impaired Spontaneous Ventilation related to major trauma and severe hypotension*	The client will breathe without assistive devices.	Maintain open airway. Initiate rescue breathing. Assist with insertion of endotracheal tube. Ventilate per CPR protocol. Maintain pulse oximetry reading at 94% to 99%. Start multiple large-bore IV lines.
▶ *Powerlessness related to the inability to sustain life without emergency interventions*	The client will survive emergency and within several hours will be able to indicate simple choices about care.	Explain all nursing/medical interventions to client. Provide emotional and physiological support to client and family as much as possible throughout resuscitation. Allow the client to make simple choices about care.

Evaluation Each goal must be evaluated to determine how it has been met by the client.

LEGAL ISSUES

Emergency medicine allows medical personnel to care for clients without obtaining informed consent. In life-threatening and emergency situations, consent is implied. In addition, the Good Samaritan Law, one of the laws and regulations enforced for the benefit of both the caregiver and the client, provides protection against malpractice to persons who stop at the scene of an accident and render care. It should be noted, however, that the Good Samaritan Law offers protection only to those who provide safe and appropriate care; it does not protect those charged with gross negligence or willful misconduct.

There are other legal issues specific to emergency care. Several injuries/illnesses must be reported to proper authorities. For instance, most states require that police be notified of MVCs, assaults, or rape. Likewise, animal control authorities require that animal bite reports be filed to facilitate follow-up on the possibility of rabies.

DEATH IN THE EMERGENCY DEPARTMENT

Death can occur in the ED at any time due to trauma, sudden illness, or even extended illness. This creates a delicate situation, as the death is usually unexpected. Family members may have a difficult time dealing with sudden death. If their loved one is being resuscitated in the ED, there is little time for health care personnel to comfort the family, as the personnel are very busy providing care to the client. In the event of sudden death, the family is usually in a state of shock and will need further assistance to cope with the death of their loved one. Special support groups are available for this assistance and should be contacted for the family.

CASE STUDY

Joe fell from a fishing boat into deep, cold water. He was wearing a life vest and was rescued within 10 minutes, at which time he was immediately dried, placed in a blanket, and brought to the ED. He is alert and oriented to person, time, and place, but is shivering uncontrollably and pale in color. His core temperature is 93°F.

The following questions will guide your development of a nursing care plan for the case study.

1. List the assessments in the order that they should be performed.
2. Identify the priority nursing diagnoses for Joe.
3. List nursing interventions in the order that they should be performed.
4. Identify the goal of treatment for Joe.

SUMMARY

- Clients in shock need immediate assessment and intervention.
- Rapid assessment and observation of ABCs is essential in treating all cardiovascular emergencies.
- Evaluation of abdominal emergencies should include taking a history of the onset of pain, as this is critical to outcome and survival.
- Ocular emergencies can be a threat to vision and thus require immediate assessment and treatment.
- Musculoskeletal and soft tissue injuries can be painful but manageable with rapid assessment and treatment.
- In cases of poisoning or overdoses, the ABCs must first be established, then the agent to which the client was exposed must be immediately identified so that prompt treatment can be initiated.
- Major trauma is a life-threatening and unexpected occurrence for both client and loved ones.
- Nurses must be aware of the legal issues related to emergency care, such as Good Samaritan Laws and mandated reporting.

Review Questions

1. Triage is a system of:
   a. identifying clients by disease.
   b. prioritizing client care.
   c. counting clients waiting for care.
   d. medical diagnosing.

2. A client with a small branch sticking out of the right mid-chest arrives at the ED during a hurricane. There is bubbling and oozing at the site. Medical personnel should first:
   a. remove the branch and save it.
   b. administer pain medication to the client.
   c. start the ABCs of CPR.
   d. stop the bleeding and take vital signs.

3. An example of a non-urgent client is:
   a. a client with CPR in progress.
   b. a client with fractures of both legs.
   c. a client with heat stroke.
   d. a client with a sprained ankle.

4. The ambulance brings a client with a large, bleeding laceration of the upper leg to the ED. Vital signs are as follows: blood pressure, 78/62; pulse, 112; and respirations, 26. A priority nursing diagnosis is:

   a. *Deficient Fluid Volume.*
   b. *Risk for Aspiration.*
   c. *Risk for Infection.*
   d. *Disturbed Body Image.*

5. Interventions for a client in shock include:

   a. pain control and assessment of vital signs.
   b. administration of oxygen and IV fluids.
   c. insertion of a nasogastric tube.
   d. calling the physician.

6. A client is brought to the ED after having run a marathon. His blood pressure is 128/78; pulse is 120; respirations are 26; and rectal temperature is 105°F. This is an example of:

   a. septic shock.
   b. runner's cramps.
   c. heat stroke.
   d. abdominal pain.

7. A method of assessing a client's neurological status is called:

   a. vital signs.
   b. pupillary response.
   c. Glasgow Coma Scale.
   d. cardiac monitor.

Critical Thinking Questions

1. On your way home from work, you come upon an MVC involving several vehicles. No emergency response vehicles have yet arrived on the scene. What steps can you take to secure the accident site and aid the victims until emergency services arrive?

2. Under what circumstances might a client present with multiple-system trauma? How would you proceed with the assessment of such a client? What immediate actions should be taken to maintain the stability of this client?

WEB FLASH!

- Compare and contrast available information on legal and ethical issues relating to emergency care found on the Web sites of various state boards of nursing.
- Locate the Emergency Nurses Association on the Internet. Share one new concept found on this Internet site that was not presented in this chapter.

CRITICAL THINKING ON MULTIPLE SYSTEMS

CHAPTER 38

MAKING THE CONNECTION

Through careful study of Chapters 1–37 critical thinking skills have been sharpened and a knowledge base developed in preparation for the exercises in this chapter. Each critical thinking exercise begins with an index of the body systems relevant to the case study. It may be useful to refer back to these chapters while working through the case study.

LEARNING OBJECTIVE

Upon completion of this chapter, you should be able to:

- *Experience critical thinking by integrating a condition to several body systems and multiple clinical problems.*

INTRODUCTION

This chapter format is different than that of the other chapters. It is an opportunity to apply critical thinking skills and problem solving techniques to several case studies that encompass more than one body system. Application of information gleaned from previous chapters is needed to develop a holistic, integrated view of multiple body systems. An example is diabetes mellitus, a condition with multiple aspects that affect other body systems such as the integumentary, nervous, musculoskeletal, cardiac, vascular, blood, gastrointestinal, urinary, and reproductive systems.

Read the case study, then analyze the relationship of the condition to other body systems. It may be helpful to first outline the condition presented in the case study by making a grid of the pathophysiology, diagnostic studies, signs and symptoms, and nursing interventions. Refer to the grid in answering the questions.

The case study questions can be completed alone, in a study group, or in a classroom setting. Once the case studies have been completed, share the answers and charts with the entire group to enhance the learning experience. Keep in mind that each student or group of students may arrive at the answers or present

the answers in a different manner. The process one takes in finding the answer is less important than the opportunity to exercise critical thinking skills, as long as sound, logical, nursing judgment is utilized in obtaining an appropriate answer. This is an opportunity to think creatively and freely.

SYSTEMS REVIEWED IN DIABETES MELLITUS EXERCISE

- Cardiovascular (Chapter 19)
- Integumentary (Chapter 21)
- Neurological (Chapter 25)
- Sensory (Chapter 26)
- Endocrine (Chapter 27)
- Urinary (Chapter 29)
- Male Reproductive (Chapter 31)

CRITICAL THINKING EXERCISE WITH DIABETES MELLITUS

Mr. Phillips, a 46-year-old insurance salesman, is admitted to the hospital with the diagnosis of type 1 diabetes mellitus.

- List the etiological risk factors for type 1 diabetes.
- Brainstorm subjective and objective data that would be included in the assessment of Mr. Phillips.
- Develop a patho-flow diagram identifying the symptoms Mr. Phillips may have been experiencing

on admission and relate the pathophysiology of diabetes mellitus to the symptoms (see the examples of a patho-flow diagram in Figure 38-1 and an interrelationship chart in Figure 38-2).

- What diagnostic tests could the physician have ordered to confirm the diagnosis of diabetes mellitus?
- Relate the possible results of the diagnostic tests to the pathophysiological cause of the results on the patho-flow diagram.
- If Mr. Phillips had been diagnosed with type 2 diabetes, how would the pathophysiology and nursing care vary?

A couple of days after Mr. Phillips was diagnosed with DM he said to the nurse, "One of my friends at work said there are a lot of future problems with diabetes. I am concerned about this. What are some of the problems? What can I do not to have these problems?"

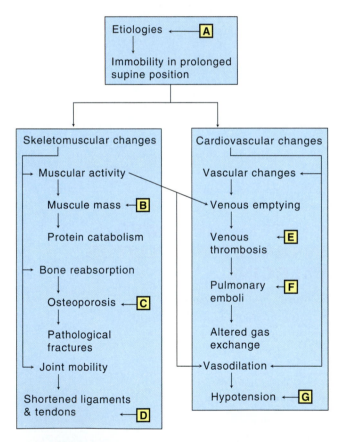

Figure 38–1 An example of a patho-flow diagram of skeletomuscular and cardiovascular changes due to immobility. Complete the following instructions corresponding to the letters located at specific points along the pathophysiological sequence of events. A. List the risk conditions that may lead to immobility. B. Name the assessment data at this point. C. List the interventions that would minimize calcium loss. D. Name the outcome criteria associated with effective nursing interventions at this point. E. State the assessment data at this point. F. List the interventions that may prevent the development of this complication. G. List the nursing interventions to minimize this consequence. (*Courtesy of the* Journal of Nursing Education)

- What would be appropriate responses of the nurse?
- List local resources or support groups where Mr. Phillips and his family could be referred.

The discharge teaching included insulin administration, diet, exercise, foot care, and eye exams.

- What is important to include in the discharge teaching regarding:

    insulin administration
    diet
    exercise
    foot care
    eye exams

- Develop a care plan for Mr. Phillips.

Eight years after Mr. Phillips was diagnosed with DM, he had a routine physical examination. At that time his BP was 174/96. The physician monitored the BP for three weeks and then placed Mr. Phillips on enalapril maleate (Vasotec). His urine had a trace of albumin.

- Physiologically what could be occurring to cause Mr. Phillips to have hypertension, which is a common complication of diabetes?
- How does the action of enalapril maleate (Vasotec) lower the BP?
- What is the rationale for placing Mr. Phillips on enalapril maleate (Vasotec) rather than propranolol hydrochloride (Inderal), verapamil (Calan), or clonidine hydrochloride (Catapres)?
- What other complications could have a circulatory etiology?

Figure 38–2 Interrelationships of Conditions and Symptoms. (*Courtesy of the* Journal of Nursing Education)

- What could be the possible long-term renal complication from diabetes mellitus?
- Explain the pathophysiology of renal complications as they relate to DM. Relate these to the patho-flow diagram previously developed.

One evening, Mr. Phillips was massaging his foot while watching television. He noticed an ulcerated area between his third and fourth toe.

- State possible reasons Mr. Phillips may not have felt pain from the ulcerated area. Relate these to the patho-flow diagram previously developed.

During a yearly physical Mr. Phillips relates difficulty obtaining an erection.

- Explain the rationale for this complication.
- What nursing interventions would be appropriate at this time?

In later years, Mr. Phillips may experience some symptoms from autonomic neuropathies.

- List symptoms that may occur and relate the symptoms to the pathophysiological etiology.

SYSTEMS REVIEWED IN CIRRHOSIS EXERCISE

- Respiratory (Chapter 18)
- Cardiovascular (Chapter 19)
- Hematologic and Lymphatic (Chapter 20)
- Integumentary (Chapter 21)
- Musculoskeletal (Chapter 24)
- Neurological (Chapter 25)
- Endocrine (Chapter 27)
- Gastrointestinal (Chapter 28)
- Urinary (Chapter 29)

CRITICAL THINKING EXERCISE WITH CIRRHOSIS

Sam Lightfoot, a 60-year-old male of American Indian descent, is admitted to the hospital with hematemesis. He has a history of alcohol abuse. Sam's wife and two daughters accompany him. Sam is 5' 10" tall and weighs 140 lbs. His vital signs are T 98.2, AP 98 and slightly irregular, R 24, BP 152/88. He is lethargic, confused, and jaundiced. When the nurse assesses his lung sounds, she hears pulmonary crackles in all lobes. His abdominal girth measures 44 inches. His wife states he has not gone to the bathroom all morning. He has +3 edema in his feet and ankles. Sam's primary diagnosis is hematemesis with a secondary diagnosis of cirrhosis.

- Brainstorm other subjective and objective data that are important to include in the assessment of Sam Lightfoot.

- Relate the pathophysiology of cirrhosis to the assessed symptoms and other symptoms Sam may have experienced. Develop a patho-flow chart relating the symptoms to the pathological cause.
- List diagnostic tests that would be appropriate for the physician to order for Sam. What abnormal laboratory results would be typical of cirrhosis?
- Relate the possible results of the diagnostic tests to the developed patho-flow chart.
- Besides alcohol abuse, what are some other causes of cirrhosis?
- List complications of cirrhosis caused by chronic alcohol abuse.
- Explain the pathophysiology of portal hypertension as it relates to cirrhosis. Relate these to the patho-flow chart previously developed.
- List diuretics that may be ordered for Sam to decrease the ascites.
- How does the action of lactulose (Cephulac) lower the level of ammonia in the blood?
- What other complications result from portal hypertension?
- Explain the rationale for the complication of pleural effusion.
- Identify possible nursing diagnoses for Sam.
- What nursing interventions would be appropriate at this time?
- Develop a care plan for Sam Lightfoot.
- If Sam's condition improved and he was scheduled for discharge, what is important to include in the discharge teaching regarding:

    bleeding tendencies
    exercise
    nutrition
    skin care

- Develop diet instructions for Sam Lightfoot. Consider cultural influence in the diet instructions.
- List local resources/support groups where Sam and his family could be referred.

Sam's daughter, Mary, says, "I wish Dad would have quit drinking years ago. I was always embarrassed by his behavior when he had too much to drink. His life could have had so much potential."

- What would be appropriate responses of the nurse?

SYSTEMS REVIEWED IN HYPERTENSION, CONGESTIVE HEART FAILURE, AND CHRONIC RENAL FAILURE EXERCISE

- Respiratory (Chapter 18)
- Cardiovascular (Chapter 19)
- Hematologic and Lymphatic (Chapter 20)

- Integumentary (Chapter 21)
- Immune (Chapter 22)
- Musculoskeletal (Chapter 24)
- Neurological (Chapter 25)
- Endocrine (Chapter 27)
- Gastrointestinal (Chapter 28)
- Urinary (Chapter 29)
- Female Reproductive (Chapter 30)

CRITICAL THINKING EXERCISE WITH HYPERTENSION, CONGESTIVE HEART FAILURE, AND CHRONIC RENAL FAILURE

Trina Brown, a 40-year-old African American female, has a twenty year history of hypertension. She has been noncompliant in taking her antihypertensive medications that were prescribed by her physician. She has recently developed symptoms of congestive heart failure and renal failure.

- Brainstorm some reasons for Trina's noncompliance.
- Name some medications that may have been prescribed to treat Trina's hypertension. List the advantage and disadvantage of each medication.
- Using Table 29–2 Chronic Renal Failure Effects on Body Systems, develop a concept map showing the relationship of hypertension to the effects of renal failure on each listed system.
- What is the relationship between hypertension, increased peripheral resistance, cardiac hypertrophy, and congestive heart failure?
- What is the relationship of blood pressure (hypotension and hypertension) and renal failure?
- What is the relationship between the heart's decreasing ability to pump blood through the blood vessels and pulmonary edema?
- Explain the relationship between fluid in the alveoli and dyspnea.
- Physiologically, what is occurring in Trina's body to cause an increased rate of respiration?
- List laboratory results that would indicate that Trina is developing chronic renal failure.
- List symptoms that would indicate Trina is developing chronic renal failure.
- List subjective and objective data for which the nurse would assess for symptoms of chronic renal failure.
- List laboratory results that would indicate that Trina is developing congestive heart failure.
- List symptoms that would indicate Trina is developing congestive heart failure? Give the cause/etiology for each symptom.
- List subjective and objective data for which the nurse would assess for symptoms of congestive heart failure.
- Identify possible nursing diagnoses for Trina.
- List nursing interventions and give rationale for each intervention.

Trina's abdomen is distended and she has lost her appetite for the last two days. She has had hiccups constantly for two hours. She says, "I am so tired of these hiccups. Why am I having them?"

- Explain to Trina the cause for her hiccups.

SYSTEMS REVIEWED IN PARKINSON DISEASE EXERCISE

- Respiratory (Chapter 18)
- Integumentary (Chapter 21)
- Musculoskeletal (Chapter 24)
- Neurological (Chapter 25)
- Sensory (Chapter 26)
- Gastrointestinal (Chapter 28)
- Urinary (Chapter 29)

CRITICAL THINKING EXERCISE WITH PARKINSON DISEASE

Mr. Gilstad is a 76-year-old man who has been exposed to several chemicals during his farming career. For the last 7 years, he has walked with his arms flexed, leaning forward with his head bowed. Recently he has had some difficulty rising from a chair and balancing himself when he walks. He fell twice when doing odd jobs around the house. He has started making a "to do list" because he has difficulty remembering. He may go to the store for three items but return with only two. His wife noticed that he has a slight tremor in his hand when he eats and often rolls his forefinger and thumb together in a circular motion.

- Use deductive reasoning and identify Mr. Gilstad's possible diagnosis.
- With these symptoms, what diagnostic tests may the doctor order?

Mr. Gilstad shared his symptoms with his family physician. After some tests were completed and results of referrals to specialists were returned, the physician told Mr. Gilstad he was suspecting Parkinson disease. Mr. Gilstad said, "Tell me about Parkinson disease."

- Relate what Mr. Gilstad could be taught about Parkinson disease.

- List objective and subjective data needed to make an appropriate and thorough assessment on Mr. Gilstad.
- List etiological causes of Parkinson disease. What possible etiological factors does Mr. Gilstad have?
- Explain the function of dopamine, a neurotransmitter, to the symptoms displayed in a client with Parkinson disease.
- List drugs that interfere in the synthesis and storage of dopamine.
- List the signs and symptoms of Parkinson disease. Think of a client with Parkinson disease, and relate his or her symptoms to the textbook symptoms.
- Develop a patho-flow map relating the pathophysiology of Parkinson disease to the systems that could be affected and the typical symptoms of that system.
- List drugs that Mr. Gilstad may receive, and relate the drugs to the symptoms that may be controlled. List the symptoms and side effects that need monitoring with each of the drugs listed.

Mr. Gilstad is becoming more rigid, having difficulty swallowing food, falling frequently, reaching for items to assist in ambulating, experiencing frequent incontinence, complaining of his eyes itching, and having severe memory loss. His voice has become soft, and his speech is slurred.

- List Mr. Gilstad's autonomic symptoms.
- Develop diet instructions for Mr. Gilstad and his wife.
- What possible surgical procedures could be done to relieve Mr. Gilstad's symptoms.
- Develop a nursing care plan for Mr. Gilstad listing nursing diagnoses, goals, and nursing interventions to address each symptom.

- Using the Internet, research new therapies for Parkinson disease, and share them with other students.

After a year, Mr. Gilstad is unable to walk and has to be lifted from his bed to his wheelchair. He is unable to verbally communicate. He no longer has bladder control. When he was fed his lunch, he started coughing and perhaps aspirated some food.

- List appropriate subjective and objective data needed in a nursing assessment.
- Re-evaluate the previously developed nursing care plan and revise appropriately.

SUMMARY

This may have been the first time facts learned in anatomy and physiology were related to a disease process, or understanding was gained as to the reason clients have particular symptoms with the disease condition. When clients are ill, they rarely have only one disorder, but several inter-related conditions. The purpose of these exercises is to provide an opportunity to think through these situations before they are encountered in a clinical situation. In applying critical thinking skills to the case studies in this chapter, pertinent questions have been asked, clinical situations evaluated and clinical decisions made, much the way it is done in the clinical environment as a student and as a nurse. In working through these questions, analyzing and synthesizing skills were utilized. Perhaps a renewed interest and awe of the complexity of the body was gained upon discovering the inter-relatedness of the body systems. Hopefully, the critical thinking experience is a catalyst to becoming a proficient, critical thinking nurse.

CHAPTER 34

References/Suggested Readings and Resources

Please note that because Internet resources are of a time-sensitive nature and URL addresses may change or be deleted, resource searches should also be conducted by association and/or topic.

CHAPTER 1
The Health Care Delivery System

REFERENCES/SUGGESTED READINGS

Aiken, L. H. (1995). Transformation of the nursing workforce. *Nursing Outlook, 43*(5), 201–209.

American Health Consultants. (1994). RNs fight PFC as hospitals struggle to cut costs—The battle is far from over. *Patient-Focused Care, 2*(11), 149–160.

American Nurses Association. (1991). *Nursing's agenda for health care reform.* Kansas City, MO: Author.

American Nurses Association. (1993a, September). *Consumers willing to see a nurse for routine "doctoring" according to Gallup poll* [news release]. Washington, DC: Author.

American Nurses Association. (1993b, September). *States with some form of nurse privileging.* Washington, DC: Author.

American Nurses Association. (1994). *Health care reform and America's nurses: Agenda for change.* Washington, DC: Author.

American Nurses Association. (1995). Managed care: Challenges and opportunities for nursing. *Nursing Facts* (Item PR-27). Washington, DC: Author.

Baker, C. M. (1994). School health: Policy issues. *Nursing and Health Care, 15*(4),178–184.

Brown, S. A., & Grimes, D. E. (1993). *A meta-analysis of process of care, clinical outcomes, and cost effectiveness of nurses in primary care roles: Nurse practitioners and nurse–midwives* [executive summary]. Washington, DC: American Nurses Association.

Centers for Disease Control and Prevention (CDC). (1998). *Combating Complacency—HIV Prevention, Geneva '98. Trends.* Available: http://www.cdcnpin.org

Chamberlain, P., Chen, Y., Osuna, E., & Yamamoto, C. (1995). Innovative culture shock prescribed for health care. *Nursing Outlook, 43*(5), 232–234.

Deparle, N. (1998). *The state of the Children's Health Insurance Program.* Health Care Financing Administration. Available: http://www.hcfa.gov/init/testm918.htm

Feldstein, P. J. (1999). *Health care economics* (5th ed.). Albany, NY: Delmar.

Friedman, E. (1997). The uninsured: From dilemma to crisis. In P. Lee & C. Estes (Eds.), *The nation's health* (5th ed.). Boston: Jones & Bartlett.

Grace, H. K. (1997). Can medical costs be contained? In J. C. McCloskey, & H. K. Grace (Eds.), *Current issues in nursing* (5th ed.). St. Louis, MO: Mosby.

Grace, H. K., & Brock, R. M. (1997). Solving the health care dilemma: What will work? In J. C. McCloskey & H. K. Grace (Eds.), *Current issues in nursing* (5th ed.). St. Louis, MO: Mosby.

Haugh, R. (1999). The new consumer. *Hospital Health Network, 73*(12), 30–34, 36.

Health Care Financing Administration (HCFA). (1998). *Medicare and Medicaid Expenses, 1997.* Available: http://www.hcfa.gov/pubforms/finance/97/ch2n1216.htm

Health Care Financing Administration (HCFA). (2000). The nation's healthcare dollar: 1998. Available: http://www.hcfa.gov/stats/nhe-oact/tables/chart.htm

Hicks, L. L., & Boles, K. E. (1997). Why health economics? In C. Harrington & C. L. Estes (Eds.), *Health policy and nursing: Crisis and reform in the U.S. health care delivery system* (2nd ed). Boston: Jones & Bartlett.

Hull, K. (1997). Hospital trends. In C. Harrington & C. L. Estes (Eds.), *Health policy and nursing: Crisis and reform in the U.S. health care delivery system* (2nd ed). Boston: Jones & Bartlett.

Kellogg Foundation. (1994, June 24). *How people view their providers. Report of a survey.* Battle Creek, MI: Author.

Kelly, L., & Joel, L. (1995). *Dimensions of professional nursing* (7th ed.). New York: McGraw-Hill.

Lee, P. R., Soffel, D., & Luft, H. (1997). Costs and coverage: Pressures towards health care reform. In P. Lee, C. Estes, & N. Ramsay (Eds.), *The nation's health* (5th ed.). Boston: Jones & Bartlett.

Levit, K. R., Lazenby, H. C., Cowan, C. A., & Letsch, S. W. (1997). National health expenditures. In C. Harrington & C. L. Estes (Eds.), *Health policy and nursing: Crisis and reform in the U.S. health care delivery system* (2nd ed). Boston: Jones & Bartlett.

Maraldo, P. J. (1997). Nursing's agenda for health care reform. In J. C. McCloskey & H. K. Grace (Eds.), *Current issues in nursing* (5th ed.). St. Louis, MO: Mosby.

McCloskey, J. C., & Grace, H. K. (Eds.). (1997). *Current issues in nursing* (5th ed.). St. Louis, MO: Mosby.

Moyer, M. E. (1997). A revised look at the number of uninsured Americans. In C. Harrington & C. L. Estes (Eds.), *Health policy and nursing: Crisis and reform in the U.S. health care delivery system* (2nd ed.). Boston: Jones & Bartlett.

News. (2000). High public esteem for nurses. *AJN 100*(1), 21.

O'Neil, E. H. (1993). *Health professions education for the future: Schools in service to the nation.* San Francisco: Pew Health Professions Commission.

Parris, N. M., & Hines, J. (1995). Payer and provider relationships: The key to reshaping health care delivery. *Nursing Administration Quarterly, 19*(3), 13–17.

Pearson, L. J. (1996). Annual update of how each state stands on legislative issues affecting advanced nursing practice. *Nurse Practitioner, 21*(1), 10–701.

Peck, S. P. (1997). Community nursing centers: Implications for health care reform. In J. C. McCloskey & H. K. Grace (Eds.), *Current issues in nursing* (5th ed.). St. Louis, MO: Mosby.

Pruitt, R. H., & Campbell, B. F. (1994). Educating for health care reform and the community. *Nursing and Health Care, 15*(6), 308–311.

Rowe, J. W. (1996). Health care myths at the end of life. *Bulletin of the American College of Surgeons, 81*(6), 11–18.

Salmon, M. E. (1995). Public health policy: Creating a healthy future for the American public. *Family & Community Health, 18*(1), 1–11.

Schieber, G. J., Poullier, J. P., & Greenwald, L. M. (1997). U.S. health expenditure performance: An international comparison and data update. In C. Harrington & C. L. Estes (Eds.), *Health policy and nursing: Crisis and reform in the U.S. health care delivery system* (2nd ed.). Boston: Jones & Bartlett.

Society for Ambulatory Care Professionals. (1994). *Glossary of managed care terms: An issue briefing*. Chicago: American Hospital Association.

Stafford, M., & Appleyard, J. (1997). Clinical nurse and nurse practitioners. In J. C. McCloskey & H. K. Grace (Eds.), *Current issues in nursing* (5th ed.). St. Louis, MO: Mosby.

Tlusty, M. (1994). Higher mortality for women with PCP [brief item]. *Nursing and Health Care, 15*(4), 211.

U.S. Department of Health & Human Services. (1993). *Medicare benefits booklet*. Washington, DC: U.S. Government Printing Office.

Vrabec, N. J. (1995). Implications of U.S. health care reform for the rural elderly. *Nursing Outlook, 43*(6), 260–265.

Washington Consulting Group. (1994, February). *Survey of certified nurse practitioners and clinical nurse specialists: December 1992, final report*. Rockville, MD: Division of Nursing.

Zerwekh, J., & Claborn, J. C. (1997). *Nursing today: Transitions and trends*. Philadelphia: W. B. Saunders Company.

RESOURCES

American Nurses Association (ANA), 600 Maryland Avenue SW, Suite 100 West, Washington, DC 20024-2571, 800-274-4ANA (262), http://www.ana.com

National Federation of Licensed Practical Nurses, Inc. (NFLPN), 1418 Aversboro Road, Garner, NC 27529, 800-948-2511, http://www.nflpn.org

Society for Ambulatory Care Professionals, One North Franklin, 31st Floor, Chicago, IL 60606, 312-422-3900, http://www.sacp-net.org

CHAPTER 2
Critical Thinking

REFERENCES/SUGGESTED READINGS

Baker, C. R. (1996). Reflective learning: A teaching strategy for critical thinking. *Journal of Nursing Education, 35*, 19–22.

Birx, E. (1993). Critical thinking and theory-based practice. *Holistic Nursing Practice, 7*(3).

Bowers, B., & McCarthy, D. (1993). Developing analytic thinking skills in early undergraduate education. *Journal of Nursing Education, 32*, 107–113.

Brigham, C. (1993). Nursing education and critical thinking: Interplay of content and thinking. *Holistic Nursing Practice, 7*(3).

Brookfield, S. (1993). On impostership, cultural suicide and owners dangers: How nurses learn critical thinking. *Journal of Continuing Education in Nursing, 24*(5), 179–205.

Center for Critical Thinking. (1997). *Critical thinking in living, working & learning (a real time video)* [On-line] Available: http://www.uncp.edu/home/vanderhoof/criticalthinking.ram

Center for Critical Thinking. (2000, January 25). *A brief history of the idea of critical thinking*. [On-line]. Available: http://www.criticalthinking.org/University/univlibrary/cthistory.nclk

Center for Critical Thinking. (2000, January 25). *Valuable intellectual traits*. [On-line] Available: http://www.criticalthinking.org/University/univlibrary/intraits.nclk

Duncan, G. (1996). An investigation of learning styles of practical and baccalaureate nursing students. *Journal of Nursing Education, 35*, 40–42.

Elder, L. & Paul, R. (2000, January 25). *Universal intellectual standards*. [On-line] Available: http://www.criticalthinking.org/University/univlibrary/unistan.nclk

Ennis, R. H. (1985). A logical basis for measuring critical thinking skills. *Educational Leadership, 43*, 44–48.

Glen, T. & Smoot, G. (1994, February/March). Critical thinking: A vital work skill. *Thrust for Educational Leadership 23*, 33–38. [On-line] Available: http://www.enc.org/reform/journals/enc2315/2315.htm

Guffey, M. E. (1998). *Five steps to better critical thinking, problem-solving and decision-making skills*. [On-line] Available: http://www.westwords.com/GUFFEY/critical.html

Heaslip, P. (1993, September). Intellectual standards: What are they? *Critical Connections* [Newsletter of the Critical Thinking Interest Group, University College of the Cariboo, Kamloops, B.C.]

Heaslip, P. (1994, November). Defining critical thinking. *Dialogue: A Critical Thinking Newsletter for Nurses, 3*.

Kurfiss, J. (1988). *Critical thinking: Theory, research, practice and possibilities*. Washington, DC: Association for the Study of Higher Education. (ASHE-ERIC Higher Education Report No. 2.)

Miller, M. A., & Malcolm, N. S. (1990). Critical thinking in the nursing curriculum. *Nursing & Health Care, 11*, 66–73.

Norris, S. P., & Ennis, R. H. (1989). *Evaluating critical thinking*. Pacific Grove, CA: Midwest Publication.

Paul, R. (1990). *Critical thinking: What every person needs to survive in a rapidly changing world*. Rohnert Park, CA: Center for Critical Thinking and Moral Critique, Sonoma State University.

Paul, R. (1992, April). Critical thinking: Basic questions and answers. *Think, 34*–38.

Paul, R. (1993). *Critical thinking: How to prepare students for a rapidly changing world*. Santa Rosa, CA: Foundation for Critical Thinking.

Paul, R. & Elder, L. (2000, January 25). *Helping students assess their thinking*. [On-line] Available: http://www.criticalthinking.org/University/univlibrary/helps.nclk

Paul, R., & Willsen, J. (1993). *Critical thinking, from an ideal evolves an imperative*. Santa Rosa, CA: The Foundation for Critical Thinking.

Scriven, M., & Paul, R. (1996). *Defining critical thinking* [On-line]. (Center for Critical Thinking at Sonoma State University, Rohnert Park, CA). Available: http://www.criticalthinking.org/University/univclass/defining.nclk

Worrell, P. J. (1990). Metacognition: Implications for instruction in nursing education. *Journal of Nursing Education, 29*(4), 170–175.

RESOURCES

California Academic Press, 217 La Cruz Avenue, Millbrae, CA 94030, 650-697-5628, http://www.calpress.com, email: info@calpress.com

Center for Critical Thinking at Sonoma State University, Box 7087, Cotati, CA 94901, 707-664-2940, http://www.criticalthinking.org

Foundation for Critical Thinking, P.O. Box 7087, Cotati, CA 94901, 410-364-5082, 800-833-3645

International Center for the Assessment of Higher Order Thinking, 707-878-9100, http://www.criticalthinking.org/icat.nclk

National Council for Excellence in Critical Thinking, 707-878-9100, http://www.criticalthinking.org/ncect.nclk

CHAPTER 3
Legal Responsibilities

REFERENCES/SUGGESTED READINGS

Badzek, L. & Gross, L. (1999). Confidentiality and privacy: At the forefront for nurses. *AJN, 99*(6), 52–54.

Beare, P., & Myers, J. (1998). *Principles and practices of adult health nursing* (3rd ed.). St. Louis, MO: Mosby.

Becker, B., & Fendler, D. (1994). *Vocational and personal adjustments in practical nursing.* (7th ed.) St. Louis, MO: Mosby.

Bernzweig, E. (1995). *The nurse's liability for malpractice: A programmed course* (6th ed.). St. Louis, MO: Mosby.

Braun, J., & Lipson, S. (1993). *Toward a restraint-free environment.* Baltimore: Health Professions Press.

Brown, S. (1999). Good Samaritan laws: Protection and limits. *RN, 62*(11), 65.

Calfee, B. (1995). Going before the board: How to prepare yourself. *Nursing95, 25*(3), 56–58.

Curtain, L. (1993). Informed consent: Cautious, calculated candor. *Nursing Management, 24*(4), 18, 20.

DeLaune, S., & Ladner, P. (1998), *Fundamentals of nursing: Standards & practice.* Albany, NY: Delmar.

Dempski, K. (2000). Serving as an expert witness. *RN, 63*(2), 65–68.

Dunn, D. (1999). Exploring the gray areas of informed consent. *Nursing99, 29*(7), 41–44.

Eggland, E. (1995). Charting smarter: Using new mechanisms to organize your paperwork. *Nursing95, 25*(9), 35–41.

Flight, M. (1998). *Law, liability, and ethics* (3rd ed.). Albany, NY: Delmar.

Green, A. (1995). Are you at risk for disciplinary action? *AJN, 95*(7), 36–42.

Hill, S., & Howlett, H. (1997). *Success in practical nursing: Personal and vocational issues* (3rd ed.). Philadelphia: W. B. Saunders Company.

Hughes, T. (1994). Is your colleague chemically dependent? *AJN, 94*(9), 31–35.

Idemoto, B., Daly, B. et al. (1993). Implementing the patient self-determination act, *AJN, 93*(1), 20, 22–25.

Joint Commission on Accreditation of Healthcare Organizations (JCAHO). (1995). *Accreditation Manual for Hospitals.* Oakbrook Terrace, IL: Author.

Lippman, H. (1992, April). Addicted nurses: Tolerated, tormented, or treated. *RN,* 36–41.

Mandell, M. (1994). Not documented, not done. *Nursing94, 24*(8), 62–63.

Mayer, T. (1995, April). *Director of nurses' attitudes toward restraint usage in long-term care.* Master's Thesis, Indiana Wesleyan University.

Meyer, C. (1993). "End-of life" care: Patients, choices, nurses' challenges. *AJN, 93*(2), 40–47.

Mitchell, P., & Grippando, G. (1993). *Nursing perspectives and issues* (5th ed.). Albany: Delmar.

Monahan, F.D., Drake, T., & Neighbors, M. (1998). *Nursing care of adults* (2nd ed.). Philadelphia: W. B. Saunders Company.

Moniz, D. M. (1998). Too few staff, too much risk. *RN, 61*(12), 63.

Sandler, R. L. (1995). Restraining devices. *American Journal of Nursing, 95*(7), 34–35.

Showers, J. (2000). What you need to know about negligence lawsuits. *Nursing 2000, 30*(2). 45–48.

Skinner, K. (1993, December). The hazards of chemical dependency among nurses. *The Journal of Practical Nursing,* 8–11.

Taylor, C., Lillis, C., & LeMone, P. (1997). *Fundamentals of nursing: The art and science of nursing care* (3rd ed.). Philadelphia: Lippincott.

Ventura, M. (1999a). Staffing issues. *RN, 62*(2), 26–30.

Ventura, M. (1999b). The great multistate licensure debate. *RN, 62*(5), 58–62.

Walsh, S. M. (1995). Resuscitation decisions: Showing a family the way. *Nursing95, 25*(8), 50–51.

Zerwekh, J., & Claborn, J. C. (1997). *Nursing today: Transitions and trends.* (2nd ed.). Philadelphia: W. B. Saunders Company.

RESOURCES

Choice in Dying, Inc., 1035 30th Street NW, Washington, D.C. 20007, 202-338-9790, 800-989-9455, http://www.choices.org

Health Privacy Project and Consumer Coalition for Health Privacy, 202-687-0880

Living Wills, Films for the Humanities and Sciences, P.O. Box 2053, Princeton, NJ 08543-2053, 800-257-5126

Medcom, Inc., 6060 Phyllis Drive, Cypress, CA 90630, 800-877-1443, http://www.medcomsolutions.com

National EMS Information Exchange, http://naemt.org/nemsie/immunity.htm

The Verdict Is, Medical Electronic Educational Services, Inc., 930 Pitner Avenue, Evanston, IL 60202, 800-323-9084

CHAPTER 4
Ethical Responsibilities

REFERENCES/SUGGESTED READINGS

American Hospital Association. (1992). *A patient's bill of rights.* Chicago: Author.

Aroskar, M. A. (1994). Politics and ethics in nursing: Implications for education. *Journal of Professional Nursing, 10*(3), 129.

Awong, L., & Miles, A. (1998a). When an adolescent wants to forgo therapy. *American Journal of Nursing, 98*(7), 67–68.

Awong, L., & Miles, A. (1998b). When the physician disregards the patient's expressed wishes. *American Journal of Nursing, 98*(2), 71.

Bandman, E. L., & Bandman, B. (1995). *Nursing ethics through the life span* (3rd ed.). Norwalk, CT: Appleton-Lange.

Beare, G., & Myers, J. (1998). *Adult health nursing* (2nd ed.) St. Louis, MO: Mosby.

Callahan, J. (1994). The ethics of assisted suicide. *Health and Social Work, 19*(4), 237–243.

Curtin, L. (1995). Nurses take a stand on assisted suicide. *Nursing Management, 26*(5), 71–76.

Daly, B. (1999). Ethics: Why a new code? *AJN, 99*(6), 64–66.

Davis, A. J., & Aroskar, M. A. (1997). *Ethical dilemmas and nursing practice* (4th ed.). Norwalk, CT: Appleton-Lange.

DeLaune, S., & Ladner, P. (1998). *Fundamentals of nursing: Standards of practice.* Albany, NY: Delmar.

Edge, R., & Groves, J.R. (1999). *The ethics of health care: A guide for clinical practice* (2nd ed.). Albany, NY: Delmar.

Fowler, M. (1999). Ethics: Relic or resource? The code for nurses. *AJN, 99*(3), 56–58.

Gordon, M., Murphy, C., Candee, D., & Hiltunen, E. (1994). Clinical judgment: An integrated model. *Advances in Nursing Science, 16*(4), 55–70.

Haddad, A. (1995). Ethics in action. *RN, 58*(5), 21–23.

Haddad, A. (1998). Ethics in action. *RN, 61*(3), 21–24.

Haddad, A. (1999a). Ethics in action, *RN, 62*(7), 23–26.

Haddad, A. (1999b). Ethics in action, *RN, 62*(1), 23–26.

International Council of Nurses. (1973). *ICN code for nurses: Ethical concepts applied to nursing.* Geneva, Switzerland: Imprimeries Populaires.

Kristoff, B., Sellin, S., & Miller, M. (1994). Patients' rights and ethical dilemmas in home care: Incorporation of psychological concepts. *Home Healthcare Nurse, 12*(5), 45–50.

Mitchell, P., & Grippando, G. (1993). *Nursing perspectives and issues.* Albany, NY: Delmar.

National Federation of Practical Nurses, Inc. (NFLPN). (1996). *Nursing practice standards for the licensed practical/vocational nurse.* Garner, NC: Author.

News (2000). Health care fraud in Hawaii. *AJN, 100*(1), 21.

Nguyen, B. (1999). Protecting nurse whistleblowers. *AJN, 99*(12), 71.

Pappas, A. (1997). Ethical issues. In J. Zerwekh & J. Claborn (Eds.), *Nursing today: Transitions and trends*. Philadelphia: W.B. Saunders Company.

Pinch, W. J. (1990). Nursing ethics: Is covering up ever harmless? *Nursing Management, 21*(9), 60–62.

Polston, M. (1999). Whistleblowing: Does the law protect you? *AJN, 99*(1), 26–31.

Raths, L., Harmin, M., & Simon, S. (1978). *Values and teaching* (2nd ed.). Columbus, OH: Merrill.

Rice, V. H., Beck, C., & Stevenson, J. S. (1997). Ethical issues relative to autonomy and personal control in independent and cognitively impaired elders. *Nursing Outlook, 45*(1), 25–34.

Salladay, S. (1995). Ethical problems. *Nursing95, 25*(2), 29–30.

Salladay, S. (1998). Ethical problems. *Nursing98, 28*(7), 30.

Schildmeier, D. (1997). Using public opinion to protect nursing practice. *AJN, 97*(3), 56–58.

Sloan, A. (1999). Whistleblowing: There are risks! *RN, 62*(7), 65–68.

Sumodi, V. (1995). Legalization of physician-assisted suicide: Point/counterpoint. *Nursing Forum 30*(1), 11–17.

Ustal, D. (1993). *Clinical ethics and values: Issues and insights*. East Greenwich, RI: Educational Resources in Health Care.

Wilson, D. M. (1996). Highlighting the role of policy in nursing practice through a comparison of "DNR" policy influences and "No CPR" decision influences. *Nursing Outlook, 44*(6), 272–279.

Wolfe, S. (1999). Ethics on the job: A survey, quality vs. cost. *RN, 62*(1), 28–33.

Zerwekh, J. V. (1997). Do dying patients really need IV fluids? *AJN, 97*(3), 26–30.

Zollo, M. B., & Derse, A. (1997). The abusive patient: Where do you draw the line? *AJN, 97*(2), 31–35.

RESOURCES

American Red Cross, Transplant Services, 2025 E Street N.W., Suite 108, Washington, DC 20006, 800-2-TISSUE (84-7783)

The Living Bank International, P.O. Box 6725, Houston, TX 77265, 800-528-2971, http://www.livingbank.org

National Association for Practical Nurse Education and Service, Inc. (NAPNES), 1400 Spring Street, Suite 330, Silver Spring, MD 20901, 301-588-2491

National Federation of Licensed Practical Nurses, Inc. (NFLPN), 1418 Aversboro Road, Garner, NC 27529, 800-948-2511, http://www.nflpn.org

United Network of Organ Sharing (UNOS), 1100 Boulders Parkway, Suite 500, P.O. Box 13770, Richmond, VA 23225-8770, 888-894-6361, 804-330-8541, http://www.unos.org

CHAPTER 5
Communication

REFERENCES/SUGGESTED READINGS

Bailey, D., & Bailey, D. (1997). *Therapeutic approaches to care of the mentally ill* (4th ed.). Philadelphia: F. A. Davis Company.

Barnsteiner, J. (1996). Newest online journal users: Clinicians. *Reflections, 22*(2), 21.

Barry, P. (1997). *Mental health and mental illness* (6th ed.). Philadelphia: Lippincott.

Brandt, M. (1995, March). Making the CPR vision a reality: Where should you start? *Journal of the American Health Information Management Association, 66*(3), 26–30.

Burtt, K. (1997, November/December). Nurses use telehealth to address rural health care needs, prevent hospitalizations. *The American Nurse, 21*.

DeLaune, S. & Ladner, P. (1998). *Fundamentals of nursing: Standards & practice*. Albany, NY: Delmar.

deWit, S. (1994). *Rambo's nursing skills for clinical practice*. Philadelphia: W. B. Saunders Company.

Dick, R., & Steen, E. (Eds.). (1991). *The computer-based patient record: An essential technology for health care*. Washington, DC: National Academy Press.

Estes, M. E. Z. (2002). *Health assessment & physical examination* (2nd ed.). Albany, NY: Delmar.

Frawley, K., & Asmonga, D. (1996). Update on the Medical Records Confidentiality Act. *Journal of the American Health Information Management Association, 67*(1), 12.

Frisch, N., & Frisch, L. (1998). *Psychiatric mental health nursing*. Albany, NY: Delmar.

Gay, K. (1993). *Getting your message across*. New York: Macmillan Publishing.

Goldsmith, J. (1996). Computers and nurses changing hospital care. *Reflections, 22*(2), 8–10.

Granade, P. (1997). The brave new world of telemedicine. *RN, 60*(7), 59–62.

Hall, E. (1959). *The silent language*. New York: Doubleday.

Jack, L. (1997). Effective communication. In J. Zerwekh, & J. Claborn (Eds.). *Nursing today: Transition and trends,* (2nd ed.). Philadelphia: W. B. Saunders Company.

Keller, V. & Baker, L. (2000). Communicate with care. *RN, 63*(1), 32–33.

Kübler-Ross, E. (1969). *On death and dying*. New York: MacMillan.

Kübler-Ross, E. (1975). *Death: The final stage of growth*. Englewood Cliffs, NJ: Prentice Hall.

Kübler-Ross, E. (1978). *To live until we say good-bye*. Englewood Cliffs, NJ: Prentice Hall.

Lorton, L., & Legler, J. (1996). A telemedicine trial. *Journal of the American Health Information Management Association, 67*(1), 40–42.

Medical Records Institute. (1994). Legality of electronic patient record systems. *Toward an electronic patient record, 2*(7).

Meranda, D. (1995). Administrative and security challenges with electronic patient record systems. *Journal of the American Health Information Management Association, 66*(3), 58–60.

Milliken, M. (1998). *Understanding human behavior* (6th ed.). Albany, NY: Delmar.

Pagano, M., & Ragan, S. (1992). *Communication skills for professional nurses*. Newbury Park, CA: Sage.

Ravitch, S. (1996). The Medical Records Confidentiality Act. *For The Record, 8*(9) 8–11.

Rhodes, A. (1995). The need for security with computerized records. *MCN, 20*(6), 299.

Roter, D., & Hall, J. (1993). *Doctors talking with patients/ patients talking with doctors*. Westport, CT: Auburn House.

Ruben, B. (1992). *Communicating with patients*. Dubuque, IA: Kendall-Hunt.

Sherman, K. (1994). *Communication and image in nursing*. Albany, NY: Delmar.

Smith, S. (1992). *Communications in nursing*. St. Louis: Mosby.

Tamparo, C., & Lindh, W. (2000). *Therapeutic communications for health professionals* (2nd ed.). Albany, NY: Delmar.

Telemedicine Research Center. (1997). *What is telemedicine?* Portland, OR: Author.

Waughfield, C. (1998). *Mental health concepts*. Albany, NY: Delmar.

Zolot, J. S. (1999). Computer-based patient records. *AJN, 99*(12), 64–69.

RESOURCES

American Health Information Management Association, 919 North Michigan Avenue, Suite 1400, Chicago, IL 60611-1683, 312-787-2672, http://www.ahima.org

CHAPTER 6
Cultural Diversity and Nursing

REFERENCES/SUGGESTED READINGS

Agre, P., & Spincola, L. (1996). Helping staff meet the needs of a culturally diverse patient population. *Nursing Forum, 23*(2), 347.

Andrews, M., & Boyle, J. S. (1998). *Transcultural concepts in nursing care* (3rd ed.). Philadelphia: Lippincott.

Andrews, M. M. (1997). Cultural diversity and community health nursing. In J. M. Swanson & M. Nics (Eds.), *Community health nursing: Promoting the health of aggregates* (2nd ed., pp. 433–458). Philadephia: W. B. Saunders Company.

Andrews, M. M., & Bolin, L. (1997). The African American community. In J. M. Swanson & M. Nies (Eds.), *Community health nursing: Promoting the health of aggregates* (2nd ed., pp. 433–458). Philadephia: W. B. Saunders Company.

Andrews, M. M., & Hanson, P. (1998). Religion, culture, and nursing. In M. M. Andrews & J. Boyle (Eds.), *Transcultural concepts in nursing care* (3rd ed.). Philadelphia: Lippincott.

Boyle, J. (1998). Culture and community. In M. M. Andrews & J. Boyle (Eds.), *Transcultural concepts in nursing care* (3rd ed.). Philadelphia: Lippincott.

Brewer, J. A., & Bonalumi, N. M. (1996). Cultural diversity in the emergency department: Health care beliefs and practices among the Pennsylvania Amish. *Journal of Emergency Nursing, 21*(6), 494–497.

Carpenito, L. J. (1999). *Nursing diagnosis: Application to clinical practice* (8th ed.). Philadelphia: Lippincott.

Clark, M. (1999). *Nursing in the community* (3rd ed.). Stamford, CT: Appleton & Lange.

Davidhizar, R., Dowd, S., & Giger, J. (1998). Educating the culturally diverse health care student. *Nurse Educator, 23*(2), 38–42.

Degazon, C. (1996). Cultural diversity and community health nursing practice. In M. Stanhope & J. Lancaster (Eds.), *Community health nursing: Promoting health of aggregates, families, and individuals* (4th ed.). St. Louis, MO: Mosby.

DeLaune, S. & Ladner, P. (1998). *Fundamentals of nursing: Standards & practice*. Albany, NY: Delmar.

Doherty, W. (1992). Private lives, public values. *Psychology Today, 25*(3), 32–27.

Doswell, W., & Erlen, J. (1998). Multicultural issues and ethical concerns in the delivery of nursing care interventions. *Nursing Clinics of North America, 33*(2), 353–361.

Edelman, C., & Mandle, C. (1998). *Health promotion throughout the lifespan* (4th ed.). St. Louis, MO. Mosby.

Edmission, K. W. (1997). Psychosocial dimensions of medical–surgical nursing. In J. M. Black & E. Matassarin-Jacobs (Eds.), *Medical surgical nursing: Clinical management for continuity of care*. Philadelphia: W. B. Saunders Company.

Estin, P. (1999). Spotting depression in Asian patients. *RN, 62*(4), 39–40.

Eshleman, J. (1992, November). Death with dignity: Significance of religious beliefs and practices in Hinduism, Buddhism, and Islam. *Today's OR Nurse,* 19–20.

Fawcett, C. (1993). *Family psychiatric nursing*. St. Louis, MO: Mosby.

Fish, S., & Shelley, J. (1988). *Spiritual care: The nurse's role* (3rd ed.). Downers Grove, IL: Inter Varsity Press.

Galanti, G. (1997). *Caring for patients from different cultures: Case studies from American hospitals* (2nd ed.). Philadelphia: University of Pennsylvania Press.

Giger, J., & Davidhizar, R. (1999). *Transcultural Nursing: Assessment and intervention* (3rd ed.). St. Louis, MO: Mosby.

Gonzalez, R. (1999). ANA advocates more diversity in nursing. *AJN, 99*(11), 24.

Grensing-Pophal, L. (1997). Dealing with diversity in the workplace. *Nursing97, 27*(9), 78.

Grossman, D. (1996). Cultural dimensions in home health nursing. *AJN, 96*(7), 33–36.

Grossman, D., & Taylor, R. (1995). Cultural diversity on the unit. *AJN, 95*(2).

Hoeman, S. (1996). Intraethnic diversity. *Home-Healthcare Nurse, 14*(7), 568.

Kelz, R. (1997). *Delmar's English–Spanish Pocket Dictionary for Health Professionals*. Albany, NY: Delmar.

Kirkpatrick, M., Brown, S., & Atkins, T. (1998). Using the internet to integrate cultural diversity and global awareness. *Nurse Educator, 23*(2), 15–17.

Lee, E. (Ed.). (1997). *Working with Asian Americans: A guide for clinicians*. San Francisco: Richman Area Multi-Services, Inc.

Leininger, M. (1996). *Transcultural nursing: Concepts, theories, research, and practices*. Columbus, OH: Greyden Press.

Lock, D. (1992). *Increasing multicultural understanding: A comprehensive model*. Newbury Park, CA: Sage.

Louie, K. B. (1999). Health promotion interventions for Asian American Pacific Islanders. In L. Zhan (Ed.) *Asian Voices* (pp 3–13). Boston: Jones and Bartlett Publishers.

Luckmann, J. (1999). *Transcultural communication in nursing*. Albany, NY: Delmar.

Malone, B. (1998). Diversity, divisiveness and divinity. *American Nurse, 30*(1), 5.

Meleis, A. I. (1997). Immigrant transitions and health care: An action plan [News]. *Nursing Outlook, 45*(1), 42.

Morley, P., & Wallis, R. (Eds.). (1978). *Culture and curing: Anthropological perspectives on traditional medical beliefs and practices*. Pittsburgh, PA: University of Pittsburgh Press.

Purnell, L. & Paulanka, B. (1997). *Transcultural health care: A culturally competent approach*. Philadelphia: F. A. Davis.

Robinson, A. (1994). Spirituality and risk: Toward an understanding. *Holistic Nursing Practice, 8*(2), 1–7.

Sherman, K. (1994). *Communication and image in nursing*. Albany, NY: Delmar.

Singelenberg, R. (1990). The blood transfusion taboo of Jehovah's Witnesses: Origins, development and function of a controversial doctrine. *Social Science Medicine, 31*(4), 515–523.

Smith, L. (1998). Concept analysis: Cultural competence. *Journal of Cultural Diversity, 5*(1), 4–10.

Spector, R. E. (1999). *Cultural diversity in health and illness*. (6th ed.). New York: Prentice-Hall.

Spradley, B. W., and Allender, J. A. (1996). *Community health nursing* (4th ed.). Philadelphia: Lippincott.

Stanhope, M., & Knollmueller, R. (1999). *Handbook of community-based and home health nursing practice* (3rd ed.). St. Louis, MO: Mosby.

Stanhope, M., & Lancaster, J. (1996). *Community Health Nursing* (4th ed.). St. Louis, MO: Mosby.

Sue, D. W., & Sue, D. (1999). *Counseling the culturally different: Theory and practice* (3rd ed.). New York: Wiley.

Talabere, L. (1996). Meeting the challenge of culture care in nursing: Diversity, sensitivity, competence, and congruence. *Journal of Cultural Diversity, 3*(2), 53–61.

U.S. Department of Commerce, Bureau of the Census. (1992). *Statistical abstract of the United States: 1999*

(112th ed.). Washington, DC: U.S. Government Printing Office.

RESOURCES

Cultural Diversity in Health Care (video), American Journal of Nursing, 345 Hudson Street, New York, NY 10014

CHAPTER 7
Wellness Concepts

REFERENCES/SUGGESTED READINGS

Baughcum, A. (1998). Mom's beliefs may cause child obesity. *Archives of Pediatric and Adolescent Medicine, 152,* 1010–1014.

Browder, S. (1998). *Attention, women over 50* [On-line]. Available: http://www.seniornews.com/new-choices/article593.html

Brown, E. (1995, August). An inexpensive and painless alternative to colonoscopy? (coprocytobiology). *Medical Update, 19,* 1.

Carey, B. (1996, July/August). The slumber solution. *Health,* 70–75.

Centers for Disease Control and Prevention (CDC). (1998). Uninsured women miss mammograms. *Morbidity and Mortality Weekly Report, 47,* 825–829.

Cerrato, P. (1999). A radical approach to heart disease. *RN, 62*(4), 65–66.

Chase, M. (1996, February 5). Simple handwashing gets new scrutiny for disease control. *The Wall Street Journal,* B1(E&W).

Dixon, B. (1995). *Good health for African Americans.* New York: Random House.

Don't overdo it: Alcohol paradox. (1996, February 5). *Industry Week, 245*(1), 19.

Eastman, P. (1996, January 17). Task force issues new screening guidelines. *Journal of the National Cancer Institute, 88*(3), 74.

Edlin, G., Golanty, E., & McCormack-Brown, K. (1997). *Essentials for Health and Wellness.* Boston: Jones and Bartlett.

Floyd, P., Mimms, S., & Yelding-Howard, C. (1995). *Personal health: A multicultural approach.* Englewood, CO: Morton Publishing Co.

Hafen, B., & Hoeger, W. (1997). *Wellness: Guidelines for a healthy lifestyle* (2nd ed.). Englewood, CO: Morton Publishing Co.

Health-club hygiene. (1995, November). *Industry Week, 244,* 31.

Hoeger, W., & Hoeger, S. (1995). *Lifetime physical fitness and wellness* (4th ed.). Englewood, CO: Morton Publishing.

Hoffman, E. (1996). *Our health, our lives.* New York: Pocket Books.

Inlander, C., & Moran, C. (1996). *77 Ways to beat colds and flu.* New York: Walker Publishing.

Lee, I., & Paffenbarger, R. (1998). Exercise can cut stroke risk 50%. *Stroke, 29,* 2049–2054.

Lyon, B. (2000). Conquering stress. *Reflections on Nursing LEADERSHIP, 26*(1), 22–23, 43.

Malaty, H. (1998). Twin study: *H pylori* tied to hygiene. *American Journal of Epidemiology, 148,* 793–797.

Matthews, K. (1998). Suppressed anger hard on women's hearts. *Psychosomatic Medicine, 60,* 633–638.

National Center for Health Statistics. (1997). *Monthly vital statistics report, 45*(11S2), 23, 40–43. [On-line] Available: http://www.youfirst.com/risks.htm

Oman, D., & Reed, D. (1998). Religious elderly tend to live longer. *American Journal of Public Health, 88,* 1469–1475.

Osteoporosis, a silent disease, finds a louder voice. (1995, November–December). *Menopause News, 5,* 1.

Payne, W., & Hahn, D. (1998). *Understanding your health* (5th ed.). St. Louis, MO: Mosby.

Poliafico, F. (1999). Abstinence is not the only answer. *RN, 62*(1), 58–60.

Quench strokes with every sip. (1995, October) *Prevention, 47,* 66.

Reed, D. (1998). Four factors predict "Healthy Aging." *American Journal of Public Health, 88,* 1463–1469.

Reichler, G. & Burke, N. (1999). *Active wellness: A personalized 10 step program for a healthy body, mind & spirit.* Time Life Custom Publishing.

Reichman, L., & Mangura, B. (1996, February). State-of-the-art tuberculosis prevention. *Chest, 109,* 301.

Robertson, J. (1996). *Peak-performance living.* New York: HarperCollins.

Seiger, L., Vanderpool, K., & Barnes, D. (1995). *Fitness and wellness strategies.* Dubuque, IA: Wm. C. Brown Communications.

Simon, H. (1992). *Staying well.* Boston: Houghton Mifflin Co.

Smith, C., & Maurer, F. (1999). *Community health nursing: Theory and practice.* (2nd ed.) Philadelphia: W. B. Saunders Company.

Social stigma of colon and rectal problems thwarts life-saving cancer screenings. (1995, October). *Executive Health's Good Health Report, 32,* 1.

U.S. Department of Agriculture, U.S. Department of Health & Human Services. (2000). *Home and Garden Bulletin No. 232* (5th ed.).

U.S. Department of Health & Human Services. (1990). *Healthy People 2000: National health promotion and disease prevention objectives.* (DHHS Publication No. [PHS] 91-50212). Washington, DC.

U.S. Department of Health & Human Services (USDHHS), Public Health Service. (1998). *Healthy people 2000: National health promotion and disease prevention objectives* and first draft *Healthy people 2010: National health promotion and disease prevention objectives.* [On-line] Available: http://web.health.gov/healthypeople

U.S. Department of Health & Human Services (USDHHS) Public Health Service (2000a). *Healthy people 2010: National health promotion and disease prevention objectives.* [On-line] Available: http://web.health.gov/healthypeople

U.S. Department of Health & Human Services (USDHHS), Public Health Service (PHS). (2000b). 1998–1999 Progress Review [On-line]. Available: http://odphp.osophs.dhhs.gov/pubs/hp2000

Wash your hands (to help prevent colds). (1996, January). *Consumer Reports on Health, 2*(1).

Weil, A. (1998). *Natural health, natural medicine.* (2nd ed.). Boston: Houghton Mifflin.

RESOURCES

Aerobics and Fitness Association of America, 15250 Ventura Boulevard, Suite 200, Sherman Oaks, CA 91403-3297, 800-446-2322, http://www.aerobics.com

American Dietetic Association, 216 West Jackson Boulevard, Suite 800, Chicago, IL 60606-6995, 800-366-1655, http://www.eatright.org

American Health Care Association, 1201 L Street, NW, Washington, DC 20005, 202-342-4444, http://www.ahca.org

American Holistic Nurses' Association, P.O. Box 2130, Flagstaff, AZ 86003-2130, 800-278-2462, http://www.ahna.org

Center for Science in the Public Interest, 1875 Connecticut Avenue, NW, Suite 300, Washington, DC 20009-5728, 202-332-9110, http://www.cspinet.org

Centers for Disease Control and Prevention, *Morbidity and Mortality Weekly Report*, http://www.cdc.gov/cdc.html

Centers for Disease Control and Prevention, 1600 Clifton Road, NE, Atlanta, GA, 30333, 404-639-3311, http://www.cdc.gov

Consumer Product Safety Commission, Washington, DC 20207, 800-638-2772, 800-638-8270 TDD, 800-492-8104 TTD in MD only

Dental Disease Prevention, Centers for Disease Control and Prevention (CDC), 1600 Clifton Road, NE, Atlanta, GA 30333

Environmental Protection Agency (EPA), Public Information Center, 401 M Street, SW, Washington, DC 20466, 800-424-9065, 202-260-2090, http://www.epa.gov

Food and Drug Administration, Office of Consumer Affairs, 5600 Fishers Lane, Rockville, MD 20857, 888-463-6332, http://www.fda.gov

Food and Nutrition Information Center, National Agricultural Library Building, Room 304, 10301 Baltimore Avenue, Beltsville, MD 20705-2351, 301-504-5719, http://www.nal.usda.gov/fnic

Healthy People 2010, Office of Disease Prevention and Health Promotion, 738-6 Humphrey Building, 200 Independence Avenue SW, Washington, DC 20201, 202-205-8583

Medic Alert Foundation International, P.O. Box 819008, Turlock, CA 95381-1009, 800-344-3226, 209-668-3333, http://www.medicalert.org

National Cholesterol Education Program Information Center, 4733 Bethesda Avenue, Room 530, Bethesda, MD 20814, 301-951-3260

National Council Against Health Fraud, Resource Center, 300 East Pink Hill Road, Independence, MO 64057, 816-228-4595, http://www.ncahf.org

National Health Information Center, P.O. Box 1133, Washington, DC 20013-1133, 800-336-4797, http://nhic-nt.health.org

National Highway Traffic Safety Administration, NES-11 HL, U.S. Department of Transportation, 400 7th Street, SW, Washington, DC 20590, 202-366-9294, Auto Hotline: 800-424-9393, http://www.nhtsa.dot.gov

National Institute for Occupational Safety and Health, Clearinghouse for Occupational Safety and Health Information, Technical Information Branch, 4676 Columbia Parkway, Cincinnati, OH 45226, 800-356-4674

The National Institute on Aging, P.O. Box 8057, Gaithersburg, MD 20898-8057, 800-222-2225, http://www.nih.gov/nia

National Institutes of Health, 9000 Rockville Pike, Bethesda, MD 20892, 301-496-1776, http://www.nih.gov

National League for Nursing, 61 Broadway New York, NY 10006, 212-363-5555, 800-669-9656, Fax 212-812-0393, http://www.nln.org

National Wellness Association/National Wellness Institute, 1300 College Court, P.O. Box 827, Stevens Point, WI 54481-0827, 715-342-2961, http://www.wellnesswi.org

National Women's Health Network, 514 Tenth Street, NW, Washington, DC 20004, 202-347-1140

U.S. Department of Agriculture, 14th & Independence Avenue, SW, Washington, DC 20250, 800-535-4555, 202-720-2791, http://www.usda.gov

U.S. Department of Health and Human Services, Office of Disease Prevention and Health Promotion, 638-East Humphrey Building, 200 Independence Avenue, SW, Washington, DC 20201, 202-690-6343, http://www.hhs.gov

World Health Organization, 525 23rd Street, NW, Washington, DC 20037, 202-974-3000, Headquarters Avenue Appia 20, 1211 Geneva 27, Switzerland, http://www.who.int

CHAPTER 8
Alternative/Complementary Therapies

REFERENCES/SUGGESTED READINGS

Achterberg, J., Dossey, B., & Kolkmeier, L. (1994). *Rituals of healing: Using imagery for health and wellness*. New York: Bantam Books.

Association of Psychophysiology and Biofeedback (AAPB). (1998). *What is biofeedback?* [On-line]. Available: http://www.aapb.org

Astin, J. A. (1998). Why patients use alternative medicine: Results of a national study. *Journal of the American Medical Association, 279*(19), 1,248.

Benson, H. (1975). *The relaxation response*. New York: William Morrow.

Borysenko, J., & Borysenko, M. (1994). *The power of the mind to heal*. Carson, CA: Hay House.

Brooke, P. (1998). Legal risks of alternative therapies. *RN, 61*(5), 53–58.

Brown, H., Cassileth, B. R., Lewis, J. P., & Renner, J. H. (1994, June 15). Alternative medicine—Or quackery? *Patient Care*, 80–98.

Budesheim, S., Neuberger, G., Kasal, S., Vogel-Smith, K., Hassanein, R., & DeViney, S. (1994). Determinants of exercise and aerobic fitness in outpatients with arthritis. *Nursing Research, 43*, 11–17.

Byers, D. C. (1983). *Better health with foot reflexology*. St. Petersburg, FL: Ingham Publishing, Inc.

Byrd, C., & Sherrill, J. (1995). The therapeutic effects of intercessory prayer. *Journal of Christian Nursing, 12*(1), 21–23.

Cerrato, P. (1998). Aromatherapy: Is it for real? *RN, 61*(6), 51–52.

Cerrato, P. (1999a). Using designer margarines to control lipid levels. *RN, 62*(10), 67–68.

Cerrato, P. (1999b). Omega-3 fatty acids: Nothing fishy here! *RN, 62*(8), 59–60.

Cerrato, P. (1999c). A radical approach to heart disease. *RN, 62*(4), 65–66.

Cerrato, P. (1999d). Tai chi: A martial art turns therapeutic. *RN, 62*(2), 59–60.

Cerrato, P. (2000). Diet and herbs for BPH? *RN, 63*(2), 63–64.

Cerrato, P. & Rowell, N. (1999). SAMe: A dietary remedy for mind and body? *RN, 62*(12), 61–64.

Chiropractic Arts Center. (1998). *Common questions about chiropractic care*. [On-line] Available: http://www.chiroarts.com/page7.html

Chopra, D. (1998). *Ageless body, timeless mind*. New York: Harmony Books.

Cousins, N. (1979). *Anatomy of an illness*. New York: Norton.

Cowens, D. (1996). *A gift for healing: How you can use therapeutic touch*. New York: Crown Trade Paperbacks.

DeLaune, S., & Ladner, P. (1998). *Fundamentals of Nursing: Standards & Practice*. Albany, NY: Delmar.

Dossey, B. M., (1995a). Imagery: Awakening the inner healer. In B. M. Dossey, L. Keegan, C. E. Guzzetta, & L. G. Kolkmeier (Eds.), *Holistic nursing: A handbook for practice* (2nd ed.). Gaithersburg, MD: Aspen.

Dossey, B. M. (1995b). The psychophysiology of bodymind healing. In B. M. Dossey, L. Keegan, C. E. Guzzetta, & L. G. Kolkmeier (Eds.), *Holistic nursing: A handbook for practice* (2nd ed.). Gaithersburg, MD: Aspen.

Dossey, B. M. (Ed.). (1997). *Core curriculum for holistic nursing*. Gaithersburg, MD: Aspen.

Dossey, L. (1997). *Healing words: The power of prayer and the practice of medicine*. San Francisco: Harper.

Dossey, L. (1999). *Prayer, healing, and medicine: An evening with Larry Dossey.* Arvada, CO: Lutheran Medical Center Community Foundation, Arvada Center.

Eisenberg, D. (1993). Medicine in a mind/body culture. In B. Moyers (Ed.), *Healing and the mind.* New York: Doubleday.

Evans, B. (1999). Complementary therapies & HIV infection. *AJN, 99*(2), 42–45.

Feuerstein, G. (1998). *Yoga and yoga therapy* [On-line]. Available: http://members.aol.com/yogaresearch/yogatherapy.htm

Fonnesbeck, B. (1998). Are you kidding? *Nursing98, 28*(3), 64.

Foster, S. (1995). Herbs for health. *The Herb Companion, 8*(1), 63–86.

Frisch, N. (1997). Changing of the guard. *Beginnings, 17*(1), 1, 11.

Frisch, N., & Frisch, L. (1998). *Psychiatric mental health nursing.* Albany, NY: Delmar.

Gagne, D., & Toye, R. C. (1994). Decreasing anxiety in psychiatric patients with therapeutic touch. *Archives of Psychiatric Nursing, 8*(3), 184–189.

Gates, R. (1997). Legal issues in alternative medicine. *Alternative Therapies in Clinical Practice, 4*(4), 143.

Guinness, A. (1993). *Family guide to natural medicine: How to stay healthy the natural way.* Pleasantville, NY: Reader's Digest.

Healing touch and energy therapy [On-line]. (1997). Available: http://www.altherapy.com/hlgtch.htm

Hodge, P. & Ullrich, S. (1999). Does your assessment include alternative therapies? *RN, 62*(6). 47–49.

Hover-Kramer, D. (1996). *Healing touch: A resource for health care professionals.* Albany, NY: Delmar.

Hutchison, C. (1999). Healing touch an energetic approach. *AJN, 99*(4), 43–48.

Japsen, B. (1995, August 21). Cost-conscious providers take to holistic medicine. *Modern Healthcare,* 138–142.

Kahn, S., & Saulo, M. (1995). *Healing yourself: A nurse's guide to self-care and renewal.* Albany, NY: Delmar.

Keegan, L. (1994). *The nurse as healer.* Albany, NY: Delmar.

Keegan, L. (1995a). Nutrition, exercise, and movement. In B. M. Dossey, L. Keegan, C. E. Guzzetta, & L. G. Kolkmeier (Eds.), *Holistic nursing: A handbook for practice* (2nd ed., pp. 257–285). Gaithersburg, MD: Aspen.

Keegan, L. (1995b). Touch: Connecting with the healing power. In B. M. Dossey, L. Keegan, C. E. Guzzetta, & L. G. Kolkmeier (Eds.), *Holistic nursing: A handbook for practice* (2nd ed., pp. 539–567). Gaithersburg, MD: Aspen.

Keegan, L. (1998). Alternative & complementary therapies. *Nursing98, 28*(4), 50–53.

Keville, K., & Green, M. (1995). *Aromatherapy: A complete guide to healing art.* Freedom, CA: Crossing Press.

King, M. O., Pettigrew, A. C., & Reed, F. C. (1999). Complementary, alternative, integrative: have nurses kept pace with their clients? *Medsurg Nursing, 8*(4), 249–56.

Kolkmeier, L. G. (1995). Relaxation: Opening the door to change. In B. M. Dossey, L. Keegan, C. E. Guzzetta, & L. G. Kolkmeier (Eds.), *Holistic nursing: A handbook for practice* (2nd ed., pp. 573–608). Gaithersburg, MD: Aspen.

Krieger, D. (1993). *Accepting your power to heal: The personal practice of therapeutic touch.* Santa Fe, NM: Bear & Company Publishing.

Lanfranco, J. (1997). *Acupressure and shiatsu information* [On-line] Available: http://www.geocities.com/HotSprings/4416/acusci.html

Long, J. (1995). Down to earth: An ancient herb for a modern garden. *The Herb Companion, 8*(1), 22.

Mackey, R. B. (1995). Discover the healing power of therapeutic touch. *AJN, 94*(4), 27–33.

Marwick, C. (1995). Should physicians prescribe prayer for health? Spiritual aspects of well-being considered. *Journal of the American Medical Association, 273*(20), 1561–1562.

Mason, J. (1999). Massage: The nursing touch. In Healing touch: An energetic approach by C. P. Hutchison. *AJN, 99*(4), 44.

McGhee, P. (1999). *Health, healing, and the amuse system.* (3rd ed.). Dubuque, IA: Kendall/Hunt.

McGhee, P. (1998). Rx: Laughter. *RN, 69*(7), 50–53.

Meehan, T. C. (1993). Therapeutic touch and postoperative pain: A Rogerian research study. *Nursing Science Quarterly, 6*(2), 69–78.

Mentgen, J. (1996). The clinical practice of healing touch. In D. Hover-Kramer (Ed.), *Healing touch: A resource for health care professionals* (pp. 155–165). Albany, NY: Delmar.

Mills, E. M. (1994). The effect of low-intensity aerobic exercise on muscle strength, flexibility, and balance among sedentary elderly persons. *Nursing Research, 43,* 206–211.

Mornhinweg, G. C., & Voignier, R. R. (1995). Holistic nursing interventions. *Orthopaedic Nursing, 14*(4), 20–24.

Moyers, B. (1995). *Healing and the mind.* New York: Doubleday.

National Institutes of Health (1998). *About the Office of Alternative Medicine* [On-line] Available: http://altmed.od.nih.gov/oam/about/general.shtml#budget

National Institutes of Health (2000). *About the Center for Complementary & Alternative Medicine* (NCCAM). [On-line] Available: http://altmed.od.nih.gov/nccam/about/general.shtml

Nightingale, F. (1969). *Nursing: What it is and what it is not.* New York: Dover Publications.

Nurse Healers-Professional Associates, Inc. (1992). *Therapeutic touch: Teaching guidelines: Beginner's level Krieger/Kunz method.* New York: Author.

Olsen, M., & Sneed, N. (1995). Anxiety and therapeutic touch. *Issues in Mental Health Nursing, 16*(2), 97–108.

O'Neil, C., Avila, J., & Fetrow, C. W. (1999). Herbal medicines: Getting beyond the hype. *Nursing99, 29*(4), 58–61.

Pert, C. (1986). The wisdom of the receptors: Neuropeptides, the emotions, and bodymind. *Advances, 3,* 8–16.

Polunin, M., & Robbins, C. (1995). Eight healing herbs, 1995–1996. *Holistic Health Directory,* 30–34.

Quinn, J. (1993). Psychoimmunologic effects of therapeutic touch on practitioners and recently bereaved recipients: A pilot study. *Advances in Nursing Science, 15*(4), 13–26.

Renner, J. H., Dillard, J. N., & Edelberg, D. (1999). Should the FDA regulate alternative medicines? *Hospital Health Network, 73*(10), 24.

Rossi, E. L. (1993). *The psychobiology of mind body healing: New concepts of therapeutic hypnosis* (rev. ed.). New York: Norton.

Schar, D. (1995). *The backyard medicine chest: An herbal primer.* Washington, DC: Elliot & Clark.

Schroeder-Shecker, T. (1994). Music for the dying. *Journal of Holistic Nursing, 12*(1), 83–99.

Simons, S. (1997). Vegetables and fruits: Natural "Phyters" against disease. Paper presented at the Texas Agricultural Extension service conference.

Snyder, J. R. (1999). Therapeutic touch in hospice care. In Healing touch: An energetic approach by C. P. Hutchison. *AJN, 99*(4), 46.

Spencer, J. W. & Jacobs, J. J. (Eds.) (1999). *Complementary/alternative medicine: An evidence-based approach.* St. Louis, MO: Mosby.

Stedman, M. (1999). Alternatives: You'd better shop around. *Health, 13*(1), 60–66.

Stevenson, C. (1994). The psychophysiological effects of aromatherapy massage following cardiac surgery. *Complementary Therapies in Medicine, 2*(1), 27.

Trevelyan, J. (1993). Aromatherapy. *Nursing Times, 89*(25), 38–40.

Vacca, V. (1998). Back to high touch. *RN, 69*(7), 88.

Walton, J. (1996). Spiritual relationships: A concept analysis. *Journal of Holistic Nursing, 14*(3), 237–250.

Weil, A. (1998). *Natural health, natural medicine: A comprehensive manual for wellness and self-care* (rev ed.). New York: Houghton Mifflin.

Weil, A. (1996). *Spontaneous healing: How to discover and enhance your body's natural ability to maintain and heal itself*. New York: Alfred A. Knopf.

Weiss, R. R., & James, W. D. (1997). Allergic contact dermatitis from aromatherapy. *American Journal of Contact Dermatology, 8*(4), 250.

Wetzel, W. (1993). Healing touch as nursing intervention. *Journal of Holistic Nursing, 11*(3), 277–285.

Wilkinson, S. (1995). Aromatherapy and massage in palliative care. *International Journal of Palliative Nursing, 1*(1), 21.

Wilson, D. F. (1995). Therapeutic touch: Foundations and current knowledge. *Alternative Health Practitioner, 1*(1), 55–63.

Zahourek, R. P., & Larkin, D. (1995). Hypnosis and therapeutic suggestion for managing pain and stress. *Alternative Health Practitioner, 1*(19), 43–55.

Zisselman, M. H., Rovner, B. W., Shmuely, Y., & Ferrie, P. (1996). A pet therapy intervention with geriatric psychiatry inpatients. *American Journal of Occupational Therapy, 50*(1), 47–51.

RESOURCES

The American Association of Therapeutic Humor, 222 South Meramec, Suite 303, St. Louis, MO 63105, 314-863-6232, http://aath.org

American Holistic Nurses' Association, P.O. Box 2130, Flagstaff, AZ 86003-2130, 800-278-AHNA (1461), http://www.ahna.org

Association for Applied Psychophysiology and Biofeedback, 10200 West 44th Avenue, Suite 304, Wheat Ridge, CO 80033-2840, 800-477-8892, 303-422-8436, http://www.aapb.org

Colorado Center for Healing Touch, 198 Union Boulevard, Suite 204, Lakewood, CO 80220, 303-989-0581, http://www.healingtouch.net

Holistic Alliance of Professional Practitioners Entrepreneurs Networkers, Inc. (HAPPEN), P.O. Box 90177, Gainesville, FL 32607, 888-8HAPPEN (42-7736)

Journal of Nursing Jocularity, P.O. Box 40416, Mesa, AZ 85274, 602-835-6165, http://www.jocularity.com, email: cardace@jocularity.com

The Laughter Remedy, 45 North Fullerton, Suite 402, Montclair, NJ 07042, 973-783-8383

Office of Alternative Medicine, OAM Clearinghouse, P.O. Box 8218, Silver Spring, MD 20907-8218, 888-644-6226, http://altmed.od.nih.gov/nccam

Patience Tai Chi Association, P.O. Box 350532, Brooklyn, NY 11235, 718-332-3477

CHAPTER 9
Loss, Grief, and Death

REFERENCES/SUGGESTED READINGS

American Nurses Association (ANA). (1992). Promotion of comfort and relief of pain in dying patients. In *Compendium of position statements on the nurse's role in end-of-life decisions*. Washington, DC: Author.

Andreas, L. (1998). Controlling pain: Keeping a dying patient comfortable. *Nursing98, 28*(1), 70.

Backer, B. A., Hannon, N. R., & Russell, N. A. (1994). *Death and dying: Understanding and care* (2nd ed.). Albany, NY: Delmar.

Barbus, A. J. (1975). The dying person's bill of rights. *AJN, 75*(1), 99.

Beckel, J. (1996). Resolving ethical dilemmas in long-term care. *Journal of Gerontological Nursing, 22*(1), 20–26.

Boon, T. (1998). Don't forget the hospice option. *RN, 61*(2), 30–33.

Boss, P. (1999). *Ambiguous loss: Learning to live with unresolved grief*. Cambridge, MA: Harvard University Press.

Bowlby, J. (1982). *Attachment and loss: Vol. 2. Separation anxiety and anger*. New York: Basic Books.

Bral, E. (1998). Caring for adults with chronic cancer pain. *AJN, 98*(4), 27–32.

Carpenito, L. J. (1997). *Handbook of nursing diagnosis* (7th ed.). Philadelphia: Lippincott.

Cerrudo, J. (1998). Letting go of Abuelo. *American Journal of Nursing, 98*(8), 53.

Corless, I., Germino, B., & Pittman, M. (Eds.). (1995). *A challenge for living: Death, dying, and bereavement*. Boston: Jones and Bartlett.

Czerwiec, M. (1996). When a loved one is dying: Families talk about nursing care. *AJN, 96*(5), 32–36.

deBlois, J. (1994, March). Changing the way we care for the dying. *Health Progress*, 48–52.

Doka, K., Rushton, C. H., & Thorstenson, T. A. (1994). HealthCare Ethics Forum '94: Caregiver distress: If it is so ethical, why does it feel so bad? *American Association Critical-Care Nurses Clinical Issues, 5*(3), 346–352.

Durham, E., & Weiss, L. (1997). How patients die. *American Journal of Nursing, 97*(12), 41–46.

Edelman, C. L., & Mandle, C. L. (1998). *Health promotion throughout the lifespan* (4th ed.). St. Louis, MO: Mosby.

Engle, G. L. (1961). Is grief a disease? *Psychosomatic Medicine, 23*, 18–22.

Engle, G. L. (1964). Grief and grieving. *AJN, 64*(9), 93–98.

Estes, M. E. Z. (2002). *Health assessment & physical examination* (2nd ed.). Albany, NY: Delmar.

Fauri, D. P., & Grimes, D. R. (1994). Bereavement services for families and peers of deceased residents of psychiatric institutions. *Social Work, 39*(2), 185–190.

Ferrell, B. (1998). End-of-life care. *Nursing98, 28*(9), 58.

Forbes, V. (1998). The dying game. *AJN, 98*(9), 50.

Haynor, P. (1998) Meeting the challenge of advance directives, *AJN, 98*(3), 27–32.

Jaffe, C. & Ehrlich, C. (1997). *All kinds of love: Experiencing hospice*. Amityville, NY: Baywood Publishing Co.

Kübler-Ross, E. (1969). *On death and dying*. New York: Macmillan.

Kübler-Ross, E. (1974). *Questions and answers on death and dying*. New York: Macmillan.

Kübler-Ross, E. (1997). *Meaning of our suffering*. Barrytown, NY: Barrytown, Ltd.

Lindemann, E. (1944). Symptomatology and management of acute grief. *American Journal of Psychiatry, 101*, 141–148.

MacGregor, P. (1994). Grief: The unrecognized parental response to mental illness in a child. *Social Work, 39*(2), 160–166.

McCaffery, M., & Pasero, C. (1999). *Pain: Clinical manual for nursing practice* (2nd ed.). St. Louis, MO: Mosby.

McClain, M. E., & Shafer, S. M. (1996). Supporting families after sudden infant death. *Journal of Psychosocial Nursing and Mental Health Services, 34*(4), 30–34.

McGowan, D. (1998). The right to say goodbye. *RN, 61*(5), 84.

North American Nursing Diagnosis Association. (2001). *Nursing diagnoses: Definitions & classification 2001–2002.* Philadelphia: Author.

Pritchett, K., & Lucas, P. (1997a). Death and dying. In B. S. Johnson (Ed.), *Psychiatric–mental health nursing: Adaptation and growth* (4th ed., pp. 206–207). Philadelphia: Lippincott.

Pritchett, K., & Lucas, P. (1997b). Grief and loss. In B. S. Johnson (Ed.), *Psychiatric–mental health nursing: Adaptation and growth* (4th ed., pp. 199–218). Philadelphia: Lippincott.

Puopolo, A. (1999). Gaining confidence to talk about end-of-life care. *Nursing99, 29*(7), 49–51.

Reese, C. D. (1996). Please cry with me: Six ways to grieve. *Nursing96, 26*(8), 56.

Rhymes, J. (1993). Hospice care in the nursing home. *Nursing Home Medicine, 1*(6), 14–16, 22–24.

Roach, S. S., & Nieto, B. C. (1997). *Healing and the grief process.* Albany, NY: Delmar.

Rodebaugh, L., Schwindt, R., & Valentine, F. (1999). How to handle grief with wisdom, *Nursing99, 29*(10), 52–53.

Smith-Stoner, M., & Frost, A. (1998). Coping with grief and loss: Bringing your shadow self into the light. *Nursing98, 28*(2), 49–50.

Smith-Stoner, M. & Frost, A. (1999). How to build your "hope skills." *Nursing99, 29*(9), 49–51

Taylor, M. (1995). Benefits of dehydration in terminally ill clients. *Geriatric Nursing, 16*(6), 271–272.

Taylor, P., & Ferszt, G. (1994). Letting go of a loved one. *Nursing94, 24*(1), 55–56.

Thompson, L. M. (1994). The future of death: Death in the hands of science. *Nursing Outlook, 42,* 175–180.

Ufema, J. (1995a). How to help dying clients feel "safe." *Nursing95, 25*(9), 59.

Ufema, J. (1995b). Insights on death and dying. *Nursing95, 25*(11,12), 19, 22–23.

Ufema, J. (1999). Reflections on death and dying. *Nursing99, 29*(6), 56–59.

Wong, M. M. (1996). *The 1996 national directory of bereavement support groups and services.* Forest Hills, NY: ADM Publishing.

Worden, J. W. (1991). *Grief counseling and grief therapy: A handbook for the mental health practitioner* (2nd ed.). New York: Springer.

RESOURCES

Association for Death Education & Counseling, 638 Prospect Ave., Hartford, CT 06105, 860-586-7503

Choice in Dying, 475 Riverside Drive, New York, NY 10115, 800-989-9455

Hospice Foundation of America, 777 17th Street, #401, Miami Beach, FL 33139, 800-854-3402, http://www.hospicefoundation.org

The National Hospice Organization, 1901 North Moore St., Suite 901, Arlington, VA 22209-1714, 703-243-5900, http://www.nho.org

CHAPTER 10
Fluid, Electrolyte, and Acid–Base Balance

REFERENCES/SUGGESTED READINGS

Bulechek, G., & McCloskey, J. (1999). *Nursing interventions: Effective nursing treatments* (3rd ed). Philadelphia: W. B. Saunders Company.

Burke, S. (1992). *Human anatomy & physiology in health and disease* (3rd ed.). Albany, NY: Delmar.

Castiglione, V. (2000). Hyperkalemia. *AJN, 100*(1), 55–56.

Clayton, K. (1997). Cancer-related hypercalcemia: How to spot it how to manage it. *AJN, 97*(5), 42–48.

Cohen, B. & Wood, D. (2000). *Memmler's the human body in health & disease* (9th ed.). Philadelphia: Lippincott.

Cook, L. (1999). The value of lab values. *AJN, 99*(5), 66–75.

DeLaune, S., & Ladner, P. (1998). *Fundamentals of nursing: Practice & standards.* Albany, NY: Delmar.

Estes, M. E. Z. (2002). *Health assessment & physical examination* (2nd ed.). Albany, NY: Delmar.

Fong, E., Scott, A., Ferris, E., & Skelley, E. (1998). *Body structures and functions* (9th ed.). Albany, NY: Delmar.

Hartshorn, J., Lamborn, M., & Noll, M. (1997). *Introduction to critical care nursing* (2nd ed.). Philadelphia: W. B. Saunders Company.

Hogstel, M. (1994). *Nursing care of the older adult* (3rd ed.). Albany, NY: Delmar.

I.V. therapy: Update97. (1997). *Nursing97, 27*(11), 60–61.

Josephson, D. L. (1999). *Intravenous infusion therapy for nurses: Principles and practice.* Albany, NY: Delmar.

Kee, J. L. (1998). *Laboratory and diagnostic tests with nursing implications.* Englewood Cliffs, NJ: Prentice Hall.

Kee, J., & Paulanka, B. (1999). *Fluids and electrolytes with clinical applications* (6th ed.). Albany, NY: Delmar.

Mader, S. (1997). *Understanding human anatomy & physiology* (3rd ed.). Dubuque, IA: Wm. C. Brown Publishers.

Marieb, E. (1997). *Essentials of human anatomy & physiology* (5th ed.). Redwood City, CA: The Benjamin/Cummings Publishing Co.

Martini, F., & Welch, K. (1997). *Fundamentals of anatomy and physiology* (4th ed.). Englewood Cliffs, NJ: Prentice-Hall.

Masoorli, S. (1995). Know the pitfalls of I.V. therapy. *NSO Risk Advisor, 20*(2), 1,4.

McConnell, E. (1999). Performing pulse oximetry. *Nursing99, 29*(11), 17.

McFarland, M., & Grant, M. (1994). *Nursing implications of laboratory tests* (3rd ed.). Albany, NY: Delmar.

Memmler, R., Cohen, B., & Wood, D. (1996). *The human body in health and disease* (8th ed.). Philadelphia: Lippincott.

Noe, D., & Rock, R. (1994). *Laboratory medicine.* Baltimore: Williams & Wilkins.

North American Nursing Diagnosis Association (NANDA). (2001). *Nursing diagnoses: Definitions & classification 2001–2002.* Philadelphia: Author.

Scanlon, V., & Sanders, T. (1999). *Essentials of anatomy and physiology* (3rd ed.). Philadelphia: F. A. Davis.

Tasota, F., & Wesmiller, S. (1998). Balancing act: Keeping blood pH in equilibrium. *Nursing98, 28*(12), 34–40.

Thibodeau, G. (1999). *Structure & function of the body* (10th ed.). St. Louis, MO: Mosby.

White, J., & Barnes, R. (1983). *Hands on biology, manual* (2nd ed.). Corpus Christi, TX: L P Enterprises.

White, V. (1997). Hyperkalemia. *AJN, 97*(6), 35.

Wong, F. (1999). A new approach to ABG interpretation. *AJN, 99*(8), 34–36.

RESOURCES

Intravenous Nurses Society, Fresh Pond Square, 10 Fawcett Street, Cambridge, MA 02138, 617-441-3008, http://www.ins1.org

CHAPTER 11
IV Therapy

REFERENCES/SUGGESTED READINGS

Asbaghi, Z. (1995). Questions and answers about blood transfusions. *Nursing95, 25*(2), 32C–32G.

Bulechek, G.M., & McCloskey, J.C. (2000). *Nursing interventions: Essential nursing treatments* (3rd ed.). Philadelphia: W. B. Saunders Company.

Charting Tips. (2000). Documenting IV therapy, part I. *Nursing2000 30*(2), 73.

Daniels, J., & Smith, L. (1999). *Clinical calculations* (4th ed.). Albany, NY: Delmar.

Drug information for the health care professional (17th ed.). (1997). Rockville, MD: USP Convention.

Ellenberger, A. (1999). Starting an IV line. *Nursing99, 29*(3), 56–59.

Fitzpatrick, L., & Fitzpatrick, T. (1997). Blood transfusion: Keeping your patient safe. *Nursing97, 27*(8), 34–41

Goldy, D. (1998). Circulatory overload secondary to blood transfusion. *American Journal of Nursing, 98*(7), 33.

Hadaway, L. C. (1999a). Choosing the right vascular access device, part I. *Nursing99, 29*(2), 18.

Hadaway, L. C. (1999b). Choosing the right vascular access device, part II. *Nursing99, 29*(7), 28–29.

Hadaway, L. C. (1999c). IV infiltration: Not just a peripheral problem. *Nursing99, 29*(9), 41–47.

Hartshorn, J., Lamborn, M., & Noll, M. (1997). *Introduction to critical care nursing* (2nd ed.). Philadelphia: W. B. Saunders Company.

I.V. therapy: Update97. (1997). *Nursing97, 27*(11), 60–61.

Josephson, D. L. (1999). *Intravenous infusion therapy for nurses: Principles and practice*. Albany, NY: Delmar.

Kee, J., & Paulanka, B. (1999). *Fluids and electrolytes with clinical applications* (6th ed.). Albany, NY: Delmar.

Larouere, E. (1999). Deaccessing an implanted port. *Nursing99, 29*(6), 60–61.

Macklin, D. (2000). Removing a PICC. *AJN, 100*(1), 52–54.

North American Nursing Diagnosis Association. (2001). *Nursing diagnoses: Definitions & classification 2001–2002.* Philadelphia: NANDA.

Pickar, G. (1999). *Dosage calculation* (6th ed.). Albany, NY: Delmar.

Rice, J. (1998). *Medications & mathematics for the nurse* (8th ed.). Albany, NY: Delmar.

Saxton, D., & O'Neill, N. (1998). *Math and meds for nurses.* Albany, NY: Delmar.

Shannon, M., Wilson, B., & Stang, C. (1990). *Appleton & Lange's 1999 drug guide.* Norwalk, CT: Appleton & Lange.

Springhouse Corporation. (2000). *Nursing2000 drug handbook.* Springhouse, PA: Author.

Wilson, B., & Shannon, M. (1997). *Dosage calculations: A simplified approach* (3rd ed.). Norwalk, CT: Appleton & Lange.

Wise, M. (1997). Understanding needle-free access devices. *Nursing97, 27*(7), 32.

Spratto, G. & Woods, A. (2000). *PDR nurse's handbook 2000.* Albany, NY: Delmar.

RESOURCES

Intravenous Nurses Society, Fresh Pond Square, 10 Fawcett Street, Cambridge, MA 02138, 616-441-3008, http://www.ins1.org

CHAPTER 12
Health Assessment

REFERENCES/SUGGESTED READINGS

American Heart Association (AHA). (1987). *Recommendations for human blood pressure determination.* (AHA Publication No. 701005). Dallas, TX: Author.

Andresen, G. (1998). Assessing the older patient. *RN, 61*(3), 46–55.

Bickley, L. S. (1999). *A guide to physical examination and history taking* (7th ed.). Phildelphia: Lippincott.

Bosley, C. L. (1995). Assessing cardiac output: Don't stop at the heart. *Nursing95, 25*(9), 43–45.

Crow, S. (1997). Your guide to gloves. *Nursing97, 27*(3), 26–28.

DeLaune, S., & Ladner, P. (1998). *Fundamentals of nursing: Standards & practice.* Albany, NY: Delmar.

Estes, M. E. Z. (2002). *Health assessment & physical examination* (2nd ed.). Albany, NY: Delmar.

Firth, P., & Watanabe, S. (1996). *Women's health.* Albany, NY: Delmar.

Fuller, J., & Schaller-Ayers, J. (1999). *Health assessment: A nursing approach.* Philadelphia: Lippincott.

Gallauresi, B. A. (1998). Pulse oximeters. *Nursing98, 28*(9), 31.

Hanson, C. (1996). *Delmar's instant nursing assessment: Gerontologic.* Albany, NY: Delmar.

Hodge, P. & Ullrich, S. (1999). Does your assessment include alternative therapies? *RN, 62*(6), 47–49.

Kirton, C. A. (1997). Assessing bowel sounds. *Nursing97, 27*(3), 64.

Klingman, L. (1999). Assessing the female reproductive system. *AJN, 99*(8), 37–43.

Klingman, L. (1999). Assessing the male genitalia. *AJN, 99*(7), 47–50.

Lazar, J. S. & O'Conner, B. B. (1997). Talking with patients about their use of alternative therapies. *Complementary and Alternative Therapies in Primary Care, 24*(4), 699.

Murray, R. B., & Zentner, J. P. (1997). *Health assessment and promotion through the lifespan* (6th ed.). Norwalk: Appleton & Lange.

O'Hanlon-Nichols, T. (1999). Neurologic assessment. *AJN, 99*(6), 44–50.

O'Hanlon-Nichols, T. (1998). Basic assessment series: Musculoskeletal system. *AJN, 98*(6), 48–52.

O'Hanlon-Nichols, T. (1998). Basic assessment series: Gastrointestinal system. *AJN, 98*(4), 48–53.

O'Hanlon-Nichols, T. (1998). Basic assessment series: The adult pulmonary system. *AJN, 98*(2), 39–45.

O'Hanlon-Nichols, T. (1997). Basic assessment series: The adult cardiovascular system. *AJN, 97*(12), 34–40.

Owen, A. (1998). Respiratory assessment revisited. *Nursing98, 28*(4), 48–49.

Rice, K. L. (1999). Measuring thigh BP. *Nursing99, 29*(8), 58–59.

Rice, K. L. (1998). Sounding out blood flow with a doppler device. *Nursing98, 28*(9), 56–57.

Taylor, C., Lillis, C., & LeMone, P. (1997). *Fundamentals of nursing: The art and science of nursing care* (3d ed.). Philadelphia: Lippincott.

Warner, P., Rowe, T., & Whipple, B. (1999). Shedding light on the sexual history. *AJN, 99*(6), 34–40.

Weber, J. (1997). *Health assessment in nursing.* Philadelphia: Lippincott.

CHAPTER 13
Diagnostic Tests

REFERENCES/SUGGESTED READINGS

Beattie, S. (1999). Cut the risks for cardiac cath patients. *RN, 62*(1), 50–54.

Cook, L. (1999). The value of lab values. *AJN, 99*(5), 66–75.

Dammel, T. (1997). Fecal occult-blood testing: Looking for hidden danger. *Nursing97, 27*(7), 44–45.

DeLaune, S., & Ladner, P. (1998). *Fundamentals of nursing: Standards & Practice*. Albany, NY: Delmar.

Ernst, D. (1999). Collecting blood culture specimens. *Nursing99, 29*(7), 56–58.

Gallauresi, B. (1998). Pulse oximeters. *Nursing98, 28*(9), 31.

Gibbar-Clements, T., Shirrell, D., & Free, C. (1997). PT and APTT: Seeing beyond the numbers. *Nursing97, 27*(7), 49–51.

Guyton, A. C. & Hall, J., (1996). *Textbook of medical physiology* (9th ed.). Philadelphia: W. B. Saunders Company.

Hill, J., & Newton, J. (1998). Contrast echo: Your role at the bedside. *RN, 61*(10), 32–35.

Hospital Nursing Section. (1995). Interpreting ECF waveform components. *Nursing95, 25*(6), 32C-32F.

Kee, J. L. (1998). *Laboratory and diagnostic tests with nursing implications*. (5th ed.). Upper Saddle River, NJ: Prentice Hall.

Laxson, C., & Titler, M. (1994). Drawing coagulation studies from arterial lines: An integrated literature review. *American Journal of Critical Care, 3*(1), 16–23.

McFarland, M., & Grant, M. (1994). *Nursing implications of laboratory tests* (3rd ed.). Albany, NY: Delmar.

Montes, P. (1997). Managing outpatient cardiac catheterization. *AJN, 97*(8), 34–37.

Siconolfi, L. (1995). Clarifying the complexity of liver function test. *Nursing95, 25*(5), 39–44.

Somerson, S., Husted, C. & Sicilia, M. (1995). Insights into conscious sedation. *AJN, 95*(6), 26–33.

Thompson, M., & Coppens, N. (1994). The effects of guided imagery on anxiety levels and movement of clients undergoing magnetic resonance imaging. *Holistic Nurse Practice, 8*(2), 59–69.

Wolfe, S. (1997). The great mammogram debate. *RN, 60*(8), 41–44.

RESOURCES

National Library of Medicine, http://www.nlm.nih.gov (then click on "Search MEDLINE")

National Network of Libraries of Medicine (NN/LM) Regional Medical Libraries, 800-338-7657

CHAPTER 14
Pain Management

REFERENCES/SUGGESTED READINGS

Acello, B. (2000). Meeting JCAHO standards for pain control. *Nursing2000, 30*(3), 52–54.

Agency for Health Care Policy and Research. (1992). *Clinical practice guideline: Acute pain management: Operative or medical procedures and Trauma*. (AHCPR Publication No. 92–0032). Rockville, MD: U.S. Department of Health and Human Services.

Agency for Health Care Policy and Research. (1994). *Clinical practice guideline: Management of cancer pain*. (AHCPR Publication No. 94–0592). Rockville, MD: U.S. Department of Health and Human Services.

American Pain Society. (1999). *Principles of analgesic use in the treatment of acute pain and cancer pain* (4th ed.). Skokie, IL: Author.

Beecher, H. K. (1956). Relationship of significance of wound to pain experienced. *JAMA, 161,* 1609–1613.

Berkowitz, C. (1997). Epidural pain control—Your job, too. *RN, 60*(8), 22–27.

Bonica, J. J. (Ed.). (1990). *The management of pain* (2d ed.). Philadelphia: Lea and Febiger.

Brand, P., & Yancey, P. (1993). *Pain: The gift nobody wants*. New York: HarperCollins.

Brown, J., Horn, J., Calbert, J., & Nolan-Goslin, K. (1999). A question of pain. *Nursing99, 29*(10), 48–51.

Chapman, G. F. (1999). Documenting a pain assessment. *Nursing99, 29*(11), 25.

Cleeland, C. S., Gonin, R., Hatfield, A. K., Edmonson, J. H., Blum, R. H., Stewart, J. A., & Pandya, K. J. (1994). Pain and its treatment in outpatients with metastatic cancer. *New England Journal of Medicine, 330,* 592–596.

Compton, P. (1999). Managing a drug abuser's pain. *Nursing99, 29*(5), 26–28.

Cousins, N. (1991). *Anatomy of an illness as perceived by the patient*. Toronto: Bantam.

Derby, S. A. (1999). Opioid conversion guidelines for managing adult cancer pain. *AJN, 99*(10), 62–65.

Donovan, M., Dillon, P., & McGuire, L. (1987). Incidence and characteristics of pain in a sample of medical-surgical inpatients. *Pain, 30,* 69–78.

Dubner, R. (1991). Pain and hyperalgesia following tissue injury: New mechanisms and new treatments. *Pain, 44,* 213–214.

Faries, J. (1997a). Taking another route to pain relief. *Nursing97, 27*(6), 28.

Faries, J. (1997b). Assessing pediatric pain. *Nursing97, 27*(8), 18.

Faries, J. (1998a). Easing your patient's postoperative pain. *Nursing98, 28*(6), 58–60.

Faries, J. (1998b). Making a smooth switch from IV analgesia. *Nursing98, 28*(7), 26.

Gordon, D., & Ward, S. (1995). Correcting patient misconceptions about pain. *AJN, 95*(7), 43–45.

Haddad, A. (2000). Ethics in action: Treating pain in substance abusers. *RN, 63*(1), 21–24.

Joint Commission on Accreditation of Healthcare Organizations (JCAHO). (1999). Joint Commission focuses on pain management. [On-line] Available: http://www.jcaho.org/news/nb207.html

Juarez, G. (1995). When culture clashes with pain control. *Nursing95, 25*(5), 90.

Kedziera, P. (1998). The two faces of pain. *RN, 61*(2), 45–46.

Liebeskind J., & Melzack, R. (1987). The International Pain Foundation: Meeting a need for education in pain management. *Pain, 30,* 1–2.

Loeb, J. L. (1999). Pain management in long-term care. *AJN, 99*(2), 48–52.

Markey, B. T., & Graham, M. (1997). Management of chronic pain with epidural steriods. *AORN Journal, 65*(4), 791.

McCaffery, M. (1979). *Nursing management of the patient with pain* (2d ed.). Philadelphia: Lippincott.

McCaffery, M. (1999a). Pain control. *AJN, 99*(8), 18.

McCaffery, M. (1999b). Understanding your patient's pain tolerance. *Nursing99, 29*(12), 17.

McCaffery, M., & Beebe, A. (1989). *Pain: Clinical manual for nursing practice*. St. Louis, MO: Mosby.

McCaffery, M. & Ferrell, B. R. (1999). Opioids and pain management. *Nursing99, 29*(3), 48–52.

McCaffery, M., & Pasero, C. (1999). *Pain: Clinical manual* (2nd ed.). St. Louis, MO: Mosby.

McDevitt, M. J. (1995). A(TENS)tion! *Nursing95, 25*(12), 46–47.

McGuire, D. B., Yarbro, C. H., & Ferrell, B. R. (1995). *Cancer pain management* (2d ed.). Boston: Jones and Bartlett.

Melzack, R., & Wall, P. D. (1965). Pain mechanisms: A new theory. *Science, 150,* 971–979.

Merskey, J., & Bogduk, N. (Eds.). (1994). *Classification of chronic pain* (2d ed., pp. 209–214). Task Force on Taxonomy. Seattle, WA: IASP Press.

North American Nursing Diagnosis Association. (2001). *Nursing diagnoses: Definitions and classification, 2001–2002.* Philadelphia: Author.

Page, G. G., Ben-Eliyahu, S., Yirmiya, R., & Liebeskind, J. C. (1993). Morphine attenuates surgery-induced enhancement of metastatic colonization in rats. *Pain, 54*(1), 21–28.

Pasero, C. (1999). Using superficial cooling for pain relief. *AJN, 99*(3), 24.

Pasero, C. (2000). Oral patient-controlled analgesia. *AJN, 100*(3), 24.

Pasero, C. & McCaffery, M. (2000). Reversing respiratory depression with naloxone. *AJN, 100*(2), 26.

Portenoy, R. K., Payne, R, et al. (1999). Oral transmucosal fentanyl citrate (OTFC) for the treatment of breakthrough pain in cancer patients: A controlled dose titration study. *Pain, 79,* 303.

Poulain, P., Langlade, A., & Goldberg, J. (1997). Cancer pain management in the home. *Pain Clinical Updates, 5*(1). Internet access http://www.halcyon.com/iasp/PCU97a.html.

Schecter, N. L., Berde, C. B., & Yaster, M. (Eds.). (1993). *Pain in infants, children, and adolescents.* Baltimore, MD: Williams & Wilkins.

Spratto, G., & Woods, A. (2000). *PDR® Nurse's Drug Handbook™.* Albany, NY: Delmar.

Stevens, B. (1994). Nursing management of pain in children. In C. L. Betz, M. M. Hunsberger, & S. Wright (Eds.), *Family-centered nursing care of children* (2nd ed.). Philadelphia: W. B. Saunders Company.

Strevy, S. (1998). Myths and facts about pain. *RN, 61*(2), 42–45.

Thomas, M., & Lundeberg, T. (1996). Does acupuncture work? *Pain Clinical Updates, 4*(3). Internet access http://www.halcyon.com/iasp/PCU96c.html

Travell, J. G., & Simons, D. G. (1983, 1998). *Travell & Simon's myofascial pain and dysfunction: The trigger point manual* (2d ed.), (Vols. 1 & 2). Baltimore: Lippincott.

Vasudevan, S. V. (1993). *Pain: A four letter word you can live with.* Milwaukee, WI: Montgomery Media.

Wong, D. L., Hockenberry-Eaton, M., Wilson, D., & Winkelstein, M. L. (1999). *Whaley & Wong's nursing care of infants and children* (6th ed.). St. Louis, MO: Mosby.

World Health Organization. (1986). *Cancer pain relief.* Geneva, Switzerland: Author.

World Health Organization. (1990). Cancer pain relief and palliative care. *Report of a WHO expert committee [World Health Organization Technical Report Series, 804].* Geneva, Switzerland: Author.

RESOURCES

Agency for Health Care Policy and Research (AHCPR), Office of Health Care Information, Executive Office Center, Suite 501, 2101 East Jefferson St., Rockville, MD 20852, http://www.ahcpr.gov

AHCPR Clearinghouse, P.O. Box 8547, Silver Spring, MD 20907-8547, 800-358-9295, http://www.ahcpr.gov

- Clinical Practice Guideline for managing acute pain. Available in three formats: (1) The clinical practice guideline (Publication No. 92-0032); (2) Quick reference guides (Adults—No. 92-0019 and Pediatric—No. 92-0020); and (3) Pain Control after Surgery: A Patient's Guide (No. 92-0021)
- Clinical Practice Guideline for managing cancer pain. Available in three formats: (1) The clinical practice guideline (Publication No. 94-0592); (2) Quick reference guides (Adults—No. 94-0593 and Pediatric—No. 92-0594); and (3) Patient's Guide (No. 94-0595)

American Chronic Pain Association, c/o P. Cowan, P.O. Box 850, Rocklin, CA 95677-0850, 916-632-0922, http://www.theacpa.org

American Pain Society (APS), 4700 W. Lake Avenue, Glenview, IL 60025, 847-375-4715, http://www.ampainsoc.org

American Society of Pain Management Nurses, 7794 Grow Drive, Pensacola, FL 32514, 888-342-7766

International Association for the Study of Pain (IASP), 909 Forty-third Street N.E., Suite 306, Seattle, WA 98105-6020, 206-547-6409, http://www.halcyon.com/iasp

Joint Commission on Accreditation of Healthcare Organizations (JCAHO), One Renaissance Boulevard, Oakbrook Terrace, IL 60181-4294, 630-792-5000, http://www.jcaho.org

National Chronic Pain Outreach Association, P.O. Box 274, Millboro, VA 24460-0274

National Committee on Treatment of Intractable Pain, P.O. Box 9553, Friendship Station, Washington, DC 20016-1553, 202-944-8140

National Headache Foundation, 428 W. St. James Place, 2nd Floor, Chicago, IL 60614-2750, 800-843-2256, http://www.headaches.org

National Hospice Organization, 1901 North Moore Street, Suite 901, Arlington, VA 22209-1714, 703-243-5900, 800-646-6460, http://www.nho.org

Nursing Research and Education/City of Hope Pain Resource Center, 1500 East Duarte Road, Duarte, CA 91010, 626-359-8111 ext. 3829, http://mayday.coh.org

Journals

Chronic Pain Letter, Box 1303, Old Chelsea Station, New York, NY 10011

The Clinical Journal of Pain, Lippincott, 2275 Washington Square, Philadelphia, PA 19106, 800-638-3030

The Journal of Pain and Symptom Management, Elsevier Publishing Co., Inc., Journal Fulfillment Department, P.O. Box 882, Madison Square Station, New York, NY 10160-0200

Pain, International Association for the Study of Pain, 909 Forty-third Street N.E., Suite 306, Seattle, WA 98105-6020, 206-547-6409

CHAPTER 15
Anesthesia

REFERENCES/SUGGESTED READINGS

American Association of Nurse Anesthetists (AANA). (2000a). Information. [On-line] Available: http://www.aana.com/information

American Association of Nurse Anesthetists (AANA). (2000b). HCFA announces it will remove physician supervision requirement for nurse anesthetists. [On-line] Available: http://www.aana.com/press/0023.asp

Ben-David, B., Vaida, S., Collins, G., Naum, M., & Gaitini, L. (1994). Transient paraplegia secondary to an epidural catheter. *Anesthesia & Analgesia, 79,* 598–600.

Berkowitz, C. (1997). Epidural pain control—Your job, too. *RN, 60*(8), 22–27.

Clinical News. (1999). "NPO after midnight" outdated? *AJN, 99*(2), 18.

Connolly, M. (1999). Postdural puncture headache. *AJN, 99*(11), 48–49.

Crenshaw, J. (1999). New guidelines for preoperative fasting. *AJN, 99*(4), 49.

Horlocker, T. T., Wedel, D. J., Schroeder, D. R., Rose, S. H., Elliott, B.A., McGregor, D. G., & Wong, G. Y. (1995). Pre-operativeantiplatelet therapy does not increase the risk of spinal hematoma associated with regional anesthesia. *Anesthesia & Analgesia, 80,* 303–309.

Kost, M. (1999). Conscious sedation: Guarding your patient against complications. *Nursing99, 29*(4), 34–39.

Liu, S., Chiu, A. A., Carpenter, R. L., Mulroy, M. F., Allen, H. W., Neal, J. M., & Pollock, J. E. (1995). Fentanyl prolongs lidocaine spinal anesthesia without prolonging recovery. *Anesthesia & Analgesia, 80,* 730–734.

Messinger, J. S., Hoffman, L. A., O'Donnell, J. M., & Dunworth, B. A. (1999). Getting conscious sedation right. *AJN, 99*(12), 44–49.

Naber, L., Jones, G., & Halm, M. (1994). Epidural analgesia: For effective pain control. *Critical Care Nurse, 14*(5), 69.

Pasero, C., & McCaffery, M. (1999). Providing epidural analgesia. *Nursing99, 29*(8), 34–39.

Scott, J. C., & Stanski, D. R. (1987). Decreased fentanyl and alfentanil dose requirements with age: A simultaneous pharmacokinetic and pharmacodynamic evaluation. *Journal of Pharmacology and Experimental Therapeutics, 240,* 159–166.

RESOURCES

American Association of Nurse Anesthetists, 222 South Prospect Avenue, Park Ridge, IL 60068-4001, 847-692-7050, Fax 847-692-6068, http://www.aana.com

American Journal of Anesthesiology, 26 Main Street, Chatham, NJ 07928-2402, 973-701-8900, http://www.amjanesthesiology.com

American Society of Anesthesiologists, 520 N. Northwest Highway, Park Ridge, IL 60068-2573, 847-825-5586, Fax 847-825-1692, http://www.asahq.org

American Society of Peri Anesthesia Nurses, 6900 Grove Road, Thorofare, NJ 08086, 856-845-5557, Fax 856-848-1881, http://www.aspan.org

American Society of Regional Anesthesia, PO Box 11086, Richmond, VA 23230-1086, 804-282-0010, Fax 804-282-0090, http://www.asra.com

Anesthesia Patient Safety Foundation, Room 9562 E. B., 1400 Locust Street, Pittsburgh, PA 15219-5166, e-mail info@apsf.org

Foundation for Anesthesia Education and Research, Charlton Building, Mayo Clinic, 200 First Street SW, Rochester, MN 55905, 507-266-6866, Fax 507-284-0120, http://www.faer.org

Society for Education in Anesthesia, 1910 Byrd Avenue, Suite 100, PO Box 11086, Richmond, VA 23230-1086, 804-282-5427, http://www.seahq.org

CHAPTER 16
Nursing Care of the Surgical Client

REFERENCES/SUGGESTED READINGS

Aldrete, J. (1995). The post-anesthesia recovery score revisited. *Journal of Clinical Anesthesiology, 7*(1), 89–91.

Association of Operating Room Nurses (1995a). *Standards and recommended practices.* Denver, CO: Author.

Association of Operating Room Nurses. (1995b) Surgical attire; recommended practices; biological monitors; sterile packages. *AORN Journal, 61*(5).

Atkinson, L., & Fortunato, N. (1996). *Berry & Kohn's operating room technique* (8th ed.). St. Louis, MO: Mosby.

Beare, P. G., & Myers, J. L. (1998). *Adult health nursing* (3rd ed.). St. Louis, MO: Mosby.

Black, J. M., & Matassarin-Jacobs, E. (1997). *Luckmann and Sorensen's medical–surgical nursing: A psychophysiologic approach* (5th ed.). Philadelphia: W.B. Saunders Company.

Brenner, Z. (1999). Preventing postoperative complications. *Nursing99, 29*(10), 34–39.

Bryant, R. A. (Ed.). (2000). *Acute and chronic wounds: Nursing management.* St. Louis, MO: Mosby.

Burden, N., Defazio-Quinn, D. M., & O'Brien, D. (2000). *Ambulatory surgical nursing.* Philadelphia: W. B. Saunders Company.

Cizzell, J. (1994). Back to basics: Test your wound assessment skills. *AJN, 94*(6), 34–35.

Erwin-Toth, P., & Hocevar, B. (1995). Wound care: Selecting the right dressing. *AJN, 95*(2), 46–51.

Fairchild, S. (1996). *Perioperative nursing: Principles and practice* (2nd ed.). Boston: Jones and Bartlett.

Gilchrist, B. (1990). Washing and dressings after surgery. *Journal of the Wound Care Society, 86*(50), 71.

Goodman, K. (1995, September). Transitional diet. *Current topics in nutrition support.* Fort Wayne, IN: Lutheran Hospital of Indiana, Inc.

Goodman, K. (1995, October). Post-op or transitional feeding. *Current topics in nutrition support.* Fort Wayne, IN: Lutheran Hospital of Indiana, Inc.

Grogan, T. (1999). Bringing bloodless surgery into the mainstream. *Nursing99, 29*(11), 58–61.

Hogstel, M. (1994). *Nursing care of the older adult* (3rd ed). Albany, NY: Delmar.

Ignatavicius, D. D., Workman, M. L., & Mishler, M. A. (1999). *Medical–surgical Nursing Across the Health Care Continuum* (3rd ed.). Philadelphia: W. B. Saunders Company.

Lewis, S. M., Collier, I. C., & Heitkemper, M. M. (1996). *Medical–surgical nursing: Assessment and management of clinical problems* (4th ed.). St. Louis, MO: Mosby.

Litwack, K. (1995). *Post anesthesia care nursing* (2nd ed.). St. Louis, MO: Mosby.

Motta, G. (1993). How moisture retentive dressings promote healing. *Nursing 93, 23*(12), 26–33.

Phillips, J. (1998). Wound dehiscence. *Nursing98, 28*(3), 33.

Phipps, W. J., Cassmeyer, V. L., Sands, J. K., & Lehman, M. K. (1999). *Medical–surgical nursing: Concepts and clinical practice* (6th ed.). St. Louis, MO: Mosby.

Smeltzer, S. C., & Bare, B. G. (1996). *Brunner and Suddarth's textbook of medical–surgical nursing* (8th ed.). Philadelphia: Lippincott.

Talabiska, D. G. (1995). Malnutrition in the elderly. *Newlines in Multi-Vitamin Infusion, 4*(2), 1, 2, 6.

Vernon, S., & Molnar-Pfeifer, G. (1997). Are you ready for bloodless surgery? *AJN, 97*(9), 40–47.

RESOURCES

American Board of Post Anesthesia Nursing Certification, 6900 Grove Road, Thorofare, NJ 08086, 609-845-5557

Association of Peri Operating Room Nurses (AORN), 2170 South Parker Road, Suite 300, Denver, CO 80231-3711, 303-755-6300, http://www.aorn.org

National Second Surgical Opinion Program, Administrative Office of Public Affairs, 330 Independence Avenue SW, Washington, DC 20201, 800-638-6833, 202-245-6183

CHAPTER 17
Nursing Care of the Oncology Client

REFERENCES/SUGGESTED READINGS

Agency for Health Care Policy and Research. (1994). *Clinical practice guidelines: Management of cancer pain* (AHCPR

Publication No. 94 0592). Rockville, MD: U.S. Department of Health & Human Services.

Alfaro-LeFevre, R., Blicharz, M., Flynn, A., & Boyer, M. (1992). *Drug Handbook: A nursing process approach.* Redwood, CA: Addison-Wesley.

American Cancer Society. (1998). Cancer facts and figures— 1998. Atlanta, GA: Author.

American Cancer Society (ACS). (2000). 2000 Facts and Figures. [On-line] Available http://www.cancer.org/statistics/cff2000/basicfacts.html

American Pain Society. (1992). *Principles of analgesic use in the treatment of acute and chronic cancer pain* (3d ed.). Skokie, IL: Author.

Baird, S., Donehower, M., Stalsbroten, V., & Ades, T. (Eds.) (1997). *A cancer source book for nurses* (7th ed.). Atlanta, GA: American Cancer Society.

Belcher, A. (1992). *Cancer nursing.* St. Louis, MO: Mosby.

Blackburn, G. (1998). Wasting away: Cancer cachexia. *Health News, 4*(4), 4. Waltham, MA: Massachusetts Medical Society.

Bral, E. (1998). Caring for adults with chronic cancer pain. *AJN, 4*(98), 27–32.

Chiramannil, A. (1998). Lung Cancer. *American Journal of Nursing, 4*(98), 46–47.

Clayton, K. (1997). Cancer-related hypercalcemia: How to spot it, how to manage it. *AJN, 97*(5), 42–48.

Erickson, J. (1994, November). Update on Hodgkin's Disease. *Nurse Practitioner,* 63–67.

Estes, M. E. Z. (2002). *Health assessment & physical examination* (2nd ed.). Albany, NY: Delmar.

Fieler, B. K. (1997). Side effects and quality of life in patients receiving high-dose rate brachytherapy. *Oncology Nursing Forum, 24*(3), 545.

Greifzu, S. (1998). Fighting cancer fatigue. *RN, 61*(8), 41–43.

Hansen, C. (1995, January). Colorectal cancer: A preventable disease. *Physician Assistant,* 15–26.

Held-Warmkessel, J. (1998). Chemotherapy complications: Helping your patient cope with adverse reactions. *Nursing98 4*(28), 41–45.

Kediziera, P. (1998). The two faces of pain. *RN, 61*(2), 45–46.

Kohr, J. (1995). Measuring your patient's pain. *RN, 58*(4), 39–40.

Lewis, S. & Collier, I. (1996). *Medical–surgical nursing: Assessment and management of clinical problems* (4th ed.). St. Louis, MO: Mosby.

McCaffery, M., & Ferrell, B. (1994, July). How to use the new AHCPR cancer pain guidelines. *AJN,* 42–47.

McCarron, E. (1995, June). Supporting the families of cancer patients. *Nursing95,* 48–51.

Myers, J. S. (2000). Chemotherapy-induced hypersensitivity reaction. *AJN, 100*(4), 53–54.

Noonan, E. (1998, May 4). Drug combination found to eliminate cancer in mice. *Corpus Christi Caller Times.*

Ottery, F. (1994, March/April). Cancer cachexia prevention, early diagnosis and management. *Cancer Practice, 2*(2), 123–131.

Otto, S. (1997). *Oncology nursing* (3rd ed.). St. Louis, MO: Mosby.

Phipps, W. J., Sands, Marek, J. F., (1999). *Medical-Surgical Nursing: Concepts and Clinical Practice* (6th ed.). St. Louis, MO: Mosby.

Porth, C. (1998). *Pathophysiology concepts of altered health states* (5th ed.), Philadelphia: Lippincott.

Researchers say new drug may boost effects of cancer radiation. (1998, May 12). *Corpus Christi Caller Times.*

Scherer, J., & Timby, B. (1999). *Introductory medical–surgical nursing* (7th ed.). Philadelphia: Lippincott.

Schweid, L., & Werner-McCullough, M. (1994, September). Will you recognize these oncological crises? *RN,* 23–27.

Smeltzer, S., & Bare, B. (1996). *Brunner and Suddarth's text book of medical–surgical nursing* (8th ed.). Philadelphia: Lippincott.

Tamoxifen for breast cancer prevention. (1998, December 15). *Healthnews, 4*(15).

Thaler-DeMers, D. (2000). The cancer survival toolbox. *AJN, 100*(4), 52.

Weber, M. (1995). Clinical snapshot: Chemotherapy-induced nausea and vomiting. *AJN, 95*(4).

White, L., & Spitz, M. (1994). Cancer risk and early detection assessment. *Capsules and Comments in Oncology Nursing, 2*(1), 2–3.

Wilkes, G. (2000). Nutrition: The forgotten ingredient in cancer care. *AJN, 100*(4), 46–51.

Woodward, W., & Thobaben, M. (1994). Special home health care nursing challenges: Patients with cancer. *Home Health Care Nurse, 12*(3), 33–37.

RESOURCES

American Cancer Society (ACS), 1599 Clifton Road, NE, Atlanta, GA 30329, 800-ACS-2345, http://www.cancer.org

National Alliance of Breast Cancer Organizations, 212-719-0154, http://www.nabco.org

National Coalition for Cancer Survivorship (NCCS), 1010 Wayne Avenue, Suite 770, Silver Spring, MD 20910-5600, 877-622-7937, http://www.cansearch.org

Office of Cancer Communications, National Cancer Institute, Building 31, Room 10A03, Bethesda, MD 20892-2580, 800-4-CANCER, http://www.nci.nih.gov

Y-ME National Organization for Breast Cancer Information and Support, 800-221-2141, http://www.y-me.org

CHAPTER 18
Nursing Care of the Client: Respiratory System

REFERENCES/SUGGESTED READINGS

American Cancer Society (ACS). (1998). *Cancer facts and figures 1998.* Atlanta, GA: Author.

American Lung Association. (2000). *Tuberculosis (TB).* [On-line] Available: http://www.lungusa.org/diseases/lungtb.html

Deglin, J. & Vallerand, A. (2001). *Davis's drug guide for nurses* (7th ed.). Philadelphia: F. A. Davis Company.

Chrisp, D. (2000). Tension pneumothorax. *Nursing2000, 30*(5), 33.

deWit, S. (1998). *Essentials of medical–surgical nursing.* (4th ed.). Philadelphia. W. B. Saunders Company.

Estes, M. E. Z. (2002). *Health assessment & physical examination* (2nd ed.). Albany, NY: Delmar.

Jones, L., & Hannum, D. (1998). Playing it safe with a particulate respirator. *Nursing98, 28*(1), 50–51.

Karch, A. (1998). *1998 Lippincott's nursing drug guide.* Philadelphia: Lippincott.

King, M. & Tomasic, D. (1999). Treating TB today. *RN, 62*(6), 26–30.

O'Hanlon-Nichols, T. (1998). Basic assessment series: The adult pulmonary system. *AJN, 98*(2), 39–45.

Owen, A. (1998). Respiratory assessment revisited. *Nursing98, 28*(4), 48–49.

Perkins, L. & Shortall, S. (2000). Ventilation without intubation. *RN, 63*(1), 34–38.

Phipps, W., Sands, J., & Marek, J. (1999). *Medical-surgical nursing: Concepts and clinical practice* (6th ed.). St. Louis, MO: Mosby.

RNWeb. (2000). *Trauma! Chest injuries.* [On-line] Available: http://www.RNWeb.com/ce/199/chestblt.html

RNWeb. (1999). *Treating TB today.* [On-line] Available: http://www.RNWeb.com/ce/699/treating.html

Shortall, S. & Perkins, L. (1999). Interpreting the ins and outs of pulmonary function tests. *Nursing99, 29*(12), 41–47

Skelskey, C., & Leshem, O. (1997). Tuberculosis surveillance in long-term care. *AJN, 97*(10), 16BBBB–16DDDD.

Spratto, G. & Woods, A. (2001). *Delmar's A–Z NDR-2001 nurse's drug reference.* Albany, NY: Delmar.

Ulrich, S. A., Canale, S. W., & Wendall, S. A. (1998). *Medical–surgical nursing care planning guides* (4th ed.). Philadelphia: W. B. Saunders Company.

Wallace, C. (1998). Emergency! Acute pulmonary edema. *RN, 61*(1), 37–40.

RESOURCES

American Cancer Society (ACS), 1599 Clifton Road, NE, Atlanta, GA 30329, 800-ACS-2345, http://www.cancer.org

American Lung Association, 1740 Broadway, New York, NY 10019, 212-315-8700, http://www.lungusa.org

American Thoracic Society, 1740 Broadway, New York, NY 10019-4374, 212-315-8808, http://www.thoracic.org

Centers for Disease Control and Prevention (CDC), Division of Tuberculosis Elimination, 1600 Clifton Road, Mailstop E-10, Atlanta, GA 30333, 404-639-8120, http://www.cdc.gov

Cystic Fibrosis Foundation, 6931 Arlington Road, Bethesda, MD 20814, 800-FIGHT-CF (344-4823), http://www.cff.org

International Association of Laryngectomies, 7440 North Shadeland Avenue, Suite 100, Indianapolis, IN 46250, 317 570-4568, http://www.larynxlink.com/ial/ial/.htm, (Lost Chord and New Voice clubs are member clubs of this organization.)

CHAPTER 19
Nursing Care of the Client: Cardiovascular System

REFERENCES/SUGGESTED READINGS

American Heart Association. (1997). "Borderline" high systolic blood pressure raises risk of stroke, heart attack, and death [On-line]. Available: http://www.americanheart.org/Whats_News/AHA_News_Release/974510.html

American Heart Association. (1999a). Cardiovascular diseases [On-line]. Available: http://www.amhrt.org/statistics/03cardio.html

American Heart Association. (1999b). Cardiovascular disease statistics [On-line]. Available: http://www.amhrt.org/Heart_and_Stroke_A_Z_Guide/cvds.html

American Heart Association. (1999c). Coronary heart disease and angina pectoris [On-line]. Available: http://www.amhrt.org/Statistics/04crnry.html

American Heart Association. (1999d). High blood pressure [On-line]. Available: http://www.americanheart.org/statistics/06/hghbld.html

American Heart Association. (1999e). Rheumatic heart disease statistics [On-line]. Available: http://www.amhrt.org/Heart_and_Stroke_A_Z_Guide/hds.html

American Heart Association. (1999f). Risk factors and coronary heart disease [On-line]. Available: http://www.amhrt.org/Heart_and_Stroke_A_Z_Guide/cvds.html

American Heart Association. (1999g). Women, heart disease and stroke [On-line]. Available: http://www.amhrt.org/Heart_and_Stroke_A_Z_Guide/women.html

Beare, P., & Myers, J. L. (1998). *Principles and practice of adult health nursing* (3d ed.). St. Louis, MO: Mosby.

Beattie, S. (1999). Cut the risks for cardio cath patients. *RN, 62*(1), 50–54.

Breen, P. (2000). DVT: What every nurse should know. *RN, 63*(4), 58–62.

Bubien, R. (2000). A new beat on an old rhythm. *AJN, 100*(1), 42–50.

Chase, S. (2000). Hypertensive crisis. *RN, 63*(6), 62–67.

Corona, G. (1999). Pacemakers: Keeping the beat today. *RN, 62*(12), 50–55.

Crumlish, C., Bracken, J., Hand, M., Keenan, K., Ruggiero, H., & Simmons, D. (2000). When time is muscle. *AJN, 100*(1), 26–35.

Halm, M., & Penque, S. (1999). Heart disease in women. *AJN, 99*(4), 26–31.

Hiller, G. (1999). Atrial fibrillation. *Nursing99, 29*(2), 27–31.

Kudenchuk, P., Maynard, C., Martin, J., Wirkus, M., & Weaver, W. D. (1996). Comparison of presentation, treatment, and outcome of acute myocardial infarction in men versus women (the Myocardial Infarction Triage and Intervention Registry). *American Journal of Cardiology, 78*, 9–14.

Lazzara, D. (1999). Shocking facts about semiautomatic defibrillation. *Nursing99, 29*(4), 55–57.

Lewis, A. M. (1999). Cardiovascular emergency. *Nursing99, 29*(6), 49–51.

Lewis, S., Heitkemper, M., & Dirksen, S. (2000). Medical–surgical nursing: Assessment and management of clinical problems (5th ed.). St. Louis, MO: Mosby.

Linton, A., Matteson, M. A., & Maebius, N. K. (2000). *Introductory nursing care of adults* (2nd ed.). Philadelphia: W. B. Saunders Company.

MacCallum, E., Hanlon, S., & Byrne, K. (1999). *Nursing99, 29*(12), 34–40.

Mancini, M. E., & Kaye, W. (1999). AEDs: Changing the way you respond to cardiac arrest. *AJN, 99*(5), 26–30.

McAvoy, J. (2000). Cardiac pain: Discovering the unexpected. *Nursing2000, 30*(3), 34–39.

McCormick, J. & Deeg, M. (2000). Pharmacologic treatment of dyslipidemia. *AJN, 100*(2), 55–60.

McGrath, A. (1997). Clinical snapshot: Raynaud's syndrome. *AJN, 97*(1), 34–35.

McKinney, B. (1999). Solving the puzzle of heart failure. *Nursing99, 29*(5), 33–39.

Metules, T. (1999). Cardiac tamponade. *RN, 62*(12), 26–31.

Monahan, F. D., Drake, T., & Neighbors, M. (1998). *Nursing care of adults* (2nd ed.). Philadelphia: W. B. Saunders Company.

Mosca, L., Manson, J. E., Sutherland, S. E., Langer, R. D., Manolio, T., & Barrett-Connor, E. (1997). Cardiovascular disease in women. American Heart Association [On-line]. Available: http://www.amhrt.org/Scientific/statements/1997/109701.html

Mosley, M., Oenning, V., & Melinik, G. (1999). Methemoglobinemia. *AJN, 99*(5), 47.

Pagana, K. D., & Pagana, T. J. (1999). *Mosby's diagnostic and laboratory test reference.* St. Louis, MO: Mosby.

Phipps, W., Sands, J., & Marek, J. (1999). *Medical–surgical nursing: Concepts and clinical practice* (6th ed.). St. Louis, MO: Mosby.

Reger, T. & Vargas, G. (1999). The return of the radial artery in CABG. *AJN, 99*(9), 26–30.

Roger, V. L., Pellikka, P. A., Bell, M. R., Chow, C. W., Bailey, K. R., & Seward, J. B. (1997). Sex and test verification bias. Impact on the diagnostic value of exercise echocardiography. *Circulation, 95*, 405–410.

Ross, G. K., & DeJong, M. J. (1999). Pericardial tamponade. *AJN, 99*(2), 35.

Ryan, D. (2000). Is it an MI? A lab primer. *RN, 63*(1), 26–30.

Scherer, J.C., & Timby, B. K. (1999). *Introductory medical–surgical nursing* (7th ed.). Philadelphia: Lippincott.

Siomko, A. (2000). Demystifying cardiac markers. *AJN, 100*(1), 36–40.

The Sixth Report of the Joint National Committee on Prevention, Detection, Evaluation, and Treatment of High Blood Pressure. (1997). NIH Publication 98-4080. Joint National Committee on Prevention, Detection, Evaluation, and Treatment of High Blood Pressure. Bethesda, MD: National Institutes of Health.

Spratto, G., & Woods, A. (2001). *2001 PDR Nurse's Drug Handbook.* Albany, NY: Delmar.

Spratto, G. R., & Woods, A. L. (1997). *RN Magazine's NDR-95: Nurse's Drug Reference.* Albany, NY: Delmar.

Swearingen, P. L. (1998). *Manual of medical–surgical nursing care: Nursing interventions and collaborative management* (4th ed.). St. Louis, MO: Mosby.

Whitaker, L., & Kelleher, A. (1994). Raynaud's syndrome: Diagnosis and treatment. *Journal of Vascular Nursing, 12*(1), 10–13.

Wigley, F. (1998). Treating Raynaud's phenomenon and its underlying causes: Cold avoidance is effective in many cases. *Journal of Musculoskeletal Medicine, 15*(9), 53–61.

Woods, A. D. (1999). Managing hypertension. *Nursing99, 29*(3), 41–46.

Zangerm, D., Solomon, A., & Gersh, B. (2000). Contemporary management of angina: Part II. Medical management of chronic stable angina. *American Family Physician, 61*(1), 129–138.

Zhang, F., Chaisson, C., Evans, S., Wilson, P., & Felson, D. (1998). The association of estrogen replacement therapy and the Raynaud phenomenon in postmenopausal women. *Annals of Internal Medicine, 15*(9), 53–61.

RESOURCES

American Heart Association, National Center, 7272 Greenville Avenue, Dallas, TX 75231-4596, 800-242-8721, http://www.amhrt.org

The Coronary Club, Inc., 9500 Euclid Avenue, Mail Code A42, Cleveland, OH 44195, 216-444-3690

The Mended Hearts, Inc., 7272 Greenville Avenue, Dallas, TX 75231, 214-706-1442, http://www.mendedhearts.org

National Cholesterol Education Program Information Center, P.O. Box 30105, Bethesda, MD 20824-0105, 301-251-1222, 301-951-3260, http://www.nhlbi.nih.gov/nhlbi

National Heart, Lung, and Blood Institute Information Center, Public Health Service, P.O. Box 30105, Bethesda, MD 20824, 301-251-1222, http://www.nhlbi.nih.gov

President's Council on Physical Fitness and Sports, Hubert Humphrey Building, Room 758H, 200 Independence Avenue S.W., Washington, DC 20201, 202-690-9000, http://www.surgeongeneral.gov/ophs

CHAPTER 20
Nursing Care of the Client: Hematologic and Lymphatic Systems

REFERENCES/SUGGESTED READINGS

Anderson, K. N., Anderson, L. & Glanze, W. (Ed.). (1998). *Mosby's medical nursing and allied health dictionary* (5th ed.). St. Louis, MO: Mosby.

Beare, P., & Myers, J. L. (1998). *Principles and practice of adult health nursing* (3d ed.). St. Louis, MO: Mosby.

Black, J. M., & Mastassarin-Jacobs, E. (1997). *Clinical Management for Continuity of Care* (5th ed.). Philadelphia: W. B. Saunders Company.

Campbell. K. (1995). Understanding acute and chronic myeloid leukaemia. *Nursing Times, 91*(47), 36–38.

Deglin, J. & Vallerand, A. (2001). *Davis's drug guide for nurses* (7th ed.). Philadelphia: F. A. Davis Company.

Fitzpatrick, L., & Fitzpatrick, T. (1997). Blood transfusion: Keeping your patient safe. *Nursing97, 27*(8), 34–41.

Gioia, K., Kleinert, D., & Hannon, M. (1999). What's wrong with this patient? *RN, 62*(2), 43–45.

Gorman, K. (1999). Sickle cell disease. *AJN, 99*(3), 38–43.

Karch, A. (1998). *1998 Lippincott's nursing drug guide.* Philadelphia: Lippincott.

Leukemia Society of America. (1998a). Facts and statistics [On-line]. Available: http://www.leukemia.org/docs/leuk_rel/facts.html

Leukemia Society of America. (1998b). Hodgkin's disease [On-line]. Available: http://www.leukemia.org/docs/leuk_rel/facts.html

Leukemia Society of America. (1998c). Lymphoma [On-line]. Available: http://www.leukemia.org/docs/leuk_rel/facts.html

Leukemia Society of America. (1998d). Myeloma [On-line]. Available: http://www.leukemia.org/docs/leuk_rel/facts.html

Lewis, S., Heitkemper, M. M., & Dirksen, S. (2000). *Medical-surgical nursing* (5th ed.). St. Louis, MO: Mosby.

Matteson, M. A., McConnell, E. J., & Linton, A. D. (1997). *Gerontological Nursing* (2nd ed.). Philadelphia: W. B. Saunders Company.

McBrien, N. (1997). Clinical snapshot: Thrombocytopenic purpura. *AJN, 97*(2), 28–29.

Mitchell, R. (1999). Sickle cell anemia. *AJN, 99*(5), 36–37.

Monahan, F. D., Drake, T., & Neighbors, M. (1998) *Nursing care of adults* (2nd ed.). Philadelphia: W. B. Saunders Company.

Pagana, K. D., & Pagana, T. J. (1999). *Mosby's diagnostic and laboratory test reference* (4th ed.). St. Louis, MO: Mosby.

Phipps, W., Sands, J., & Marek, J. (1999). *Medical-surgical nursing: Concepts and clinical practice* (6th ed.). St. Louis, MO: Mosby.

Spratto, G., & Woods, A. (2000). *PDR® Nurse's drug handbook™.* Albany, NY: Delmar.

Thibodeau, G. A., & Patton, K. T. (1999). *Anatomy and physiology* (4th ed.) St. Louis, MO: Mosby.

Thomas, C. L. (Ed.). (1997). *Taber's cyclopedic medical dictionary* (18th ed.). Philadelphia: F. A. Davis.

Warmkessel, J. H. (1997). Caring for patients with non-Hodgkin's lymphoma. *Nursing97, 27*(6), 48–49.

Williams, L. & Hopper, P. (1999). *Understanding medical surgical nursing.* Philadelphia: F. A. Davis Company.

RESOURCES

American Cancer Society (ACS), 1599 Clifton Road, N.E., Altanta, GA 30329, 800-ACS-2345, http://www.cancer.org

Aplastic Anemia Foundation, Inc., P.O. Box 613, Annapolis, MD 21404, 800-247-2820, http://www.aplastic.org

BMT (Bone Marrow Transplant) Newsletter, 1985 Spruce Ave., Highland Park, IL 60035, 708-831-1913, http://www.bmtnews.org

Cancer Information Service (CIS), 800-4-CANCER

Center for Sickle Cell Disease, 202-806-7930

Cooley's Anemia Foundation, 105 E. 22nd St., Room 911, New York, NY 10010, 800-221-3571

Cure for Lymphoma Foundation, 215 Lexington Ave., New York, NY 10016, 800-CFL-6848, http://www.cfl.org

The Leukemia Society of America, Inc. (LSA), 600 Third Ave., New York, NY 10016, 800-955-4LSA, 212-573-8484, http://www.leukemia.org

National Association for Sickle Cell Disease, 4221 Wilshire Boulevard, Suite 360, Los Angeles, CA 90010, 213-936-7205, 800-421-8453

National Heart, Lung, and Blood Institute, 9000 Rockville Pike, Bethesda, MD 20892, 301-496-4236

The National Hemophilia Foundation, SOHO Building, Suite 406, 110 Greene St., New York, NY 10012, 212-219-8180

National Marrow Donor Program, 3433 Broadway St. N.E., Minneapolis, MN 55413, http://www.marrow.org

Office of Cancer Communications, National Cancer Institute, Building 31, Room 10A24, Bethesda, MD 20892, 800-4-CANCER

Sickle Cell Disease Foundation of Greater New York, 1 West 125th St., Room 206, New York, NY 10027

CHAPTER 21
Nursing Care of the Client:
Integumentary System

REFERENCES/SUGGESTED READINGS

Ashburn, M. A. (1995). Burn pain: The management of procedure-related pain. *Journal of Burn Care and Rehabilitation, 16*(3. Pt. 2): Supplement. 365–71.

Barczak, C., Barnett, R., Childs, E., & Bosley, L. (1997, July/August). Fourth national pressure ulcer prevalence survey. *Advances in Wound Care,* 10–14.

Beare, P., & Myers, J. L. (1998) *Principles and practice of adult health nursing* (3rd ed.). St. Louis, MO: Mosby.

Bjorgen, S. (1998). Herpes zoster. *AJN, 98*(2), 46–47.

Bozinko, G., Lowe, K., & Reigart, C. (1998). A new option for burn victims. *RN, 61*(11), 37–39.

Bryant, R. A. (1999). *Acute and chronic wounds: Nursing management* (2nd ed.). St. Louis, MO: Mosby.

Carpenito, L. J. (1997). *Nursing diagnosis: Application to clinical practice* (7th ed.). Philadelphia: Lippincott.

Carroll, P. (1995). Bed selection: Help patients rest easy. *RN, 58*(5), 44–50

Dennison, P. D., & Black, J. M. (1997). Nursing care of clients with peripheral vascular disorders. In J. M. Black & E. Matassarin-Jacobs (Eds.), *Luckmann and Sorensen's medical-surgical nursing: A psychophysiologic approach* (5th ed.). 1253–1313. Philadelphia: W. B. Saunders Company.

Deters, G. E. (1996). Management of patients with dermatologic problems. In S. C. Smeltzer & B. G. Bare (Eds.), *Brunner and Suddarth's textbook of medical-surgical nursing* (8th ed.). 1445–1500. Philadelphia: Lippincott.

Erwin-Toth, P., & Hocevar, B. (1995). Wound care: Selecting the right dressing. *AJN, 95*(2), 46–51.

Estes, M. E. Z. (2002). *Health assessment & physical examination* (2nd ed.). Albany, NY: Delmar.

Fritsch, D. E., & Yurko, L. C. (1995). Management of persons with burns. In W. J. Phipps, V. L. Cassmeyer, J. K. Sands, & M. K. Lehman (Eds.), *Medical-surgical nursing: Concepts and clinical practice* (5th ed.). 2358–2397. St. Louis, MO: Mosby.

Hill, M. (1998). Nursing management of adults with skin disorders. In P. G. Beare & J. L. Myers (Eds.), *Principles and practice of adult health nursing* (3rd ed.). 2089–2115. St. Louis, MO: Mosby.

Jackson, L. (1995). Quick response to hypothermia and frostbite. *AJN, 95*(3), 52.

Kornfeld, H. S. (1995). Co-meditation: Guiding patients through the relaxation process. *RN, 58*(11), 57–59.

Kovach, T. (1995). The barrier defense: Skin hydration as infection control. *The Journal of Practical Nursing, 45*(1), 13–19.

Maklebust, J. (1995). Pressure ulcers: What works. *RN, 58*(9), 46–50.

Martini, F., & Bartholomew, E. (2000). *Essentials of anatomy and physiology* (3rd ed.).). Englewood Cliffs, NJ: Prentice-Hall.

McCain, D., & Sutherland, S. (1998). Skin grafts for patients with burns. *AJN, 98*(7), 34–39.

Mendez-Eastman, S. (1998). When wounds won't heal. *RN, 61*(1), 20–23.

Morykwas, M., & Argenta, L. (1995, May). An update on the use of negative pressure to promote healing of pressure sores and chronic wounds. *Proceedings of the 27th annual conference, Wound Ostomy and Continence Nurses,* Denver, CO.

National Decubitus Foundation. (1998). Cost savings through bedsore avoidance [On-line]. Available: http://www.decubitus.org/cost/cost.html

National Pressure Ulcer Advisory Panel (NPUAP). (1999). PUSH Tool [On-line]. Available: http://www.npuap.org/pushins.htm

Nicol, N. H. (1997). Nursing care of clients with integumentary disorders. In J. M. Black & E. Matassarin-Jacobs (Eds.), *Luckmann and Sorensen's medical-surgical nursing: A psychophysiologic approach* (5th ed.). 1955–1982. Philadelphia: W. B. Saunders Company.

Ogden, B. L. (1998). Nursing management of adults with burns. In P.G. Beare & J. L. Myers (Eds.), *Principles and practice of adult health nursing* (3rd ed.). 2117–2142. St. Louis, MO: Mosby.

Sabatini, M. M. (1995). Skin cancer: The silent pandemic. *Dermatology Nursing, 7*(1), 45–50.

Schwartz, S., Shires, G., & Spencer, F. (1994). *Principles of surgery* (6th ed.). New York: McGraw-Hill.

Seeley, R. R., Stephens, T. D., & Tate, P. (1995) *Anatomy and physiology* (3rd ed.). St. Louis, MO: Mosby.

Seymour, J. (1995). Skin care: Sun protection. *Nursing Times, 91*(25), 61, 63.

United States Department of Health and Human Services (USDHHS). (1992). *Pressure ulcers in adults: Prediction and prevention* (Publication Nos. 92-0047 and 92-0050). Rockville, MD: Public Health Service, Agency for Health Care Policy and Research.

Vermette, E. (1998). Emergency! Malignant hyperthermia. *AJN, 98*(4), 45.

Weaver, V. (1995). Management of persons with problems of the skin. In W. J. Phipps, V. L. Cassmeyer, J.K. Sands, & M. K. Lehman (Eds.), *Medical-surgical nursing: Concepts and clinical practice* (5th ed.). 2317–2357. St. Louis, MO: Mosby.

Wiebelhaus, P., & Hansen, S. (1999). Burns: Handle with care. *RN, 62*(11), 52–57.

RESOURCES

American Burn Association, 65 North Michigan Avenue, Suite 1530, Chicago, IL 60611, 800-548-2876, http://ameriburn.org/home.htm

American Hair Loss Council, 401 North Michigan Avenue, Chicago, IL 60611, 312-321-5128, 888-873-9714, http://www.ahlc.org

Dermatology Foundation, 1560 Sherman Avenue, Suite 870, Evanston, IL 60201-4802, 847-328-2256, http://www.dermfnd.org

National Burn Victim Foundation, 246A Madisonville Road, P.O. Box 409, Basking Ridge, NJ 07920, 908-953-9091, http://www.nbvf.org

National Decubitus Foundation, 4255 South Buckley Road, Suite 228, Aurora, CO 80013, http://www.decubitus.org

National Pressure Ulcer Advisory Panel (NPUAP), 11250 Roger Bacon Drive, Suite 8, Reston, VA 20190-5202, 703-464-4849, http://www.iglou.com/npuap

National Psoriasis Foundation, 6600 SW 92nd, Suite 300, Portland, OR 97223, 503-244-7404, http://www.psoriasis.org

Skin Cancer Foundation, 245 Fifth Avenue, Suite 1403, New York, NY 10016, 212-725-5176, http://www.skincancer.org

CHAPTER 22
Nursing Care of the Client: Immune System

REFERENCES/SUGGESTED READINGS

Arthritis Foundation. (1999a). *Arthritis types and prevalence* [On-line] Available: http://www.arthritis.org/resource/fs/arthritis%5Fprevalence.asp

Arthritis Foundation. (1999b). *Getting a grip on rheumatoid arthritis* [On-line]. Available: http://www.arthritis.org/resource/RAcampaign

Arthritis Foundation. (1999c). *Rheumatoid arthritis* [On-line]. Available: http://www.arthritis.org/offices/ae/about/rheumatoid.asp

Arthritis Foundation. (1999d). *Rheumatoid arthritis fact sheet* [On-line]. Available: http://www.arthritis.org/resource/fs/rheumatoid.asp

Barbarito, C. (1999). Emergency anaphylaxis. *AJN, 99*(1), 33.

Bertino, L. S., & Lu, L. C. (1993). The bite of the wolf: Systemic lupus erythematosus. *Rehabilitation Nursing, 16*(3), 173–178.

Burt, S. (1998). What you need to know about latex allergy. *Nursing98, 28*(10), 33–39.

Carpenito, L. J. (1997). *Nursing diagnosis: Application to clinical practice*. Philadelphia: Lippincott.

Carroll, P. (1999). Latex allergy: What you need to know. *RN, 62*(9), 40–46.

Cunning, S. (2000). When the Dx is myasthenia gravis. *RN, 63*(4), 26–30.

Gritter, M. (1998). The latex threat. *AJN, 98*(9), 26–32.

Guyton, A. C., & Hall, J. E. (1996). *Textbook of medical physiology* (9th ed.). Philadelphia: W.B. Saunders Company.

Hausman, K. A. (1995). Interventions for clients with problems of the peripheral nervous system. In D. D. Ignatavicius, M. L. Workman, & M. A. Mishler (Eds.), *Medical-surgical nursing: A nursing process approach*. Philadelphia: W. B. Saunders Company.

Howard, J. (1997). *Myasthenia gravis: A summary* [On-line]. Available: http://www.myasthenia.org/information/summary.htm

Ignatavicius, D. D. (1999). Interventions for clients with connective tissue disease. In D. B. Ignatavicius, M.L. Workman, & M. A. Mishler (Eds.), *Medical-surgical nursing across the health-care continuum* (3d ed., pp. 405–445). Philadelphia: W. B. Saunders Company.

Johnson, B. (1999). Systemic lupus erythematosus. *AJN, 99*(1), 40–41.

Jurewicz, M. (2000). Anaphylaxis: When the body overreacts. *Nursing2000, 30*(7), 58–61.

Lupus Foundation of America (LFA). (1995). *Causes, symptoms, testing, treatment* [On-line]. Available: http://www.lupus.org

Mahot, G. (1998). Rheumatoid arthritis. *AJN, 98*(12), 42–43.

Myers, J. S. (2000). Chemotherapy: Induced hypersensitivity reaction. *AJN, 100*(4), 53–54.

National Heart, Lung, and Blood Institute (NHLBI). (1999, July) *Use of autologous blood* [On-line]. Available: http://www.nhlbi.nih.gov/nhlbi/blood/transf/prof/transhc.htm

National Institute of Allergy and Infectious Diseases (NIAID). (1999a, July). *Asthma and allergy statistics* [On-line]. Available: http://www.niaid.gov/factsheets/allergystat.htm

National Institute of Allergy and Infectious Diseases (NIAID). (1999b, July). *Transplantation* [On-line]. Available: http://www.niaid.nih.gov/publications/womenshealth/transplant.htm

National Institute of Arthritis, Musculoskeletal, and Skin Diseases (NIAMS). (1999). *Systemic lupus erythematosus* [Online]. Available: http://www.nih.gov/niams/healthinfo/slehandout

National Institute of Neurological Disorders and Stroke (NINDS). (1999a). *Myasthenia gravis* [On-line]. Available: http://www.ninds.nih.gov/patients/Disorders/myasthenia/myasthenia.htm

National Institute of Neurological Disorders and Stroke (NINDS). (1999b). *Neurological sequelae of lupus* [On-line]. Available: http://www.ninds.nih.gov/patients/Disorders/lupus/lupus.htm#moreinfo

Pagana, K. D., & Pagana, T. J. (1999). *Mosby's diagnostic and laboratory test reference* (4th ed.). St. Louis, MO: Mosby.

Stewart, K. (1998). Myasthenia gravis cholinergic crisis. *Nursing98, 28*(12), 33.

Thomson, J. M., McFarland, G. K., Hirsch, J. E., & Tucker, S. M. (Eds.) (1997). *Mosby's clinical nursing* (4th ed.). St. Louis, MO: Mosby.

RESOURCES

The American Academy of Allergy, Asthma, and Immunology, 611 E. Wells Street, Milwaukee, WI 53202, 414-272-6071, http://www.aaaai.org

American Association of Blood Banks, 8101 Glenbrook Road, Bethesda, MD 20814-2749, 301-907-6977, http://www.aabb.org

Arthritis Foundation, 1330 West Peachtree Street, Atlanta, GA 30309, 800-283-7800, http://www.arthritis.org

Asthma and Allergy Foundation of America, 1233 Twentieth Street, N.W., Suite 402, Washington, DC 20036, 800-7ASTHMA, http://www.aafa.org

Foundation for Latex Allergy Research and Education, Long Beach Memorial Hospital, 2501 Cherry Avenue, Suite 350, Long Beach, CA 90806, 562-997-7888, http://www.flare.org

Latex Allergy News, 860-482-6869

Latex Allergy Web Ring, http://www.webring.org

Lupus Foundation of America, Inc., 1300 Piccard Drive, Suite 200, Rockville, MD 20850-4303, 800-558-0121, 301-670-9292, http://www.lupus.org

Myasthenia Gravis Foundation, Inc., 123 West Madison, Suite 800, Chicago, IL 60602-4503, 800-541-5454, http://www.myasthenia.org

CHAPTER 23
Nursing Care of the Client: HIV and AIDS

REFERENCES/SUGGESTED READINGS

Aids Treatment Data Network. (1999, May). *Viral load tests* [On-line]. Available: http://www.aidsinfonyc.org/network/simple/viral.html

Carpenito, L. J. (1997). *Nursing diagnosis: Application to clinical practice*. Philadelphia: Lippincott.

Centers for Disease Control and Prevention. (1996a). Update: Mortality attributable to HIV infection among persons aged 25–44 years—United States, 1994. *Morbidity and Mortality Weekly Report, 45*(6), 10–14.

Centers for Disease Control and Prevention. (1996b). Continued sexual risk behavior among HIV-seropositive, drug-using men—Atlanta; Washington, D.C.; and San Juan, Puerto Rico, 1993. *Morbidity and Mortality Weekly, 15*(7), 13–15.

Centers for Disease Control and Prevention. (1996c). AIDS associated with injecting drug use—United States, 1995. *Morbidity and Mortality Weekly Report, 45*(19), 37–42.

Centers for Disease Control and Prevention. (1995a). Questions and Answers: CDC DRAFT guidelines for HIV counseling and voluntary testing for pregnant women. *CDC HIV/AIDS prevention.* 1–5.

Centers for Disease Control and Prevention. (1995b). USPHS/IDSA Guidelines for the prevention of opportunistic infections in persons infected with human immunodeficiency virus: A summary. *Morbidity and Mortality Weekly Report, 44*(RR–8), 1–33.

Centers for Disease Control and Prevention. (1994). Guidelines for preventing the transmission of Mycobacterium tuberculosis in health-care facilities, 1994. *Morbidity and Mortality Weekly, 43*(RR–13), 1–132.

Finkelstein, D. M., Williams, P. L., Molenberghs, G., Feinberg, J., Powderly, W. G., Kahn, J., Dolin, R., & Cotton, D. (1996). Patterns of opportunistic infections in patients with HIV infection. *Journal of Acquired Immune Deficiency Syndromes and Human Retrovirology, 12,* 38–45.

Flaskerud, J. H., & Ungvarski, P. J. (1995). *HIV/AIDS: A guide to nursing care* (3d ed.). Philadelphia: W.B. Saunders Company.

Guyton, A. C., & Hall, J. E. (1996). *Textbook of medical physiology* (9th ed.). Philadelphia: W.B. Saunders Company.

Kaplan, L. D. (1999). The malignancies associated with AIDS. In M.A. Sande & P. A. Volberding (Eds.), *The medical management of AIDS* (2d ed., pp. 339–364). Philadelphia: W.B. Saunders Company.

Kirsten, V., & Whipple, B. (1998). Treating HIV disease: Hope on the horizon. *Nursing98, 28*(11), 34–39.

Lindberg, C.E. (1995). Perinatal transmission of HIV: How to counsel women. *Maternal Child Nursing, 20,* 207–212.

Lisanti, P., & Zwolski, K. (1997). Understanding the devastation of AIDS. *AJN, 97*(7), 27–34.

Mumu, R. D., Lyons, D. A., Borucki, M. J., & Pollard, R. B. (1997). *HIV manual for health care professionals.* Norwalk, CT: Appleton & Lange.

National Institute of Allergy and Infectious Diseases (NIAID) and National Institutes of Health (NIH). (1999, May). *HIV/AIDS statistics* [On-line]. Available: http://www.niaid.nih.gov/factsheets/hivstat.htm

National Institute of Allergy and Infectious Diseases (NIAID) and National Institutes of Health (NIH). (1999, March). *HIV infection and AIDS* [On-line]. Available: http://www.niaid.nih.gov/factsheets/hivinf.htm

National Institute of Allergy and Infectious Diseases (NIAID) and National Institutes of Health (NIH). (1997, May). *HIV wasting syndrome* [On-line]. Available: http://www.niaid.nih.gov/factsheets/hivwasting.htm

Paar, D. P. (1997). Hepatitis. In R.D. Mumu, M. J. Borucki, D. A. Lyons. & R. B. Pollard (Eds.), *HIV manual for health care professionals* (pp. 77–86). Norwalk, CT: Appleton & Lange.

Pagana, K. D., & Pagana, T. J. (1999). *Mosby's diagnostic and laboratory test reference* (4th ed.). St. Louis, MO: Mosby.

Thomson, J. M., McFarland, G. K., Hirsch, J. E., & Tucker, S. M. (Eds.) (1997). *Mosby's clinical nursing* (4th ed.). St. Louis, MO: Mosby.

Ventura, M. (1999). The realities of HIV/AIDS. *RN, 62*(4), 26–30.

RESOURCES

AIDS Treatment Data Network: The Network, 611 Broadway, Suite 613, New York, NY 10012, 800-734-7104, http://www.aidsinfonyc.org/network

The American Academy of Allergy, Asthma, and Immunology, 611 E. Wells Street, Milwaukee, WI 53202, 414-272-6071, http://www.aaaai.org

CHAPTER 24
Nursing Care of the Client: Musculoskeletal System

REFERENCES/SUGGESTED READINGS

Altizer, L. (1995). Total hip arthroplasty. *Orthopaedic Nursing, 4,* 7–17.

Arthritis Foundation. (1998). Gout fact sheet [On-line]. Available: http://www.arthritis.org/resource/fs/gout.asp

Beare, P. G., & Myers, J. L. (1998). *Adult health nursing* (3rd ed.). St. Louis, MO: Mosby.

Carpenito, L. J. (1999). *Nursing care plans and documentation* (3rd ed.). Philadelphia: Lippincott.

Darovic, G. (1997). Caring for patients with osteoporosis. *Nursing97, 27*(5), 50–51.

deWit, S. C. (1998). *Essentials of medical surgical nursing* (4th ed.). Philadelphia: W. B. Saunders Company.

Dowd, R. & Cavalieri, R. J. (1999). Help your patient live with osteoporosis. *AJN, 99*(4), 55–60.

Huston, C. (1998). Emergency! Cervical spine injury. *AJN, 98*(6), 33.

Johnson, J., Anderson, C., Barrett, A., Duke, K., & Sharp, D. (1995). Roller traction: Mobilizing patients with acetabular fractures. *Orthopaedic Nursing, 1,* 21–24.

Leslie, M. (2000). When the ache is not arthritis. *RN, 63*(3), 38–40.

Lewis, A. M. (1999). Orthopedic and vascular emergencies. *Nursing99, 29*(12), 54–56.

Monahan, F. D.,& Neighbors, M. (1998). *Medical-surgical nursing: Foundations for clinical practice* (2nd ed.). Philadelphia: W. B. Saunders Company.

National Institute of Allergies and Infectious Diseases (NIAID). (1999). Lyme disease [On-line]. Available: http://www.niaid.nih.gov/publications/lyme

National Institute of Arthritis and Musculoskeletal and Skin Diseases (NIAMS). (1998, May). Genetics of osteoarthritis panel discussion [On-line]. Available: http://www.nih.gov.niams/reports/oabrief3.htm

National Institute of Arthritis and Musculoskeletal and Skin Diseases (NIAMS). (1998, October). Osteoporosis: progress and promise [On-line]. Available: http://www.nih.gov/niams/healthinfo/opbkgr/htm

National Institute of Arthritis and Musculoskeletal and Skin Diseases (NIAMS). (1999, January). Questions and answers about gout [On-line]. Available: http://www.nih.gov/niams/healthinfo/gout/htm

National Institute of Neurological Disorders and Stroke (NINDS). (1999, July). Carpal tunnel syndrome [Online]. Available: http://www.ninds.nih.gov/patients/Disorder/CARPAL/carpal/HTM#moreinfo

National Osteoporosis Foundation (NOF). (1999a). Osteoporosis: Bone health [On-line]. Available: http://www.nof.org/osteoporosis/bonehealth.htm

National Osteoporosis Foundation (NOF). (1999b). Osteoporosis: Bone mass measurement [On-line]. Available: http://www.nof.org/osteoporosis/bonemass.htm

National Osteoporosis Foundation (NOF). (1999c). Osteoporosis: Fast facts [On-line]. Available: http://www.nof.org/osteoporosis/stats.htm

National Osteoporosis Foundation (NOF). (1999d). Osteoporosis: Men and osteoporosis [On-line]. Available: http://www.nof.org/osteoporosis/men_and_osteo.htm

National Osteoporosis Foundation (NOF). (2000). Prevention: How can I prevent osteoporosis? [On-line] Available: http://www.nof.org/prevention/prevention.htm

O'Hanlon-Nichols, T. (1998). Basic assessment series: Musculoskeletal system. *AJN, 98*(6), 48–52.

Phipps, W. J., Sands, J. K., & Marek, J. F. (1999). *Medical-surgical nursing: Concepts and clinical practice* (6th ed.). St. Louis, MO: Mosby.

Sipos, D. A. (1995). Carpal tunnel syndrome. *Orthopaedic Nursing, 1,* 17–20.

Smeltzer, S. C., & Bare, B. G. (1996). *Brunner and Suddarth's textbook of medical-surgical nursing* (8th ed.). Philadelphia: Lippincott.

Sparks, S. M., & Taylor, C. M. (1999). *Nursing diagnosis reference manual* (4th ed.). Springhouse, PA: Springhouse Corporation.

Sullivan, M. P., & Sharts-Hopko, N. C. (2000). Preventing the downward spiral. *AJN, 100*(8), 26–31.

Taber, C. W. (1997). *Taber's cyclopedic medical dictionary* (18th ed.). Philadelphia: F. A. Davis Company.

Timby, B. K., Scherer, J. C., & Smith, N. E. (1999). *Introductory medical surgical nursing* (7th ed.). Philadelphia: Lippincott.

The TMJ Association. (1998). Changing the face of TMJ [On-line]. Available: http://www.tmj.org

Wade, C. F. (2000). Keeping lyme disease at bay. *AJN, 100*(7), 26–31.

Yarnold, B. (1999). Hip fracture. *AJN, 99*(2), 36–40.

RESOURCES

American Occupational Therapy Association, Inc., 4720 Montgomery Lane, P.O. Box 31220, Bethesda, MD 20824-1220, 301-652-2682, Fax 301-652-7711, http://www.aota.org

American Physical Therapy Association, 1111 North Fairfax Street, Alexandria, VA 22314, 703-684-2782, Fax 703-684-7343, 800-999-2782, http://www.apta.org

Arthritis Foundation, 1330 West Peachtree Street, Atlanta, GA 30309, 800-283-7800, http://www.arthritis.org

National Amputation Foundation, 38-40 Church Street, Malverne, NY 11565, 516-887-3600, Fax 516-887-3667, http://www.va.gov/uso/naf.htm

National Easter Seal Foundation, Development Department, Easter Seal Society of Metropolitan Chicago, 14 E. Jackson Boulevard, Suite 900, Chicago, IL 60604, 312-939-5115, http://www.eastersealchicago.org

National Institute of Arthritis and Musculoskeletal and Skin Diseases (NIAMS), NIAMS/National Institutes of Health, Bethesda, MD 20892, 301-495-4484, http://www.nih.gov/niams

National Osteoporosis Foundation, 1232 22nd Street N.W., Washington, DC 20037-1292, 202-223-2226, http://www.nof.org

Osteoporosis and Related Bone Diseases, National Resource Center, 1150 17th Street N.W. Suite 500, Washington, DC 20036-4603, 800-624-2663, http://www.osteo.org

The TMJ Association, Ltd., P.O. Box 26770, Milwaukee, WI 53226-0770, 414-259-3223, http://www.tmj.org

CHAPTER 25
Nursing Care of the Client: Neurological System

REFERENCES/SUGGESTED READINGS

American Academy of Neurology (AAN). (1997a). *Headache* [On-line], Available: http://www.aan.com/public/head/html

American Academy of Neurology (AAN). (1997b). *Tourette's syndrome* [On-line], Available: http://www.aan.com/public/head/html

Andersen, G. (1998). DX dementia: But what kind? *RN, 61*(6), 26–30.

Barinaga, M. (1995). Neurotrophic factors enter the clinic. *Science, 264,* 772–774.

Barinaga, M. (1995). Researchers broaden the attack on Parkinson's disease. *Science, 267,* 455–456.

Barker, E. (1999). Brain attack! A call to action. *RN, 62*(5), 54–57.

Barr, M. L., & Kiernan, J. A. (1998). *The human nervous system: An anatomical viewpoint* (7th ed.). Philadelphia: Lippincott.

Beare, P. G., & Myers, J. L. (Eds.). (1998). *Principles and practice of adult health nursing* (3rd ed.). St. Louis, MO: Mosby.

Carpenito, L. J. (1997). *Handbook of nursing diagnosis* (7th ed.). Philadelphia: Lippincott.

Costa, M. (1998). Clinical snapshot: Trigeminal neuralgia. *AJN, 98*(6), 42–43.

Cox, H. C., Hinz, M. D., Lubno, M. A., Newfield, S. A., Ridenour, N.A., Slater, M. M., & Sridaramont, K. (1997). *Clinical applications of nursing diagnosis: Adult, child, women's, mental health, geriatric, and home health considerations.* (3rd ed.). Philadelphia: F.A. Davis.

Crigger, N., & Forbes, W. (1997). Assessing neurologic function in older patients. *AJN, 97*(3), 37–40.

Evans, M. J. (Ed.). (1995). (2nd ed.). *Neurological–neurosurgical nursing.* Springhouse, PA: Springhouse.

Frozena, C. (1997). Multiple Sclerosis. *AJN, 97*(11), 48–49.

Gumm, S. L. (2000). Straight talk about MS. *Nursing2000, 30*(1), 50–51.

Halper, J., & Holland, N. (1998a). Meeting the challenge of multiple sclerosis (Part I). *AJN, 98*(10), 26–31.

Halper, J., & Holland, N. (1998b). Meeting the challenge of multiple sclerosis (Part II). *AJN, 98*(11), 39–46.

Hickey, J. V. (1997). *The clinical practice of neurological and neurosurgical nursing* (4th ed.). Philadelphia: Lippincott.

Huston, C. (1998). Emergency! Cervical spine injury. *AJN, 98*(6), 33.

Huston, C. J., & Boelman, R. (1995). Autonomic dysreflexia. *AJN, 95*(6), 55.

Hyde, T. M., & Weinberger, D. R. (1995). Tourette's syndrome: A model neuropsychiatric disorder. *Journal of American Medical Association, 273,* 498–501.

Kalbach, L. R. (1991). Unilateral neglect: Mechanism and nursing care. *Journal of Neuroscience Nursing, 23,* 25–129.

Kurlan, R. (1998). *Current pharmacology of Tourette's Syndrome.* Bayside, NY: Tourette Syndrome Association. [On-line]. Available: http://www.2mgh.harvard.edu/lsa/medsci/medicationsanddosages.html

Lewis, A. M. (1999). Neurologic emergency! *Nursing99, 29*(10), 54–56

McCance, K. L., & Huether, S. E. (1998). *Pathophysiology: The biological basis for disease in adults and children* (3rd ed.). St. Louis, MO: Mosby.

Meissner, J. E. (1994). Caring for clients with multiple sclerosis. *Nursing94, 24*(8), 60–61.

Mitiguy, J. (1991). The brain under attack. *HEADline,* 2–8, 10.

Mitsumoto, H., Ikeda, K., Klinlosz, B., Cedarbaum, J.M., Wong, V., & Lindasy, R. M. (1994). Arrest of motor neuron disease in wobbler mice cotreated with CNTF and BDNF. *Science, 265,* 1107–1110.

Monlus-Swift, C. (1998). Neurological disorders. In P.L. Swearingen (Ed.), *Manual of medical–surgical nursing care:*

Nursing interventions and collaborative management (4th ed., pp. 181–319). St. Louis, MO: Mosby.

Nadler-Moodie, M., & Wilson, M. (1998). Latest approaches in Alzheimer's care. *RN, 61*(7), 42–46.

National Spinal Cord Injury Statistical Center. (1998). *Spinal cord injury fact and figures.* Birmingham, AL: University of Alabama at Birmingham. (Supported by Grant No. HI33N-50009-95A from National Institute on Disability and Rehabilitation Research, United States Department of Education.)

National Stroke Association Press Release. (March 13, 1995). *Stroke deaths increase for first time in 35 years.*

National Stroke Association. (1998a). *Stroke in America Campaign* [On-line], Available: http://www.stroke.org

National Stroke Association. (1998b). *Stroke prevention guidelines* [On-line], Available: http://www.stroke.org

New treatment for stroke victims. (1997, January). *The Journal Gazette.*

O'Hanlon-Nichols, T. (1999). Neurologic assessment. *AJN, 99*(6), 44–50.

Raine, M. (1997, May 12). New technology eases the tremors caused by Parkinson's disease. *Corpus Christi Caller Times.* Corpus Christi, TX: Caller Times Publishing Co.

Reiman, E. M., Caselli, R. J., Yun, L. S., Chen, K., Bandy, D., Minoshima, S., Thibodeau, S. N., & Osborne, D. (1996). Preclinical evidence of Alzheimer's disease in person homozygous for the ε allele for apolipoprotein ε. *New England Journal of Medicine, 334,* 752–758.

Rudick, R. (1997). New approaches to multiple sclerosis. *Health News, 3*(17), 1–2. Waltham, MA: Massachusetts Medical Society.

Samuels, M. A. (Ed.). (1995). *Manual of neurological therapeutics* (5th ed.). Boston: Little Brown.

Schweiger, J. L. (1999). Alzheimer's disease. *Nursing99, 29*(6), 34–41.

Smeltzer, S. C., & Bare, B. G. (Eds.). (1996). *Brunner and Suddarth's textbook of medical surgical nursing* (8th ed.). Philadelphia: Lippincott.

Taggart, H. M. (1998, March/April). Multiple sclerosis update. *Orthopaedic Nursing.*

Thelan, L. A., Davie, J. K., & Urden, L. D. (1998). *Critical care nursing: Diagnosis and management* (3rd ed.). St. Louis, MO: Mosby.

RESOURCES

Alzheimer's Association, 919 North Michigan Avenue, Suite 1000, Chicago, IL 60611, 800-272-3900, http://www.alz.org

Alzheimer's Disease Education and Referral Center, P.O. Box 8250, Silver Spring, MD 20907-8250, 800-438-4380, http://www.alzheimer.org

American Academy of Neurology, 1080 Montreal Avenue, St. Paul, MN 55116, 612-695-1940, http://www.aan.com

American Association of Spinal Cord Injury Nurses (AASCIN), 75-20 Astoria Boulevard, Jackson Heights, NY 11370-1177, 718-803-3782

American Council for Headache Education, 800-255-ACHE (2243), e-mail: achehg@talley.com

American Parkinson's Disease Association, Inc., 1250 Hylan Boulevard, Staten Island, NY 10305, 718-981-8001, 800-223-2732, http://neurosurgery.mgh.harvard.edu/pd-suprt.htm#APDA

American Spinal Injury Association, 250 East Superior, Room 619, Chicago, IL 60611, 312-908-6207

Brain Injury Association, Inc., 105 North Alfred Street, Alexandria, VA 22314, 703-236-6000, http://www.biausa.org

Epilepsy Foundation, 1000 Elmwood Avenue, Rochester, NY 14620, 800-724-7930

Epilepsy Foundation of America, 4351 Garden City Drive, Suite 406, Landover, MD 20785, 301-459-3700, 800-332-1000, http://www.efa.org

Guillain-Barré Foundation, International, P.O. Box 262, Wynnewood, PA 19096, 610-667-0131, http://www.webmast.com/gbs

Huntington's Disease Society, 140 West 22 Street, 6th Floor, New York, NY 10011-2420, 212-242-1968, 800-532-7667, http://neuro~www2msh.harvard.edu/hdsa/society.nclk

National Headache Foundation, 800-843-2256, http://www.headache.org

National Institute of Neurological Disorders and Stroke, Office of Scientific Health Reports, P.O. Box 5801, Bethesda, MD 20824, 301-496-5751, 800-352-9424, http://www.ninds.nih.gov

National Multiple Sclerosis Society, 733 Third Avenue, New York, NY 10017, 212-986-3240, 800-344-4867, http://www.nmss.org

National Parkinson's Foundation, 1501 N.W. Ninth Avenue, Miami, FL 33136, 305-547-6666, 800-327-4545, http://www.parkinson.org

National Spinal Cord Injury Association, 545 Concord Avenue, Suite 29, Cambridge, MA 02138, 617-441-8500, http://www.spinalcord.org

National Spinal Cord Injury Hotline, 800-526-3456

National Stroke Association, 96 Inverness Drive East, Suite 1, Englewood, CO 80112-5112, 800-STROKES (787-6537), http://www.strokes.org

Parkinson's Disease Foundation, William Black Medical Res. Building, Columbia-Presbyterian Medical Center, 710 West 168th Street, New York, NY 10032, 212-923-4700, http://www.pdf.org

Tourette Syndrome Association, 42-40 Bell Boulevard, Suite 205, Bayside, NY 11361, 718-244-2999, http://www.2mgh.harvard.edu/tse/tsamain.nclk

CHAPTER 26
Nursing Care of the Client: Sensory System

REFERENCES/SUGGESTED READINGS

Cavendish, R. (1998). Clinical snapshot: Hearing loss. *AJN, 98*(8), 50–51.

Dana, R. (1998, January 27). Dry eye syndrome. *Health News* 1, 3.

Kearney, K. (1997). Retinal detachment. *AJN, 97*(8), 50.

Ramponi, D. (2000). Go with the flow during an eye emergency. *Nursing2000, 30*(8), 54–56.

Shelp, S. (1997). Your patient is deaf, now what? *RN, 60*(2), 37–40.

Smeltzer, S. C., & Bare, B. G. (1996). *Brunner and Suddarth's Textbook of Medical-Surgical Nursing* (8th ed.). Philadelphia: Lippincott.

Sparks, S. M. & Taylor, C. M. (1998). *Nursing diagnosis reference manual* (4th ed.). Springhouse, PA: Springhouse Corporation.

Spencer, J. (1998, February 17). Coping with hearing loss. *Health News* 2, 1–2.

Tupper, S. (1999). When the inner ear is out of balance. *RN, 62*(11), 36–40.

Walbecker, J. (1997). Knowing the signs. *RN, 60*(2), 40–41.

RESOURCES

Alexander Graham Bell Association for the Deaf, 3417 Volta Place NW, Washington, DC 20007, 202-337-5220, http://www.agbell.org

American Academy of Ophthalmology, 655 Beach Street, San Francisco, CA 94109, 415-561-8500, http://www.eyenet.org

American Academy of Otolaryngology, Head and Neck Surgery, 1 Prince Street, Alexandria, VA 22314, 703-836-4444, http://www.entnet.org

American Council of the Blind, 1155 15th Street NW, Suite 720, Washington, DC 20005, 202-467-5081, 800-424-8666, http://acb.org

American Foundation for the Blind, Inc., 11 Penn Plaza, Suite 300, New York, NY 10011, 212-502-7600, http://www.afb.org, e-mail: afbinfo@afb.org

American Speech-Language-Hearing Association, 10801 Rockville Pike, Rockville, MD 20852, 800-498-2071, 301-897-5700, http://www.asha.org

American Tinnitus Association, P.O. Box 5, Portland, OR 97207, http://www.ata.org, 503-248-9985

Better Hearing Institute, 515 King St., Suite 420, Alexandria, VA 22314, 800-327-9355

Better Vision Institute, Inc., 1655 North Fort Myer Drive, Suite 200, Arlington, VA 22209, 703-243-1528, http://www.visionsite.org

Braille Institute, 741 N. Vermont Avenue, Los Angeles, CA 90029-3594, 213-663-1111, 800-272-4553, http://www.healthy.net/pan/cso/cioi/BI.HTM, http://www.brailleinstitute.org

Guide Dogs for the Blind, P.O. Box 15200, San Rafael, CA 94915, 415-499-4000, 800-295-4050, http://www.guidedogs.com

Guide Dog Users, Inc., 12 Riverside St., Apt. 1-2, Watertown, MA 02172, 617-926-9198

Guiding Eyes for the Blind, 611 Granite Springs Road, Yorktown Heights, NY 10598, 914-245-4024, http://www.guiding-eyes.org

International Hearing Dog Inc., 5901 East 89th Avenue, Henderson, CO 80640, 303-287-3277, http://www.ihdi.org

Leader Dogs for the Blind, 1039 South Rochester Road, Rochester, MI 48307, 248-651-9011, http://www.leader-dog.org

Lion's International, 300 22nd St., Oak Brook, IL 60523-8842, 630-571-5466, http://www.lionsclub.org

National Association for the Deaf, 814 Thayer Avenue, Silver Spring, MD 20910, 301-587-1788 (TTY 301-587-1789), http://www.nad.org, e-mail: nadhg@juno.com

National Association for Visually Handicapped, 22 West 21st Street, New York, NY 10010, 212-889-3141, http://www.navh.org

National Board for Certification and Hearing Instruments, National Hearing Aid Helpline, 16880 Middlebelt Rd, Suite 4, Livonia, MI 48154, 734-522-7200, 800-521-5247, http://www.hearingihs.org

National Society to Prevent Blindness, 500 East Remington Rd., Schaumburg, IL 60173, 800-221-3004, http://www.preventblindness.org

Recording for the Blind, Inc., 20 Roszel Rd., Princeton, NJ 08540, 609-452-0606, http://www.rfbd.org

Self Help for Hard of Hearing, 7910 Woodmont Avenue, Suite 1200, Bethesda, MD 20814, 301-657-2248, http://www.shhh.org

CHAPTER 27
Nursing Care of the Client: Endocrine System

REFERENCES/SUGGESTED READINGS

American Diabetes Association. (1996). Nutrition recommendations and principles for people with diabetes mellitus.

Position Statement: American Diabetes Association. *Diabetes Care, 19*(1), 16–19.

American Diabetes Association. (1995). American Diabetes Association: Clinical practice recommendations 1995. *Diabetes Care, 18*(1).

Angelucci, P. A. (1995). Caring for patients with hypothyroidism. *Nursing, 25*(5), 60–61.

Baer, C. L., & Williams, B. R. (1996). *Clinical pharmacology and nursing* (3rd ed.). Springhouse, PA: Springhouse Corp.

Beare, P. G., & Myers, J. L. (Eds.). (1998). *Adult health nursing* (3rd ed.). St. Louis, MO: Mosby.

Betz, J. L. (1995). Fast-acting human insulin analogs: A promising innovation in diabetes care. *The Diabetes Educator, 21*(3), 195–197.

Burton, M. (1997). Pheochromocytoma. *AJN, 97*(11), 57.

Centers for Disease Control and Prevention (CDC). (1999). The public health of diabetes in the United States [On-line]. Available: http://www.cdc.gov/diabetes/survl/surveil.htm

Centers for Disease Control and Prevention (CDC). (1998). Diabetes facts [On-line]. Available: http://www.cdc.gov/diabetes/pubs/facts98.htm

Chase, S. (1997). Oral hypoglycemics. *RN, 60*(12), 45–49.

Clayton, L., & Dilley, K. (1998). Cushing's syndrome. *AJN, 98*(7), 40–41.

Depree, P. (1998). Lispro insulin. *Nursing98, 28*(11), 54–55.

5 tips for finger sticks. (1999). 5 tips for finger sticks. *Nursing99, 29*(5), 59.

Fleming, D. (1999). Challenging traditional insulin injection practices. *AJN, 99*(2), 72–74.

Freeland, B. (1998). Diabetic ketoacidosis. *AJN, 98*(8), 52.

Halpin-Landry, J., & Goldsmith, S. (1999). Feet first: Diabetes care. *AJN, 99*(2), 26–33.

Heater, D. (1999a). If ADH goes out of balance: Diabetes insipidus. *RN, 62*(7), 42–46.

Heater, D. (1999b). If ADH goes out of balance: SIADH. *RN, 62*(7), 47–49.

Hernandez, D. (1998). Microvascular complications of diabetes. *AJN, 98*(6), 26–31.

Hutchinson, C., & Peppard, C. (1998). Hypoglycemia. *Nursing98, 28*(8), 68–69.

Ignatavicius, D. D., Workman, M. L., & Mishler, M.A. (1999). *Medical-surgical nursing across the health care continuum* (3rd ed.). Philadelphia: W. B. Saunders Company.

Jaffe, M. S. (1996). *Medical-surgical nursing care plans: Nursing diagnoses & interventions* (3d ed.). Stanford, CT: Appleton & Lange.

Knight, J. (1998). Inserting an insulin catheter. *Nursing98, 28*(2), 58–60.

LeMone, P., & Burke, K. M. (1996). *Medical-surgical nursing: Critical thinking in client care*. New York: Addison-Wesley Nursing.

McCance, K. L., & Huether, S. E. (1998). *Pathophysiology: The biologic basis for disease in adults and children* (3d ed.). St. Louis, MO: Mosby.

Monahan, F. D., & Neighbors, M. (1998). *Medical-surgical nursing: Foundations for clinical practice* (2d ed.). Philadelphia: W. B. Saunders Company.

Norris, J. (Senior Ed.). (1998). *Handbook of medical-surgical nursing* (2d ed.). Springhouse, PA: Springhouse Corp.

Pagana, K. D., & Pagana, T. J. (1999). *Mosby's diagnostic and laboratory test reference* (4th ed.). St. Louis, MO: Mosby.

Pickar, G. D. (1999). *Dosage calculations* (6th ed.). Albany, NY: Delmar.

Reising, D. (1995, February). Acute hyperglycemia. *Nursing95, (2)*, 33–40.

Reising, D. (1995, February). Acute hypoglycemia. *Nursing95, (2)*, 41–48.

Robertson, C. (1998). When your patient is on an insulin pump. *RN, 61*(3), 30–33.

Smeltzer, S. C., & Bare, B. G. (1996). *Brunner & Suddarth's textbook of medical-surgical nursing* (8th ed.). Philadelphia: Lippincott.

Spratto, G. R., & Woods, A. L. (2000). *PDR® nurses handbook*. Albany, NY: Delmar.

Springhouse. (1999). *Illustrated guide to diagnostic tests* (2d ed.). Springhouse, PA: Springhouse Corp.

Strowig, S. M. (1995, June). Insulin therapy. *RN*, 30–37.

The Expert Committee on the Diagnosis and Classification of Diabetes Mellitus. (1997). Report of the expert committee on the diagnosis and classification of diabetes mellitus. *Diabetes Care, 20*(7), 1183–1197.

Thibodeau, G. A., & Patton, K. T. (1997). *The human body in health & disease* (2d ed.). St. Louis, MO: Mosby.

Tomky, D. (1997). Diabetes: Taking a new look at an old adversary. *Nursing97, 27*(11), 41–45.

U.S. Department of Health and Human Services, National Center for Chronic Disease Control and Prevention, Division of Diabetes Translation (1992). *Diabetes in the United States: A strategy for prevention*. Washington, DC: U.S. Public Health Service.

Walpert, N. (1998). The highs and lows of autoimmune thyroid disease. *Nursing98, 28*(12), 58–60.

Young, J. (1999). Myxedema coma. *Nursing99, 29*(5), 59.

RESOURCES

American Association of Diabetes Educators, 444 N. Michigan Avenue, Suite 1240, Chicago, IL 60611, 800-832-6874, 312-644-2233

American Diabetes Association, ADA National Service Center, 1660 Duke Street, Alexandria, VA 22314, 800-232-3472, 703-549-1500, http://www.diabetes.org

American Dietetic Association, 216 W. Jackson Boulevard, Chicago, IL 60606-6995, 800-877-1600, 312-899-0040, http://www.eatright.org

Juvenile Diabetes Foundation International, 120 Wall Street, New York, NY 10005-4001, 800-223-1138, 212-785-9500

National Diabetes Information Clearinghouse (NDIC), 1 Information Way, Bethesda, MD 20842-3560, http://www.niddk.nih.gov

National Institutes of Health, 9000 Rockville Pike, Bethesda, MD 20892, 301-496-4000, http://www.nih.gov/science/campus

CHAPTER 28
Nursing Care of the Client: Gastrointestinal System

REFERENCES/SUGGESTED READINGS

Boekhold, K. (2000). Who's afraid of hepatitis C? *AJN, 100*(5), 26–31.

Bradley, M., & Pupiales, M. (1997). Essential elements of ostomy care. *AJN, 97*(7), 38–45.

Brietfeller, J. (1999). Peritonitis. *AJN, 99*(4), 33.

Cameron, J. L. (1998). *Current surgical therapy* (6th ed.). St. Louis, MO: Mosby.

Carpenito, L. J. (2000). *Nursing diagnosis: Application to clinical practice* (8th ed.). Philadelphia: Lippincott.

Carroll, P. (1999). Monitoring the gut to prevent MODS. *RN, 62*(10), 34–37.

Centers for Disease Control and Prevention (2000). Viral hepatitis A. [On-line] Available: http://www.cdc.gov/ncidod/diseases/hepatitis/a/index.htm

Centers for Disease Control and Prevention (2000). Viral hepatitis B. [On-line] Available: http://www.cdc.gov/ncidod/diseases/hepatitis/b/index.htm

Centers for Disease Control and Prevention (2000). Viral hepatitis C. [On-line] Available: http://www.cdc.gov/ncidod/diseases/hepatitis/c/index.htm

Centers for Disease Control and Prevention (2000). Viral hepatitis D. [On-line] Available: http://www.cdc.gov/ncidod/diseases/hepatitis/d/hep00051

Centers for Disease Control and Prevention (2000). Viral hepatitis E. [On-line] Available: http://www.cdc.gov/ncidod/diseases/hepatitis/e/hep00058

Giacchino, S., & Houdek, D. (1998). Ruptured varices! Act fast. *RN, 61*(5), 33–36.

Klonowski, E. & Masoodi, J. (1999). The patient with Crohn's disease. *RN, 62*(3), 32–37.

Krupp, K., & Heximer, B. (1998). Going with the flow: How to prevent feeding tubes from clogging. *Nursing98, 28*(4), 54–55.

Lau, D. T., Kleiner, D. E., Park, Y., DiBisceglie, A. M. & Hoofnagle, J. H. (1999). Resolution of chronic delta hepatitis after 12 years of interferon alpha therapy. *Gastroenterology, 117*(5), 1229–33.

Martin, F. (1997). Ulcerative colitis. *AJN, 97*(8), 38–39.

McConnell, E. (1998). Giving medications through an enteral feeding tube. *Nursing98, 28*(3), 66.

Metheny, N., Wehrle, M. A., Wiersema, L., & Clark, J. (1998). pH, color, and feeding tubes. *RN, 61*(1), 25–27.

Metheny, N., Wehrle, M. A., Wiersema, L., & Clark, J. (1998). Testing feeding tube placement: Ascultation vs. pH method. *AJN, 98*(5), 37–42.

National Institute of Diabetes and Digestive and Kidney Diseases (1997). What I need to know about hepatitis A [On-line] Available: http://www.niddk.nih.gov/health/digest/pubs/hep/hepa/hepa.htm

National Institute of Diabetes and Digestive and Kidney Diseases (1998). What I need to know about hepatitis B. [On-line] Available: http://www.niddk.nih.gov/health/digest/pubs/hep/hepb/hepb.htm

National Institute of Diabetes and Digestive and Kidney Diseases (1999). What I need to know about hepatitis C. [On-line] Available: http://www.niddk.nih.gov/health/digest/pubs/hep/hepc/hepc.htm

National Institute of Diabetes and Digestive and Kidney Diseases (2000). Chronic hepatitis C: Current disease management. [On-line] Available: http://www.niddk.nih.gov/health/digest/pubs/chrnhepc/chrnhepc.htm

National Institute of Diabetes and Digestive and Kidney Diseases (2000). The digestive diseases dictionary: E–K. [On-line] Available: http://www.niddk.nih.gov/health/digest/pubs/dddctnry/pages/e-k.htm

O'Brien, B., Davis, S. & Erwin-Toth, P. (1999). G-tube site care: A practical guide. *RN, 62*(2), 52–56.

O'Hanlon-Nichols, T. (1998). Basic assessment series: Gastrointestinal system. *AJN, 98*(4), 48–53.

Phipps, W., Sands, J., & Marek, J. (1999) *Medical-surgical nursing: Concepts and clinical practice* (6th ed.). St. Louis, MO: Mosby.

Rayhorn, N. (1999). Understanding inflammatory bowel disease. *Nursing99, 29*(12), 57–61.

RNWeb. (2000). *The patient with Crohn's disease* [On-line] Available: http://www.RNWeb.com/ce/199/chestblt.html

RNWeb. (2000). *Oncology today: Colorectal colon* [On-line] Available: http://www.RNWeb.com/ce/199/chestblt.html

Springhouse Corporation. (1999). *Illustrated guide to diagnostic tests*. Springhouse, PA: Author.

Spratto, G., & Woods, A. (2001). *2001 PDR Nurse's Drug Handbook*. Albany, NY: Delmar.

SpringNet (2000). *Caring for a patient with colon cancer* [On-line] Available: http://www.springnet.com/ce/j801a.htm

SpringNet (2000). *Irritable bowel syndrome* [On-line] Available: http://www.springnet.com/ce/j801a.htm

SpringNet (2000). *Pancreatitis: Managing a flare-up* [On-line]. Available: http://www.springnet.com/ce/j801a.htm

RESOURCES

American Liver Foundation, 75 Maiden Lane, Suite 603, New York, NY 10038, 800-GO-LIVER (465-4837), http://liverFoundation.org

Crohn and Colitis Foundation of America, Inc., 386 Park Avenue South, 17th Floor, New York, NY 10016-8804, 212-685-3440, http://www.ccfa.org

National Digestive Diseases Clearinghouse, 2 Information Way, Bethesda, MD 20892, 301-654-3810, http://www.niddk.nih.gov

National Foundation for Ileitis and Colitis, 386 Park Avenue South, New York, NY 10016, 212-685-3440, http://www.ccfa.org

United Ostomy Association, 19772 McArthur Boulevard, Suite 200, Irvine, CA 92612, http://www.uoa.org

CHAPTER 29
Nursing Care of the Client: Urinary System

REFERENCES/SUGGESTED READINGS

American Cancer Society (ACS). (1999a). Basic facts [On-line]. Available: http://www.cancer.org/statistics/basicfacts.html

American Cancer Society (ACS). (1999b). Selected cancers—bladder cancer [On-line]. Available: http://www.cancer.org/statistics/cff99/selectedcancers.html

American Society of Nephrology (ASN). (1999). Kidney disease facts & statistics [On-line]. Available: http://www.asn_online.com/facts/prevalence.html

Hayes, D. (2000). Caring for your patient with a permanent hemodialysis access. *Nursing2000, 30*(3), 41–46.

Johnson, S. (2000). From incontinence to confidence. *AJN, 100*(2), 69–76.

Kearney, K. (2000). Dialysis disequilibrium syndrome. *AJN, 100*(2), 53–54.

Kelly, M. (1997). Acute renal failure. *AJN, 97*(3), 32–33.

King, B. (1997). Preserving renal function. *RN, 60*(8), 34–39.

Lewis, S., Heitkemper, M., & Dirksen, S. (2000). *Medical-surgical nursing: Assessment and management of clinical problems* (5th ed.). St. Louis, MO: Mosby.

Loughrey, L. (1999). Taking a sensitive approach to urinary incontinence. *Nursing99, 29*(5), 60–61.

Marchiondo, K. (1998). A new look at urinary tract infection. *AJN, 98*(3), 34–38.

National Institute of Allergies and Infectious Diseases (NIAID). (1998, December). Biologic differences [On-line]. Available: http://www.niaid.nih.gov/publications/transplant/bio.htm

National Institute of Diabetes and Digestive and Kidney Diseases (NIDDK). (1998). Urinary incontinence in women [On-line]. Available: http://www.niddk.nih.gov/health/urolog/pubs/uiwomen/uiwomen.htm

National Institute of Diabetes and Digestive and Kidney Diseases (NIDDK). (1998a, February). Kidney stones in adults [On-line]. Available: http://www.niddk.nih.gov/health/kidney/pubs/stonadult/stonadult.htm

National Institute of Diabetes and Digestive and Kidney Diseases (NIDDK). (1998b, February). Polycystic kidney disease [On-line]. Available: http://www.niddk.nih.gov/health/kidney/pubs/polycyst/polycyst.htm

National Institute of Diabetes and Digestive and Kidney Diseases (NIDDK). (1999, January). Urinary tract infection in adults [On-line]. Available: http://www.niddk.nih.gov/health/kidney/pubs/utiadult/utiadult.htm

National Institute of Diabetes and Digestive and Kidney Diseases (NIDDK). (1999, May). Glomerular diseases [On-line]. Available: http://www.niddk.nih.gov/health/kidney/pubs/glomer/glomer.htm

National Kidney Foundation (NKF). (1997). About kidney disease [On-line]. Available: http://www.kidney.org/general/aboutdisease/index.cfm

National Kidney Foundation (NKF). (1998a, November). Ten facts about African-Americans and kidney disease [On-line]. Available: http://www.kidney.org/general/news/african-american.cfm

National Kidney Foundation (NKF). (1998b, November). The problem of kidney and urologic disease [On-line]. Available: http://www.kidney.org/general/news/problem.cfm

National Kidney Foundation (NKF). (1999, January). New study explains why cranberry juice may help UTI sufferers [On-line]. Available: http://www.kidney.org/general/news/cranberry.cfm

National Kidney Foundation (NKF). (1999, May). National Kidney Foundation releases nutrition guidelines for dialysis patients [On-line]. Available: http://www.kidney.org/general/news/nutguide.cfm

National Kidney Foundation (NKF). (1999a). End-stage renal disease in the United States [On-line]. Available: http://www.kidney.org/general/news/esrd.cfm

National Kidney Foundation (NKF). (1999b). Six warning signs of kidney and urinary tract disease [On-line]. Available: http://www.kidney.org/general/aboutdisease/warningsigns.cfm

PDR Nurse's Handbook. (1999). Albany, NY: Delmar and Montvale, NJ: Medical Economics Company.

Rice, J. (1998). *Medications and mathematics for the nurse* (8th ed.). Albany NY: Delmar.

Sasso, K. (1998). New options for stress incontinence. *RN, 61*(9), 36–39.

Scherer, J. C., & Timby, B. K. (1995). *Introductory medical-surgical nursing* (6th ed.). Philadelphia: Lippincott.

Smith, D. (1999). Gauging bladder volume without a catheter. *Nursing99, 29*(12), 52–53.

Sosa-Guerrero, S., & Gomez, N. (1997). Dealing with end-stage renal disease. *AJN, 97*(10), 44–50.

Stockert, P. (1999). Getting UTI patients back on track. *RN, 62*(3), 49–52.

Townsend, C. (2000). *Nutrition and diet therapy* (7th ed.). Albany, NY: Delmar.

Williams, L. & Hopper, P. (1999). *Understanding medical surgical nursing*. Philadelphia: F. A. Davis Company.

Zellner, K. (1999). Acute tubular necrosis. *RN, 62*(10), 42–46.

RESOURCES

American Association of Kidney Patients, 100 South Ashley Drive, Suite 280, Tampa, FL 33602, 800-749-2257, http://www.aakp.org

American Society of Nephrology, 1200 19th Street N.W. #300, Washington, DC 20036, 202-857-1190, http://www.asn-online.com

Bard Urological Division, C.R. Bard, Inc., Covington, GA 800-526-2687, http://www.crbard.com

Bladder Health Control, c/o American Foundation for Urologic Disease, 1128 North Charles Street, Baltimore, MD 21201, 410-468-1800, 800-242-2383, 877-OVERACT (877-683-7228), 410-468-1800, http://www.afud.org/oab

Interstitial Cystitis Association, 51 Monroe Street, Suite 1402, Rockville, MD 20850, 301-610-5300, 800-HELP-ICA, http://www.ichelp.org

Medic Alert® Foundation, 2323 Colorado Avenue, Turlock, CA 95382-2018, 209-668-3333, 800-IDALERT (800-432-5378), http://www.medicalert.org

National Association for Continence (NAFC), P.O. Box 8310, Spartanburg, SC 29305-8310, 864-579-7900, 800-BLADDER (800-252-3337), http://www.nafc.org

National Kidney and Urologic Diseases Information Clearinghouse, 3 Information Way, Bethesda, MD 20892-3580, 301-468-6345

National Kidney Foundation, 30 East 33rd Street, Suite 1100, New York, NY 10016, 212-889-2210, 800-622-9010, http://www.kidney.org

Polycystic Kidney Research Foundation, 4901 Main Street, Suite 320, Kansas City, MO 64112, 800-753-2873

The Simon Foundation for Continence, P.O. Box 835-F, Wilmette, IL 60091, 847-864-3913 (Headquarters), 800-23-SIMON (Patient Information), http://www.simonfoundation.org

CHAPTER 30
Nursing Care of the Client:
Female Reproductive System

REFERENCES/SUGGESTED READINGS

American Cancer Society (ACS) (1998). *Cancer facts and figures—1998*. Atlanta: Author.

Angelucci, P. (1997). Benign prostatic hyperplasia. *Nursing97, 27*(11), 54–55.

Baird, S., Donehower, M., Stalsbroten, V., & Ades, T. (Eds.). (1997). *A cancer source book for nurses* (7th ed.). Atlanta: American Cancer Society.

Crandall, L. (1997). Menopause made easier. *RN, 60*(7), 46–50.

Estes, M. E. Z. (2002). *Health assessment & physical examination* (2nd ed.). Albany, NY: Delmar.

Gordon, S., Brenden, J., Wyble, J., & Ivey, C. (1997). When the Dx is penile cancer. *RN, 60*(3), 41–44.

Hoskins, C. & Haber, J. (2000). Adjusting to breast cancer. *AJN, 100*(4), 26–31.

Kessenich, C. (1999). Myths & facts about menopause. *Nursing99, 29*(4), 67.

Klingman, L. (1999). Assessing the female reproductive system. *AJN, 99*(8), 37–43.

MacDermott, B. L., Deglin, J. H. (1995). *Understanding basic pharmacology: Practical approaches for effective application*. Philadelphia: F. A. Davis.

Marieb, E. N. (1999). *Human anatomy and physiology* (4th ed.). Redwood City, CA: Benjamin/Cummings Publishing.

Martini, F. & Bartholomew, E. (2000). *Essentials of anatomy and physiology* (4th ed.). Englewood Cliffs, NJ: Prentice Hall.

Mazmanian, C. (1999). Hysterectomy: Holistic care is the key. *RN, 62*(6), 32–35.

Mogus, M. (1997). Pelvic floor surgery? *RN, 60*(4), 36–41.

Moore, A. (1999). Emergency contraceptive options. *RN, 62*(12), 43–45.

North American Nursing Diagnosis Association. (1999). *NANDA nursing diagnoses: Definitions and classification 1999–2000*. Philadelphia: Author.

Otto, S. (1997). *Oncology nursing* (3rd ed.). St. Louis, MO: Mosby.

Pickar, G. D. (1999). *Dosage calculations* (6th ed.). Albany, NY: Delmar.

Schnore, S., & Matsuda, K. (1997). Today's contraceptive choices. *RN, 60*(12), 30–37.

Scura, K. & Whipple, B. (1997). How to provide better care for the post menopausal woman. *AJN, 97*(4), 36–44.

Shurpin, K. (1997). Ovarian cancer. *AJN, 97*(4), 34–35.

Smeltzer, S., & Bare, B. (2000). Management of patients with female reproductive system disorders. In *Brunner and Suddarth's Medical-Surgical Nursing* (9th ed., pp. 1225–1404). Philadelphia: Lippincott.

Spratto, G., & Woods, A. (2000). *PDR for Nurses*. Albany, NY: Delmar.

Taber, C. W. (1997). *Taber's cyclopedic medical dictionary* (18th ed.). Philadelphia: F. A. Davis.

Tamoxifen for breast cancer prevention. (1998, December 15). *Healthnews, 4*(15).

Thomas, S. & Greifzu, S. (2000). Breast cancer. *RN, 63*(4), 40–45.

Warner, P., Rowe, T., & Whipple, B. (1999). Shedding light on the sexual history. *AJN, 99*(6), 34–40.

Wasaha, S., & Angelopoulos, F. (1996). What every woman should know about menopause. *AJN, 96*(1), 25–33.

Weber, E. (1997). Questions and answers about breast cancer diagnosis. *AJN, 97*(10), 34–38.

Wolfe, S. (1997). The great mammogram debate, *RN, 60*(8), 41–44.

RESOURCES

American Association of Sex Educators, Counselors, and Therapists, P.O. Box 238, Mount Vernon, IA 52314, fax 319-895-6203, AASECT@worldnet.att.net

American Cancer Society, Inc., 1599 Clifton Road, NE, Atlanta, GA 30329, 404-320-3333, 800-ACS-2345, http://www.cancer.org

American College of Obstetricians and Gynecologists (ACOG), 409 12th Street SW, P.O. Box 96920, Washington, DC 20090-6920, http://www.acog.org

American Society of Reproductive Medicine, 1209 Montgomery Highway, Birmingham, AL 35216-2809, http://www.asrm.org

Association of Women's Health, Obstetrical, and Neonatal Nursing (AWHONN), 2000 L. Street NW, Suite 740, Washington, DC 20036, http://www.awhonn.org

Cancer Information Service, National Cancer Institute, Building 31 Room 10 A 07, Bethesda, MD 20892, (301) 496-5583, http://www.aoa.dhhs.gov

National Breast Cancer Hotline, 212 West Van Buren, Chicago, IL 60016, 800-221-2141, http://www.y-me.org

National Osteoporosis Foundation (NOF), 1232 22nd St. NW, Washington, DC 20037-1292, 202-223-2226, http://www.nof.org

North American Menopause Society (NAMS), Wolf H. Utain, M.D., 5900 Landerbrook Dr., Suite 195, Mayfield Heights, OH 44124, 440-442-7550, e-mail: info@menopause.org, http://www.menopause.org

Older Women's League, 666 11th Street, N.W., Suite 700, Washington, DC 20001, 202-783-6686

RESOLVE, Inc., 5 Water Street, Arlington, MA 02174-4814, 617-643-2424

CHAPTER 31
Nursing Care of the Client:
Male Reproductive System

REFERENCES/SUGGESTED READINGS

American Cancer Society (ACS) (1998). *Cancer facts and figures—1998*. Atlanta: Author.

Angelucci, P. (1997). Benign prostatic hyperplasia. *Nursing97, 27*(11), 54–55.

Baird, S., Donehower, M., Stalsbroten, V., & Ades, T. (Eds.). (1997). *A cancer source book for nurses* (7th ed.). Atlanta: American Cancer Society.

Cummings, J. M., Parra, R. O., & Boullier, J. A. (1995). Laser prostatectomy: Initial experience and urodynamic follow-up. *Urology, 45*(3), 414–19.

Estes, M. E. Z. (2002). *Health assessment & physical examination* (2nd ed.). Albany, NY: Delmar.

Gordon, S., Brenden, J., Wyble, J., & Ivey, C. (1997). When the Dx is penile cancer. *RN, 60*(3), 41–44.

Greifzu, S. (2000). Prostate cancer. *RN, 63*(6), 26–31.

Held-Warmkessel, J. (1999). How to care for men with prostate cancer. *Nursing99*(11), 51–53.

Klingman, L. (1999). Assessing the male genitalia. *AJN, 99*(7), 47–50.

Lafrades, A. R. (1999). Homemade male incontinence pouch. *Urologic Nursing, 19*(3), 199.

Little, C. (2000). Testicular torsion. *Nursing2000, 30*(4), 33.

Marieb, E. N. (1999). *Human anatomy and physiology* (4th ed.). Redwood City, CA: Benjamin/Cummings Publishing.

Martini, F. H. & Bartholomew, E. F. (2000). *Essentials of anatomy and physiology* (4th ed.). Englewood Cliffs, NJ: Prentice Hall.

Miller, K. (1999). Testicular torsion. *AJN, 99*(6), 33.

North American Nursing Diagnosis Association. (1999). *NANDA nursing diagnoses: Definitions and classification 1999–2000.* Philadelphia: Author.

Otto, S. (1997). *Oncology nursing* (3rd ed.). St. Louis, MO: Mosby.

Pickar, G. D. (1999). *Dosage calculations* (6th ed.). Albany, NY: Delmar.

Smeltzer, S., & Bare, B. (2000). Management of patients with female reproductive disorders. In *Brunner and Suddarth's Medical-Surgical Nursing* (9th ed., pp. 1225–1404). Philadelphia: Lippincott.

Spratto, G., & Woods, A. (2000). *PDR for Nurses.* Albany, NY: Delmar.

Taber, C. W. (1997). *Taber's cyclopedic medical dictionary* (18th ed.). Philadelphia: F. A. Davis.

Warner, P., Rowe, T., & Whipple, B. (1999). Shedding light on the sexual history. *AJN, 99*(6), 34–40.

Zaccognini, M. (1999). Prostate cancer, *AJN, 99*(4), 34–35.

RESOURCES

American Association of Sex Educators, Counselors, and Therapists, P.O. Box 238, Mount Vernon, IA 52314, Fax 319-895-6203, e-mail: AASECT@worldnet.att.net

American Cancer Society, Inc., 1599 Clifton Road, NE, Atlanta, GA 30329, 404-320-3333, 800-ACS-2345, http://www.cancer.org

American Society of Reproductive Medicine, 1209 Montgomery Highway, Birmingham, AL 35216-2809, http://www.asrm.org

Cancer Information Service, National Cancer Institute, Building 31 Room 10 A 07, Bethesda, MD 20892, (301) 496-5583, http://www.aoa.dhhs.gov

Recovery of Male Potency, Grace Hospital, 18700 Meyers Rd., Detroit, MI 48235

RESOLVE, Inc., 5 Water Street, Arlington, MA 02174-4814, 617-643-2424

CHAPTER 32
Nursing Care of the Client: Sexually Transmitted Diseases

REFERENCES/SUGGESTED READINGS

Centers for Disease Control and Prevention (CDC). (1999a, July). *Hepatitis B—Fact sheet* [On-line]. Available: http://www.cdc.gov/ncidod/diseases/hepatitis/b/fact.htm

Centers for Disease Control and Prevention (CDC). (1999b, July). *Hepatitis B vaccine—Fact sheet* [On-line]. Available: http://www.cdc.gov/ncidod/diseases/hepatitis/b/factvax.htm

Hadley, J. (1999). *Culturally relevant behavioral intervention dramatically reduces STDs* [On-line]. Available: http://www.niaid.nih.gov/newsroom/std.htm

Jagger, J., & Perry, J. (1999). Power in numbers: Reducing your risk of blood borne exposures. *Nursing99, 29*(1), 51–52.

Lammon, C. B., Foote, A. W., Leli, P. G., Ingle, J., & Adams, M. H. (1995). *Clinical nursing skills.* Philadelphia: W. B. Saunders Company.

National Institute of Allergy and Infectious Diseases (NIAID) and National Institutes of Health (NIH). (1998a, June). *An introduction to sexually transmitted diseases* [On-line]. Available: http://www.niaid.nih.gov/factsheets/stdinfo.htm

National Institute of Allergy and Infectious Diseases (NIAID) and National Institutes of Health (NIH). (1998b, June). *Chlamydial infection* [On-line]. Available: http://www.niaid.nih.gov/factsheets/stdclam.htm

National Institute of Allergy and Infectious Diseases (NIAID) and National Institutes of Health (NIH). (1998c, June). *Gonorrhea* [On-line]. Available: http://www.niaid.nih.gov/factsheets/stdgon.htm

National Institute of Allergy and Infectious Diseases (NIAID) and National Institutes of Health (NIH). (1998d, June). *Vaginitis due to vaginal infections* [On-line]. Available: http://www.niaid.nih.gov/factsheets/stdvag.htm

National Institute of Allergy and Infectious Diseases (NIAID) and National Institutes of Health (NIH). (1998e, June). *Other important STDs* [On-line]. Available: http://www.niaid.nih.gov/factsheets/stdother.htm

National Institute of Allergy and Infectious Diseases (NIAID) and National Institutes of Health (NIH). (1998a, July). *Genital herpes* [On-line]. Available: http://www.niaid.nih.gov/factsheets/stdherp.htm

National Institute of Allergy and Infectious Diseases (NIAID) and National Institutes of Health (NIH). (1998b, July). *Human papillomavirus and genital warts* [On-line]. Available: http://www.niaid.nih.gov/factsheets/stdhpv.htm

National Institute of Allergy and Infectious Diseases (NIAID) and National Institutes of Health (NIH). (1998c, July). *Syphilis* [On-line]. Available: http://www.niaid.nih.gov/factsheets/stdsyph.htm

National Institute of Allergy and Infectious Diseases (NIAID) and National Institutes of Health (NIH). (1998, December). *Sexually transmitted diseases statistics* [On-line]. Available: http://www.niaid.nih.gov/factsheets/stdstats.htm

Sharts-Hopko, N. (1997). STDs in women: What you need to know. *AJN, 97*(4), 46–54.

RESOURCES

American College of Obstetricians and Gynecologists (ACOG), 409 Twelfth Street S.W., P.O. Box 96920, Washington, DC 20090-6920, 202-863-2518, http://www.acog.org

American Public Health Association (APHA), 1015 Fifteenth Street N.W., Washington, DC 20005, 202-789-5600, Fax 202-789-5661, e-mail: comments@apha.org, http://www.apha.org

American Social Health Association (ASHA), P.O. Box 13827, Research Triangle Park, NC 27709-9940, 800-230-6089, Herpes Hotline: 919-361-8488, http://www.ashastd.org

Centers for Disease Control and Prevention (CDC), 1600 Clifton Road N.E., Atlanta, GA 30333, 404-329-1388, http://www.cdc.gov

National Foundation for Infectious Diseases, 4733 Bethesda Avenue, Suite 750, Bethesda, MD 20814

National Institute of Allergy and Infectious Diseases, National Institutes of Health, NIAID Office of Public Liaison, Building 31, Room 7A-50, 31 Center Drive MSC 2520, Bethesda, MD 20892, http://www.niaid.nih.gov

Planned Parenthood Federation of America, Inc., 810 Seventh Avenue, New York, NY 10019, 212-541-7800, http://www.plannedparenthood.org

U.S. Department of Health and Human Services (USD-HHS), Public Health Service, 200 Independence Avenue S.W., Washington, DC 20201, 877-696-6775, http://www.os.dhhs.gov

World Health Organization (WHO), Avenue Appia, CH 1211 Geneva 27, Switzerland, http://www.who.int

CHAPTER 33
Nursing Care of the Client: Mental Illness

REFERENCES/SUGGESTED READINGS

Aguilera, D. C. (1997). *Crisis intervention theory and methodology* (8th ed.). St. Louis, MO: Mosby.

American Psychiatric Association. (2000). *Diagnostic and statistical manual of mental disorders* (4th ed.). (DSM-IV-TR [text-revision]) Washington, DC: Author.

Andresen, G. (1998). Assessing the older patient. *RN, 61*(3), 46–55.

Badger, J. M. (1995). Reaching out to the suicidal patient. *AJN, 95*(3), 24–31.

Bailey, K. P. (1998). *Lippincott's need-to-know psychotropic drug facts*. Philadelphia: Lippincott.

Clark, C. C. (1997). Posttraumatic stress disorder: How to support healing. *AJN, 97*(8), 27–32.

Clark, M. J. (1999). Violence. In *Nursing in the community* (3rd ed.). Stamford, CT: Appleton & Lange.

Cole, M. (1999). Bipolar disorder: Illness or eccentricity? *Nursing Spectrum (NY NJ), 11A*(2), 4–5.

Cole, M. (1999). Bridging the great divide: Management of the patient with bipolar disorder. *Nursing Spectrum (NY NJ), 11A*(3), 8–9.

Constantino, R. E., & Bricker, P. L. (1997). Social support, stress, and depression among battered women in the judicial setting. *Journal of the American Psychiatric Nurses Association, 3*(3), 81–88.

Deglin, J. H., & Vallerand, A. H. (1999). *Davis's drug guide for nurses* (6th ed.). Philadelphia: F. A. Davis.

DiVitto, S. (1998). Empowerment through self-regulation: Group approach for survivors of incest. *Journal of the American Psychiatric Nurses Association, 4*(3), 77–86.

Eskreis, T. R. (1998). Seven common legal pitfalls in nursing. *AJN, 98*(4), 34–41.

Eskreis-Nelson, T. R. (1997). Shedding some light on psychiatric care issues. *RN, 60*(2), 57–60.

Flowers, E. M. (1997). Recognition and psychopharmacologic treatment of geriatric depression. *Journal of the American Psychiatric Nurses Association, 3*(2), 32–39.

Frisch, N. C., & Frisch, L. E. (1998). *Psychiatric mental health nursing*. Albany, NY: Delmar.

Garcia, G., & Ghani, S. (2000). Pharmacology update: Newer medications and indications used in psychiatry. *Lippincott's Primary Care Practice, 4*(2), 207–220.

Glod, C. A. (1997). Attention deficit hyperactivity disorder throughout the lifespan: Diagnosis, etiology, and treatment. *Journal of the American Psychiatric Nurses Association, 3*(3), 89–92.

Gorman, L. M., Sultan, D. F., & Raines, M. (1996). *Davis's manual of psychococial nursing for general patient care*. Philadelphia: F. A. Davis.

Hargreaves, W. A., & Shumway, M. (1989). Effectiveness of mental health services for the severely mental ill. In C. A. Taube & A. Hohmann (Eds.), *The future of mental health services research*. Washington, DC: U. S. Government Printing Office.

Harrison, B., & Kaarsemaker, B. (2000). Continuous quality improvement to an electroconvulsive therapy delivery system. *Journal of Psychosocial Nursing Mental Health Services, 38*(3), 27–37.

Hinkle, P. (2000). Bipolar illness in primary care: An overview. *Lippincott's Primary Care Practice, 4*(2), 163–173.

Hyman, A., Schillinger, D., & Lo, B. (1995). Laws mandating reporting of domestic violence: Do they promote patient well-being? *JAMA, 273*(22), 1781–1787.

Isaacs, A. (1998). Depression & your patient. *AJN, 98*(7), 26–31.

Johnson, L., & Cheffer, N. D. (1996). Child sexual abuse: A case of intrafamilial abuse. *Journal of the American Psychiatric Nurses Association, 2*(4), 108–114.

Ladebauche, P. (1997). Childhood trauma: When to suspect abuse. *RN, 60*(9), 38–42.

Lynch, S. H. (1997). Elder abuse: What to look for, how to intervene. *AJN, 97*(1), 27–32.

McCloskey, J. C., & Bulechek, G. M. (1996). *Nursing interventions classification (NIC)* (2nd ed.). St. Louis, MO: Mosby.

McEnany, G. (1998). Sexual dysfunction in the pharmacologic treatment of depression: When "Don't Ask, Don't Tell" is an unsuitable approach to care. *Journal of the American Psychiatric Nurses Association, 4*(1), 24–29.

Medical Education Group Learning Systems. (1995). *Domestic violence: A practical guide for physicians* [On-line]. Available: http://www.cme.edu/phydom/domes.html

Mohr, W. (1998). Updating what we know about depression in adolescents. *Journal of Psychosocial Nursing and Mental Health Services, 36*(9), 12–19.

Morris, R. (1998). Elder abuse: What the law requires. *RN, 61*(8), 52–53.

NIMH funds study of drugs for schizophrenia and Alzheimer's. (1999). *Journal of Psychosocial Nursing Mental Health Services, 37*(12), 7.

Osgood, N. (1992). *Suicide in later life*. San Francisco, CA: Jossey-Bass, Inc.

Peplau, H. E. (1962). Interpersonal techniques: The crux of psychiatric nursing. *AJN, 62*(6), 50–54.

Peplau, H. E. (1963). A working definition of anxiety. In S. Burd & M. Marshall (Eds.), *Some clinical approaches to psychiatric nursing*. New York: Macmillan.

Peplau, H. E. (1991). *Interpersonal relations in nursing*. New York: Springer.

Physician Desk Reference. (53rd ed.). (1999). Montvale, NY: Medical Economics.

Ponech, S. (2000). Telltale signs. *Nursing Management, 31*(5), 32–38.

Ravetti, L. (2000). Patient education: For the recovering individual. *Lippincott's Primary Care Practice, 4*(2), 341–343.

Romme, M. (1998). Listening to the voice hearers. *Journal of Psychosocial Nursing and Mental Health Services, 36*(9), 40–44.

Sajo, E. (2000). Pharmacology update: Pharmacology of substance abuse. *Lippincott's Primary Care Practice, 4*(2), 319–335.

Schaffer, S. (2000). Patient education: Patient's guide to medication used for depression. *Lippincott's Primary Care Practice, 4*(2), 237–239.

Sexual assault glossary of terms [On-line]. (1996, December 27). Available: http://asucd.ucdavis.edu/organizations/other/rpep/terms.htm

Shea, C. A., Mahoney, M., & Lacey, J. M. (1997). Breaking through the barriers to domestic violence intervention. *AJN, 97*(6), 26–34.

Sullivan, G. H. (1998). Getting informed consent. *RN, 61*(4), 59–62.

Sundeen, S., Stuart, G. W., Rankin, E. A. D., & Cohen, S. A. (1998). *Nurse–Client interaction: Implementing the nursing process* (6th ed.). St. Louis, MO: Mosby.

Townsend, M. C. (2000). *Psychiatric mental health nursing: Concepts of care* (3rd ed.). Philadelphia: F. A. Davis.

Townsend, M. C. (1997). *Nursing diagnoses in psychiatric nursing: A pocket guide for care plan construction* (4th ed.). Philadelphia: F. A. Davis.

United States Code Annotated, Title 42, The Public Health and Welfare, Chapter 67, Child Abuse Prevention and Treatment and Adoption Reform; Subchapter 1, Child Abuse Prevention and Treatment; Definitions; Title II, Victims of Child Abuse Act of 1990; Subtitle D, Federal Victims' Protection and Rights; Section 226, Child Abuse Reporting. St. Paul, MN: West.

U. S. House of Representatives, Select Committee on Aging, (1981, April 3). *Elder Abuse (an examination of a hidden problem)* (Comm. Pub. No. 97–277). Washington, DC: U. S. Government Printing Office.

Walton-Moss, B., & Becker, K. (2000). Women and substance use disorders. *Lippincott's Primary Care Practice, 4*(2), 290–301.

Ward-Collins, D. (1998). "Noncompliant": Isn't there a better way to say it? *AJN, 98*(5), 27–32.

Wilkinson, L. K. (1996). The martial arts: A mental health intervention? *Journal of the American Psychiatric Nurses Association, 2*(6), 202–206.

Women's Issues and Social Empowerment (W.I.S.E.). (1997, April 15). The dynamics of domestic violence [Online]. Available: http://www.infoxchange.net.au/wise/DVIM/DVDynamics.htm

Wuerker, A. (2000). The family and schizophrenia. *Issues of Mental Health Nursing, 21*(1), 127–141.

Yamashita, M., & McNally-Forsyth, D. (1998). Family coping with mental illness: An aggregate from two studies, Canada and United States. *Journal of the American Psychiatric Nurses Association, 4*(1), 1–8.

RESOURCES

American Anorexia/Bulimia Association, 165 W 46th Street, S. 1108, New York, NY 10036, 212-575-6200, http://www.aabainc.org

American Psychiatric Association, 1400 K Street N.W., Washington, DC 20005, 202-682-6000, http://www.psych.org

American Psychiatric Nurses Association, 1200 19th Street N.W., Suite 300, Washington, DC 20036-2422, 202-857-1133, http://www.apna.org

Anorexia/Bulimia Support, 3049 E. Genesee Street, Syracuse, NY 13224, 315-445-1975

Anxiety Disorders Association of America, 11900 Parklawn Drive, Suite 100, Rockville, MD 20852, 301-231-9350, http://www.adaa.org

NARSAD Research (National Alliance for Research on Schizophrenia and Depression), 60 Cutter Mill Road, Suite 404, Great Neck, NY 11021, 516-829-0091, Fax 516-487-6930, http://www.mhsource.com/narsad.html

National Alliance for the Mentally Ill (NAMI), 200 N. Glebe Road, Suite 1015, Arlington, VA 22203-3754, 800-950-NAMI (6264), 703-524-7600, http://www.nami.org

National Association of Anorexia Nervosa and Associated Disorders, P.O. Box 7, Highland Park, IL 60035, 847-831-3438, http://www.anad.org

National Center on Elder Abuse, American Public Welfare Association, 8101 1st Street N.E., Suite 500, Washington, DC 20002, 202-682-2470, http://www.aoa.dhhs.gov/aoa/dir/143.html

National Depressive and Manic-Depressive Association, 730 North Franklin Street, Suite 501, Chicago, IL 60610-3526, 800-826-3632, http://www.ndmda.org

National Institute of Mental Health, 6001 Executive Boulevard, Room 8184, MSC 9663, Bethesda, MD 20892-9663, http://www.nimh.nih.gov

Parents Anonymous, The National Organization, 675 W. Foothill Blvd., Suite 200, Claremont, CA 91711-3475, 909-621-6184, http://www.parentsanonymous-natl.org

Recovery, Inc.: The Association of Nervous and Former Mental Patients, 802 N. Dearborn Street, Chicago, IL 60610, 312-337-5661, http://www.recovery-inc.com

Victims of Incest Can Emerge Survivors (VOICES), P.O. Box 148309, Chicago, IL 60614, 800-786-4238, http://www.voices-action.org

CHAPTER 34
Nursing Care of the Client: Substance Abuse

REFERENCES/SUGGESTED READINGS

Alcoholics Anonymous. (1939). *Alcoholics Anonymous.* New York: Alcoholics Anonymous World Services.

American Psychiatric Association. (2000). *Diagnostic and statistical manual of mental disorders* (4th ed.). T-R (text revision). Washington, DC: Author.

Anderson, N. (1996). Decisions about substance abuse among adolescents in juvenile detention. *Image, 28*(1), 65–70.

Antai-Otong, D. (1995). Helping the alcoholic patient recover. *AJN, 95*(8), 22–29.

Biggs-Stewart, K., & Richards, A. (2000). Recognizing and managing your patient's alcohol abuse. *Nursing2000, 30*(2), 56–59.

Brent, M. (1997). Unexpected alcohol withdrawal. *AJN, 97*(6), 52–53.

Crigger, N. (1998). Defying denial: Clues to detecting alcohol abuse. *AJN, 98*(8), 20–21.

Haack, M. (1998). Treating acute withdrawal from alcohol and other drugs. *Nursing Clinics of North America, 33*(1), 75–92.

Haddad, A. (2000). Ethics in action: Treating pain in substance abusers. *RN, 63*(1), 21–24.

Johnson, V. (1973). *I'll quit tomorrow.* New York: Harper & Row.

Johnson, V. (1988). *Intervention: How to help someone who doesn't want help.* New York: New American Library.

Johnston, L., O'Malley, P., & Bachman, J. (1991). *Drug use among American high school seniors, college students and young adults 1975–1990.* Rockville, MD: National Institute on Drug Abuse, U.S. Department of Health and Human Services, Alcohol Drug Abuse, and Mental Health Administration.

Johnston, L., O'Malley, P., & Bachman, J. (1998). Drug use by American young people begins to turn downward [Online]. Available: http://www.isr.umich.edu/src/mtf

Kendig, S. (1995). Women at risk for infection: The woman who is chemically dependent. *Journal of Obstetric, Gynecologic, and Neonatal Nursing, 24*(8), 776–781.

Kleber, H. (1994). Opioids detoxification. In M. Galanter & H. Kleber, *Textbook of substance abuse treatment.* Washington, DC: American Psychiatric Press.

Landau, E. (1995). *Hooked: Talking about addictions.* Brookfield, CT: The Millbrook Press.

Langone, J. (1995). *Tough choices.* Boston: Little, Brown and Company.

National Institute on Alcohol Abuse and Alcoholism (NIAAA). (1999a). Age-specific number of deaths for cirrhosis with and without mention of alcohol, United States, 1970–95 [On-line]. Available: http://silk.nih.gov/silk/niaaa/database/cirmrt3a.txt

National Institute on Alcohol Abuse and Alcoholism (NIAAA). (1999b). Traffic crashes, traffic crash fatalities, and alcohol-related traffic crash fatalities, United States, 1977–96 [On-line]. Available: http://silk.nih.gov/silk/niaaa/database/crash01.txt

National Institute on Alcohol Abuse and Alcoholism (NIAAA). (1999c). Updated cost estimates for 1992 and inflation- and population-adjusted costs of alcohol and drug abuse for 1995 [in millions of current-year dollars] [On-line]. Available: http://silk.nih.gov/silk/niaaa/database/cost7.txt

National Institute on Drug Abuse (NIDA). (1997). Diagnosis and treatment of drug abuse in family practice [On-line]. Available: http://165.112.78.61/Diagnosis-Treatment/Diagnosis6.html

National Institute on Drug Abuse (NIDA). (1998a). Criteria for substance dependence diagnosis [On-line]. Available: http://www.nida.nih.gov/DSR.html

National Institute on Drug Abuse (NIDA). (1998b). Nicotine addiction [On-line]. Available: http://www.nida.nih.gov/researchreports/nicotine/nicotine.html

National Institute on Drug Abuse (NIDA). (1999a). Commonly abused drugs [On-line]. Available: http://www.nida.nih.gov/DrugsofAbuse.html

National Institute on Drug Abuse (NIDA). (1999b). Cigarettes and other nicotine products [On-line]. Available: http://www.nida.nih.gov/Infofax/tobacco.html

National Institute on Drug Abuse (NIDA). (1999c). Cocaine abuse and addiction [On-line]. Available: http://www.nida.nih.gov/ResearchReports/Cocaine/cocaine.html

National Institute on Drug Abuse (NIDA). (1999e). Ecstasy [On-line]. Available: http://www.nida.nih.gov/Infofax/ecstasy.html

National Institute on Drug Abuse (NIDA). (1999f). Heroin [On-line]. Available: http://www.nida.nih.gov/Infofax/heroin.html

National Institute on Drug Abuse (NIDA). (1999g). Heroin: Abuse and addiction [On-line]. Available: http://www.nida.nih.gov/ResearchReports/Heroin/heroin.html

National Institute on Drug Abuse (NIDA). (1999h). Inhalants [On-line]. Available: http://www.nida.nih.gov/Infofax/inhalants.html

National Institute on Drug Abuse (NIDA). (1999i). LSD [On-line]. Available: http://www.nida.nih.gov/Infofax/lsd.html

National Institute on Drug Abuse (NIDA). (1999j). Marijuana [On-line]. Available: http://www.nida.nih.gov/Infofax/marijuana.html

National Institute on Drug Abuse (NIDA). (1999k). Methamphetamine: Abuse and addiction [On-line]. Available: http://www.nida.nih.gov/ResearchReports/Methamph/methamph.html

National Institute on Drug Abuse (NIDA). (1999l). PCP (Phencyclidine) [On-line]. Available: http://www.nida.nih.gov/Infofax/pcp.html

National Institute on Drug Abuse (NIDA). (1999m). Steroids (Anabolic) [On-line]. Available: http://www.nida.nih.gov/Infofax/steroids.html

Navarra, T. (1995). Enabling behavior: The tender trap. *AJN, 95*(1), 50–52.

Powell, A. (1999). Alcohol withdrawal in critical care. *Dimensions of Critical Care Nursing, 18*(6), 24–28.

Santomier, J., & Hogan, P. (1991). Health implications of alcohol and other drug use. In M. Naegle (Ed.), *Substance abuse education in nursing* (Vol.1). New York: National League for Nursing.

Waugfield, C. (1998). *Mental health concepts* (4th ed.). Albany, NY: Delmar.

RESOURCES

Al-Anon Al-Ateen Family Intergroup, 200 Park Avenue S., Room 814, New York, NY 10003, 212-254-7236, 212-254-7230, 800-344-2666, 800-939-2770 (Spanish), http://www.al-anon.org

Alcoholics Anonymous (AA), P.O. Box 459, Grand Central Station, New York, NY 10017, 212-870-3400, http://www.alcoholics-Anonymous.org

American Council for Drug Education, 164 W. 74th Street, New York, NY 10023, 800-488-DRUG, 301-294-0600, http://www.acde.org

Cocaine Helpline, 800-662-HELP, http://www.nd.edu

Codependents Anonymous (CODA), P.O. Box 33577, Phoenix, AZ 85607-3577, 602-277-7991, http://www.codependents.org

Drug Abuse Resistance Education (DARE), Local Police Department, http://www.dare-america.com

Drug Enforcement Administration (DEA), Information Services Section (CPI), 700 Army-Navy Drive, Arlington, VA 22202, 202-307-1000, http://www.usdoj.gov/dea

Families Anonymous, (Families of Substance Abusers), Box 3475, Culver City, CA 90231-3415, 800-736-9805, http://www.escape.ca

Mothers Against Drunk Driving (MADD), 511 E. John Carpenter Freeway, No. 700, Irving, TX 75062, 214-744-6233, or, 3601 SW 29th, Topeka, KS 66614, 800-443-6233, http://www.madd.org

Narcotics Anonymous (NA), World Service Office, P.O. Box 9999, Van Nuys, CA 91409, 818-773-9999, http://www.na.org

National Clearinghouse for Alcohol and Drug Information, Box 2345, Rockville, MD 20857, 301-468-2600, http://www.health.org

National Clearinghouse for Tobacco and Health, 170 Laurier Avenue West, Suite 1000, Ottawa, Ontario, Canada K1P 5V5, 800-267-5234, http://www.health.org

National Cocaine Hotline, 800-COCAINE (262-2463), http://www.viser.net

National Council on Alcoholism, Inc., 12 West 21st Street, New York, NY 10010, 212-206-6770, http://www.ncadd.org

National Nurses Society on Addictions, 5700 Old Orchard Road, First Floor, Skokie, IL 60077, 847-966-5010, http://www.nnsa.org

National Self-Help Clearinghouse, 33 West 42nd Street, New York, NY 10036, 212-840-1259, http://www.mhselfhelp.org

Office of Substance Abuse Prevention, 5600 Fishers Lane, Rockwall II, Rockville, MD 20857, 301-443-0373, http://www.ed.gov/offices

Students Against Driving Drunk (SADD) Inc., P.O. Box 800, Marlboro, MA 01752, 508-481-3568, http://www.sadd.org

Toughlove, P.O. Box 1069, Doylestown, PA 18901, 215-348-7090, http://www.toughlove.org

CHAPTER 35
Nursing Care of the Older Client

REFERENCES/SUGGESTED READINGS

Administration on Aging (AoA). (2000). The Administration on Aging and the Older American's Act. [On-line] Available: http://www.aoa.dhhs.gov/aoa/pages/aoafact.html

American Association of Retired Persons (AARP). (1998). *A profile of older Americans*. Washington, DC: Department of Health and Human Services.

Andersen, C. (1999). *Antecedents, correlates, and impact of violent behaviors in the elderly VA client*. Unpublished thesis, University of Iowa, Iowa City, IA.

Andersen, C. F. (1999). *Nursing student to nursing leader: The critical path to leadership development*. Albany, NY: Delmar.

Bahr, Sr. R. T. (1994). An overview of gerontological nursing. In M. Hogstel (Ed.), *Nursing care of the older adult* (3rd ed., pp. 2–25). Albany: Delmar.

Fetters, C. (1994). *Standard of care on wandering*. Knoxville, IA: Department of Veterans Affairs Medical Center, Division of Nursing.

Gallo, J., Fulmer, T., Paveza, G., & Reichel, W. (1999). *Handbook of geriatric assessment* (3rd ed.). Gaithersburg, MD: Aspen Publishers.

Hogstel, M. (Ed.). (1994). *Nursing care of the older adult* (3rd ed.). Albany, NY: Delmar.

Maas, M., Buckwalter, K., & Hardy, M. (1991). *Nursing diagnosis and new interventions for the elderly*. Redwood City, CA: Addison-Wesley.

McCloskey, J., & Bulechek, G. (1999). *Nursing interventions classifications (NIC)* (3rd ed.). St. Louis, MO: Mosby.

National Council on Aging (NCOA) (2000). Facts about older Americans. [On-line] Available: http://www.ncoa.org/news/mra_2000/factsheet.html

Needham, J. F. (1995). *Gerontological nursing*. Albany, NY: Delmar.

Peskin, B. (1999). *Beyond the zone*. Houston, TX: Noble Publishing.

Social Security Administration (SSA). (2000). The president signs the "Senior Citizens' Freedom to Work Act of 2000." [On-line] Available: http://www.ssa.gov/legislation/legis_bulletin_040700.html

Wilkinson, J. (1999). *A family caregiver's guide to planning and decision making for the elderly*. Minneapolis, MN: Fairview Press.

Yen, P. K. (1995). Maximizing calcium intake. *Geriatric Nursing, 16*(2), 92–93.

RESOURCES

Administration on Aging (AoA), U.S. Department of Health and Human Services, 330 Independence Avenue S.W., Washington, DC 20201, 202-619-0724, http://www.aoa.dhhs.gov

American Association of Geriatric Psychiatry, 7910 Woodmont Avenue, Suite 1050, Bethesda, MD 20814-3004, 301-654-7850, http://www.aagpgpa.org

American Association of Retired Persons (AARP), 601 East Street N.W., Washington, DC 20049, 800-424-3410, http://www.aarp.org

American Nurses Association (ANA), Council on Gerontological Nursing Practice, 600 Maryland Avenue S.W., Suite 100W, Washington, DC 20024, 800-274-4262, http://www.nursingworld.org

Department of Health and Human Services, Public Health Service, Agency for Healthcare Research and Quality, Executive Office Center, 200 Independence Avenue, S.W., Washington, DC 20201, 202-619-0257, 877-696-6775, http://www.dhhs.gov, www.ahcpr.gov

National Council on Aging, Inc. (NCOA), 409 3rd Street, S.W., Washington, DC 20024, 800-424-9046, http://www.ncoa.org

CHAPTER 36
Rehabilitation, Home Health, Long-Term Care, and Hospice

REFERENCES/SUGGESTED READINGS

Abrams, W. B., Beers, M. H., & Berkow, R. (Eds.). (2000). *The Merck manual of geriatrics* (3rd ed.). Whitehouse Station, NJ: Merck Research Laboratories.

American Association of Retired Persons (AARP). (1998). *A profile of older Americans*. Washington, DC: U.S. Department of Health and Human Services.

American Health Care Association (AHCA). (1998). The looming crisis [On-line]. Available: http://www.ahca.org

American Health Care Association (AHCA). (2000). Nursing facility subacute care: The quality and cost-effective alternative to hospital care. [On-line] Available: http://www.ahca.org/who/pubsubac.htm

Assisted Living Federation of America (ALFA). (1999). What is assisted living [On-line]. Available: http://www.alfa.org

Barker, E. (1999). Life care planning. *RN, 62*(3), 58–61.

Benefield, L. (1996). Making the transition to home care nursing. *AJN, 96*(10), 47–49.

Boon, T. (1998). Don't forget the hospice option. *RN, 61*(2), 30–33.

Bral, E. (1998). Caring for adults with chronic cancer pain. *AJN, 98*(4), 26–32.

Diaz, D. (1995). Geriatric UPDATE 95. *Nursing95, 25*(3), 62–64.

Gresham, G. E., Duncan, P. W., Stason, W. B., et al. (1995, May). *Post stroke rehabilitation*. Clinical Practice Guideline, No. 16, Rockville, MD: U.S. Department of Health and Human Services. Public Health Service Agency for Health Care Policy and Research. AHCPR Publication No. 95–0062.

Grove, N. (1997). Helping families select a nursing home. *RN, 60*(3), 37–40.

Health Care Financing Administration (HCFA). (2000a). Highlights: National Health Care Expenditures, 1998. [On-line] Available: http://www.hcfa.gov/stats/nke-oact/hilites.htm

Health Care Financing Administration (HCFA). (2000b). National Health Expenditures Projection. [On-line] Available: http://www.hcfa.gov/stats/NHE-Proj/proj1998/tables

Health, Education, and Human Services Division. (1994). *Long-term care reform*. (GAO)/HEHS–94–227). Washington DC: U.S. General Accounting Office.

Hospice Education Institute (1999). Definition of palliative care [On-line]. Available: http://www.hospiceworld.org

Kazanowski, M. (1997). A commitment to palliative care: Could it impact assisted suicide? *Journal of Gerontologic Nursing, 23*(3), 36–42.

Kennison, M. (1999). A case study in care. *RN, 62*(1), 46–48.

Lasky, W. F. (1995). Assisted living: A brand new world. *Nursing Homes, 44*(7), 40–41.

Lattanzi-Licht, M. E. (1998). *The hospice choice: In pursuit of a peaceful death*. New York: Simon and Schuster/Fireside.

Millea, K. (1995). Home health care UPDATE 95. *Nursing95, 25*(7), 57–59.

National Adult Day Services Association (NADSA). (2000). Adult day services fact sheet. [On-line] Available: http://www.ncoa.org/nadsa/ADS_factsheet.htm

National Association for Home Care (NAHC). (1999). Hospice [On-line]. Available: http://www.nahc.org/HAA

National Association for Home Care (NAHC). (2000). Basic statistics about home care. [On-line] Available: http://www.nahc.org/consumer/hcstats.html

National Hospice Organization (NHO). (1999). The basics of hospice [On-line]. Available: http://www.nho.org

National Institute on Aging (NIA). (1996). Planning for long-term care [On-line]. Available: http://www.nih.gov/nia/health/pubpub/longterm.htm

Puopolo, A. (1999). Gaining confidence to talk about end-of-life care. *Nursing99, 29*(7), 49–51.

Ufema, J. (1999). Reflections on death and dying. *Nursing99, 29*(6), 56–59.

Waid, M. O. (1998). Brief summaries of Medicare and Medicaid. [On-line] Available: http://www.hcfa.gov/medicare/ormedmed.htm

RESOURCES

American Association of Homes and Services for the Aging (AAHSA), Suite 500, 901 E Street N.W., Washington, DC 20004-2011, 202-783-2242, http://www.aahsa.org

American Association of Retired Persons (AARP), 601 E Street N.W., Washington, DC 20049, 202-434-6190, 800-424-3410, http://www.aarp.org

American Health Care Association (AHCA), 1201 L Street N.W., Washington, DC 20005, 202-842-4444, http://www.ahca.org

American Hospital Association (AHA), Chicago Headquarters (CH), One North Franklin, Chicago, IL 60606, 312-422-3000, http://www.aha.org

American Hospital Association (AHA), Washington Office (WO), 325 Seventh Street N.W., Washington, DC 20004, 202-638-1100, 800-424-4301, http://www.aha.org

Assisted Living Federation of America, Suite 400, 10300 Eaton Place, Fairfax, VA 22030, 703-691-8100, http://www.alfa.org

Association of Rehabilitation Nurses (ARN), 4700 W. Lake Avenue, Glenview, IL 60025-1485, 800-229-7530, 847-375-4710, http://www.rehabnurse.org

Department of Health and Human Services (DHHS), 200 Independence Avenue, S.W., Washington, DC 20201, 202-619-0257, 877-696-6775, http://www.hhs.gov

Foundation for Hospice & Home Care, 519 C Street N.E., Washington, DC 20002, 302-547-6586

Health Care Financing Administration (HCFA), 7500 Security Boulevard, Baltimore, MD 21244, 800-638-6833, http://www.hcfa.gov

Home Healthcare Nurses Association, 7794 Grow Drive, Pensacola, FL 32514, 850-474-1066, 800-558-4462, http://www.hhna.org

Hospice Association of America (HAA), 228 Seventh Street S.E., Washington, DC 20003, 202-546-4759, http://www.nahc.org/HAA

Hospice Education Institute, 190 Westbrook Road, Essex, CT 06426-1510, 860-767-1620, 800-331-1620, http://www.hospiceworld.org

Hospice Foundation of America (HFA), 2001 S Street N.W. #300, Washington, DC 20009, 800-854-3402, http://www.hospicefoundation.org

National Adult Day Services Association (NADSA), 409 Third Street, S.W., Washington, DC 20024, 202-479-6682, http://www.ncoa.org/nadsa

National Association for Home Care (NAHC), 228 Seventh Street S.E., Washington, DC 20003, 202-547-7424, http://www.nahc.org

National Citizens' Coalition for Nursing Home Reform, Suite 202, 1424 16th Street N.W., Washington, DC 20036-2211, 202-332-2275, http://www.nccnhr.org

National Hospice and Palliative Care Organization (NHPCO), 1700 Diagonal Road, Suite 300, Alexandria, VA 22314, 703-243-5900, http://www.nhpco.org

National Rehabilitation Association, 633 S. Washington Street, Alexandria, VA 22314, 703-836-0850, http://nationalrehab.org

National Rehabilitation Information Center (NARIC), 1010 Wayne Avenue, Suite 800, Silver Spring, MD 20910-5633, 301-562-2400, 800-346-2742, http://www.naric.com

Nursing Home Information Service, National Council of Senior Citizens, 8403 Colesville Road, Suite 1200, Silver Spring, MD 20910, 310-578-8800, 888-3-SENIOR, http://www.ncscinc.org

CHAPTER 37
Nursing Care of the Client: Responding to Emergencies

REFERENCES/SUGGESTED READINGS

American Heart Association. (1997). *Advanced cardiac life support*. Dallas, TX: Author.

Arbour, R. (1998). Aggressive management of intracranial dynamics. *Critical Care Nurse, 18,* 30–40.

Armstrong, J. F. (1998). Bombs and other blasts. *RN, 61*(11), 26–29.

Blank-Reid, C. (1999). Strangulation. *RN, 62*(2), 32–35.

Bowen, T., & Bellamy, R. (Eds.). (1998). *Emergency war surgery. United States Department of Defense.* Washington, DC: United States Government Printing Office.

Campolo, S. (1997). Emergency! Spontaneous pneumothorax. *AJN, 97*(2), 30.

Carroll, P. (1999). Chest injuries. *RN, 62*(1), 36–43.

Hayes, L. (2000). Poison emergency. *Nursing2000, 30*(9), 34–39.

Keep, N., & Gilbert, C. (1995). How safe is your ED? *AJN, 95*(9), 44–51.

Laskowski-Jones, L. (1995). Meeting the challenge of chest trauma. *AJN, 95*(9), 22–30.

Laskowski-Jones, L. (2000a). Responding to summer emergencies. *Nursing2000, 30*(5), 34–39.

Laskowski-Jones, L. (2000b). Responding to winter emergencies. *Nursing2000, 30*(1), 34–39.

Lewis, A. M. (1999). Neurologic emergency. *Nursing99, 29*(10), 54–56.

Miller-Keane, (1997). *Encyclopedia and dictionary of medicine, nursing, and allied health*. (6th ed.). Philadelphia: W.B. Saunders Company.

National Association of Emergency Medical Technicians. (1998). *PHTLS. Basic and advanced pre-hospital trauma life-support* (4th ed.). St. Louis, MO: Mosby.

Pettinicchi, T. A. (1998). Lightning strike. *Nursing98, 28*(7), 33.

Polaski, A., & Tatro, S. (1996). *Luckmann's core principles and practice of medical–surgical nursing*. Philadelphia: W. B. Saunders Company.

Quinn, S. (1998). ED triage. *RN, 61*(9), 53–60.

Ramponi, D. (2000). Go with the flow during an eye emergency. *Nursing2000, 30*(8), 54–56.

Schulmerich, S. C. (1999). When nature turns up the heat. *RN, 62*(8), 35–38.

Sommers, M. (1998). Missed injuries. *RN, 61*(10), 28–31.

Stacy, P. (1998). On-scene care. *RN, 61*(9), 50–52.

TRAUMA! (1998). *RN, 61*(9), 49.

Sullivan, E., & Decker, P. (1997). *Effective leadership and management in nursing*. Menlo Park, CA: Addison Wesley.

Talbert, S., & Talbert, P. (1998). Flight nursing: Summary of strategies for managing severe traumatic brain injury during early posttraumatic phase. *Journal of Emergency Nursing, 24,* 254–257.

RESOURCES

American Association of Critical Care Nurses (AACN), 101 Columbia, Aliso Viejo, CA 92656, 949-362-2000, http://www.aacn.org

American Red Cross, Attn: Public Inquiry Office, 11th Floor, 1621 North Kent Street, Arlington, VA 22209, 703-248-4222, http://www.redcross.org

Emergency Nurses Association (ENA), 915 Lee Street, Des Plaines, IL 60016, 800-243-8362, http://www.ena.org

Salvation Army World Service Office, 615 Slaters Lane, Alexandria, VA 22313, 703-684-5528

CHAPTER 38
Critical Thinking on Multiple Systems

REFERENCES/SUGGESTED READINGS

Beare, P., & Myers, J. (1998). *Adult health nursing* (3rd ed.). St. Louis, MO: Mosby.

Cerrato, P. (1997). New acute MI guidelines. *RN, 60*(1).

Hernandez, D. (1998). Assessing microvascular complications of diabetes. *AJN, 98*(6), 26–32.

Hurley, M. (1998). New hypertension guidelines. *RN, 61*(3), 25–28.

Ignatavicius, D., Workman, M., & Mishler, M. (Eds.). (1999). *Medical-surgical nursing across the health-care continuum* (3rd ed.). Philadelphia: W. B. Saunders Company.

Janowski, M. (1997). Managing health failure. *RN, 59*(2), 34–39.

King, B. (1997). Preserving renal function. *RN, 60*(8), 43–40.

Little, C. (2000). Renovascular hypertension. *AJN, 100*(2), 46–52.

O'Hanlon-Nichols, T. (1997). Basic assessment series: The adult cardiovascular system. *AJN, 97*(12), 34–40.

RESOURCES

The Center for Critical Thinking and Moral Critique, Sonoma State University, 4656 Sonoma Mountain Road, Santa Rosa, CA 95404, 800-833-3645, http://www.criticalthinking.org

The Foundation for Critical Thinking, 4655 Sonoma Mountain Road, Santa Rosa, CA 95404, 410-364-5082

The International Center for the ASsessment of Higher Order Thinking, 707-664-4082

The National Council for Excellence in Critical Thinking, 707-664-4275

Renal Links, http://www.albany.net/907Erubcrgd/renalink.html

Appendix A: NANDA Nursing Diagnoses 2001–2002

Activity Intolerance

Risk for Activity Intolerance

Impaired Adjustment

Ineffective Airway Clearance

Latex Allergy Response

Risk for Latex Allergy Response

Anxiety

Death Anxiety

Risk for Aspiration

Risk for Impaired Parent/Infant/Child Attachment

Autonomic Dysreflexia

Disturbed Body Image

Risk for Imbalanced Body Temperature

Bowel Incontinence

Effective Breastfeeding

Ineffective Breastfeeding

Interrupted Breastfeeding

Ineffective Breathing Pattern

Decreased Cardiac Output

Caregiver Role Strain

Risk for Caregiver Role Strain

Impaired Verbal Communication

Decisional Conflict (Specify)

Parenteral Role Conflict

Acute Confusion

Chronic Confusion

Constipation

Perceived Constipation

Risk for Constipation

Ineffective Coping

Ineffective Community Coping

Readiness for Enhanced Community Coping

Defensive Coping

Compromised Family Coping

Disabled Family Coping

Readiness for Enhanced Family Coping

Ineffective Denial

Impaired Dentition

Risk for Delayed Development

Diarrhea

Risk for Disuse Syndrome

Deficient Diversional Activities

Disturbed Energy Field

Impaired Environmental Interpretation Syndrome

Adult Failure to Thrive

Risk for Falls

Dysfunctional Family Processes: Alcoholism

Interrupted Family Processes

Fatigue

Fear

Deficient Fluid Volume

Excess Fluid Volume Risk for Deficient Fluid Volume

Risk for Imbalanced Fluid Volume

Impaired Gas Exchange

Anticipatory Grieving

Dysfunctional Grieving

Delayed Growth and Development

Risk for Disproportionate Growth

Ineffective Health Maintenance

Health-Seeking Behaviors (Specify)

Impaired Home Maintenance

Hopelessness

Hyperthermia

Hypothermia

Disturbed Personal Identity

Functional Urinary Incontinence

Reflex Urinary Incontinence

Stress Urinary Incontinence

Total Urinary Incontinence

Urge Urinary Incontinence

Risk for Urge Urinary Incontinence

Disorganized Infant Behavior

Risk for Disorganized Infant Behavior

Readiness for Enhanced Organized Infant Behavior

Ineffective Infant Feeding Pattern

Risk for Infection

Risk for Injury

Risk for Perioperative-Positioning Injury

Decreased Intracranial Adaptive Capacity

Deficient Knowledge

Risk for Loneliness

Impaired Memory

Impaired Bed Mobility

Impaired Physical Mobility

Impaired Wheelchair Mobility

Nausea

Unilateral Neglect

Noncompliance

Imbalanced **N**utrition: Less than Body Requirements

Imbalanced **N**utrition: More than Body Requirements

Risk for Imbalanced **N**utrition: More than Body Requirements

Impaired **O**ral Mucous Membrane

Acute **P**ain

Chronic **P**ain

Impaired **P**arenting

Risk for Impaired **P**arenting

Risk for **P**eripheral Neurovascular Dysfunction

Risk for **P**oisoning

Post-Trauma Syndrome

Risk for **P**ost-Trauma Syndrome

Powerlessness

Risk for **P**owerlessness

Ineffective **P**rotection

Rape-Trauma Syndrome

Rape-Trauma Syndrome: Compound Reaction

Rape-Trauma Syndrome: Silent Reaction

Relocation Stress Syndrome

Risk for **R**elocation Stress Syndrome

Ineffective **R**ole Performance

Bathing/Hygiene **S**elf-Care Deficit

Dressing/Grooming **S**elf-Care Deficit

Feeding **S**elf-Care Deficit

Toileting **S**elf-Care Deficit

Chronic Low **S**elf-Esteem

Situational Low **S**elf-Esteem

Risk for Situational Low **S**elf-Esteem

Self-Mutilation

Risk for **S**elf-Mutilation

Disturbed **S**ensory Perception (Specify: Visual, Auditory, Kinesthetic, Gustatory, Tactile, Olfactory)

Sexual Dysfunction

Ineffective **S**exuality Patterns

Impaired **S**kin Integrity

Risk for Impaired **S**kin Integrity

Sleep Deprivation

Disturbed **S**leep Pattern

Impaired **S**ocial Interaction

Social Isolation

Chronic **S**orrow

Spiritual Distress

Risk for **S**piritual Distress

Readiness for Enhanced **S**piritual Well-Being

Risk for **S**uffocation

Risk for **S**uicide

Delayed **S**urgical Recovery

Impaired **S**wallowing

Effective **T**herapeutic Regimen Management

Ineffective **T**herapeutic Regimen Management

Ineffective Community **T**herapeutic Regimen Management

Ineffective Family **T**herapeutic Regimen Management

Ineffective **T**hermoregulation

Disturbed **T**hought Processes

Impaired **T**issue Integrity

Ineffective **T**issue Perfusion (Specify Type: Renal, Cerebral, Cardiopulmonary, Gastrointestinal, Peripheral)

Impaired **T**ransfer Ability

Risk for **T**rauma

Impaired **U**rinary Elimination

Urinary Retention

Impaired Spontaneous **V**entilation

Dysfunctional **V**entilatory Weaning Response

Risk for Other-Directed **V**iolence

Risk for Self-Directed **V**iolence

Impaired **W**alking

Wandering

From *Nursing Diagnoses: Definitions & Classification, 2001–2002,* by North American Nursing Diagnosis Association, 2001. Philadelphia: Author. Copyright 2001 by North American Nursing Diagnosis Association. Reprinted with permission.

Appendix B: Abbreviations, Acronyms, and Symbols

AA	Alcoholics Anonymous	**ATG**	antithymocytic globulin
AAA	abdominal aortic aneurysm	**ATN**	acute tubular necrosis
AAP	American Academy of Pediatrics	**ATP**	adenosine triphosphatase
AARP	American Association of Retired Persons	**ATSDR**	Agency for Toxic Substances and Disease
AAN	American Academy of Neurology		Registry
AANA	American Association of Nurse Anesthetists	**A-V**	arteriovenous
ABC	airway, breathing, circulation	**AWS**	alcohol withdrawal syndrome
ABG	arterial blood gases	**BAER**	brainstem auditory-evoked response
a.c.	before meals	**BBA**	Balanced Budget Act
ACE	angiotensin-converting enzyme	**BCG**	bacilles *Calmette-Guérin*
ACKD	acquired cystic kidney disease	**bid**	twice a day
ACS	American Cancer Society	**BMD**	bone mineral density
ACTH	adrenocorticotropic hormone	**BMT**	bone marrow transplantation
AD	Alzheimer's disease	**B&O**	belladonna and opium
ADA	American Diabetes Association	**BP**	blood pressure
ADA	Americans with Disabilities Act	**BPH**	benign prostatic hypertrophy
ADAMHA	Alcohol, Drug Abuse, and Mental Health	**BRM**	biologic response modifier
	Administration	**BSE**	breast self examination
ADC	AIDS dementia complex	**BUN**	blood urea nitrogen
ADH	antidiuretic hormone	**C**	Celsius
ADHD	attention deficit hyperactivity disorder	**CA**	cancer antigen
ADL	activities of daily living	**Ca$^+$**	calcium ion
AFB	acid-fast bacillus	**CABG**	coronary artery bypass graft
AHA	American Hospital Association	**CaCl$_2$**	calcium chloride
AHCA	American Health Care Association	**CAD**	coronary artery disease
AHCPR	Agency Health Care Policy and Research	**C & S**	culture and sensitivity
AHNA	American Holistic Nurses' Association	**CARF**	Commission on Accreditation of Rehabilita-
AICD	automatic implantable cardioverter-defibrillator		tion Facilities
AIDS	acquired immunodeficiency syndrome	**CAT**	computed axial tomography
AJN	*American Journal of Nursing*	**CATT**	computerized axial transverse tomography
AL-ANON	Alcoholic self-help group or adults	**CBC**	complete blood count
AL-ATEEN	Alcoholic self-help group for teens	**CBD**	common bile duct
AL-ATOT	Self-help group for younger children in the	**cc**	cubic centimeter
	family of an alcoholic	**CCNS**	cell-cycle nonspecific
ALFA	Assisted Living Federation of America	**CCRC**	continuing care retirement community
ALG	antilymphocytic globulin	**CCS**	cell-cycle specific
ALL	acute lymphocytic leukemia	**CCU**	coronary care unit
ALS	amyotrophic lateral sclerosis	**CDC**	Centers for Disease Control and Prevention
ALT	alanine aminotransferase	**CEA**	carcinoembryonic antigen
AMA	against medical advice	**CEPN-LTC™**	Certification Examination for Practical and
AMA	American Medical Association		Vocational Nurses in Long-Term Care
AML	acute myelocytic leukemia	**CHAP**	community health accreditation program
ANA	American Nurses Association	**CHD**	coronary heart disease
ANA	antinuclear antibody	**CHF**	congestive heart failure
ANS	autonomic nervous system	**CHIP**	Children's Health Insurance Program
AoA	Administration on Aging	**CIN**	cervical intraepithelial neoplasia
AORN	Association of Operating Room Nurses	**CK or CPK**	creatine kinase or creatine phosphokinase
APA	American Psychiatric Association	**Cl$^-$**	chloride ion
APRN	advance practice registered nurse	**CLL**	chronic lymphocytic leukemia
APS	Adult Protective Services	**CLTC**	certified in long-term care
APS	American Pain Society	**CML**	chronic myelocytic leukemia
APTT	activated partial thromboplastin time	**CMV**	cytomegalovirus
ARDS	adult respiratory distress syndrome	**CNM**	certified nurse midwife
ARF	acute renal failure	**CNO**	community nursing organization
ASN	American Society of Nephrology	**CNS**	central nervous system
ASO	antireptolysin-O	**CNS**	clinical nurse specialist
AST	aspartate aminotransferase	**CO$_2$**	carbon dioxide
ATC	around the clock	**CO$_2^-$**	carbon dioxide ion

COLD	chronic obstructive lung disease	**ERG**	electroretinogram
COOH	carboxyl group	**ERT**	estrogen replacement therapy
COPD	chronic obstructive pulmonary disease	**ESR**	erythrocyte sedimentation rate
CPAP	continuous positive airway pressure	**ESRD**	end-stage renal disease
CPM	continuous passive motion	**ESU**	electrical surgical unit
CPR	cardiopulmonary resuscitation	**ESWL**	extracorporeal shock wave lithotripsy
CPR	computerized patient record	**ET**	endotracheal
CPS	Child Protective Services	**ETT**	endotracheal tube
CRNA	Certified Registered Nurse Anesthetist	**EVAD**	explantable venous access device
CRP	C-reactive protein	**F**	Fahrenheit
CRP	C-reactive protein test	**FAE**	fetal alcohol effects
CSF	cerebrospinal fluid	**FAS**	fetal alcohol syndrome
CSM	circulation, movement, sensation	**FBD**	fibrocystic breast disease
CT	computed tomography	**FBS**	fasting blood sugar
CVA	cerebrovascular accident	**FCA**	False Claims Act
CVC	central venous catheter	**FDA**	Food and Drug Administration
CVP	A combination of chemotherapy drugs: cyclophosphamide (Cytoxan), vincristine (Oncovin), prednisone (Deltasone)	**FeSO$_4$**	iron sulfate
		FOBT	fecal occult blood test
D$_5$W	dextrose 5% in water	**4 Ps**	passage, passenger, powers, pysche
DAI	diffuse axonal injury	**FSBG**	finger stick blood glucose
D & C	dilatation and curettage	**FSH**	follicle-stimulating hormone
DDS	doctor of dental surgery	**GAD**	generalized anxiety disorder
DEA	Drug Enforcement Agency	**GCS**	Glasgow Coma Scale
DES	diethylstilbestrol	**GDM**	gestational diabetes mellitus
DET	diethyltriptamine	**GERD**	gastroesophageal reflux disease
DETOX	detoxification	**GFR**	glomerular filtration rate
DEXA	dual energy x-ray absorptiometry	**GGT**	gammaglutamy transpeptidase
DHHS	Department of Health and Human Services	**GGTP**	gamma-glutamyl transpeptidase
DIC	disseminated intravascular coagulation	**GH**	growth hormone
DICC	dynamic infusion cavernosometry and cavernosography	**GHb**	glycosylated hemoglobin
		GI	gastrointestinal
DJD	degenerative joint disease	**GIFT**	gamete-intrafallopian transfer
DKA	diabetic ketoacidosis	**GTT**	glucose tolerance test
DMD	doctor of dental medicine	**h**	hour(s)
DMT	dimethyltriptamine	**H$^+$**	hydrogen ion
DNA	deoxyribonucleic acid	**H$_2$CO$_3$**	carbonic acid
DNR	do not resuscitate	**H$_2$O**	water
DO	doctor of osteopathy	**H&H**	hemoglobin and hematocrit
DOM	dimethyl-4-ethylamphetamine	**HAV**	hepatitis A virus
DPA	dual photon absorptiometry	**HB$_5$AG**	hepatitis B surface antigen
DPAHC	durable power of attorney for health care	**HBIG**	hepatitis B immune globulin
DRG	diagnosis-related group	**HBV**	hepatitis B virus
DSM-IV	*Diagnostic and Statistical Manual of Mental Disorders,* 4th edition	**HCFA**	Health Care Financing Administration
		hCG	human chorionic gonadotropin
		HCl	hydrochloric acid
DST	dexamethasone suppression test	**HCO$_3^-$**	bicarbonate ion
DVT	deep vein thrombosis	**Hct**	hematocrit
DXA	duel energy x-ray absorptionetry	**HCV**	hepatitis C virus
EABV	effective arterial blood volume	**HD**	Hodgkin's Disease
ECF	extended care facility	**HDL**	high density lipoprotein
ECF	extracellular fluid	**HDV**	hepatitis D virus
ECG (EKG)	electrocardiogram	**HELP**	Herpetics Engaged in Living Productively
ECT	electroconvulsive therapy	**Hep B**	hepatitis B
ED	emergency department	**Hgb F**	fetal hemoglobin
EEG	electroencephalograph	**Hgb**	hemoglobin
EENT	eyes, ears, nose, and throat	**HGH**	Human Growth Hormone
EGD	esophagogastroduodenoscopy	**HHNK**	hyperosmolar hyperglycemic nonketotic syndrome
EKG	electrocardiogram		
ELISA	enzyme-linked immunosorbent assay	**Hib**	*haemophilus influenzae* type B
EMG	electromyogram	**HICPAC**	Hospital Infection Control Practices Advisory Committee
EMLA	eutectic (cream) mixture of local anesthetics		
EMS	emergency medical services	**HIV**	human immunodeficiency virus
EMT	emergency medical technician	**HLA-DW4**	human leukocyte antigen DW4
EPA	Environmental Protection Agency	**HMO**	health maintenance organization
EPO	exclusive provider organization	**HPV**	human papillomavirus
EPS	extrapyramidal symptom	**HR**	heart rate
ERCP	endoscopic retrograde cholangiopancre-atogram	**HRSA**	Health Resources and Services Administration
		HSV	herpes simplex virus

HSV-2	herpes simplex virus type 2	**MCNS**	minimal charge nephrotic syndrome
IABP	intra-aortic balloon pump	**MD**	doctor of medicine
IADL	instrumental activities of daily living	**MDI**	metered-dose inhaler
I&O	intake and output	**MDMA**	methylene dioxyamphetamine
IASP	International Association for the Study of Pain	**MDR**	multidrug-resistant
		MDR-TB	multidrug-resistant tuberculosis
IBD	inflammatory bowel disease	**MDS**	minimum data set
ICF	intermediate care facility	**mEq**	milliequivalent
ICF	intracellular fluid	**mEq/L**	milliequivalents per liter
ICN	International Council of Nurses	**mg**	milligram
ICU	intensive care unit	**MG**	myasthenia gravis
ID	intradermal	**Mg^{++}**	magnesium ion
IDDM	insulin-dependent diabetes mellitus	**MgCl**	magnesium chloride
IFG	impaired fasting glucose	**Mg/dL**	milligrams per deciliter
IgG	immunoglobulin G	**mg/kg**	milligram per kilogram
IgM	immunoglobulin M	**MgSO$_4$**	magnesium sulfate
IGT	impaired glucose tolerance	**MI**	myocardial infarction
IHCT	interdisciplinary health care team	**min**	minute
IHS	Indian Health Service	**mL**	milliliter
IM	intramuscular	**mL/hr**	milliliter per hour
in	inch	**mm^3**	cubic millimeter
INR	International Normalized Ratio	**mm Hg**	millimeters of mercury
IOL	intraocular lens	**MOM**	Milk of Magnesia
IOM	Institute of Medicine	**MOPP**	A combination of chemotherapy drugs: mechlorethamine or nitrogen mustard (Mustargen), vincristine (Oncovin), procarbazine hydrochloride (Matulane), prednisone (Deltasone)
IOP	intraocular pressure		
ITP	idiopathic thrombocytopenic purpura		
ITT	insulin tolerance test		
IUD	intrauterine device		
IV	intravenous	**mOsm/kg**	milliosmoles/kilogram
IVAD	implantable vascular access device	**MRI**	magnetic resonance imaging
IVF-ER	*in vitro* fertilization and embryo replacement	**MRSA**	methicillin-resistant *staphylococcus aureus*
IVP	intravenous push, intravenous pyelogram	**MS**	morphine sulfate
		MS	multiple sclerosis
IVPB	intravenous piggyback	**MSG**	monosodium glutamate
JCAHO	Joint Commission on Accreditation of Healthcare Organizations	**MSH**	melanocyte-stimulating hormone
		MUGA	multi-gated acquisition
K$^+$	potassium ion	**MVC**	motor vehicle collision
kcal	kilocalorie	**NA**	Narcotics Anonymous
KCl	potassium chloride	**Na$^+$**	sodium ion
kg	kilogram	**NaOH**	Sodium hydroxide
KS	Kaposi's Sarcoma	**Na$_2$SO$_4$**	sodium sulfate
KS	ketosteroids	**NaCl**	sodium chloride
KUB	kidneys/ureters/bladder	**NaH$_2$PO$_4$**	sodium dihydrogen phosphate
KVO	keep vein open	**Na$_2$HPO$_4$**	disodium phosphate
L	liter	**NADSA**	Natinoal Adult Day Services Association
LAAM	levo-alpha-acetyl-methadol	**NAHC**	National Association for Home Care
lb	pound	**NaHCO$_3$**	sodium bicarbonate
LDH	lactic dehydrogenase	**NaHPO$_4$**	sodium monohydrogen phosphate
LDL	low density lipoprotein	**NANDA**	North American Nursing Diagnosis Association
LE	lupus erythematosus		
LES	lower esophageal sphincter	**NaOH**	sodium hydroxide
LH	luteinizing hormone	**NAPNES**	National Association of Practical Nurse Education and Service Inc.
LLQ	left lower quadrant		
LMP	last menstrual period	**NCCAM**	National Center for Complementary and Alternative Medicine
LOC	level of consciousness		
LP	lumbar puncture		
LP/VN	licensed practical/vocational nurse	**NCHS**	National Center for Health Statistics
LPN	licensed practical nurse	**NCLEX**	National Council Licensure Examination
LSD	lysergic acid diethylamide	**NCLEX-PN**	National Council Licensure Examination—Practical Nurse
LTB	laryngotracheobronchitis		
LUQ	left upper quadrant	**NCLEX-RN**	National Council Licensure Examination—Registered Nurse
LVN	licensed vocational nurse		
MAC	*myobacterium avium* complex	**NCOA**	National Council on Aging
MADD	Mothers Against Drunk Driving	**NCSBN**	National Council of State Boards of Nursing
MAO	monoamine oxidase	**NFLPN**	National Federation of Licensed Practical Nurses, Inc.
MAOI	monoamine oxidase inhibitor		
MAP	mean arterial pressure	**NG**	nasogastric
MAR	medication administration record	**NGT**	nasogastric tube
mcg (or μg)	microgram	**NH$_2$**	amino group

NHL	non-Hodgkin's lymphoma		**PID**	pelvic inflammatory disease
NHO	National Hospice Organization		**PKD**	polycystic kidney disease
NIA	National Institute on Aging		**PKU**	phenylketonuria
NIAAA	National Institute on Alcohol Abuse and Alcoholism		**PLMD**	periodic limb movement disorder
NIAID	National Institute of Allergies and Infectious Diseases		**PMI**	point of maximum intensity
			PMN	polymorphonuclear leukocyte
NIAMS	National Institute of Arthritis and Musculo-skeletal and Skin Diseases		**PMR**	progressive muscle relaxation
			PMS	premenstrual syndrome
NIC	Nursing Interventions Classification		**PNI**	psychoneuroimmunology
NIDA	National Institute on Drug Abuse		**PNS**	peripheral nervous system
NIDDK	National Institute of Diabetes and Digestive and Kidney Diseases		**po**	*per os,* Latin for "by mouth"
			PO₂ (PaO₂)	partial pressure of oxygen
NIDDM	non insulin-dependent diabetes mellitus		PO_4^{--}	phosphate ion
NIH	National Institute of Health		**PPBS**	post prandial blood sugar
NKF	National Kidney Foundation		**PPG**	post prandial glucose
NLN	National League for Nursing		**PPO**	preferred provider organization
NMS	neuroleptic malignant syndrome		**PPS**	prospective payment system
NNRTI	nonnucleoside reverse transcriptase inhibitor		**PRA**	plamsa renin assay
			PRL	prolactin level
NOC	Nursing Outcomes Classification		**PRN**	*pro re nata,* Latin for "as required"
NOF	National Osteoporisis Foundation		**PRO**	peer review organization
NP	nurse practitioner		**PROM**	passive range of motion
NPO	*nil per os,* Latin for "nothing by mouth"		**PSA**	prostate specific antigen
NPUAP	National Pressure Ulcer Advisory Panel		**PSDA**	Patient Self-Determination Act
NRTI	nucleoside analog reverse transcriptase inhibitor		**PSP**	phenolsulfonphtalein
			PSVT	paroxysmal supraventricular tachycardia
NSAID	nonsteroidal anti-inflammatory drug		**pt**	pint
NSR	normal sinus rhythm		**PT**	physical therapist
O₂	oxygen		**PT**	prothrombin time
OAM	Office of Alternative Medicine		**PTCA**	percutaneous transluminal coronary angioplasty
O&P	ova and parasite			
OBRA	Omnibus Budget Reconciliation Act		**PTH**	parathyroid hormone
OCD	obsessive compulsive disorder		**PTSD**	post-traumatic stress disorder
OHCS	hydroxycorticosteroids		**PTT**	partial thromboplastin time
OHL	oral hairy leukoplakia		**PTU**	propylthiouracil
OR	operating room		**PUSH Tool**	Pressure Ulcer Scale for Healing
ORIF	open reduction/internal fixation		**PVC**	premature ventricular contraction
OSHA	Occupational Safety and Health Adminis-tration		**PVD**	peripheral vascular disease
			q	*quaque,* Latin for "every"
OT	occupational therapist		**qd**	every day
OTC	over-the-counter		**qh**	every hour
oz	ounce		**qid**	four times a day
p̄	after		**qod**	every other day
P	pulse		**qs**	quantity sufficient
PA	physician's assistant		**q2h**	every 2 hours
PAC	premature atrial contractions		**qt**	quart
PaCO₂	partial pressure of carbon dioxide		**R**	respiration
PACU	postanesthesia care unit		**RA**	rheumatoid arthritis
PaO₂	partial pressure of oxygen		**RAD**	reactive airway disease
Pap	Papanicolaou test		**RAIU**	radioactive iodine uptake
PAT	paroxysmal atrial tachycardia		**RAST**	radio allergosorbent test
PBI	protein bound iodine		**RBC**	red blood count, red blood cell
PCA	patient-controlled analgesia		**RD**	registered dietician
PCO₂ (PaCO₂)	partial pressure of carbon dioxide		**RDS**	respiratory distress syndrome
PCP	phencyclidine		**Resp**	respirations
PCP	*pneumocystis carinii* pneumonia		**RF**	rheumatoid factor
PCP	primary care provider		**RIA**	radio immuno assay
PCR	polymerase chain reaction		**RICE**	rest, ice, compression, elevation
PDA	patent ductus arteriosis		**RLQ**	right lower quadrant
PDPH	postdural puncture headache		**RN**	registered nurse
PEG	percutaneous endoscopic gastrostomy		**RNA**	ribonucleic acid
PERRLA	pupils equal, round, reactive to light and accommodation		**RNFA**	registered nurse first assistant
			ROM	range of motion
PET	positron emission tomography		**ROM**	rupture of membranes
PFT	pulmonary function test		**ROS**	review of systems
pH	potential hydrogen		**RPCH**	rural primary care hospital
PHS	Public Health Services		**RPh**	registered pharmacist
PICC	peripherally inserted central catheter		**RPR**	rapid plasma reagin

RR	recovery room
RSV	respiratory syncytial virus
R/T	related to
RT	respiratory therapist
RTI	respiratory tract infection
RUGS	resource utilization group system
RUQ	right upper quadrant
s̄	without
SA	sinoatrial
SADD	Students Against Drunk Driving
SAME	S-adenosylmathionine
SaO₂	oxygen saturation
SBC	school-based clinic
SBP	systolic blood pressure
SC/SQ	subcutaneous
SCA	sickle-cell anemia
SCD	sequential compression device
SCI	spinal cord injury
SGOT	serum glutamate oxaloacetate transaminase
SH	somatotropin hormone
SIADH	syndrome of inappropriate antidiuretic hormone
SL	sublingual
SLE	systemic lupus erythematosus
SMBG	self-monitor blood glucose
SNF	skilled nursing facility
SOP	standard operating procedure
SPECT	single photon emission computed tomography
SPF	sun protection factor
s̄s̄	one half
SSA	Social Security Administration
SSRI	selective serotonin reuptake inhibitor
STAT	statim, Latin for "immediately"
STD	sexually transmitted disease
SW	social worker
SXA	single energy x-ray absorbtiometry
T	temperature
TAC	tetracaine, adrenaline, cocaine
TB	tuberculosis
Tbsp	tablespoon
TD	tardive dyskinesia
TDD	telecommunication device for the deaf
TEE	transesophageal echocardiography
TEFRA	Tax Equity Fiscal Responsibility Act
TENS	transcutaneous electrical nerve stimulation
T4	throxine
THA	total hip arthroplasty
TIA	transient ischemic attack
TIBC	total iron binding capacity
t.i.d.	three times a day
TIG	tetanus immune globulin
TIPS	transjugular intrahepatic portosystemic shunt
TKA	total knee arthroplasty
TM	tympanic membrane
TMD	temporomandibular joint disease/disorder
TMJ	temporomandibular joint
TNM	tumor, node, metastasis

t.o.	telephone order
TOF	tetralogy of Fallot
TPN	total parenteral nutrition
TPR	temperature, pulse, respirations
Tr or tinct	tincture
TRAM	transplantation of the rectus abdominis muscle
TRF	thyrotropin-releasing factor
TSE	testicular self examination
TSH	thyroid-stimulating hormone
TSI	thyroid-stimulating immunoglobulin
tsp	teaspoon
TSS	toxic shock syndrome
T3	triiodothyronine
TULIP	transurethral ultrasound-guided laser-induced prostatectomy
TURP	transurethral resection of the prostate
U	unit
UA	routine urinalysis
UAP	unlicensed assistive personnel
UC	ulcerative colitis
UGI	upper gasrointestinal tract
UIS	Universal Intellectual Standards
UTI	urinary tract infection
UL	upper intake level
UMLS	Universal Medical Language System
U-100	100 units insulin per cc
UPP	urethra pressure profile
UPSIT	University of Pennsylvania Smell Identification Test
URQ	upper right quadrant
USDHHS	United States Department of Health and Human Services
USPHS	United States Public Health Service
UTI	urinary tract infection
UV	ultraviolet
VA	Veterans Administration, Veterans Affairs
VAC	vacuum assisted closure
VAD	ventricular assist device, vascular access device
VAS	Visual Analog Scale
VCD	vacuum constriction device
VDRL	venereal disease research laboratory
VF	ventricular fibrillation
VLDL	very low-density lipoprotein
VMA	vanillylmandelic acid
VS	vital signs
VSD	ventricular septal defect
VT	ventricular tachycardia
WASP	white, Anglo-Saxon, Protestant
WBC	white blood cell, white blood count
WHO	World Health Organization
WISE	Women's Issues and Social Empowerment
WNL	within normal limits
WPM	words per minute
wt	weight
ZIFT	zygote-intra-fallopian transfer

Appendix C: English/Spanish Words and Phrases

Being able to say a few words or phrases in the client's language is one way to show that you care. It lets the client know that you as a nurse are interested in the individual. There are three rules to keep in mind regarding the pronunciation of Spanish words.

- If a word ends in a vowel, or in *n* or *s,* the accent is on the next to the last syllable.
- If the word ends in a consonant other than *n* or *s,* the accent is on the last syllable.
- If the word does not follow these rules, it has a written accent over the vowel of the accented syllable.

Courtesy phrases, names of body parts, and expressions of time and numbers are included in this section for quick reference. The English version will appear first, followed by the Spanish translation and Spanish pronunciation.

Courtesy Phrases

Please	Por favor	Por fah-**vor**
Thank-you	Grácias	**Grah**-the-as
Good morning	Buénos dias	Boo-**ay**-nos **dee**-as
Good afternoon	Buénas tardes	Boo-**ay**-nas **tar**-days
Good evening	Buénas noches	Boo-**ay**-nas **no**-chays
Yes/No	Si/no	See/no
Good	Bien	Be-en
Bad	Mal	Mahl
How many?	Cuántos?	Coo-**ahn**-tos?
Where?	Dónde?	**Don**-day?
When?	Cuándo?	Coo**ahn**-do?

Body Parts

abdomen	el abdomen	el ab-doh-men
ankle	el tobillo	el to-**beel**-lyo
anus	el ano	el **ah**-no
anvil (incus)	el yunque	el **yoon**-kay
appendix	el apéndice	el ah-**pen**-de-thay
aqueous humor	el humor acuoso	el oo-**mor** ah-coo-**o**-so
bladder	la vejiga	lah vay-**nee**-gah
brain	el cerebro	el thay-**ray**-bro
breast	el pecho	el **pay**-cho
buttock	la nalga	lah **nahl**-gah
calf	la pantorrilla	lah pan-tor-**reel**-lyah
cervix	la cerviz	lah ther-**veth**
cheek	la mejilla	lah may-**heel**-lyah
chin	la barbilla	lah bar-**beel**-lyah
choroid	la coroidea	lah co-ro-e-**day**-ah
ciliary body	el cuerpo ciliar	el coo-**err**-po the-le-**ar**
clitoris	el clítoris	el **clee**-to-ris
coccyx	el coxis	el **coc**-sees
conjunctiva	la conjuntiva	lah con-hoon-**tee**vah
cornea	la córnea	lah **cor**-nay-ah
penis	el pene	el **pay**-nay
prostrate gland	la próstata	lah **pros**-ta-tah
pupil	la pupila	lah poo-**pee**-lah
rectum	el recto	el **rec**-to
retina	la retina	lah ray-**tee**-nah
sclera	la esclerótica	lah es-clay-**ro**-te-cah

scrotum	el escroto	el es-**cro**-to
seminal vesicle	la vesícula seminal	lah vay-**see**-coo-lah say-me-**nahl**
shoulder	el hombro	el **om**-bro
small intestine	el intestino delgado	el in-tes-**tee**-no del-**gah**-do
spinal cord	la médula espinal	lah **may**-doo-lah es-pe-**nahl**
spleen	el bazo	el **bah**-tho
stirrup (stapes)	el estribo	el es-**tree**-bo
stomach	el estómago	el es-**toh**-mah-go
temple	la sien	lah se-**ayn**
testis	el testículo	el tes-**tee**-coo-lo
thigh	el muslo	el **moos**-lo
thorax	el tórax	el **to**-rax
tongue	la lengua	lah **len**-goo-ah
trachea	la tráquea	lah **trah**-kay-ah
upper extremities	las extremidades superiores	las ex-tray-me-**dahd**-es soo-pay-re-**or**-es
ureter	el uréter	el oo-**ray**-ter
uterus	el útero	el **oo**-tay-ro
vagina	el vagina	lah vah-**hee**-nah
vitreous humor	el humor vítreo	el oo-**mor vee**-tray-o
wrist	la muñeca	lah moo-**nyay**-cah

Expressions of Time, Calendar, and Numbers

after meals	después de comer	des-poo-**es** day co-**merr**
at bedtime	al acostarse	al ah-cos-**tar**-say
before meals	antes de comer	**ahn**-tes day co-**merr**
daily	el diario	el de-**ah**-re-o
date	la fecha	lah **fay**-chah
day	el dia	el **dee**-ah
every hour	a cada hora	ah **cah**-dah **o**-rah
hour (time)	la hora	lah **o**-rah
how often	cada cuánto tiempo	**cah**-dah coo-**ahn**-to te-**em**-po
noon	el mediodia	el may-de-o-**dee**-ah
now	ahora	ah-**o**-rah
once	una vez	**oo**-nah veth
today	hoy	**oh**-e
tomorrow	mañana	mah-**nyah**-nah
tonight	esta noche	**es**-tah **no**-chay
week	la semana	lah say-**mah**-nah
year	año	**a**-nyo
Sunday	el domingo	el do-**meen**-go
Monday	el lunes	el **loo**-nes
Tuesday	el martes	el **mar**-tes
Wednesday	el miércoles	el me-**err**-co-les
Thursday	el jueves	el hoo-**ayves**
Friday	el viernes	el ve-**err**-nes
Saturday	el sábado	el **sah**-bah-do
zero	cero	**thay**-ro
one	uno	**oo**-no
two	dos	dose
three	tres	trays
four	cuatro	coo-**ah**-tro
five	cinco	**theen**-co
six	seis	**say**-ees
seven	siete	se-**ay**-tay
eight	ocho	**o**-cho
nine	nueve	noo-**ay**-vay
ten	diez	de-**eth**

Nursing Care Sentences and Questions

What is your name?
¿Como se llama usted?
¿**Co**-mo say **lyah**-mah oos-**ted?**

I am a student nurse.
Soy estudiente enfermera(o).
Soy es-too-de-**ahn**-tay en-fer-**may**-ra(o).

My name is . . .
Mi nombre es . . .
Mee **nom**-bray es . . .

Do you need a wheelchair?
¿Necesita usted una silla de rueda?
¿Nay-thay-**se**-ta oos-**ted oo**-nah **seel**-lyah day
    roo-**ay**-dah?

How do you feel?
¿Como se siente?
¿**Co**-mo say se-**ayn**-tah?

When is your family coming?
¿Cuándo viene su familia?
¿Coo-**ahn**-do vee-**en**-nah soo fah-**mee**-le-ah?

This is the call light.
Esta es la luz para llamar a la enfermera.
Es-tah es lah looth **pah**-ra lyah-**mar** a lah
    en-fer-**may**-ra.

If you need anything, press the button.
Si usted necesita algo, oprima el botón.
See oos-**ted** nay-thay-**se**-ta **ahl**-go o-pre-**ma** el
    bo-**tone.**

Do not turn without calling the nurse.
No se voltee sin llamar a la enfermera.
No say **vol**-tay seen lyah-**mar** a lah en-fer-**may**-ra.

The side rails on your bed are for your protection.
Los rieles del costado están para su protección.
Los re-**el**-es del cos-**tah**-do es-**tahn pah**-ra soo
    pro-tec-the-**on.**

Please do not try to lower or climb over the side rail.
Por favor no pretenda bajarlos (barjarlas) o treparse
    sobre ellos.
Por fah-**vor** no pray-**ten**-dah ba-**har**-los o
    tray-**par**-say **so**-bray **ayl**-lyos.

The head nurse is . . .
La jefa de enfermeras es . . .
La **hay**-fay day en-fer-**may**-ras es . . .

Do you need more blankets or another pillow?
¿Necesita usted más frazadas u orta almohada?
¿Nay-thay-**si**-ta oos-**ted** mahs frah-**thad**-dahs oo
    o-trah al-mo-**ah**-dah?

You may not smoke in the room.
No se puede fumar en el cuarto.
No say poo-**ay**-day foo-**mar** en el coo-**ar**-to.

Do you want me to turn on (turn off) the lights?
¿Quiere usted que encienda (apague) la luz?
¿Ke-**ay**-ray oos-**ted** day en-the-**en**-dah (a-**pah**-gay)
    lah looth?

Are you thirsty?
¿Tiene usted sed?
¿Tee-**en**-nah oos-**ted** sayd?

Are you allergic to any medication?
¿Es usted alérgico(a) a alguna medicina?
¿Es oos-**ted** ah-**lehr**-hee-co(a) ah ah-**goo**-nah nay-de-
    thee-nah?

You may take a bath.
Usted puede bañarse.
Oos-**ted** poo-**ay**-day bah-**nyar**-say.

Do not lock the door, please.
No cierre usted la puerta con llave, por favor.
No the-**err**-ray oos-**ted** lah poo-**err**-tah con **lyah**-vay
    por fah-**vor.**

Call if you feel faint or in need of help.
Llame si usted se siente débil o si necesita ayuda.
Lyah-mah see oos-**ted** say se-**ayn**-tah **day**-bil o see
    nay-thay-**se**-ta ah-**yoo**-dah.

Call when you have to go to the toilet.
Llame cuando tenga que ir al inodoro.
Lyah-mah coo-**ahn**-do **ten**-gah kay eer al in-o-**do**-ro.

I will give you an enema.
Le pondré una enema.
Lay pon-**dray oo**-nah ay-**nay**-mah.

Turn on your left (right) side.
Voltese a su lado izquierdo (derecho).
Vol-**tay**-say ah soo **lah**-do ith-ke-**er**-do(dah) (day-**ray**-
    cho[cha]).

Here is an appointment card.
Aqui tiene usted una tarjeta con la información
    escrito.
Ah-**kee** tee-**en**-nah oos-**ted oo**-nah tar-**hay**-tah con
    lah in-for-mah-the-**on** es-**cree**-to.

You are going to be discharged (released) today.
A usted le van a dar de alta hoy.
Ah oos-**ted** lay vahn ah dar day **ahl**-tah **oh**-e.

How did this illness begin?
¿Como empezó esta enfermedad?
¿**Co**-mo em-pa-**tho es**-tah en-fer-may-**dahd**?

Is the pain better after the medicine?
¿Siente usted alivio depués de tomar la medicina?
¿Se-**ayn**-tah oos-**ted** al-**lee**-ve-o des-poo-**es** day to-**mar** lah may-de-**thee**-nah?

Where is the pain?
¿Que la duele? (or) Dónde le duele?
¿**Kay** lah doo-**ay**-le? (or) **Don**-day lay doo-**ay**-le?

Do you have pains in your chest?
¿Tiene usted dolores in el pecho?
¿Tee-**en**-nah oos-**ted** do-**lor**-es en el **pay**-cho?

Are you in pain now?
¿Tiene usted dolores ahora?
¿Tee-**en**-nah oos-**ted** do-**lor**-es ah-**o**-rah?

Is it constant pain or does it come and go?
¿Es un dolor constante o va y vuelve?
¿Es oon do-**lor** cons-**tahn**-tay o vah ee voo-**el**-vah?

Is there anything that makes the pain better?
¿Hay algo que lo alivie?
¿**Ah**-ee **ahl**-go kay lo al-**le**-ve?

Is there anything that makes the pain worse?
¿Hay algo que lo aumente?
¿**Ah**-ee **ahl**-go kay lo ah-oo-**men**-tay?

Where do you feel the pain?
¿Dónde siente usted el dolor?
¿**Don**-day se-**ayn**-tah oos-**ted** el do-**lor**?

Point to where it hurts.
Apunte usted por favor, adonde le duele.
Ah-**poon**-tay oos-**ted** por fah-**vor** ah-**don**-day lay doo-**ay**-le.

Show me where it hurts.
Enséñeme usted donde le duele.
En-**say**-nah-may oos-**ted** don-day lay doo-**ay**-le.

Is the pain sharp or dull?
¿Es agudo o sordo el dolor?
¿Es ah-**goo**-do o **sor**-do el do-**lor**?

Do you know where you are?
¿Sabe usted donde esta?
¿Sah-**bay** oos-**ted** don-day es-**tah**?

You are in the hospital.
Usted está en el hospital.
Oos-**ted** es-**tah** en el os-pee-**tahl**.

You will be okay.
Usted va a estar bien.
Oos-**ted** vah a es-**tar be**-en.

Do you have any drug reactions?
¿Tiene usted alguna sensibilidad a productos químicos?
¿Te-**en**-nah oos-**ted** al-**goo**-nah sen-se-be-le-**dahd** a pro-**dooc**-tos **kee**-me-cos?

Have you seen another doctor or native healer for this problem?
¿Ha visto usted a otro médico o curandero tocante a este problema?
¿Ah **vees**-to oos-**ted** a o-tro **may**-de-co o coo-ran-**day**-ro to-**cahn**-tay a **es**-ah pro-**blay**-mah?

Have you vomited?
¿Ha vomitado usted?
¿Ah vo-me-**tah**-do oos-**ted**?

Do you have any difficulty in breathing?
¿Tiene usted alguna dificultad para respirar?
¿Te-**en**-nah oos-**ted** ah-**goo**-nah de-fe-cool-**tahd pah**-ra res-pe-**rar**?

Do you smoke?
¿Fuma usted?
¿Foo-**mar** oos-**ted**?

How many per day?
¿Cuántos al dia?
¿Coo-**ahn**-tos al **dee**-ah?

For how many years?
¿Por cuántos años?
¿por coo-**ahn**-tos **a**-nyos?

Do you awaken in the night because of shortness of breath?
¿Se despierta usted por la noche por falta de respiración?
¿Say des-pee-**err**-tah oos-**ted** por lah **no**-chay por **fahl**-tah day res-pe-rah-the-**on**?

Is any part of your body swollen?
¿Tiene usted alguna parte del cuerpo hinchada?
¿Te-**en**-nah oos-**ted** ah-**goo**-nah **par**-tay del coo-**err**-po in-**chah**-da?

How much water do you drink daily?
¿Cuántos vasos de agua bebe usted diariamente?
¿Coo-**ahn**-tos **vah**-sos day **ah**-goo-ah **bay**-be oos-**ted** de-ah-re-ah-**men**-tay?

Are you nauseated?
¿Tiene náusea?
¿Te-**en**-nah **nah**-oo-say-ah?

Are you going to vomit?
¿Va a vomitar?
¿Vah a vo-me-**tar**?

When was your last bowel movement?
¿Cuánto tiempo hace que evacúa usted?
¿Coo-**ahn**-to te-**em**-po **ah**-the kay ay-vah-**coo**-ah oos-**ted**?

Do you have diarrhea?
¿Tiene usted diarrea?
¿Te-**en**-nah oos-**ted** der-ar-**ray**-ah?

How much do you urinate?
¿Cuánto orina usted?
¿Coo-**ahn**-to o-**re**-nah oos-**ted**?

Did you urinate?
¿Orinó usted?
¿O-re-**no** oos-**ted**?

What color is your urine?
¿De qué color es la orina?
¿Day kay co-**lor** es lah o-**re**-nah?

Call when you have to go to the toilet.
Llame usted cuando tenga que ir al inodoro.
Lyah-mah oos-**ted** coo-**ahn**-do **ten**-gah kay eer al in-o-**do**-ro.

I need a urine specimen from you.
Necesito una muestra de orina de usted.
Nay-thay-**se**-to **oo**-nah moo-**ays**-trah day o-**re**-nah day oos-**ted**.

We will put a tube in your bladder so that you can urinate.
Le pondremos un tubo en la vejiga para que puede orinar.
Lay pon-**dray**-mos un **too**-be en lah vay-**hee**-gah **pah**-rah kay poo-**ay**-day o-re **nar**.

When was your last menstrual period?
¿Cuándo fue se última menstruación?
¿Coo-**ahn**-do foo-**ay** soo **ool**-te-mah mens-troo-ah-the-**on**?

Are you bleeding heavily?
¿Está sangrando mucho?
¿Es-**tah** san-**grahn**-do **moo**-cho?

Take off your clothes, please
Desvístase usted, por favor.
Des-**ves**-tah-say oos-**ted** por-fah-**vor**.

Just relax.
Relaje usted el cuerpo.
Ray-**lah**-he oos-**ted** el coo-**err**-po.

I am going to listen to your chest.
Voy a escucharle el pecho.
Voye a es-coo-**char**-lay el **pay**-cho.

Let me feel your pulse.
Déjeme tomarle el pulso.
Day-ha-me to-**bar**-lay el **pool**-so.

I am going to take your temperature.
Voy a tomarle la temperatura.
Voye a to-**mar**-lay lah tem-pay-rah-**too**-rah.

Lie down, please.
Acuéstese, por favor.
Ah-coo-**es**-tah-say por fah-**vor**.

Do you understand?
¿Me comprende usted?
¿May com-**pren**-day oos-**ted?**

That's right.
Así. Bien.
Ah-**see**. Be-en.

You are doing very well.
Usted va muy bien.
Oos-**ted** vah **moo**-e be-en.

Do not take any medicine from home.
No tome usted ninguna medicina traída de su casa.
No **to**-may oos-**ted** nin-**goon**-ay may-de-**thee**-nah trah-**ee**-dah day soo **cah**-sah.

I am going to give you an injection.
Voy a ponerle ana inyección.
Voye a po-**nerr**-lay **oo**-nah in-yec-the-**on**.

Take a sip of water.
Tome usted un traguito de agua.
To-may oos-**ted** un trah-**gee**-to day **ah**-goo-ah.

Very good. That was fine.
Muy bien. Excelente.
Moo-e **be**-en. Ex-thay-**len**-tay.

Don't be nervous.
No se ponga nervioso(a).
No say **pon**-gah ner-ve-o-so(ah).

Do you feel dizzy?
¿Se siente vertigo?
¿**Say** see-**ayn**-tah **verr**-to-go?

Please lie still.
Quédese inmóvil, por favor.
Kay-day-say in-**mo**-veel por fah-**vor.**

You must drink lots of liquids.
Usted debe tomar muchos líquidos.
Oos-**ted day**-bay to-**mar moo**-chos **lee**-ke-dos.

References

Kelz, R.K. *Conversational Spanish for Medical Personnel.* Albany, N.Y.: Delmar Publishers, 1982. Velazquez de la Cadena, M., E. Gray, and J. Iribas. *New Revised Velazquez Spanish and English Dictionary.* Clinton, N.J.: New Win Publishing, Inc., 1985.

Glossary

Abortion Termination of pregnancy before the age of fetal viability, usually 24 weeks.

Abuse Incident involving some type of violation to the client; Misuse, excessive, or improper use of a substance, the absence of which does not cause withdrawal symptoms.

Accreditation Process by which a voluntary, nongovernmental agency or organization appraises and grants accredited status to institutions and/or programs or services that meet predetermined structure, process, and outcome criteria.

Acculturation Process of learning norms, beliefs, and behavioral expectations of a group.

Acid Any substance that in a solution yields hydrogen ions bearing a positive charge.

Acidosis Condition characterized by an excessive number of hydrogen ions in a solution.

Acoustic Neuroma A slow-growing and usually benign tumor of the vestibular portion of the inner ear involving the cranial nerve VIII.

Acquired Immunodeficiency Syndrome (AIDS) Progressively fatal disease that destroys the immune system and the body's ability to fight infection; caused by the human immunodeficiency virus (HIV).

Active Euthanasia Process of taking deliberate action that will hasten a client's death.

Active Listening Process of hearing spoken words and noting nonverbal behaviors.

Actively Suicidal Descriptor of an individual intent upon hurting or killing self and who is in imminent danger of doing so.

Activities of Daily Living Basic care activities that include mobility, bathing, hygiene, grooming, dressing, eating, and toileting.

Acupressure Technique of releasing blocked energy within an individual when specific points (tsubas) along the meridians are pressed or massaged by the practitioner's fingers, thumbs, and heel of the hands.

Acupuncture Technique of application of heat and needles to various points on the body to alter the energy flow.

Acute Pain Discomfort identified by sudden onset and relatively short duration, mild to severe intensity, and a steady decrease in intensity over several days or weeks.

Addiction Overwhelming preoccupation with obtaining and using a drug for its psychic effects; used interchangeably with dependence.

Adhesion Internal scar tissue from previous surgeries or disease processes.

Adjuvant Medication Drug used to enhance the analgesic efficacy of opioids, treat concurrent symptoms that exacerbate pain, and provide independent analgesia for specific types of pain.

Administrative Law Law developed by those persons who are appointed to governmental administrative agencies and who are entrusted with enforcing the statutory laws passed by the legislature.

Adult Day Care Provision of a variety of services in a protective setting for adults who are unable to stay alone, but who do not need 24-hour care.

Advance Directive Written instruction for health care that is recognized under state law and is related to the provision of such care when the individual is incapacitated.

Adventitious Breath Sound Abnormal sound, including sibilant wheezes (formerly wheezes), sonorous wheezes (formerly rhonchi), fine and course crackles (formerly rales), and pleural friction rubs.

Affect Outward expression of mood or emotions.

Afferent Nerve Pathway Ascending spinal cord pathway that transmits sensory impulses to the brain.

Afferent Pain Pathway Ascending spinal cord.

Agglutination Clumping together of red blood cells.

Agglutinin Specific kind of antibody whose interaction with antigens is manifested as agglutination.

Agglutinogen Any antigenic substance that causes agglutination by the production of agglutinin.

Agnosia Inability to recognize, either by sight or sound, familiar objects such as a hairbrush.

Agnostic Individual who believes that the existence of God cannot be proved or disproved.

Agranulocytosis Acute condition causing a severe reduction in the number of granulocytes (basophils, eosinophils, and neutrophils).

Aldrete Score Scoring system for objectively assessing the physical status of clients recovering from anesthesia; serves as a basis for dismissal from the postanesthesia care unit (PACU) and ambulatory surgery; also known as the postanesthetic recovery score.

Algor Mortis Decrease in body temperature after death, resulting in lack of skin elasticity.

Alkalosis Condition characterized by an excessive loss of hydrogen ions from a solution.

Allergen Type of antigen commonly found in the environment.

Alopecia Partial or complete baldness or loss of hair.

Alternative Therapy Therapy used instead of conventional or mainstream medical practices.

Ambulatory Surgery Surgical operation performed under general, regional, or local anesthesia and involving fewer than 24 hours of hospitalization.

Amenorrhea Absence of menstruation.

Amnesia Inability to remember things.

Amphiarthrosis Articulation of slightly movable joints such as the vertebrae.

Amputation Removal of all or part of an extremity.

Analgesia Pain relief without producing anesthesia.

Analgesic Substance that relieves pain.

Analyte Substance that is measured.

Anaphylaxis Type I systemic reaction to allergens.

Anasarca Generalized edema.

Anesthesia Absence of normal sensation.

Anesthesiologist Licensed physician educated and skilled in the delivery of anesthesia who also adds to the knowledge of anesthesia through research or other scholarly pursuits.

Anesthetist Qualified RN, dentist, or medical doctor who administers anesthetics.

Aneurysm Weakness in the wall of a blood vessel.

Anger Control Assistance Nursing intervention aimed at facilitating the expression of anger in an adaptive and nonviolent manner.

Angina Pectoris Chest pain caused by a narrowing of the coronary arteries.

Angiocatheter Intracatheter with a metal stylet.

Angioedema Allergic reaction consisting of edema of subcutaneous tissue, mucous membranes, or viscera.

Angiogenesis Formation of new blood vessels.

Angiography Visualization of the vascular structures through the use of fluoroscopy with a contrast medium.

Angioma Benign vascular tumor involving skin and subcutaneous tissue: most are congenital.

Anion Ion bearing a negative charge.

Annulus Valvular ring in the heart.

Anorexia Loss of appetite.

Anorexia Nervosa Psychiatric disorder of self-imposed starvation that results in a 15% or more loss of body weight.

Anosognosia Lack of awareness of own neurological deficits.

Antibiotic Resistance Resistance to a previously effective antimicrobial agent.

Antibody Immunoglobulin produced by the body in response to bacteria, viruses, or other antigenic substances.

Anticipatory Grief Occurrence of grief work before an expected loss actually occurs.

Anticipatory Guidance Information, teaching, and guidance given to a client in anticipation of an expected event.

Antigen Any substance identified by the body as nonself.

Antineoplastic Agent that inhibits the growth and reproduction of malignant cells.

Antioxidant Substance that prevents or inhibits oxidation, a chemical process wherein a substance is joined to oxygen.

Anxiety Subjective response that occurs when a person experiences a real or perceived threat to well-being; a diverse feeling of dread or apprehension.

Anxiolytic Antianxiety medication.

Aphasia Inability to communicate; often the result of a brain lesion.

Apheresis Removal of unwanted blood components.

Appendicitis Inflammation of the vermiform appendix.

Appropriate for Gestational Age Infant's weight falls between the 90th and 10th percentile for gestational age.

Areflexia Absence of reflexes.

Aromatherapy Therapeutic use of concentrated essences or essential oils that have been extracted from plants and flowers.

Arousal State of wakefullness and alertness.

Arterial Blood Gases Measurement of levels of oxygen, carbon dioxide, pH, partial pressure of oxygen (PO_2 or PaO_2), partial pressue of carbon dioxide (PCO_2 or $PaCO_2$), saturation of oxygen (SaO_2), and bicarbonate (HCO_3) in arterial blood.

Arteriography Radiographic study of the vascular system following the injection of a radiopaque dye through a catheter.

Arteriosclerosis Cardiovascular disease wherein plaque forms on the inside of artery walls, reducing the space for blood flow.

Arthroplasty Replacement of both articular surfaces within a joint capsule.

Ascites Abnormal accumulation of fluid in the peritoneal cavity.

Asepsis Absence of pathogenic microorganisms.

Aseptic Technique Collection of principles used to control and/or prevent the transfer of pathogenic microorganisms from sources within (endogenous) and outside (exogenous) the client.

Aspiration Procedure performed to withdraw fluid that has abnormally collected or to obtain a specimen; also inhalation of regurgitated gastric contents into the pulmonary system.

Assault Threat to do something that may cause harm or be unpleasant to another person.

Assisted Living Combination of housing and services for persons who require assistance with activities of daily living.

Assisted Suicide Situation wherein another person provides a client with the means to end his own life.

Asthma Condition characterized by intermittent airway obstruction due to antigen–antibody reaction.

Astigmatism Asymmetric focus of light rays on the retina.

Ataxia Inability to coordinate voluntary muscle action.

Atelectasis Collapse of a lung or a portion of a lung.

Atheist Individual who does not believe in God or any other deity.

Atherosclerosis Cardiovascular disease of fatty deposits on the inner lining, the tunica intima, of vessel walls.

Atom Smallest unit of an element which still retains the properties of that element and which cannot be altered by any chemical change.

Audible Wheeze Wheeze that can be heard without the aid of a stethoscope.

Auditory Hallucination Perception by an individual that someone is talking when no one in fact is there.

Aura Peculiar sensation preceding a seizure or migraine; may be a taste, smell, sight, sound, dizziness, or just a "funny feeling."

Auscultation Physical examination technique that involves listening to sounds in the body that are created by movement of air or fluid.

Autoimmune Disorder Disease wherein the body identifies its own cells as foreign and activates mechanisms to destroy them.

Autologous From the same organism (person).

Automatic Implantable Cardioverter-defibrillator (AICD) Implantable device that senses a dysrythmia and automatically sends an electrical shock directly to the heart to defibrillate it.

Automatism Mechanical, repetitive motor behavior performed unconsciously.

Autonomic Nervous System That part of the peripheral nervous system consisting of the sympathetic and parasympathetic nervous systems and controlling unconscious activities.

Autonomy Self-direction; Ethical principle based on the individual's right to choose and the individual's ability to act on that choice.

Autopsy Examination of a body after death by a pathologist to determine cause of death.

Autosomal Pertaining to a condition transmitted by a non-sex chromosome.

Awareness Capacity to perceive sensory impressions through thoughts and actions.

Azotemia Nitrogenous wastes present in the blood.

Bacteremia Condition of bacteria in the blood.

Bactericide Bacteria-killing chemicals; found in tears.

Balanced Budget Act Federal law enacted in 1997 that replaced cost-based reimbursement for care in skilled nursing facilities with a prospective payment system based on client assessment within a resource utilization group system.

Bands Immature neutrophils.

Barium Chalky-white contrast medium.

Base Substance that when dissociated produces ions that will combine with hydrogen ions.

Baseline Level Lab value that serves as a reference point for future value levels.

Battery Unauthorized or unwanted touching of one person by another.

Behavioral Tolerance Compensatory adjustments of behavior made under the influence of a particular substance.

Beneficence Ethical principle based on the duty to promote good and prevent harm.

Benign Not progressive; favorable for recovery.

Bereavement Period of grief following the death of a loved one.

Bioethics Application of general ethical principles to health care.

Biofeedback Measurement of physiological responses that yields information about the relationship between the mind and body and helps clients learn the way to manipulate these responses through mental activity.

Biologic Response Modifier Agent that destroys malignant cells by stimulating the body's immune system.

Biopsy Excision of a small amount of tissue.

Blanching White color of the skin when pressure is applied.

Blastic Phase Intensified phase of leukemia that resembles an acute phase in which there is an increased production of white blood cells.

Body Image Individual's perception of physical self, including appearance, function, and ability.

Bodymind Inseparable connection and operation of thoughts, feelings, and physiological functions.

Borborygmi High-pitched, loud, rushing sounds produced by the movement of gas in the liquid contents of the intestine.

Bradycardia Heart rate less than 60 beats per minute in an adult.

Bradykinesia Slowness of voluntary movement and speech.

Bradypnea Respiratory rate of 10 or fewer breaths per minute.

Breakthrough Pain Sudden, acute, temporary pain that is usually precipitated by a treatment, a procedure, or unusual activity of the client.

Brief Dynamic Therapy Short-term psychotherapy that focuses on resolving core conflicts deriving from personality and living situations.

Bronchial Breath Sound Loud, tubular, hollow-sounding breath sound normally heard over the sternum.

Bronchiectasis Lung disorder characterized by chronic dilation of the bronchi.

Bronchitis Inflammation of the bronchial tree accompanied by hypersecretion of mucus.

Bronchovesicular Breath Sound Breath sound normally heard in the area of the scapula and near the sternum; medium in pitch and intensity, with inspiratory and expiratory phases of equal length.

Bruxism Grinding of teeth during sleep.

Buffer Substance that attempts to maintain pH range, or hydrogen ion concentration, in the presence of added acids or bases.

Bulimia Nervosa Psychiatric disorder characterized by episodic binge-eating followed by purging.

Butterfly Needle Wing-tipped needle.

Cachectic Being in a state of malnutrition and wasting.

Cachexia State of malnutrition and protein wasting.

Calculus Concentration of mineral salts in the body leading to the formation of stone.

Cancer Disease resulting from the uncontrolled growth of cells, which causes malignant cellular tumors.

Capitated Rate Preset fee based on membership rather than services provided; payment system used in managed care.

Carcinogen Substance that initiates or promotes the development of cancer.

Carcinoma Cancer occurring in epithelial tissue.

Cardiac Cycle Cycle of an impulse going completely through the conduction system of the heart, and the ventricles contracting.

Cardiac Output Volume of blood pumped per minute by the left ventricle.

Cardiac Tamponade Collection of fluid in the pericardial sac hindering the functioning of the heart.

Caseation Process whereby the center of the primary tubercle formed in the lungs as a result of tuberculosis becomes soft and cheese-like due to decreased perfusion.

Cataract Condition in which the lens of the eye loses its transparency and becomes opaque.

Categorical Imperative Concept that states that one should act only if the action is based on a principle that is universal.

Cation Ion bearing a positive charge.

Cavitation Process whereby a cavity is created in the lung tissue through the liquefaction and rupture of a primary tubercle.

Ceiling Effect Medication dosage beyond which no further analgesia occurs.

Cellular Immunity Type of acquired immunity involving T-cell lymphocytes.

Centering Process of bringing oneself to an inward focus of serenity; done before beginning an energetic touch therapy treatment.

Central Line Venous catheter inserted into the superior vena cava through the subclavian or internal or external jugular vein.

Central Nervous System System of the brain and spinal cord.

Cephalalgia Headache; also known as cephalgia.

Certification Voluntary process that establishes and evaluates standards of care; mandatory for any health care services receiving federal funds.

Cerumen Ear wax.

Chain of Custody Documentation of the transfer of evidence (of a crime) from one worker to the next in a secure fashion.

Chalazion Cyst of the meibomian glands.

Chancre Clean, painless, syphilitic primary ulcer appearing 2 to 6 weeks after infection at the site of body contact.

Chemoreceptor Receptor that monitors the levels of carbon dioxide, oxygen, and pH in the blood.

Chemotherapy Use of drugs to treat illness, especially cancer.

Cheyne-Stokes Respirations Breathing characterized by periods of apnea alternating with periods of dyspnea.

Chlamydia Sexually transmitted disease caused by the spherical bacterial organism *Chlamydia trachomatis*.

Cholecystitis Inflammation of the gallbladder.

Cholelithiasis Presence of gallstones or calculi in the gallbladder.

Chorea Condition characterized by abnormal, involuntary, purposeless movements of all musculature of the body.

Chronic Acute Pain Discomfort that occurs almost daily over a long period, has the potential for lasting months or years, and has a high probability of ending; also known as progressive pain.

Chronic Nonmalignant Pain Discomfort that occurs almost daily, has been present for at least 6 months, and ranges in intensity from mild to severe; also known as chronic benign pain.

Chronic Pain Discomfort generally identified as long term (lasting 6 months or longer) that is persistent, nearly constant, or recurrent, and that produces significant negative changes in a person's life.

Chronobiology Science of studying biorhythms.

Chvostek's Sign Abnormal spasm of the facial muscles in response to a light tapping of the facial nerve.

Chyme Acidic, semi-fluid paste found in the gastrointestinal tract.

Circadian Rhythm Biorhythm that cycles on a daily basis.

Circulating Nurse RN responsible and accountable for management of personnel, equipment, supplies, the environment, and communication throughout a surgical procedure.

Cirrhosis Chronic degenerative changes in the liver cells and thickening of surrounding tissue.

Civil Law Law that deals with relationships between individuals.

Client Advocate Person who speaks up for or acts on behalf of the client.

Closed Reduction Repair of a fracture done without surgical intervention.

Coarse Crackle Moist, low-pitched crackling and gurgling lung sound of long duration.

Codependent Description for persons who live based on what others think of them.

Cognition Intellectual ability to think.

Cognitive Behavior Therapy Treatment approach aimed at helping a client identify stimuli that cause the client's anxiety, develop plans to respond to those stimuli in a non-anxious manner, and problem-solve when unanticipated anxiety-provoking situations arise.

Colic Condition of acute abdominal pain.

Colostomy Surgically created opening from the colon through the abdominal wall.

Combination Chemotherapy Administration of a combination of chemotherapy drugs over a set period of time.

Command Hallucination Perception by an individual of a voice or voices telling the individual to do something, usually to himself and/or someone else.

Communication The sending and receiving of a message.

Comorbidity Simultaneous existence of more than one disease process within an individual.

Complementary Therapy Therapy used in conjunction with conventional medical therapies.

Complicated Grief Grief associated with traumatic death such as death by homicide, violence, or accident; survivors suffer emotions of greater intensity than those associated with normal grief.

Compound Combination of atoms of two or more elements.

Computed Tomography Radiological scanning of the body with x-ray beams and radiation detectors to transmit data to a computer that transcribes the data into quantitative measurement and multidimensional images of the internal structures.

Concept Mental picture of abstract phenomena that serves to organize observations related to those phenomena.

Conductive Hearing Loss Condition characterized by the inability of sound waves to reach the inner ear.

Confabulation The making up of information to fill in memory gaps.

Confidential Private or secret.

Confidentiality Nondisclosure of the identity of or personal information about an individual.

Congruence Agreement between two things.

Conjunctivitis Inflammation of the conjunctiva.

Conscious Sedation Minimally depressed level of consciousness during which the client retains the ability to maintain a continuously patent airway and to respond appropriately to physical stimulation or verbal commands.

Consciousness State of awareness of self, others, and surrounding environment.

Constipation Condition characterized by hard, infrequent stools that are difficult or painful to pass.

Constitutional Law Law that defines and limits the power of government.

Contraception Measure taken to prevent pregnancy.

Contract Law Enforcement of agreements among private individuals.

Contracture Permanent shortening of a muscle.

Contrast Medium Radiopaque substance that facilitates roentgen (x-ray) imaging of the body's internal structures.

Crackle Abnormal breath sound that resembles a popping sound, heard on inhalation and exhalation; not cleared by coughing.

Crenation Condition wherein cells decrease in size, shrivel and wrinkle, and are no longer functional when in a hypertonic solution.

Crepitus Grating or crackling sensation or sound.

Cretinism Congenital lack of thyroid hormones causing defective physical development and mental retardation.

Criminal Law Law concerning acts of offense against the welfare or safety of the public.

Crisis Acute state of disorganization that occurs when the individual's usual coping mechanisms are no longer effective. Stressor that forces an individual to respond and/or adapt in some way.

Critical Thinking Mode of thinking—about any subject, content, or problem—whereby the thinker improves the quality of his or her thinking by skillfully taking charge of the structures inherent in thinking and imposing intellectual standards (or a level of degree of quality) upon them.

Cross-Tolerance Decreased sensitivity to other substances in the same category.

Cryptorchidism Failure of one or both testes to descend.

Cultural Assimilation Process whereby individuals from a minority group are absorbed by the dominant culture and take on the characteristics of the dominant culture.

Cultural Diversity Differences among people that result from racial, ethnic, and cultural variables.

Culture Dynamic and integrated structures of knowledge, beliefs, behaviors, ideas, attitudes, values, habits, customs, languages, symbols, rituals, ceremonies, and practices that are unique to a particular group of people. Growing of microorganisms to identify a pathogen.

Curative To heal or restore to health.

Curing Ridding one of disease.

Cutaneous Pain Discomfort caused by stimulation of the cutaneous nerve endings in the skin.

Cyanosis Bluish discoloration of the skin and mucous membranes observed in lips, nail beds, and earlobes.

Cycling Alteration in mood between depression and mania.

Cystitis Inflammation of the urinary bladder.

Cystocele Downward displacement of the bladder into the anterior vaginal wall.

Cytology Study of cells.

Cytomegalovirus One of the herpes type viruses: inhabits saliva, urine, blood, semen, and vaginal secretions.

Dawn Phenomenon Early morning glucose elevation produced by the release of growth hormone.

Death Rattle Breathing sound in the period preceding death caused by a collection of secretions in the larynx.

Debride To remove dead or damaged tissue or foreign material from a wound.

Decomposition Chemical reaction wherein the bonding between atoms in a molecule is broken and simpler products are formed.

Defamation Use of words to harm or injure the personal or professional reputation of another person.

Dehiscence Complication of wound healing wherein the wound edges separate.

Dehydration Condition wherein more water is lost from the body than is being replaced.

Delirium Cognitive changes or acute confusion of rapid onset (less than 6 months).

Delusion False belief that misrepresents reality.

Dementia Organic brain pathology characterized by losses in intellectual functioning and a slow onset (longer than 6 months).

Deontology Ethical theory that considers the intrinsic significance of an act as the criterion for determination of good.

Dependence Reliance on a substance to such a degree that abstinence causes functional impairment, physical withdrawal symptoms, and/or psychological craving for the substance. See also addiction.

Depolarization Contraction of the heart.

Depression State wherein an individual experiences feelings of extreme sadness, hopelessness, and helplessness.

Detoxification Elimination of a substance from the body.

Dialysate Solution used in dialysis, designed to approximate the normal electrolyte structure of plasma and extracellular fluid.

Dialysis Mechanical means of removing nitrogenous waste from the blood by imitating the function of the nephrons; involves filtration and diffusion of wastes, drugs, and excess electrolytes and/or osmosis of water across a semipermeable membrane into a dialysate solution.

Diarthrosis Freely movable joint.

Differentiation Acquisition of characteristics or functions different from those of the original.

Diffusion Process whereby a substance moves from an area of higher concentration to an area of lower concentration.

Digestion Mechanical and chemical processes that convert nutrients into a physically absorbable state.

Diplopia Double vision.

Discipline Branch of learning, field of study, or occupation requiring specialized knowledge.

Disciplined Trained by instruction and exercise.

Disenfranchised Grief "Grief that is not openly acknowledged, socially sanctioned, or publicly shared" (Doka, Rushton, & Thorstenson, 1994).

Dislocation Injury in which the articular surfaces of a joint are no longer in contact.

Disorientation State of mental confusion in which awareness of time, place, self, and/or situation is impaired.

Distraction Technique of focusing attention on stimuli other than pain.

Diverticula Sac-like protrusion of the intestinal wall that results when the mucosa herniates through the bowel wall.

Diverticulitis Inflammation of one or more diverticula.

Diverticulosis Condition in which multiple diverticula are present in the colon.

Domestic Violence Aggression and violence involving family members.

Dominant Culture Group whose values prevail within a society.

Drug Incompatibility Undesired chemical or physical reaction between a drug and a solution, between two drugs, or between a drug and the container or tubing.

Drug Interaction Effect one drug can have on another drug.

Durable Power of Attorney for Health Care Legal document designating who may make health care decisions for a client when that client is no longer capable of decision making.

Dysarthria Difficult and defective speech due to a dysfunction of the muscles used for speech.

Dysfunctional Grief Persistent pattern of intense grief that does not result in reconciliation of feelings.

Dysmenorrhea Painful menstruation.

Dyspareunia Painful intercourse.

Dysphasia Impairment of speech resulting from damage to the speech center in the brain.

Dyspnea Difficulty breathing as observed by labored or forced respirations through the use of accessory muscles in the chest and neck.

Dysrhythmia Irregularity in the rate, rhythm, or conduction of the electrical system of the heart.

Dysuria Difficult or painful urination.

Ecchymosis Large, irregular hemorrhagic area on the skin; also called a bruise.

Edema Detectable accumulation of increased interstitial fluid.

Efferent Nerve Pathway Descending spinal cord pathway that transmits sensory impulses from the brain.

Efferent Pain Pathway Descending spinal cord.

Effluent Liquid output from an ileostomy.

Electrocardiogram Graphic recording of the heart's electrical activity.

Electroconvulsive Therapy Procedure whereby clients are treated with pulses of electrical energy sufficient to cause brief convulsions or seizures.

Electroencephalogram Graphic recording of the brain's electrical activity.

Electrolyte Element or compound that, when dissolved in water or another solvent, dissociates (separates) into ions (electrically charged particles).

Element Basic substance of matter.

Embolus Mass, such as a blood clot or an air bubble, that circulates in the bloodstream.

Emergency Medical or surgical condition requiring immediate or timely intervention to prevent permanent disability or death.

Emergency Medical Technician Health care professional trained to provide basic lifesaving measures prior to arrival at the hospital.

Emergency Nursing Care of clients who require emergency interventions.

Emotional Lability Loss of emotional control.

Empathy Capacity to understand another person's feelings or perception of a situation.

Emphysema Lung disease wherein air accumulates in the tissues of the lungs.

Encephalitis Inflammation of the brain.

Endocrine Group of cells secreting substances directly into the blood or lymph circulation and affecting another part of the body.

Endometriosis Growth of endometrial tissue on structures outside of the uterus, within the pelvic cavity.

Endorphins Group of opiate-like substances produced naturally by the brain which raise the pain threshold, produce sedation and euphoria, and promote a sense of well-being.

Endoscopy Visualization of a body organ or cavity through a scope.

Energetic-Touch Therapy Technique of using the hands to direct or redirect the flow of the body's energy fields and thus enhance balance within those fields.

Enzyme Globular protein produced in the body that catalyzes chemical reactions within the cells by promoting the oxidative reactions and synthesis of various chemicals.

Enzyme-Linked Immunosorbent Assay (ELISA) Basic screening test currently used to detect antibodies to HIV.

Epidural Analgesia Analgesics administered via a catheter that terminates in the epidural space.

Epistaxis Hemorrhage of the nares or nostrils; also known as nosebleed.

Erythema Redness of the skin that may be caused by inflammation of tissues or by sunburn.

Erythrocytapheresis Procedure that removes abnormal red blood cells and replaces them with healthy ones.

Erythropoiesis Production of red blood cells and their release by the red bone marrow.

Eschar Dry, dark, leathery scab composed of denatured protein.

Ethical Dilemma Situation wherein there is a conflict between two or more ethical principles.

Ethical Principle Widely accepted code, generally based on the humane aspects of society, that directs or governs actions.

Ethical Reasoning Process of thinking through what one ought to do in an orderly, systematic manner based on principles.

Ethics Branch of philosophy concerned with determining right from wrong on the basis of a body of knowledge.

Ethnicity Cultural group's perception of itself or a group identity.

Ethnocentrism Assumption of cultural superiority and an inability to accept other cultures' ways of organizing reality.

Euphoric Characterized by elation out of context to the situation.

Eupnea Easy respirations with a rate of breaths per minute that is age-appropriate.

Euthanasia Intentional action or lack of action that causes the merciful death of someone suffering from a terminal illness or incurable condition; derived from the Greek word *euthanatos,* which literally means "good or gentle death."

Evisceration Complication of wound healing characterized by a complete separation of wound edges accompanied by visceral protrusion.

Exacerbation Increase in the symptoms of a disease.

Exclusive Provider Organization Organization wherein care must be delivered by the plan in order for clients to receive reimbursement for health care services.

Excretion Elimination of drugs or waste products from the body.

Expected Outcome Detailed, specific statement that describes the methods through which a goal will be achieved and that includes aspects such as direct nursing care, client teaching, and continuity of care.

Exposure Contact with an infected person or agent.

Expressed Contract Conditions and terms of a contract given in writing by the concerned parties.

External Respiration Exchange of gases between the atmosphere and the lungs.

Extracellular Fluid Fluid outside of the cells; includes interstitial, intravascular, synovial, cerebrospinal, and serous fluids; aqueous and vitreous humor; and endolymph and perilymph.

Extravasation Escape of fluid into the surrounding tissue.

False Imprisonment Situation wherein a person is made to wrongfully believe that he cannot leave a place.

Fasciculation Involuntary twitching of muscle fibers.

Fee for Service System in which the health care recipient directly pays the provider for services as they are provided.

Feedback Response from the receiver of a message so that the sender can verify the message.

Felony Crime of a serious nature that is usually punishable by imprisonment in a state penitentiary or by death.

Fibrinolysis Process of breaking fibrin apart.

Fidelity Ethical concept based on faithfulness and keeping promises.

Filtration Process of fluids and the substances dissolved in them being forced through the cell membrane by hydrostatic pressure.

Fine Crackle Dry, high-pitched crackling and popping lung sound of short duration.

First Assistant Associate of the surgeon, referring physician, or surgical resident who assists the surgeon to retract tissue, aids in the removal of blood and fluids at the operative site, and assists with hemostasis and wound closure.

Flashback Rushing of blood back into intravenous tubing when a negative pressure is created on the tubing. Reliving of an original trauma as if the individual were currently experiencing it.

Flow Rate Volume of fluid to infuse over a set period of time.

Fluoroscopy Immediate, serial images of the body's structure or function.

Formal Contract Written contract that cannot be changed legally by an oral agreement.

Fracture Break in the continuity of a bone.

Fraud Wrong that results from a deliberate deception intended to produce unlawful gain.

Free Radical Unstable molecule that alters genetic codes and triggers the development of cancer growth in cells.

Friction Force of two surfaces moving against one another.

Fulguration Procedure to destroy tissue with long, high-frequency electric sparks.

Gastric Ulcer Erosion in the stomach.

Gastritis Inflammation of the stomach mucosa.

Gate Control Pain Theory Theory that proposes that the cognitive, sensory, emotional, and physiologic components of the body can act together to block an individual's perception of pain.

General Anesthesia Method of producing unconsciousness; complete insensibility to pain; amnesia; motionlessness; and muscle relaxation.

Genuineness Sincerity.

Gerontological Nursing Specialty within nursing that addresses and advocates for the special care needs of older adults.

Gerontologist Specialist in gerontology in advanced practice nursing, geriatric psychiatry, medicine, and social services.

Gerontology Study of the effects of normal aging and age-related diseases on human beings.

Glasgow Coma Scale Neurological screening test that measures a client's best verbal, motor, and eye response to stimuli.

Glaucoma A disorder characterized by an abnormally high pressure of fluid inside the eyeball.

Glucagon Hormone secreted by the alpha cells of the pancreas which stimulate release of glucose by the liver.

Glycogenesis Conversion of glucose into glycogen.

Glycogenolysis Conversion of glycogen into glucose.

Glycosuria Presence of excessive glucose in the urine.

Goiter Enlargement of the thyroid gland.

Gonorrhea Sexually transmitted disease caused by the gram-negative bacterial organism *Neisseria gonorrhea.*

Good Samaritan Law Law that provides protection to health care providers by assuring them of immunity from civil liability when care is provided at the scene of an emergency and the caregiver does not intentionally or recklessly cause the client injury.

Granulation Tissue Delicate connective tissue consisting of fibroblasts, collagen, and capillaries.

Graphesthesia Ability to identify letters, numbers, or shapes drawn on the skin.

Grief Series of intense physical and psychological responses that occurs following a loss; a normal, natural, necessary, and adaptive response to a loss.

Grief Work Process whereby the bereaved experiences freedom from attachment to the deceased, becomes reoriented to the environment where the deceased is no longer present, and establishes new relationships.

Gynecomastia Abnormal enlargement of one or both breasts in males.

Hallucination Sensory perception that occurs in the absence of external stimuli and that is not based on reality.

Haustra Sac-like pouches of the colon.

Healing Process that activates the individual's recovery forces from within.

Healing Touch Energy-based therapeutic modality that alters the energy fields through the use of touch, thereby affecting physical, mental, emotional, and spiritual health.

Health According to the World Health Organization, the state of complete physical, mental, and social well-being, not merely the absence of disease or infirmity.

Health Care Delivery System Mechanism for providing services that meet the health-related needs of individuals.

Health Care Financing Agency Federal agency in charge of administering the Medicare program.

Health Care Surrogate Law Law enacted by some states that provides a legal means for decision making in the absence of advance directives.

Health History Review of the client's functional health patterns prior to the current contact with a health care agency.

Health Maintenance Organization Prepaid health plan that provides primary health care services for a preset fee and focuses on cost-effective treatment methods.

Hearing Act or power of receiving sounds.

Heart Sound S_1 and S_2 sound heard by auscultating the heart.

Heberden's Nodes Enlargement and characteristic hypertrophic spurs in the terminal interphalangeal finger joints.

Hemarthrosis Bleeding into the joints.

Hematemesis Vomiting of blood.

Hematocrit Percentage of red blood cells in a given volume of blood.

Hematopoiesis Process of blood cell production and development.

Hematuria Blood in the urine.

Hemiparesis Weakness of one side of the body.

Hemiplegia Paralysis of one side of the body.

Hemolysis Breakdown of red blood cells and the release of hemoglobin.

Hemopneumothorax Presence of blood and air within the pleural space.

Hemorrhagic Exudate Discharge that has a large component of red blood cells.

Hemorrhoid Swollen vascular tissue in the rectal area.

Hemothorax Condition wherein blood accumulates in the pleural space of the lungs.

Hepatitis Chronic or acute inflammation of the liver.

Hesitancy Difficulty initiating the urinary stream.

Hindmilk Follows foremilk, is higher in fat content, leading to weight gain, and is more satisfying.

Hirsutism Excessive body hair in a masculine distribution.

Histamine Substance released during allergic reactions.

HIV-Wasting Syndrome Unexplained weight loss of more than 10% of body weight accompanied by weakness, chronic diarrhea, and fever in those infected with HIV.

Homan's Sign Test to check for the presence of clots in the leg.

Homeostasis Balance or equilibrium among the physiologic, psychological, sociocultural, intellectual, and spiritual needs of the body.

Homologous From the same species.

Homonymous Hemianopia Loss of vision in half of the visual field on the same side of both eyes.

Hormone Substance that initiates or regulates activity of another organ, system, or gland in another part of the body.

Hospice Humane, compassionate care provided to clients who can no longer benefit from curative treatment, and have 6 months or less to live.

Human Immunodeficiency Virus (HIV) Retrovirus that causes AIDS.

Human Leukocyte Antigen Antigen present in human blood.

Humoral Immunity Type of immunity dominated by antibodies.

Hydrostatic Pressure Pressure that a fluid exerts against a membrane; also called filtration force.

Hypergylcemia Condition wherein the blood glucose level becomes too high as a result of the absence of insulin.

Hyperopia Farsightedness.

Hypersensitivity Excessive reaction to a stimulus.

Hypersomnia Alteration in sleep pattern characterized by excessive sleep, especially in the daytime.

Hyperthermia Condition in which the core body temperature rises above 106°F.

Hypertonic Solution Solution that has a higher molecular concentration than the cell; also called a hyperosmolar solution.

Hypertrophy Increase in muscle mass.

Hyperuricemia Increased uric acid blood level.

Hyperventilation Breathing characterized by deep, rapid respirations.

Hypervigilant Condition of constantly scanning the environment for potentially dangerous situations.

Hypervolemia Increased circulating fluid volume.

Hypnosis Altered state of consciousness or awareness resembling sleep and during which a person is more receptive to suggestion.

Hypoglycemia Condition wherein the blood glucose level is exceedingly low.

Hypomania Mild form of mania without significant impairment.

Hypothermia Condition in which the core body temperature drops below 95°F.

Hypotonic Solution Solution that has a lower molecular concentration than the cell; also called hypo-osmolar solution.

Hypoventilation Breathing characterized by shallow respirations.

Hypovolemia Abnormally low circulatory blood volume.

Hypoxemia Decreased oxygen level in the blood.

Iatrogenic Caused by treatment or diagnostic procedures.

Idiopathic Occuring without a known cause.

Ileal Conduit Implantation of the ureters into a piece of ileum, which is attached to the abdominal wall as a stoma so urine can be removed from the body.

Ileostomy Opening created in the small intestine at the ileum. specific signs and symptoms of an infectious agent.

Illusion Inaccurate perception or misinterpretation of sensory stimuli.

Imagery Relaxation technique of using the imagination to visualize a pleasant, soothing image.

Immune Response Body's reaction to substances identified as nonself.

Immunity Body's ability to protect itself from foreign agents or organisms.

Immunotherapy Treatment to suppress or enhance immunological functioning.

Impaired Nurse Nurse who is habitually intemperate or is addicted to the use of alcohol or habit-forming drugs.

Implantable Port Device made of a radiopague silicone catheter and a plastic or stainless steel injection port with a self-sealing silicone-rubber septum.

Implied Contract Contract that recognizes a relationship between parties for services.

Impotence Inability of an adult male to have an erection firm enough, or to maintain it long enough, to complete sexual intercourse.

Incidence Frequency of disease occurrence.

Incident Report Risk-management tool used to describe and report any unusual event that occurs to a client, visitor, or staff member.

Incubation Period Time interval between the entry of an infectious agent in the host and the onset of symptoms.

Induction Dose Initial dose of chemotherapy.

Infertility Inability or diminished ability to produce offspring.

Infiltration Seepage of foreign substances into the interstitial tissue, causing swelling and discomfort at the IV site.

Inflammation Nonspecific cellular response to tissue injury.

Informed Consent Legal form signed by a competent client and witnessed by another person that grants permission to the client's physician to perform the procedure described by the physician and that demonstrates the client's understanding of the benefits, risks, and possible complications of the procedure, as well as alternate treatment options.

Insomnia Difficulty in falling asleep initially or in returning to sleep once awakened.

Inspection Physical examination technique that involves thorough visual observation.

Instrument of Healing Means by which healing can be achieved, performed, or enhanced.

Insulin Pancreatic hormone that aids in both the diffusion of glucose into the liver and muscle cells, and the synthesis of glycogen.

Internal Respiration Exchange of oxygen and carbon dioxide at the cellular level.

Interstitial Fluid Fluid in tissue spaces around each cell.

Intoxication Reversible effect on the central nervous system soon after the use of a substance.

Intracath Plastic tube for insertion into a vein.

Intracellular Fluid Fluid within the cells.

Intraoperative Phase Time during the surgical experience that begins when the client is transferred to the operating room table and ends when the client is admitted to the postanesthesia care unit.

Intrathecal Analgesia Administration of analgesics into the subarachnoid space.

Intravascular Fluid Fluid consisting of the plasma in the blood vessels and the lymph in the lymphatic system.

Intravenous (IV) Therapy Administration of fluids, electrolytes, nutrients, or medications by the venous route.

Intravesical Within the urinary bladder.

Intussusception Telescoping of one part of the intestine into another.

Invasive Accessing the body tissues, organs, or cavities through some type of instrumentation procedure.

Ion Atom bearing an electrical charge.

Ischemia Oxygen deprivation, usually due to poor perfusion.

Ischemic Pain Discomfort resulting when the blood supply of an area is restricted or cut off completely.

Isotonic Solution Solution that has the same molecular concentration as does the cell; also called an isosmolar solution.

Isotopes Atoms of the same element that have different atomic weights (i.e., different numbers of neutrons in the nucleus).

IV Push (bolus) Method of administering a large dose of medication in a relatively short time, usually 1–30 minutes.

Jaundice Yellow discoloration of the skin, sclera, mucous membranes, and body fluids that occurs when the liver is unable to fully remove bilirubin from the blood.

Johnsonian Intervention Confrontational approach to a client with a substance problem that lessens the chance of denial and encourages treatment before the client "hits bottom."

Judgment Ability to evaluate alternatives to arrive at an appropriate course of action. Conclusion based on sound reasoning and supported by evidence.

Justice Ethical principle based on the concept of fairness extended to each individual.

Justify To prove or show to be valid.

Kaposi's Sarcoma Vascular malignancy that can occur any place in the body, including internal organs.

Keloid Abnormal growth of scar tissue that is elevated, rounded, and firm with irregular, clawlike margins.

Keratin Tough, fibrous protein produced by cells in the epidermis called keratinocytes.

Keratitis Inflammation of the cornea.
high level of bilirubin (jaundice).

Kernig's Sign Diagnostic test for inflammation in the nerve roots; the inability to extend the leg when the thigh is flexed against the abdomen.

Ketone Acidic byproduct of fat metabolism.

Ketonuria Presence of ketones in the urine.

Kyphosis Increased roundess of the thoracic spinal curve.

Law That which is laid down or fixed.

Lethargy Decreased energy level.

Leukemia Cancer occurring in blood-forming tissues.

Leukocytosis Increased number of white blood cells.

Leukopenia Decreased number of white blood cells.

Liability Obligation one has incurred or might incur through any act or failure to act.

Libel Written words that harm or injure the personal or professional reputation of another person.

Libido Sexual energy.

Licensure Mandatory system of granting licenses according to specified standards.

Life Review Form of reminiscence wherein a client attempts either to come to terms with conflict or to gain meaning from life and die peacefully.

Ligation Application of a band or tie around a structure.

Lipodystrophy Atrophy or hypertrophy of subcutaneous fat.

Lipoma Benign tumor consisting of mature fat cells.

Lipoprotein Blood lipid bound to protein.

Liquefaction Necrosis Death and subsequent change of tissue to a liquid or semi-liquid state; often descriptive of a primary tubercle.

Listening Interpreting the sounds heard and attaching meaning to them.

Litholapaxy Procedure involving crushing of a bladder stone and immediate washing out of the fragments through a catheter.

Lithotripsy Method of crushing a calculus any place in the urinary system with ultrasonic waves.

Liver Mortis Bluish-purple discoloration of the skin, usually at pressure points, that is a by-product of red blood cell destruction.

Living Will Legal document that allows a person to state preferences about the use of life-sustaining measures should she be unable to make her wishes known.

Locomotor Pertaining to movement or the ability to move.

Logic Formal principles of a branch of knowledge (such as nursing).

Long-Term Care Facility Health care facility that provides services to individuals who are not acutely ill, have continuing health care needs, and cannot function independently at home.

Lordosis Exaggeration of the curvature of the lumbar spine.

Loss Any situation, either actual, potential, or perceived, wherein a valued object or person is changed or is no longer accessible to the individual.

Lumbar Puncture Aspiration of cerebrospinal fluid from the subarachnoid space.

Lung Stretch Receptor Receptor that monitors the patterns of breathing and prevents overexpansion of the lungs.

Lymphoma Tumor of the lymphatic system.

Macular Degeneration Atrophy or deterioration of the macula, the point on the retina where light rays meet as they are focused by the cornea and lens of the eye.

Magnetic Resonance Imaging Imaging technique that uses radiowaves and a strong magnetic field to make continuous cross-sectional images of the body.

Maintenance Therapy Small doses of chemotherapy given every 3 to 4 weeks to maintain remission.

Malignant Becoming progressively worse and often resulting in death.

Malpractice Negligent acts on the part of a professional; relates to the conduct of a person who is acting in a professional capacity.

Managed Care System of providing and monitoring care wherein access, cost, and quality are controlled before or during delivery of services.

Mania Extremely elevated mood with accompanying agitated behavior.

Material Principle of Justice Rationale for determining those times when there can be unequal allocation of scarce resources.

Matter Anything that occupies space and possesses mass.

Maturational Loss Loss that occurs as a result of moving from one developmental stage to another.

Median Survival Time Average length of life.

Medicaid Government title program (XIX) that pays for health services for the aged, poor, disabled, and low-income families with dependent children.

Medical Model Traditional approach to health care wherein the focus is on treatment and cure of disease.

Medicare Amendment (Title XVIII) to the Social Security Act that helps finace the health care of persons over 65 years old and for permanently disabled younger persons who receive Social Security disability benefits.

Medigap Insurance Insurance plan for persons with Medicare that pays for health care costs not covered by Medicare.

Meditation Quieting of the mind by focusing the attention.

Melanin Pigment that gives skin its color.

Melena Stool containing partially broken down blood; usually black, sticky, and tar-like.

Ménière's Disease State of hearing loss characterized by tinnitus and vertigo.

Meningitis Inflammation of the meninges.

Menopause Cessation of menstruation.

Menorrhagia Excessively heavy menstrual flow.

Mental Disorder Clinically significant behavior or psychological syndrome or pattern that occurs in an individual and is associated with present distress or disability or with a significantly increased risk of suffering, death, pain, disability, or an important loss of freedom (APA, 1994).

Mental Illness Condition wherein an individual has a distorted view of self, is unable to maintain satisfying personal relationships, and is unable to adapt to the environment.

Mentation Ability to concentrate, remember, or think abstractly.

Metastasis Spread of cancer cells to distant areas of the body by way of the lymph system or bloodstream.

Metrorrhagia Vaginal bleeding between menstrual periods.

Microthrombi Very small clots.

Micturition Process of expelling urine from the urinary bladder; also called urination or voiding.

Minority Group Group of people that constitute less than a numerical majority of the population and who, because of their cultural, racial, ethnic, religious, or other characteristics, are often labeled and treated differently from others in the society.

Misdemeanor Offense that is less serious than a felony and may be punished by a fine or by sentence to a local prison for less than 1 year.

Misuse Use of a legal substance for which it was not intended, or exceeding the recommended dosage of a drug.

Mixed Agonist-Antagonist Compound that blocks opioid effects on one receptor type while producing opioid effects on a second receptor type.

Mixture Substances combined in no specific way.

Modulation Central nervous system pathway that selectively inhibits pain transmission by sending signals back down to the dorsal horn of the spinal cord.

Molecule Atoms of the same element that unite with each other.

Mood Subjective report of the way an individual is feeling.

Mortuary Funeral home.

Mourning Period of time during which grief is expressed and resolution and integration of the loss occur.

Myasthenia Gravis Autoimmune disease characterized by extreme muscle weakness and fatigue due to the body's inability to transmit nerve impulses to voluntary muscles.

***Mycobacterium Avium* Complex** Two closely related mycobacteria, *mycobacterium avium* and *mycobacterium intracellulare,* that are grouped together.

Myocardial Infarction Necrosis (death) of the myocardium caused by an obstruction in a coronary artery; commonly known as heart attack.

Myocarditis Inflammation of the myocardium of the heart.

Myofascial Pain Syndrome Group of muscle disorders characterized by pain, muscle spasm, tenderness, stiffness, and limited motion.

Myopia Nearsightedness.

Myringotomy Surgical incision of the eardrum.

Myxedema Severe hypothyroidism in adults.

Necrosis Tissue death as the result of disease or injury.

Neglect Situation wherein a basic need of the client is not being provided.

Negligence General term referring to careless acts on the part of an individual who is not exercising reasonable or prudent judgement.

Neoplasm Any abnormal growth of new tissue.

Nephrotoxic Quality of a substance that causes kidney tissue damage.

Neuralgia Paroxysmal pain that extends along the course of one or more nerves.

Neurogenic Shock Hypotensive situation resulting from the loss of sympathetic control of vital functions from the brain.

Neuropeptide Amino acid produced in the brain and other sites in the body that acts as a chemical communicator.

Neurotransmitter Chemical substance produced by the body that facilitates nerve-impulse transmission.

Nevi Pigmented areas in the skin; commonly known as birthmarks or moles.

Nociceptor Receptive neuron for painful sensations.

Nocturia Awakening at night to void.

Nocturnal Enuresis Incontinence that occurs during sleep.

Noninvasive Descriptor for procedure wherein the body is *not* entered with any type of instrument.

Nonmaleficence Ethical principle based on the obligation to cause no harm to others.

Nonshivering Thermogenesis Metabolism of brown fat; process unique to the newborn.

Nonverbal Communication Sending a message without words; sometimes called body language.

Nosocomial Originating in the hospital.

Nosocomial Infection Infection that is acquired in the hospital or other health care facility and was not present or incubating at the time of the client's admission.

Noxious Stimulus Underlying pathology that causes pain.

Nuchal Cord Condition of the umbilical cord being wrapped around the baby's neck.

Nuchal Rigidity Pain and rigidity in the neck.

Nullipara Condition of never having delivered an infant after 24 weeks' gestation.

Nursing An art and a science that assists individuals to learn to care for themselves whenever possible; also involves caring for others when they are unable to meet their own needs.

Nursing Audit Process of collecting and analyzing data to evaluate the effectiveness of nursing interventions.

Nursing Care Plan Written guide that organizes data about a client's care into a formal statement of the strategies that will be implemented to help the client achieve optimal health.

Nursing Diagnosis Second step in the nursing process; a clinical judgement about individual, family, or community (aggregate) responses to actual or potential health problems/life processes.

Nursing Intervention Action performed by a nurse that helps the client achieve the results specified by the goals and expected outcomes.

Nursing Intervention Classification Standardized language for nursing interventions.

Nursing Minimum Data Set Elements contained in clinical records and abstracted for studies on the effectiveness and costs of nursing care.

Nursing Outcomes Classification Standardized language for nursing outcomes.

Nursing Practice Act Statute that is enacted by the legislature of a state and that outlines the scope of nursing practice in that state.

Nursing Process Systematic method of providing care to clients, consisting of five steps: assessment, diagnosis, outcome identification and planning, implementation, and evaluation.

Nutrition All of the processes (ingestion, digestion, absorption, metabolism, and elimination) involved in consuming and utilizing food for energy, maintenance, and growth.

Nystagmus Constant, involuntary movement of the eye in various directions.

Obesity Weight that is 20% or more above the ideal body weight.

Objective Data Observable and measurable data that are obtained through standard assessment techniques performed during the physical examination and through laboratory and diagnostic tests.

Occult Blood Blood in the stool that can be detected only through a microscope or by chemical means.

Occult Blood Test (Guaiac) Test for microscopic blood done on stool.

Older Adulthood Developmental stage occurring from the age of 65 years until death.

Oligomenorrhea Decreased menstrual flow.

Oliguria Diminished production of urine.

Omnibus Budget Reconciliation Act Federal law first enacted in 1989 to provide for rights and clinical guidelines to ensure quality health services for older Americans.

Oncology Study of tumors.

Ongoing Assessment Type of assessment that includes systematic monitoring and observation related to specific problems.

Ongoing Planning Continuous updating of the client's plan of care.

Onset of Action Time it takes the body to respond to a drug after administration.

Oophoritis Inflammation of the ovary.

Open Reduction Surgical procedure that enables the surgeon to reduce (repair) a fracture under direct visualization.

Opinion Subjective belief.

Opioid Morphine-like compound that produces bodily effects such as pain relief, sedation, constipation, and respiratory depression.

Opisthotonos Complete arching of the body with only the head and feet on the bed.

Opportunistic Infection Infection in persons with a defective immune system that rarely causes harm in healthy individuals.

Oppression Condition wherein the rules, modes, and ideals of one group are imposed on another group.

Orchiectomy Removal of a testis.

Orientation Person's awareness of self in relation to person, place, time, and, in some cases, situation.

Orthopedics (Orthopaedics) Branch of medicine that deals with the prevention or correction of the disorders and diseases of the musculoskeletal system.

Orthopnea Difficulty breathing while lying down.

Orthostatic Hypotension Significant decrease in blood pressure that results when a person moves from a lying or sitting (supine) position to a standing position.

Osmolality Measurement of the total concentration of dissolved particles (solutes) per kilogram of water.

Osmolarity Concentration of solutes per liter of cellular fluid.

Osmosis Movement of a solvent, usually water, through a semipermeable membrane, from a region of higher concentration to a region of lower concentration.

Osmotic Pressure Pressure exerted against the cell membrane by the water inside a cell.

Osteoporosis Increase in the porosity of bone.

Otitis Externa Bacterial infection of the external ear canal.

Otitis Media Inflammation of the middle ear.

Otosclerosis Conductive hearing loss secondary to a pathologic change of the bones in the middle ear.

Overflow Incontinence Leaking of urine when the bladder becomes very full and distended.

Oxidation Chemical process of combining with oxygen.

Oxidized Joined with oxygen.

Pain Unpleasant sensory and emotional experience associated with actual or potential tissue damage or described in terms of such.

Pain Threshold Level of intensity at which a person feels pain.

Pain Tolerance Level of intensity or duration of pain that a person is willing to endure.

Palliative Relief of symptoms, such as pain, without altering the course of disease.

Palliative Care Care that relieves symptoms, such as pain, but does not alter the course of disease.

Pallor Abnormal paleness of the skin, seen especially in the face, conjunctiva, nail beds, and oral mucous membranes.

Palpation Physical examination technique that uses the sense of touch to assess texture, temperature, moisture, organ location and size, vibrations and pulsations, swelling, masses, and tenderness.

Palpitation Fluttering or pounding sensation in the chest.

Pancreatitis Acute or chronic inflammation of the pancreas.

Papanicolaou Test Smear method of examining stained exfoliative cells.

Paracentesis Aspiration of fluid from the abdominal cavity.

Paradoxical Reaction Opposite effect of that which would normally be expected.

Paramedic Specialized health care professional trained to provide advanced life support to the client requiring emergency interventions.

Paraplegia Paralysis of lower extremities.

Paresthesia Abnormal sensation such as burning, prickling, or tingling.

Paroxysmal Descriptor for a symptom that begins and ends abruptly.

Paroxysmal Nocturnal Dyspnea Condition of suddenly awakening, sweating, and having difficulty breathing.

Passive Euthanasia Process of cooperating with the client's dying process.

Patient-Controlled Analgesia Device that allows the client to control the delivery of intravenous or subcutaneous pain medication in a safe, effective manner through a programmable pump.

Peer Assistance Program Rehabilitation program that provides an impaired nurse with referrals, professional and peer counseling support groups, and assistance and monitoring back into nursing.

Peptic Ulcer Erosion formed in the esophagus, stomach, or duodenum resulting from acid/pepsin imbalance.

Perception Ability to experience, recognize, organize, and interpret sensory stimuli.

Percussion Physical examination technique that uses short, tapping strokes on the surface of the skin to create vibrations of underlying organs.

Percutaneous Balloon Valvuloplasty Insertion of a balloon in a stenosed valve to expand the narrowed valvular space.

Perfusion Blood flow through an organ or body part.

Pericardial Friction Rub Short, high-pitched squeak heard as two inflamed pericardial surfaces rub together.

Pericardiocentesis Removal of fluid from the pericardial sac.

Pericarditis Inflammation of the membrane sac surrounding the heart.

Perioperative Period of time comprising the preoperative, intraoperative, and postoperative phases of surgery.

Peripheral Nervous System System of the cranial nerves, spinal nerves, and the autonomic nervous system.

Peripheral Resistance Pressure within a vessel that resists the flow of blood such as plaque buildup or vasoconstriction.

Peristalsis Coordinated, rhythmic, serial contraction of the smooth muscles of the gastrointestinal tract.

Peritonitis Inflammation of the peritoneum, the membranous covering of the abdomen.

Permeability Ability of a membrane to permit substances to pass through it.

Petechiae Pinpoint hemorrhagic spots on the skin.

Phantom Limb Pain Neuropathic pain that occurs after amputation with pain sensations referred to an area in the missing portion of the limb.

Phlebitis Inflammation in the wall of a vein without clot formation.

Phlebothrombosis Formation of a clot because of blood pooling in the vessel, trauma to the vessel's endothelial lining, or a coagulation problem with little or no inflammation in the vessel.

Phlebotomist Individual who performs venipuncture.

Phlebotomy Removal of blood from a vein.

Physically Aggressive Descriptor of an individual who threatens or actually harms someone.

Phytochemical Physiologically active compound present in plants in very small amounts that gives plants flavor, odor, and color.

Piggyback Addition of an intravenous solution to infuse concurrently with another infusion.

Pleural Effusion Collection of fluid within the pleural cavity.

Pleural Friction Rub Abnormal breath sound that is creaky and grating in nature and is heard on inspiration and expiration.

Pleurisy Condition arising from inflammation of the pleura, or sac, that encases the lung.

***Pneumocystis Carinii* Pneumonia** The most common opportunistic infection associated with advanced HIV.

Pneumonia Inflammation of the bronchioles and alveoli accompanied by consolidation, or solidification of exudate, in the lungs.

Pneumothorax Condition wherein air or gas accumulates in the pleural space of the lungs, causing the lungs to collapse.

Polydipsia Excessive thirst.

Polymenorrhea Menstrual periods that are abnormally frequent, generally less than every 21 days.

Polyp Abnormal growth of tissue.

Polyphagia Increased hunger.

Polypharmacy Problem of clients taking numerous prescription and over-the-counter medications for the same or various disease processes, with unknown consequences from the resulting combinations of chemical compounds and cumulative side-effects.

Polyuria Increased urination.

Port-a-Cath Port that has been implanted under the skin with a catheter inserted into the superior vena cava or right atrium through the subclavian or internal jugular vein.

Post Void Residual Urine that remains in the bladder after urination.

Post-mortem Care Care given immediately after death before the body is moved to the mortuary.

Postoperative Phase Time during the surgical experience that begins at the end of the surgical procedure and ends when the client is discharged from medical care by the surgeon, in addition to being discharged from the hospital or institution.

Postprandial After eating.

Preferred Provider Organization Type of managed care model wherein member choice is limited to providers within the system.

Preoperative Phase Time during the surgical experience that begins when the client decides to have surgery and ends when the client is transferred to the operating table.

Presbycusis Sensorineural hearing loss associated with aging.

Presbyopia Inablility of the lens of the eye to change curvature to focus near objects.

Prescriptive Authority Legal recognition of the ability to prescribe medications.

Pressured Speech Rapid, intense style of speech.

Prevention Hindering, obstructing, or thwarting a disease or illness.

Priapism Prolonged erection that does not occur in response to sexual stimulation.

Primary Care Care focused on promoting wellness and preventing illness or disability.

Primary Care Provider Health care provider whom a client sees first for health care, typically a family practitioner (physician/nurse), internist, or pediatrician.

Primary Health Care Client's point of entry into the health care system; includes assessment, diagnosis, treatment, coordination of care, education, prevention services, and surveillance.

Primary Hypertension High blood pressure, the cause of which is unknown; also known as essential hypertension.

Primary Prevention All practices designed to keep health problems from developing.

Primary Tubercle Nodule that contains tubercle bacilli and forms within lung tissue.

Privacy Right to be left alone, to choose care based on personal beliefs, to govern body integrity, and to choose when and how sensitive information is shared.

Progressive Muscle Relaxation Stress management strategy in which muscles are alternately tensed and relaxed.

Prolapsed Uterus Downward displacement of the uterus into the vagina.

Prospective Payment Predetermined rate paid for each episode of hospitalization based on the client's age and principle diagnosis and the presence or absence of surgery or comorbidity.

Proxemics Study of the space between people and its effect on interpersonal behavior.

Psychoanalysis Therapy focused on uncovering unconscious memories and processes.

Psychomotor Domain Area of learning that involves performance of motor skills.

Psychoneuroimmunology Study of the complex relationship among the cognitive, affective, and physical aspects of humans.

Psychoprophylaxis Mental and physical preparation for childbirth; synonymous with Lamaze.

Psychosis State wherein an individual has lost the ability to recognize reality.

Psychotherapy Treatment of mental and emotional disorders through psychological rather than physical methods.

Ptosis Drooping upper eyelid.

Public Law Law that deals with an individual's relationship to the state.

Pulse Amplitude Measurement of the strength or force exerted by the ejected blood against the arterial wall with each contraction.

Pulse Deficit Condition in which the apical pulse rate is greater than the radial pulse rate.

Pulse Rate Indirect measurement of cardiac output obtained by counting the number of peripheral pulse waves over a pulse point.

Pulse Rhythm Regularity of the heart beat.

Purpura Reddish-purple patches on the skin indicative of hemorrhage.

Purulent Exudate Discharge that occurs with severe inflammation accompanied by infection; also called pus.

Pyelonephritis Bacterial infection of the renal pelvis, tubules, and interstitial tissue of one or both kidneys.

Pyuria Pus in the urine.

Quadriplegia Dysfunction or paralysis of both arms, both legs, and bowel and bladder.

Race Grouping of people based on biological similarities such as physical characteristics.

Radiography Study of x-rays or gamma ray-exposed film through the action of ionizing radiation.

Radiotherapy Treatment of cancer with high-energy radiation.

Rapport Bond or connection between two people that is based on mutual trust.

Reasoning Use of the elements of thought to solve a problem or settle a question.

Reconstructive To rebuild or reestablish.

Rectocele Anterior displacement of the rectum into the posterior vaginal wall.

Recurrent Acute Pain Discomfort marked by repetitive painful episodes that may recur over a prolonged period or throughout a client's lifetime.

Referred Pain Discomfort from the internal organs that is felt in another area of the body.

Reflective Introspective.

Reframing Technique of monitoring negative thoughts and replacing them with positive ones.

Regional Anesthesia Method of temporarily rendering a region of the body insensible to pain.

Rehabilitation Process designed to assist individuals to reach their optimal level of physical, mental, and psychosocial functioning.

Relapse Return to a previous behavior or condition.

Relaxation Technique Method used to decrease anxiety and muscle tension.

Religious Support System Group of ministers, priests, rabbis, nuns, or lay persons who are able to meet clients' spiritual needs in the health care setting.

Remission Decrease or absence of symptoms of a disease.

Renal Colic Severe pain in the kidney that radiates to the groin.

Repolarization Recovery phase of the cardiac muscle.

Residual Urine Urine remaining in the bladder after the individual has urinated.

Respect Acceptance of an individual as is and in a nonjudgmental manner.

Respiration Process of exchanging oxygen and carbon dioxide.

Respite Care Care and service that provides a break to caregivers and is utilized for a few hours a week, for an occasional weekend, or for longer periods of time.

Responsiveness Person's ability to perceive environmental stimuli and body reactions and then to respond with thought and action.

Restraint Protective device used to limit the physical activity of a client or to immobilize a client or extremity.

Résumé Tool that summarizes employment qualifications.

Resuscitation Support measures implemented to restore consciousness and life.

Reticulocyte Immature red blood cell.

Retroperitoneal Behind the peritoneum outside the peritoneal cavity.

Reverse Tolerance Phenomenon whereby a smaller amount of substance will elicit the desired psychic effects.

Review of Systems Brief account of any recent signs or symptoms related to any body system.

Rheumatoid Arthritis Chronic, systemic auto-immune disease characterized by joint stiffness.

Rigor Mortis Stiffening of the body that occurs 2 to 4 hours after death as a result of contraction of skeletal and smooth muscles.

Salt Product formed when an acid and a base react with each other.

Sarcoma Cancer occurring in connective tissue.

Sclerotherapy Treatment which involves injecting a chemical into the vein, causing the vein to become sclerosed (hardened) so blood no longer flows through it.

Sclerotic Hardened tissue.

Scoliosis Lateral curvature of the spine.

Scrub Nurse RN, LP/VN, or surgical technologist who provides services under the direction of the circulating nurse and who is qualified by training or experience to prepare and maintain the integrity, safety, and efficiency of the sterile field throughout an operation.

Sebaceous cyst Sebaceous gland filled with sebum.

Sebum Oily substance secreted by the sebaceous glands of the skin.

Seclusion Confinement of a client to a single room.

Secondary Care Care focused on diagnosis and treatment after the client exhibits symptoms of illness.

Secondary Hypertension High blood pressure occurring as a sequel to a pre-existing disease or injury.

Secondary Prevention Early detection, diagnosis, screening, and intervention, generally before symptoms appear, to reduce the consequences of a health problem.

Sedation Reduction of stress, excitement, or irritability via some degree of central nervous system depression.

Semipermeable Membrane Membrane that allows passage of only certain substances.

Sensation Ability to receive and process stimuli received through the sensory organs.

Sensitivity Susceptibility of a pathogen to an antibiotic.

Sensorineural Hearing Loss Condition in which the inner ear or chochlear portion of cranial nerve VIII is abnormal or diseased.

Sensory Deficit Change in the perception of sensory stimuli; can affect any of the senses.

Sensory Deprivation State of reduced sensory input from the internal or external environment, manifested by alterations in sensory perception.

Sensory Overload State of excessive and sustained multisensory stimulation manifested by behavior change and perceptual distortion.

Seroconversion Evidence of antibody formation in response to disease or vaccine.

Serosanguineous Exudate Discharge that is clear with some blood tinge; seen with surgical incisions.

Serous Exudate Discharge composed primarily of serum; is watery in appearance and has a low protein level.

Serum Lithium Level Laboratory test done to determine whether the client's lithium level is within a therapeutic range.

Shaman Folk healer-priest who uses natural and supernatural forces to help others.

Shamanism Practice of entering altered states of consciousness with the intent of helping others.

Shearing Force exerted against the skin by movement or repositioning.

Shock Condition of profound hemodynamic and metabolic disturbance characterized by inadequate tissue perfusion and inadequate circulation to the vital organs.

Shroud Covering for the body after death.

Sibilant Wheeze Abnormal breath sound that is high pitched and musical in nature and is heard on inhalation and exhalation.

Sickled Condition in which red blood cells become crescent-shaped and elongated.

Single-Payer System Health care delivery model wherein the government is the only entity to reimburse.

Single Point of Entry Common feature of HMOs wherein the client is required to enter the health care system through a point designated by the plan.

Situational Loss Loss that occurs in response to external events that are usually beyond the individual's control.

Slander Words that are communicated verbally to a third party and that harm or injure the personal or professional reputation of another.

Snellen Chart Chart containing various-sized letters with standardized numbers at the end of each line of letters.

Somatic Nervous System Nerves that connect the central nervous system to the skin and skeletal muscles and control conscious activities.

Somatic Pain Nonlocalized discomfort originating in tendons, ligaments, and nerves.

Somnambulism Sleepwalking.

Somogyi Phenomenon In response to hypoglycemia, the release of glucose-elevating hormones (epinephrine, cortisol, glucose) which produces a hyperglycemic state.

Sonorous Wheeze Abnormal breath sound that is low pitched and snoring in nature and is louder on expiration.

Spermatogenesis Production of sperm.

Spinal Shock Cessation of motor, sensory, autonomic, and reflex impulses below the level of injury; characterized by flaccid paralysis of all skeletal muscles, loss of spinal reflexes, loss of sensation, and absence of autonomic function below the level of injury.

Spiritual Care Recognition of spiritual needs and the assistance given toward meeting spiritual needs.

Spiritual Need Individual's desire to find meaning and purpose in life, pain, and death.

Sprain Injury to ligaments surrounding a joint caused by a sudden twist, wrench, or fall.

Stable Alert with vital signs within the client's normal range.

Standard Level or degree of quality.

Standard of Practice Guidelines established to direct nursing care.

Startle Response Overreaction to minor sounds or noises.

Stasis Dermatitis Inflammation of the skin due to decreased circulation.

Status Asthmaticus Persistent, intractable asthma attack.

Statutory Law Law enacted by legislative bodies.

Steatorrhea Fatty stool.

Stent Tiny metal tube with holes in it that prevents a vessel from collapsing and keeps the atherosclerotic plaque pressed against the vessel wall; any material used to hold tissue in place or provide support.

Stereognosis Ability to recognize an object by feel.

Stereotyping Beliefs that all people within the same racial, ethnic, or cultural group act alike and share the same beliefs and attitudes.

Sterile Without microorganisms.

Sterile Conscience Individual's personal sense of honesty and integrity with regard to adherence to the principles of aseptic technique, including prompt admission and correction of any errors and omissions.

Sterile Field Area surrounding the client and the surgical site that is free from all microorganisms; created by draping of the work area and the client with sterile drapes.

Stoma Surgical opening between a cavity and the surface of the body.

Stomatitis Inflammation of the oral mucosa.

Strabismus Inability of the eyes to focus in the same direction.

Strain Injury to a muscle or tendon due to overuse or overstretching.

Stress Incontinence Leakage of urine when a person does anything that strains the abdomen, such as coughing, laughing, jogging, dancing, sneezing, lifting, making a quick movement, or even walking.

Stress Test Measure of a client's cardiovascular response to exercise.

Stridor High-pitched, harsh sound heard on inspiration when the trachea or larynx is obstructed.

Stroke Volume Volume of blood pumped by the ventricle with each contraction.

Stye Pustular inflammation of an eyelash follicle or sebaceous gland on the eyelid margin.

Subacute Care Short-term, aggressive care for clients who are out of the acute stage of illness but who still require skilled nursing, monitoring, and ongoing treatment.

Subluxation Partial separation of an articular surface.

Substance A drug, legal or illegal, that may cause physical or mental impairment.

Suicidal Ideations Thoughts of hurting or killing oneself.

Suicide Purposefully taking one's own life.

Surfactant Phospholipids that are present in the lungs and lowers surface tension to prevent collapse of the airways.

Surgery Treatment of injury, disease, or deformity through invasive operative methods.

Synarthrosis Immovable joint.

Synergism Result of two or more agents working together to achieve a greater effect than either could produce alone.

Synergy Two or more agents working together to achieve more than either could alone.

Synthesiasis Hearing colors and seeing sounds.

Synthesis Chemical reaction when two or more atoms, called reactants, bond and form a more complex molecular product. Putting data together in a new way.

Syphilis Sexually transmitted disease caused by the spirochete *Treponema pallidum*.

Systemic Lupus Erythematosus Chronic, progressive, incurable autoimmune disease affecting multiple body organs.

Tachycardia Heart rate in excess of 100 beats per minute in an adult.

Tachypnea Respiratory rate greater than 24 beats per minute.

Telangiectasia Permanent dilation of groups of superficial capillaries and venules; commonly known as "spider veins."

Telemedicine Use of communications technology to transmit health information from one location to another.

Teleology Ethical theory that states that the value of a situation is determined by its consequences.

Tenesmus Spasmodic contradiction of the anal or bladder sphincter, causing pain and a persistent urge to empty the bowel or bladder.

Teratogenic Causing abnormal development of the embryo.

Tertiary Care Care focused on restoring the client to the state of health that existed before the development of an illness; if unattainable, then care directed to attaining the optimal level of health possible.

Tertiary Prevention Treatment of an illness or disease after symptoms have appeared so as to prevent further progression.

Tetany Sharp flexion of the wrist and ankle joints, involving muscle twitching or cramps, caused by decreased blood calcium level.

Therapeutic Communication Communication that is purposeful and goal directed, creating a beneficial outcome for the client.

Therapeutic Massage Application of pressure and motion by the hands with the intent of improving the recipient's well-being.

Therapeutic Touch Technique of assessing alterations in a person's energy fields and using the hands to direct energy to achieve a balanced state.

Thoracentesis Aspiration of fluid from the pleural cavity.

Thrombectomy Surgical removal of a clot.

Thrombocytopenia Decrease in the number of platelets in the blood.

Thrombophlebitis Formation of a clot due to an inflammation in the wall of the vessel.

Thrombosis Formation of a clot in a vessel.

Thrombus Formed clot that remains at the site where it formed.

Tinnitus Ringing sound in the ear.

Tolerance Decreased sensitivity to subsequent doses of the same substance; an increased dose of the substance is needed to produce the same desired effect.

Tophi Subcutaneous nodules of sodium urate crystals.

Tort Civil wrong committed by a person against another person or property.

Tort Law Enforcement of duties and rights among individuals and independent of contractual agreements.

Touch Means of perceiving or experiencing through tactile sensation.

Toxic Poisonous.

Transcutaneous Electrical Nerve Stimulation Process of applying a low-voltage electrical current to the skin through cutaneous electrodes.

Transducer Instrument that converts electrical energy to sound waves.

Transduction Noxious stimulus that triggers electrical activity in the endings of afferent nerve fibers (nociceptors).

Transesophageal Echocardiography Diagnostic ultrasonic imaging of the cardiac structures through the esophagus.

Transmission Process whereby the pain impulse travels from the receiving nociceptors to the spinal cord.

Trauma Wound or injury.

Triage Classification of clients to determine priority of need and proper place of treatment.

Trichomoniasis Sexually transmitted disease caused by a parasitic protozoan *Trichomonas vaginalis*.

Trocar Sharply pointed surgical instrument contained in a cannula.

Trousseau's Sign Carpal spasm caused by inflating a blood pressure cuff above the client's systolic pressure and leaving it in place for 3 minutes.

Trust Ability to rely on an individual's character and ability.

Tumor Marker Substance found in the serum that indicates the possible presence of malignancy.

Turgor Normal resiliency of the skin.

Type and Cross-Match Laboratory test that identifies the client's blood type (e.g., A or B) and determines the compatibility of the blood between potential donor and recipient.

Ultrasound Use of high-frequency sound waves to visualize deep body structures; also called an echogram.

Uncomplicated Grief Grief reaction that normally follows a significant loss.

Unilateral Neglect Failure to recognize or care for one side of the body.

Urethrocele Downward displacement of the urethra into the vagina.

Urethrostomy Formation of a permanent fistula opening into the urethra.

Urge Incontinence Inability to suppress the sudden urge or need to urinate.

Urinary Incontinence Involuntary loss of urine from the bladder.

Urinary Retention Inability to void when there is an urge to void.

Urobilinogen Colorless derivative of bilirubin formed by the normal bacterial action of intestinal flora on bilirubin.

Urolithiasis Calculus or stone formed in the urinary tract.

Urticaria Allergic reaction causing raised pruritic, red, nontender wheals on the skin; also called hives.

Utility Ethical principle that states that an act must result in the greatest degree of good for the greatest number of people involved in a given situation.

Value System Individual's collection of inner beliefs that guides the way the person acts and helps determine the choices the person makes.

Values Principles that influence the development of beliefs and attitudes.

Values Clarification Process of analyzing one's own values to better understand those things that are truly important.

Varicosities Visibly prominent, dilated, and twisted veins.

Vasectomy Surgical resecton of the vas deferens.

Vasoconstrict Decrease in the diameter of a vessel.

Vasodilate Increase in the diameter of a vessel.

Vein Ligation Tying off an involved section of a vein with suture.

Vein Stripping Introducing a wire into a vein to strip the walls of the vein.

Venereal Disease Disease usually acquired as a result of sexual contact; the preferred term currently in use is sexually transmitted disease.

Venipuncture Puncturing of a vein with a needle to aspirate blood.

Ventilation Movement of gases into and out of the lungs.

Veracity Ethical principle based on truthfulness (neither lying nor deceiving others).

Verbal Communication Using words, either spoken or written, to send a message.

Verbally Aggressive Descriptor of an individual who says things in a loud and/or intimidating manner.

Vertigo Dizziness.

Vesicant Solution capable of causing tissue injury or destruction when it escapes into surrounding tissue.

Vesicular Breath Sound Soft, low breath sound heard over the majority of lung tissue.

Vesicular Sound Soft, breezy, low-pitched sound heard longer on inspiration than expiration that results from air moving through the smaller airways over the lung periphery, with the exception of the scapular area.

Villi Finger-like projections that line the small intestine.

Viral Load Test Test that measures copies of HIV RNA.

Virchow's Triad Three factors (pooling of blood, vessel trauma, and a coagulation problem) that lead to the formation of a clot.

Visceral Pain Discomfort felt in the internal organs.

Visual Hallucination Perception by an individual that something is present when nothing in fact is.

Vitiligo Depigmentation of the skin caused by destruction of melanocytes; appears as milk-white patches on the skin.

Void Process of urine elimination.

Volvulus Twisting of a bowel on itself.

Wellness State of optimal health wherein an individual moves toward integration of human functioning, maximizes human potential, takes responsibility for health, and has greater self-awareness and self-satisfaction.

Western Blot Test Confirmatory test used to detect HIV infection.

Whistleblowing Calling attention to unethical, illegal, or incompetent actions of others.

Windowing Cutting a hole in a plaster cast to relieve pressure on the skin or a bony area and to permit visualization of the underlying body part.

Withdrawal Symptoms produced when a substance on which an individual has dependence is no longer used by that individual.

Word Salad Nonsensical combination of words that is meaningless to others.

Wound Disruption in the integrity of body tissue.

Yin and Yang Opposing forces that, when in balance, yield health.

Index

Note: Page numbers in *italics* indicate illustrations; page numbers followed by a "t" indicate a table.

sprain, 591
strain, 591
systemic disorders
gout, 610
lyme disease, 610
Music, culture and, 140
Music therapy, 140
MVCs. *See* motor vehicle collisions (MVCs)
Myasthenia gravis (MG), 562–65
assessment, 562–63
medical-surgical management, 562
nursing diagnoses, 563
sample nursing care plan, 563–65
Mycobacterium avium complex (MAC), 575
Mycosis funcoides, 528–29
Myelogram, 261t
Myocardial infarction, 452–55
assessment, 454
medical-surgical management, 453–54
nursing diagnoses, 454–55
Myocarditis, 444–45
medical-surgical management, 445
nursing management, 445
Myofacial pain syndromes, 285
Myopia, 683, 685, *686*
Myxedema, 722

N

NA. *See* Narcotics Anonymous (NA)
Nails (finger and toe), 510, 513, *514*
Naltrexone, 935
NANDA. *See* North American Nursing Diagnosis Association (NANDA)
Narcotics Anonymous (NA), 936
National Center for Complementary and Alternative Medicine (NCCAM), 127
National Collegiate Athletic Association, 936
National Council Licensure Exam (NCLEX), 36
National Federation of Licensed Practical Nurses (NFLPN), 5, 37, 59
National Institute on Alcohol Abuse and Alcoholism (NIAAA), 924
National Kidney Foundation, 775
National League for Nursing (NLN), 5
National Pressure Ulcer Advisory Panel (NPUAP), 541
Native Americans
end-stage renal disease, 797
health beliefs, 95
hypertension, 468
religions, 100
rituals following death, 150
Nausea
chemotherapy and, 370
postoperative, 348

NCCAM. *See* National Center for Complementary and Alternative Medicine (NCCAM)
NCLEX. *See* National Council Licensure Exam (NCLEX)
Near-drowning, fresh-water versus salt-water, 994t
Nebulizer use, 413
Neck assessment. *See* head and neck assessment
Necrosis, 239, 462
Neglect, 913–15
assessment, 914–15
medical-surgical management, 914
nursing diagnoses, 914–15
Negligence, 40, *41*
Neonatal death, 151t
Neoplasms, 360–61
Nephropathy. *See* chronic renal failure
Nephrotoxic substance, 793
Nerve block, 301, 311
Neuralgia, 285, 659
Neurogenic shock, 639
Neurological assessment, 224
Neurological flow sheet, *995*
Neurological/neurosurgical emergencies, 995–96
assessment, 996
medical-surgical management, 995–96
nursing diagnoses, 996
Neurological system, 613–63
anatomy and physiology, 614–18
central nervous system, 614–16
peripheral nervous system, 616–17
assessment, 618–24
cerebral function, 618–21
communication, 620–21
emotional status, 620
intellectual function, 619–20
level of consciousness, 618–19
mental status, 619
pupil reaction, 620
cranial nerve function, 621
health history, 618
motor function, 621–22
balance, 622
coordination, 621, 622
muscle size and symmetry, 621
muscle strength, 621
muscle tone, 621
posturing, 622
reflexes, 623–24
abnormal, 624
examination, 623
grading scale, 624t
sensory function, 622–23
graphesthesia, 623
integration of sensation, 623
pain and temperature, 622
proprioception, 622
stereognosis, 622–23

tactile sensation, 622
vibration, 622, *623*
case study, 614–18
diagnostic tests, 624t
disorders
Alzheimer's disease, 652–55, 961–62
amyotrophic lateral sclerosis, 651–52
brain tumor, 629–30
cerebrovascular accident, 630–33
encephalitis, 660
epilepsy/seizure disorder, 633–35
Guillain-Barré syndrome, 655–57
headaches, 657–59
head injuries, 624–29
herniated intervertebral disk, 635–37
Huntington's disease/chorea, 660–61
meningitis, 660
multiple sclerosis, 646–51
Parkinson's disease, 642–45
spinal cord injury, 637–42
transient ischemic attacks, 630–33, 962
trigeminal neuralgia, 659–60
Neuron, *615*
Neuropeptides, 127
Neurophils, 240t
Neurosurgery, 301
Neurotransmitters, 127, 615
Nevi, 508
NFLPN. *See* National Federation of Licensed Practical Nurses (NFLPN)
NIAAA. *See* National Institute on Alcohol Abuse and Alcoholism (NIAAA)
Nicotine abuse, 931–32
associated problems/disorders, 931
incidence, 931
potential for addiction, 931
signs and symptoms, 931
treatment/rehabilitation, 932
withdrawal, 932
Nightingale, Florence, 136
Nightingale Pledge, 56t
Nitrosureas, 366, 367t
NLN. *See* National League for Nursing (NLN)
Nociceptors, 285
No Code. *See* do not resuscitate (DNR)
Nocturia, 851
Nocturnal enuresis, 779
Nocturnal tumescence penile monitoring, 275t
Non-Hodgkin's lymphoma, 501–2, 583
assessment, 502
medical-surgical management, 501
nursing diagnoses, 502
Nonmaleficence, 55